Maged Argalious • Ehab Farag •
Deepak Sharma
Editors

Basic Sciences in Anesthesia

Second Edition

Springer

Editors
Maged Argalious
Multispecialty Anesthesiology, Department of Anesthesiology, Integrated Hospital Care Institute
Cleveland Clinic, Cleveland Clinic Lerner College of Medicine of Case Western Reserve University
Cleveland, OH, USA

Ehab Farag
Multispecialty Anesthesiology, Department of Anesthesiology, Integrated Hospital Care Institute
Cleveland Clinic, Cleveland Clinic Lerner College of Medicine of Case Western Reserve University
Cleveland, OH, USA

Deepak Sharma
Department of Anesthesiology and Pain Medicine
University of Washington
Seattle, WA, USA

ISBN 978-3-031-60202-3 ISBN 978-3-031-60203-0 (eBook)
https://doi.org/10.1007/978-3-031-60203-0

This Springer imprint is published by the registered company Springer Nature Switzerland AG
The registered company address is: Gewerbestrasse 11, 6330 Cham, Switzerland

To my late parents whose passion for research and scientific discovery proved to be contagious. To my wife Nermine, for her unrelenting faith, her unconditional love, and her impressive emotional intelligence. To my children Daniel and Sandra, for their cheerful and joyous personalities and their genuine love of family.

Maged Argalious

To my beloved wife Abeer, my constant companion and greatest love. To my cherished daughters, Monica and Rebecca, the lights of my life.

To my son-in-law George, whose presence in our family brings us great joy. And to my family, whose guidance and love have been my foundation.

With deepest gratitude,

Ehab Farag

My sincerest thanks to my parents Mrs. Renu and Col. PC Sharma, and my dear wife Madhu, and my daughters Deeya and Drishti for their constant support, love, and encouragement.

Deepak Sharma

Foreword to the Second Edition

Dear readers,

I am pleased to introduce the second edition of *Basic Sciences in Anesthesia*. This updated edition gives you the most recent evidence-based information, following the outstanding achievement of the original text, which had more than 135,000 chapter downloads globally.

The chapters in this textbook are authored by nationally recognized anesthesiologists, including more than twenty contributing authors from Cleveland Clinic. They have generously offered their expertise and experience on the most foundational topics—serving the needs of clinicians in training and in practice.

Understanding the basic science is a cornerstone of innovation. New perioperative pharmacologic agents have been shown to improve outcomes, reduce pain, and enhance patient experience. These advances further empower surgical innovation and make it possible to deliver safer care to patients.

I am confident that anesthesiologists at all stages of their careers will find this textbook to be an invaluable resource. Thank you to the authors and editors for their hard work in updating the excellent second edition..

Tomislav Mihaljevic MD
CEO and President
Cleveland Clinic
Cleveland, USA

Preface to the First Edition

The basic sciences are the essence of Anesthesiology. Therefore, the American Board of Anesthesiology (ABA) includes an examination on the basic sciences for the ABA certification. The lack of a specific book dedicated to the basic sciences in anesthesiology has driven us to compose this book. We tried our best to follow the syllabus of the ABA basic sciences examination in order to create an accurate resource for study. The motto of this book is to follow Alexander Pope's advice in 1709: "A little learning is a dangerous thing; drink deep, or taste not the Pierian spring: there shallow droughts intoxicate the brain, and drinking largely sobers us again." This message is still relevant today in the field of anesthesiology.

The content of each chapter of the book is presented in a comprehensive manner and is conducive for successful study. Every chapter highlights key topics and includes questions testing comprehension of the respective subject matter. Moreover, suggested references are included for further research in the basic sciences.

We would like to thank our colleagues for their hard work and dedication in writing the book. In addition, we would like to thank Ms. Maureen K. Pierce and Joanna Renwick from Springer International Publishing for their perseverance during the process.

At the end, we hope this book will be helpful in preparation for the ABA basic science examination as well as serve as a tool for practicing anesthesiologists who would like to refresh their knowledge in basic sciences.

Cleveland, USA — Ehab Farag
Cleveland, USA — Maged Argalious
Cleveland, USA — John E. Tetzlaff
Seattle, USA — Deepak Sharma

Contents

Contributors

Mohamed Abdalla Department of Anesthesiology, University Hospitals of Cleveland, Cleveland, OH, USA;
Case Western Reserve University, Cleveland, OH, USA

Basem Abdelmalak Departments of General Anesthesiology and Outcomes Research, Cleveland Clinic, Anesthesia for Bronchoscopic Surgery and Center for Procedural Sedation, Cleveland, OH, USA

Ahmad Maher Adi Department of Cardiothoracic Anesthesiology and Critical Care, Cleveland Clinic, Cleveland, OH, USA

Maged Argalious Division of Multispecialty Anesthesiology, Department of Anesthesiology, Integrated Hospital Care Institute, Cleveland Clinic, Cleveland, OH, USA;
Cleveland Clinic Lerner College of Medicine of Case Western Reserve University, Cleveland, OH, USA

Maria Bauer Department of Anesthesiology and Critical Care Medicine, The Johns Hopkins Hospital, Baltimore, MD, USA

Sekar S. Bhavani Cleveland Clinic Lerner College of Medicine, Anesthesiology Institute, Cleveland Clinic, Cleveland, OH, USA

Siddhant Bhoir Department of Anesthesiology and Perioperative Medicine, MD Anderson Cancer Center, The University of Texas, Austin, TX, USA;
Anesthesiology and Surgical Oncology Research Group., Houston, TX, USA

Ravi Bhoja Department of Anesthesiology and Pain Management, University of Texas Southwestern Medical Center, Dallas, TX, USA

Andrew Bowdle Department of Anesthesiology, University of Washington, Seattle, WA, USA

Sorin J. Brull Department of Anesthesiology and Perioperative Medicine, Mayo Clinic College of Medicine and Science, Jacksonville, FL, USA

Jack Buckley Department of Anesthesiology, UCLA Medical Center, Los Angeles, CA, USA

Arne O. Budde Department of Anesthesiology and Perioperative Medicine, Penn State Health, Milton S. Hershey Medical Center, Hershey, PA, USA

G. Burkhard Mackensen Division of Cardiothoracic Anesthesiology, Department of Anesthesiology and Pain Medicine, University of Washington, Seattle, WA, USA

Anthony Cartwright Practice Plus Group, The University of Sheffield, Plymouth, UK

Juan P. Cata Department of Anesthesiology and Perioperative Medicine, The University of Texas – MD Anderson Cancer Center, Houston, TX, USA;
Anesthesiology and Surgical Oncology Research Group, Houston, TX, USA

Verghese T. Cherian Department of Anesthesiology and Perioperative Medicine, Penn State Health, Milton S. Hershey Medical Center, Hershey, PA, USA

Maria-Jose Corrales-Martinez Department of Outcomes Research, Cleveland Clinic, Cleveland, OH, USA

Kenneth C. Cummings Integrated Hospital Care Institute, Cleveland Clinic Foundation, Cleveland, OH, USA

Jacek B. Cywinski Multi-Specialty Anesthesiology, Integrated Hospital-Care Institute, Cleveland Clinic, Cleveland, OH, USA

Laurie S. Daste Department of Anesthesiology, LCMC Health, New Orleans, LA, USA

Aaron J. Douglas Department of Anesthesiology, Saint Luke's Health System, Kansas City, MO, USA

D. John Doyle Department of General Anesthesiology, Cleveland Clinic, Cleveland, OH, USA

Siddharth Pawan Dugar Respiratory Institute, Cleveland Clinic Foundation, Cleveland, OH, USA

Ehab Farag Anesthesiology, Department of General Anesthesiology, Cleveland Clinic Lerner College of Medicine, Case Western University, Cleveland, OH, USA;
Departments of General Anesthesia and Outcomes Research, Cleveland Clinic, Cleveland, OH, USA

Myroslav Figura Department of Anesthesiology, UCLA Medical Center, Los Angeles, CA, USA

Elizabeth A. M. Frost Department of Anesthesiology, Icahn Medical Center at Mount Sinai, New York, NY, USA

Maged Guirguis Department of Anesthesiology and Critical Care Medicine, Ochsner Health Systems, Louisiana State University School of Medicine, New Orleans, USA

Sam D. Gumbert Department of General Anesthesia, Anesthesiology Institute, Cleveland Clinic, Cleveland Clinic Lerner College of Medicine of Case Western Reserve University, Cleveland, OH, USA

Nathan J. Harrison Department of Anesthesiology and Pain Management, Ochsner Health Systems, Covington, LA, USA

Aaron Hawke Anesthesiology Residency Program, Cleveland Clinic Foundation, Anesthesia Institute, Cleveland, OH, USA

Srdjan Jelacic Department of Anesthesiology, University of Washington, Seattle, WA, USA

Brian K. Johnson Department of Anesthesia and Perioperative Medicine, University Hospitals Cleveland Medical Center, Cleveland, OH, USA

Daniel Katz Icahn Medical Center at Mount Sinai, New York, NY, USA

Allen Keebler Department of General Anesthesiology, Cleveland Clinic, Cleveland, OH, USA

Marta Kelava Division of Cardiothoracic and Vascular Anesthesiology, Department of Anesthesiology, Integrated Hospital-Care Institute Cleveland Clinic, Cleveland, OH, USA

Robert J. Kerris Anesthesiology and Perioperative Medicine, Penn State Health, Milton S. Hershey Medical Center, Hershey, PA, USA

Sandeep Khanna Division of Multi-Specialty Anesthesiology, Cleveland Clinic Foundation, Cleveland, OH, USA;
Division of Cardiothoracic Anesthesiology, Cleveland Clinic Foundation, Cleveland, OH, USA;
Outcomes Research Consortium®, Houston, TX, USA

Reem Khatib Department of General Anesthesiology, Cleveland Clinic, Cleveland, OH, USA

Sree Kolli Department of MultiSpeciality Anesthesiology, Cleveland Clinic, Cleveland, OH, USA

Jonathan Korets Department of Anesthesiology, SUNY Upstate Medical University, Syracuse, NY, USA

Swamy Kurra Department of Anesthesiology, SUNY Upstate Medical University, Syracuse, NY, USA

Andrzej P. Kwater Department of Anesthesiology and Perioperative Medicine, The University of Texas – MD Anderson Cancer Center, Houston, TX, USA

Mani Latifi Respiratory Institute, Cleveland Clinic Foundation, Cleveland, OH, USA

Elizabeth Demers Lavelle Department of Anesthesiology, SUNY Upstate Medical University, Syracuse, NY, USA

Fenghua Li Department of Anesthesiology, SUNY Upstate Medical University, Syracuse, NY, USA

Melanie Liu Division of Cardiothoracic Anesthesiology, Department of Anesthesiology and Pain Medicine, University of Washington, Seattle, WA, USA

Kamal Maheshwari Departments of General Anesthesiology and Outcomes Research, Cleveland Clinic Foundation, Anesthesia Institute, Cleveland, OH, USA

Crystal Manohar Anesthesiology and Critical Care Medicine, Department of Anesthesiology, University of Texas Health San Antonio, San Antonio, TX, USA

Edward J. Mascha Section of Biostatistics, Full Staff Biostatistician, Department of Quantitative Health Sciences, Cleveland Clinic, Cleveland, OH, USA;
Anesthesiology, Cleveland Clinic Lerner College of Medicine at Case Western Reserve University, Cleveland, OH, USA

Piyush Mathur Divisions of General Anesthesiology and ICR, Department of Anesthesiology, Cleveland, OH, USA

Gary S. McDaniel Baton Rouge Orthopedic Clinic, Baton Rouge, LA, USA

David L. McDonagh Department of Anesthesiology and Pain Management, University of Texas Southwestern Medical Center, Dallas, TX, USA

Trisha McGinnis Department of Intensive Care and Resuscitation, Anesthesiology Institute, Cleveland Clinic, Cleveland, OH, USA;
Department of General Anesthesiology, Anesthesiology Institute, Cleveland Clinic, Cleveland, OH, USA

Ashley Miller Department of Intensive Care and Resuscitation, Anesthesiology Institute, Cleveland Clinic, Cleveland, OH, USA;
Department of General Anesthesiology, Anesthesiology Institute, Cleveland Clinic, Cleveland, OH, USA

Eduardo Mireles-Cabodevila Respiratory Institute, Cleveland Clinic Foundation, Cleveland, OH, USA

Yulia Obelcz Department of Anesthesiology & Pain Medicine, Harborview Medical Center, University of Washington, Seattle, WA, USA

Adeeb Oweidat Department of Anesthesiology, University of Iowa, Iowa, USA;
Anesthesia Department, University of Iowa Hospitals, Iowa City, IA, USA

Matthew E. Patterson Department of Anesthesiology and Critical Care Medicine, Ochsner Health Systems, Louisiana State University School of Medicine, New Orleans, USA

Silvia Perez-Protto Department of Intensive Care and Resuscitation, Department of General Anesthesiology, Cleveland Clinic, Cleveland, OH, USA

Maria F. Ramirez Department of Anesthesiology and Perioperative Medicine, MD Anderson Cancer Center, The University of Texas, Austin, TX, USA;
Anesthesiology and Surgical Oncology Research Group., Houston, TX, USA

Ihab Adly Riad Cleveland Clinic Lerner College of Medicine, Cleveland, OH, USA;
Regional Anesthesia, Cleveland Clinic, Cleveland, OH, USA;
Department of Regional Anesthesiology, Lutheran Hospital, Cleveland, OH, USA

Jia W. Romito Department of Anesthesiology and Pain Management, University of Texas Southwestern Medical Center, Dallas, TX, USA

J. Ross Renew Department of Anesthesiology and Perioperative Medicine, Mayo Clinic College of Medicine and Science, Jacksonville, FL, USA

Kurt Ruetzler Department of Outcomes Research and General Anesthesiology, Anesthesiology Institute, Cleveland Clinic Foundation, Cleveland, OH, USA

Joe Salloum Divisions of General Anesthesiology and ICR, Department of Anesthesiology, Cleveland, OH, USA

Joanna Schindler Department of Anesthesiology, Emory University School of Medicine, Grady Memorial Hospital, Atlanta, GA, USA

Jay D. Shah Department of Anesthesiology and Critical Care Medicine, Ochsner Health Systems, Louisiana State University School of Medicine, New Orleans, USA

Dmitry Sharakou Department of General Anesthesiology and ICR, Cleveland Clinic, Cleveland, OH, USA

Ian R. Slade Department of Anesthesiology & Pain Medicine, Harborview Medical Center, University of Washington, Seattle, WA, USA

Roshni Sreedharan Division of Multi-Specialty Anesthesiology, Cleveland Clinic Foundation, Cleveland, OH, USA;
Department of Intensive Care and Resuscitation, Anesthesiology Institute, Cleveland Clinic, Cleveland, OH, USA;
Department of General Anesthesiology, Anesthesiology Institute, Cleveland Clinic, Cleveland, OH, USA

Carlos Trombetta Division of Multi-Specialty Anesthesiology, Cleveland Clinic Foundation, Cleveland, OH, USA;
Division of Cardiothoracic Anesthesiology, Cleveland Clinic Foundation, Cleveland, OH, USA

Matthew K. Whalin Department of Anesthesiology, Emory University School of Medicine, Grady Memorial Hospital, Atlanta, GA, USA

Part I
Applied Anatomy

Contents

Peripheral Nerve Block Anesthesia

1

Sree Kolli and Adeeb Oweidat

Abstract

Peripheral nerve is composed of axons of multiple neurons bundled together in fascicles. Performing a successful block requires the local anesthetic to be deposited near the nerve or in the same fascial plane in which the nerve lies. Advances in ultrasound technology allow real-time visualization of needle advancement toward the nerve, potentially avoiding critical structures. It also allows to visualize the spread of local anesthetic around the nerve or the fascial plane desired. Ultrasound and peripheral nerve stimulators facilitate nerve blockade and improve success rate, but their use does not eliminate the risk of nerve injury.

Keywords

Peripheral nerve block • Nerve anatomy • Upper limb blocks • Interscalene block • Supraclavicular block • Infraclavicular block • Axillary block • Lower limb blocks • Femoral nerve block • Adductor canal block • Sciatic nerve block • Suprainguinal Fascia Iliaca (SIFI) Plane Block • Pericapsular nerve group (PENG) Block • Popliteal sciatic nerve block • Ankle block • Transversus abdominis plane (TAP) block • Rectus sheath Block • External oblique intercostal block • Quadratus lumborum Block

Key Points

1. Peripheral nerve is composed of axons of multiple neurons bundled together in fascicles.
2. To achieve good block, local anesthetic should be injected near the nerve or in the same fascial plane in which the nerve lies.
3. Advances in ultrasound technology allowed real-time visualization of needle advancement toward the nerve, potentially avoiding critical structures. It also allows to visualize the spread of local anesthetic around the nerve.
4. Ultrasound and peripheral nerve stimulators facilitate nerve blockade, but their use does not eliminate the risk of nerve injury.
5. Anesthesia of the shoulder and upper extremity can be obtained by blockade of the brachial plexus (C5-T1).
6. Supraclavicular block does not eliminate the risk of phrenic nerve paralysis. The incidence depends on the volume of local anesthetic injected.
7. Interscalene and supraclavicular block can miss the lower trunk; hence, axillary approach to brachial plexus is most optimal for procedures on forearm and hand.
8. Infraclavicular block avoids the risk of phrenic nerve paralysis, making it an excellent choice in patients with respiratory issues.
9. Combined suprascapular nerve block and axillary nerve block can be utilized as alternative technique to provide analgesia for shoulder surgery in patients with risk of respiratory complications.
10. Femoral nerve block is easy to learn, low risk with minimal complications. It is useful for surgery on the anterior thigh and knee, quadriceps tendon repair, and postoperative pain management of femur and knee surgery.
11. Adductor canal block for knee surgery provides comparable analgesia to femoral nerve block with motor sparing effect facilitating early ambulation.
12. Sciatic nerve block is useful for surgical procedures involving hip, knee, and distal lower extremity. It can be blocked at multiple locations by multiple approaches.

S. Kolli (✉)
Department of MultiSpeciality Anesthesiology, Cleveland Clinic, Cleveland, OH, USA
e-mail: KOLLIS@ccf.org

A. Oweidat
Anesthesia Department, University of Iowa Hospitals, Iowa City, IA, USA

M. Argalious et al. (eds.), *Basic Sciences in Anesthesia*,
https://doi.org/10.1007/978-3-031-60203-0_1

13. PENG block targeting the articular branches of the femoral, obturator and accessory obturator nerve is a newer technique for analgesia in hip fractures and surgery.
14. Popliteal nerve block is useful for surgery on foot and ankle, combined with saphenous nerve block can provide complete anesthesia of the limb distal to the knee.
15. Transversus abdominis plane (TAP) block provides postoperative analgesia for surgeries on anterior abdominal wall. It is relatively easy and safe block to perform under ultrasound guidance.
16. Rectus sheath block covers the anterior cutaneous branches of the intercostal nerves, and therefore, it is well suited for postoperative analgesia for surgery with midline (or paramedian) abdominal incisions.
17. External Oblique Intercostal (EOIFP) block is a superficial block that provides coverage to the lateral upper abdominal area, by blocking the thoracolumbar nerves T7-T11.
18. Quadratus lumborum (QL) block is achieved by placing the local anesthetic adjacent to the QL muscle and obtaining visceral analgesia is an advantage of the block.

1.1 Anatomy of the Nerve

A peripheral nerve trunk is composed of axons of multiple neurons bundled together in connective tissue and endoneurial fluid (◘ ◉ Fig. 1.1). Each axon is surrounded by endoneurium, which is made up of glycocalyx and a mesh of collagen. Axons are bundled together into groups called fascicles, and each fascicle is wrapped in a layer of connective tissue called perineurium. All the fascicles are finally ensheathed in a connective tissue layer called epineurium. The blood vessels run between the fascicles and supply oxygen and nutrients to the axons.

1.2 Upper Limb Blocks

The brachial plexus is a neural bundle that provides sensory and motor innervation to the upper extremity. Nerve roots of C5-T1 undergo complex congregation forming components named roots, trunks, divisions, and cords, before forming the terminal nerves of the upper extremity (◘ ◉ Fig. 1.2). The plexus can be blocked at several locations, depending on the required region of the upper limb to be blocked.

The interscalene space is a potential space between the anterior and middle scalene muscles. The 5 roots of the cervical and the first thoracic spinal nerves give rise to 3 trunks (superior, middle, and inferior) that emerge between the medial and anterior scalene muscles to lie on the floor of the posterior triangle of the neck. The roots of the plexus lie deep to the prevertebral fascia, whereas the trunks are covered by its lateral extension, the axillary sheath. Each trunk divides into an anterior and a posterior division behind the clavicle, at the apex of the axilla. The divisions combine to produce the 3 cords, which are named lateral, median, and posterior according to their relationship to the axillary artery. Individual nerves are formed as these neuronal elements descend distally.

1.2.1 Interscalene Block

This is a technique of anesthetizing the roots or trunks of the brachial plexus in the neck between the anterior and middle scalene muscles. The procedure was first well described and popularized by Alon Winnie in 1970 [1].

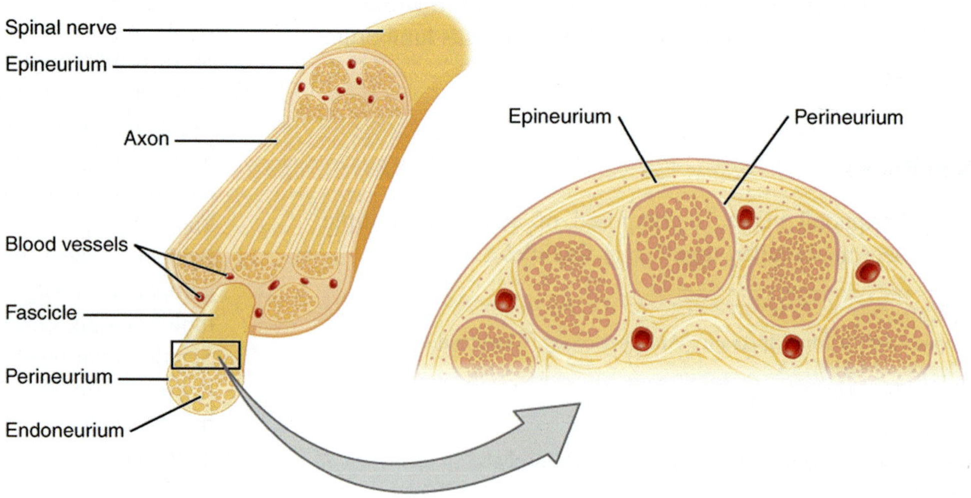

Fig. 1.1 Anatomy of a nerve (Reprinted under Creative Commons Attribution 4.0 International License from OpenStax, Anatomy & Physiology. Houston, TX, OpenStax, Rice University. 2016. Download for free at ► http://cnx.org/content/col11496/latest/)

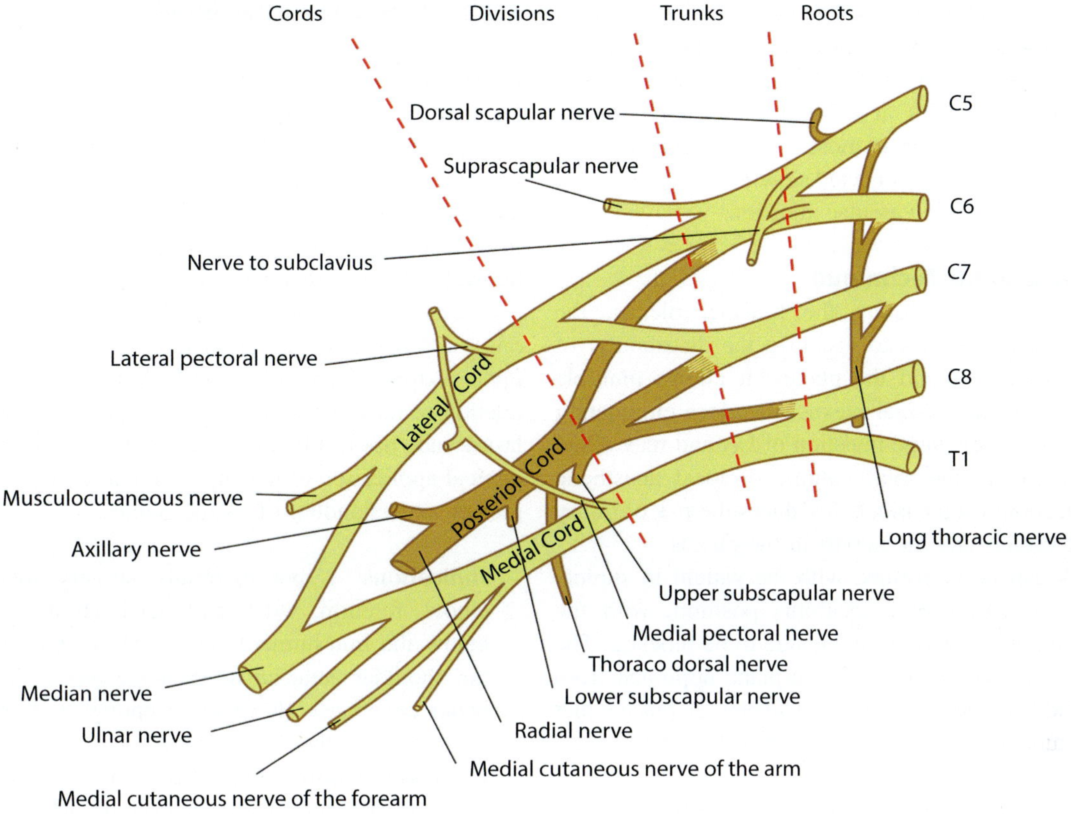

Fig. 1.2 Brachial plexus anatomy

Interscalene nerve block is typically performed to provide anesthesia or analgesia for surgery of the shoulder and upper arm. A successful block at this level anesthetizes the shoulder and upper arm, but does not reliably block nerve roots innervating the forearm, as the inferior trunk is often not included into the block.

- **Indications**: Shoulder surgeries, such as rotator cuff repair, acromioplasty, hemiarthroplasty, total shoulder arthroplasty, humerus fractures, and elbow surgery.
- **Contraindications**: Patient refusal, infection at planned injection site, preexisting neurologic defects, local anesthetic allergy, coagulopathy, contralateral phrenic nerve dysfunction, and severe chronic obstructive pulmonary disease.
- **Complications**: Diaphragmatic paralysis, pneumothorax, hoarseness, Horner's syndrome, epidural/intrathecal injection, local anesthetic (LA) toxicity, infection, hematoma, and allergic reaction.

1.2.1.1 Landmark/Nerve Stimulator Technique

The landmarks used for the block are the clavicular head of the sternocleidomastoid muscle, clavicle, and external jugular vein. The patient can be positioned supine or with the back mildly elevated and head rotated away from the side to be blocked. Palpate the sternocleidomastoid that overlies the superior aspects of the scalene muscles. Having the patient lift his or her head off the bed will help define the lateral border of the sternocleidomastoid muscle. The anterior scalene muscle emerges from under the sternocleidomastoid muscle and runs inferiorly and laterally toward the first rib.

By placing the fingers under the sternocleidomastoid muscle and inferior to the external jugular vein, sliding them laterally will identify anterior scalene muscle. The interscalene groove separates the anterior from the middle scalene muscle. This groove sometimes is obvious during palpation, but frequently is subtle and more like a cleft.

Once the groove is palpated, several maneuvers can be performed to confirm the groove. During deep inspiration, the groove often is accentuated because the scalenes are accessory muscles of respiration, which tense during inspiration. The groove also can be tracked down toward the first rib and palpate for the subclavian artery, which emerges between the scalenes.

Once the interscalene groove is identified, the palpating fingers should be gently but firmly pressed between the anterior and middle scalene muscles and should not be moved during the entire block procedure to allow for precise redirection of the needle when necessary. The needle is inserted 3–4 cm above the clavicle and advanced at an angle almost perpendicular to the skin plane. The nerve stimulator should be initially set to deliver 0.8–1.0 mA. The needle is advanced slowly until stimulation of the brachial plexus is obtained—seen as twitch of the pectoralis, deltoid, arm, forearm, or hand muscles at 0.2–0.5 mA. This typically occurs at a depth of 1–2 cm in most of the patients and 25–35 mL of local anesthetic is injected slowly with intermittent aspiration to rule out intravascular injection.

1.2.1.2 Ultrasound Technique

Apart from precisely locating the brachial plexus, the ultrasound guidance allows to visualize the distribution of the local anesthetic around the plexus. It allows multiple injections around the brachial plexus, therefore eliminating the reliance on a single large injection of LA and may allow for the reduction in the total volume of local anesthetic required to accomplish the block. It reduces the risk of injury to the blood vessels and the nerves in the plexus.

The block can be performed with the patient in supine, semi-sitting, or semi-lateral decubitus position, with the patient's head facing away from the side to be blocked. The latter position is more suitable for in-plane approach from the lateral side, especially when a catheter is placed that needs to be tunneled away from the surgical drapes.

- **Scanning Technique 1 (Transverse Sweep)**: The transducer is positioned in the transverse plane just below the level of cricoid. Start by identifying the hyperechoic arc of the trachea and moving the probe posterolaterally until sternocleidomastoid muscle is identified. This muscle is triangular shaped and located anteriorly to the carotid artery and internal jugular vein. Once the great vessels are identified, slide the probe more laterally to identify the scalene muscles and the brachial plexus that lies in between them appearing as hypoechoic trunks.
- **Scanning Technique 2 (Backtracking)**: The other scanning technique is to identify the brachial plexus in the supraclavicular fossa and then track cephalad into the interscalene space. The transducer is placed over the sternocleidomastoid, 1–2 cm superior to the head of the clavicle. Move laterally to identify the subclavian artery and immediately superior and posterior to the artery, the brachial plexus is seen as a grouping of small hyperechoic circles with hypoechoic centers, like a cluster of grapes. The plexus is then traced cephalad to the preferred block region at the level of C6.

Once the plexus is identified, the needle is inserted in-plane—typically in a lateral-to-medial direction. As the needle passes through the prevertebral fascia, a certain loss of resistance is often felt. Inject 1–2 ml of local anesthetic to confirm correct location before the rest of the dose (15–25 cc in adults) is injected, visualizing the spread around the plexus.

1.2.2 Supraclavicular Block

Often called the "spinal anesthesia of the upper extremity," the supraclavicular block is a technique of anesthetizing the brachial plexus at distal trunks and origin of the divisions, where the brachial plexus is confined to its smallest surface area. The first percutaneous supraclavicular block was performed by Kulenkampff in Germany in 1911, reportedly on himself [2]. The advantages of a supraclavicular technique over other brachial plexus block approaches are its rapid onset and complete and predictable anesthesia for the entire upper extremity and particularly hand surgery. The introduction of ultrasound guidance to regional anesthesia in the last decade has resulted in significant renewed interest in the clinical application of the supraclavicular block, as well as a greater understanding of its mechanics.

- **Indications**: Upper extremity surgery including arm, elbow, forearm, wrist, and hand. (It is best for areas below the mid-humerus level. Above the mid-humerus, the shoulder area, an interscalene block would provide better coverage). However, if enough volume is used it can diffuse to the shoulder area.
- **Contraindications**: Patient refusal, infection at planned injection site, preexisting neurologic defects, local anesthetic allergy, coagulopathy, contralateral phrenic nerve dysfunction, and severe chronic obstructive pulmonary disease.
- **Complications**: Diaphragmatic paralysis, pneumothorax, hoarseness, Horner's syndrome, LA toxicity, infection, hematoma, and allergic reaction.

1.2.2.1 Landmark/Nerve Stimulator Technique Classic Approach

The most common supraclavicular technique is the subclavian perivascular approach, described by Winnie and Collins [3]. The interscalene groove is palpated and followed distally until the pulsation of the subclavian artery is felt. This should be at the midpoint of the clavicle, about 1 cm posterior to it. It is important to note that the dome of the lung is medial to the insertion point of the needle. Entry to the sheath can be identified by a "click" as the needle pierces the tough fascia, by paresthesia, or by an appropriate motor response when a nerve stimulator is used.

For vertical supraclavicular block, also called the "plumb bob" technique, identify the lateral border of the sternocleidomastoid as it inserts onto the clavicle by asking the patient to raise the head slightly off the bed. The needle entry site is immediately superior to the clavicle, just lateral to the identified lateral border of the sternocleidomastoid. The needle is inserted vertically at 90° to the bed and would result in contact with the brachial plexus in most patients.

1.2.2.2 Ultrasound Technique

The patient can be positioned anywhere from supine to sitting upright with their head rotated away from the block site. The probe is placed in the supraclavicular fossa and oriented perpendicular to the subclavian artery. The subclavian artery is identified by its thick wall and brisk pulsations. Immediately superior and posterolateral to the artery, the brachial plexus is seen as a grouping of small hyperechoic circles with hypoechoic centers, similar to a bunch of grapes. Alternatively, the plexus can be found in the interscalene space and followed distally to its association with the subclavian artery. Deep to the artery, the structures of note are the dome of the lung (identified by its characteristic movement and scatter) and the first rib (identified by its hyperechoic surface with dense posterior shadowing).

Once the plexus is identified, the needle is inserted in-plane from a lateral-to-medial direction. The entrance of the needle into the brachial plexus sheath is often associated with a palpable "pop" as the needle passes through the paravertebral fascia/ brachial plexus sheath. After a careful aspiration, 1–2 mL of local anesthetic is injected to confirm the proper needle placement. When the injection displaces the brachial plexus away from the needle, an additional advancement of the needle 1–2 mm deeper may be required to accomplish adequate spread of the local anesthetic. When injection of the local anesthetic does not appear to result in a spread in and around the brachial plexus, additional needle repositioning and injections may be necessary.

1.2.3 Infraclavicular Block

The infraclavicular brachial plexus block is another way of blocking the brachial plexus below the level of the clavicle. It is functionally similar to the supraclavicular block and is useful for distal arm, elbow, wrist, and hand surgery. Infraclavicular block avoids the risk of phrenic nerve block, making it an excellent choice in patients with respiratory issues.

In the infraclavicular fossa, the brachial plexus separates into individual cords that are named medial, lateral, and posterior based on their locations relative to the axillary artery. These cords bundle around the axillary artery as it travels inferior to the coracoid and into the axilla. The cords lie deep to the pectoralis muscles and superficial to the lung while the axillary vein runs inferior to the artery.

- **Indications**: Surgery on the distal arm, elbow, wrist, and hand.
- **Contraindications**: Patient refusal, infection at planned injection site, presence of pacemaker at the site (U/S technique may not be possible due to limitation of probe placement), preexisting neurologic defects, local anesthetic allergy, coagulopathy.
- **Complications**: LA toxicity, infection, bleeding, hematoma, pneumothorax, and nerve injury.

1.2.3.1 Landmark Technique

Vertical Infraclavicular Block

The landmarks required for the block are anterior process of the acromion, jugular notch, and the subclavian artery; and coracoid process and the medial clavicular head. The patient is positioned supine with the head tuned to the opposite side and arm abducted and flexed at the elbow. The coracoid process can be identified by palpating the bony prominence just medial to the shoulder by elevating and lowering the arm. The coracoid process meets the fingers of the palpating hand as the arm is lowered. Mark the medial clavicular head and draw a line joining these 2 points. The needle insertion point is 3 cm caudal to the mid point of the line joining the coracoid process and the medial clavicular head. The goal is to achieve a hand twitch using a current of 0.2–0.5 mA.

1.2.3.2 Ultrasound Technique

The patient can be positioned anywhere from supine to sitting position, and abduction of the arm will bring the artery and plexus closer to the skin. The transducer is placed just medial to the coracoid process with its cranial end below the clavicle. The pectoralis major and minor muscles are identified just above the plexus and vessels. The probe is rotated and moved as needed to obtain a transverse image of the artery. The 3 cords of the brachial plexus appear as hyperechoic circles surrounding the artery. The lateral cord is the closest to the coracoid; the posterior cord is deep to the artery, while the medial cord is the furthest from the coracoid and sometimes lies between the artery and the vein.

Once the structures of interest are identified, the needle is inserted in-plane from the superior or inferior end of the transducer. The aim of the block is to surround each cord with local anesthetic, often achieved by injecting local anesthetic around the artery. Appropriate needle position is confirmed by the spread of the local anesthetic around the artery, dissecting the cords away from the artery. The steep angle of the needle for this deep block severely compromises the needle visualization. This can be improved by applying extra pressure on the probe and often injecting small amount of local anesthetic solution also improves needle visualization.

1.2.4 Axillary Block

The axillary block is one of the most commonly used regional anesthesia techniques. This block aims to block the terminal branches of the brachial plexus, which include the median, radial, ulnar, and musculocutaneous nerves. It is achieved by injecting local anesthetic around the axillary artery as median, ulnar, and radial nerves are all located within the neurovascular sheath. A separate injection is needed to block the musculocutaneous nerve.

- **Indications**: Surgeries on hand, elbow, and some forearm operations.
- **Contraindications**: Patient refusal, infection at planned injection site, preexisting neurologic defects, local anesthetic allergy, coagulopathy.
- **Complications**: LA toxicity, infection, bleeding, hematoma, and allergic reaction.

1.2.4.1 Landmark Technique

Surface landmarks required for the axillary brachial plexus block are the axillary artery pulsation, coracobrachialis muscle, and the pectoralis major muscle. With the patient positioned supine and arm abducted at 90° and the axillary arterial pulsation as a point of reference, the median nerve is positioned superficially and immediately above the pulse; the ulnar nerve is found superficial slightly deeper than the median nerve; the radial nerve is located behind the pulse. The musculocutaneous nerve can be found 1–3 cm deeper and above the pulse, often outside the brachial plexus sheath as it moves distally away from the axillary fossa.

Once the axillary artery pulse is felt, the artery is fixed between the index and middle finger, pressed firmly against the humerus. The needle is advanced directly below the pulse until a radial nerve twitch is obtained, and local anesthetic is injected. The needle is withdrawn and reinserted above the artery and advanced slowly; median nerve twitch should be encountered first and on further advancement ulnar twitch should appear. Inject local anesthetic at both these points. The needle is finally brought back to skin and redirected into the coracobrachialis muscle until the tip is close to the musculocutaneous nerve. This is confirmed by the disappearance of the local coracobrachialis twitch and appearance of biceps twitch. Inject the last portion of the local anesthetic dose here.

1.2.4.2 Ultrasound-Guided Technique

The patient position is the same as the landmark technique. Palpate the pectoralis major muscle at its insertion into the humerus and place the transducer immediately distal to it and perpendicular to the axis of the arm. Slide the transducer to locate the axillary artery and brachial plexus if not already visualized. Identify the individual nerves and insert the needle in-plane from the cephalad direction toward the posterior aspect of the axillary artery. Local anesthetic should be deposited posterior to the artery first covering the radial nerve. The needle is then withdrawn and redirected superior to the artery, and local anesthetic is injected around the median and ulnar nerves. Finally, the musculocutaneous nerve is anesthetized by injecting local anesthetic around it in the coracobrachialis muscle. Frequent aspiration, slow administration of local anesthetic, and avoiding injection at high pressure are critical to decrease the risk of intravascular injection and nerve injury.

1.2.5 Superior Trunk Block

The superior trunk block, first described in 2014, has emerged as a promising alternative to the interscalene and supraclavicular brachial plexus blocks.

The superior trunk is formed by the fusion of C5 and C6 nerve roots of the brachial plexus in the exit of the interscalene groove. Traveling more distally, it bifurcates into anterior and posterior divisions and in to the suprascapular nerve (SSN). The SSN then travels posteriorly and caudally to the supraspinous fossa under the omohyoid muscle. Thus, local anesthetic injection around the superior trunk should produce similar analgesia of the shoulder as the interscalene block because all the terminal nerves innervating the shoulder (axillary nerve, suprascapular nerve, and lateral pectoral nerve) arise distal to the superior trunk. In addition, the site of injection is further away from the phrenic nerve, and this should theoretically reduce the risk of hemi-diaphragmatic paresis.

1.2.5.1 Ultrasound-Guided Technique

Using a high frequency linear transducer (10–15 MHz), the C5 and C6 roots are identified in the interscalene groove; however, they are traced distally until they form the superior trunk, which is visible as a single hypoechoic structure with a hyperechoic connective tissue boundary lying just below the deep cervical fascia. The SSN identified as a small hypoechoic circle that separates from the lateral aspect of the superior trunk and courses laterally under the omohyoid muscle away from the brachial plexus [4].

The targeted level of insertion for the injection is just proximal to the suprascapular nerve diverging from the superior trunk. Local infiltration of 1% lidocaine up to 2 mL will be used to anesthetize the skin for needle insertion using a 25-gauge needle. A 20-gauge, 4-inch stimuplex needle will be inserted lateral to medial under the deep cervical fascia and superficial to the middle scalene muscle, using in-plane technique. The tip of the needle will be placed adjacent to the lateral boundary of the superior trunk. At this location, 10-15 ml of Ropivacaine 0.5% local anesthetic will be injected under ultrasound guidance. An out-of-plane approach may also be used if preferred.

1.2.5.2 Pros and Cons of the Block

Supraclavicular brachial plexus approach, near the upper trunk, has demonstrated a high analgesic efficacy after shoulder surgery with less incidence of phrenic nerve palsy and as a result of the high proportion of connective tissue in this area, persistent postoperative neurological symptoms could be less risky than in the classical interscalene approach.

A limitation of this technique is the risk of puncturing the subclavian artery because of its proximity to the anterior division of the upper trunk and the difficulty in ultrasound visualization of the suprascapular nerve in some patients, as a result of the angle required to achieve a good ultrasound resolution. Care should be taken to avoid injuring the transverse cervical artery and dorsal scapular artery that cross over the brachial plexus and can overlie the superior trunk (4).

1.2.6 Suprascapular Nerve (SSN) Block

The sensory innervation of the shoulder joint is complex and involves contributions from the axillary, suprascapular (SSN), subscapular, musculocutaneous, and lateral pectoral nerves. Of those listed, the axillary and SSN are considered the most important. The SSN receives 70% of the sensory fibers from the shoulder joint. The other 30% are innervated by the axillary nerve, musculocutaneous, and the lateral pectoral nerve.

The SSN arises from the ventral rami of the C5 and C6 nerve roots and emerges off the lateral aspect of the superior trunk of the brachial plexus and runs through the posterior triangle under the inferior belly of the omohyoid and trapezius muscles. It enters the supraspinous fossa under the suprascapular transverse ligament. The suprascapular artery and vein pass above this ligament. In the supraspinous fossa, the nerve is in close proximity to the bone and exits the suprascapular fossa to the infrascapular fossa lateral to the spinoglenoid notch. The nerve is susceptible to injury and impingement at the level of the notch as it passes beneath the suprascapular transverse ligament. This site represents an attractive region for SSN blockade as the nerve has not divided yet.

The traditional ultrasound (US)-guided approach to block the SSN is at the suprascapular notch where the SSN enters the supraspinous fossa (posterior approach). In this location, the SSN is located deeply and is difficult to visualize by US. Numerous anatomical variations in the sensory branching from the SSN exist. In around 50% of the cases, sensory branches already separate from the main stem before the main stem enters the suprascapular notch.

A more desirable supraclavicular approach (anterior approach) has been shown to be more effective as it ensures that all sensory branches of the SSN are blocked. This is done by placing the transducer over the supraclavicular region, where C5 and C6 roots are again identified in the interscalene groove and are traced distally until they form the superior trunk, which is visible as a single hypoechoic structure with a hyperechoic connective tissue boundary lying just below the deep cervical fascia. The suprascapular nerve is seen as a small hypoechoic circle that separates from the lateral aspect of the superior trunk and courses laterally under the omohyoid muscle away from the brachial plexus.

– *Technical description of the block:*

Suprascapular nerve (anterior approach):

With the patient in a supine position, a linear US probe is placed over the supraclavicular area. After identifying the superior trunk, you trace the SSN more distally as it is seen branching off and traveling beneath the omohyoid muscle. After infiltration with 1 ml of 1% lidocaine, a 4-inch 20-gauge stimuplex needle is inserted in line with the probe in a lateral-to-medial orientation toward the SSN. After negative aspiration, Ropivacaine 0.5% solution is then injected in 5-ml aliquots.

Suprascapular nerve (Posterior approach):

The patient is placed in sitting position in order to gain access to the suprascapular area. After skin and transducer preparation, place a linear high frequency 8–13 MHz transducer on the scapula to obtain a transverse view of the SSN and suprascapular vessels. Ask the patient to place the hand over to the contralateral shoulder. This will serve two purposes, first this will move the scapula laterally to provide more space for SSN scanning, and second, it will move the target SSN injection site more laterally away from the thorax. Position the transducer oblique (not parallel) to the spine of the scapula in the supraspinous fossa because the SSN runs an oblique course between the suprascapular notch and the spinoglenoid notch. Place one end of the transducer over the scapular spine and the other end directing toward the coracoid process. The suprascapular notch is identified below the trapezius and supraspinatus muscles. The SSN is then identified beneath the superior transverse scapular ligament. The needle is inserted in plane, and 10 mL of 0.2% ropivacaine is injected close to the SSN [5].

1.2.7 Axillary (AN) Nerve Block

Axillary nerve (AN) contains fibers from the ventral rami of C5 and C6. It is one of the terminal branches of the posterior cord of the brachial plexus. It is formed at the lateral border of the subscapularis muscle as the nerve runs posteriorly, beneath the shoulder joint toward the surgical neck of the humerus. It passes through the quadrangular space in close relation with the posterior circumflex humeral artery (PCHA) and splits into an anterior and a posterior branch either within the quadrangular space or later within the deltoid muscle (DM).

Anatomically, the quadrilateral space is bordered superiorly by the teres minor, laterally by the proximal humerus, medially by the long head of the triceps tendon, and inferiorly by the teres major. These borders create the compartment that the distal branch of the axillary nerve and posterior circumflex humeral artery navigate through.

In the anterior approach, the SSN is blocked in the supraclavicular fossa. A linear array transducer (8–13 MHz, Sonosite) is placed in the transverse plane to visualize the superior trunk in the short-axis view. The suprascapular nerve is visualized as it branches off from the superior trunk and courses beneath the inferior belly of the omohyoid muscle.

Ultrasound-Guided Technique:

The patient is placed in a beach chair position, with the shoulder in neutral position but rotated 45 degrees inward with the hand resting on the ipsilateral thigh. After proper disinfection, using a linear ultrasound transducer (13–6 MHz) positioned parallel to the longitudinal axis of the shaft of the humerus and approximately 2 cm below the posterolateral part of the acromion on the dorsal side of the arm, identify the surgical neck and the shaft of the humerus and the cross section of the PCHA, using ultrasound Doppler. Important landmarks are the deltoid muscle (DM) in longitudinal section, the head of the humerus (HH), the humeral shaft (SH), the teres minor muscle (TM) in transverse section, and the triceps muscle in longitudinal section.

Using the in-line technique, the needle is advanced piercing the deltoid muscle with the needle tip below the fascia caudal to the teres minor muscle (TM) and just cranial to the posterior circumflex humeral artery. You should identify the neurovascular quadrangular space, locate the AN, and inject aliquots of 0.5% ropivacaine 10–15 mL.

– Clinical discussion including the pros and cons of the block:

The potential advantages of a combined SSN-AN block are that it spares the motor function of the upper limb while avoiding the potential serious complications associated with IBPB, such as phrenic nerve palsy and vertebral artery/epidural injection. Nevertheless, it should be noted that SSN block + AN block may cause diaphragmatic palsy when the anterior approach for the SSN block is performed.

The limitation of the combined approach is the difficulty in direct visualization of the axillary nerve as well as the suprascapular nerve (both anterior and posterior approach). It requires superior technical skills, and sometimes nerve stimulation may be needed to help locate the nerve.

1.3 Lower Limb Blocks

1.3.1 Femoral Nerve Block

The femoral nerve block is an essential block that is easy to learn, low risk with minimal complications. It is useful for surgery on the anterior thigh and knee, quadriceps tendon repair, and postoperative pain management of femur and knee surgery. It is frequently combined with other lower extremity blocks, such as sciatic and obturator blocks, to achieve anesthesia of almost the entire lower extremity.

- **Anatomy**: The femoral nerve is the largest branch of the lumbar plexus and travels through the pelvis in the groove between the psoas and iliacus muscle. It emerges beneath the inguinal ligament, posterolateral to the femoral vessels (Fig. 1.3). At the femoral crease, the nerve is on the surface of the iliacus muscle and covered by the fascia iliaca or sandwiched between 2 layers of fascia iliaca. It divides into its branches at or above the level of the inguinal ligament.
- **Indications**: Surgery on anterior thigh, knee, quadriceps tendon, and in combination with sciatic and obturator blocks for distal limb and foot surgery.

1.3.1.1 Landmark Technique

The patient is positioned supine with both legs extended, and the operator should stand on the same side of the patient. Identify the landmarks anterior superior iliac spine and the pubic tubercle, and draw a line joining the 2 points (Fig. 1.4). Palpate the femoral artery on this line and insert the needle perpendicularly, just lateral to the femoral artery pulsations. A visible or palpable twitch of the quadriceps muscle or the patella at 0.2–0.4 mA is the most reliable nerve stimulator response. It is very common to get a sartorius muscle twitch as the nerve to the sartorius muscle branch from the anteromedial aspect of the femoral nerve may be lying outside the iliacus fascia. When injecting local

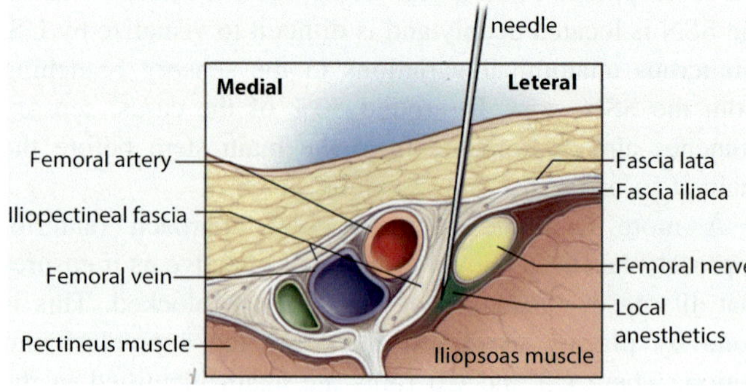

Fig. 1.3 Femoral nerve anatomy (Reprinted with permission from Farag and Brown [6])

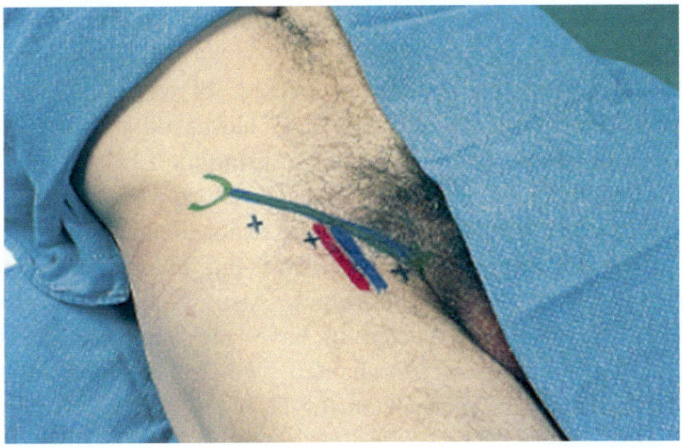

Fig. 1.4 Femoral nerve block—landmark technique (Reprinted with permission from Farag and Brown [4])

anesthetic, accepting the sartorius muscle twitch results in inconsistent block success; hence, it should not be accepted in landmark/nerve stimulation technique.

1.3.1.2 Ultrasound Technique

The patient is positioned supine, and the ultrasound probe is placed parallel to the inguinal crease. Sliding the transducer medially and laterally, identify the femoral artery and trace upward to the common femoral artery if profunda femoris branch is seen on the initial scan. Immediately lateral to the vessel, and deep to the fascia iliaca is the femoral nerve, which is typically hyperechoic and roughly triangular or oval in shape. Once the femoral nerve is identified, the needle is inserted in-plane from a lateral-to-medial orientation. The goal is to place the needle tip below the fascia iliaca, immediately adjacent to the lateral aspect of the femoral nerve. The correct placement is confirmed by the spread of the local anesthetic in the wedge-shaped tissue space lateral to the femoral artery, either lifting the femoral nerve off the iliopsoas or the spread above the nerve lateral to the artery.

Adductor Canal Block

The adductor canal also called hunter's canal/sub-sartorial canal was first described in the eighteenth century by John Hunter. It is defined as a musculoaponeurotic tunnel extending from the apex of the femoral triangle to adductor hiatus. The canal is bounded laterally by vastus medialis, medially by adductor magnus and adductor longus, and superiorly by sartorius. The canal consistently contains the superficial femoral vessels, saphenous nerve (sensory), and the nerve to vastus medialis (NVM) (motor and sensory)). However, it may contain the medial femoral cutaneous nerve (sensory) 61% of the time and the anterior cutaneous branch of obturator nerve (sensory) 21% of the time. The motor branches from the obturator nerve leave before entering into the adductor canal. The NVM in conjunction with the saphenous nerve contributes to substantial innervation to the anteromedial aspect of the knee joint including the joint capsule and the medial retinaculum. The sole motor nerve to potentially be anesthetized during ACB is the NVM. Thus, the unique possibility of performing a predominantly sensory block with minimal motor blockade has attracted many providers to perform ACB [7].

The ACB has been performed at the mid-thigh level, approximately halfway between the ASIS and the superior border of the patella. The superficial femoral artery (SFA) is identified at the mid-thigh level underneath the sartorius muscle. Typically, the saphenous nerve is usually visible as a hyperechoic structure anterolateral to the artery. However, the nerve does cross the SFA and becomes located medially as one traverses the adductor canal more distally. The vastus medialis is visible lateral to neurovascular bundle.

The adductor canal block (ACB) can often spare quadriceps muscle strength; however due to its predominantly anteromedial coverage of the peripatellar and intra-articular aspects of the knee, ACB fails to alleviate posterior knee pain which may be severe in intensity.

– *Technical description of the block*

With the patient in supine position, the probe is placed midway between the ASIS and the superior border of the patella. The sartorius muscle, the deeper SFA, and saphenous nerve are identified. Using an in-plane technique, a 4-inch needle for a single shot or a Touhy needle is introduced from the lateral side of the probe if a catheter is to be placed. The target of the needle tip is at the 9'oclock of the SFA nerve. Here, LA showing spread inside the adductor canal and surrounding the SFA. The femoral vein lies beneath the saphenous nerve, below the SFA, and hence can be injured if significant pressure is placed on the probe. The success of the block depends on being able to accurately inject local anesthetic and fill up the adductor canal to anesthetize saphenous nerve and NVM.

– *Clinical discussion including the pros n cons of the block*

Apart from reports of muscle weakness following ACB due to proximal spread into the femoral triangle, no major complications have been reported with the block. It is considered a very safe regional technique. Similar to a femoral block, the posterior part of the knee will not be covered by an ACB. Supplementation with a sciatic nerve block or iPACK block is recommended.

Lateral Femoral Cutaneous Nerve (LFCN)

– *Relevant anatomy and Sonoanatomy:*

The LFCN is a branch of the posterior division of the L2 and L3 spinal nerves. It is a predominantly sensory branch of the lumbar plexus. It travels within the retroperitoneum, enters the pelvis lateral to the margin of the psoas muscle, courses obliquely across the iliacus, emerges deep to the inguinal ligament (IL) medial to the ASIS, and crosses the superficial surface of the sartorius muscle (Sa). Block of the lateral femoral cutaneous nerve provides anesthesia or analgesia in the anterolateral thigh.

The LFCN typically is located between the tensor fasciae latae (TFLM) and sartorius (SaM) muscles, 1–2 cm medial and inferior to the ASIS, and 1.0 cm deep to the skin surface. Ultrasound imaging of the lateral femoral cutaneous nerve yields an oval hypoechoic structure in cross-sectional view. The lateral edge of the sartorius muscle is a useful landmark, and as such, it can be relied on throughout the procedure. The LFCN branches sometimes may be seen across the anterior margin of the TFL. With the patient in the supine or lateral position, palpation of the ASIS provides the target for transducer placement. It is positioned at 2 cm inferior and medial to the ASIS. Typically, the nerve is identified slightly more distally in its course. If nerve stimulator is used, precise identification of the LFCN may be confirmed by eliciting a tingling sensation on the lateral side of the thigh.

– *Technical description of the block:*

The patient is positioned supine with the probe placed immediately inferior to the ASIS, parallel to the inguinal ligament. Initially, the tensor fasciae latae and the sartorius muscle should be identified. The branches of the lateral femoral cutaneous nerve are sometimes visualized in the hypoechoic fat-filled subfascial space between the sartorius muscle medially and the TFLM laterally in the short-axis view. A skin wheal is then made on the lateral aspect of the transducer, and the needle is inserted in-plane in a lateral-to-medial orientation, through the subcutaneous tissue and the tensor fasciae latae muscle. A pop may be felt as the needle tip enters the plane between the tensor fascia latae and sartorius muscles. After gentle aspiration, 1–2 mL of LA is injected to verify the needle tip position, then a total of 5–10 ml of 0.5% Ropivacaine to have a successful blockade.

The lateral femoral cutaneous nerve has been targeted as part of multimodal analgesia for surgical incisions involving the proximal part of the lateral thigh (hip surgeries, autologous skin harvesting) as well as in patients diagnosed with Meralgia paresthetica, which is a disorder related to the entrapment of the LFCN.

– *Clinical discussion including the pros n cons of the block*

The LFCN provides adequate coverage of any lateral skin incision involving the thigh. PENG blocks do not provide coverage to this area of the skin, so using the LFCN in conjunction with a PENG block seems to have some added benefit. The LFCN is considered a very safe regional technique.

The limitation of the LFCN is the inconsistency in identifying the nerve ultrasound. Also, blockade of the LFCN cannot be expected to have any analgesic effect proximal to the greater trochanter, so there is limited anesthesia of the surgical incision for THA.

1.3.2 Sciatic Nerve Block

The sciatic nerve is the largest nerve trunk in the body and arises from the sacral plexus. It exits the pelvis posteriorly via the greater sciatic notch and descends into the thigh between the greater trochanter and the ischial tuberosity. The sciatic nerve provides sensory and motor supply to most of the lower leg via its terminal branches (tibial and common peroneal).

1.3.2.1 Landmark/Nerve Stimulator Techniques

Posterior Approach (Labat) [8]

The patient is placed in Sim's position (lateral decubitus position with the upper operative leg flexed to 90° at hip and knee. The landmarks are the greater trochanter (GT), posterior superior iliac spine (PSIS), and the sacral hiatus. Draw the first line joining the greater trochanter and the PSIS and mark a midpoint on the line. Draw a second line joining the greater trochanter and the sacral hiatus. Now drop a line perpendicularly from the midpoint of the first line, and the point of needle insertion is where it crosses the second line. The needle is inserted perpendicular to the skin surface and any motor stimulation of the sciatic nerve (hamstring, calf foot, or toe twitches) is acceptable and inject local anesthetic.

Inferior Approach (Raj)

The patient is positioned supine, and the hip and knee are flexed to 90°. Identify and draw a line joining the greater trochanter and the ischial tuberosity. Mark a point half way in the groove between the hamstrings and the adductor muscles. Insert the needle perpendicular to the skin with a slight medial intent to get the sciatic motor response.

Anterior Approach (Beck)

The anterior sciatic nerve block can be performed when the patient cannot be positioned laterally due to postoperative

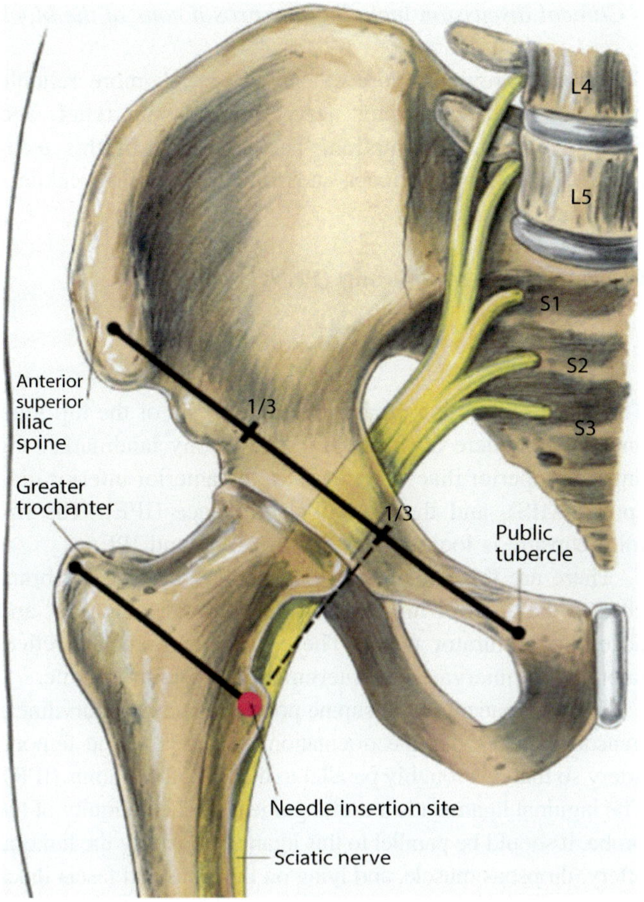

Fig. 1.5 Anterior sciatic nerve block (Reprinted with permission from Farag and Brown [9])

pain, trauma, or the presence of external fixation devices. The patient is positioned supine. Identify and draw a line joining the anterior superior iliac spine and the pubic tubercle. Draw another line parallel to the first one from the greater trochanter (◘ ◉ Fig. 1.5). The point of needle insertion is where a perpendicular line from the junction of the medial and middle third of the first line meets the second line. Insert the needle perpendicularly until it contacts the femur. Now redirect slightly medially to slide off the femur and advance a few centimeters to get a motor response. In a few patients, the sciatic nerve lies immediately posterior to the femur and may be inaccessible. A slight external rotation of the limb can overcome this problem.

1.3.2.2 Ultrasound Technique

The use of ultrasound guidance facilitated multiple approaches at several convenient levels to block the sciatic nerve. The common sites are the transgluteal/subgluteal and the anterior approaches.

Anterior Approach

The anterior sciatic nerve block is ideally suited for postoperative patients requiring additional block as positioning them laterally is not easy. The ultrasound guidance not only reduces the risk of vascular injury, but also eliminates the need for use of precise geometry to identify the needle entry point. The patient is positioned supine with slight abduction and external rotation of the thigh. The sciatic nerve is imaged approximately at the level of the minor trochanter. At this location, a curved transducer placed over the anteromedial aspect of the thigh will reveal the musculature of all 3 fascial compartments of the thigh: anterior, medial, and posterior. Beneath the superficial sartorius muscle is the femoral artery, and deep and medial to this vessel is the profunda femoris artery. Both of these can be identified with color Doppler ultrasound for orientation. The femur is easily seen as a hyperechoic rim with the corresponding shadow beneath the vastus intermedius. Medial to the femur is the body of the adductor magnus muscle, separated by the fascial plane(s) of the hamstrings muscles. The sciatic nerve is visualized as a hyperechoic, slightly flattened oval structure sandwiched between these 2 muscle planes and is typically visualized at a depth of 6–8 cm. The needle is inserted in-plane or out of plane from the medial aspect of the thigh and advanced toward the sciatic nerve avoiding the femoral vessels. Once the needle tip is close to the nerve or in the fascial plane between the adductors and the hamstrings when the nerve is not clearly visualized, 1–2 mL of local anesthetic is injected to confirm the adequate distribution of the local anesthetic and the rest of the dose in injected in divided doses after negative aspiration.

Posterior Approach (Transgluteal/Subgluteal)

The sciatic nerve can be easily identified between the greater trochanter and ischial tuberosity, beneath a well-defined muscle plane. The nerve also can be traced backward from the popliteal region in difficult cases. The approach and the actual site of the block is based on the patient's anatomic characteristics and personal preference.

A low-frequency curvilinear probe is used to identify the bony landmarks at the transgluteal level. The sciatic nerve is located deep to the gluteus muscle, slightly closer to the ischial tuberosity, and appears as an oval or triangular hyperechoic structure. At the subgluteal level, the nerve is located deep to the long head of the biceps muscle and the posterior surface of the adductor magnus. The needle is inserted in-plane typically from the lateral side and advancer toward the nerve. Once in the desired location 1–2 cc of local anesthetic is injected after negative aspiration. Often the nerve is better visualized after the initial injection of local anesthetic and moves away from the needle. The rest of the local anesthetic is injected in divided doses after negative aspiration and absence of high resistance to injection.

Suprainguinal Fascia Iliaca (SIFI) Plane Block

– *Relevant anatomy and Sonoanatomy*

The fascia iliaca is a fascial sheath that overlies the iliacus and psoas major muscle in the pelvis. It continues beneath the inguinal ligament where it becomes continuous with the epimysium to the iliopsoas muscle group. Three nerves, the lateral femoral cutaneous nerve (LFTN), femoral nerve (FN), and obturator nerve (ON), are bound down to iliopsoas muscle in the pelvis by the fascia iliaca. The anterior superior iliac spine (ASIS) is palpated and the ultrasound probe is placed slightly inferior and medial to it, perpendicular to the inguinal ligament between ASIS and the pubic symphysis. The iliacus muscle is identified superficial to the ilium, and the hyperechoic fascia iliaca is identified on the superficial border of the muscle. Superficial to the fascia iliaca, the abdominal wall muscles meet those of the lower extremity at the inguinal ligament (Fig. 1.4). The tapered confluence of the internal oblique (cephalad) and the sartorius (caudad) at the inguinal ligament has been described as a bow tie or horizontal hourglass sitting atop the iliacus muscle at the level of the anterior inferior iliac spine (AIIS). The deep circumflex iliac artery may be identified between the internal oblique and fascia iliaca, and serves as both a landmark and structure to avoid.

– *Technical description of the block*

In the supine position with the inguinal area exposed, a linear transducer is placed in parasagittal orientation just medial to ASIS. Slide the probe toward and away from the ASIS, along the inguinal ligament, until the bow tie or hourglass of the sartorius and internal oblique are visualized.

A 20G 10 mm needle is advanced in plane from caudal to cranial direction with an aim of piercing the fascia iliaca north of the inguinal ligament. The needle can enter inferior or at the level of the ligament and pointed cephalad. One important landmark is the deep circumflex iliac artery, which is lateral to the femoral artery on top of the fascia iliaca and serves as a good landmark if your needle is in the right plane. After the "pop" through fascia iliaca, 1–2 mL of saline or local anesthetic is injected to hydro dissect between hyperechoic fascia iliaca and iliacus muscle beneath it. The needle is further advanced in the cephalad direction separating those two components more proximally. Approximately 30–40 ml of 0.2% ropivacaine is most commonly utilized.

– *Clinical discussion including the pros n cons of the block*

SIFI block provides more extensive spread, more reliable blockade of the obturator nerve, greater pain relief, and reduced opioid consumption. The downside of this technique is causing quadriceps and adductor muscle weakness impairing ambulation.

Pericapsular Nerve Group (PENG) Block

– *Relevant anatomy and Sonoanatomy*

The PENG block is a periarticular analgesia of the hip joint and pelvis. There are three important bony landmarks: the anterior superior iliac spine (ASIS), the anterior inferior iliac spine (AIIS), and the ilio-pubic eminence (IPE). The hip joint capsule is located between the AIIS and IPE.

There are three main nerves that give off articular branches to the anterior hip capsule: the femoral, obturator, and accessory obturator nerve. These articular branches reflect laterally to innervate the anteromedial hip joint capsule.

With the patient in the supine position, place the curvilinear transducer in an oblique orientation over area of the femoral artery so that it is roughly parallel to the ilio-pubic ramus (IPR). The inguinal ligament is a useful guide as to the obliquity of the probe, it should be parallel to this ligament. Identify the femoral artery, iliopsoas muscle, and lying on iliopsoas and fascia iliaca is the femoral nerve. Increase the depth as needed to visualize the hyperechoic line of the underlying bone. If this line has a curved appearance, it represents the femoral head and the hip joint. If this is seen, slide the probe in a cranial direction, the curved line of the hip joint will transition into a flat line that represents the IPR. The AIIS is often seen as a prominence at the lateral end. The IPE lies at the medial end but with a linear probe its often not possible to see in the same view. Ensure that you identify femoral neurovascular bundle, so that it can be avoided during needle insertion.

– *Technical description of the block*

With the patient in supine position, a curvilinear low-frequency ultrasound probe (2–5 MHz) was initially placed in a transverse plane over the AIIS and then aligned with the pubic ramus by rotating the probe counterclockwise approximately 45 degrees. In this view, the IPE, the iliopsoas muscle and tendon, the femoral artery, and pectineus muscle were observed. Plan a safe needle trajectory with 10 mm 21G stimuplex needle from lateral to medial that will contact the IPE under femoral artery just lateral to the psoas tendon. 20 ml of desired local anesthetic is injected under muscle lifting it up off the bone [10].

PENG block is a new regional analgesia technique for hip fractures and surgeries. It is a promising alternative to other regional nerve blocks, such as femoral nerve blocks or fascia iliaca nerve block.

– Clinical discussion including the pros n cons of the block

An ideal block technique should provide complete analgesia of the hip joint without muscle weakness. In general, PENG block avoids the femoral nerve block and thus quadriceps weakness; however, a large volume of local anesthetic greater than 20 cc can reach femoral nerve and cause motor weakness.

The PENG block does not provide coverage or analgesia for surgical incisions in hip fracture surgery. Thus, a separate block for LFTN is often needed to cover the lateral incision. Beware that both the femoral nerve and the LFCN can be injured as the needle is inserted to reach the target.

1.3.3 Popliteal Sciatic Nerve Block

The popliteal block is essentially a block of the sciatic nerve in the popliteal fossa. Sciatic nerve is a nerve bundle that consists of 2 separate nerve trunks: the tibial and the common peroneal nerves. They diverge in the popliteal fossa about 4–10 cm above the popliteal crease (◘ ◉ Fig. 1.6). It is a commonly performed block for surgery on the ankle and foot. The addition of saphenous nerve block to cover the medial lower leg and ankle gives complete analgesia for ankle and foot surgery.

– **Indications**: Ankle and foot surgery, Achilles tendon repair.

1.3.3.1 Landmark Techniques

Lateral Popliteal Approach

The landmarks are popliteal fossa crease, vastus lateralis, and biceps femoris muscles. This block is performed with the patient supine and thus has the advantage of not requiring to place the position prone. The foot on the side to be blocked is positioned elevated to facilitate easy visualization of muscle twitch.

The groove between the vastus lateralis and the biceps femoris muscles is palpated and a point in the groove, approximately 7 cm above the popliteal crease or at the level of superior border of patella, is marked for needle point. The needle is inserted perpendicular to the leg into the groove and advanced to contact the femur. The needle is withdrawn to skin and redirected 30° posteriorly to locate the nerve with nerve stimulator. Once the desired muscle twitch is obtained, the calculated dose of local anesthetic is injected after negative aspiration.

Posterior Approach

The landmarks used are the popliteal crease, semimembranosus, and the biceps femoris. The patient is positioned prone for this approach with the leg resting on a pillow. The

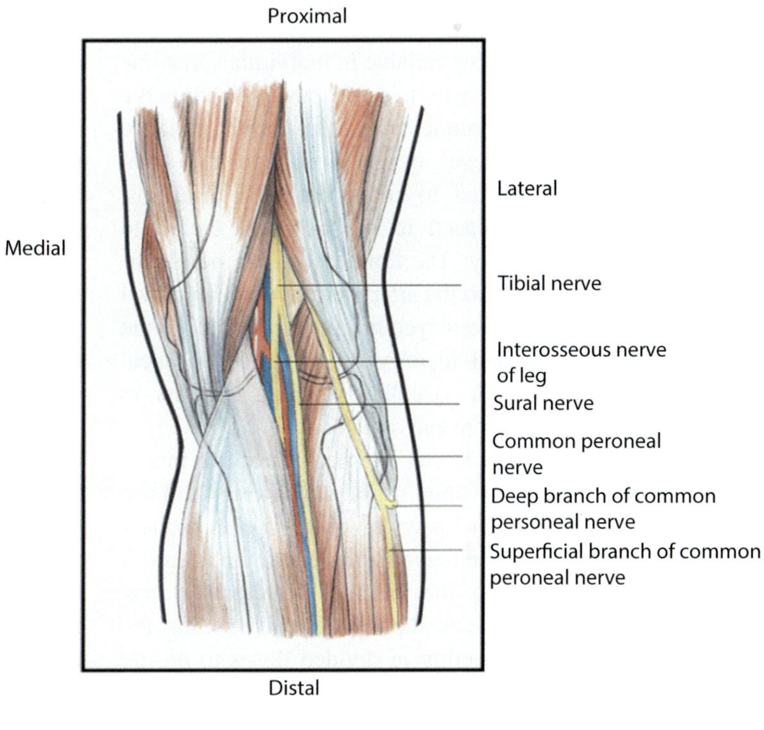

Fig. 1.6 Popliteal sciatic nerve block (Reprinted with permission from Yared and Brown [11])

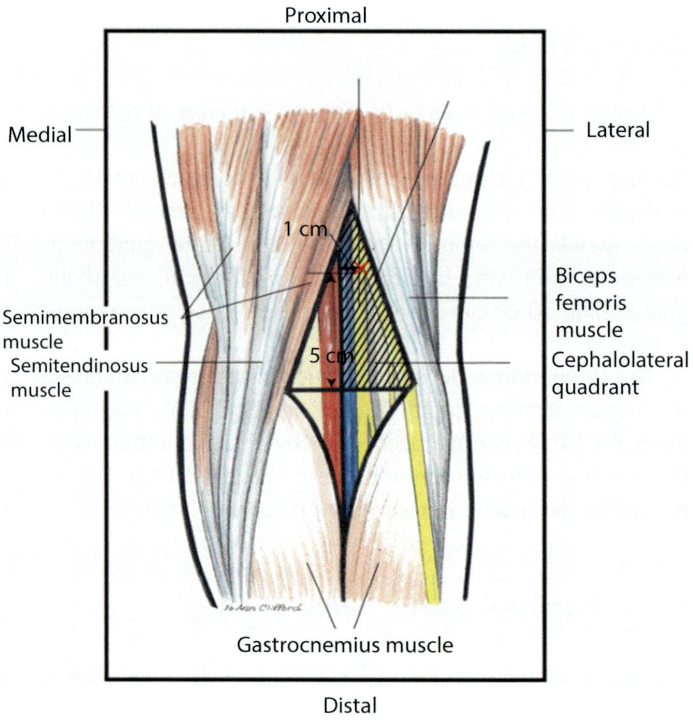

Fig. 1.7 Popliteal sciatic nerve block—posterior approach (Reprinted with permission from Yared and Brown [11])

knee is flexed to mark the popliteal crease. Trace the biceps femoris laterally and semimembranosus medially and find the apex of the popliteal fossa. Drop a line from the apex of the fossa to the middle of the popliteal crease and mark a point 5–7 cm proximal and 1 cm lateral to popliteal crease for needle entry (◘ ◉ Fig. 1.7).

1.3.3.2 Ultrasound-Guided Technique

The level at which the sciatic nerve divides into tibial and common peroneal nerve is so variable in individuals that one of the components can be easily missed in the isolated nerve stimulation/landmark technique. The ultrasound guidance correctly identifies the level of division, and the local anesthetic can be deposited to cover both the divisions. A linear transducer is placed in the popliteal crease to identify the popliteal artery. The tibial nerve can be identified superficial and lateral to the artery as a hyperechoic oval or round structure with honeycomb pattern. Sliding the transducer proximally will identify the common peroneal nerve laterally and can be visualized coming together to form the sciatic nerve before the division.

Ultrasound-guided block can be performed in prone, lateral, or supine (with elevation of the leg/flexing the knee and hip to create enough space to place the transducer beneath the knee). Once the nerve is identified, the needle is inserted in-plane avoiding the vascular structures. Local anesthetic is injected close to the nerve, repositioning the needle as needed, and injecting in divided doses to ensure adequate circumferential spread around the nerve.

1.3.4 Ankle Block

Ankle block is a simple, easy-to-perform procedure that is highly effective for surgeries involving the foot and toes. It involves blocking the 4 terminal branches of the sciatic nerve (deep and superficial peroneal, tibial, and sural) and the terminal branch of the femoral nerve (saphenous). The ankle block will not provide analgesia/anesthesia for the ankle itself; a popliteal nerve block supplemented by saphenous nerve block is required for surgery on the ankle.

The posterior tibial and the deep peroneal are the 2 deep nerves that need injection underneath the fascia, while the 3 superficial nerves (saphenous, sural, and the superficial peroneal) are anesthetized by subcutaneous infiltration.

- **Indications**: Surgery on the foot and toes including podiatry surgery, foot/toe debridement/amputation.
- **Complications**: Bleeding/hematoma, nerve injury, vascular injury.

1.3.4.1 Landmark Technique

The deep peroneal nerve is located immediately lateral to the tendon of the extensor hallucis longus muscle (between the extensor hallucis longus and the extensor digitorum longus). The pulsations of the dorsalis pedis artery are felt here; the nerve is positioned immediately lateral to the artery. With the finger positioned in the groove just lateral to the extensor hallucis longus, the needle is inserted under the skin and advanced until the bone is contacted. From the bone, the needle is withdrawn 1–2 mm, and 2–3 mL of local anesthetic is injected (◘ ◉ Fig. 1.8).

From the same needle entry point, advance the needle subcutaneously laterally and medially to the malleoli, injecting 3–5 ml in each direction. These lateral and medial infiltrations block the superficial peroneal and the saphenous nerves, respectively. The sural nerve is blocked by infiltrating local anesthetic between the lateral malleolus and the Achilles tendon.

The posterior tibial nerve is located just behind and distal to the medial malleolus. The pulse of the posterior tibial artery can be felt at this location; the nerve is just posterior to the artery. The needle is inserted in the groove behind the medial malleolus below the pulse of the tibial artery and advanced to contact the bone. Once bone is contacted, the needle is withdrawn 1–2 mm and local anesthetic is injected after negative aspiration.

1.3.4.2 Ultrasound-Guided Technique

The tibial nerve is the largest of the 5 nerves to be blocked and can be easily identified using ultrasound. A linear transducer placed just proximal to the medial malleolus will identify the tibial nerve immediately posterior to the tibial artery. In difficult cases, color Doppler can identify the artery and injecting local anesthetic just behind the artery will block the tibial nerve.

The deep peroneal nerve can be identified with a transducer placed transversely at the level of the ankle and appears as a small hyperechoic structure. It is small and often not easily identified, but the dorsalis pedis artery can be identified and local anesthetic injected next to it to achieve the block. Sural nerve and saphenous nerve are small hyperechoic structures that may be seen next to the saphenous veins.

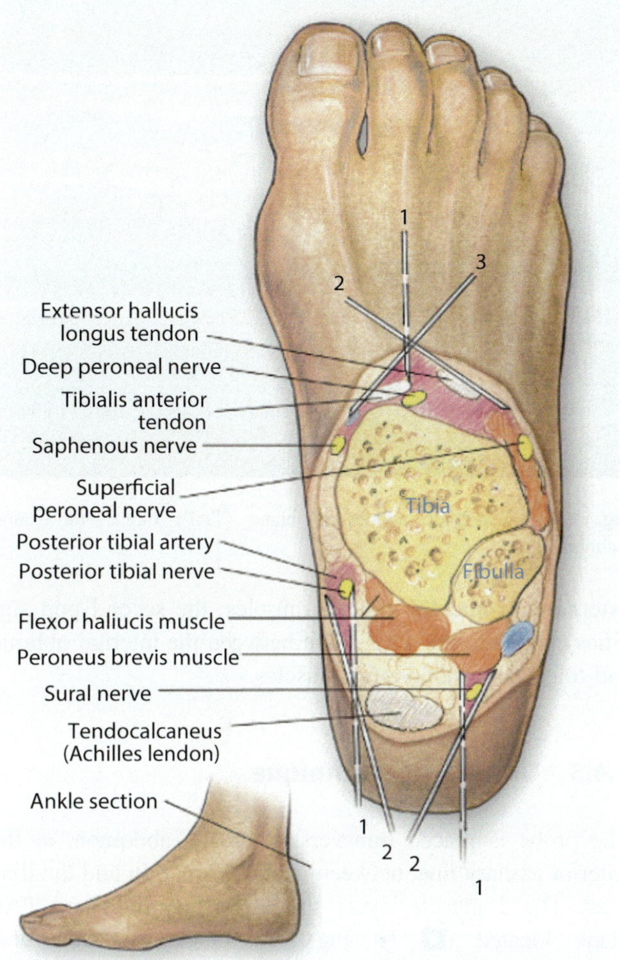

Fig. 1.8 Ankle block (Reprinted with permission from Brown [12])

1.4 Fascial Plane Blocks

1.4.1 Transversus Abdominis Plane (TAP) Block

The transversus abdominis plane (TAP) block was first described as a landmark-guided technique involving needle insertion at the triangle of Petit. It has been shown to provide good postoperative analgesia for a variety of procedures.

- **Indications**: Postoperative analgesia for laparotomy, appendectomy, laparoscopic surgery, ileostomy closure, abdominoplasty, and cesarean delivery; as an alternative to epidural anesthesia for operations on the abdominal wall.
- **Complications**: Bowel perforation/hematoma, infection, intravascular injection, liver laceration. The complications are very rare, and the use of ultrasound has further minimized the complications.

The anterior abdominal wall (skin, muscles, and parietal peritoneum) is innervated by the anterior rami of the lower 6 thoracic nerves (T7-T12) and the first lumbar nerve (L1). Terminal branches of these somatic nerves course through the lateral abdominal wall within a plane between the internal oblique muscle (IOM) and transversus abdominis muscle. This intermuscular plane is called the transversus abdominis plane. Injection of local anesthetic within the TAP can result in unilateral analgesia to the skin, muscles, and parietal peritoneum of the anterior abdominal wall.

1.4.2 Landmark Technique

The triangle of Petit is an area bounded by the latissimus dorsi muscle posteriorly, the external oblique muscle (EOM) anteriorly, and the iliac crest inferiorly. A needle is inserted perpendicular to all planes, looking for a tactile endpoint of 2 pops. The first pop indicates penetration of the external oblique fascia and entry into the plane between

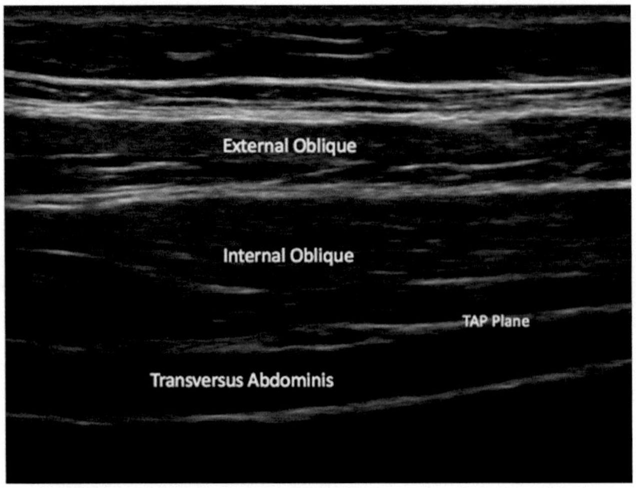

Fig. 1.9 Transversus abdominis plane (TAP) block—ultrasound technique

external and internal oblique muscles; the second pop signifies entry into the TAP plane between the internal oblique and transversus abdominis muscles.

1.4.3 Ultrasound Technique

The probe is placed transversely on the abdomen, at the anterior axillary line, between the costal margin and the iliac crest. The 3 muscle layers should be identified and TAP plane located (◘ ◉ Fig. 1.9). Once the transverse abdominal plane is identified, a skin wheal is made 2–3 cm medial to the medial aspect of the transducer, and the needle is inserted in-plane in a medial to lateral orientation. The needle penetrates through the subcutaneous tissue, EOM, and IOM. As the needle enters the TAP plane, a "pop" may be felt. After gentle aspiration, 1–2 mL of local anesthetic is injected to verify the location of the needle tip. When injection of the local anesthetic appears to be intramuscular, the needle is advanced or withdrawn carefully 1–2 mm and another bolus is administered. This gesture is repeated until the correct plane is achieved. At least 20 cc of LA is required to achieve a satisfactory block.

1.4.4 Rectus Sheath Block

The rectus sheath is formed from the aponeuroses of the fascial sheaths of all three lateral abdominal wall muscles. The external oblique (EOM), internal oblique (IOM), and transversus abdominis (TAM) muscles each form a bilaminar aponeurosis at its medial border converging to form the lateral border of the RAM, termed the *linea semilunaris.* The sensorimotor innervation of the anterior abdominal wall is supplied by the ventral rami of the thoracolumbar spinal (T7-L1) segmental nerves. The thoracolumbar nerves course along the anterolateral wall within the transversus abdominis plane (TAP), and continue anteromedial, eventually encroaching upon the lateral aspect of the rectus sheath. The nerves then enter the lateral aspect of RAM and contribute to the formation of a nerve plexus that runs craniocaudally within the muscle in close relation to the lateral branch of the deep epigastric artery. The thoracolumbar nerves typically pierce the posterior border and/or lateral border of the RAM approximately 1.5–2.5 cm from the lateral edge of the RAM. Performing a bilateral rectus sheath block provides analgesia to the anteromedial abdominal wall and periumbilical area (spinal dermatomes T9, T10, and T11). The technique blocks the anterior cutaneous branches of the intercostal nerves, and therefore, it is well suited for postoperative analgesia for surgery with midline (or paramedian) abdominal incision. Rectus sheath block does not provide analgesia for the lateral abdomen nor visceral analgesia.

1.4.4.1 Ultrasound Technique

The rectus muscle is imaged with the ultrasound probe in short-axis orientation above the level of the umbilicus with the patient supine. A broadband (5–12 MHz) linear array probe is used, with an imaging depth of 4–6 cm. Typically, a 21-gauge, 100 mm needle is inserted in-plane 3–8 cm lateral to the lateral edge of the transducer The needle is advanced in-plane from lateral to medial and superficial to deep. The needle should penetrate through the lateral aspect of the linea semilunaris and enter the lateral aspect of the RAM. The needle is further advanced until it is positioned deep to the potential space between the deepest (posterior) border of the RAM, but superficial to the posterior rectus sheath. This target site will be referred to as the "posterior rectus sheath compartment." 15–20 ml of local anesthetic is incrementally injected while observing for the expanding anechoic fluid collection. As the local anesthetic is injected, it will often result in clear separation of the deep border of the RAM from the posterior rectus sheath. The same procedure is repeated on the contralateral side.

1.4.5 Ilioinguinal/Iliohypogastric Nerve Block

The iliohypogastric (IH) and ilioinguinal (II) nerves arise from L1 and emerge from the upper part of the lateral border of the psoas major muscle. The ilioinguinal nerve is a smaller nerve and courses caudad to the iliohypogastric nerve. Both nerves cross obliquely anterior to the quadratus lumborum and iliacus muscles and perforate the transverse abdominis muscle near the anterior part of the iliac crest. In the anterior abdominal trunk, the nerves travel between the transverse abdominis and the internal oblique muscles. The iliohypogastric nerve supplies the skin over the inguinal region. The ilioinguinal nerve runs anteroinferiorly to the superficial inguinal ring, where it emerges to supply the skin on the superomedial aspect of the thigh. Blockade of both nerves is indicated for analgesia following inguinal hernia repair.

1.4.5.1 Ultrasound Technique

Place the patient in the supine position. Identify the iliac crest and the groin area. Mark the anterior superior iliac spine (ASIS). After skin and transducer preparation, place a linear 10–12 MHz transducer oblique along a line joining the ASIS and the umbilicus immediately superior and medial to the ASIS. Insert a 21G 100 mm needle from medial to lateral. Here, you will identify the layers of the abdominal wall attaching to the ASIS from superficial to deep: external oblique, internal oblique (IO), and transverse abdominus muscle. Watch out for the deep circumflex iliac artery in the plane between IO and transverse abdominus muscle. Injection medial and lateral to artery will provide successful block of both nerves. 20 ml of 0.5% Ropivacaine usually provides reliable analgesia for the inguinal region.

1.4.6 External Oblique Intercostal (EOI) Block

External abdominal oblique muscle is an abdominal muscle but there is an important part of it that lies over the thoracic cage. It originates from the external surfaces of ribs 5–12 running down and medial to insert to the linea semilunaris. The attaching fibers interdigitate with those of serratus anterior and latissimus dorsi on the lateral side of thorax. At the midclavicular line medially and inferiorly, the external abdominal oblique continues as an aponeurosis via which it inserts to the linea alba, pubic tubercle, and anterior half of iliac crest.

The thoracoabdominal nerves originate from the anterior rami of spinal nerves T7–T11. About the middle of their course through the intercostal space anterior to the midclavicular line, they give off a lateral cutaneous branch, which pierces the external intercostal and external oblique muscle to subsequently divide into anterior and posterior branches that innervate the skin of the lateral thorax and abdominal wall as far as the margin of the rectus abdominis muscle anteriorly. Thus, effective analgesia for incisions involving the upper lateral abdomen requires blockade of the lateral cutaneous branches of T7–T11 that could potentially be achieved by instilling local anesthetic solution above the costal margin in the thoracic fascial plane either deep or superficial to the external oblique muscle.

1.4.6.1 Ultrasound Technique

The block is performed with the patient in the supine position with their ipsilateral arm abducted. The linear ultrasound probe will be placed on the chest wall in the sagittal orientation between the midclavicular and anterior axillary lines at the level of sixth rib. This is followed by identifying rib six either by placing the ultrasound transducer at the level of lower costal margin (10th rib) and counting up or by identifying the seventh rib at the level of the xiphoid process and then moving the transducer one rib cranially. The transducer is then rotated so the cranial end is directed slightly medially and the caudal end laterally to produce a paramedian sagittal oblique view with a short-axis view of the ribs, approximately 1–2 cm medial to the anterior axillary line. The external oblique muscle is identified at the level ribs 6 and 7 in line with the xiphoid process. The layers that can be identified from superficial to deep include: subcutaneous tissue, external oblique muscle, intercostal muscles between ribs, pleura, and lung (Fig A). The skin entry point for the injection is cranial to the sixth rib level just medial to the anterior axillary line, with needle advanced in plane from a superomedial-to-inferolateral direction, through the external oblique muscle. The needle tip endpoint was the tissue plane between the external oblique and intercostal muscles at the caudal end of the sixth rib and between the sixth and seventh ribs. In our practice, we usually inject 20 mL of a mixture of bupivacaine 0.25% with liposomal bupivacaine in each side of the bilateral block. The mixture is injected between the external oblique and the intercostal muscles, dissecting the tissue plane between the sixth and seventh ribs, and then, the needle is directed caudally toward the eighth rib [13].

1.4.6.2 Clinical Discussion Including Pros and Cons of the Block

The potential advantages of the EOIFP block is that it is a superficial block, it provides coverage to the lateral upper abdominal area, and the needle/catheter insertion site is distant from the site of surgery. Thus, this block is a huge advantage for liver transplant patients who are coagulopathic and deserving of high-quality analgesia.

The limitation of the EOI block, like other fascial plane blocks, is that it lacks visceral analgesic coverage. The EOIFP block also does not reliably extend below the umbilicus. There is a potential risk of pneumothorax and local anesthetic systemic toxicity.

Indications:

Surgeries above the umbilicus: chevron incisions for hepatobiliary surgery, open nephrectomy, splenectomy, and open cholecystectomy.

Complications: Pneumothorax, infection, bleeding, LAST.

1.4.7 Quadratus Lumborum Block

Ultrasound-guided quadratus lumborum (QL) block is a fascial plane block where local anesthetic is injected adjacent

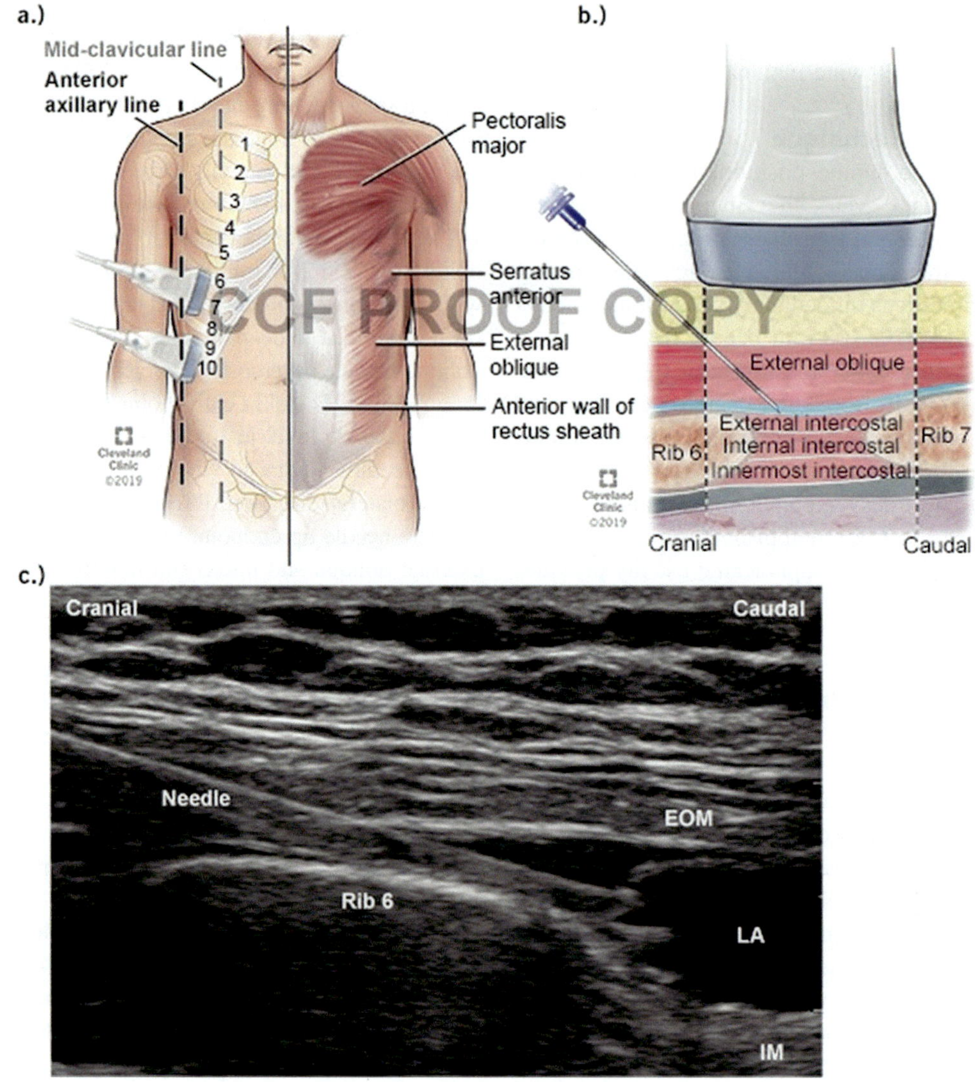

to the QL muscle to anesthetize the thoracolumbar nerves [14]. The QL muscle is a posterior abdominal wall muscle, dorsal to the iliopsoas muscle. It originates from the medial half of the iliac crest and inserts into the lower medial border of the 12th rib. It also has four small tendinous insertions to the apices of the transverse processes of the upper four lumbar vertebrae. The QL muscle is surrounded by thoracolumbar fascia. The ventral rami of the spinal nerve roots including the subcostal and iliohypogastric nerves traverse on the ventral surface of the QL.

Ultrasound Scanning technique:

Pt is positioned in lateral decubitus position, preferred by most as it gives more exposure to the neuraxial structures, more stability in handling the ultrasound probe and needle. Some proceduralists prefer supine position with slight tilt using a bump especially if performing bilateral blocks.

With the patient positioned in the lateral position, start scanning at the midaxillary line between the iliac crest and subcostal margin, identify the three abdominal muscle layers moving the probe posteriorly until they taper and fascia transversalis and QL muscle appears.

Scanning can also be done beginning posteriorly 4–5 cm lateral to the lumbar spinous process at the L3–4 level or higher. At this level, the transverse process of lumbar vertebrae, erector spinae muscle, psoas major muscle, and QL can be identified as a Shamrock sign.

Depending on the final endpoint of the needle, three different variations are described:

Lateral QL Block: The needle is directed from anterior to posterior toward the junction of tapered abdominal muscle layers and QL muscle. Local anesthetic is injected in the anterolateral border of QL muscle at the junction with the transversalis fascia (Fig B).

Posterior QL Block: The needle is advanced in similar fashion to the first technique, but needle tip is advanced further posterior to the QL muscle. The local anesthetic is deposited between the QL muscle and the erector spinae, latissimus dorsi muscle (Fig B).

Anterior QL Block: The needle is advanced from anterior to posterior through the erector spinae muscle and QL to deposit the local anesthetic at the space between the fascial layers of the QL and psoas major muscles (Fig B) Similar to other fascial plane blocks, it requires a large volume of local anesthetic to obtain a reliable spread and block. Volumes of 20–30 mL are usually recommended.

Complications. Inadvertent puncture of intra-abdominal structures, such as the kidney, liver, and spleen. Extra caution should be taken especially for the right sided block as the right kidney is slightly lower than the left. Due to the vascularity of the area, bleeding risks are high especially with anterior approach to the QL block.

Questions and Answers

Questions (Choose the Most Appropriate Answer)

1. A 36-year-old female complains of pain along her medial forearm and hand postoperatively after open reduction internal fixation (ORIF) of a humerus fracture. She received a preoperative interscalene block. Which nerve would have possibly been missed in the block?
   A. Radial nerve
   B. Ulnar nerve
   C. Intercostobrachial nerve
   D. Median nerve
   E. Musculocutaneous nerve
2. A 46-year-old male received an interscalene block for a left shoulder arthroplasty resulting in a dense block along his arm, hand, and the majority of his shoulder except the upper portion. What can be done to supplement the block?
   A. Injecting LA around the C3 to C4 nerve roots
   B. Injecting LA around C8 to T1 nerve roots
   C. Perform an intercostobrachial block
   D. Repeating the interscalene block
   E. None of the above
3. What patient population is most susceptible to the adverse events from an interscalene nerve block?
   A. 62-year-old male smoker with severe chronic obstructive pulmonary disease (COPD)
   B. 37-year-old male with sickle cell trait
   C. 21-year-old female with exercise-induced asthma
   D. 75-year-old male with mild coronary artery disease
   E. 25-year-old female in her first trimester of pregnancy
4. A 76-year-old patient fractured her proximal humerus after a fall. A peripheral nerve block was planned for post-op pain after ORIF. In an ultrasound-guided supraclavicular approach to the brachial plexus, where are the plexus trunks/divisions in relation to the subclavian artery?
   A. Anterior and lateral
   B. Superior and lateral
   C. Superior and medial
   D. Superior and posterior
   E. Anterior and medial
5. A supraclavicular brachial plexus block is placed for shoulder surgery. For optimal postoperative analgesia, the catheter should be placed_______.
   A. Anterior to the subclavian artery
   B. Posterior to the subclavian artery
   C. Superior to the subclavian artery
   D. As close as possible to the first rib
   E. Under the first rib
6. What is the most common complication associated with a brachial plexus block using the supraclavicular approach?
   A. Intravascular injection into the subclavian artery
   B. Phrenic nerve palsy
   C. Intravascular injection into the vertebral artery
   D. Pneumothorax
   E. Block failure
7. Which of the following is the best indication for a supraclavicular nerve block?
   A. Shoulder arthroplasty
   B. Surgery on fifth digit
   C. Upper limb and hand surgery
   D. Shoulder arthroscopy
   E. First rib excision
8. Which portion of the upper extremity may not be completely anesthetized after performing a supraclavicular brachial plexus block?
   A. Lateral portion of the hand
   B. Elbow
   C. Medial portion of the hand
   D. Posterior medial portion of the forearm
   E. Anterior lateral portion of the arm
9. Inadequate anesthesia of the lateral part of the forearm following an axillary block is most likely the result of inadequate block of which nerve?
   A. Ulnar nerve
   B. Radial nerve
   C. Intercostobrachial nerve
   D. Median nerve
   E. Musculocutaneous nerve
10. Complications of the axillary block include:
    A. Nerve injury
    B. Vascular puncture

C. Hematoma
D. Local anesthetic toxicity
E. All of the above

11. To avoid nerve injury while performing axillary block, which of the following should be taken into consideration?
 A. Avoid injection of local anesthetic when high resistance is encountered
 B. Avoid injection of local anesthetic when stimulation is obtained with intensity of less than 0.2 mA
 C. Stop injecting the local anesthetic when the patient complains of severe pain during the injection
 D. All of the above

12. All of the following statements are true about axillary brachial plexus block except:
 A. Under ultrasound, the median nerve is a rounded hyperechoic structure
 B. A curvilinear transducer probe should be used for deeper penetration.
 C. The structures of interest when performing the block are superficial, 1–3 cm from the skin.
 D. The axillary artery can be associated with one or more axillary veins and are usually located medial to the artery

13. A patient receives an infraclavicular block for distal radial fracture fixation, and complete anesthesia of hand and forearm are noted. Upon inflation of the surgical tourniquet, the patient complains of pain under the axilla. Which of the following nerves was not blocked?
 A. Musculocutaneous nerve
 B. Radial nerve
 C. Medial brachial cutaneous nerve
 D. Intercostobrachial nerve

14. Infraclavicular catheter is placed for analgesia in a patient after elbow arthroplasty and the patient received a bolus followed by continuous infusion. Approximately 12 h after the block, the patient complains of severe pain on the lateral side of the elbow. Motor function in the hand is diminished. All tubing is connected and the pump is working. What is the most likely cause?
 A. Radial nerve injury from the block
 B. Normal postoperative pain
 C. Secondary block failure
 D. Incorrect drug choice

15. Advantages of infraclavicular block over axillary block include all of the following except:
 A. Single needle entry
 B. Block of medial brachial cutaneous and antebrachial cutaneous nerves
 C. Easier catheter placement for continuous analgesia
 D. Easy needle visualization with ultrasound

16. In a typical transverse scan of the inguinal region, the femoral nerve is immediately deep to the following structure:
 A. The fascia of the iliopsoas muscle
 B. The fascia iliaca
 C. The fascia lata
 D. The femoral artery

17. While performing a femoral nerve block using nerve stimulation, all of the following are reliable responses ensuring successful block except:
 A. A quadriceps muscle twitch
 B. Stimulation of the femoral nerve at 0.4 mA
 C. A sartorial muscle twitch
 D. A patellar twitch

18. A femoral nerve block can be used as an adjunct to control pain in each of these surgeries except:
 A. Proximal femur surgery
 B. Knee surgery
 C. Medial foot surgery
 C. Proximal anterior thigh surgery

19. Which of the following statements is true regarding the transversus abdominis plane block using ultrasound-guided technique?
 A. Coagulopathy is an absolute contraindication
 B. Low volume, high concentration of local anesthetic solution is used ideally
 C. Saline can be used to identify and open the TAP fascial plane prior to injecting local anesthetic
 D. It can be reliably used as the sole mode of analgesia after abdominal surgery

20. All of the following statements are true regarding the TAP block except:
 A. The anterior abdominal wall is innervated by T7 to L1
 B. The nerves lie in the plane between the internal oblique and the transversus abdominis muscles
 C. The aim of the block is to deposit local anesthetic in the plane between the internal oblique and transversus abdominis muscles
 D. A single injection of 20 cc of local anesthetic will reliably block all the nerves on one side of the abdomen.

21. Sciatic nerve block performed by posterior approach (Labat [9]), all of the following statements are true except:
 A. The landmarks used are the greater trochanter and the sacral hiatus
 B. The patient is placed in Sim's position

C. The posterior superior iliac spine and sacral hiatus are the bony landmarks
D. The landmarks include the greater trochanter and ischial tuberosity

22. Regarding an ultrasound-guided transgluteal approach to a sciatic nerve block, all of the following statements are true except:
A. It is indicated for surgery on the tibia, ankle, and foot
B. The landmarks used are the greater trochanter and the posterior superior iliac spine
C. Combined with a lumbar plexus block, anesthesia of the entire lower extremity can be achieved
D. In contrast to common belief, it is a relatively easy block to perform with a high success rate

Answers

1. **B**. The interscalene block is most utilized for shoulder and humeral fracture surgeries but is not sufficient for surgeries involving the hand because the lower nerve roots and trunk of the brachial plexus are missed.
2. **A**. Injecting local anesthetic around C3 to C4 nerve roots would give a superficial cervical plexus bock and help this patient since these nerve roots supply some sensation to upper part of the shoulder.
3. **A**. Due to the almost 100% involvement of the ipsilateral phrenic nerve with an interscalene block, it is advisable to be cautious with patients with limited pulmonary function, such as patients with severe COPD.
4. **D**. When using the ultrasound, in the supraclavicular approach for the brachial plexus, the trunks and the divisions appear as compact bunch of grapes superior and posterior to the artery.
5. **C**. The catheter is usually inserted superior to the subclavian artery in the case of shoulder surgery or in the corner pocket between the artery and the first rib in the case of hand surgery. The correct position of catheter can be confirmed under ultrasound by injecting local anesthetic or 1 ml of air into the catheter and observing the distribution in relation to the artery.
6. **B**. To minimize phrenic nerve paralysis, try not to inject above the plexus to avoid exposing the nerve to toxic high concentration of local anesthetics. In addition, avoiding injection above the plexus might decrease the incidence of phrenic nerve palsy after the block.
7. **C**. The supraclavicular block is very efficient for upper limb and hand surgeries.
8. **C**. Supraclavicular block can be used for shoulder, elbow, or hand surgery; however, it can miss the lower portion of the brachial plexus, thus sparing the ulnar nerve distribution of the medial side of the hand.
9. **E**. The musculocutaneous nerve is a terminal branch of the lateral cord of the brachial plexus. Without blockade of the musculocutaneous nerve, adequate anesthesia of the lateral forearm is unlikely. Classic teaching is that the musculocutaneous nerve blockade can be accomplished by the injection of local anesthetic into the belly of the coracobrachialis muscle. Ultrasound studies have shown that the musculocutaneous nerve is not in the coracobrachialis muscle in approximately 20% of patients.
10. **E**. A hematoma can occur during an axillary block, especially if the patient was on anticoagulants or if there are multiple needle punctures to the veins or axillary artery. The most common cause of local anesthetic toxicity during axillary block is inadvertent intravascular injection. To avoid systemic toxicity during an axillary block, avoid fast forceful injection, perform careful frequent aspiration during the injection, and adjust the dose and volume of local anesthetic injected in the elderly and frail patients.
11. **D**. To avoid nerve injury during any peripheral nerve block, never inject local anesthetic when abnormally high resistance is encountered on injection. Stop injecting local anesthetic when patient complains of severe pain on injection and when stimulation is obtained with current intensity less than 0.2 mA. Withdraw the needle slightly to obtain the same response with current greater than 0.2 mA before injecting the local anesthetic.
12. **B**. In order to obtain the best image when performing the axillary brachial plexus block, a linear transducer with high frequency should be used. A higher penetration is not needed as the structures of interest are superficial, 1–3 cm from the skin. A curved low-frequency probe should be used when imaging deeper structures as it allows higher penetration at the expense of lower resolution.
13. **D**. The intercostobrachial nerve arises from T2 and is not blocked by any approach to brachial plexus. It may be blocked by subcutaneous infiltration of local anesthetic under the ventral side of the proximal arm.
14. **C**. The patient most likely had sufficient local anesthetic spread from the initial bolus. With resolution of the initial block, the lateral cord was not adequately blocked by the infusion, leading to pain in the musculocutaneous nerve distribution.
15. **D**. The infraclavicular approach has many advantages, including single needle entry and the included block of the medial brachial cutaneous and medial antebrachial cutaneous nerves. It is also a good location for catheter placement. Needle visualization

with ultrasound is often more difficult due to the steep angle of the needle and the depth of the plexus.

16. **B**. While all the given structures can be found in a typical transverse scan of the inguinal region, the femoral nerve is typically superficial to the iliopsoas muscle and lateral to the femoral artery. The fascia lata is superficial and can be found in the subcutaneous layer.
17. **C**. A twitch of the sartorius muscle can be commonly seen when using nerve stimulation for locating the femoral nerve. A band-like contraction of the thigh without movement of the patella is often how sartorius muscle stimulation manifests and can be mistaken for femoral nerve stimulation. Sartorius muscle twitch is not a reliable response because the nerve branches to the sartorius muscle coming off the femoral nerve may be outside the femoral sheath.
18. **D**. The proximal portion of the anterior thigh is innervated by the ilioinguinal and genitofemoral nerves but not the femoral nerve.
19. **C**. Coagulopathy is a relative contraindication for the TAP block. The TAP bock depends on the spread of LA in a large plane, and hence, it is a high-volume block. It is used as an adjunct for anterior abdominal wall incisions/drains. It does not provide adequate analgesia as a sole analgesia as it does not block the visceral component. The spread of local anesthetic in TAP block depends on the volume and the site of injection. Saline can be used to hydrodissect and identify the TAP plane without wasting the local anesthetic while trying to identify the TAP plane.
20. **D**. The anterolateral abdominal wall is innervated by the anterior rami of the lower 6 thoracic nerves (T7 to T12) and the first lumbar nerve (L1). The nerves lie in the fascial plane between the internal oblique and the transverse abdominis muscles. Injection of LA within the TAP can provide unilateral analgesia to the skin, muscles, and parietal peritoneum of the anterior abdominal wall from T7 to L1 depending on the volume and the site of the injection.
21. **D**. The posterior sciatic nerve block described by Labat [9] involves placing the patient in Sim's lateral position with hip and leg flexed to 90°. The anatomical landmarks used are the posterior superior iliac spine (PSIS), the greater trochanter (GT), and the sacral hiatus (SH). Draw 2 lines joining the 3 bony landmarks. From the midpoint of the PSIS and GT, drop a perpendicular line and mark where it crosses the line joining the GT and SH. This is the point of needle insertion for the block.
22. **B**. An ultrasound-guided transgluteal sciatic nerve block is relatively easy to perform with a high success rate. It utilizes the greater trochanter and the ischial tuberosity as the bony landmarks. Combined with a lumbar plexus block, anesthesia of the entire lower extremity can be achieved. Combined with a femoral/saphenous nerve block, anesthesia of the lower limb below the knee can be achieved.

References

1. Winnie AP. Interscalene brachial plexus block. Anesth Analg. 1970;49(3):455–66.
2. Kulenkampff D. "Zur anästhesierung des plexus brachialis" [On anesthesia of the brachial plexus]. Zentralblatt für Chirurgie (in German). 1911;38:1337–40.
3. Winnie AP, Collins VJ. The subclavian perivascular technique of brachial plexus anesthesia. Anesthesiology. 1964;25:353–63.
4. Aguirre O, Tobos L, Reina MA, Sala-Blanch X. Upper trunk block: description of a supraclavicular approach of upper trunk at the points of its division. Br J Anaesth. 2016;117(6):823–4. https://doi.org/10.1093/bja/aew366. PMID: 27956682.
5. Chan CW, Peng PW. Suprascapular nerve block: a narrative review. Reg Anesth Pain Med. 2011;36(4):358–73. https://doi.org/10.1097/AAP.0b013e3182204ec0. PMID: 21654552.
6. Farag E, Brown DL. Chapter 14 Femoral block. In: Farag E, Mounir-Soliman L, editors. Brown's atlas of regional anesthesia. 5th ed. Philadelphia: Elsevier; 2016.
7. Jaeger P, Nielsen ZJ, Henningsen MH, Hilsted KL, Mathiesen O, Dahl JB. Adductor canal block versus femoral nerve block and quadriceps strength: a randomized, double-blind, placebo-controlled, crossover study in healthy volunteers. Anesthesiology. 2013;118(2):409–15. https://doi.org/10.1097/ALN.0b013e318279fa0b. PMID: 23241723.
8. Labat G. Regional anesthesia: its technique and clinical applications. 2nd ed. Philadelphia: W. B. Saunders Publishers; 1924. p. 45–55.
9. Farag E, Brown DL. Chapter 13 Sciatic block. In: Farag E, Mounir-Soliman L, editors. Brown's atlas of regional anesthesia. 5th ed. Philadelphia: Elsevier; 2016.
10. Girón-Arango L, Peng PWH, Chin KJ, Brull R, Perlas A. Pericapsular nerve group (PENG) block for hip fracture. Reg Anesth Pain Med. 2018;43(8):859–63. https://doi.org/10.1097/AAP.0000000000000847. PMID: 30063657.
11. Yared M, Brown DL. Chapter 17 Popliteal and saphenous block. In: Farag E, Mounir-Soliman L, editors. Brown's atlas of regional anesthesia. 5th ed. Philadelphia: Elsevier; 2016.
12. Brown DL. Chapter 19 Ankle block. In: Farag E, Mounir-Soliman L, editors. Brown's atlas of regional anesthesia. 5th ed. Philadelphia: Elsevier; 2016.
13. Elsharkawy H, Kolli S, Soliman LM, Seif J, Drake RL, Mariano ER, El-Boghdadly K. The External Oblique intercostal block: anatomic evaluation and case series. Pain Med. 2021;22(11):2436–42. https://doi.org/10.1093/pm/pnab296. PMID: 34626112.
14. Elsharkawy H, El-Boghdadly K, Barrington M. Quadratus Lumborum block: anatomical concepts, mechanisms, and techniques. Anesthesiology. 2019;130:322–35.

Central Neuraxial Anatomy and Anesthetic Application (Central Neuraxial Blockade)

2

Nathan J. Harrison, Laurie S. Daste, Gary S. McDaniel, Matthew E. Patterson, Jay D. Shah, and Maged Guirguis

Abstract

Epidural, spinal, and caudal anesthesia comprises the most commonly used regional anesthetic techniques referred to as neuraxial anesthesia. These techniques may not only provide a means for the primary anesthetic during surgery but are commonly used for perioperative and postoperative analgesia in addition to its widespread use in controlling labor pain. While the clinician may have performed these techniques for years, it is helpful to review the important concepts in order to safely and effectively deliver the best care for the patient undergoing neuraxial anesthesia. This chapter reviews relevant anatomy, pharmacology, and standard techniques as well as newer approaches using ultrasound guidance for neuraxial blockade. Finally, this chapter covers indications for providing neuraxial techniques and complications that may arise, and presents the latest guidelines for treating the anticoagulated patient when considering neuraxial anesthesia.

N. J. Harrison
Department of Anesthesiology and Pain Management, Ochsner Health Systems, Covington, LA, USA
e-mail: nharrison@ochsner.org

L. S. Daste
Department of Anesthesiology, LCMC Health, New Orleans, LA, USA
e-mail: ldaste@ochsner.org

G. S. McDaniel
Baton Rouge Orthopedic Clinic, Baton Rouge, LA, USA

M. E. Patterson · J. D. Shah · M. Guirguis (✉)
Department of Anesthesiology and Critical Care Medicine, Ochsner Health Systems, Louisiana State University School of Medicine, New Orleans, USA
e-mail: mguirguis@ochsner.org

M. E. Patterson
e-mail: mpatterson@ochsner.org

J. D. Shah
e-mail: v-jayshah@ochsner.org

Keywords

Neuraxial anesthesia • Epidural anesthesia • Spinal anesthesia • Combined spinal epidural • Caudal anesthesia • Neuraxial blockade • Spinal anatomy • Landmarks • Ultrasound guidance

Key Points

1. Neuraxial anesthesia can be used as a primary anesthetic, an adjunct anesthetic for intraoperative pain control in addition to general anesthesia or postoperative pain control for surgeries involving the abdomen, perineum, or lower extremities.
2. Absolute contraindications to neuraxial anesthesia include patient refusal, bleeding diathesis, elevated intracranial pressure (except pseudotumor cerebri), infection at site of injection, hypovolemia, and indeterminate neurologic disease.
3. Neuraxial anesthesia can be achieved by injection of local anesthetics (lidocaine, bupivacaine, chloroprocaine, etc.) with or without additives into the intrathecal space (spinal) or the epidural space (epidural).
4. As a fetus, the spinal cord spans the entire length of the spine. The spinal cord ends at the L3 level in early childhood, and in adulthood, the spinal cord extends from the foramen magnum to the L1-2 level.
5. Local anesthetics exert their effects at the level of the nerve root, producing numbness in a dermatomal distribution.
6. Additives can be used to alter the length (epinephrine, clonidine) and onset (sodium bicarbonate) of blockade.
7. Hypotension is the most common adverse effect of neuraxial anesthesia. It is caused by sympathetic blockade, which can decrease systemic venous resistance, venous return, and cardiac output. This sympathetic blockade extends 2 dermatomes above and below the sensory/motor blockade and is treated with crystalloid bolus and vasopressors.

M. Argalious et al. (eds.), *Basic Sciences in Anesthesia*,
https://doi.org/10.1007/978-3-031-60203-0_2

8. Epidural hematoma is the most feared complication of neuraxial anesthesia. Particular attention needs to be paid to the coagulation status and platelet functioning of the patient, including medications that may affect these functions. Treatment is surgical decompression and magnetic resonance imaging (MRI) should be obtained early so as not to delay surgery.
9. Post-dural puncture headache (PDPH) is a relatively common adverse effect of neuraxial anesthesia. Risk factors include female sex, young age, pregnancy, and history of previous PDPH and the use of cutting-point, large-bore needles. Treatment includes adequate hydration, caffeine, analgesics, and, if warranted, epidural blood patch.
10. Many situations exist in which neuraxial anesthesia and anticoagulation would both be appropriate for a patient at the same time. The American Society of Regional Anesthesia (ASRA) guidelines exist as expert opinion to help guide the practitioner in risk benefit analysis and should be referenced whenever neuraxial anesthesia is considered on an anticoagulated patient.

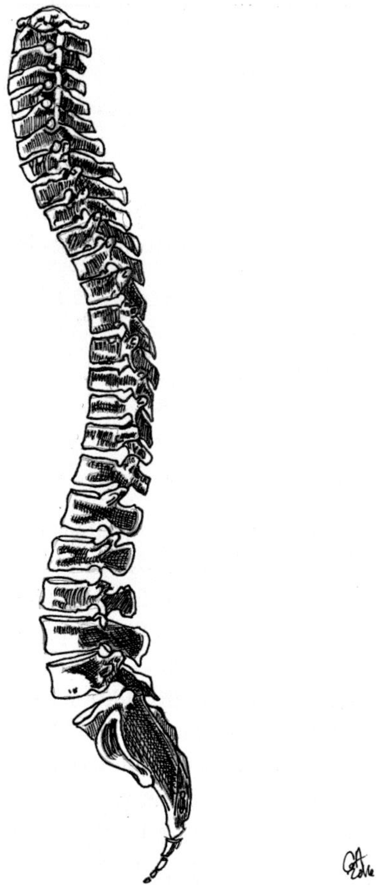

Fig. 2.1 Sagittal view of spine demonstrating lumbar and cervical lordosis and thoracic kyphosis. Note spinous process angles, which change according to level of the spine (Reprinted with permission Ochsner Health Systems © 2016. All Rights Reserved)

2.1 Anatomy

2.1.1 The Vertebral Column

The vertebral column consists of the bony vertebral bodies, their posterior elements, and the intervertebral disks that form the boundaries of the vertebral canal in which lies the spinal cord and exiting nerve roots. The vertebral canal provides structural support to the body as well as protection for the spinal cord and nerve roots within the spine. The spine consists of 33 vertebrae from the base of the skull to the coccyx. There are 7 cervical, 12 thoracic, 5 lumbar, and 5 sacral vertebrae. The 5 sacral vertebrae are fused to form the sacrum, which is attached to the coccygeal vertebrae, or coccyx. A sagittal view of the spine reveals a double-C shape in which the cervical and lumbar regions exhibit a concave curvature (lordosis), and the thoracic region appears convex (kyphosis) (◘ ◉ Fig. 2.1) [1].

Although the shape of the anatomy of the spine varies at each level, a vertebra generally consists of a vertebral body connected to the vertebrae above and below it by intervertebral disks. At the thoracic and lumbar levels, the vertebral body is a large circular structure connected to a posterior vertebral arch [1]:

- The vertebral body is joined to 2 pedicles that course ventral to dorsal, which are each fused with a laterally extending transverse process.
- The laminar elements extend medially and dorsally and fuse posteriorly to form a single spinous process.
- The vertebral body, 2 pedicles, transverse processes, 2 laminae, and spinous process connect to form a hollow circle, which, when stacked with other vertebrae, form a cylinder that encases the spinal cord and its covering.
- While the vertebral bodies connect to each other by disks anteriorly, each vertebra connects posteriorly by facet joints. The facet joints are formed on each side by a superior articular process from the caudally located vertebra and an inferior articular process from the cephalad vertebra.
- Intervertebral foramina, or neural foramina, are lateral openings between cephalad and caudal vertebral pedicles through which the nerve roots leave the spinal cord and exit to each side (◘ ◉ Fig. 2.2).

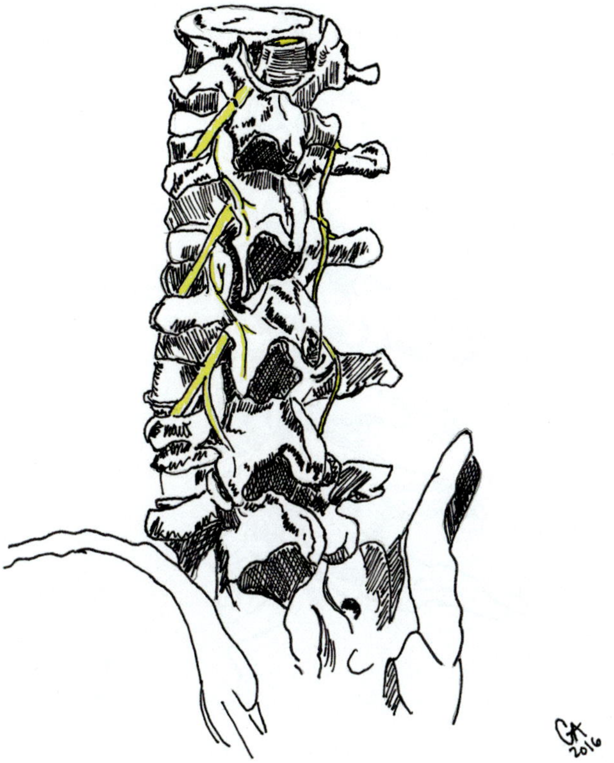

Fig. 2.2 Left oblique view of lumbar spine. Note nerve roots exiting neural foramen beneath pedicles (Reprinted with permission Ochsner Health Systems © 2016. All Rights Reserved)

The cervical vertebrae differ from the thoracic and lumbar spine by the presence of bilateral transverse foramina, which contain the vertebral arteries as they pass superiorly through C6 and upward to the foramen magnum. The first cervical vertebrae, or the atlas, lacks a body but instead connects with the C2 vertebra, also called the axis. The atlas has a superiorly extending odontoid process, or dens, which essentially exists as the embryologic C1 body. The dens of C2 articulate with the posterior surface of the anterior arch of C1 [2]. The atlas and axis allow increased range of motion of the head and neck. The joint between the occipital bone and C1 forms the atlanto-occipital joint, which allows movement of the head, and the atlanto-axial joint between the atlas and axis allows for the twisting motion of the neck. The cervical spine also differs from the remaining vertebrae in that all the spinous processes, except for C7, are bifid. (Figs. 2.3 and 2.4).

The thoracic vertebrae are each connected to bilateral corresponding ribs. The spinous processes of the cervical and lumbar spine are shorter and appear to be in a more horizontal axis, allowing for a more direct trajectory during spinal and epidural needle placement (Fig. 2.5). The spinous processes of the mid-thoracic spine on the other hand are more caudally angulated, which requires a compensatory angulation when performing spinal and epidural needle placement. The interlaminar spaces are larger in the lumbar area than in the thoracic spine [3].

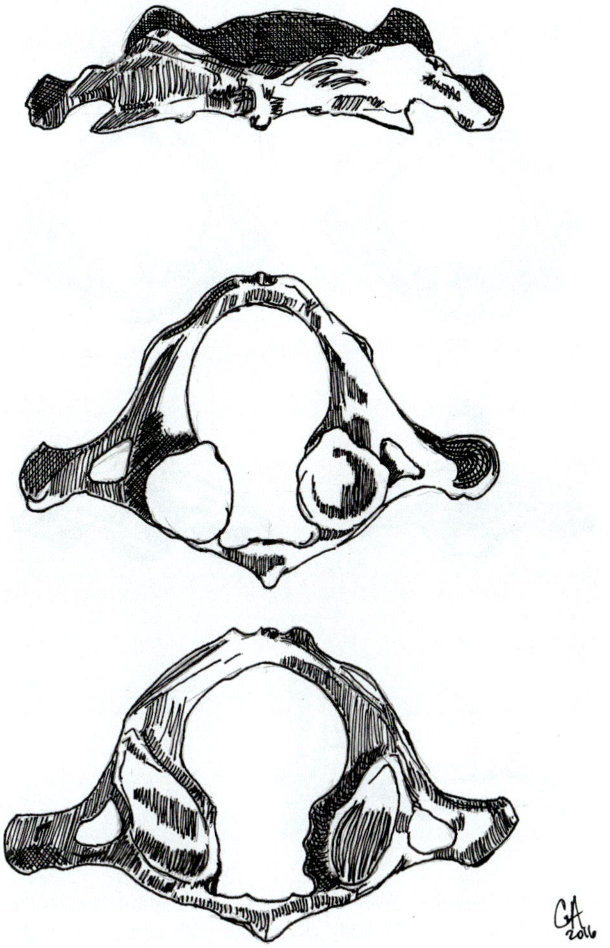

Fig. 2.3 C1 vertebra (atlas) with superior view, inferior view, and anterior view (Reprinted with permission Ochsner Health Systems © 2016. All Rights Reserved)

The 5 sacral vertebrae fuse prior to birth to form the sacrum:

- Each sacral vertebral level contains paired anterior and posterior intervertebral foramen from which the sacral nerve roots exit.
- The transverse and costal processes of S1 fuse to form the bilateral sacral ala, the wing-like lateral processes located superiorly at the base of the sacrum. The sacral alae articulate bilaterally with the ilium to form the sacroiliac joints.
- The sacrum also joins superiorly with the L5 vertebrae (via the L5/S1 intervertebral disk) and inferiorly with the coccyx (via the sacrococcygeal ligament).
- The sacrum contains a central canal, which is a continuation of the vertebral canal. The canal terminates at the sacral hiatus, a fissure located in the posterior sacrum where the laminae of the fifth vertebrae do not fuse.

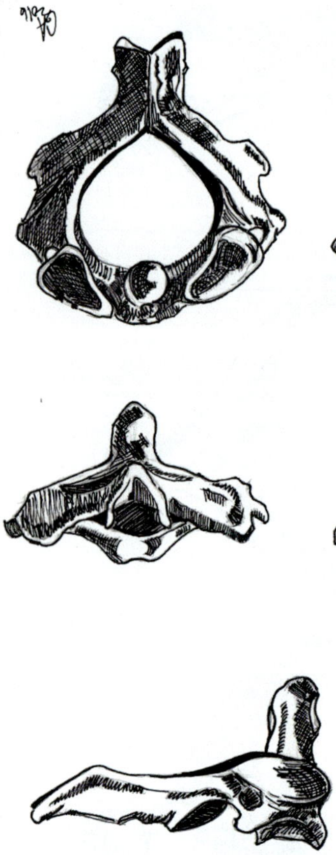

Fig. 2.4 C2 vertebra (axis) with views from multiple angles. Note dens, which serves as C1 body (Reprinted with permission Ochsner Health Systems © 2016. All Rights Reserved)

- The sacral cornu, a landmark for caudal anesthesia, can be found here as bilateral projections on either side of the sacral hiatus [3].
- The filum terminale, the most caudal extension of the pia mater, extends to the sacral hiatus. Although the dural sac typically ends at the S2 level in adults, the epidural fat continues to the hiatus, which is what allows access to the epidural space at this level during caudal techniques [4, 5].

2.1.2 Ligaments

Several ligaments surround the vertebral column and, together with the paraspinous muscles, provide support and structure to the spine:

- The vertebral bodies and intervertebral disks are bound together anteriorly and posteriorly by the anterior and posterior spinal ligaments, respectively, in a cephalad to caudal direction along the length of the cervical, thoracic, and lumbar spine.

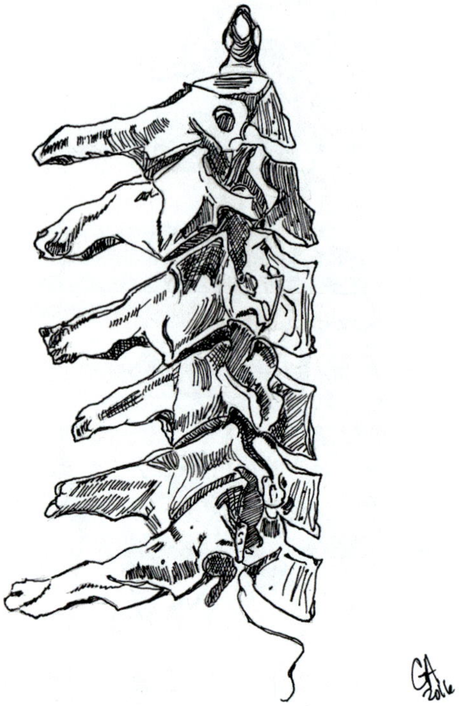

Fig. 2.5 Cervical spine spinous processes have a relatively horizontal angle (Reprinted with permission Ochsner Health Systems © 2016. All Rights Reserved)

- Dorsal to the vertebral canal, the ligamentum flavum is a thick layer of tissue connecting the lamina along the spinal column immediately posterior to the epidural space. When placing an epidural needle, this ligament is used as a landmark to help determine entrance to the epidural space. In some individuals, the ligamentum flavum is absent, which can place the patient at a higher risk for unintended dural puncture.
- The interspinous ligament connects adjacent spinous processes, and the supraspinous ligament is the most superficially located ligament along the posterior surface of the spinous processes.
- Therefore, using a midline approach, the order of structures encountered during an epidural placement is skin, subcutaneous tissue, supraspinous ligament, interspinous ligament, ligamentum flavum, and, finally, epidural space.

2.1.3 Landmarks

When trying to locate the appropriate vertebral level in order to perform neuraxial anesthesia without the assistance of fluoroscopy, it is necessary to know surface landmarks:

- The C7 spinous process is the most prominent bony landmark in the base of the neck, whereas a line drawn between the lower edges of the scapulae denotes the T7 interspace. These 2 landmarks are useful for locating the desired interspaces for thoracic epidurals and paravertebral blocks [6].

- The most important landmarks for labor epidurals and spinal anesthesia are the iliac crests. A horizontal line drawn between the crests (Tuffier's line) generally will traverse the L4/5 interspace, which is below the spinal cord in most adults [6].
- Finally, the bilateral posterior superior iliac spines designate the level of the S2 vertebral body, which is the inferior border of the dural sac in adults [6].

2.1.4 The Spinal Cord

As a fetus, the spinal cord spans the entire length of the spine. As the infant ages, the spine lengthens at a faster rate compared to the growth of the spinal cord. As a result, the spinal cord ends at the L3 level in early childhood, and in adulthood, the spinal cord extends from the foramen magnum to the L1-2 level.

As the spinal cord approaches L1, it tapers off into the conus medullaris and eventually becomes the cauda equina, or "horse's tail," a bundle of nerve roots that float relatively freely in the cerebrospinal fluid (CSF) of the spinal canal. A spinal anesthetic performed below L1 would be in the territory of the cauda equina and decrease the potential for spinal cord trauma as the needle theoretically displaces the nerve roots to the side.

There are 31 pairs of spinal nerves (8 cervical, 12 thoracic, 5 lumbar, and 5 sacral). The nerve roots exit the spinal column through bilateral intervertebral foramen. In the cervical spine, the nerve roots exit above their corresponding vertebral body. At the C7 body, the C7 root exits above and the C8 root exits below (between C7 and T1). Starting at T1, the nerve roots then exit below their respective vertebral bodies [2].

The dural sac, as well as the subarachnoid space, extends below the cauda equina to S2 in adults and S3 in children. The dura often continues to sheath the nerve roots as they exit the spinal canal into the intervertebral foramen. As such, there is a risk of subdural or subarachnoid injection even when approaching from a caudal or transforaminal approach. Although the dura mater extends to S2, the pia mater continues as a thin strand of tissue to form the filum terminale, which connects the conus to the coccyx [4].

2.1.5 Meninges

The meninges are the 3 layers of connective tissue surrounding the spinal cord composed of the outermost dura mater, the arachnoid mater, and the innermost pia mater. Superficial to these layers, the epidural space exists as a potential space between the dura mater and the ligamentum flavum. It contains fat, lymphatics, and blood vessels, and it is in this space that local anesthetic can be instilled for epidural anesthesia (◘ ◉ Fig. 2.6). The epidural space communicates freely with the adjacent paravertebral spaces by the intervertebral foramen. Closely adherent to the dura mater is the arachnoid mater. Beneath the arachnoid layer is the subarachnoid space, where cerebrospinal fluid is contained within the spinal column. The innermost layer is known as the pia mater, which is closely adherent with the spinal cord. The pia will extend laterally above T12 to form a dense triangular band between the dorsal and ventral roots known as the denticulate ligament [4]. Radiographic studies also suggest the presence of dorsal median connective tissue or septa within the epidural space, which may lead to an unintentional unilateral neuraxial anesthetic [7].

2.1.6 Cerebrospinal Fluid

The major function of cerebrospinal fluid is to insulate and protect the brain and spinal nerves against trauma. It is found in cerebral ventricles and the subarachnoid space of the brain and spinal cord. It flows freely across the foramen magnum, allowing for introduction of local anesthetic to the brain in the event of a complete or high spinal. CSF is mostly formed in the choroid plexus of the cerebral ventricles. In adults, normal CSF production is 500 cc/day, yet total CSF volume is only about 150 cc secondary to continuous reabsorption into arachnoid granulations.

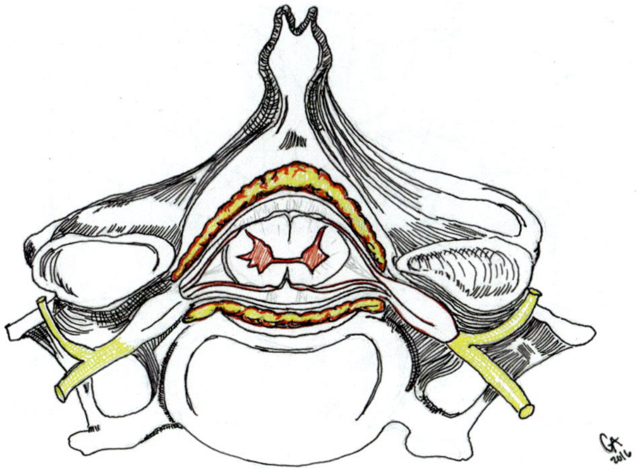

Fig. 2.6 Axial view of spine reveals a cross-section of spinal cord and exiting nerve roots, which lie between anterior and posterior epidural space. Spinal nerve roots exit through intervertebral foramen (Reprinted with permission Ochsner Health Systems © 2016. All Rights Reserved)

2.1.7 Blood Supply

The spinal cord is supplied by a single anterior spinal artery and 2 paired posterior arteries. The anterior spinal artery arises from the vertebral artery in the cervical region and supplies the anterior two-thirds (motor innervation) of the spinal cord. The posterior arteries are formed from the posterior inferior cerebellar arteries and cover the posterior one-third (sensory innervation) of the cord (◘ ◉ Fig. 2.7). Below the cervical level, the spinal cord also receives additional blood supply from segmental or radicular arteries, which feeds the anterior spinal artery in the thoracic and lumbar region. The anterior spinal artery receives variable contributions from these arteries and relies heavily on the large artery of Adamkiewicz or great radicular artery (GRA). The GRA typically branches off the aorta around T9-T12, but can be anywhere from T5-L5, and it is almost always on the left [2]. If this artery is damaged, a patient may present with bilateral lower extremity motor deficits from a process called anterior spinal artery syndrome. This syndrome occurs as a result of decreased spinal cord perfusion pressure, which is equal to mean arterial pressure (MAP)—spinal cord pressure. Anterior spinal artery syndrome, therefore, may occur secondary to either a decrease in MAP (hypotension, damaged GRA) or an increased spinal cord pressure (from a variety of factors including increased CSF pressure or mechanical pressure).

The venous drainage from the spinal cord flows through the vertebral venous plexus. The plexus can be enlarged in situations that obstruct abdominal venous return, such as increased intra-abdominal pressure secondary to gravid uterus or tumors compressing the vena cava. This may result in an increased likelihood of intravascular injection during epidural anesthesia as well as increase the spread of local anesthetic by decreasing the volume of the epidural space.

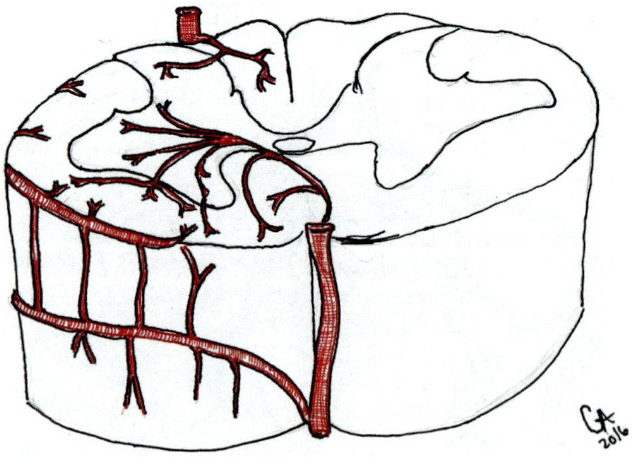

Fig. 2.7 Cross-section of the spinal cord with the midline anterior spinal anatomy and one of the 2 paired posterior spinal arteries on the left side (Reprinted with permission Ochsner Health Systems © 2016. All Rights Reserved)

2.2 Neuraxial Anesthesia

2.2.1 Preoperative Considerations

2.2.1.1 Indications

Neuraxial anesthesia may be indicated as the primary anesthetic for major or minor surgeries or as an adjunctive anesthetic for intraoperative pain control in addition to general anesthesia. It is most useful as the primary anesthetic in surgeries involving the abdomen, perineum, or lower extremities. Neuraxial anesthesia is also an option for thoracic and upper abdominal surgeries, although it may not be the optimal choice for a patient with respiratory insufficiency or during prolonged surgeries resulting in compromised respiratory function (such as pneumoperitoneum). This is related to the fact that these patients rely heavily on accessory muscles of inspiration, which are often weakened with high neuraxial anesthesia, despite minimal changes in tidal volume. In these situations, an epidural or spinal may be useful to supplement general anesthesia in providing postoperative pain relief. Continuous epidural anesthesia is also widely used in labor analgesia [6].

2.2.1.2 Contraindications

Absolute contraindications to neuraxial anesthesia include patient refusal, bleeding diathesis, elevated intracranial pressure (except pseudotumor cerebri), infection at site of injection, hypovolemia, and indeterminate neurologic disease [6].

Other disease processes are discussed as relative contraindications, and clinical judgment should be used in these situations. Severe aortic or mitral stenosis or left ventricular outflow obstruction when combined with spinal or rapidly achieved epidural anesthesia may result in sudden, severe hypotension and possible cardiac ischemia. These effects are secondary to a sympathetic blockade, leading to vasodilation, venous pooling, and ultimately decreased preload. However, neuraxial anesthesia can be used safely with close monitoring, and when possible, a slowly dosed epidural would be preferred over spinal anesthesia to avoid the abrupt decline in blood pressure.

Sepsis or distant infections have been implicated in predisposing the patient to meningitis, epidural abscess, or central nervous system (CNS) infection via hematogenous spread following neuraxial anesthesia. While it is recommended to exercise caution in such patients, it is generally not contraindicated to perform a neuraxial block as it may actually be a better choice for some sick patients.

Chronic back pain or preexisting neurological deficits and paresthesia due to prior neurologic disease are generally not contraindications; however, prior symptoms or exacerbations of a disease state may mask or imitate side effects or complications associated with the procedure itself. Some practitioners would defer from performing neuraxial or regional anesthesia on such patients. It is, therefore, important to thoroughly interview and examine the patient and document reported findings prior to performing the neuraxial blockade. Also, in many patients with prior lumbar surgeries the ligamentum flavum may not be intact. Therefore, the provider should not rely on loss of resistance technique to find the epidural space and consideration should be made to enter at a level remote from previous surgery.

Previously, there were concerns that neuraxial anesthesia in a human immunodeficiency virus (HIV)-infected patient would hasten central nervous system manifestations of the disease. However, it is now understood that CNS involvement occurs early during the course of HIV infection and introduction of HIV into a previously virus-free CNS after is not a concern.

2.2.1.3 Preparation

Preparation for neuraxial anesthesia, like general anesthesia, should begin with a discussion with the patient and obtaining informed consent. The patient interview should include specific questions, such as whether there is a history of anesthetic complications, prior difficult placement of epidural or spinal anesthesia, history of bleeding disorders or thrombocytopenia, whether the patient is taking any anticoagulant medications, and history of spine disorders (i.e., scoliosis) or surgeries. The provider should then discuss the benefits and potential complications associated with neuraxial blockade. These include the rare but serious complications, such as bleeding, infection, or temporary nerve damage, as well as more common but less severe risks, such as post dural puncture headache and mild pain.

2.2.1.4 Location, Monitors, and Additional Equipment

Generally, a neuraxial blockade should only be performed in a facility with appropriate emergency equipment, medications, and personnel available in the event of an urgent situation requiring intubation or resuscitation. The procedure can be performed in an operating room or in an outside area with the above requirements. Patients should have frequent monitoring of blood pressure and pulse oximetry. Supplemental oxygen via nasal cannula or face mask with end tidal CO2 (EtCO2) monitoring is recommended if sedation is provided. Patients should have an adequately functioning intravenous line prior to the procedure. Although an ultrasound machine is typically unnecessary for neuraxial blockade, it may facilitate a difficult placement in a patient with poor surface landmarks, as discussed later in this chapter. Required practice for sterile technique includes hat, mask, and gloves.

2.2.1.5 Premedication and Sedation

Lumbar neuraxial anesthesia may be performed completely awake, with minimal sedation or under general anesthesia. Performing this block under general anesthesia, however, remains controversial. The reasoning is that the patient would be unable to verbalize pain or paresthesia during injection, symptoms that are associated with intraneural injection and postoperative neurological deficits. On the other hand, providing deep sedation or general anesthesia would reduce sudden patient movement, allowing for easier needle placement and less chance of nerve damage. Epidurals and spinals of the thoracic and particularly of the cervical spine should be placed in awake patients. The exception to this is the pediatric population, in which case neuraxial anesthesia is often performed under general anesthesia secondary to poor patient cooperation.

Pharmacological premedication, typically in the form of midazolam and fentanyl, is often beneficial prior to performing regional anesthesia. Premedication is avoided for labor epidurals, so it is essential to discuss expectations and verbally guide the patient through the procedure if desired. In situations where premedication is not used, patients should be provided with ample local anesthetic skin infiltration.

2.2.2 Patient Positioning

A patient can be positioned in either the sitting, prone, or lateral position for neuraxial anesthesia. Regardless of the type of position chosen, the goal is to flex the spine in order to draw apart the adjacent spinous processes and expand the interlaminar foramen.

2.2.2.1 Sitting

The sitting position is the most commonly encountered arrangement for spinal and epidural placement. In this position, the patient is curled forward, pressing the chin into the chest and the buttocks into the bed to form a C shape with the spine. This allows the spinous processes to be pressed closer to the skin where they are more easily palpated and also promotes the most expansion of the interlaminar space. The midline is also the most recognizable in the sitting position, which is of significant value in the obese population. This position is not ideal for a heavily sedated patient (◘ ◉ Fig. 2.8) [6].

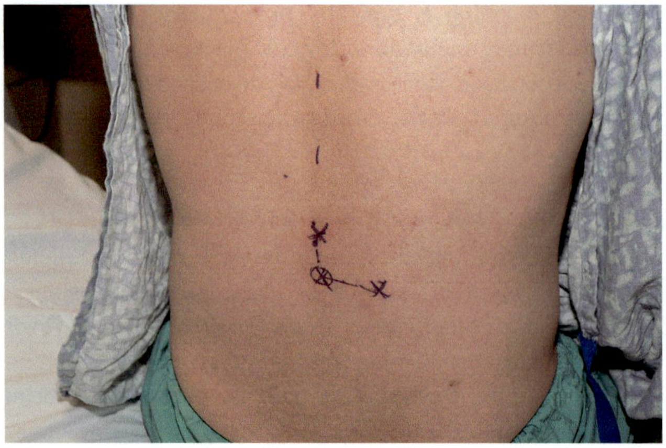

Fig. 2.8 Marks are made on patient's skin at midpoint of probe's long and short sides. Needle insertion site should be intersection of these 2 marks

2.2.2.2 Lateral Decubitus

This position is preferable in a patient under general anesthesia or in the elderly, sick population in which the patient is unable to sit upright without generous assistance. In the lateral decubitus position, the patient would lie on his or her side with the neck and knees flexed forward and pulled into the patient's chest.

2.2.2.3 Prone

The prone position is most often used for chronic pain procedures under the guidance of fluoroscopy. Rarely, the prone position is also used as the jackknife position for perineal procedures. In the prone position, the midline surface landmarks are not as easily appreciated. Because CSF pressure is lower than when the patient is upright, CSF aspiration is typically necessary to confirm subarachnoid injection as the CSF will not be free flowing.

2.2.3 Needles

Several different types of needles are available for spinal anesthesia, varying in overall size and the contour of their tips. In general, a smaller needle gauge decreases the incidence of post-dural puncture headaches (PDPH). The tapered pencil-point needles (Whitacre, Sprotte) are most commonly selected as their blunt tips are designed to ease the dural fibers apart versus cutting needles, such as a Quincke. Pencil-point needles also produce a ragged-edged hole in the dura, which provokes a more robust inflammatory response. Both the cutting of less dural fibers and the increased inflammatory response are thought to contribute to a smaller CSF leak and subsequently a lower risk of PDPH. These needles contain a side port that allows for directed injection of local anesthetic. Since these pencil-tip needles require more force to push through the dura, a more pronounced popping sensation can be appreciated by the operator. The other basic type of needle is the open-ended beveled needle (Quincke). Such open-ended beveled needles cut through the dura, which is associated with more dural trauma and elevated risk of PDPH.

One recent cadaver study evaluated needle type (pencil point vs. cutting), needle gauge, and angle of dural puncture (30° vs. 90°) and found that a large-bore cutting needle was associated with a larger dual leak over 1 h than blunt-tip smaller bore needles. No correlation was found between dura leak and angle of puncture [8].

The most commonly used epidural needle is the blunt-tipped Tuohy needle, which is designed to push the dura outward and away rather than penetrate through it. This needle features a curved edge that gently directs the epidural catheter in the direction of the curve for optimal placement in the epidural space.

All needles contain a removable, smaller-gauged inner stylet, which occludes the center of the needle to prevent lodging of bone fragments or subcutaneous tissue, which if present can lead to a false sense of resistance and possibly result in dural puncture in epidural placement. Such an inner stylet also serves to prevent the transfer of epithelial cells and possible surface contaminants into the intrathecal space.

2.3 Spinal Anesthesia

2.3.1 Indications

Spinal anesthesia is commonly indicated for surgical procedures involving the mid to lower abdomen, perineum, and lower extremities. It is becoming more regularly encountered in orthopedic surgeries including total hip and knee replacements. Benefits of regional anesthesia over general anesthesia in this population include reduced postoperative pain, decreased opioid consumption, reduced incidence of pulmonary embolism and deep venous thrombosis, decreased hospital length of stay, and increased rehabilitation—although there is no consensus on whether it results in decreased morbidity and mortality [9, 10].

2.3.2 Contraindications

As previously mentioned, absolute contraindications for neuraxial anesthesia include patient refusal, bleeding diathesis, elevated intracranial pressure, infection at site of injection, severe hypovolemia, and indeterminate neurologic disease [11].

More specific to spinal anesthesia, the risk of sudden and severe hypotension following injection of local anesthetic into the intrathecal space is significantly more pronounced and immediate than in epidural anesthesia. This is likely due to the direct injection of local anesthetic into the CSF and the subsequent bathing of nerve roots. Spinal anesthesia is therefore contraindicated in many patients with hypovolemia and cardiac outflow obstructions, such as aortic stenosis or hypertrophic obstructive cardiomyopathy (HOCM).

2.3.3 Technique

2.3.3.1 Midline Approach

For the midline approach, the patient is placed in the preferred position (can be in seated or lateral decubitus) and the spine is palpated to identify the midline and individual spinous processes. The interspinous spaces may be palpated as a depression between the bony spinous processes. Using the surface landmarks discussed earlier, the desired level can be identified by counting the number of spaces above or below these landmarks. Skin should then be cleaned with chlorhexidine or a similar solution, with subsequent application of a sterile fenestrated drape. A small-gauge needle, such as a 25-gauge 1.5-in. needle, is used to anesthetize the skin and subcutaneous tissue through the creation of a skin wheal with local anesthetic infiltration. This smaller needle also can be advanced deeper to act as a finder needle, identifying the superior and inferior borders of the space.

Next, an introducer needle, such as an 18G 1.5-in. hollow-bore needle, is placed into the space along the superior surface of the inferior spinous process. This thicker, shorter needle breaks the skin and assists in the guidance of the thin spinal needle. The spinal needle is then advanced through the introducer needle in slow, gradual movements in a slightly cephalad direction. The needle will easily pass through the subcutaneous tissue and then transverse the supraspinous and interspinous ligaments before encountering the thicker ligamentum flavum. The needle is further advanced until it penetrates the dura, which is accompanied by a characteristic popping sensation. Once the spinal needle is in the intrathecal space, the stylet is then removed to confirm the return of cerebrospinal fluid (CSF) into the hub of the needle (◘ ◉ Fig. 2.9). If no fluid is apparent, the stylet should be replaced and the needle slowly advanced, again removing the stylet to check for return of fluid. With visible confirmation of CSF, a syringe containing local anesthetic is firmly attached to the needle. Aspiration of the syringe should reveal a swirl of clear CSF. The local anesthetic can then be slowly injected through the needle, reconfirming the correct location by a second aspiration near the end of the injection. Once complete, the needle and syringe are withdrawn and removed from the patient's back [11].

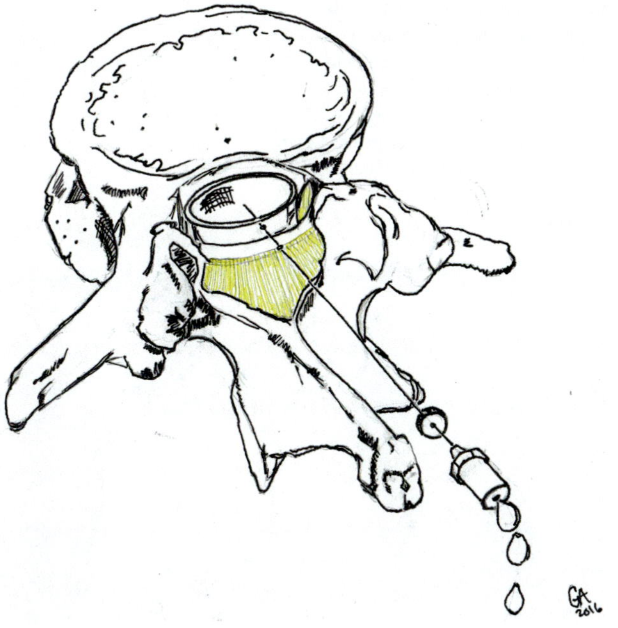

Fig. 2.9 View of spinal needle traversing ligamentum flavum and dura mater (Reprinted with permission Ochsner Health Systems © 2016. All Rights Reserved)

If the needle encounters bone superficially, the introducer and spinal needles should be slightly withdrawn and redirected either superiorly or inferiorly as it is likely contacting a neighboring spinous process. If the needle contacts bone at a deeper level, this likely indicates that the needle is not midline, so the needle should be withdrawn and redirected to the left or right of the previous location to avoid contacting the lamina. If the appearance of blood-tinged CSF is present on aspiration and does not clear immediately, the needle should be withdrawn and reinserted at a different interspace. Finally, if the patient reports transient paresthesia at any time (unilateral burning or shooting pain in buttocks, legs or perineum), local anesthetic should not be injected; instead, the operator should redirect the needle, as the paresthesia may indicate possible needle contact with a nerve or nerve root.

2.3.3.2 Paramedian Approach

Although the midline approach may be easier to perform for most patients, the paramedian approach can be selected if a neuraxial anesthetic is difficult to place because of a patient's spinal anatomy (e.g., severe spinal stenosis or prior spine surgery). This approach is also more commonly chosen for thoracic epidural placement given the angulated nature of the thoracic spinous processes. In this approach, the needle is inserted 1–2 cm lateral to the midline of the inferior surface of the superior spinous process and directly slightly medial and cephalad (◘ ◉ Fig. 2.10). The needle then passes through skin and subcutaneous tissue and directly

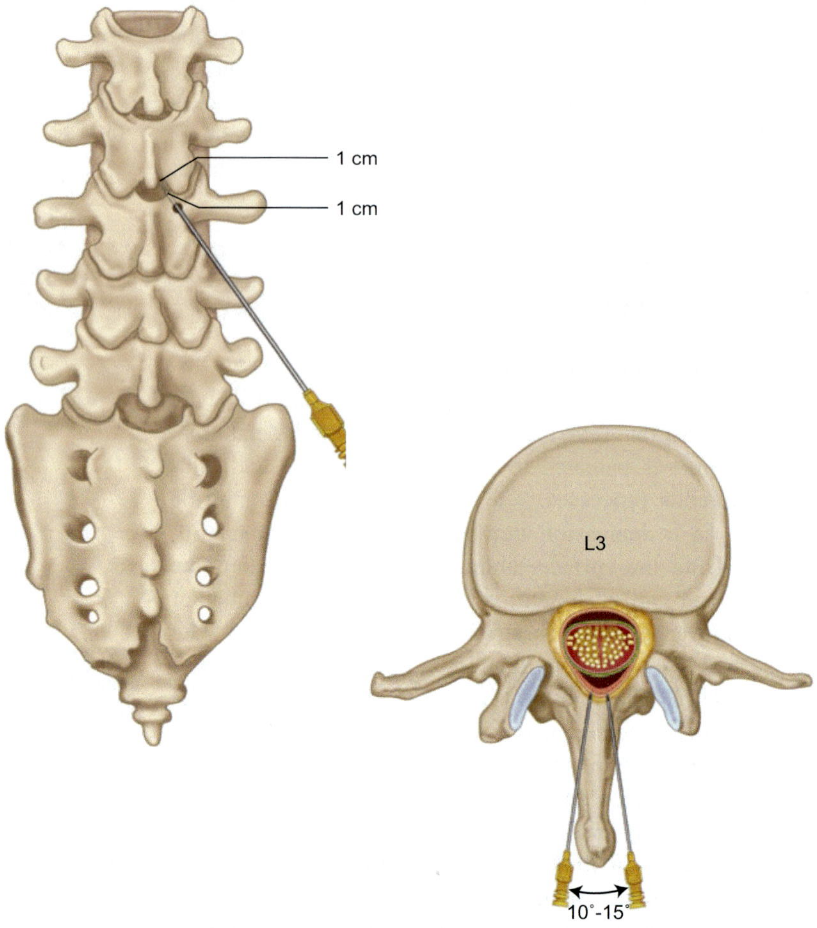

Fig. 2.10 Paramedian approach for spinal anesthesia uses an entry point 1 cm lateral and inferior to superior spinous process and directed at a 15-degree angle medially and cephalad (Reprinted with permission Ochsner Health Systems © 2016. All Rights Reserved)

encounters the ligamentum flavum, thus bypassing the medially located supraspinous and interspinous ligaments. If the needle contacts the lamina superficially, the needle should be redirected to walk off the bone in a cephalad direction. The operator should be mindful to avoid directing the needle too medially in this approach as it could potentially cross the midline [11].

2.3.4 Assessment of Neuraxial Blockade

Once injected, the local anesthetic bathes the nerve roots, blocking the small and unmyelinated nerve fibers (sympathetic, temperature/proprioception) first, followed by the large, myelinated fibers (sensory/motor). Since there is a differential in the density of neural blockade depending on the fiber type, the sympathetic blockade is typically at least 2 dermatomes levels higher than the sensory blockade, and the sensory blockade is 2 levels higher than the motor blockade.

The small C-type nerve fibers responsible for temperature change are the first to be affected, so one can test the adequacy of a spinal block within the first few minutes by wiping a wet alcohol pad over the patient's skin bilaterally. One can also test the adequacy of the sensory blockade by gently pricking the patient's skin with a blunt needle or the broken, sharp edge of a tongue depressor.

For intra-abdominal procedures, the minimum dermatome level should be approximately T4 (level of the nipples). For perineal, vaginal, and hip surgeries, a T10 level (at the umbilicus) should be adequate.

2.3.5 Pharmacokinetics and Pharmacodynamics of Spinal Anesthesia

The largest determinants of anesthetic spread include patient position during and immediately after injection and the dosage and baricity of the local anesthetic injected. A larger injected total *dose* (not volume or concentration alone) of local anesthetic will result in further spread in either direction [12]. The baricity of a local anesthetic basically refers to the relative density of the drug in relation to that of CSF. A hyperbaric drug is denser, and thus heavier, than CSF and will migrate in a direction consistent with gravity (i.e., it will sink with gravity). A hypobaric solution is lighter than CSF and will spread in a direction opposite to gravity (rise against gravity). An isobaric anesthetic has the same density as CSF and will likely remain where it is injected [13]. For example, if a patient is injected with a solution while seated in an upright position, a hyperbaric solution will spread caudally, a hypobaric solution will spread cephalad, and an isobaric solution will remain at the site of injection. Dextrose is typically added to a solution to make it hyperbaric whereas fentanyl or sterile water added to a solution will make it hypobaric.

Patient positioning after injection will also determine spread [13]. If a patient is placed in Trendelenburg position, the anesthetic will travel cephalad, and if the patient is in reverse-Trendelenburg, the solution will travel caudally. This is not true for isobaric solutions, however, as gravity does not play a role in these cases.

When a hyperbaric solution is used for a thoracic neuraxial in a patient in the supine position, the injected drug will migrate to the most dependent region of the spine. The natural curvature of the spine dictates that the most posterior and dependent curvature of the thoracic spine occurs at the T4-T8 level, therefore producing an anesthetic level toward T4.

The spread and distribution of any spinal anesthetic is also highly dependent on the volume of CSF in the spinal column. In general, increased CSF volume is associated with decreased spread of local anesthesia, and decreased volume results in increased spread [13]. Patient factors affecting CSF volume include patient height (taller patients require more local anesthetic), intra-abdominal pressure including pregnancy or large intra-abdominal tumors, and individual anatomic variations of the spinal column. In the case of pregnancy, the thought is that the increased intra-abdominal pressure leads to engorgement of epidural veins, thereby decreasing CSF volume. Thus, parturients would require less anesthetic solution to achieve the same spread.

Some recent studies have indicated that obesity may prolong the effects of spinal anesthesia, possibly due to a reduction in CSF volume as a result of epidural fat or extradural vein distention, although controversy still exists regarding the effects of obesity on duration and spread of spinal anesthesia [14].

Age also may be an independent determinant in that the elderly have decreased CSF volume, possibly due to severe kyphosis, and require smaller doses of local anesthetic.

The height of the injection site and the direction of injection through the needle are also factors that may affect the level of anesthesia obtained.

2.3.5.1 Spinal Anesthetic Agents

One of the more commonly used local anesthetics for spinal anesthesia is hyperbaric 0.75% bupivacaine. This has a relatively slow onset of about 5–10 min with a prolonged duration of 90–120 min. The addition of epinephrine may modestly prolong the duration to 100–150 min. The typical dosage for hyperbaric bupivacaine is 8–10 mg for lower abdominal surgeries (up to T10 level), and 14–20 mg for a T4 level [14].

Other local anesthetics that are less commonly used include 5% lidocaine and 10% procaine (60–90 min), and 0.25–1% ropivacaine and 1% tetracaine (90–120 min). All solutions must be preservative-free to avoid neurotoxicity.

Years ago, lidocaine was the most commonly used local anesthetic for spinal anesthesia. However, in recent years it is typically avoided secondary to the concern for transient neurological symptoms (TNS) and cauda equina syndrome (CES) encountered more commonly with lidocaine. These syndromes are discussed in further detail later.

More specific details on mechanism of action and side effects of local anesthetics can be found in the pharmacology chapter on these agents.

2.3.5.2 Additives to Local Anesthetics

Vasoconstrictors (epinephrine 1:200,000), opioids (fentanyl), and alpha-2-adrenergic agonists (clonidine) are often added to the local anesthetic solution to prolong the duration and intensify the effect of a spinal anesthetic [6].

The addition of epinephrine or phenylephrine is thought to benefit in multiple ways. First, the vasoconstriction of nearby tissue limits the redistribution of local anesthetic away from the intended site of action, prolonging the duration of anesthetic by keeping the drug in contact with the nerve fibers. This vasoconstriction also prevents systemic reabsorption of local anesthetic, decreasing the incidence of local anesthetic systemic toxicity (LAST) [15]. And finally, the presence of epinephrine, if accidentally injected intravascularly, will alert the provider to the incorrect needle placement by the accompanying hypertension and tachycardia.

The effects of vasoconstrictors are not the same for all local anesthetics. This has the most apparent effect on tetracaine and the least significant effect on bupivacaine. The increased duration of action is more pronounced in anesthetics with shorter intrinsic duration as well as the degree of spinal cord vasodilation associated with the drug. For example, tetracaine is associated with the most vasodilation of spinal cord vasculature, and the addition of epinephrine to tetracaine has the most effect on prolongation of duration.

Opioids, such as fentanyl and morphine, also can be added to enhance surgical analgesia and improve postoperative pain without prolonging motor or sympathetic blockade. These opioids work at receptors located in the dorsal horn of the spinal cord. Fentanyl, a lipophilic agent, provides a more localized effect with a shorter onset and approximately 6-h duration of effect due to its rapid vascular uptake. Morphine, on the other hand, is hydrophilic, and provides roughly 6–24 h of analgesic effect.

Respiratory depression may be seen with the addition of opioids. With fentanyl, respiratory depression would occur early with the rostral spread of opioid in the CSF and immediate vascular uptake. On the contrary, respiratory depression with morphine often presents in a biphasic manner. It may first occur within 30 min due to vascular absorption, but it also may occur later (6–18 h) due to slow penetration of the brainstem with delayed rostral spread.

Pruritus and nausea are also common side effects associated with the addition of opioids. The treatment for pruritus consists of opioids antagonists or agonist/antagonists; however, given in large doses it may also reverse the analgesic effects [16].

2.4 Epidural Anesthesia

Epidural anesthesia is regional blockade of spinal nerves achieved by placing local anesthetics and sometimes adjuvants, such as epinephrine or sodium bicarbonate, into the epidural space surrounding the dural sac. The epidural space is the potential space between the ligamentum flavum posteriorly and the dura mater anteriorly and contains epidural fat and veins.

In contrast to the limited duration of spinal anesthesia, the duration of anesthetic blockade can be controlled by placing a catheter in the epidural space and providing a bolus and subsequent continuous infusion. Epidural anesthesia also can be utilized in conjunction with spinal anesthesia in a technique known as combined spinal epidural injection (CSE). A single shot technique without a catheter may be used, but generally this technique is used to deliver steroids to spinal nerves for the treatment of chronic pain, not as a regional anesthetic.

2.4.1 Indications

Epidural anesthesia can be used as a primary anesthetic for surgeries involving the abdomen and lower extremities and also for postoperative pain control in surgeries involving the thorax, abdomen, and lower extremities. It is particularly helpful when used in a patient who has comorbidities that may preclude or limit the use of general anesthesia. Lumbar epidural anesthesia is commonly used in the management of labor pain in the parturient. Thoracic epidural anesthesia is frequently used for postoperative pain control after surgery, such as a thoracotomy. Pain management specialists can inject steroid around nerve roots for the treatment of radiculopathy and other chronic pain conditions along almost the entire length of the vertebral column [11].

2.4.2 Contraindications

Absolute contraindications to epidural anesthesia are similar to those in spinal anesthesia and include patient refusal, inability to remain still, or evidence of increased intracranial pressure. Some patients may not be able to maintain proper positioning or remain still throughout the procedure; this exposes the patient to greater risk of neurological complications, such as spinal cord/nerve root trauma or inadvertent dural puncture. Relative contraindications to epidural anesthesia include coagulopathy, including iatrogenic coagulopathy secondary to anticoagulation, thrombocytopenia, local infection over the selected site, and hypovolemia. Risks, benefits, and alternatives must be carefully considered when relative contraindications are present [11].

2.4.3 Technique

As in spinal anesthesia, there are 3 positions utilized in the delivery of epidural anesthesia: sitting, lateral, and prone. The most common position for lumbar and thoracic epidurals is the sitting position. The lateral position can be used if the patient cannot sit upright or if there is a contraindication to the sitting position. The prone position is used exclusively by pain management specialists in conjunction with fluoroscopy. With all positions except the prone position, the patient is asked to flex the spinal column, thereby increasing the space between the spinous processes and facilitating placement. In a similar fashion to spinal anesthesia, the patient's back is prepped and draped in a sterile fashion.

There are 4 approaches used in accessing the epidural space. Two of the approaches are interlaminar: midline and paramedian. The others are caudal and transforaminal—the latter being used for chronic pain management when selectivity is required for blocking one nerve root at a time. The 2 interlaminar approaches are described as follows since epidural catheters are commonly left in place using these approaches. The caudal and transforaminal approach will be discussed later.

2.4.3.1 Midline Approach

The midline approach is generally used for lumbar epidural placement. As discussed previously, a line connecting the bilateral iliac crests crosses the L4 vertebra and the spinous process can be palpated. Entering at L3/4 or L4/5 allows safe entry below the conus medullaris, which typically ends at the level of the L1 or L2 vertebral body in adults. The spinous processes are palpated to identify the intraspinous space. Once the space is identified, a skin wheal is made in the midline with local anesthetic. A 17 or 18 gauge epidural needle (most commonly a Tuohy needle) is then placed into the skin wheal and directed perpendicular to the coronal plane with a slight cephalad tilt and advanced until an increase in resistance is felt. This should indicate contact with the supraspinous ligament and continued advancement is made into the intraspinous ligament. At that point, the stylet is removed and the needle is advanced in an incremental or continuous fashion using the loss of resistance or hanging drop technique to identify the epidural space [6, 11].

2.4.3.2 Paramedian Approach

The paramedian approach is most often utilized with epidural placement in the thoracic spine as the spinous processes in this area are at a steeper angle in relation to the coronal plane making the midline approach difficult. As in the midline approach, the initial step is the identification of the spinous processes of the desired level. A skin wheal is then made about 1–2 cm lateral and 2 cm inferior to the midline of the desired level. The epidural needle is then inserted through the skin wheal and advanced medially and cephalad at an angle of 15–20° until lamina is contacted. The stylet is then removed and the needle is "walked off" the lamina medially and cephalad employing loss of resistance or hanging drop technique to identify the epidural space. When placing an epidural using the paramedian approach, the epidural needle penetrates the paraspinous muscles then enters the ligamentum flavum en route to the epidural space. While the supraspinous and interspinous ligaments are penetrated during a midline approach the epidural space, the paramedian approach is lateral to these ligaments [6, 11].

2.4.3.3 Catheter Placement and Test Dose

Once the epidural space has been identified, a catheter is advanced though the epidural needle. Typically, 3–5 cm is added to the depth of the epidural needle in order to leave the catheter in the epidural space. At this time, the catheter is aspirated in order to detect intrathecal or intravascular placement. If no CSF or blood is aspirated, which would indicate intrathecal or intravascular placement respectively, a test dose of lidocaine with epinephrine can be administered. Intravascular injection of the test dose may produce a metallic taste in the mouth secondary to the lidocaine and a rapid increase in heart rate secondary to the epinephrine. Sudden motor blockade of the lower extremities indicates an intrathecal injection of local anesthetic. While absence of these findings is not 100% sensitive for aberrant placement, the epidural catheter can now be used with reasonable confidence of correct placement.

2.4.3.4 Caudal Approach

In the caudal approach to epidural anesthesia, the sacral hiatus is the access point for the epidural space. This approach takes advantage of the fact that the epidural fat continues caudally through the sacral canal even beyond the distal-most point of the thecal sac, which generally terminates around S1-S3, depending on age. In children, the thecal sac ends around S3 and with increasing age moves proximally toward S1 and S2. The sacral hiatus is a natural defect of S5 dorsal midline and can be identified by palpating the 2 sacral cornu, which border the hiatus laterally and lie about 3–5 cm above the coccyx. The caudal epidural anesthesia technique is primarily used in pediatrics and pain management. Caudal epidural injection is used in pediatric anesthesia as part of an intraoperative anesthetic plan and postoperative pain control for urologic and lower extremity surgery, such as inguinal hernia repair and hypospadias correction. In pain management, the caudal approach is used to deliver steroids to the sacral nerve roots and lumbar canal. A catheter also can be employed and threaded up to the lower lumbar vertebra in order to treat pain arising from the lumbar nerve roots. This is often done in the setting of prior surgery where accessing the lumbar epidural space with an interlaminar technique would be technically difficult or impossible due to a surgically absent ligamentum flavum. Caudal injection is performed with the patient in the prone position. After cleaning and draping in the usual fashion, the skin over the hiatus is anesthetized and a 22 gauge spinal needed is introduced through the sacrococcygeal ligament and advanced until it contacts the sacrum. It is then slightly withdrawn, the angle of entry flattened, and subsequently advanced. Flushing the needle with saline and observing for the absence of tissue swelling will confirm placement within the epidural space. If swelling is noted, this indicates that the needle lies posterior to the sacrococcygeal ligament and it must be redirected [6].

2.4.4 Pharmacokinetics and Pharmacodynamics of Epidural Anesthesia

The principle site of action for epidural anesthesia is the spinal nerve root. Local anesthetic instilled into the epidural fat then crosses the dural layer and affects impulse conduction. To a lesser extent, local anesthetics will diffuse into the subarachnoid space and exert some effect.

Three of the more common local anesthetics used in epidural anesthesia include **2-chloroprocaine**, **lidocaine**, and **bupivacaine**. Duration of local anesthetic action in epidural anesthesia is not as important as in spinal anesthesia since use of a catheter allows continuous administration. In general terms, duration can be remembered by the 1-2-3 rule: 1 h for chloroprocaine, 2 h for lidocaine, and 3 h for bupivacaine. Speed of onset mirrors duration with chloroprocaine having the fastest onset, lidocaine slightly longer, and bupivacaine having the longest duration.

In addition to local anesthetics, several other medications can be added to the epidural space in order to modify the effects of the block. **Sodium bicarbonate** is often added to the local anesthetic and can decrease the time to onset of the block. Only the uncharged form of the local anesthetic penetrates the nerve fiber and blocks sodium conduction. However, with the addition of sodium bicarbonate, the pH is lowered and as the local anesthetics used in neuraxial anesthesia are weak bases, this forces more of the solution to the un-ionized form, thus leading to a greater fraction penetrating the nerve fiber and halting conduction. Sodium bicarbonate can be used with a variety of local anesthetics but is not added to bupivacaine as it can precipitate at a high pH. Another example of an additive includes **epinephrine**, which can be added to local anesthetic to increase the duration of blockade. This occurs because the vasoconstricting effects of epinephrine limits absorption into the vasculature and thus delays metabolism of the drug. The addition of epinephrine extends the duration of chloroprocaine and lidocaine by about 50%. The decreased absorption also decreases the likelihood of local anesthetic systemic toxicity (LAST). **Clonidine** also can be injected into the epidural space as an adjuvant. As an α(alpha)2 agonist, clonidine increases the reuptake of norepinephrine at the pre- and post-synaptic terminal of the neuromuscular junction. This mimics the action of inhibitory neuropathways on pain signal transmission in the dorsal horn of the spinal column. Additionally, clonidine has been shown to inherently block transmission of pain signals in C and A delta fibers and cause local vasoconstriction, thereby reducing the washout of local anesthetic in the same manner as epinephrine [17].

2.5 Combined Spinal Epidural

The combined spinal epidural (CSE) technique combines the rapid onset of spinal anesthesia with the ability to control duration of epidural anesthesia via an epidural catheter. Additionally, the dural puncture adds an element of reassurance that the catheter is, in fact, in the epidural space. Also, there is the theoretical benefit of a denser block as epidural medication migrates intrathecally though the dural puncture. A CSE is done in the same manner as an epidural injection, but after the epidural space is accessed, instead of immediately placing a catheter a spinal needle is advanced through the epidural needle until it penetrates the dura. CSF is aspirated to confirm placement and medication then can be injected into the intrathecal space. The spinal needle is withdrawn leaving the epidural needle in place, and a catheter is placed through the needle into the epidural space.

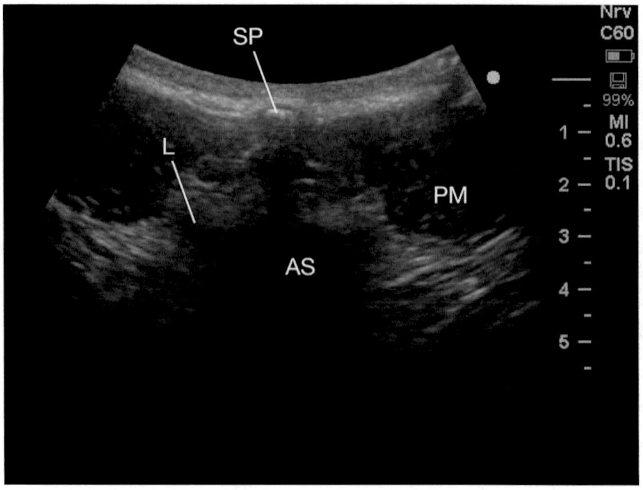

Fig. 2.11 Midline transverse probe placement: Spinous view. (*SP* spinous process, *AS* acoustic shadow behind spinous process and laminae, *PM* paraspinous muscle)

2.6 Ultrasound-Guided Neuraxial Procedures

Traditionally, landmarked-guided techniques are utilized in the delivery of spinal and epidural anesthesia. However, ultrasound guidance can aid in the ease and success of these procedures. It can be beneficial in all patients but there are specific situations where ultrasound guidance may be most helpful: patients with poorly identifiable surface landmarks, morbid obesity, lumbar spinal instrumentation, scoliosis, and ankylosing spondylitis. Advantages of ultrasound guidance include identifying correct vertebral level, identifying midline, identifying depth of various structures (spinous processes, lamina, epidural and subarachnoid spaces), identifying the optimal interspace, and identifying anatomical abnormalities (scoliosis, prior laminectomy, and instrumentation). A low-frequency curvilinear ultrasound probe (2–5 MHz) is often used for better penetration to these deeper structures.

With the probe in a transverse plane (perpendicular to the vertebral column) on the approximate center of the patient's back, identify the dropout (acoustic shadow) of the spinous process with its characteristic acoustic outline (◘ ◉ Fig. 2.11). Slide the probe cephalad or caudal to obtain a transverse interspinous view (◘ ◉ Fig. 2.12). The acoustic shadow of the spinous process will give way to an echogenic interspinous ligament. A slight cephalad tilt of the probe may be necessary. The ligamentum flavum is visualized as a horizontal hyperechoic line running between the articular processes and facet joints. It is common to see a single hyperechoic line representing the ligamentum flavum/dura complex. Deep to this is the hypoechoic

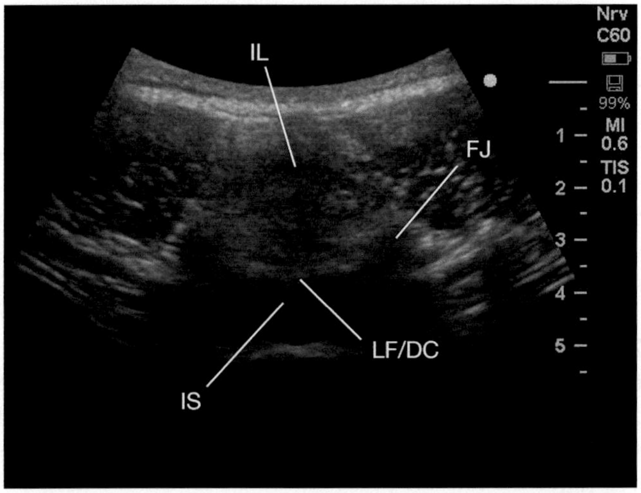

Fig. 2.12 Midline transverse probe placement: interspinous view. (*IL* interspinous ligament, *FJ* facet joint, *LF/DC* ligamentum flavum/dura complex, *IS* intrathecal space)

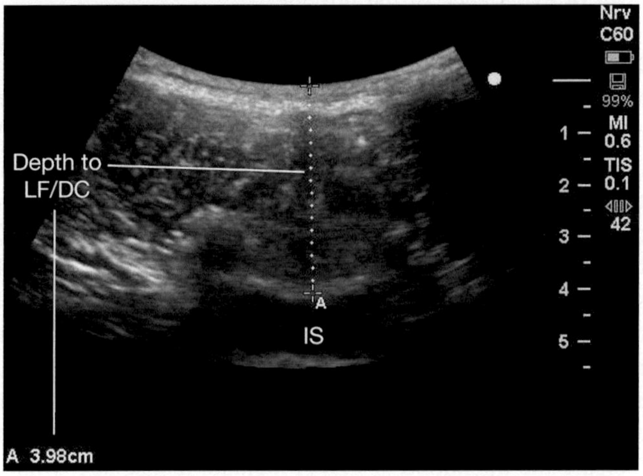

Fig. 2.13 Ultrasound machine's electronic caliper function measures depth from skin to ligamentum flavum to provide expected depth of needle insertion. (*IS* intrathecal space, *LF/DC* ligamentum flavum/dura complex)

intrathecal space that appears gray or black due to its weaker spectral reflection. Once this view is obtained, a mark on the patient's skin can be made at the midpoint of the probe's long and short sides. The needle insertion site should be the intersection of these 2 marks (◘ ◉ Fig. 2.8). At this point, it is beneficial to freeze the image on the ultrasound image. The ultrasound machine's electronic calipers can be used to measure the depth from skin to the ligamentum flavum to provide the expected depth of needle insertion (◘ ◉ Fig. 2.13). The spinal or epidural needle should be inserted at the respective mark on the skin and the initial angle should attempt to reproduce the cephalad angulation used with the ultrasound probe needed to obtain the interspinous view. A loss of resistance to air or saline technique should still be employed for epidural procedures to confirm entry into the epidural space and to avoid dural puncture [18, 19].

2.7 Complications Associated with Neuraxial Anesthesia

2.7.1 Cardiovascular

2.7.1.1 Hypotension

Cardiovascular manifestations of neuraxial anesthesia are largely due to the blockade of small, unmyelinated sympathetic nerve roots. This sympathetic blockade usually extends 2 dermatomes above and below the sensory/motor blockade. Hypotension immediately following spinal anesthesia is a common side effect occurring as a result of sympathetic blockade, thereby decreasing systemic venous resistance and often decreasing venous return and cardiac output as well. The severity of hypotension is related to the level of the spinal block as well as degree of coexisting hypovolemia. Treatment involves restoring preload by placing the patient in slight Trendelenburg, providing intravenous (IV) fluids and vasopressors. Some practitioners will routinely administer 1 L of fluid as a preload before or during spinal or epidural anesthesia as prophylaxis against hypotension [20].

2.7.1.2 Bradycardia

Many patients experience modest bradycardia following a spinal, although rarely bradycardia can progress to asystole and cardiac arrest without appropriate treatment. The underlying cause for bradycardia is believed to result from a blockade of the T1-T4 cardio accelerator fibers. This may also occur as a result of the Bezold–Jarisch reflex in which bradycardia occurs in response to decreased venous return. Treatment for minor bradycardia and hypotension may begin with IV ephedrine; more severe, persistent bradycardia may be treated with atropine and/or epinephrine [11].

2.7.2 Respiratory

2.7.2.1 Dyspnea

While true hypoventilation can occur with epidural and spinal anesthesia if it extends into the thoracic and cervical regions, a much more common occurrence is the feeling of dyspnea secondary to loss of proprioception in the intercostal muscles [20].

2.7.3 Gastrointestinal and Genitourinary

2.7.3.1 Nausea

Nausea after spinal or epidural anesthesia is often caused by 1 of 2 mechanisms: hypotension and subsequent decreased cerebral perfusion. Once the hypotension is treated and cerebral perfusion pressure is restored, the nausea usually resolves. Alternatively, nausea can be caused by a predominance of parasympathetic tone. After spinal or epidural anesthesia produces sympathetic blockade, the patient is left with a predominance of parasympathetic tone and resulting nausea. Ondansetron or promethazine are good choices for treating nausea due to parasympathetic overstimulation [11].

2.7.3.2 Urinary Retention

S2-S4 nerve roots innervate the bladder. Blockade of these nerve roots inhibits the voiding reflex and sensation of a full bladder. Addition of opioids can also increase the incidence of urinary retention. Foley catheterization should be routinely used in the presence of spinal or epidural anesthesia.

2.7.4 Neurologic

2.7.4.1 Transient Neurologic Symptoms

Transient neurologic symptoms (TNS) is defined as pain in the back or buttocks that can radiate to the legs within a few hours of spinal anesthesia, which is not associated with any other neurologic dysfunction and resolves within 24 h. TNS has the greatest association with lidocaine but is also seen with other local anesthetics as well [21].

2.7.4.2 High Spinal Blockade

Exaggerated spread of local anesthetic secondary to the administration of a large or disproportionate dose of local or an unusual distribution secondary to patient anatomy may lead to a high or complete spinal blockade. The spread of local anesthetic into the cervical levels and sometimes even beyond the foramen magnum affecting the cranial nerves can lead to severe outcomes.

The patient likely will first complain of weakness and numbness of the upper extremities and nausea. Dyspnea may be a common side effect once the phrenic nerve (C3-C5) supplying the diaphragm is affected, in addition to the effects resulting from the loss of proprioception from the intercostal musculature. As the anesthetic continues to spread cephalad to surround the cranial nerves, the patient will experience severe hypovolemia and bradycardia, progressing to syncope and loss of consciousness. Respiratory insufficiency may develop as a result of ischemia to the ventilation centers of the brainstem secondary to hypovolemia and decreased perfusion.

Treatment for a high spinal consists of cardiopulmonary support. Hypotension can be treated with intravenous fluids and vasopressors plus placement of the patient in Trendelenburg positioning, which act to increase venous return and systemic venous resistance. The operator should not attempt to block further spread of anesthetic by placing the patient in head-up position for this reason. Support of the patient's airway is warranted once respiratory distress is present. Tracheal intubation and mechanical ventilation are often necessary, particularly in patients at increased risk for aspiration [11, 20].

2.7.4.3 Failed Spinal

Occasionally, a spinal anesthetic may not provide adequate analgesia and anesthesia even though the technique appeared seemingly successful. This may result from subdural injection (injection into the potential space between the dura and arachnoid layers instead of the subarachnoid layer), incomplete penetration of the needle opening into the intrathecal space resulting in only partial injection, or movement of the needle during injection. Failure rate is often related to the level of experience of the provider.

2.7.4.4 Post-dural Puncture Headache

Puncture of the dura during spinal anesthetic, lumbar puncture, or an epidural wet tap can result in a post-dural puncture headache (PDPH). The proposed mechanism for this headache is a direct result of CSF loss through the open dural puncture site faster than the rate of CSF production, leading to a downward displacement of the brain and stretching of supporting structures (meninges, tentorium, and cranial nerves). Traction and tension on the blood vessels may also contribute to pain. There have been case reports, especially in young patients, of cerebral hemorrhage after dural puncture secondary to this tension. Factors that increase the likelihood of PDPH include: female sex, young age, pregnancy, and history of previous PDPH and the use of cutting-point, large-bore needles [8, 20].

Symptoms often present 12–48 h following the procedure, although occasionally symptoms can appear as early as immediately post-procedure or sometimes as long as several weeks later. The hallmark presentation is a positional headache, which intensifies when the patient is in an upright posture and is relieved while lying flat. The headache is typically bilateral, frontal, or occipital (sometimes extending to the neck) and described as a throbbing or constant pain. It is commonly associated with nausea and photophobia.

Treatment is typically conservative with caffeine, analgesics (nonsteroidal anti-inflammatory drugs, acetaminophen, opioids), rest and supine positioning, and fluids. Caffeine acts as a vasoconstrictor to decrease dilation and traction of intracranial vasculature. Caffeine, as well as fluid resuscitation, aids to increase CSF production. Recumbent positioning helps to prevent further loss of CSF through the dural defect.

If the headache persists after conservative treatment, the patient may be offered an epidural blood patch, which is typically very effective, offering immediate results. This procedure involves removing roughly 20 ml of autologous blood and reinjecting it into the epidural space at or below the level of the dural puncture. This is believed to work by sealing the dural puncture to prevent further leakage of CSF.

2.7.4.5 Nerve Root/Spinal Cord Trauma or Compression

Nerve root or spinal cord trauma can occur during needle or catheter placement. Usually, this results in transient paresthesias that resolve immediately either spontaneously or with removal of the needle or catheter. Some paresthesias may be associated with postoperative neurologic problems but most of these problems resolve spontaneously.

It is of paramount importance while performing spinal or epidural anesthesia never to inject in the presence of a paresthesia. Should the needle/catheter be located within an area of restricted spread (thus causing increased pressure on nearby nerve roots or spinal cord), the spinal cord or nerve root the damage may be much more severe.

2.7.4.6 Epidural Hematoma

An epidural hematoma can cause spinal cord compression resulting in severe neurological deficits and paralysis. Epidural hematomas may be caused by rupture of the veins of the epidural venous plexus. Clinically significant epidural hematomas occur at a rate of 1:150,000 epidural procedures and 1:220,000 for spinal procedures. The majority of these have occurred in the presence of anticoagulation or intrinsic defects of coagulation. Thus, neuraxial anesthesia is relatively contraindicated in patients on anticoagulation, a known coagulation defect, thrombocytopenia (less than 60 K), and severe platelet dysfunction. An epidural hematoma can present at the time of the procedure but also has been known to present on catheter removal. Symptoms of an epidural hematoma include back pain, motor deficits, and bowel or bladder incontinence. Treatment consists of surgical decompression so urgent MRI is indicated as not to delay surgery. In the setting of a spinal hematoma, surgical decompression of the hematoma in less than 8 h from the onset of symptoms is crucial to provide the best long-term neurological outcome [22, 23].

2.7.4.7 Epidural Abscess

Epidural abscesses can also cause significant spinal cord compression in a similar fashion to epidural hematomas. The presentation of an epidural abscess can occur as early as 5 days after spinal or epidural anesthesia but presentation can be delayed up to several weeks. An epidural abscess can be a complication of spinal or epidural anesthesia, neurosurgical procedures or can occur spontaneously in the absence of a neuraxial procedure. Those occurring in the absence of recent procedures are thought to be secondary to systemic infection seeding the epidural space. Symptoms of an epidural abscess include fever, chills, back pain, increased with percussion, radicular pain, bowel and bladder dysfunction, and paralysis. Elevated white blood cell (WBC) count also can be seen. Urgent MRI or computed tomography (CT) is indicated as definitive treatment consists of surgical decompression. Additionally, antimicrobial antibiotics with particular attention to covering for *Staphylococcus aureus* and *Staphylococcus epidermidis* should be initiated [24].

2.8 American Society of Regional Anesthesia Guidelines

Many situations exist in which neuraxial anesthesia and anticoagulation would both be appropriate for a patient at the same time; the most common scenario being deep vein thrombosis (DVT) prophylaxis in a postoperative patient. The American Society of Regional Anesthesia (ASRA) has developed guidelines to assist the practitioner in making decisions concerning regional and neuraxial anesthesia in patients on anticoagulation with their fourth edition being published in 2018. These guidelines are consensus opinions by experts in the fields of anticoagulation and neuraxial anesthesia. They also represent a thorough review of case reports and the literature surrounding epidural hematomas since they are such rare events, they do not lend themselves to study by randomized control trial. Thus, this is the strongest level of evidence available to guide practitioners. The ASRA guidelines for regional anesthesia list items for each drug: how long to discontinue the drug before receiving neuraxial anesthesia, when the next dose of the drug can be given after needle placement, when the catheter can be removed, and how long after removal before restarting the anticoagulant or antiplatelet therapy. ◉ Table. 2.1 consists of the latest ASRA recommendations for planning regional anesthesia in relation to various anticoagulants. ◉ Since these ASRA guidelines relate to perioperative neuraxial anesthesia and do not adequately apply to the variety of interventional spine procedures, other guidelines have been created. In 2018, ASRA published a second edition of recommendations from numerous pain and spine societies regarding anticoagulation and interventional spine and pain procedures. Table. 2.2 covers the stratification of various interventional spine procedures into high, intermediate, or low risk. High risk procedures include invasive procedures, such as spinal cord stimulator (SCS) trial, intrathecal pump placement, and vertebroplasty. Intermediate risk procedures include epidural steroid injections and sympathetic blockade. Low risk procedures include sacroiliac (SI) joint injections and peripheral

Table 2.1 ASRA guidelines for regional anesthesia

Drug	Amount of time drug must be discontinued before procedure	Amount of time medication must be delayed after procedure	Catheter removal	Time interval between removing catheter and restarting medication
Apixaban Eliquis	3 days	Catheters should be removed 6 h before dosing	Do not recommend restarting with indwelling catheter If unanticipated administration, hold 26–30 h	6 h
Aspirin	No restrictions	No restrictions	No restrictions	No restrictions
Dabigatran Pradaxa	Highly dependent on renal function: If unknown: 5 days If CrCl > 80: 3 days	Catheters should be removed 6 h before dosing	Do not recommend restarting with indwelling catheter If unanticipated administration, hold 34–36 h	6 h
Enoxaparin Lovenox (prophylactic dosing) (h)	12	> 12	12	4
Enoxaparin Lovenox (treatment dosing) (h)	24	> 12	24	4
Heparin (prophylactic dosing SQ)	4–6 h (5000 U BID or TID)	1 h	4–6 h	1 h
Heparin (treatment dosing)	4–6 h IV 8–12 h for SQ (<10,000 U BID) 12 h (7500–10,000 U BID) 24 h (>10,000 U BID) If on heparin > 5 days check PLT CT	1 h	Hold for 4 h (ideally 6 h) If on heparin > 5 days check PLT CT	1 h
Rivaroxaban Xarelto	3 days	Catheters should be removed 6 h before dosing	Do not recommend restarting with indwelling catheter If unanticipated administration, hold 22–26 h	6 h
Warfarin Coumadin	5 days + Normal INR Consider 1–2 mg oral Vitamin K if INR > 1.5 at 24-48 h mark prior to procedure For 1st dose 24 h before surgery or if second dose then check INR	No delay If catheter left in place 1) Low dose 2) Daily INR 3) Routine neuro checks 4) Minimize sensory and motor block 5) Hold is INR > 3.0	INR < 1.5 remove and neuro checks × 24 h 1.5- < 3.0 Assess all medication that alter coagulation and remove with caution continue neuro checks until INR stabilizes at therapeutic level > 3.0 hold or reduce warfarin do not pull Therapeutic INR No recommendation	No recommendation on time to hold Continue neurological assessment for 24 h following catheter removal
Edoxaban Novel selective Xa inhibitor	72 h	Catheters should be removed 6 h before dosing	Do not recommend restarting with indwelling catheter If unanticipated administration, hold 20–28 h	6 h
Betrixaban Novel selective Xa inhibitor	72 h If CrCl < 30 mL/min, avoid neuraxial block	Catheter should be removed before dosing	Do not recommend restarting with indwelling catheter If unanticipated administration, hold 72 h	5 h
Fondaparinux Arixtra Anti-facto xa	36–42 h	6–12 h	36–42 h	6–12 h
Thienopyridines/P2Y12 inhibitors				
Clopidogrel Plavix	5–7 days If within 5–7 must show normal PLT function	Immediately (if no Loading Dose) 6 h (if Loading Dose)	Neuraxial catheters may be maintained for 1–2 days prior to removal	Immediately (if no Loading Dose) 6 h (if Loading Dose)

(continued)

Table 2.1 (continued)

Drug	Amount of time drug must be discontinued before procedure	Amount of time medication must be delayed after procedure	Catheter removal	Time interval between removing catheter and restarting medication
Ticagrelor Brilinta	5–7 days	Do not recommend restarting with indwelling catheter	Do not recommend restarting with indwelling catheter	24 h
Ticlopidine Ticlid	10 days	Immediately (if no loading dose) 6 h (if loading dose)	Neuraxial catheters may be maintained for 1–2 days prior to removal	Immediately
Prasugrel	7–10 days	Do not recommend restarting with indwelling catheter	Do not recommend restarting with indwelling catheter	Immediately
Cangrelor Kengreal IV P2Y12 inhibitor	3 h	Do not recommend restarting with indwelling catheter	Do not recommend restarting with indwelling catheter	8 h

PLT platelet, *BID* twice daily, *DVT* deep vein thrombosis, *LMH* low molecular weight heparin, *SQ* subcutaneous, *INR* international normalized ratio

Table 2.2 Neuraxial and pain guidelines

High risk	Intermediate risk	Low risk
Spinal cord stimulation trial and implant Dorsal root ganglion stimulation trial and implant Intrathecal catheter and pump placement Vertebroplasty, kyphoplasty, epiduroscopy, and epidural decompression Percutaneous decompression laminotomy	Interlaminar and transforaminal ESI Cervical facet MBNB and RFA Paravertebral nerve block Intradiscal procedures Sympathetic blocks Trigeminal and sphenopalatine ganglia blocks	Peripheral nerve blocks Peripheral joint and musculoskeletal injections Trigger point injections including piriformis Sacroiliac joint injection and sacral lateral branch blocks Thoracic facet MBNB and RFA Pocket revision and generator/pump replacement

Patients with high risk for bleeding (multiple anticoagulants, old age, history of bleeding or bleeding tendency, advanced liver or renal disease) undergoing low or intermediate risk procedures should be elevated to next higher stratification
SCS spinal cord stimulator, *ESI* epidural steroid injection, *MBNB* medial branch nerve block, *RFA* radiofrequency ablation, *IPG/ITP* internal pulse generator/intrathecal pump, *SI* sacroiliac

Table 2.3 Guidelines advising how long patients should stop taking their medications before the procedure and when to restart after the procedure

Drug	When to stop			When to restart
	High risk	Intermediate risk	Low risk	
ASA	Primary prophylaxis 6 days Secondary prophylaxis shared assessment and risk stratification	Shared assessment and risk stratification	No	24 h
Nonsteroidal anti-inflammatory drugs (NSAIDs)				
NSAIDs	5 half-lives	No (consider stopping for certain procedures such as cervical ESI)	No	24 h
Diclofenac Ketorolac Ibuprofen	1 day			
Etodolac Indomethacin	2 days			
Naproxen Meloxicam	4 days			
Nabumetone	6 days			
Oxaprozin Piroxicam	10 days			24 h

(continued)

Table 2.3 (continued)

Drug	When to stop			When to restart
	High risk	Intermediate risk	Low risk	
Phosphodiesterase inhibitors				
Cilostazol	2 days	No	No	24 h
Dipyridamole	2 days	No	No	24 h
ASA combinations	Follow ASA recommendations	No Shared assessment and risk stratification	No	
Anticoagulants				
Coumadin	5 days Normal INR	5 days Normal INR	No Shared assessment and risk stratification	24 h
Acenocoumarol	3 days Normal INR	3 days Normal INR	No Shared assessment and risk stratification	24 h
IV heparin	6 h	6 h	6 h	2 h (if moderate or high risk and involved bleeding the 24 h)
SQ heparin (BID & TID)	24 h	6 h	Shared assessment and risk stratification	2 h for low risk, 6–8 h for intermediate and high risk
LMWH prophylactic	12 h	12 h	12 h	4 h (low risk) > 12 h medium to high risk
LMWH therapeutic	24 h	24 h	24 h	4 h (low risk) > 12 h medium to high risk
Fibrinolytic agents	48 h	48 h	48 h	N/A
Fondaparinux	4 days	4 days	Shared assessment and risk stratification	6 h for low risk, 24 h for intermediate and high risk
New anticoagulants				
Dabigatran	4–6 days (dependent on renal function)	5 days (dependent on renal function)	Shared assessment and risk stratification	24 h
Rivaroxaban	3 days	3 days	Shared assessment and risk stratification	24 h
Apixaban	3 days	3 days	Shared assessment and risk stratification	24 h
Edoxaban	3 days	3 days	Shared assessment and risk stratification	24 h
Gp iib/iia inhibitors				
Abciximab	5 days	5 days	2 days	8–12 h
Eptifibatide	24 h	24 h	8 h	8–12 h
Tirofiban	24 h	24 h	8 h	8–12 h
Thienopyridines/P2Y12 inhibitors				
Clopidogrel	7 days	7 days	Assess risk of discontinuation	12 h, 24 h if loading dose given
Prasugrel	7–10 days	7–10 days	Assess risk of discontinuation	24 h
Ticagrelor	5 days	5 days	Assess risk of discontinuation	24 h
Cangrelor	3 h	3 h	Assess risk of discontinuation	No recommendation

IV intravenous, *SQ* subcutaneous, *BID* twice daily, *TID* three times a day nerve blocks. The duration to hold and then restart each antiplatelet and anticoagulant medication is then compared against the level of risk of the procedure. ◘ Tables ◉ 2.2 and ◉ 2.3 summarize these guidelines [25, 26].

2.9 Summary Questions (Choose the Most Appropriate Answer)

1. The primary mechanism of prescription opioid-induced analgesia is exerted by:
   a. **The mu-opioid receptor**
   b. The delta-opioid receptor
   c. The sigma-opioid receptor
   d. The kappa-opioid receptor

The mu-opioid receptor is the main mechanism of action by which opioids cause analgesia

2. Opioid-related adverse effects are primarily mediated by:
   a. Mu-opioid receptor type 1
   b. **Mu-opioid receptor type 2**
   c. Serotoninergic receptors
   d. Dopaminergic receptor type 1

The mu-opioid receptor type 2 is responsible for most of the adverse effects related to opioids (i.e., respiratory depression, sedation, pruritus, prolactin release, dependence, anorexia, and sedation).

3. The following opioid is considered a biased agonist of the mu-opioid receptor:
   a. Oxycodone
   b. Methadone
   c. Hydromorphone
   d. Oliceridine

Oliceridine is a biased agonist of mor that has been recently approved for acute postoperative pain.

4. Which route of administration should be considered to provide reliable and rapid-onset opioid-induced analgesia:
   a. Transdermal
   b. Oral
   c. **Intravenous**
   d. Rectal

The intravenous route of administration provides reliable and rapid onset of analgesia and should be considered for the treatment of acute pain

5. The liver is responsible for:
   a. Phase I metabolism
   b. Phase II metabolism
   c. Definite drug excretion
   d. **A and b**

Most opioids undergo liver metabolism in 2 phases. In phase I, opioids change their chemical structure to produce a more water-soluble and less active metabolite. Phase II involves reactions that couple opioids with another polar molecule, such as glucuronic acid, sulfate, or glycine, in a process called conjugation.

6. Remifentanil is considered:
   a. A long-acting opioid
   b. A short-acting opioid
   c. An intermediate-acting opioid
   d. **An ultra-short-acting opioid**

Remifentanil is the only ultra-short-acting opioid clinically available.

7. The longest-acting opioid—after single-dose intravenous administration—to treat acute pain is:
   a. **Methadone**
   b. Sufentanil
   c. Hydromorphone
   d. Fentanyl

Methadone has a half-life between 8–60 h. it is available in oral and intravenous formulations.

8. Opioids:
   a. Increase gastric emptying
   b. Stimulate small bowel propulsion
   c. Decrease fluid reabsorption
   d. **None of the above**

Opioids decrease gastric emptying (gastroparesis), inhibit small bowel propulsion, and increase fluid reabsorption and the tone of the anal sphincter, which are the physiological bases of opioid-induced constipation.

9. The following molecules are approved for opioid-induced constipation, except:
   a. Alvimopan
   b. Naloxegol
   c. **Oxymorphone**
   d. Methylnaltrexone

Oxymorphone is a mu-opioid receptor agonist. alvimopan, naloxegol, and methylnaltrexone are peripheral antagonists of the mu-opioid receptor approved for the treatment of opioid-induced constipation.

10. A 55-year-old man is diagnosed with opioid-induced respiratory depression, which of the following can be administered for treatment:
    a. Alvimopan
    b. **Naloxone**
    c. Naloxegol
    d. Methylnaltrexone

Naloxone is an opioid antagonist and the first choice for life-threatening opioid-induced respiratory failure.

References

1. Afton-Bird G. Atlas of regional anesthesia. In: Miller RD, editor. Miller's anesthesia. Philadelphia: Elsevier; 2005.
2. Agur A, Dalley A. Grant's atlas of anatomy. 12th ed. Philadelphia: Lippincott Williams & Wilkins; 2009.
3. Brown DL. Atlas of regional anesthesia. Philadelphia: WB Saunders; 1992.
4. Reynolds F, Speedy HM. The subdural space: the third place to go astray. Anesthesia. 1990;45:120–3.
5. Crighton IM, Barry BP, Hobbs GJ. A study of the anatomy of the caudal space using magnetic resonance imaging. Br J Anaesth. 1997;78:391–5.
6. Butterworth JF IV, Mackey DC, Wasnick JD. Chapter 45. Spinal, epidural, and caudal blocks. In: Butterworth IV JF, Mackey DC, Wasnick JD, editors. Morgan & mikhail's clinical anesthesiology. 5th ed. New York: McGraw-Hill; 2013.
7. Savolaine ER, Pandya JB, Greenblatt SH, Conover SR. Anatomy of the human lumbar epidural space: new insights using CT-epidurography. Anesthesiology. 1988;68(2):217–20.
8. O'Connor G, Gingrich R, Moffat M. The effect of spinal needle design, size and penetration angle on dural puncture cerebrospinal fluid loss. AANA J. 2007;75(2):111–6.
9. Macfarlane AJ, Govindarajulu AP, Vincent WS, Brull R. Does regional anesthesia improve outcome after total knee arthroplasty? Clin Orthop Relat Res. 2009;467(9):2379–402.
10. Ballantyne JC. Does epidural analgesia improve surgical outcome? Br J Anesthesia. 2004;92:4–6.
11. Miller DM, Pardo MC. Basics of anesthesia. Philadelphia: Elsevier; 2011.
12. Hocking G, Wildsmith JA. Intrathecal drug spread. Br J Anaesth. 2004;93:568–78.
13. Breivik H, Niemi G, Haugtomt H, Högström H. 6 Optimal epidural analgesia: importance of drug combinations and correct segmental site of injection. Best Pract Res Clin Anesthesiol. 1995;9(3):493–512.
14. Sheskey MC, Rocco AG, Bizzari-Schmid M, Francis DM, Edstrom H, Covino BG. A dose-response study of bupivacaine for spinal anesthesia. Anesth Analg. 1983;62:931–5.
15. Neal JM, Bernards CM, Butterworth JF 4th, Di Gregorio G, Drasner K, Hejtmanek MR, et al. ASRA practice advisory on local anesthetic systemic toxicity. Reg Anesth Pain Med. 2010;35(2):152–61.
16. Kumar K, Singh S. Neuraxial opioid-induced pruritus: an update. J Anesthesia Clin Pharmacol. 2013;29(3):303–7.
17. Elia N, Culebras X, Mazza C, Schiffer E, Tramèr MR. Clonidine as an adjuvant to intrathecal local anesthetics for surgery: systematic review of randomized trials. Reg Anesth Pain Med. 2008;33:159–67.
18. Gray AT. Ultrasound-guided regional anesthesia: current state of the art. Anesthesiology. 2006;104:368–73.
19. Grau T, Leipold RW, Conradi R, Martin E, Motsch J. Efficacy of ultrasound imaging in obstetric epidural anesthesia. J Clin Anesth. 2002;14:169–75.
20. Horlocker TT. Complications of spinal and epidural anesthesia. Anesthesiol Clin North America. 2000;18:461–85.
21. Freedman JM, Li DK, Drasner K, Jaskela MC, Larsen B, Wi S. Transient neurologic symptoms after spinal anesthesia: an epidemiologic study of 1,863 patients. Anesthesiology. 1998;89(3):633–41.
22. Moen V, Dahlgren N, Irestedt L. Severe neurological complications after central neuraxial blockades in Sweden 1990–1999. Anesthesiology. 2004;101:950–9.
23. Shroll J, Guirguis M, D'Mello A, Mroz T, Lin J, Farag E. Epidural hematoma with atypical presentation. A A Case Rep. 2014;2(7):75–7.
24. Practice advisory for the prevention, diagnosis, and management of infectious complications associated with neuraxial techniques: a report by the American society of anesthesiologists task force on infectious complications associated with neuraxial techniques. Anesthesiology. 2010;112(3):530–45.
25. Narouze S, Benzon HT, Provenzano DA, Buvanendran A, De Andres J, Deer TR, et al. Interventional spine and pain procedures in patients on antiplatelet and anticoagulant medications: guidelines from the American society of regional anesthesia and pain medicine, the European society of regional anaesthesia and pain therapy, the American academy of pain medicine, the international neuromodulation society, the North American neuromodulation society, and the world institute of pain. (Second Edition) Reg Anesth Pain Med. 2018;43(3):225–262.
26. Horlocker TT, Wedel DJ, Rowlingson JC, Enneking FK, Kopp SL, Gogarten W, Leffert LR, Benzon HT. Regional anesthesia in the patient receiving antithrombotic or thrombolytic therapy: American society or regional anesthesia and pain medicine evidence-based guidelines (Fourth Edition). Reg Anesth Pain Med. 2018;43(3):263–309.

Anatomy of the Brain and Spinal Cord

3

Matthew K. Whalin and Joanna Schindler

Abstract

The anatomy of the brain and spinal cord has important implications for the manifestations of neurological disease, perioperative monitoring of the nervous system, and the actions of drugs administered during anesthesia. The geographic organization of sensory and motor pathways leads to predictable symptom patterns for lesions in a particular area. Even in the absence of injury, the management of several reflex responses that occur during surgery requires an understanding of the underlying anatomy. Knowledge of the anatomy of the spine is also important for the safe and effective practice of neuraxial anesthesia.

Keywords

Brain • Spinal cord • Autonomic nervous system • Sympathetic • Parasympathetic • Baroreceptor reflex • Epidural • Subdural

Key Points

1. The brain receives 15% of the body's cardiac output and accounts for 25% of the body's total oxygen consumption. The brain has no glucose or oxygen stores making it susceptible to ischemic damage within minutes.
2. The Circle of Willis is an anastomosis of the left and right internal carotid and vertebrobasilar systems. The majority of healthy individuals do not have a complete Circle of Willis.
3. The cranial epidural space is created when significant force leads to high-pressure bleeding. Bleeding in the cranial subdural space requires much less force to injure the small bridging veins.
4. The spinal epidural space is continuous from the sacral level to the cranial base and allows medications to be injected into the epidural space at one level in order to provide analgesia and anesthesia for a broad range of dermatomes.
5. The sympathetic nervous system arises from the thoracolumbar spine and mediates fight-or-flight responses, while the parasympathetic system arises from the craniosacral region and promotes rest-and-digest functions.
6. The autonomic nervous system modulates cardiovascular and respiratory function through several reflex arcs.

3.1 Anatomy of the Brain

The brain can be divided into 3 components: the cerebrum, the cerebellum, and the brainstem. The cerebrum, or forebrain, has 2 components: the telencephalon and the diencephalon. The outer portion of the telencephalon is known as the cerebral cortex, whereas the inner (subcortical) regions include portions of the basal ganglia. The diencephalon contains the thalamus and hypothalamus.

3.1.1 Cerebral Cortex

The cerebral cortex is folded into gyri and separated by sulci. This folded structure allows the expansive cortex to fit into the cranial vault in a compact fashion. The lateral surfaces of each hemisphere are traditionally divided into 4 lobes: frontal, parietal, temporal, and occipital. The different lobes

M. K. Whalin (✉) · J. Schindler
Department of Anesthesiology, Emory University School of Medicine, Grady Memorial Hospital, Atlanta, GA, USA
e-mail: mwhalin@emory.edu

J. Schindler
e-mail: jlavi@emory.edu

M. Argalious et al. (eds.), *Basic Sciences in Anesthesia*,
https://doi.org/10.1007/978-3-031-60203-0_3

are separated from each other by sulci with overall organization consistent across individuals.

The frontal lobe consists of areas responsible for initiative, judgment, abstract reasoning, and creativity. The central sulcus separates the motor cortex in the posterior frontal lobe from the somatosensory cortex in the parietal lobe. Damage to the parietal lobe can result in hemineglect highlighting its importance in the integration of sensory information. The occipital lobe is posterior to the parietal lobe and contains the visual cortex. The temporal lobe contains the auditory cortex and houses key regions for memory formation and language.

Deep within the lateral sulcus lies the insula which plays roles in consciousness, emotion, and homeostasis. (◉ Fig. 3.1). The cerebral hemispheres communicate with each other via a bundle of myelinated and unmyelinated fibers called the corpus callosum.

3.1.2 Basal Ganglia

The basal ganglia are a collection of nuclei in the telencephalon, diencephalon, and midbrain that control motor function. The striatum is part of the telencephalon. Striatal damage is an early feature of the autosomal-dominant movement disorder Huntington's chorea. The substantia nigra is a midbrain structure. Dopaminergic efferents from the substantia nigra are critical for motor control, and damage to this area leads to Parkinson's disease. In addition to their role in motor function, the basal ganglia are an important component of the reward pathway and may play a role in addiction.

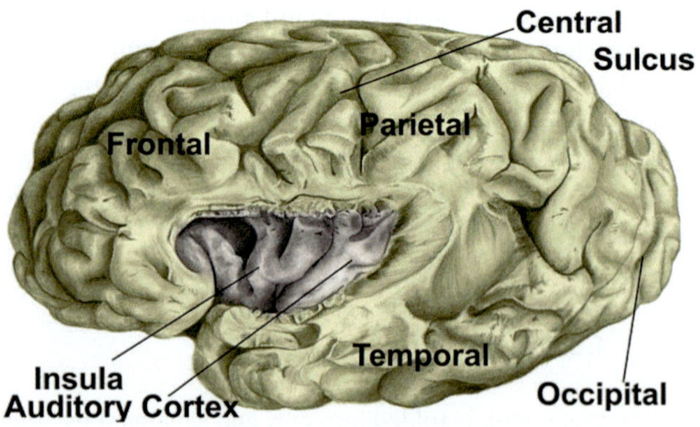

Fig. 3.1 Lobes of brain. Frontal and parietal lobes are separated by central sulcus. Some sources identify limbic and insula as additional lobes. In this diagram, lateral portions of the brain have been cut away to demonstrate the insula deep in the lateral sulcus (Reprinted with permission from Jacobson and Marcus [1])

3.1.3 Cerebellum

The cerebellum arises from the hindbrain and lies in the posterior fossa of the skull. It is separated from the brainstem by the fourth ventricle and from the cerebrum by the tentorium. The cerebellum plays a key role in balance and the coordination of movement. Cerebellar deficits may lead to ataxia or intention tremor. Patients with cerebellar disease may have difficulty with finger-nose-finger (dysmetria) or rapid alternating movements (dysdiadochokinesia). In contrast to lesions of the cerebrum, unilateral cerebellar damage usually manifests on the same side of the body.

3.2 Anatomy of the Brainstem

The brainstem is made up of the midbrain, pons, and medulla and is located ventral to the cerebellum. The cranial nerves (CN) are numbered based on their place of exit from the brainstem from rostral to caudal (◉ Fig. 3.2). The brainstem contains essential ascending and descending tracts and nuclei that are involved with consciousness as well as cardiac, respiratory, sensory, and motor functions. The brainstem houses these critical parts in a densely compact arrangement such that even very small lesions can have devastating effects.

3.2.1 Midbrain

The midbrain is a transition from the cerebrum to the brainstem. It houses the nuclei for cranial nerves III (oculomotor) and IV (trochlear). The base of the midbrain contains the corticospinal, corticobulbar, and corticopontine pathways which together form the crus cerebri. It also houses the substantia nigra.

The tegmentum portion of the midbrain contains the ascending tracts of the spinal cord and lower brainstem and many of the descending pathways as well. The red nucleus interacts with these tracts playing an important role in motor coordination. The locus coeruleus nuclei located here have norepinephrine-containing neurons that connect to multiple other brain structures to regulate the sleep-wake cycle and arousal. The midbrain also houses the periaqueductal gray matter with descending autonomic tracts which are targets in emerging chronic pain treatments.

3.2.2 Pons

The pons contains nuclei for CN V (trigeminal), VI (abducens), VII (facial), and VIII (vestibulocochlear) near its junction with the medulla. The corticospinal tract, medial lemniscus, and spinothalamic tracts all travel through the

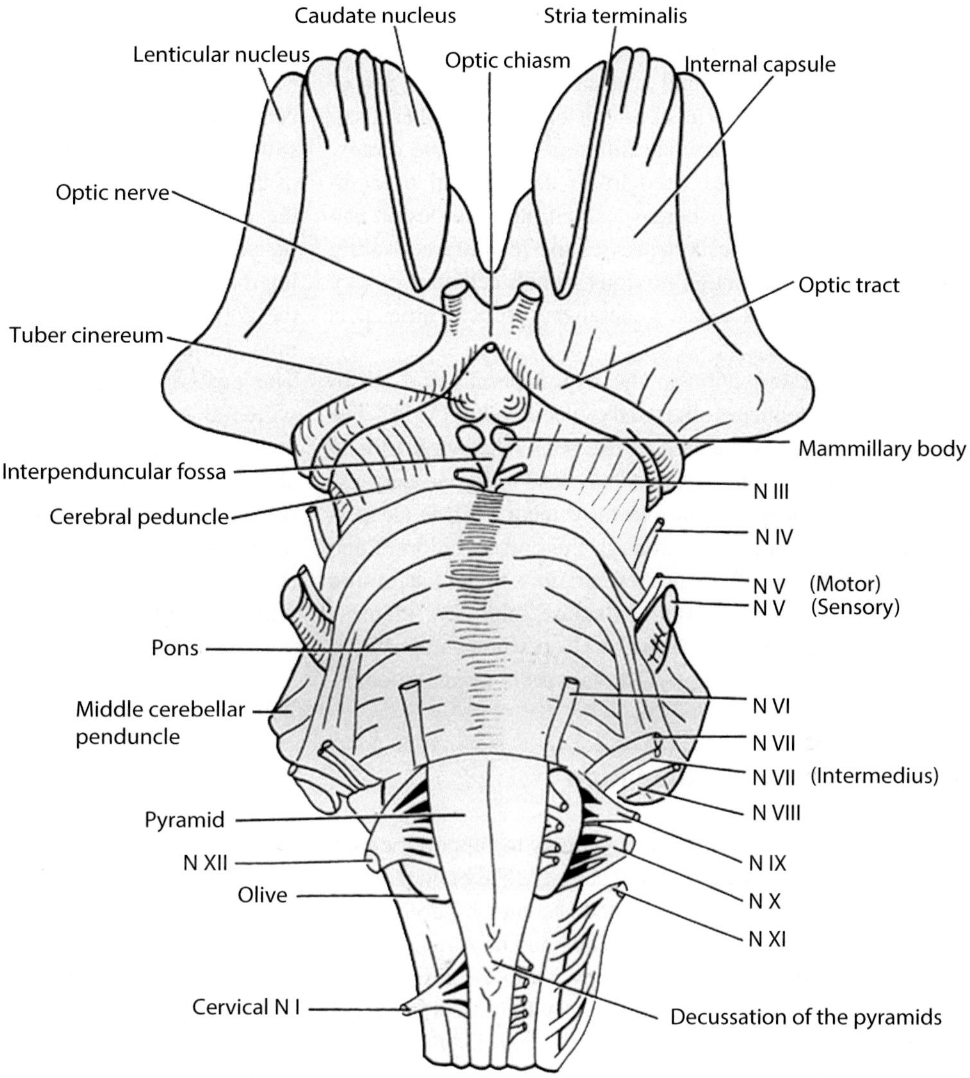

Fig. 3.2 Brainstem and cranial nerves. Cranial nerves exit ventral surface of brainstem and are numbered from rostral to caudal. Cranial nerves III and IV originate in midbrain, V-VII come from pons, and VIII-XII emerge from medulla (Reprinted with permission from Jacobson and Marcus [1])

pons. The raphe nuclei extend from the middle of the pons into the medulla and modulate arousal, sleep-wake cycles, and pain sensory input. Rapid correction of hyponatremia may lead to extensive demyelination of the base of the pons known as central pontine myelinolysis. This presents clinically as locked-in syndrome.

3.2.3 Medulla

The medulla contains nuclei for CN IX (glossopharyngeal), X (vagus), XI (accessory), and XII (hypoglossal). These nuclei control taste, salivation, lacrimation, tongue movement, swallowing, and vocalization. The medulla also houses many ascending and descending tracts that connect the spinal cord to the cortex.

3.2.4 Role of the Brainstem in Respiration and Consciousness

Several key processes are controlled by brainstem circuits. Areas of respiratory control span from the pons to the caudal medulla. The pons, retrotrapezoid nucleus, and raphe modulate respiratory drive, while the solitary nucleus and ventral lateral medulla receive feedback from peripheral areas, such as the lungs, carotid bodies, and respiratory muscles. As a result, acute herniation of the ventrolateral medulla causes changes in respiration, such as Cheyne–Stokes breathing with intermittent apnea.

The reticular activating system is a set of nuclei and circuits that play an important role in arousal. The system has ascending projections as well as a descending reticulospinal tract. This tract modulates spinal reflex activity, spinal autonomic activity, and sensory input. The system is a functional classification based on its nonspecific role in regulating consciousness and arousal. A variety of types of stimuli can modulate the level of consciousness and arousal. Since different stimuli activate different parts of the cortex, large areas of the cortex need to be damaged in order to decrease consciousness whereas a small midbrain lesion can result in coma. Anesthesia depresses the reticular activating system so that even though noxious stimuli activate sensory thalamic and cortical areas, generalized cortical arousal is inhibited.

The reticular formation in the hypothalamus and brainstem actively regulates the daily sleep-wake cycle. The reticular formation structures of the pons discharge prior to sleep and certain pontine lesions may lead to hyper-alertness and decreased sleep. Rapid eye movement (REM) sleep is specifically triggered by neurons in the dorsal midbrain and pontine tegmentum. Many of these neurons release serotonin or norepinephrine. Monoamine oxidase inhibitors increase norepinephrine and decrease REM sleep whereas decreased serotonin levels can promote wakefulness in animal models.

3.3 The Cerebral Circulation

The brain has an extensive vascular supply to support the high metabolic needs of constant neural activity. The brain receives 15% of the body's cardiac output and accounts for 25% of the body's total oxygen consumption. The brain has no glucose or oxygen stores so if blood flow stops it can be permanently damaged within minutes. As shown in ◉ Fig. 3.3, the burden of this constant blood supply is placed on two internal carotid arteries and two vertebral arteries which form a complex anastomosis known as the Circle of Willis. Venous blood drains into the dural venous sinuses.

3.3.1 Arterial Supply to the Brain

The internal carotid arteries pierce the cavernous sinus to enter the subarachnoid space. Here, the ophthalmic, posterior communicating, and anterior choroidal arteries branch off before each internal carotid artery divides into an anterior and middle cerebral artery. The anterior cerebral artery (ACA) passes above the optic chiasm and forms an arch around the corpus callosum. As shown in ◉ Fig. 3.4, it supplies the medial surface of the hemisphere and contributes to the blood supply of the internal capsule and caudate nucleus. The middle cerebral artery (MCA) receives the majority of blood flow (between 60 and 80%) from the internal carotid artery. It supplies the frontal, parietal, and temporal lobes, part of the optic radiation, and two-thirds of the lateral surface of the brain. The MCA provides branches to the corpus striatum and internal capsule. MCA occlusion leads to contralateral hemiplegia.

The 2 vertebral arteries fuse to form the basilar artery between the medulla and pons, and the basilar artery quickly splits into the 2 posterior cerebral arteries at the upper border of the pons. Because the posterior cerebral arteries arise from the internal carotid arteries during embryogenesis, 25% of people receive most of their posterior circulation from their internal carotid arteries. The posterior circulation supplies the corpus callosum, occipital and temporal cortices, thalamus, subthalamic nucleus, optic radiation, and midbrain. The posterior inferior cerebellar artery is a branch of the vertebral artery that provides blood supply to the medulla and cerebellum. The anterior and posterior spinal arteries also branch from the vertebral artery and supply parts of the medulla before continuing to the spinal cord via the foramen magnum. The basilar artery gives rise to the anterior inferior cerebellar and superior cerebellar arteries which supply the pons, cerebellum, and inner ear.

3.3.2 The Circle of Willis

The Circle of Willis is a system of anastomoses linking the left and right internal carotid and vertebrobasilar systems (◉ Fig. 3.5). It lies in the deep interpeduncular cistern of the subarachnoid space and provides collateral flow in the event of arterial occlusion. The anterior portion of the circle consists of the anterior cerebral arteries and the small anterior communicating artery. The posterior communicating artery provides an anastomosis between the internal carotid and vertebrobasilar systems. Dozens of perforating arteries branch from the Circle of Willis. All arteries of the Circle of Willis contribute to the short perforating branches, and they provide the blood supply to the optic nerve, chiasm, tract, and hypothalamus. Long perforating branches are formed from the 3 cerebral arteries and supply the thalamus, corpus striatum, and internal capsule. There is extensive anatomic variation, and a complete Circle of Willis is present in less than 50% of normal individuals. Roughly 15% of patients are at risk for insufficient collateral flow because of deficits in both the anterior communicating artery and one or both posterior communicating arteries.

3.3.3 Venous Drainage of the Brain

Superficial and deep veins form a complex drainage system. The thin-walled veins have no valves or surrounding muscle. They traverse the arachnoid mater and empty into the dural venous sinuses. Specifically, the superficial cerebral veins drain the cerebral cortex and underlying white matter into the superior sagittal sinus, cavernous sinus, and transverse sinus.

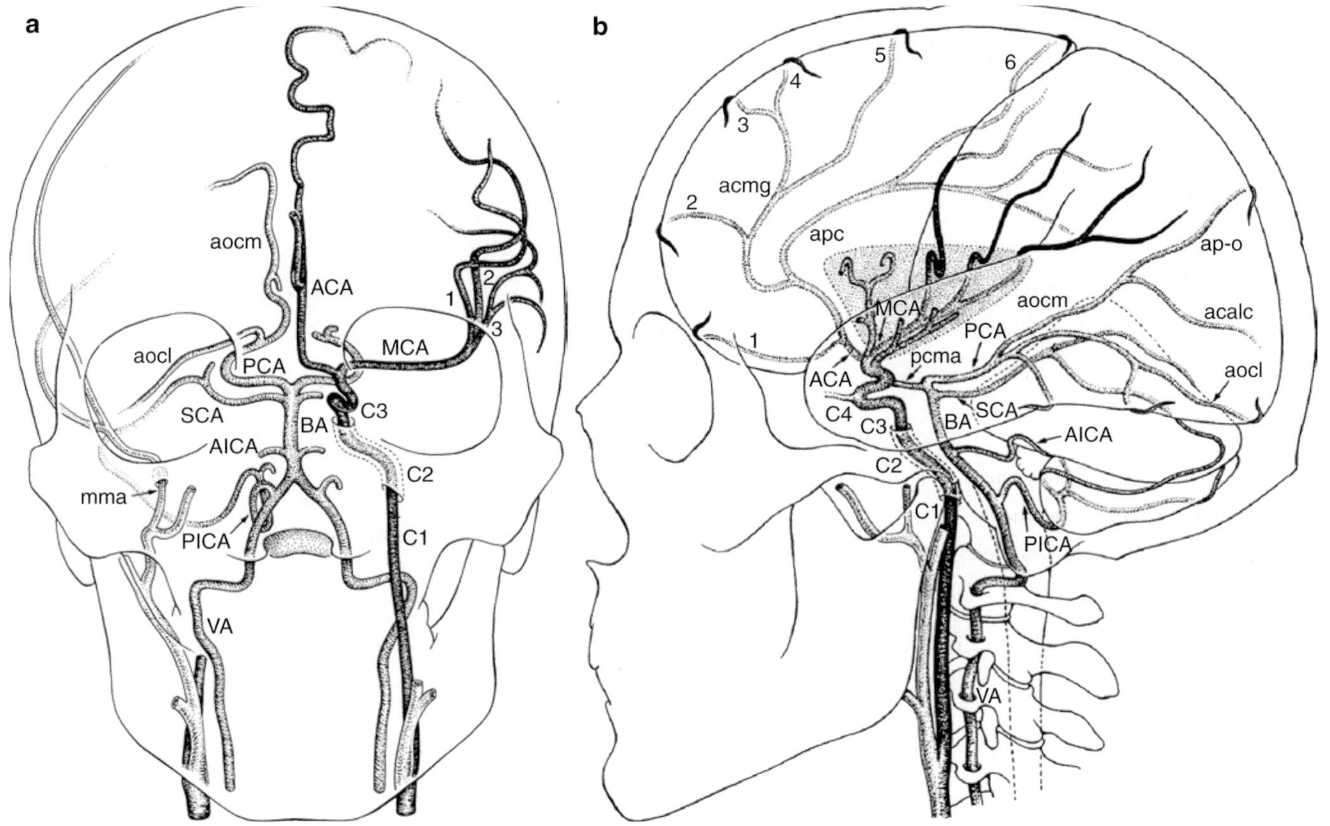

Fig. 3.3 Frontal **a** and lateral **b** views of the arterial supply of the brain. Internal carotid and vertebral arteries deliver oxygenated blood to brain. In these images, only the left carotid (*darker shading*) and right vertebrobasilar system (*lighter shading*) are shown within the skull to minimize overlap. Abbreviations: *ACA* anterior cerebral artery, *AICA* anterior inferior cerebellar artery, *BA* basilar artery, *C1–C4* cervical, petrous, cavernous and cerebral parts of internal carotid artery, *MCA* middle cerebral artery, *mma* middle meningeal artery, *PCA* posterior cerebral artery, *pcma* posterior communicating artery, *PICA* posterior inferior cerebellar artery, *SCA* superior cerebellar artery, *VA* vertebral artery, in **a** 1–3 refer to the trifurcation of the MCA; in **b** 1–6 are branches of the ACA (Reprinted with permission from ten Donkelaar [2])

The deep vertebral veins drain the corpus striatum, thalamus, and choroid plexuses into various larger veins that eventually form the great cerebral vein. The great cerebral vein unites with the inferior sagittal sinus and forms the straight sinus which eventually empties into the transverse sinus.

Ultimately, all the venous sinuses drain into the internal jugular veins (IJV) which comprise the superior and inferior jugular venous bulbs. On average, two-thirds of the blood from a single internal carotid artery is drained by the ipsilateral IJV, and one-third is drained by the contralateral jugular vein. Although the jugular venous blood is derived from both cerebral hemispheres, the venous drainage is usually asymmetrical, with the majority of patients draining cerebral venous blood dominantly into the right-sided jugular bulb. Cerebral oxygenation is often monitored in patients with brain injury by measuring jugular venous saturation ($SjvO_2$). The normal $SjvO_2$ ranges from 55 to 70% with values below and above this threshold reflecting cerebral ischemia and hyperemia, respectively.

3.4 Anatomy of the Spinal Cord and Spine

The spinal cord is an extension of the central nervous system (CNS) that links the brain to the peripheral nervous system. In humans, as in all vertebrates, the spinal cord is protected by the bony spine. Early in fetal development, the spinal cord initially spans the entire length of the vertebral column. As development continues, the tip of the spinal cord known as the conus medullaris becomes more cephalic as the bony spine grows at a faster rate. At birth, the spinal cord terminates around L3 with the more cephalic "adult" position reached at 2 years. A magnetic resonance imaging (MRI) study of 504 adults found a mean termination of the conus in the lower third of L1 which agrees with pooled cadaveric studies [4]. The cord ended above the L2/3 disk in almost 99% of the modern MRI cohort. These data support the safety of therapeutic and diagnostic dural puncture at L3/4 level or below.

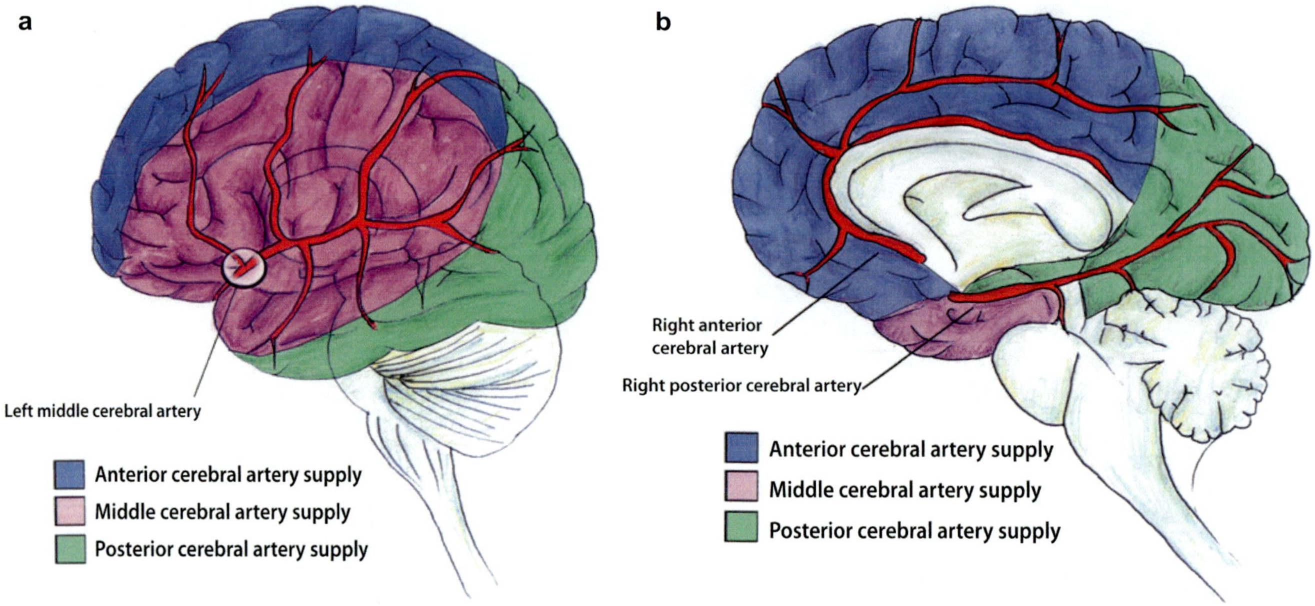

Fig. 3.4 Vascular territories of cerebral cortex. The color-coded regions show the predominant arterial supply to the lateral surface of the left cortex **a** and the medial surface of the right cortex **b** (Reprinted with permission from Jacobson and Marcus [1])

3.4.1 Variations in Vertebral Configuration

Other anatomic features of the spine have relevance to neuraxial anesthesia. ◉ Fig. 3.6 shows the typical arrangement of the human vertebral column into 7 cervical, 12 thoracic, and 5 lumbar vertebrae as well as the 5 fused vertebrae of the sacrum and coccyx. The acute angles of the spinous processes in the thoracic region can make paramedian neuraxial approaches more successful than midline attempts. Additionally, the normal curvature of the spine shown in the figure has implications for the spread of intrathecal medications (see ► Chap. 2). Nearly 90% of patients have 24 presacral vertebrae, as shown in ◉ Fig. 3.6, but one study reported 25 presacral vertebrae in 5% and 23 vertebrae in 6% of a North American cohort [6]. These differences arise from variation in the fusion of vertebrae around L5 and S1. In addition to variable fusion of the sacrum, there also can be incomplete fusion of the neural arch of one or more vertebrae. Such an isolated cleft spine, or *spina bifida*, is present in 10–20% of the population and should be considered a normal variant. These are often asymptomatic, and there may or may not be exterior evidence for closed defects, such as a tuft of hair in the sacral area (hence the term *spina bifida occulta*). Open forms are usually associated with neurologic deficits.

3.4.2 Spinal Nerves

The relationships of the vertebrae to the cord and spinal nerves are shown in ◉ Fig. 3.7. At a basic level, the cord can be divided into gray and white matter. As in the brain, the white matter is composed primarily of myelinated axons that are organized into tracts that ascend or descend in the spinal cord (◉ Fig. 3.8). The cellular gray matter contains a sensory dorsal horn and a somatomotor ventral horn which come together via the intermediate zone to give an H-shaped appearance. In the thoracolumbar region, there is also an intermediolateral portion of the gray matter that forms part of the sympathetic nervous system. Projections to and from the gray matter horns give rise to dorsal and ventral roots which unite to form the spinal nerves.

Cervical spinal nerves C1–7 emerge above their respective vertebrae, and C8 exits between the C7 and T1 vertebrae. The thoracic, lumbar, and sacral nerves course through foramina below their respective vertebrae. The relative ascension of the spinal cord discussed previously means that the sacral and lower lumbar spinal nerves travel some distance caudad before exiting the vertebral canal. This area is termed the *cauda equina* because of its resemblance to a horse's tail. Together with the coccygeal nerve, there are 31 pairs of spinal nerves. ◉ Fig. 3.9 shows the approximate sensory distribution of these spinal nerves. Although such

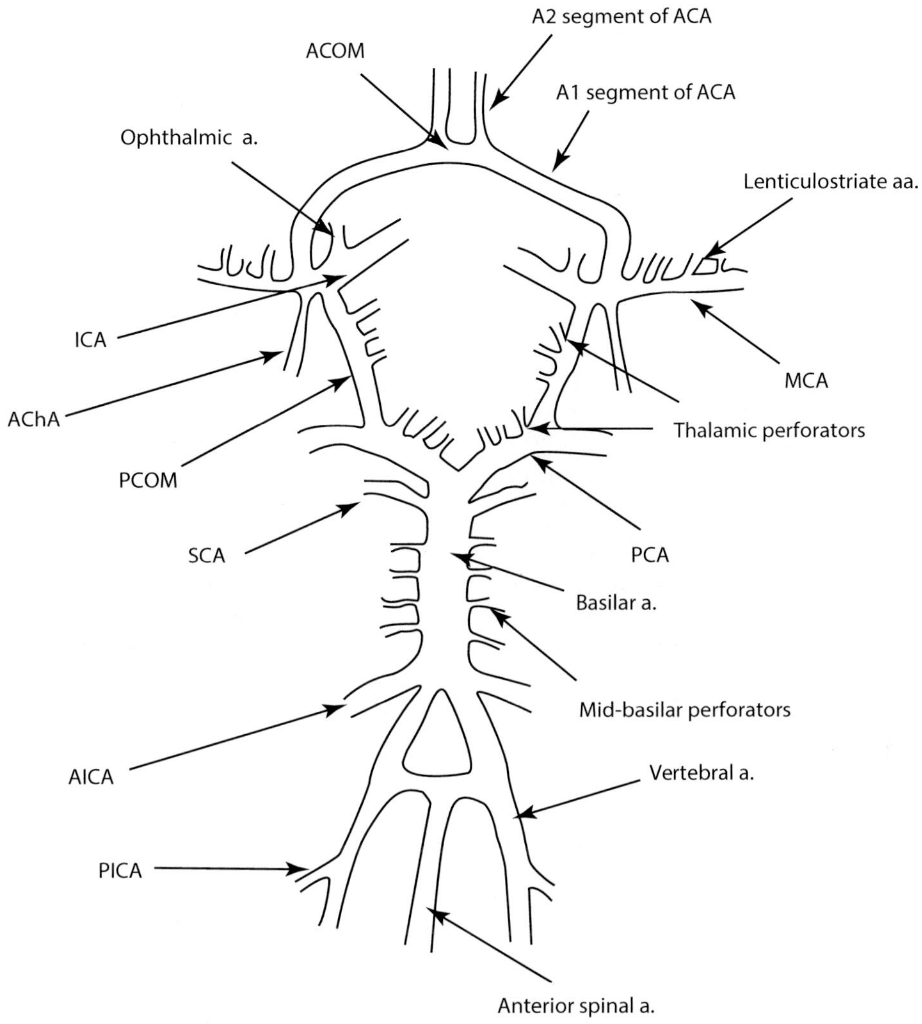

Fig. 3.5 Circle of Willis. Abbreviations: *ACA* anterior cerebral artery, *ACha* anterior choroidal artery, *ACOM* anterior communicating artery, *AICA* anterior inferior cerebellar artery, *ICA* internal carotid artery, *MCA* middle cerebral artery, *PCA* posterior cerebral artery, *PCOM* posterior communicating artery, *PICA* posterior inferior cerebellar artery, *SCA* superior cerebellar artery (Reprinted with permission from Tarulli [3])

dermatome maps are useful for assessing neuraxial blocks, there can be some variation and overlap of this innervation.

3.4.3 Arterial Supply of the Spinal Cord

The spinal cord receives blood from a pair of posterior spinal arteries and a single anterior spinal artery (◉ Fig. 3.10). The anterior spinal artery is formed by branches of each vertebral artery and supplies the anterior two-thirds of the cord. The posterior spinal arteries arise either from the vertebral arteries or from the posterior inferior cerebellar arteries and supply the remainder of the spinal cord. These three longitudinal arteries receive additional blood from feeders known as radicular, medullary, or radiculo-medullary arteries. These radicular arteries are particularly important to blood flow in the thoracic region and below. They are variable, but there are typically eight that feed the anterior spinal artery and twelve that feed the posterior spinal arteries. The artery of Adamkiewicz is the largest anterior radicular artery and can be disrupted during aortic surgeries. In most people, this is a left-sided vessel that originates from an intercostal branch off the aorta between T8 and L1, but its origin can be quite variable.

3.5 Meninges: Epidural, Subdural, and Subarachnoid Spaces

The CNS is surrounded by 3 protective membranes known as the meninges. The most external is the dura mater. The arachnoid and pia mater lie below the dura and are collectively referred to as the leptomeninges due to many shared characteristics. The cranial meninges pass through the foramen magnum to continue as the spinal meninges.

3.5.1 Dura Mater

The dura mater is a tough fibrous connective tissue that fuses with the inner periosteum of the cranium and creates

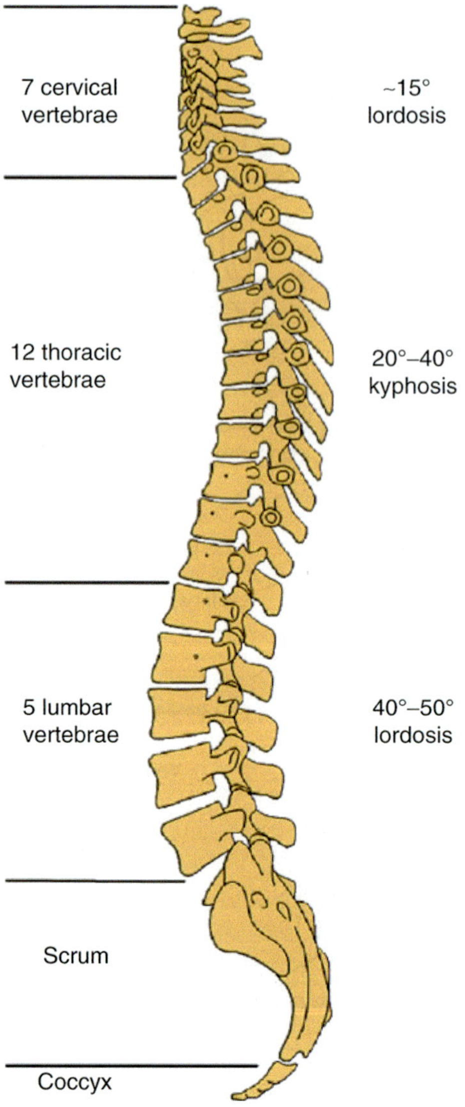

Fig. 3.6 Divisions of human spine. This sagittal view shows the normal distribution of vertebrae into cervical, thoracic, and lumbar segments (Reprinted with permission from Patel et al. [5])

compartments within the brain to separate the cerebrum from the cerebellum (*Tentorium cerebelli*), the cerebral hemispheres (*Falx cerebri*), cerebellar hemispheres (*Falx cerebelli*), and the pituitary gland (*Diaphragma sellae*). The cranial dura is comprised of an inner meningeal layer and an outer endosteal layer. These two layers separate only to enclose the venous sinuses. Although the dura adheres to the cranial bones, the meningeal layer surrounds the cranial nerves and fuses with the epineurium as they exit the cranium.

The cranial dura is continuous with the dural sac surrounding the spinal cord and becomes continuous with the periosteum of the coccyx. The spinal dura then surrounds the spinal roots and nerves as they exit the intervertebral foramina and eventually fuses with the epineurium.

3.5.2 Subdural and Epidural Spaces

The cranial epidural and subdural spaces become clinically significant with trauma and aging. The epidural space is created when significant force leads to high-pressure bleeding, which then causes separation of the periosteum and dura. The majority of cases involve middle meningeal artery injury and 75–95% are associated with skull fracture. The classic presentation is a lucid interval followed by gradual deterioration as intracranial pressure increases. As expected, an epidural hematoma does not cross cranial suture lines because the dura is tightly attached to the skull at the suture lines. The only treatment for an epidural hematoma is emergent surgery for evacuation.

In contrast to epidural bleeds, enlargement of the cranial subdural space by separation of the dura and arachnoid mater requires much less force. Injury to small bridging veins can easily lead to a subdural hematoma. Acute subdural hematomas are most commonly found in children, whereas chronic subdural hematomas are more common in older people whose bridging veins have already become fragile and stretched due to brain shrinkage. Subacute subdural hematomas can occur after injury in any age group. Signs and symptoms of increased intracranial pressure may develop up to three weeks post-injury due to slower blood accumulation.

The spinal epidural space contains connective tissue, fat, a venous plexus, small arterial branches, and lymphatics. Contrast studies have shown that fluid injected into the epidural space at the sacral level will spread up to the cranial base. As a result, medications can be injected into the epidural space at one level to provide analgesia and anesthesia for a broad range of dermatomes. Although the spinal subdural space does not normally exist due to the close apposition of the dura and arachnoid, it is a potential space that has been inadvertently accessed during attempts at epidural catheter placement. Subdural injection may lead to spinal cord damage as a result of direct toxicity or compressive effects.

3.5.3 Arachnoid Mater and the Subarachnoid Space

The outermost cell layer of the arachnoid mater consists of tight junctions that contain the cerebrospinal fluid (CSF) that is secreted by the choroid plexuses of the cerebral ventricles. The arachnoid mater is closely opposed to the pia mater and underlying brain except at concavities of the brain where the pia adheres to the brain's surface while the arachnoid spans the area. Therefore, the subarachnoid space varies in depth with deeper portions at the concavities forming cisterns of CSF. The cisterns house much of the cerebral vasculature

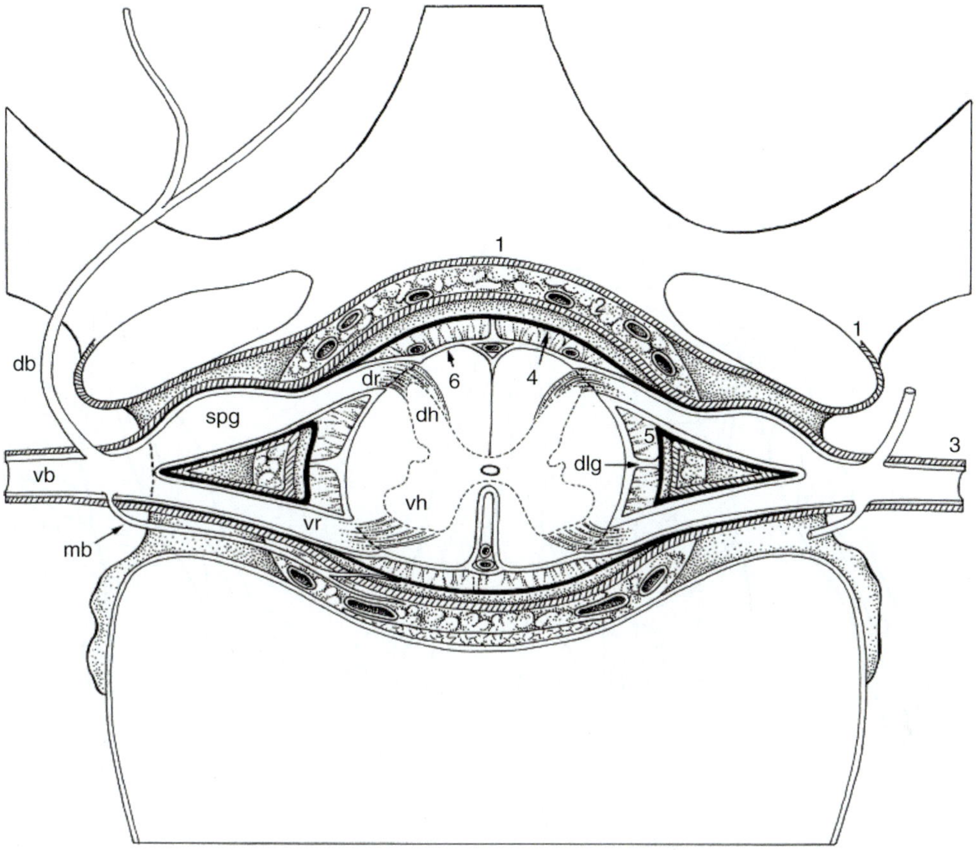

Fig. 3.7 Cross section of vertebral column at level of a spinal nerve. The spinal nerve has dorsal, ventral, and meningeal branches (*db*, *vb*, and *mb*, respectively). It divides into a ventral root (*vr*) and a dorsal root (dr). The dorsal root ganglion is also known as a spinal ganglion (*spg*). The roots enter the spinal cord and connect to the dorsal and ventral horns (*dh* and *vh*). Structures of the meninges are indicated by numbers as follows: (*1*) periost, (*2*) epidural space, (*3*) dura mater, (*4*) arachnoid mater, (*5*) subarachnoid space, and (*6*) pia mater. The pia mater also gives rise to the denticulate ligaments (*dlg*) which tether the spinal cord (Reprinted with permission from ten Donkelaar [2])

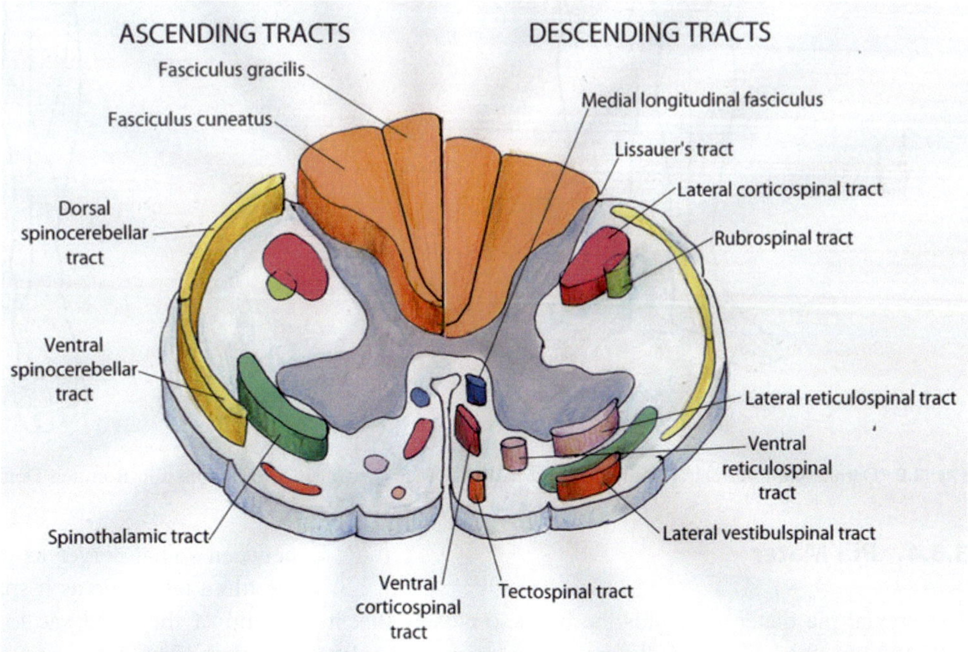

Fig. 3.8 Major spinal cord pathways. Ascending tracts are shown as elevated components on the *left* side of the figure, whereas descending tracts are shown as elevated components on the *right* side of the figure (Reprinted with permission from Jacobson and Marcus [1])

including the MCA, basilar artery, ACA, Circle of Willis, and the great cerebral vein. The cerebral subarachnoid space drains CSF into the fourth ventricle via three connections. The arachnoid membranes also form villi and granulations that aid CSF reabsorption into the venous system from the higher pressure ventricular system via the lower pressure venous sinuses. The cranial arachnoid is continuous with the spinal arachnoid mater.

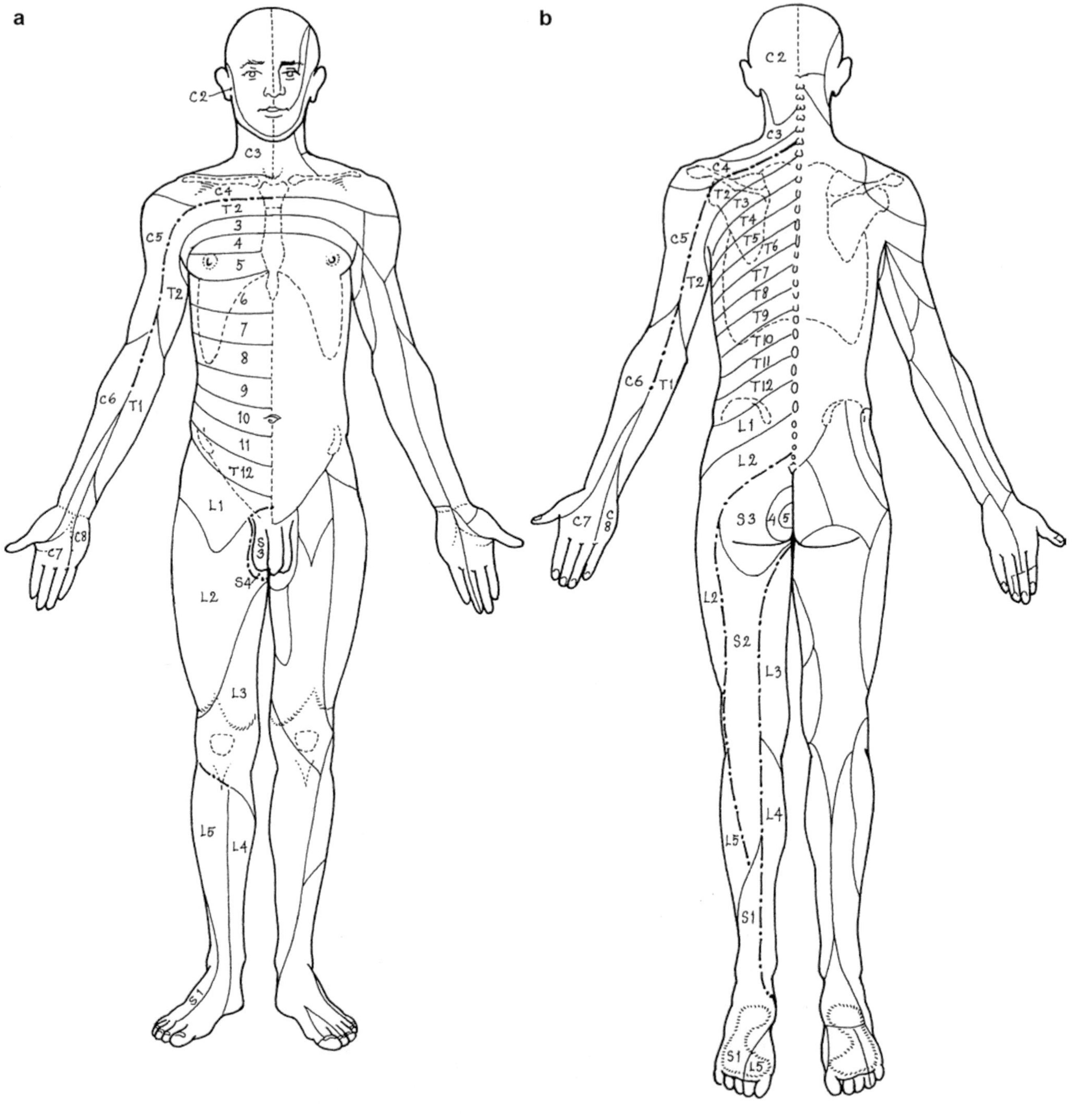

Fig. 3.9 Dermatomes of ventral **a** and dorsal **b** body surfaces (Reprinted with permission from ten Donkelaar [2])

3.5.4 Pia Mater

The cranial pia mater surrounds the brain so closely that it follows into the sulci and fissures. The spinal pia also closely encases the spinal cord and forms denticulate ligaments that help secure the spinal cord to the dura between spinal nerves as they exit. The pia extends around the filum terminale as it spans from the *conus medullaris* to the tip of the dural sac to further stabilize the spinal cord and dura. The pia continues to the perineurium of cranial and spinal nerves and attaches to the blood vessels as they enter and exit the CNS.

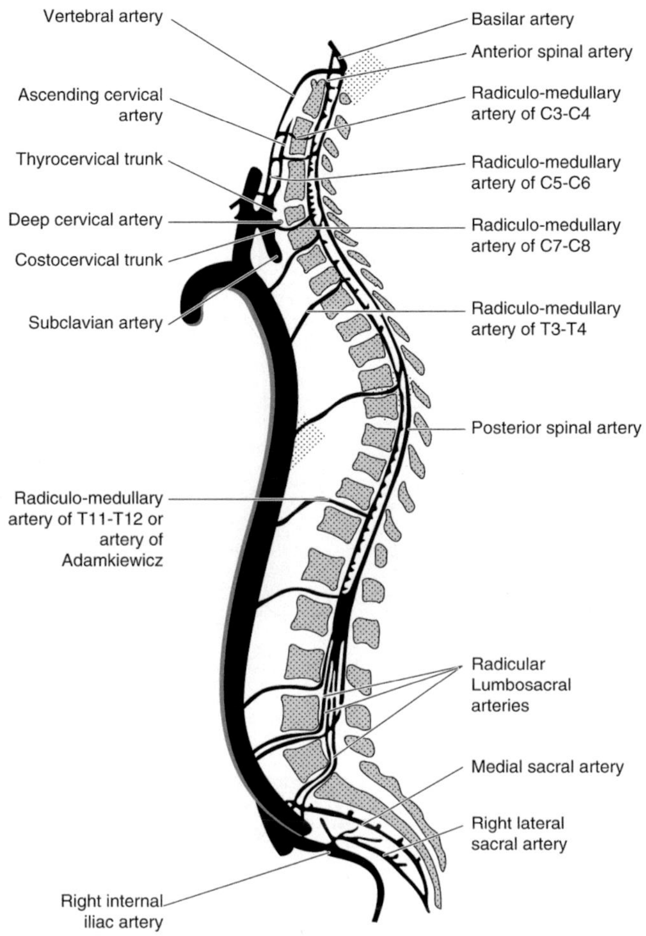

Fig. 3.10 Blood supply of spinal cord (Reprinted with permission from Brambrink et al. [7])

3.6 Anatomy of the Autonomic Nervous System

The autonomic nervous system (ANS) is broadly divided into the sympathetic and parasympathetic nervous systems. Managing the physiology of this system is key to the practice of anesthesiology. One may think of the sympathetic nervous system (SNS) as mediating fight-or-flight responses and the parasympathetic nervous system (PNS) as mediating rest-and-digest responses. The efferent components of both arms are characterized by preganglionic and postganglionic neurons activated by specific neurotransmitters.

3.6.1 The Sympathetic Nervous System

The sympathetic ANS is also known as the thoracolumbar system because its preganglionic cell bodies are found in the intermediolateral gray column from T1-L3. Myelinated axons from these neurons exit via the ventral root and briefly travel along the spinal nerve before exiting via the white communicating branch of the rami communicantes (◉ Fig. 3.11). The rami communicantes link the spinal nerves to the 22 paired ganglia of the sympathetic chain. Each preganglionic axon can take one of three possible routes from the white communicating ramus: (1) synapse in the sympathetic ganglion at that level, (2) travel caudad or cephalad within the sympathetic chain before synapsing at another ganglion in the chain, or (3) travel some distance in the chain before exiting it without synapsing. Those axons that leave the sympathetic chain without synapsing travel either to one of several large unpaired ganglia or go directly to the adrenal medulla.

The sympathetic chain ganglia, also known as paravertebral ganglia, lie anterolateral to the spinal cord. They contain postganglionic cell bodies with nicotinic acetylcholine receptors. Postganglionic axons are frequently unmyelinated and give rise to the gray communicating ramus when they rejoin the spinal nerves. Those axons that terminate at sweat glands release acetylcholine, while those traveling to the heart and blood vessels release norepinephrine. Most ganglia in the chain are unnamed, but the three cervical paravertebral ganglia are referred to as the superior, middle, and inferior cervical ganglia. In 80% of patients, the inferior cervical ganglia are fused with the first thoracic ganglia and termed the stellate or cervicothoracic ganglia. The stellate ganglion is sometimes the target for regional sympathetic nerve blockade to treat painful conditions of the ipsilateral head, neck, and arm.

Many preganglionic axons that leave the sympathetic chain without synapsing are destined for large, unpaired ganglia also known as prevertebral, preaortic, or collateral ganglia (◉ Fig. 3.12). These are named the celiac, superior mesenteric, aorticorenal, and inferior mesenteric ganglia. The postganglionic neurons are activated by acetylcholine via nicotinic receptors and release norepinephrine at their targets in the pelvic and abdominal organs. Other preganglionic axons travel from the sympathetic chain to the adrenal medulla. The chromaffin cells of the adrenal medulla are modified neuronal cells that function as postganglionic cells which release epinephrine and norepinephrine into the blood.

3.6.2 The Parasympathetic Nervous System

The parasympathetic ANS is also known as the craniosacral system because its preganglionic efferents arise from the brainstem and sacral spinal cord. It utilizes acetylcholine at both the preganglionic and postganglionic synapses. In contrast to the sympathetic ANS, many of the postganglionic neurons lie near their target organs and fewer appear as discrete ganglia on a gross anatomic level. The sacral portion

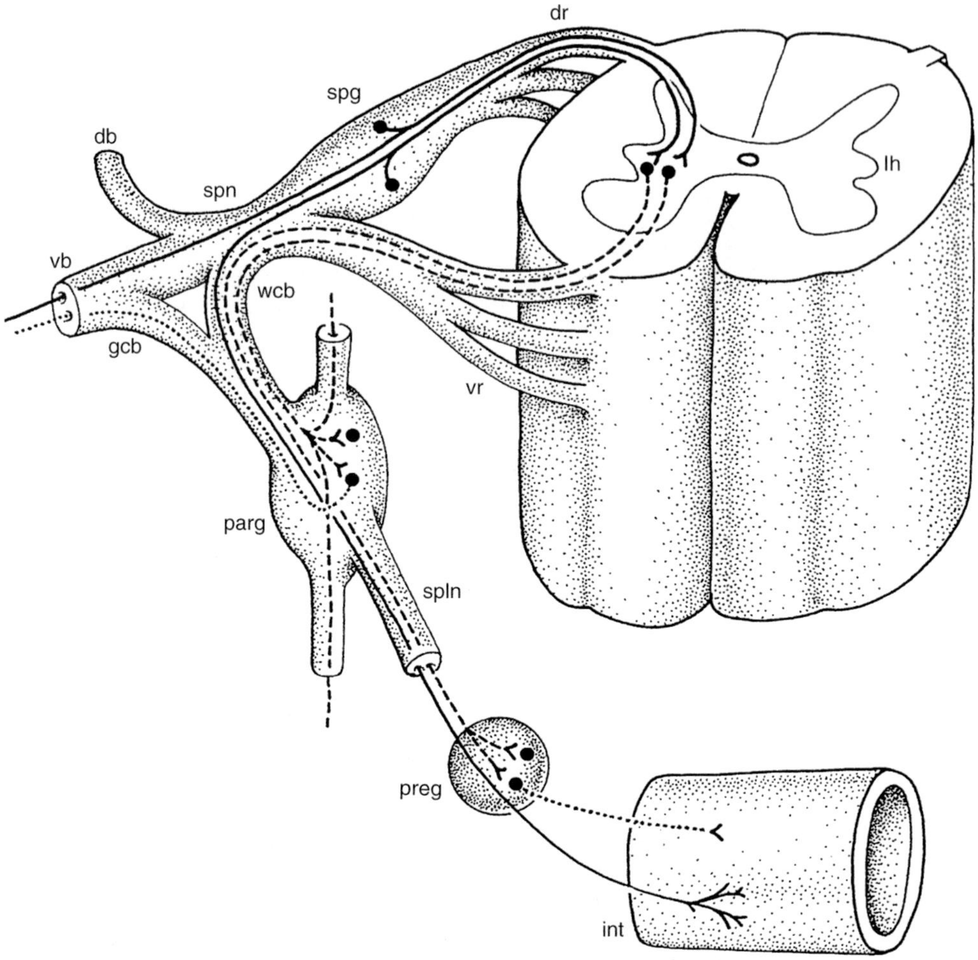

Fig. 3.11 Arrangement of preganglionic and postganglionic neurons of the sympathetic nervous system. Afferents are shown as solid lines and efferents as dotted lines. Preganglionic neurons are located in the intermediolateral gray column, which is shown here as the lateral horn (*lh*). After exiting the cord via the ventral root and spinal nerve the axons of these preganglionic neurons depart via the white ramus communicantes which is also known as the white communicating branch (*wcb*). They then either synapse in a paravertebral ganglion (*parg*), continue to an unpaired prevertebral ganglion (*preg*) via the thoracic splanchnic nerves (*spln*) or continue to the adrenal medulla. Postganglionic neurons in the paravertebral ganglion give rise to the gray communicating branch (*gcb*) as the rejoin the spinal nerve (*spn*) (Reprinted with permission from ten Donkelaar [2])

of the parasympathetic ANS arises from S2-S4 and innervates the distal colon and rectum as well as genitourinary structures via the pelvic splanchnic nerves. It works in concert with the sympathetic ANS to coordinate micturition and sexual responses. Somatic innervation to pelvic structures also arises from S2–4 and travels via the pudendal nerves.

The cranial portion of the parasympathetic ANS is associated with CN III, VII, IX, and X. Preganglionic efferents from the Edinger–Westphal nucleus travel via CN III to the ciliary ganglia where they synapse with neurons that innervate the sphincter pupillae and ciliary muscle. The other parasympathetic innervation of the eye travels via CN VII to synapse at the pterygopalatine ganglion before continuing to the lacrimal glands. The pterygopalatine ganglion is also known as the sphenopalatine ganglion, and it also sends fibers to mucous glands of the nose, mouth, and pharynx. Part of the digestion function of the parasympathetic ANS is promoted by the stimulation of saliva production via CN VII and IX. Facial nerve fibers synapse in the submandibular ganglion before postganglionic fibers continue to the submandibular and sublingual glands, while parasympathetic tracts in the glossopharyngeal nerve synapse in the otic ganglion *en route* to the parotid glands.

The vagus nerve (CN X) carries the most clinically significant components of the parasympathetic nervous system. It projects efferents to key structures and organs in the neck, chest, and abdomen down to the transverse colon. Although its preganglionic axons sometimes pass through sympathetic ganglia, they do not synapse in those structures. Rather they continue to synapse in or near the walls of their target organs.

3.6.3 Autonomic Control of Hemodynamics and Respiration

The vagus nerve carries parasympathetic outflow from the medulla to the heart and plays a critical role in cardiovascular homeostasis. The carotid sinus reflex is an important homeostatic mechanism that modulates blood pressure. As shown in ◉ Fig. 3.13, high pressure is detected by baroreceptors in the carotid sinus. This signal travels to the nucleus of the solitary tract via the glossopharyngeal nerve, and the

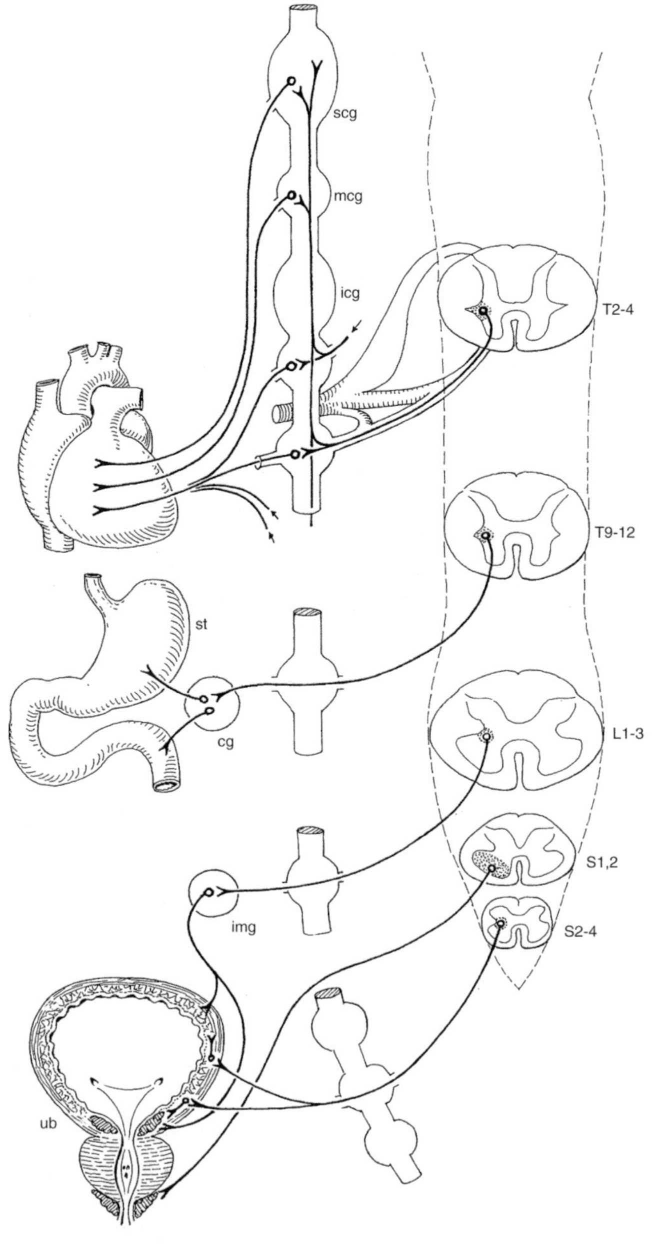

Fig. 3.12 Sympathetic and parasympathetic innervation of major organs. The heart receives sympathetic innervation from *upper* thoracic levels (T2-4) as well as from cervical ganglia (shown as *scg*, *mcg*, and *icg* for superior, middle and inferior cervical ganglia). Lower thoracic levels (T9-12) innervate the upper gut via the celiac ganglion (*cg*) whereas neurons in the lumbar region (L1-3) synapse in the inferior mesenteric ganglion (*img*). Parasympathetic innervation from sacral levels synapse with postganglionic neurons in the walls of organs, such as the urinary bladder (*ub*) (Reprinted with permission from ten Donkelaar [2])

efferent reflex limb decreases heart rate by increasing vagal parasympathetic tone. This reflex also leads to vasodilation and decreased cardiac contractility by inhibiting sympathetic outflow as part of a coordinated response to decrease blood pressure. Similar baroreceptors in the aortic arch send afferent reflex information via the vagus nerve itself. The vagus also forms the efferent arm of other bradycardic reflexes, such as the oculocardiac reflex. The vagus nerve may mediate both arms of the reflex in cases, such as laparoscopic insufflation or peritoneal stretch, though the afferent pathways of these reflexes are not well characterized.

Chemoreceptors located near the carotid bifurcation and aortic arch also play a role in regulating respiration. Activation of these receptors by increased pCO_2 or decreased pH leads to an increase in respiratory drive. Signals from the carotid bodies travel via CN IX, and those from the aortic bodies return to the brainstem via CN X.

3.7 Nociception

The process of nociception illustrates how the anatomic organization of the CNS provides for both localized and integrated responses to noxious stimuli. Receptors on free nerve endings of A-δ and unmyelinated C fibers are activated by heat, cold, extreme pressure, or other irritants. The response can be amplified by the release of substance P. The resulting action potentials travel to bipolar cell bodies located in the dorsal root ganglia. Axons from these bipolar neurons travel through the dorsal root to the dorsal horn. These signals trigger responses within the spinal cord and travel through ascending pathways to the brain. Within the cord, painful stimuli trigger a withdrawal reflex that helps protect the body from injury. This spinal reflex involves interneurons in the gray matter that form a bridge in the reflex arc between the sensory information entering the dorsal horn and motor neurons located in the ventral horn. For simplicity, such reflex arcs are often diagrammed as occurring within a single spinal level, but in reality, the signals travel short distances up and down to activate the muscle groups responsible for withdrawal of the affected limb. In cases, such as stepping on something sharp, these painful stimuli also trigger motor responses in the contralateral limb (crossed extensor reflex) and core muscle groups to facilitate shifting a person's weight onto the other leg. Pain signals reach the brain via the spinothalamic tract shown in ◉ Fig. 3.14. They also trigger responses of the autonomic nervous system.

Blocking the withdrawal reflex is a hallmark of anesthesia and represents the output of studies of minimum alveolar concentration (MAC) for volatile anesthetics. It is important to remember that these responses are independent of brain activity and can occur even when the patient is unconscious. Indeed, elegant studies by Antognini and Rampil revealed that general anesthetics act primarily in the spinal cord to produce immobility (reviewed by Antognini [8]). Therefore,

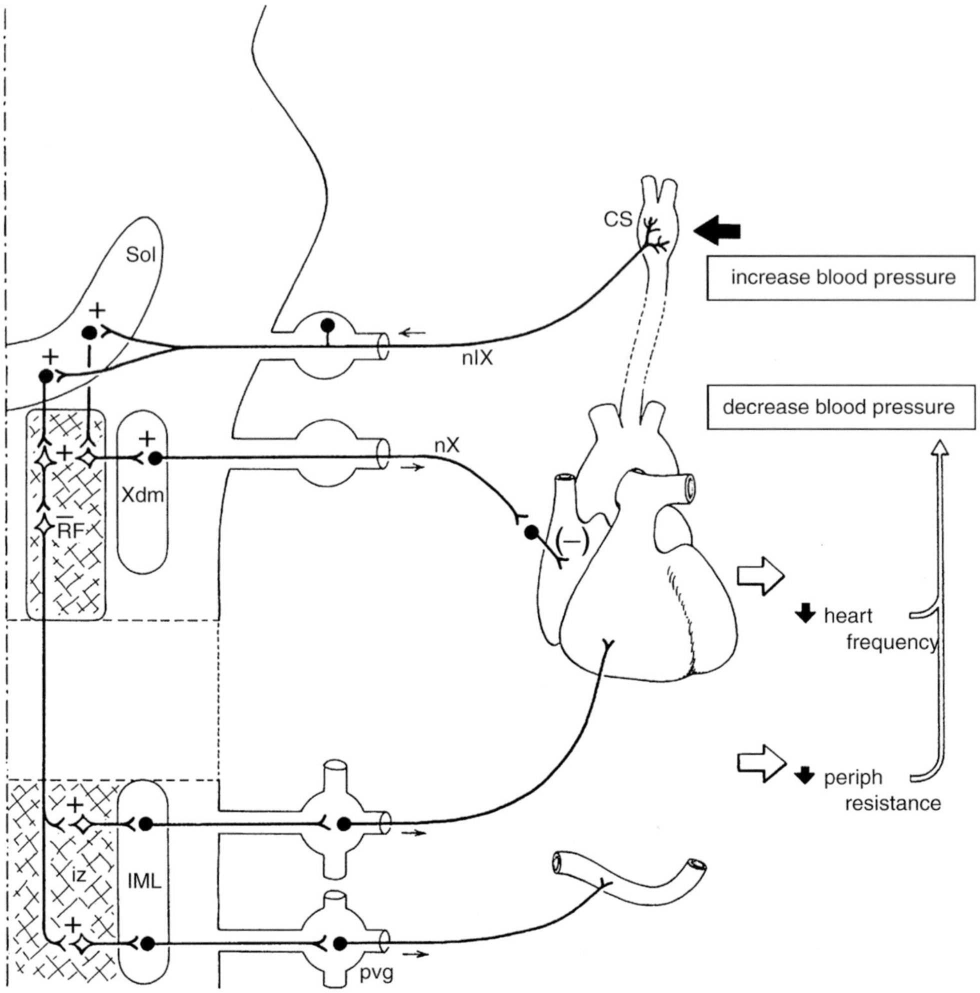

Fig. 3.13 Baroreceptor reflex. Stretch receptors in the carotid sinus (*CS*) transmit signals via afferents in the glossopharyngeal nerve (*nIX*) to the nucleus of the solitary tract (*Sol*). After traveling through the reticular formation (*RF*) the signal passes through the dorsal motor nucleus of the vagus (*Xdm*) and then the vagus nerve itself (*nX*) on the way to the nodal tissue of the heart. The sympathetic arm of the response travels to the paravertebral ganglia (*pvg*) via the intermediate zone of spinal gray matter (*iz*) and the intermediolateral nucleus (*IMZ*). Postganglionic nerves then continue on to the heart and blood vessels (Reprinted with permission from ten Donkelaar [2])

withdrawal response to surgical stimulation in an anesthetized patient does not indicate that the patient is "awake."

3.8 Implications for Intraoperative Neuromonitoring

Knowledge of brain and spinal cord anatomy is fundamental to the proper use of intraoperative neuromonitoring. One technique to monitor the integrity of the posterior columns of the spinal cord is somatosensory evoked potentials (SSEPs). Peripheral sensory nerves are stimulated with electrodes. The response to stimulation is then recorded over the somatosensory cortex and possibly the cervical spine. SSEPs monitor the integrity of the pathway that transmits vibration and proprioception, including the posterior columns of the spinal cord (labeled as fasciculus cuneatus and gracilis in ◉ Fig. 3.8).

The anterior portion of the spinal cord can be monitored with motor evoked potentials (MEPs). Stimulation over the motor cortex leads to activation of the corticospinal tract and a compound muscle action potential that is recorded in the periphery. In addition to utility in brain and spine surgery, MEPs may be used to detect ischemia during aortic procedures that may disrupt supply of the anterior spinal artery.

Evoked potentials also can be used to monitor specific cranial nerves. For example, brainstem auditory evoked potentials (BAEPs) travel along CN VIII to the brainstem and activate the cochlear nucleus, superior olivary complex, inferior colliculus, and auditory radiation. Visual evoked potentials (VEPs) are an analogous technique in which light stimuli are transmitted along CN II to the optic chiasm and eventually to the visual cortex where responses are measured over the occipital lobe.

Other cranial nerves can be monitored using electromyography (EMG) either by recording spontaneous or stimulated activity. For example, the facial nerve (CN VII) is commonly monitored during acoustic neuroma resection and other operations in the cerebellopontine angle as well as during parotid surgery. Specialized endotracheal tubes with electrodes that contact the vocal cords can be used to monitor the integrity of the recurrent laryngeal nerve during thyroid surgery.

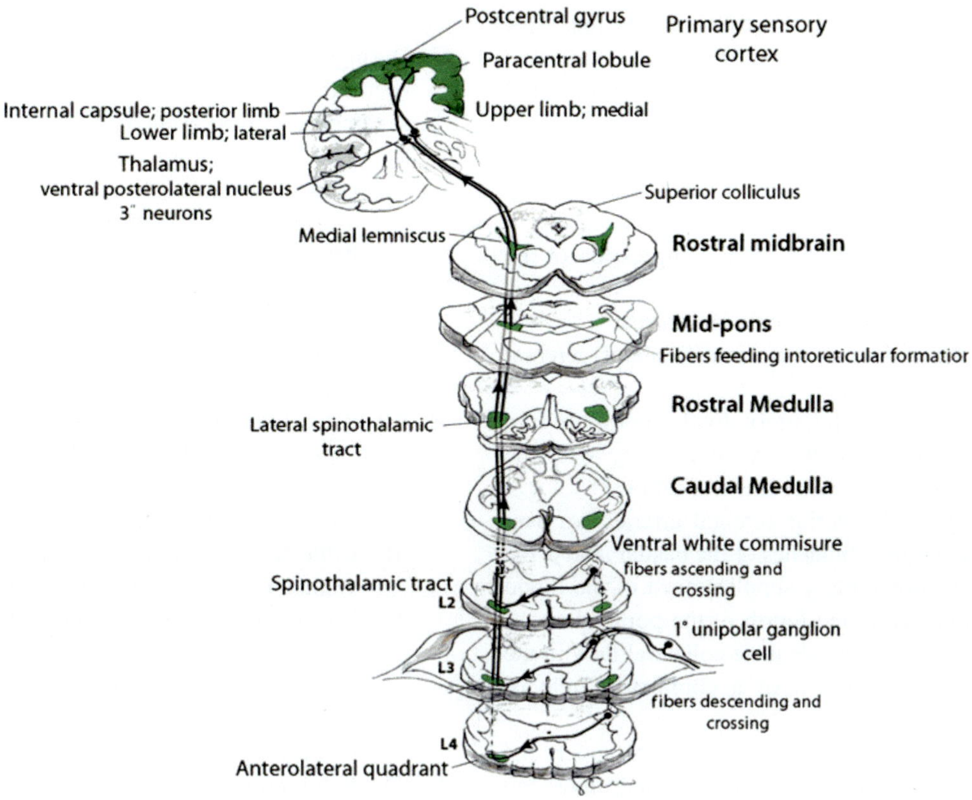

Fig. 3.14 Spinothalamic/anterolateral system for pain and temperature transmission. Note that incoming fibers may synapse at level of entry or travel up or down a few levels before synapsing (Reprinted with permission from Jacobson and Marcus [1])

3.9 Conclusion

Oliver Wendell Holmes famously suggested that the state Morton induced with ether be called anesthesia, meaning "without sensation." Just as the anatomy of the brain and spinal cord is central to the process of sensation, so too, is it central to the practice of anesthesiology. Advancing our knowledge of brain and spinal cord anatomy has led to improved surgical procedures, anesthetic techniques, intraoperative monitoring, and pain management. This has fostered dramatic increases in patient safety but there is more work ahead. As we learn more about brain and spinal cord anatomy, we may develop drugs and techniques that allow more specific and targeted anesthetics that further improve patient care and safety.

3.10 Questions and Answers

Questions (Choose the Most Appropriate Answer)

1. A patient presents to the angiography suite for removal of a thrombus in the proximal portion of her right middle cerebral artery. Which of the following symptoms is she **LEAST** likely to display?
   A. Paralysis of the left arm
   B. Symmetric wrinkling of the forehead
   C. Expressive aphasia
   D. Inability to recognize her left hand
2. Which of the following statement(s) is/are true regarding the brainstem?
   A. The brainstem houses critical parts that control cardiac, respiratory, sensory, and motor functions in a densely compact arrangement which can lead to clinically devastating deficits with very small lesions.
   B. The bilateral locus coeruleus nuclei have norepinephrine-containing neurons that connect to the cortex, hippocampus, thalamus, midbrain, pons, medulla, cerebellum, and spinal cord to regulate the sleep–wake cycle and arousal.
   C. The raphe nuclei lie from the middle of the pons extending into the medulla and its neurons also contain norepinephrine and modulate arousal, sleep–wake cycle, and pain sensory input.
   D. A and B
   E. A and C
3. An expanding cranial mass lesion is causing the medial aspect of the temporal lobe to herniate across

the tentorium. Which of the following is the most accurate statement about this process?

A. The ipsilateral pupil may be fixed and dilated because of compression of sympathetic fibers in cranial nerve III.

B. Compression of the posterior cerebral artery may cause visual field defects.

C. Motor weakness occurs from compression of the middle cerebral artery.

D. All of the above statements are correct.

4. Which of the following statement(s) about cerebral circulation is **NOT** true:

A. Each internal carotid artery divides unevenly into an anterior and middle cerebral artery with the latter receiving most of the blood flow.

B. Although the posterior cerebral arteries are usually the terminal branches of the basilar artery, the internal carotid artery supplies most of the blood to this vessel in one fourth of the population.

C. Most patients have adequate collateral flow in the brain because they have a complete Circle of Willis.

D. Cerebral venous drainage consists of superficial and deep veins that are thin-walled, have no valves or surrounding muscle, and empty into the dural venous sinuses.

E. All are true.

5. Which of the following scenarios, if any, is most likely to lead to cortical ischemia?

A. Left carotid occlusion in a patient with a hypoplastic anterior communicating artery

B. Proximal basilar artery occlusion in a patient with a hypoplastic left posterior communicating artery

C. A clip placed on the right anterior cerebral artery just distal to its origin in a patient with hypoplasia of both posterior communicating arteries

D. Anterograde perfusion of the right axillary artery when there is no flow through the left carotid or vertebral arteries during aortic arch surgery in a patient with hypoplasia of the anterior communicating and right posterior communicating artery

E. None of the above: Collateral flow should be adequate in all four cases.

6. You have just extubated a patient after emergency repair of an aortic dissection. The patient complains that he is unable to move his legs. Which of the following is **LEAST** likely to be noted on exam?

A. Decreased rectal tone

B. Intact biceps tendon reflex

C. Impaired vibratory sensation in the feet

D. Loss of pinprick sensation in the thigh

E. Absent patellar tendon reflexes

7. During placement of a carotid stent, the patient becomes abruptly bradycardic. Which of the following statements is most accurate regarding this response?

A. The efferent limb travels along the glossopharyngeal nerve.

B. The resulting increase in vagal tone decreases heart rate and contractility.

C. The nucleus of the solitary tract is a key relay point for the reflex.

D. It leads to increased release of acetylcholine and norepinephrine.

8. All of the following are true about epidural and subdural spaces **EXCEPT**:

A. Chronic subdural hematomas are common in children due to their delicate cerebral veins.

B. Little force is required to damage small bridging veins and cause a subdural hematoma.

C. The continuity of the epidural space from the sacrum to the cranial vault means that medications can be injected into the epidural space at one level to provide analgesia and anesthesia for a broad range of dermatomes.

D. Subdural injection of local anesthesia may lead to spinal cord damage as a result of direct toxicity or compressive effects.

E. Both the spinal epidural and subdural spaces are only potential spaces that are iatrogenically created.

9. Responses to stepping on a nail include all of the following **EXCEPT**:

A. Primary activation of a cell in the dorsal root ganglion without a prior synapse

B. A spinal reflex arc occurs that involves multiple spinal levels.

C. Ascending pain signals cross in the brainstem to activate the contralateral cortex.

D. It triggers responses of the opposite leg as well as core muscles in the trunk.

10. Which of the following is **NOT** true about cranial epidural hematomas?

A. The epidural space is created when significant force leads to high-pressure bleeding, which then causes separation of the periosteum and dura.

B. The majority of cases involve middle meningeal artery injury and the hematoma crosses cranial suture lines.

C. They commonly present with a lucid interval followed by gradual deterioration as intracranial pressure.

D. The only treatment for an epidural hematoma is emergent surgery for evacuation.
E. Seventy-five to ninety-five percent of epidural hematomas are associated with skull fractures.

Answers

1. **C**. The middle cerebral artery supplies two-thirds of the lateral surface of the brain and is a common site for ischemic strokes. Because motor and sensory pathways decussate (cross the midline), many symptoms are contralateral to the affected hemisphere. Common findings include contralateral sensory loss and weakness, but each side of the upper portion of the face has motor innervation from both hemispheres. For this reason, an upper motor neuron deficit in the face often spares the forehead. MCA ischemia of the language-dominant hemisphere may lead to aphasia. The left hemisphere is dominant for language in 99% of right-handed individuals and roughly 70% of left-handed individuals. It is therefore very unlikely the patient in question would have a language issue with a right-sided lesion. Not recognizing one's own hand is a type of hemineglect and is classically associated with right MCA stroke.
2. **D**. The brainstem is made up of the midbrain, pons, and medulla and is located just ventral to the cerebellum. It contains essential ascending and descending tract and nuclei that are involved with consciousness as well as cardiac, respiratory, sensory, and motor functions. In addition, the brainstem houses these critical parts in a densely compact arrangement that can lead to clinically devastating deficits with very small lesions.
   The bilateral locus ceruleus nuclei located here have norepinephrine containing neurons that connect to the cortex, hippocampus, thalamus, midbrain, pons, medulla, cerebellum, and spinal cord to regulate the sleep-wake cycle and arousal. The raphe nuclei lie from the middle of the pons extending into the medulla. Its neurons contain *serotonin* and modulate arousal, sleep-wake cycle, and pain sensory input by projecting to the cortex, hippocampus, basal ganglia, thalamus, cerebellum, and spinal cord.
3. **B**. Uncal herniation can be rapidly fatal unless the pressure is relieved. The medial portion of the temporal lobe is forced through the tentorium and puts pressure on the midbrain. The posterior cerebral artery may be compressed and cause homonymous hemianopia. Hemiplegia and sensory loss may result from compression of the crus cerebri of the midbrain, which contain key sensory and motor tracts. The course of the oculomotor nerve (CN III) places it at risk for compression and a "blown pupil" results when its *parasympathetic* fibers are injured.
4. **C**. Each internal carotid artery divides unevenly into an anterior and middle cerebral artery. The middle cerebral artery receives roughly 60–80% of blood delivered by the internal carotid artery. The vertebral arteries form the basilar artery between the medulla and pons and then the basilar artery quickly splits into the 2 posterior cerebral arteries at the upper border of the pons. Although the posterior cerebral arteries are usually the terminal branches of the basilar artery, they arise from the internal carotid artery during embryogenesis. In about 25% of individuals, this "fetal" supply is preserved and the majority of blood flow to the posterior cerebral artery comes from the internal carotid via the posterior communicating artery.
   The Circle of Willis is an anastomosis of the internal carotid and vertebrobasilar systems for both hemispheres that provides collateral flow in the event of arterial occlusion. The anterior communicating artery provides a collateral from one internal carotid to the other, and the posterior communicating arteries on each side link the carotids to the vertebrobasilar system. Less than half the population has a complete circle, but most have adequate collateral flow because having one of the two pathways is sufficient.
   Superficial and deep veins form a complex drainage system. The thin-walled veins have no valves or surrounding muscle. They traverse the arachnoid mater and eventually empty into the dural venous sinuses. Specifically, the superficial cerebral veins drain the cerebral cortex and underlying white matter into the superior sagittal sinus, cavernous sinus, and transverse sinus. The deep vertebral veins drain the corpus striatum, thalamus, and choroid plexuses into various larger veins that eventually form the great cerebral vein. The great cerebral vein unites with the inferior sagittal sinus and forms the straight sinus, which eventually empties into the transverse sinus.
5. **E**. The full Circle of Willis provides two routes for collateral flow but having just one of two pathways is generally sufficient to provide adequate collateral flow. All of the scenarios listed have one patent route for flow so the risk for ischemia should be low. In the case of the left carotid occlusion with a hypoplastic anterior communicating artery, the posterior communicating arteries provide a path for flow from the vertebrobasilar system or the right carotid. Similarly, for a proximal basilar occlusion with a hypoplastic left posterior communicating artery the left posterior cerebral artery should be able to fill from the right carotid via the right posterior communicating artery. A clip on the proximal portion of the anterior cerebral

artery should still allow perfusion from the opposite side via the anterior communicating artery.

Right axillary cannulation is a perfusion strategy for replacement of the aortic arch. Blood from the bypass machine enters the right axillary artery and can travel up the right carotid and vertebral arteries. Even if both the right posterior and anterior communicating arteries are hypoplastic, blood should be able to reach the left side of the brain by traveling from the right vertebral artery to the left vertebral artery and then on to the left MCA and ACA via the left posterior communicating artery.

6. **C**. The anterior spinal artery relies on radicular arteries to augment supply of blood to the thoracic and lumbar spine. The artery of Adamkiewicz is the largest anterior radicular artery and can be disrupted during aortic surgeries. This can lead to an anterior spinal artery syndrome that features ischemia of the anterior two-thirds to three-fourths of the spinal cord from the thoracic region and below (thus sparing the arms in this scenario). Disruption of the spinothalamic tract would decrease pinprick sensation and the descending motor pathways are frequently compromised. Vibratory sensation is likely to be intact because the posterior columns are usually supplied by the posterior spinal arteries.
7. **C**. Treatment of carotid stenosis may trigger the baroreceptor reflex whether the approach is open or endovascular. The *afferent* limb of the reflex travels via the glossopharyngeal nerve to the nucleus of the solitary tract. The efferent responses are mediated by the vagus nerve and sympathetic nervous system. Heart rate decreases through increased acetylcholine release by vagal terminals in the sinoatrial node, whereas contractility decreases via inhibition of the *sympathetic* innervation of the ventricles. Decreased catecholamine release from this sympathetic inhibition also triggers vasodilation and may contribute to hypotension.
8. **A**. Small bridging vein injury can lead to a subdural hematoma with less force than that required to cause an epidural bleed in the brain. Acute subdural hematomas are most commonly found in children, whereas chronic subdural hematomas are more common in older people whose bridging veins have already become fragile and stretched due to brain shrinkage. Subacute subdural hematomas can occur after injury in any age group and signs and symptoms of increased intracranial pressure develops up to three weeks post-injury due to slower blood accumulation.

   The spinal epidural space contains connective tissue, fat, a venous plexus, small arterial branches, and lymphatics. Contrast media has shown that fluid injected into the epidural space at the sacral level will spread up to the cranial base. As a result, medications can be injected into the epidural space at one level to provide analgesia and anesthesia for a broad range of dermatomes. Although the spinal subdural space does not normally exist due to the close apposition of the dura and arachnoid, it is a potential space that has been inadvertently accessed during attempts at epidural catheter placement. Subdural injection may lead to spinal cord damage as a result of direct toxicity or compressive effects.
9. **C**. The afferent limb of a spinal reflex involves primary activation of bipolar neurons whose cell bodies reside in the dorsal root ganglion. This triggers a coordinated response to a painful stimulus. Withdrawal of the limb in question often requires that the reflex pathway travels to different spinal levels to activate the appropriate motor neurons. In the case of stepping on something sharp, weight is shifted away from the affected leg by activating core muscles and extensor muscles in the contralateral leg (crossed extensor response). In contrast to the posterior column system, which decussates in the brainstem, pain signals traveling through the spinothalamic tract cross in the spinal cord itself. This difference leads to characteristic pattern of deficits if one half of the spinal cord is damaged (Brown-Séquard syndrome): paralysis and loss of proprioception of the ipsilateral limb below the lesion with loss of pain and temperature sensation contralateral to the lesion.
10. **B**. The epidural space is created when significant force leads to high-pressure bleeding, which then causes separation of the periosteum and dura. The majority of cases involve middle meningeal artery injury and 75–95% are associated with skull fracture. A lucid interval followed by gradual deterioration as intracranial pressure increases is the classic presentation. An epidural hematoma does not cross cranial suture lines because the dura is tightly attached to the skull at the suture lines. The only treatment for an epidural hematoma is emergent surgery for evacuation.

References

1. Jacobson S, Marcus EM. Neuroanatomy for the neuroscientist. Boston: Springer; 2011. Available from: MyiLibrary http://www.myilibrary.com?id=346989 or SpringerLink. https://doi.org/10.1007/978-1-4419-9653-4
2. ten Donkelaar HJ. Clinical neuroanatomy: brain circuitry and its disorders. Heidelberg/New York: Springer; 2011.

3. Tarulli A. Neurology: a clinician's approach. Cham: Springer International Publishing; 2016. Available from: http://sfx.ethz.ch/sfx_locater?sid=ALEPH:EBI01&genre=book&isbn=9783319296326. Online via SFX.
4. Saifuddin A, Burnett SJ, White J. The variation of position of the conus medullaris in an adult population. A magnetic resonance imaging study. Spine (Phila Pa 1976). 1998;23(13):1452–6.
5. Patel VV, Patel A, Harrop JS, Burger E. Spine surgery basics. 1st ed. Berlin: Springer, Berlin; 2013.
6. Bornstein PE, Peterson RR. Numerical variation of the presacral vertebral column in three population groups in North America. Am J Phys Anthropol. 1966;25(2):139–46.
7. Brambrink A, Kirsch JR. Essentials of neurosurgical anesthesia & critical care : strategies for prevention, early detection, and successful management of perioperative complications. New York: Springer; 2012.
8. Antognini JF, Carstens E. In vivo characterization of clinical anaesthesia and its components. Br J Anaesth. 2002;89(1):156–66.

Anatomy of the Airway/Airway Management

4

Sekar S. Bhavani and Basem Abdelmalak

Abstract

This chapter reviews upper airway anatomy and airway management. One of the most challenging aspects in clinical anesthesia is the consistent identification of patients in whom airways are likely to be challenging to secure for failure to do so can result in a wide spectrum of complications including injury to the upper or lower airway, larynx or at worst, hypoxia, hypercapnia, neurological injury that can potentially lead to neurological injury or even death. The act of securing the airway involves multiple steps, viz.: initial airway assessment, patient positioning for optimization of visualization of the upper airway and vocal cords, face mask ventilation, placement of an upper airway device or an advanced airway to secure the airway and finally extubation or removal of the airway device safely. A failure to accomplish any one of these steps would constitute a "difficult airway" scenario.

Keywords

Airway anatomy • Airway management • Anatomical landmarks • Inspiration • Expiration • Difficult airway • Intubation • Muscle relaxants • Drug selection • Blocks • Upper airway anesthesia • Sedation • Bronchoscopy • Endotracheal tube • Combitube • Surgical airway

S. S. Bhavani · B. Abdelmalak (✉)
Cleveland Clinic, Cleveland Clinic Lerner College of Medicine Anesthesiology Institute, Cleveland, OH, USA
e-mail: abdelmb@ccf.org

S. S. Bhavani
e-mail: bhavans@ccf.org

B. Abdelmalak
Departments of General Anesthesiology and Outcomes Research, Cleveland Clinic, Anesthesia for Bronchoscopic Surgery and Center for Procedural Sedation, Cleveland, OH, USA

M. Argalious et al. (eds.), *Basic Sciences in Anesthesia*,
https://doi.org/10.1007/978-3-031-60203-0_4

Key Points

1. The airway starts at the nares and extends down to the alveoli and they all contribute to the physiology and the difficulties that one might face during airway management.
2. The nose serves multiple functions including olfactory, humidification, filtration, and phonation in addition to being a pathway to respiration.
3. The larynx has 3 paired and 3 unpaired cartilages and its position in relation to the cervical spine varies in adults and children.
4. The extrinsic muscles of the larynx act as elevators and depressors of the larynx.
5. The epiglottis serves the function of protecting the airway and preventing aspiration and its shape and size determines the type of laryngoscopy blade one might need to use in order to visualize the vocal cords.
6. The larynx is supplied by the superior and recurrent laryngeal nerves and the function and position of the vocal cords is affected by its integrity.
7. The cricothyroid membrane, which can often be easily identified, serves as an entry point for emergent access to the airway below the vocal cords.
8. The upper airway is intimately associated with major vascular and nerves in the neck and may be involved in a pathology that arises from these structures.
9. Inspiration is an active process. Normal exhalation is predominantly a passive process. The diaphragm contributes almost 70% to a normal tidal volume.
10. The intercostal and accessory muscles come into play during forced inspiration and expiration.
11. There is no single test that would consistently identify patients at a high risk for difficulties in securing their airway.
12. Multiple scoring techniques have been suggested that might facilitate identifying patients at a risk.
13. Use of muscle relaxants might facilitate ventilation in patients with a difficult mask ventilation.

14. There are an increasing number of techniques and devices that are available to facilitate visualization and control of the airway and one must invest the time and learn the skills involved.
15. Asleep and awake intubation using a flexible intubating scope (fiberoptic) is an underused tool due to lack of experience, unfamiliarity with the technique, and presumed patient dissatisfaction.
16. Mastering of the techniques of airway topicalization techniques and use of adjunct medications will facilitate an awake intubation (with a flexible bronchoscope or other devices) and increase its success rate.
17. Bronchial blockers and double lumen tubes offer the opportunity to isolate the lungs and can be lifesaving in some instances.

4.1 Part 1: Anatomy

4.1.1 Topographical Anatomy as Landmarks

4.1.1.1 Nose

The airway functionally begins at the nares and the mouth, where air first enters the body. Breathing preferentially occurs through the nose in the newborns. The nose and the nasal passages provide the least resistance to inspiration in children because:

- The oral cavity in the child is smaller.
- The muscles are less mature.
- The tongue is proportionately larger and closer to the soft palate compared to adults.

The differences become less significant as the child grows older. In an adult, resistance to airflow through the nasal passages is twice the resistance through the mouth. Therefore, during exercise or respiratory distress, mouth breathing occurs to facilitate a reduction in airway resistance and increased airflow.

The nose serves a number of functions:

- Respiration,
- Olfaction,
- Humidification and filtration of inspired air,
- Phonation.

The nasal cavity extends from the nostrils to the nasopharynx. It measures about 10–14 cm back to front in an adult and is separated into 2 passages by the nasal septum.

The nasal septum is composed of both a bony and a cartilaginous component and is the main support for the external nose. It is not uncommon to find that it is deviated to one side to produce two unequal passages. It has a rich blood supply, is highly convoluted, and provides a large surface area for humidifying and warming the inspired air.

Superiorly, it is bound by the cribriform plate that separates the nasal cavity from the anterior cranial fossa. Disrupted of this, due to facial trauma, can result in direct communication with the anterior cranial fossa and CSF leak if the dura is also damaged. A misdirected nasogastric tube, nasal airways, or nasotracheal tubes can also be accidently introduced into the subarachnoid space in trauma patients if care is not taken.

Laterally, the nasal fossa is bound by 3 turbinates: the superior, middle, and inferior. The paired paranasal sinuses—frontal, ethmoidal, sphenoidal, and maxillary—drain through apertures into the lateral wall of the nose. Prolonged nasotracheal intubation, particularly in children, may lead to infection of the ipsilateral maxillary sinus due to obstruction to the sinus drainage.

The nasal cavity derives its blood supply from a rich plexus of arteries including the ethmoid branches of the ophthalmic artery, the sphenopalatine and greater palatine branches of the maxillary artery, and the superior labial and lateral nasal branches of the facial artery. These arteries all communicate anteriorly at the "Little's area"—the site commonly involved in epistaxis.

The nasal cavity has both autonomic and sensory innervation. The autonomic nervous system is involved through a complex reflex mechanisms in the regulation of the blood flow, congestion, and secretions from the nasal passages. This allows the nasal passages to shrink and swell quickly in response to certain inciting events. The olfactory area is located in the upper third of the nasal cavity and is innervated by the olfactory nerve. The rest of the nasal cavity is supplied by the first 2 divisions of the trigeminal nerve. Trigeminal nerve fibers are involved in transmitting sensations of pain, temperature, and touch, and pass through the sphenopalatine ganglion to the midbrain.

4.1.1.2 The Pharynx

The pharynx extends from the base of the skull superiorly to the level of the cricoid cartilage antero-inferiorly and the inferior border of the sixth cervical vertebra postero-inferiorly (◉ Fig. 4.1). It measures about 12–15 cm in length in an adult. It is divided into 3 subdivisions—the nasopharynx, the oropharynx, and the laryngopharynx (hypopharynx):

- The nasopharynx starts at the termination of the turbinates and nasal septum and extends down to the soft

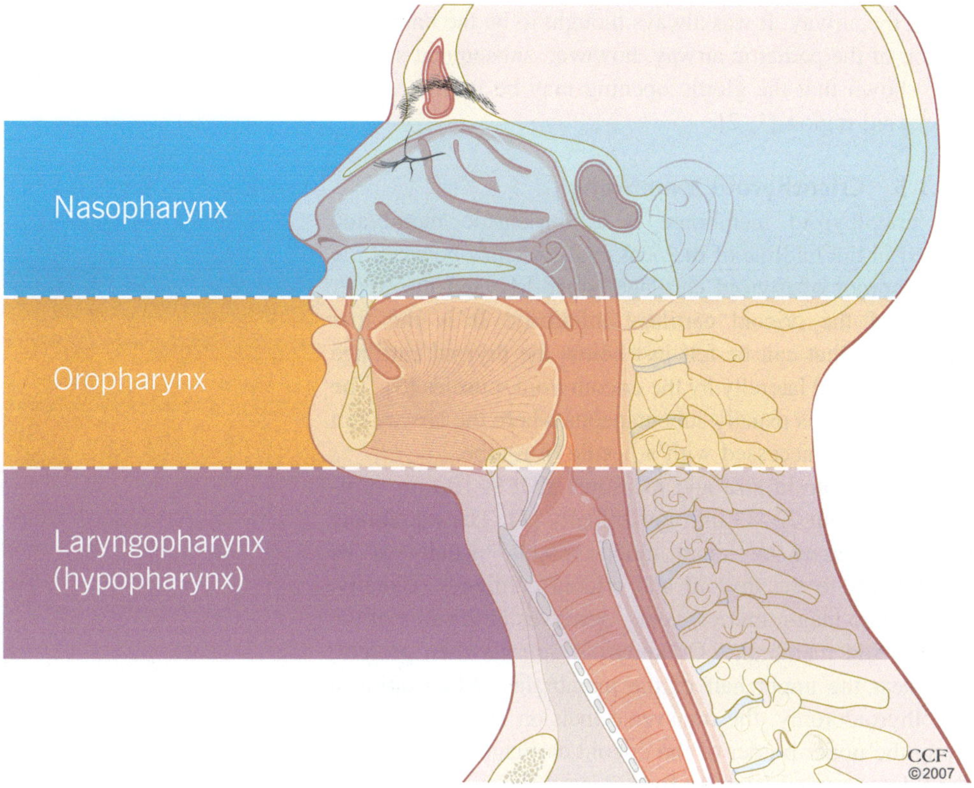

Fig. 4.1 The 3 subdivisions of the pharynx (Reprinted with permission, Cleveland Clinic Center for Medical Art and Photography © 2007–2017. All Rights Reserved)

palate. It is innervated by the pharyngeal branch of the trigeminal nerve-V2.

- The oropharynx starts below the soft palate and extends inferiorly to the superior edge of the epiglottis. It is innervated by Cranial Nerve IX.
- The laryngopharynx starts at the superior border of the epiglottis and extends inferiorly to the inferior border of the cricoid cartilage, where it becomes continuous with the esophagus. It is innervated by Cranial Nerve X.

4.1.1.3 Epiglottis

The epiglottis is composed of fibroelastic cartilage and maintains some flexibility throughout life. Its shape and flexibility changes with age but it never calcifies. It prevents the entry of food into the airway during swallowing. It is attached to the thyroid and hyoid cartilages by the thyroepiglottic and the hyoepiglottic ligaments.

The angle between the base of the tongue and the epiglottis is called the vallecula. The tip of the Macintosh blade placed in this angle can help push the tongue and the surrounding soft tissue anteriorly and pull up the epiglottis, bringing the vocal cords into view during direct laryngoscopy (DL).

4.1.1.4 Larynx

The larynx is formed by 3 unpaired—the thyroid, cricoid, and epiglottis—and 3 paired— the arytenoids, corniculates, and cuneiforms cartilages. They normally lie opposite C3–C5 in adults. The thyroid, arytenoids, and cricoid cartilages contain hyaline and ossify with advanced age. They are connected to each other by ligaments, muscles, and membranes.

The thyroid cartilage is formed by 2 laminae, which fuse anteriorly in the midline of the neck, forming a protuberance. The shape of the thyroid cartilage differs in males and females. The more acute angle of fusion between the 2 sides in some males results in the prominent "Adam's apple."

Superiorly, the inlet is formed by the upper edge of the epiglottis, a fold of mucous membrane stretched between the 2 arytenoid cartilages, and aryepiglottic folds.

For simplicity, the anatomical space around the larynx is divided into 3 spaces—the supraglottic, glottic, and subglottic spaces:

- The supraglottic space extends from the inlet of the larynx to the lower margin of the false vocal cords.
- The glottis is formed by the true vocal folds and the space between the vocal cords.
- The subglottic space extends below the glottis to the first tracheal ring.

Cricoid Cartilage

The cricoid cartilage supports the lower limit of the larynx. It is shaped like a ring. It is the only complete cartilaginous ring in the airway. It was always thought to be the narrowest portion of the pediatric airway, however, subsequent studies have shown that the glottic opening may be narrower than the cricoid region [1, 2].

4.1.1.5 Cricothyroid Membrane

The cricothyroid membrane is a fibroelastic membrane located in the midline of the neck that stretches between the lower border of thyroid cartilage superiorly and the upper border of the cricoid cartilage inferiorly. It is the first indentation that can be felt just below the thyroid cartilage and is bordered laterally by the cricothyroid muscles [3]. The central portion is usually subcutaneous where the airway can be emergently accessed with a needle or a tube.

It is variable in size and measures abut 9–10 mm vertically and about 22–33 mm horizontally [3]. The membrane may be pierced by small blood vessels, usually at its attachments to the thyroid and cricoid cartilages. Usually, there are no major arteries, veins, or nerves in the area of the cricothyroid membrane. Cricothyroid artery, when present, runs near the upper half of the membrane. When doing a cricothyroidotomy, the transverse incision should be made along the upper border of the cricoid cartilage. The incision should not extend laterally for > 1 cm [3].

Though it is well described, it may be difficult to identify, especially in female and/or obese patients [4, 5]. When the surface identification is challenging, an ultrasound may prove to be a valuable bedside tool in identifying this structure in an emergency [6, 7].

Muscles of the Larynx

The muscles of the larynx are divided into extrinsic and intrinsic muscles (◉ Fig. 4.2). The extrinsic muscles act as elevators or depressors of the larynx.

The extrinsic muscles are divided into suprahyoid and infrahyoid muscle groups. The suprahyoid muscles attach the larynx to the hyoid bone and serve as elevators of the larynx. They include:

- Thyrohyoid,
- Stylohyoid,
- Mylohyoid,
- Geniohyoid,
- Digastric,
- Stylopharyngeus,
- Palatopharyngeus.

The infrahyoid group acts as depressors of the larynx and includes:

- Omohyoid,
- Sternohyoid,

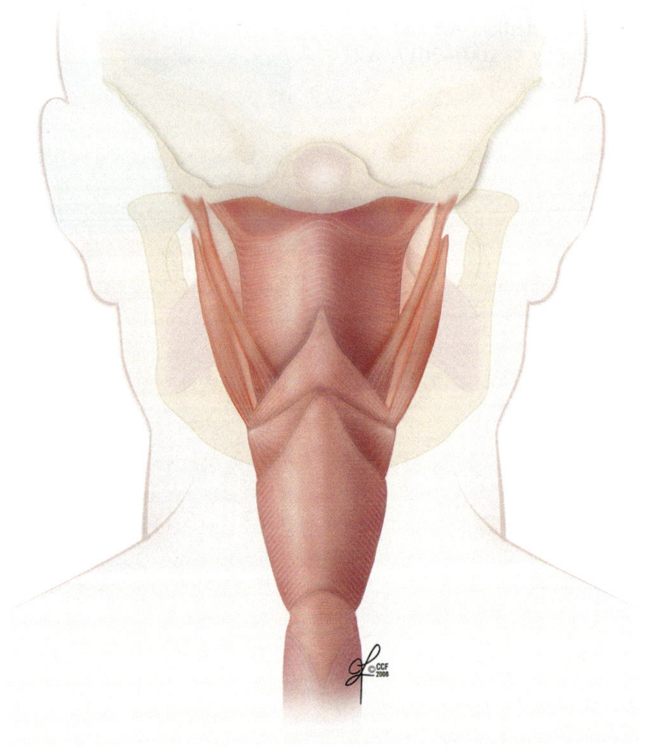

Fig. 4.2 Muscles of the larynx (Reprinted with permission, Cleveland Clinic Center for Medical Art & Photography © 2007–2017. All Rights Reserved)

- Sternothyroid.

The intrinsic muscles of the larynx are involved in phonation and protection of the airway during deglutition. They bring this about by opening the airway (abductors), closing the airway (adductors) or by changing the tension (tensors). The intrinsic muscles of the larynx include the:

- Posterior cricoarytenoid,
- Lateral cricoarytenoid,
- Arytenoids (transverse and oblique),
- Thyroarytenoid,
- Cricothyroid.

All the intrinsic laryngeal muscles, except the cricothyroid muscle, are supplied by the recurrent laryngeal nerve. The latter is supplied by the external branch of the superior laryngeal nerve.

Laryngeal Competence

The laryngeal inlet can be closed at 3 levels (◉ Fig. 4.3):

- At the level of the aryepiglottic folds—by aryepiglottic and oblique arytenoid muscles.

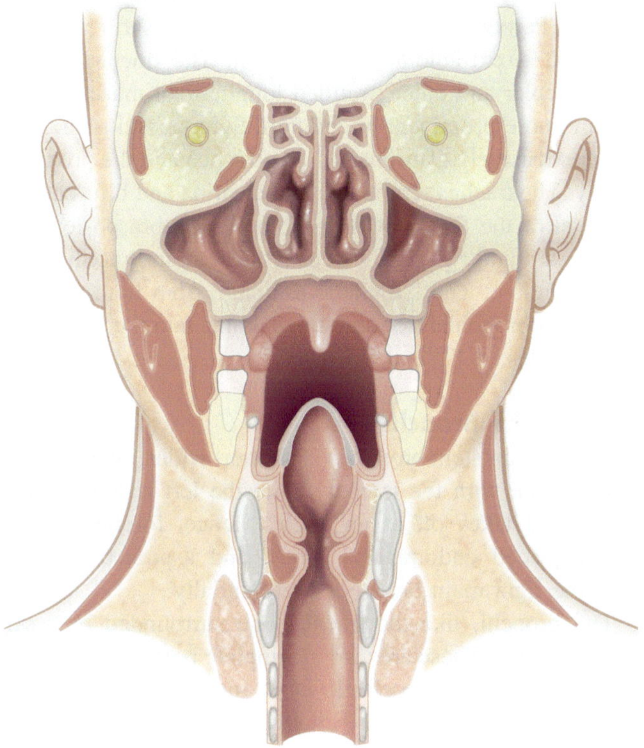

Fig. 4.3 Anatomy of the upper respiratory tract (Reprinted with permission, Cleveland Clinic Center for Medical Art & Photography © 2007–2017. All Rights Reserved)

- At the level of the false vocal cords—by lateral thyroarytenoids.
- At the level of true vocal cords—by interarytenoids, the lateral cricoarytenoids, and the cricothyroid.

During laryngeal spasm, both true and false vocal cords lie tightly in the midline opposite each other.

Blood Supply of the Larynx

Blood supply to the larynx is derived from the superior and inferior laryngeal arteries on each side. The former is derived from the superior thyroid artery, which originates from the external carotid artery. The superior laryngeal artery supplies the tissues from the epiglottis down to the vocal cords. The inferior thyroid artery ascends with the recurrent laryngeal nerve from its origin with the thyrocervical trunk and enters the larynx at the lower border of the inferior constrictor and supplies the laryngeal muscles and mucosa. The inferior laryngeal artery supplies the region around the cricothyroid. These 2 branches communicate extensively with each other and with those of the contralateral side.

Venous return from the larynx parallels the arteries. The superior and inferior laryngeal veins drain into the superior and inferior thyroid veins, respectively. The superior thyroid vein drains into the internal jugular vein and the inferior thyroid vein usually drains into the left brachiocephalic vein.

Innervation of the Larynx

The larynx is supplied by the paired recurrent laryngeal nerves and the internal and external branches of the superior laryngeal nerves. The superior laryngeal and recurrent laryngeal nerves are branches of the vagus nerve.

All the intrinsic muscles of the larynx, except the cricothyroid muscle, are supplied by the recurrent laryngeal nerve. The cricothyroid muscle derives its motor innervation from the external branch of the superior laryngeal nerve.

- **Superior Laryngeal Nerve**: The superior laryngeal nerve exits the cranium just outside of the jugular foramen. At the level of the hyoid bone, it divides into an external and an internal branch. The external branch accompanies the superior thyroid artery to the cricothyroid muscle, giving off a branch to the inferior constrictor of the pharynx along the way. The internal branch pierces the thyrohyoid membrane laterally between the thyroid cartilage and greater cornu of the hyoid bone. The nerve provides sensory innervation from the back of the base of the tongue to the level of the vocal cords.
- **Recurrent Laryngeal Nerve**: The left recurrent laryngeal nerve branches out of the vagus nerve in the thorax and courses cephalad after looping around the arch of the aorta. On the right, the nerve loops beneath the subclavian artery and then follows a cephalad course to the larynx. Both nerves lie in the tracheoesophageal groove before they reach the larynx. The recurrent laryngeal nerve supplies all the intrinsic muscles of the larynx except the cricothyroid. It also provides sensory innervation to the larynx below the vocal cords.

The recurrent laryngeal nerve may be injured by trauma or during surgery in the head and neck and upper chest. It can also be affected by pressure from an endotracheal tube (ETT) or a supraglottic airway (SGA). The left recurrent laryngeal nerve may be involved by tumors in the chest or aneurysm of the aortic arch.

4.1.1.6 Vocal Cords, Positions with Paralysis

Normally, the vocal cords meet in the midline during phonation but move apart with inspiration. Injury to the adductors of the vocal cords (recurrent laryngeal nerves) results in failure for the vocal cords to return to the midline with expiration, resulting in a small gap between the edges. The left nerve is likely to be paralyzed twice as frequently as the right side. This is in part due to its proximity to the intrathoracic structures during its course from the neck into the chest before it loops back around the left subclavian artery.

Superior Laryngeal Nerve

The superior laryngeal nerve innervates the tensor of the vocal cord and its damage can lead to change in voice. The hoarseness might improve with time due to compensation from the other side. When there is unilateral injury, on endoscopy, the cords may appear wavy.

With total bilateral paralysis of the superior laryngeal nerves, the vocal cords are relaxed, abducted, and appear wavy (cadaveric position). On administration of muscle relaxants, a similar picture may be seen.

Recurrent Laryngeal Nerve

The recurrent laryngeal nerves supply both the adductors and the abductors of the vocal cords. The abductor fibers are more vulnerable to damage as compared to the adductors. It is thus possible to have pure abductor palsy or both adductor and abductor palsy.

Unilateral Vocal Cord Paralysis

In the case of unilateral abductor palsy, the cords will continue to meet in the midline on phonation; however, during inspiration only the normal cord will move away from the midline. In the case of complete unilateral palsy, however, the unaffected cord will try and compensate and will cross the midline to meet its paralyzed counterpart. On inspiration, the unaffected cord will move to full abduction. Thus, there will be no respiratory distress.

Bilateral Vocal Cord Paralysis

Bilateral vocal cord paralysis can be complete or incomplete. When there is a complete paralysis of both adductors and abductors, the vocal cords tend to be midway between abduction and adduction and a reasonable opening exists for breathing. However, when there is an incomplete paralysis, the adductors will tend to draw the vocal cords together and thus produce severe respiratory distress. Thus, incomplete paralysis is more dangerous than complete bilateral recurrent nerve paralysis.

4.1.1.7 Trachea

Structure of the Trachea in Neck and Chest

The trachea begins at the cricoid cartilage (at the level of C5–6) and ends at the bifurcation of the trachea into the left and right main bronchi (level of T5 posteriorly, Angle of Louis anteriorly). It is made up of 16–20 incomplete horseshoe-shaped cartilaginous rings whose posterior edges are connected by membrane and fibroelastic tissue. There is some variation in the size and shape of the tracheal rings, but they usually measure about 4 mm in width and 1 mm in thickness. They tend to calcify and lose their compliance with age resulting in less tolerance to blunt trauma.

The trachea is 10–20 cm long and 12 mm in diameter in an adult. Part of it is intrathoracic (beyond the sixth ring) and part of it is extrathoracic in location. The trachea has an inner circular and outer stratified longitudinal muscle layers that are more prominent in children. Submucosal glands are found extensively distributed in the trachea and the proximal airway. The trachea terminates in the carina and bifurcates at the level of the fourth or fifth thoracic vertebra posteriorly, into the left and right main stem bronchi slightly to the right of the midline. The lymphatic drainage from both sides of the tracheobronchial tree and lungs drains into the subcarinal lymph nodes.

4.1.1.8 The Bronchi

The right main stem bronchus is shorter, wider, and takes off more in line with the trachea while the left is longer, narrower, and takes off at an angle. Hence, foreign bodies, deeply placed endotracheal tubes, and aspirated material enter the right main bronchus preferentially.

The bronchi, like the trachea, are surrounded by cartilaginous rings. These are also incomplete posteriorly and are connected by a fibroelastic and muscular tissue. This incomplete ring architecture allows for change in the size of the airway with the respiratory cycle. Identification of the membrane facilitates orientation and identification of the trachea and the bronchi during flexible (fiberoptic) bronchoscopy. The rings become discrete plates once they enter the substance of the lung. The right main stem bronchus gives rise to 3 lobar bronchi, and the left gives rise to 2. Both the main bronchi and the lower lobe bronchi are situated outside the lung substance. These then divide to give rise to the bronchopulmonary segments that supply the respective lobules. Airways become smaller as they divide inside the lungs and the cartilaginous plates disappear when the airway diameter becomes less than 0.6 mm. Although the diameter of each new division of the airway decreases progressively, the aggregate cross-sectional area increases, thus increasing the overall area available for air exchange.

The airway smooth muscles are supplied by the autonomic nervous system. They are stimulated by the vagus nerve and inhibited by sympathetic innervation from the upper thoracic ganglia. They maintain the bronchomotor tone. Though the muscles progressively decrease in thickness, their ratio to the bronchial wall increases with each division. Hence, the small bronchioles can be effectively cut off during bronchospasm. They also play a protective role in closure of non-perfused portions of the lung when a ventilation-perfusion mismatch occurs.

4.1.1.9 Airway Anatomical Relationships in the Neck and Chest

The upper part of the trachea is covered by the thyroid gland and its isthmus. The recurrent laryngeal nerves usually run in the tracheoesophageal groove. The left nerve tends to run its entire course along the tracheoesophageal groove after its origin below the aortic arch. The right nerve loops around the right subclavian artery and courses medially to lie in the tracheoesophageal groove. Both of these nerves are in close proximity to the inferior thyroid artery branches.

The esophagus is usually directly posterior to the trachea but in some instances may lie partially to the left of the trachea. The anterior wall of the esophagus with the membranous segment of the trachea may be connected by loose connective tissue. The brachiocephalic artery lies in front of and in close apposition to the trachea. The aortic arch wraps around the lower part of the trachea on the left side and the left main bronchus courses under the arch.

The trachea and the esophagus are enveloped by the deep layer of the deep cervical fascia. This facial layer fused with the pericardium and visceral pleura. This fusion allows infections to descend from the neck and the air to ascend to the neck producing subcutaneous emphysema from tracheobronchial tree or lung disruptions. There are no arteries traversing this plane and this facilitates entry into the mediastinum from the neck for mediastinoscopy.

4.1.2 Muscles of Respiration, Accessory Muscles

Respiration involves the act of inspiration and expiration. Inspiration is an active process. Normal exhalation is predominantly a passive process, associated with little to no muscle contraction and is primarily driven by the elastic recoil of the thoracic wall.

4.1.2.1 Inspiration

During active inspiration, there is a change in all the 3 planes of the thoracic cavity—the vertical, horizontal, and antero-posterior. This is brought about by an upward and outward movement of the ribs combined with a downward displacement of the diaphragm. The muscles involved in inspiration are as follows.

Diaphragm

The diaphragm is a fibromuscular structure that separates the thoracic and abdominal cavities and serves as the primary organ of respiration. During normal quiet breathing, the predominant muscle of respiration in the diaphragm is responsible for almost 70% of the tidal volume in a normal breath. It increases all the 3 diameters of thorax.

The diaphragm arises from 3 distinct sites:

- The sternal part arises as 2 fleshy slips from the posterior aspect of the xiphoid process.
- The costal part arises from the lower 6 or 7 ribs and their costal cartilages.
- The posterior part arises from the medial and lateral arcuate ligaments and the median arcuate ligament, and these attach the diaphragm to the upper lumbar vertebra.

From their origin, these fibers converge to the central tendon. The central tendon is pierced by 3 important structures: the inferior vena cava, the aorta, and the esophagus. The right dome separates the liver from the chest and is higher than the left dome.

Blood Supply

The diaphragm derives its blood supply from lower 5 intercostal and subcostal arteries, the superior and inferior phrenic arteries, and the pericardiophrenic and musculophrenic arteries.

Nerve Supply

- The phrenic nerve is the motor supply to the diaphragm. It also serves as the sensory supply to the central tendon. It arises in the neck from the 3rd, 4th, and 5th cervical ventral rami.
- Sensory fibers accompany the lower 6 thoracic intercostal nerves.

Mechanism of Action

When the diaphragm contracts, initially the dome only descends, pushing the abdominal contents away. As inspiration continues, due to pressure from the abdominal organs, the central dome gets fixed and the transverse and antero-posterior diameters are increased by elevation of the lower ribs. The zone of apposition between the diaphragm and the lateral chest wall at the initiation of the breath is very important and determines to a large extent the inspiratory capacity. When we take a maximal breath, the zone of apposition is almost zero.

Intercostal Muscles

There are 3 intercostal muscles:

- The external intercostal,
- The internal intercostal,
- The innermost intercostal.

External Intercostals:

- The external intercostals arise from the inferior border of the rib above and are inserted into the superior border of the rib below a given intercostal space. They are incomplete anteriorly and are replaced by the anterior

intercostal membrane between the sternal border and the costochondral junction bilaterally.
- The muscle fibers are directed downward and medially in the anterior part and downward and laterally in the posterior part.
- Contraction of these fibers results in an upward and outward movement of the ribs resulting in an increase in the antero-posterior and transverse diameters of the chest.

Internal Intercostals:

- The internal intercostals arise from the lower part of the inner surface of the rib above and are inserted into the upper border of the rib below a given intercostal space.
- These muscles are in a deeper plane as compared to the external intercostal muscles. Beyond the angle of the rib, posteriorly, they are replaced by posterior intercostal membrane from angle of the rib to the body of the corresponding vertebra bilaterally.
- The muscle fibers are directed at right angle to those of the externus muscles. When these fibers contract, they pull the ribs together and inward, thus facilitating forced expiration.

Innermost Intercostals:

- They represent an incomplete muscle layer and often extend beyond 1 rib thus covering more than 1 intercostal space. They arise from the costal grove above and are inserted into the superior edge of the rib below.
- They have a more supportive role and they assist both the external and internal intercostal muscles.

Nerve Supply
All the intercostal muscles are supplied by intercostal nerves.

Accessory Muscles of Inspiration
Accessory muscles involved in forced inspiration are:

- Pectoralis major and minor.
- Serratus anterior.
- Scalene group of muscles.
- Sternocleidomastoid.

The accessory muscles only come into play when the patient develops respiratory failure. They elevate and fix the first and second ribs and allow the chest to increase its antero-posterior and transverse diameters.

4.1.2.2 Accessory Muscles of Expiration
The muscles that contribute to forced expiration include:

- Muscles of anterior abdominal wall
  - Rectus abdominus,
  - External oblique,
  - Internal oblique,
  - Transversus abdominus.
- Quadratus lumborum.
- Latissimus dorsi.
- Serratus posterior inferior.

Flat muscles of anterior abdominal wall compress the lower part of the thorax and increase the intra-abdominal pressure. The quadratus lumborum stabilizes the 12th rib. The latissimus dorsi and serratus posterior inferior help in forced expiration by depressing the ribs.

4.1.3 Differences Between Infant and Adult

An understanding of the subtle but significant anatomical and physiological features of the pediatric airway that differentiates it from the adult airway would facilitate the development of a rational set of strategies to manage both normal and difficult pediatric airways.

4.1.3.1 Anatomical Differences
Size of the Occiput:

- Larger in children as compared to adults.
- In infants, it is often necessary to place a small roll under the shoulder to bring the airway in a better alignment for direct visualization by a laryngoscope.
- In children, sometimes it may not be necessary to place any pillow, while in an adult, one may need to place a pillow under the occiput to bring it in alignment.
- Nasopharynx.
- Infants are obligate nasal breathers for the first 3–5 months.
- Children develop adenoid hypertrophy that leads to nasopharyngeal obstruction in the first decade more often than adults.
- These adenoidal tissue can be very fragile and so caution should be exercised when placing a nasal airway in infants as they can bleed.
- Drainage of the sinuses can get blocked when a nasal airway is inserted for a prolonged period.
- Oral Cavity.
- Mouth opening in children is smaller.
- The ratio of the tongue to the volume of the oral cavity is proportionately larger than in children as compared to adults. Hence, the tongue is more prone to fall back and obstruct the airway in children. It is thus important to pull the mandible forward opening up the oropharyngeal space following induction.

- Tonsillar hypertrophy is also very common in children and may obscure the view of the larynx during laryngoscopy.

Shape of the Epiglottis:

- In infants, it is narrow, omega-shaped, angled over the airway and stiffer. It will need to be retracted with the tip of the laryngoscope blade in order to visualize the laryngeal inlet. Unlike the adult epiglottis, hyoepiglottic ligament is more elastic in young children; thus, a laryngoscope blade tip in the vallecula may not elevate the epiglottis out of view in order to visualize the vocal cords.
- The adult epiglottis is larger, flat, broad, in line with the trachea, and can usually be moved by pressure in the anterior vallecula.

Pediatric Larynx:

- Sits at a higher level at C3–4 in a neonate as compared to C5–6 in an adult.
- The tongue is also closer to the hyoid bone making visualization of laryngeal structures more difficult as it produces a more acute angle between the plane of the tongue and the glottic opening plane.
- The higher attachment of the larynx is also often misdescribed as "anterior." The adult airway, in contrast, appears to descend vertically down from the epiglottis.
- The larynx of the pediatric patient has often been described to be funnel shaped with the narrowest portion being at the level of the cricoid cartilage (subglottic); however, this has been shown to be untrue in more recent studies. The adult airway is often described as being a straight tube with the narrowest point being defined by the vocal cords. The transition from pediatric to adult airway is completed by the age of 5 years.
- The thyroid cartilage is quite prominent in an adult but is not so in a child.
- The cartilages that form the larynx are soft, very pliable, and easily compressible from the outside in infants and young children.

Trachea:

- The trachea is shorter in children than it is in adults. This becomes important in determining the depth to which one needs to place the endotracheal tube. With flexion and extension of the neck, the tube can travel significantly, resulting in inadvertent extubation or bronchial intubation.

Airway Resistance:

- Resistance in the airway is indirectly related to the diameter of the airway. Due to the small size of the airway, even a small change in the luminal diameter can significantly affect the resistance to airflow, thus increasing the work of breathing.
- The laryngeal structures are soft and pliable so that external laryngeal manipulation of the airway makes intubation much easier than expected.

4.2 Part 2: Airway Management

4.2.1 Assessment/Identification of Difficult Airway

One of the most difficult aspects in clinical anesthesia is the identification of patients in whom airways are likely to be challenging to secure. This is in part due to the fact that they are not very common and even when they are encountered they are not reported consistently.

Over time, multiple qualitative and quantitative assessments have been proposed to identify patients preoperatively. Unfortunately, none of these parameters alone have consistently been able to identify the subset of patients with difficult airways. When taken together, however, they have a better predictive value.

The act of securing the airway involves multiple steps, viz.: positioning, face mask ventilation, visualization of the vocal cords, and securing the airway or intubation. A failure to accomplish any one of these acts would constitute a "difficult airway" scenario.

4.2.1.1 A History of Difficult Airway

It cannot be emphasized enough that a good history and physical examination goes a long way in identifying patients with a difficult airway. A history of a prior difficult airway should always be taken seriously. A history of facial trauma, tumors, radiation to the head and neck, acute and chronic infections, obvious facial deformities, and congenital syndromes should alert one to the possibility of associated airway malformations and difficult access.

The presence of a beard, morbid obesity, advanced age, marked cachexia, overhanging incisors, micrognathia, and retrognathia could give us an inkling regarding the possibility of a difficult mask ventilation.

4.2.1.2 Diabetes Mellitus

The incidence of difficult airway is thought to be almost 10 times higher in patients with long-standing diabetes mellitus as compared to patients without diabetes. The limited joint mobility syndrome occurs in 30–40% of insulin-dependent diabetics and is thought to be due to glycosylation of tissue proteins that occurs in patients with chronic hyperglycemia.

4.2.1.3 Mallampati Classification

Mallampati et al. in 1985 suggested that "the size of the base of the tongue is an important factor determining the degree of difficulty of direct laryngoscopy" [8]. He proposed a classification based on the ability to visualize the faucial pillars, soft palate, and base of uvula in a seated patient whose mouth is opened wide and the tongue is maximally protruded (◉ Fig. 4.4).

Important Points:

- The patient sits upright with the head in a neutral position [9].
- The observer should sit opposite the patient at the eye level.
- The mouth must be opened as widely as possible.
- The tongue should be protruded maximally.
- The pharyngeal structures are visualized.

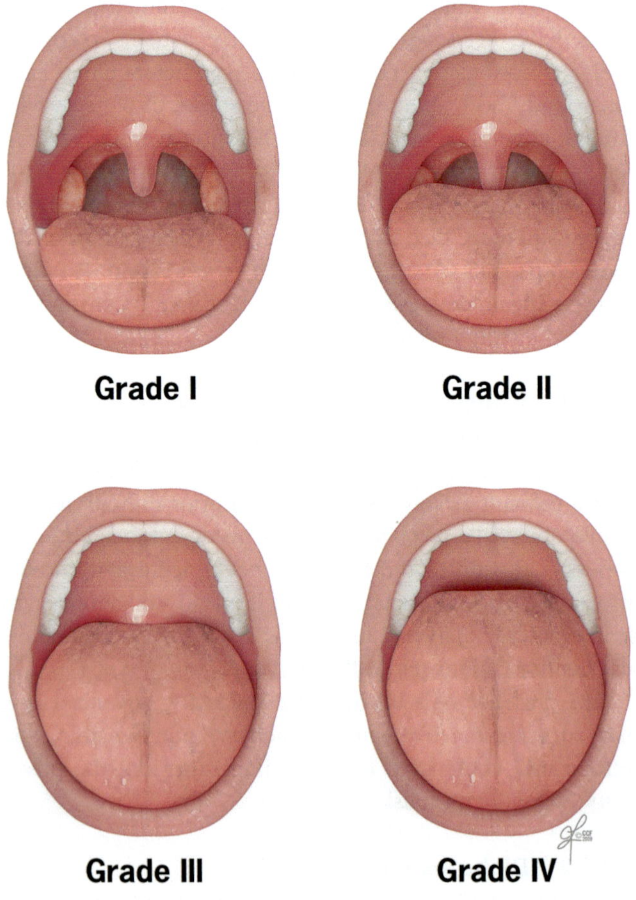

Fig. 4.4 Mallampati classification (Reprinted with permission, Cleveland Clinic Center for Medical Art & Photography © 2007–2017. All Rights Reserved)

They are classified according to the structures seen. Mallampati initially proposed 3 grades:

- Class 1—Faucial pillars, soft palate, and uvula could be visualized.
- Class 2—Faucial pillars and soft palate could be visualized, but uvula was masked by the base of the tongue.
- Class 3—Only soft palate can be visualized.

Later, Samsoon and Young [10] in 1987 added a fourth grade to the original classification:

- Class 4—Soft palate not visible.

Not uncommonly, when we do the test, we tend to ask our patients to phonate. This was not alluded to in the initial work of Mallampati et al. [8, 11]. It was Lewis et al. who introduced this concept and recommended that the Mallampati test be performed with the patient in the sitting position, the head fully extended, the tongue protruded and phonating [11, 12]. Khan et al. in 2013 showed that a Mallampati score in the supine position without phonation has better predictive value for difficult mask ventilation than for intubation [11, 13].

4.2.1.4 Inter-incisor Gap

In order to assess the inter-incisor gap, with the patient sitting in front of you at eye level, ask the patient to maximally open his or her mouth. Measure the distance between the upper and the lower incisors in the midline. It should normally measure about 30–40 mm or 2 fingers breath. It indirectly indicates movement at the temporomandibular joint. The cutoff is arbitrary and there is conflicting evidence regarding its usefulness as a single parameter.

4.2.1.5 Upper Lip Bite Test

The upper lip bite test (ULBT), [14] introduced as a simple beside test by Khan et al. [15] was based on the premise that it could predict difficult laryngoscopic intubation. With this test, we test the range and freedom of anterior advancement of the mandibular joint and the lower jaw in general. By this, it indirectly predicts the amount of space that can be potentially available in the oropharynx and the ease of visualization of the laryngeal inlet. It is classified as:

- Class 1—Lower incisors can bite upper lip above vermilion line.
- Class 2—Lower incisors can bite upper lip below vermilion line.
- Class 3—Lower incisors cannot bite upper lip.

This evaluation has been found to be fairly specific without great sensitivity [15–17].

4.2.1.6 Neck Circumference

The neck circumference is measured at the level of the thyroid cartilage. The cutoff neck circumference related to difficult intubation has not been clearly identified. Brodsky et al., in 2002, showed that the probability of difficult intubation increased from 5% (in patients with a neck circumference of 40 cm) to 35% in patients with a neck circumference of 60 cm [18]. This increase in the neck circumference has also been associated with a higher incidence of obstructive sleep apnea (OSA) [18]. The neck circumference was identified as a better predictor of difficult intubation in obese patients rather than the degree of obesity nor the presence of OSA [19].

4.2.1.7 Thyromental Distance

The thyromental distance (TMD) is measured from the thyroid notch to the lower border of the mandibular mentum with the patient's head fully extended. This indirectly gives us a clue regarding the submandibular space.

During laryngoscopy, the tongue is usually displaced into this space. In a patient with a short TMD or a non-compliant submandibular space, the tongue would tend to be displaced posteriorly, thus obstructing a clear view of the vocal cords and potentially increasing the degree of difficulty of securing the airway. An exact cutoff value at which it would have a significant predictive value is still elusive [11, 20]. Most anesthesiologist use a distance of less than 6 cm between the thyroid cartilage and the mandible to indicate a decreased TMD [21].

TMD has been shown to vary with the patient's size. Hence, Schmitt et al. in 2002 suggested that "the ratio of the patient's height to TMD (ratio of height to TMD = RHTMD) would improve the accuracy of predicting difficult laryngoscopy compared with TMD alone." And should be used instead of TMD for predicting difficulty in visualizing the vocal cords.

4.2.1.8 Thyromental Height

The thyromental height is measured between the anterior border of the thyroid cartilage and the anterior border of the mental protuberance of the patient lying supine with her/his mouth closed [22]. The test has not yet been validated in a large population and the actual cutoff has not been defined.

4.2.1.9 Hyomental Distance

Hyomental distance (HMD) is measured as the distance from the symphysis of the mandible to the body of the hyoid bone. This measurement, like the thyromental height, also gives the anesthesiologist a clue to the space where the tongue would normally be displaced during laryngoscopy.

This distance may be more challenging to discern in an obese patient as the hyoid bone may be difficult to identify.

4.2.1.10 Sternomental Distance

The sternomental distance is measured from the top of the sternum to the symphysis of the mandible. It is measured with the patient lying supine, the head in a neutral position, and neck fully extended. The sternomandibular distance is a good indicator of maximum neck extension.

4.2.1.11 Radiological Measurements

For over half a century, multiple radiological signs have been suggested that could indicate a difficult intubation. Multiple authors have suggested measuring different anatomical distances that could predict difficult intubation. Lateral neck X-rays are usually taken in a sitting position with the jaw relaxed and the head in a neutral position. The predictive value can be enhanced by adding views with extreme head extension. Measurements used that may indicate the potential for difficult airway include:

- Reduced angle of the mandible [23].
- Shortened distance from the upper incisors to the posterior border of the ramus of the mandible.
- Short ramus of the mandible [24, 25].
- Increase in the posterior depth of the mandible [24].
- Increase in the anterior depth of the mandible [24].
- Reduction in the distance between the occiput and the spinous process of C1 [24].
- Reduction in the C1–C2 interspinous gap [24].
- Reduced mobility of the mandible because of temporomandibular joint dysfunction or trismus [23].
- High arched palate associated with a long narrow mouth [23].
- Premaxillary overgrowth [23].
- Increased alveolar mental distance.
- Reduced mandibulo hyoid distance [25].

However, before recommending routine X-rays of the neck, the risk of X-rays should be balanced against the perceived benefits of being able to predict a difficult airway. Munster et al. suggested that anatomical location of the vocal cords in relation to cervical vertebrae could predict the degree of difficulty in visualizing the vocal cords [26]. They suggested that a higher position of the vocal cords was associated with an increasing difficulty of direct laryngoscopy and a higher Cormack–Lehane score.

4.2.1.12 Computerized Facial Analysis

Using facial profile pictures to predict difficulty in visualization of the vocal cords and therefore difficulty in intubation has been proposed in the past [27]. A simpler, noninvasive method of computerized facial analysis was proposed in 2011 by Conner et al. [28]. In their study, they analyzed the digital photographs (frontal and left and right sided views) of patients postoperatively and correlated it to the degree of difficulty met with intraoperatively using a facial structure analysis software. They suggested that "the model presented significantly outperformed the current standard of the combination of MP and TMD examinations, and is based on quantification of facial anatomy performed by an unbiased computer algorithm" [28]. These findings have to be validated by larger studies.

4.2.1.13 Range of Motion

While questioned by some, it has been widely accepted that visualization of the vocal cords for intubation is facilitated by proper alignment of the oral, pharyngeal, and laryngeal axes. When we fail to align these axes, difficult intubation can be anticipated. This can be illustrated in patients with diabetes mellitus, ankylosing spondylitis, or post-radiation and burn contracture of soft tissue in the neck where the impact of these conditions on the anatomical structures limits this alignment. In general, however, if there is no limitation to neck extension, there is a less likelihood for difficulty during intubation.

4.2.1.14 Wilson Score

Wilson [29] identified 5 factors—patient weight, head and neck movement, jaw movement, mandibular size, and prominence of the upper incisors—as factors that contribute to a difficult visualization of the laryngeal hiatus during routine laryngoscopy. The factors were each graded as 0, 1, and 2, depending on set criteria and a sum total was determined. A composite score of 5 or less would indicate easy laryngoscopy. A score of > 8 would indicate a high probability of difficult laryngoscopy.

Use of Ultrasound (US):

It has been suggested to use ultrasound (US) examination to help predicting airway difficulty, however, the authors believe that the most value for using US in airway management is for identifying and marking cricothyroid membrane to facilitate invasive elective or emergency airway access especially in obese patients.

4.2.2 Description of the Difficulty with Laryngoscopy/Intubation

4.2.2.1 Cormack–Lehane Classification

The Cormack–Lehane classification is a grading system commonly used to describe laryngeal view during direct laryngoscopy [30]:

- **Grade 1**—"If most of the glottis is visible."
- **Grade 2**—"If only the posterior part extremity of the glottis is visible—Light pressure on the larynx will nearly always bring at least the arytenoids into view, if not the cords."
- **Grade 3**—"If no part of the glottis can be seen, but only the epiglottis."
- **Grade 4**—"If not even the epiglottis can be exposed."

However, despite its widespread use, the CL classification has not been fully validated and often there is a lot of confusion between the different grades even among anesthesiologists [30]. Multiple modifications have been proposed to the CL classification, such as dividing grade 2 and/or grade 3 into grade 2a/2b and 3a/3b, respectively, [31] and classifying the grade of difficulty as easy restricted and difficult depending on the need of alternate techniques.

4.2.2.2 POGO Scoring System

Percentage of glottic opening (POGO) visualized has been used to assess the difficulty of intubation. A score of 100 denotes complete from the anterior commissure to the interarytenoid notch, and if the interarytenoid commissure cannot even be visualized, a score of 0 is given [32]. Because the POGO score differentiates between varying degrees of partial glottic visibility, it might provide a better assessment tool than the more commonly used Cormack–Lehane system.

4.2.2.3 Intubation Difficulty Score

The Intubation Difficulty Score (IDS) developed by Adnet et al. [33] uses 7 variables to determine the IDS score. The IDS score is the sum of N1 through N7. They include:

- N1—first attempt = 0, further attempts = 1.
- N2—need for additional operators.
- N3—alternative intubation techniques used; e.g., patient reposition, change of blade, or tube change approach.
- N4—Cormack and Lehane grade on initial attempt; grade 1 = 0.
- N5—lifting force applied during laryngoscopy; need for increased force gets 1 point.
- N6—need for external laryngeal pressure or manipulation to improve view gets a point.
- N7—the position of the vocal cords during laryngoscopy (open- 0, closed 1).

A score of 0 indicates easy intubation; a score from 1 to 5 indicates slight difficulty; and a score greater than 5 indicates moderate to major difficulty [34].

Of note, the prior discussion was for the most part referencing the use of the commonly used direct laryngoscopy blades such as Macintosh and Miller. However, with the advent of the videolaryngoscopy more than a decade ago, clinicians are trying to figure out a scoring system that would accurately predict and/or quantify the difficult videolaryngoscopy intubation scenarios.

4.2.3 Techniques for Managing Airway

4.2.3.1 Awake Versus Asleep

Awake intubation is often underused due to lack of experience, unfamiliarity with the technique, and presumed patient dissatisfaction. A well-executed awake intubation is both safe and well-tolerated and accepted by patients. It should be noted that while awake intubation is the conventionally used term for intubating a patient before induction of general anesthesia, most of these procedures are performed under sedation with maintenance of spontaneous ventilation. When the issue is primarily a difficult intubation rather than mask ventilation, the asleep technique may be used in certain situations. It is appropriate to master the flexible intubating scope-assisted intubations in simulation training labs and an asleep patient (electively, when difficult intubation is not anticipated) initially before having to resort to the technique in an awake patient. While flexible intubating (Fiberoptic) scope is commonly used and the best tolerated and versatile device for "awake" intubation, any other device can be used to accomplish this task including videolaryngoscope, direct laryngoscope, light-wand, etc.

Absolute Contraindications to Awake Technique

The cited contraindications for awake intubation include:

- Patient refusal.
- Patient's inability to comply with instructions.

However, in the authors' clinical practice, such contraindications are extremely rarely encountered. Proper patient discussion and education of the benefits and risks of such a technique is almost always met with acceptance, and mastery of the technique can overcome the lack of patient compliance with instructions if encountered.

Relative Contraindications:

- Inexperience.
- Allergy to local anesthetics
- Airway bleeding that might preclude a proper visualization, however proper suctioning, and/or placement of a supraglottic airway awake, and intubation through it has been utilized successfully in these situations.

It Should Be Used with Caution:

- Patients with very large and occlusive upper airway tumors and stridor due to an increased risk of complete airway obstruction. In this group of patients, an awake tracheostomy may be considered.

4.2.3.2 Retrograde Intubation Techniques

Retrograde intubation is useful for patients who have an anatomic problem that makes orotracheal intubation impossible or dangerous using conventional techniques. It has an application not only for elective use in patients with an unstable cervical spine or face trauma but also when the view is obscured by secretions or blood. It has been successfully used in awake, sedated, spontaneously breathing, or apneic patients. This technique can be successful in both children and adults, but the neck should allow for identification of landmarks and the cricothyroid membrane.

A guide wire is introduced into the larynx through a Tuohy needle that is placed through the cricothyroid membrane or membranous space between the cricoid cartilage and the first tracheal ring. The wire is gently guided upward to emerge in the mouth or nostril. An endotracheal tube is then guided antegrade into the airway using the wire as a guide. Multiple techniques have been described including the classical railroading technique using the guidewire, using a guiding catheter, using a fiberoptic bronchoscope and silk pull-through techniques [35]. Once the endotracheal tube is passed through the larynx, the wire is removed and the tube is passed further into the trachea. The position of the tube is confirmed by capnography and auscultation and by fiberoptic bronchoscopy if required.

4.2.4 Drug Selection

4.2.4.1 Anti-sialogogues

Glycopyrrolate 0.2 mg is usually given intravenously due to its lack of central nervous system (CNS) effects and relatively less likelihood of producing tachycardia when compared to atropine. The onset of action after an intravenous (IV) administration is usually within a minute, but after intramuscular (IM) injection, the onset may be delayed by 15–30 min. It dries the mucus membranes facilitating the efficacy of topical anesthesia and improves visualization. That said, the authors of this chapter tend not to use glycopyrrolate routinely due to the potential detrimental effect of tachycardia in some of our patients with coronary artery disease (CAD). In addition, secretions are rarely of a quantity that creates a concern, except for certain situations such as in patients with esophageal strictures who cannot handle their secretions well.

4.2.4.2 Local Anesthetics

Lidocaine is the most commonly used agent for topical airway anesthesia. The maximum described dose for topical administration in the context of airway topicalization has been 9 mg/kg. The dose should be decreased in patients with liver disease. Topically lidocaine can be atomized, nebulized, or can be used as a "spray as you go". It can be administered by a cricothyroid puncture or transtracheal puncture to augment the airway anesthesia. Lidocaine also can be used to produce a local nerve block. In experienced hands, such nerve blocks can provide excellent anesthesia and intubating conditions.

Cocaine can also be used as an alternate to lidocaine. It has the added benefit of producing local vasoconstriction. Usually, a 4% solution is used for topicalization for fiberoptic (FO) intubation, particularly when a nasal route is chosen. It has become less popular due to its cardiac and central nervous system side effects (tachycardia, hypertension, coronary artery spasm, and dysrhythmia), potential for abuse, and is not easily available.

Three blocks are used to provide anesthesia to the upper airway:

- Glossopharyngeal (oropharynx).
- Superior laryngeal (larynx above the cords).
- Translaryngeal (trachea below the cords).

Glossopharyngeal Block

Glossopharyngeal block can be performed by using 2 different approaches: intraoral and peristyloid (Figs. 4.6 and 4.7).

Intraoral Block

For intraoral block, adequate topical anesthesia must be provided to the tongue and tonsillar mucosa so that the patient will allow manipulation of this sensitive area (◉ Fig. 4.6a). The tongue is displaced to visualize the posterior palatopharyngeal fold (posterior tonsillar pillar) and about 5 ml of lidocaine is injected submucosally just caudal to the pillar after ensuring a negative aspiration for blood using a bent 22-gauge needle (◉ Fig. 4.6b). The process is repeated on the contralateral side.

This block also can be achieved by applying pressure to this area using a local anesthetic soaked gauze. This latter approach has a lower success rate but avoids the possibility of intravascular injection.

Peristyloid Approach

In the peristyloid approach, bony landmarks (mastoid process and the angle of the mandible) are identified on the lateral aspect of the neck. The tip of the styloid process ideally lies at the midpoint of the line joining these 2 landmarks. Using a 22-gauge needle, the styloid process is then identified and then the needle is walked off the process posteriorly and about 5–7 ml of local anesthetic is injected in this area (◉ Fig. 4.7). The process is repeated on the contralateral side.

Both these blocks carry the risk of intravascular injection due to the proximity of the great vessels in the neck.

Superior Laryngeal Nerve Block

The superior laryngeal nerve is blocked just before it penetrates the thyrohyoid membrane between the greater cornu of the hyoid bone and the superior cornu of the thyroid cartilage (◉ Fig. 4.8). Identification of the hyoid bone can be difficult in patients with short, thick, or edematous necks. After negative aspiration, 2–3 mL of local anesthetic is then injected at the site. This block also can be associated with intravascular injection of the local anesthetic.

Translaryngeal

By this method, the trachea and larynx can be anesthetized. The local anesthetic is injected by going through the cricothyroid membrane (◉ Fig. 4.9). It is invasive and carries potential risks to the airway. As the patients usually tend to cough after injection of the local anesthetic in the trachea, it also provides some spotty anesthesia to the supraglottic structures.

4.2.5 Sedation

Although awake intubation can be achieved using local anesthesia alone, some form of sedation is often used to facilitate patient tolerance. Anxiolytic or analgesic drugs are most commonly used, but it is important to realize that safety of awake intubation relies on the maintenance of spontaneous breathing. Over-sedation may result in respiratory depression, apnea, or loss of airway muscle tone resulting in airway obstruction. There are several medications that are commonly used to facilitate awake (sedated) intubation, and one should choose one that they are most familiar with and can result in a reliable, reproducible safe sedation plane.

4.2.5.1 Midazolam and Fentanyl

Midazolam is a benzodiazepine that can be given as a bolus in incremental doses starting at 0.5–1.0 mg increments up to about 5 mg. As it lacks analgesic properties, it is often used in conjunction with fentanyl. The main advantage of this technique is the availability of the medications, simplicity in execution, extensive experience in using and managing the side effects, availability of medications to reverse the effects, antegrade amnesia (midazolam), and low cost. Large frequent boluses can still result in respiratory arrest.

American Society of Anesthesiologists®

DIFFICULT AIRWAY ALGORITHM

1. Assess the likelihood and clinical ompact of basic management problems:
   - Difficulty with patient cooperation or consent
   - Difficult mask ventilation
   - Difficult supraglottic airway placement
   - Difficult laryngoscopy
   - Difficult intubation
   - Difficult surgical airway access
2. Actively pursue opportunities to deliver supplemental oxygen throughout the process of difficult airway management.
3. Consider the relative merits and deasibility of basic management choices:
   - Awake intubation vs. intubation after induction of general anesthesia
   - Non-invasive technique vs. invasive techniques for the initial approach to intubation
   - Video-assisted technique vs. invasive techniques for the initial approach to intubation
   - Preervation vs. ablation of spontaneous ventilation
4. Develop primary and alternative strategies:

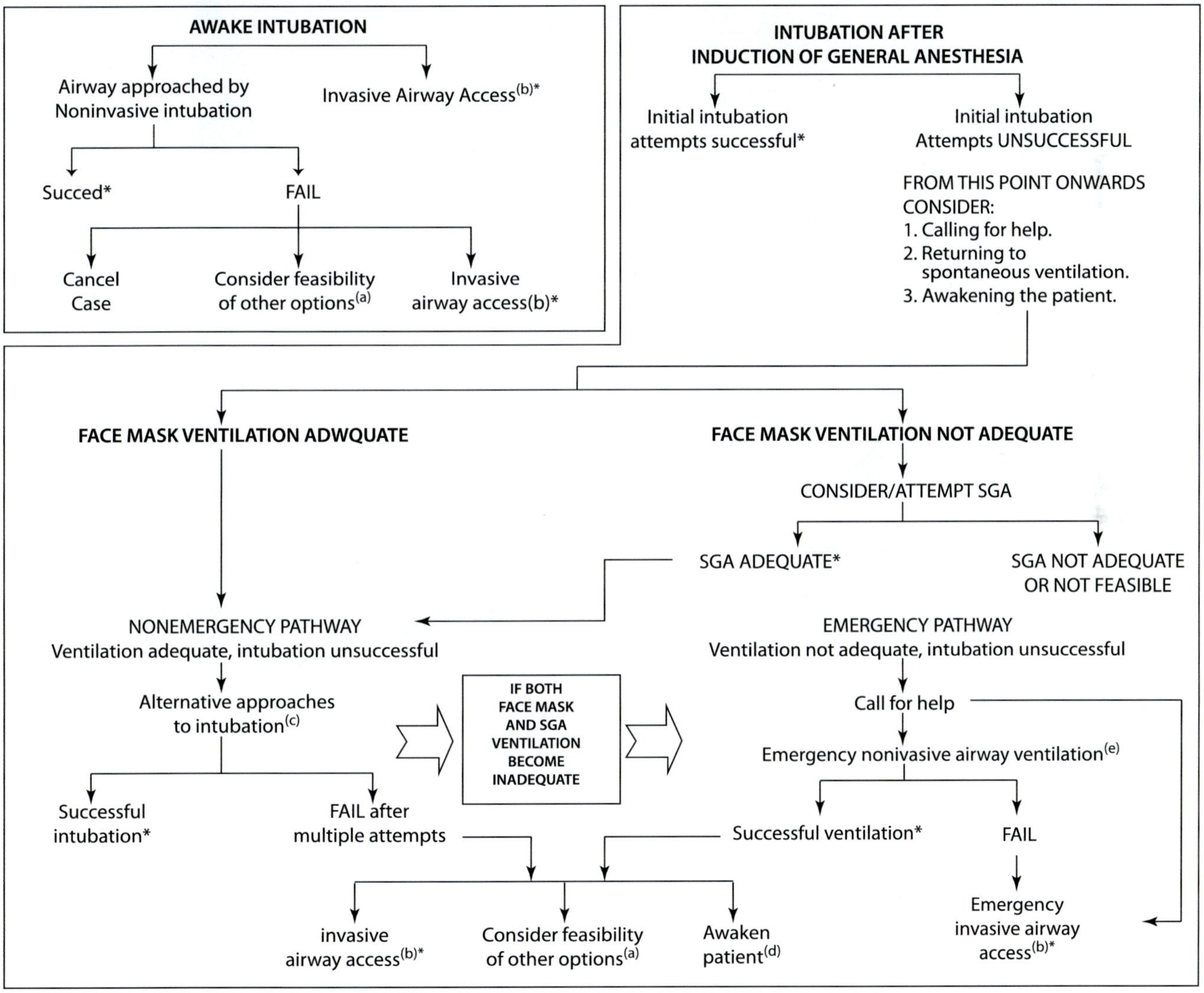

Fig. 4.5 ASA difficult airway algorithm

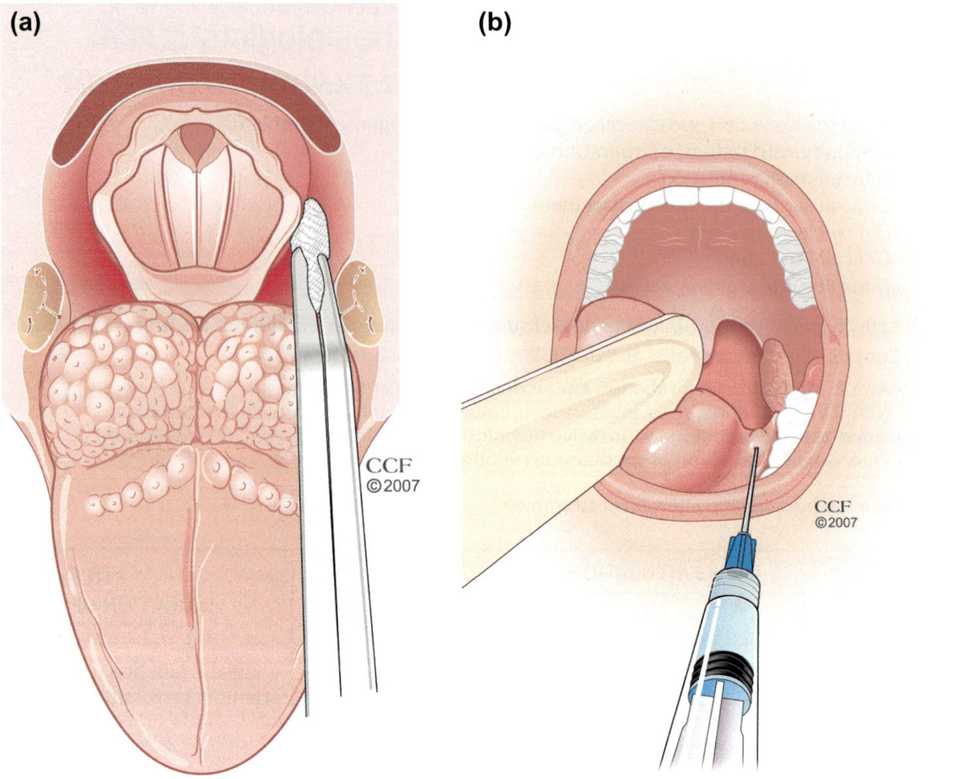

Fig. 4.6 Intraoral approach for glossopharyngeal block. (**a**) Local anesthesia is applied to the tongue and tonsillar mucosa using anesthesia-soaked gauze. (**b**) Just caudal to the posterior tonsillar pillar, 5 ml of lidocaine is injected submucosally (Reprinted with permission, Cleveland Clinic Center for Medical Art & Photography © 2007–2017. All Rights Reserved)

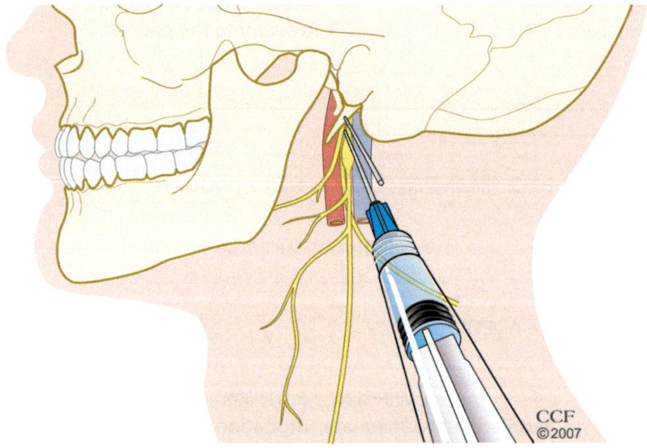

Fig. 4.7 Peristyloid approach for glossopharyngeal block (Reprinted with permission, Cleveland Clinic Center for Medical Art & Photography © 2007–2017. All Rights Reserved)

4.2.5.2 Remifentanil

Remifentanil has a very rapid onset and offset of action. Its metabolism is independent of renal and hepatic function. It has excellent anti-tussive and analgesic properties. It can be used in conjunction with a small dose of midazolam to reduce recall. Remifentanil is commonly associated with bradycardia, hypotension, apnea, hypoxia, and may cause chest wall rigidity.

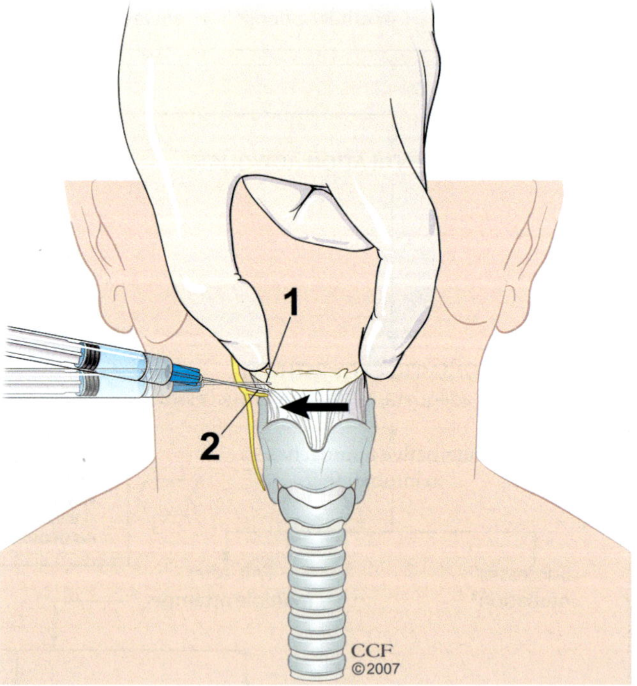

Fig. 4.8 Superior laryngeal nerve block (Reprinted with permission, Cleveland Clinic Center for Medical Art & Photography © 2007–2017. All Rights Reserved)

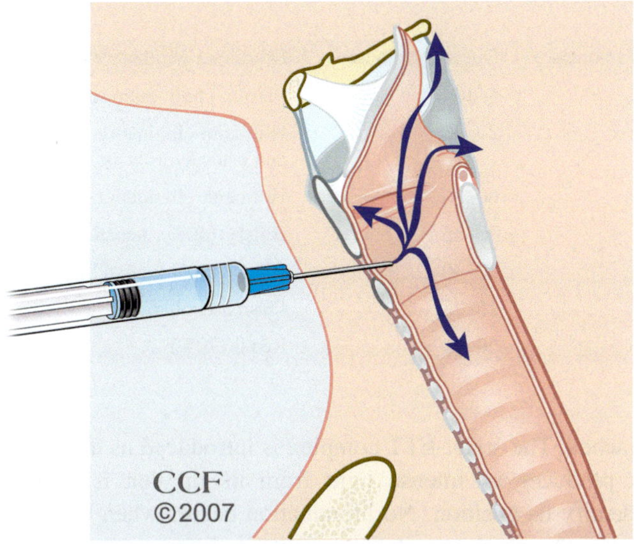

Fig. 4.9 Translaryngeal block (Reprinted with permission, Cleveland Clinic Center for Medical Art & Photography © 2007–2017. All Rights Reserved)

4.2.5.3 Propofol

Propofol can be used in small incremental boluses, as an infusion, or as a target-controlled infusion (TCI). It may be challenging to achieve the correct balance between under-sedation and over-sedation due to its narrow therapeutic index when used for sedation. It can also be supplemented with opioids or benzodiazepines, but the addition of the latter will increase the risk of over-sedation.

4.2.5.4 Dexmedetomidine

Dexmedetomidine is an alpha-2 adrenoceptor agonist. It produces sedation, amnesia, anxiolysis, and has some analgesic properties. It has minimal effect on respiration. It can be started as a loading bolus of 1 mcg/kg over 10 min followed by an infusion of 0.3–0.7 mcg/kg/h.

4.2.5.5 Use Versus Avoidance of Muscle Relaxants

Patient-related factors alluded to earlier, anesthesiologist's technical skills, knowledge of airway management, anesthesia technique, use of muscle relaxants [36], facilities and support [37] available all dictate success of airway management in both an emergent and planned intubation of the airway [38]. Normally, tracheal intubation follows administration of a muscle relaxant to supplement the drugs given for the induction of general anesthesia and relaxes the jaw and the vocal cords, thus facilitating endotracheal intubation. It has been the common dogma to administer a neuromuscular blocking agent after establishing or confirming face mask ventilation following induction of anesthesia [39]. This has been based on the fear that muscle paralysis would worsen ventilation in a patient with a difficult mask ventilation [39].

There is increasing evidence that such a "conservative" approach is not warranted [40]. There are multiple caveats to this argument. The muscle relaxants when they take full effect may actually turn a difficult mask situation scenario into an easy one, and even if the difficult ventilation persists after muscle relaxation, intubation may prove to be an easy task. Please note that in the American Society of Anesthesiologists (ASA) difficult airway algorithm (◉ Fig. 4.5), [41] it addresses waking the patient up when we cannot intubate, and cannot ventilate the patient and not following a failed mask ventilation.

We should be aware that even with only induction agent and no muscle relaxants used, we may not have enough time to prevent dangerously low levels of prolonged hypoxia before the patient wakes up [40, 42]. With the increasing availability of Sugammadex which facilitates rapid reversal of rocuronium and vecuronium, there has been less hesitation in using muscle relaxants. However, such ability to readily reverse muscle relaxation should not replace or impact the decision to perform awake versu asleep intubation. The time it takes to recognize difficult, acquire the muscle reversal agent in quantities sufficient to reverse such deep muscle relaxation may not be enough to prevent neurologic damage from hypoxemia.

Thus, in a seemingly normal airway with no anticipated difficulty with either mask ventilation or intubation, administering the muscle relaxants immediately following the induction agent seems reasonable. However, when difficulties with either mask ventilation or intubation is anticipated, an awake technique should be considered.

4.2.5.6 Dose of Muscle Relaxants

See ◘ ◉ Table 4.1 for dosages for muscle relaxants [43–46].

4.2.5.7 Effect of Priming

In general, depolarizing neuromuscular agents have an earlier onset of action as compared to the non-depolarizing muscle relaxants. By administering a sub-paralyzing dose of non-depolarizing agent followed a few minutes later by the intubating dose of a depolarizing agent (succinylcholine), the onset of the blockade has been shown to be earlier than if the agent had been given without the priming dose [47]. Such a dosing strategy also helps to eliminate the defasciculation phenomenon observed after administration of the succinylcholine without the priming dose, that is why it is often referred to as a defasciculating dose. Fasciculations could result in postoperative myalgias, and, in extreme very rare conditions, can result in rhabdomyolysis, hemoglobinuria, and renal dysfunction.

Table 4.1 Dosages of muscle relaxants

Drug	Ed95 mg/Kg	Intubation dose mg/Kg	Onset minutes	Duration minutes	Dominant elimination pathway
Succinylcholine	0.3–0.6	1–1.5	1–1.5	5–10	Plasma cholinesterase
Atracurium	0.2	0.4–0.6	3-5	20–35	Hofmann elimination and ester hydrolysis
Cisatracurium	0.05	0.15–0.2	1-2	60	Hofmann elimination
Vecuronium	0.05	0.1–0.2	3–5	20–36	Biliary (60%), hepatic (20%)
Rocuronium	0.3–0.6	0.6–1.2	1-2	30–40	Biliary (70%), renal? (30%)
Mivacurium	0.07–0.08	0.15–0.2	3–5	15–25	Plasma cholinesterase
Pancuronium	0.07	0.08–0.12	3-5	60–90	Renal (70%)

4.2.6 Devices

4.2.6.1 Flexible Fiberoptic

Flexible intubating scope (formerly known as fiberoptic bronchoscopy) not only allows us to visualize the tracheobronchial tree but also can be used to facilitate the placement of an ETT or offer therapeutic modalities through the various access ports. A standard adult bronchoscope has 3 channels: one for light source; one for the optics; and the third is a working channel that allows for suctioning, obtaining biopsies, and instrumentation.

4.2.6.2 Rigid Bronchoscopy

Rigid bronchoscopy is a hollow metal tube, available in several sizes (diameter and lengths), that facilitates direct visualization of the trachea and the proximal bronchus. Due to its rigid nature and inability to flex the tip, it can be used only in the trachea and the proximal bronchi.

The lumen may be cylindrical and of a uniform diameter through most of its length. Occasionally, they taper toward the tip. The tip is usually beveled and occasionally has a lip with which one can lift the epiglottis and facilitate its introduction into the airway. The accessory channels are for administration of oxygen, suction, and instrumentation. Ventilating bronchoscopes are available that allow us to administer positive pressure or jet ventilation during airway surgery.

It is most commonly used in patients who have obstruction of either their trachea or a proximal bronchus, since the rigid bronchoscope's large lumen facilitates suctioning and the removal of debris, or for interventional procedures such as insertion of silicon airway stents.

4.2.6.3 Transillumination

Light Wands

The lighted stylet uses the principle of transillumination first described in 1959 by Yamamura et al. for nasotracheal intubation [48]. The airway is never directly visualized but the characteristic of the illumination of the soft tissue of the neck (midline) is used to direct the end of the stylet to the trachea. The stylet-ETT complex is introduced as a unit and it produces an intense light from its tip that is used to identify its position. No illumination occurs when the stylet enters the esophagus. It is available in different sizes for use in children and adults. Success rate is variable [48–51] and varies dependent on the operator's experience and skill rather than on the intubation device itself.

Advantages:

- It is a simple and easy to learn technique.
- Allows intubation under suboptimal illumination [48].

Technique:

- Load the ETT onto a well-lubricated stylet with the tip of the stylet just at the end of the ETT.
- Bend the stylet to an acute 90° angle proximal to the cuff of the ETT.
- Place the head in a neutral position with the neck slightly extended [48].
- Stand at the head end or the side of the patient as appropriate.
- Dim the room lights if required, particularly in obese patients.
- Administer the induction medications if you are planning to do under a general anesthesia (GA).
- Gently open the mouth and advance the stylet-ETT complex in the midline.
- If you get any resistance, gently "rock" the stylet backward and redirect it toward he thyroid prominence.
- Now direct the illumination anteriorly and gently advance the stylet until you see a more focused light through the glottis opening (coning) and glow below the thyroid prominence.
- When the tip of the ETT-TL enters the trachea, a well-defined circular glow can be seen in the suprasternal notch or just above it slightly below the thyroid prominence.
- Advance the ETT off the stylet and confirm placement of ETT.

Complications:

- Trauma to the larynx.
- Subluxation of the cricoarytenoids.
- Disconnection of the distal light source [48, 49].

Limitations:

- Operator dependent.
- Difficult in patients with large tongue and long epiglottis.
- Avoided in patients with anatomical variations of the upper airway, tumor, trauma, infection, or suspected foreign bodies that might increase the risk of complications or failed intubation
- Very obese patients with a short neck who do not lend themselves to transillumination technique.
- Uncooperative unsedated patient [48, 49].

4.2.6.4 Laryngoscope Blades

The choice of laryngoscope can influence the chance of successful tracheal intubation. Regular practice is required to ensure that we can not only successfully visualize the airway but also perform a successful intubation. The 2 most commonly used blades for intubation are the Macintosh and the Miller blades. They are available in different sizes and there have been multiple modifications to enhance their usefulness in different clinical scenarios.

When using the Macintosh blade (left-handed), the tongue is usually swept and the blade is advanced into the vallecula and the tongue is displaced anteriorly to expose the epiglottis. The Miller blade is introduced into the oral cavity and the channel created by the blade allows for visualization of the glottis when the epiglottis is elevated using the tip. Its lower profile allows it to be used in patients with a limited jaw opening, temporomandibular joint (TMJ) disease, anterior larynx, micrognathia, and children and adults with a long floppy epiglottis. The drawback of the Miller blade is the inability to sweep the tongue, thus limiting the maneuvering space in the oral cavity and sometimes making identification of the landmarks difficult. The glottis is, in general, viewed better with the straight blades while tracheal intubation is easier with the curved blades [52]. However, the most important factor in the choice of any airway device should be the operator's past experience and familiarity with the equipment [53].

Modifications

There are more than 50 different modifications of both the Macintosh and Miller blades that have been introduced in clinical practice. Some of the commonly used are:

- Polio laryngoscope blade.
- McCoy blade.
- Wisconsin blade.
- Wis-Hipple.
- Henderson laryngoscope blade.

In addition, laryngoscope blades have also been enhanced with accessory devices such as oxygen (Oxyscope) [54], suction channel (Khan and Tull) [54], ultraviolet light source (Intubrite) [54], and ultralight weight (Trulite) [54].

Disposable Versus Reusable Blades

One of the potential risks of reusing laryngoscope handles and blades is contamination with blood and oral secretions. Standard cleaning techniques may fail to sanitize some contaminations and the risk of cross-infection is real, but there is no consensus in current guidelines regarding cleaning and disinfection of this equipment [55]. Single-use disposable blades could offer protection from such a transmission of disease. Most disposable blades use the indirect fiber transmitted lighting system and thus offer better illumination as compared to conventional tungsten incandescent light bulbs.

4.2.6.5 Alternative Intubating Devices

Videolaryngoscopes

Since the introduction of the Bullard laryngoscope in the late 1980s, there has been several new "videolaryngoscopes" that have been introduced into the market. All of these share the same common feature of capturing the image of the glottis using a camera that is mounted near the tip of the blade and transferring it to a video screen, [56] either mounted onto the handle or an external device. As these devices have a more acute angle of the tip, visualization of the glottis opening is facilitated with minimal external laryngeal manipulation [56]. A number of studies have shown that videolaryngoscopes offer a better view of the glottis as compared with direct laryngoscopy [57–59]. The videolaryngoscopic blade may conform to the shape of the Macintosh blade, or carry a more acute angulated blade, or may be "anatomically" shaped with or without a tube channel guide to facilitate intubation.

Some of the commonly used videolaryngoscopes include [60]:

- Storz C-Mac (based on Macintosh and Miller).
- Storz C-Mac D blade (more angulated).
- McGrath (based on Macintosh).
- McGrath Series 5 (more angulated).
- Glidescope (based on Macintosh).
- Glidescope with angulated blades (Ranger, Cobalt).
- Pentax Airway Scope (anatomically shaped).
- AirTraq Optical Laryngoscope (with a tube channel).
- Res-Q-Scope.

- King Vision.

There have been number of studies comparing the different videolaryngoscopes. The design of the blade appears to play a significant role in visualization of the vocal cords [61, 62].

Indications

- Difficult visualization of the glottic opening.
- As part of the difficult airway algorithm.
- Limited mobility of the cervical spine.
- Micrognathia and retrognathia.
- Morbid obesity.
- As an adjunct to placement of a gum elastic bougie or use of fiberoptic bronchoscope to enter the vocal cords.
- Demonstration of anatomy and as an educational tool.

Disadvantages

Some of the disadvantages following routine use of a videolaryngoscope include:

- Increased intubation time.
- Loss of skill set with Direct Laryngoscopy.
- Lack of depth perception leading to trauma.
- Inability to use in the face of lots of secretions or bleeding in the back of throat.
- Fogging of camera lens.
- Expense.

Complications

- Perforation of the soft palate, posterior pharyngeal wall, and tonsillar pillars [63, 64].
- Failure to intubate in spite of good visualization.

For uncomplicated airways, videolaryngoscopes are not superior to direct laryngoscopy. It is a good teaching tool as it allows the instructor to simultaneously visualize what the trainee is seeing and thus can be used as a teaching tool. They can prove challenging to introduce into a small oral cavity and the distal camera can get fogged, thus resulting in poor visualization. In addition, we need to understand that though we might have a good view of the glottis, intubation can still be challenging as it utilizes a virtual reality principle versu direct visualization as is the case with direct laryngoscopy.

4.2.7 Alternatives and Adjuncts

4.2.7.1 Supraglottic Airway (Traditional and Modified)

The first one invented of this category is the laryngeal mask airways (LMAs) in the 1980s by a British anesthesiologist, Dr. Archie Brain. It was introduced as a safe alternative to endotracheal intubation and as a fallback mechanism when confronted with a cannot ventilate-cannot intubate situation. With increasing familiarity and use of the device, it has come to play an important role in the available options of routine airway management.

Indications

- Airway management in both routine and emergency surgery when control of the airway is required with or without neuromuscular blockade.
- Rescue following a failed attempt at endotracheal intubation as part of the difficult airway algorithm.
- Situations when there are contraindications to an endotracheal intubation.
- Patients in whom one wants to avoid manipulations of the cervical spine, or the disease process limits the movement of the cervical spine making endotracheal intubation difficult or fraught with danger.

Contraindications

- No absolute contraindication.
- Use with caution
  - Patient with increased aspiration risk
    - Full stomach.
    - Gastric outlet obstruction.
    - severe reflux disease.
    - Gastroparesis and delayed gastric emptying.
    - Intestinal obstruction.
    - Morbid obesity.
    - Increased intra-abdominal pressure.
  - Patients in need of increased airway pressures for assuring adequate ventilation
    - Reduced pulmonary compliance.
    - Severe uncontrolled reactive bronchopulmonary disease.
  - Unusual surgical positioning.
  - Need for manipulation of the head and neck resulting in inadequate seal.
  - Need for pulmonary isolation.

Difficulties with Supraglottic Insertion

- Difficulty in supraglottic airway (SGA) insertion can be encountered when faced with small mouth opening and/or obstruction at the level of the vocal cords as well as limited neck movement.

Complications

Complications are rare but the most common complaint is sore throat. Some of the more serious complications include:

- During the procedure
  - Malposition and inability to ventilate.
  - Laryngospasm.
  - Damage to the arytenoid cartilages.
  - Aspiration of the gastrointestinal contents.
- Postoperative
  - Sore throat.
  - Postoperative dysphagia, dysarthria, or dysphonia.
  - Temporomandibular joint dislocation.
  - Soft tissue injury to the lips, tongue, epiglottis, palate, tonsils, and oropharynx leading to bleeding.
  - Esophageal rupture.
  - Lingual nerve injury.
  - Recurrent laryngeal nerve injury.

All SGAs share the same design of having a hollow shaft or tube connected to a cuff or sealing device that is designed to sit in the hypopharynx facing the glottis. The tip of the SGA is designed to sit at the esophageal inlet, and some of them (second generation) have a channel through which an orogastric tube can be inserted to decompress the stomach. They may be reusable or for 1 time use only. Most routinely used SGAs have a fenestrated diaphragm at the laryngeal inlet to prevent entry of the epiglottis in the shaft. Those used as a conduit for intubation, however, do not have this diaphragm. Some of them are soft and floppy and take the shape of the oropharynx, while others are preformed, stiff, and cannot be deformed. Some also have a stiff bite guard to prevent bite down into the lumen. They are available in different sizes and usually the patient's weight and form of the oral cavity dictates the size selected. It is safer to use larger size with an underfilled cuff rather than a small size with an overinflated cuff, as they will be associated with increased incidence of mucosal ischemia.

There are many types of SGAs available and the commonly used ones include:

- Classic LMA.
- LMA Supreme.
- Intubating LMA.
- Fast-track.
- I-Gel.
- King Tube.

4.2.7.2 Combitube

Combitube combines the lumen of an endotracheal tube with an esophageal obturator airway. It is designed to permit ventilation whether placed in the trachea or esophagus. It facilitates airway management for both the skilled or novice operator. It can be inserted into the trachea as a conventional tube, or blindly or using direct laryngoscopy. If the Combitube resides in the esophagus, the blue lumen should be used to ventilate the patient.

Indications

- Emergent prehospital settings.
- In-hospital emergencies and airway rescue.
- "Cannot intubate-cannot ventilate" situations.

Procedure

In most instances, the tube is placed blindly. One can use a laryngoscope if available to displace the tongue. The Combitube is then placed blindly by passing it over the tongue until the patient's teeth rest between the 2 black lines. A jaw thrust can facilitate its placement. At this time, we have 2 options.

If the Combitube enters the trachea, inflation of the distal cuff (white pilot balloon) will produce the seal and ventilation can be initiated. If the Combitube enters the esophagus, both balloons should be inflated and the device creates 2 seals: (1) proximally in the pharynx with the pharyngeal cuff (blue pilot balloon) and (2) distally in the esophagus with the distal cuff (white pilot balloon). Ventilation occurs via the side ports of the blue-topped lumen. The distal lumen can be used to decompress the stomach.

The distal cuff has a capacity of 12 ml while the proximal lumen has a capacity of 85 ml.

Complications

- Inability to ventilate the patient.
- Tongue engorgement.
- 9th and 12th cranial nerve dysfunction.
- Esophageal perforation.
- Pyriform sinus perforation.
- Stomach insufflation, regurgitation.

The next generation of the tube includes the King LT, LT-D, LTSD tubes and the Easytube.

4.2.8 Transcutaneous or Surgical Airway

4.2.8.1 Cricothyroidotomy

This procedure involves gaining access to the trachea through the cricothyroid membrane that stretches between the inferior border of the thyroid cartilage and the superior border of the cricoid cartilage. Access through this space can be achieved using:

- A needle or catheter placed directly though the membrane.
- A guidewire placed through this space through a needle and following dilatation, a larger cannula railroaded in.
- Open cricothrotomy—wherein access is obtained surgically by cutting down to this membrane.

This procedure may be elective, planned, or emergently performed. The technique used would depend on the indication and the urgency. As the cricothyroid membrane is superficial and there are no major vascular structures crossing it (see earlier Anatomy section), it can be accomplished quickly, safely, and with low risk for bleeding.

Indications

Modified from *Benumof and Hagberg's Airway Management* ("Percutaneous Dilational Cricothyrotomy and Tracheostomy") [65]:

- As part of the management for control of the airway when orotracheal or nasotracheal intubation and fiberoptic approaches have failed.
- Airway management in trauma patients (injury to the head and neck, face, cervical spine) in whom endotracheal intubation is impossible or likely to be associated with significant morbidity or mortality.
- Emergently, when airway devices or intubation devices are not readily available.
- As an alternate to emergent tracheostomy in patients with a recent sternotomy.

Contraindications

Modified from *Benumof and Hagberg's Airway Management* ("Percutaneous Dilational Cricothyrotomy and Tracheostomy") [65]:

- Trauma to the thyroid or cricoid cartilage.
- Inability to discern anatomy due to
  - Obesity.
  - Edema.
  - Subcutaneous emphysema.
  - Trauma to the front of neck.
  - Bleeding.
- Pediatric patients (less than 10 years of age) due to difficulty in identifying anatomy and loose connective tissue.
- Pre-existing laryngeal diseases, such as cancer, acute or chronic inflammation, or epiglottitis.
- Lack of experience or knowledge of technique.

Procedure

- Immobilize the larynx between the thumb and the index finger of the non-dominant hand.
- Identify the cricothyroid membrane.
- Infiltrate the skin and subcutaneous tissue with a local anesthetic.
- Make a horizontal stab incision through both skin and cricothyroid membrane.
- Stabilize the larynx by placing a cricoid hook under the cricoid cartilage.
- Insert the tracheotomy or endotracheal tube into the trachea.

Complications

- Early [65]
  - Misplacement.
  - Loss of airway control.
  - Subcutaneous or mediastinal emphysema due to false passage.
  - Bleeding.
  - Infection.
  - Main stem intubation.
  - Pneumothorax/pneumomediastinum.
  - Dissection of the mucosa resulting in airway obstruction.
  - Damage to the larynx, thyroid cartilages, vocal cords, or the trachea..
  - Esophageal perforation.
- Delayed [65]
  - Accidental decannulation resulting in respiratory embarrassment and death.
  - Subglottic stenosis.
  - Voice change.
  - Infection.
  - Bleeding.

4.2.8.2 Tracheostomy

Tracheostomy involves access to the airway below the cricothyroid membrane either surgically or percutaneously. Open tracheostomy is considered the golden standard against which all the other access procedures are compared.

Indications

Indications are the same as those for a cricothyrotomy as alluded to earlier. In addition, it is also indicated in the following situations:

- Prolonged intubation.
- Prolonged mechanical ventilatory support.
- Facilitate pulmonary toilet.
- Cannot ventilate-cannot intubate situation.

It provides a more stable platform for mechanical ventilator support as compared to a cricothyrotomy.

Contraindications

- Contraindications to surgical tracheostomy [65]
  - Short thick neck as evidenced by
    - Inability to identify landmarks in spite of extension of the neck and proper positioning.
    - Inability to palpate the cricoid cartilage above the sternal notch.
  - Inability to discern anatomy due to
    - Obesity.
    - Edema.
    - Subcutaneous emphysema.
    - Trauma to the front of neck.
    - Bleeding.
    - Tumor or mass overlying the proposed site of stoma.
  - High levels of positive end-expiratory pressure (PEEP) (> 15 cm of H_2O).
- Relative contraindication for percutaneous tracheostomy [65]:
  - Large thyroid gland.
  - High innominate artery.
  - Uncorrected coagulopathies.
  - Young children (less than 15 years).
  - Unintubated patients in severe respiratory distress.

Percutaneous Versus Surgical

See ◉ Table 4.2 for overview of percutaneous versus surgical tracheostomy [66–69].

Procedure

Tracheostomies can be performed through an open or percutaneous technique. Open tracheostomy is one of the oldest procedures described in the literature and is still the procedure of choice for some trauma centers. However, the use of percutaneous tracheostomy has been increasing since its introduction in the 1980s.

Studies have supported percutaneous over open tracheostomies. However, the final technique depends on the surgeon's experience and abilities, in addition to guidelines of the facility where this procedure is to be performed. It is important to prepare for and anticipate any problems and be proactive in managing any complications.

Complications

- Early [65]
  - Bleeding.
  - Loss of airway control.
  - Trauma to the trachea, larynx, esophagus.
  - Tracheoesophageal fistula.
  - Injury to the great vessels.
  - Airway fire.
  - Pneumomediastinum, subcutaneous emphysema, or pneumothorax.
  - Cardiac arrest.
- Late [65]
  - Bleeding.
  - Stomal infection.
  - Mediastinal infection.
  - Fistula between the trachea and the esophagus, great vessels, innominate artery, innominate vein, skin.
  - Displacement and loss of airway control.
  - Obstruction of the tube.
  - Granuloma.
  - Subglottic stenosis.

4.2.8.3 Translaryngeal or Transtracheal Jet Ventilation

Translaryngeal or transtracheal jet ventilation is a method of providing ventilation in an open system, with high frequency and low tidal volumes. In this technique, the oxygen is delivered as a pulsed breath through a jet nozzle (◉

Table 4.2 Percutaneous versus surgical tracheostomy

	Percutaneous	Surgical
Time to accomplish	Less time	More time
Expense	Less expensive	More expensive
Infection	Less common	More common
Bleeding	Less common	More common
Anterior tracheal injury	More common	Less common
Posterior tracheal perforation	More common	Less common

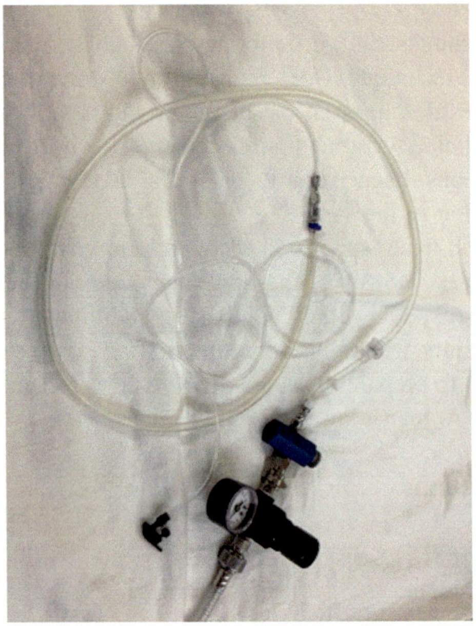

Fig. 4.10 Translaryngeal or transtracheal jet ventilation device

Fig. 4.10). This pulse of air can be delivered manually or by automatic devices. Due to the "Venturi effect," there is entrainment of air from the surrounding that allows for administration of an effective tidal volume. It can be used in the presence of a partial laryngeal obstruction that permits exhalation.

The jet ventilation rate is usually high (12–20 breaths/min). Faster rates can result in some air-trapping and "auto-PEEP." These effects allow air exchange by generating higher airway pressures and splinting the airway and alveoli open, thus optimizing V/Q matching.

This is different from high frequency jet ventilation, which is a mechanical ventilation mode that can be delivered through an endotracheal tube by a mechanical ventilator and has proven beneficial in the pediatric population, for example, in premature babies suffering from acute respiratory distress syndrome (ARDS).

Indications

Jet ventilation is ideally suited for patients with normal, unobstructed airways and normal lung and chest wall compliance. It is dependent on driving pressure and the entrainment of air for providing an adequate tidal volume. It is crucial that the patient exhale completely between each administered breath to prevent barotrauma.

Indications:

- As part of management during a shared airway surgical procedure.
- As part of difficult airway management in a "cannot intubate-cannot ventilate" scenario
- Inability to maintain a patient's airway utilizing non-invasive means.
- Upper airway partial obstruction with an obscured view due to uncontrolled bleeding or vomiting.
- Severe facial trauma.
- Mandibular fracture making jaw manipulation impossible.
- Partial obstruction to the larynx and upper airway due to
  - Infection, such as epiglottitis or Ludwig's angina.
  - Allergic or immunologic reaction.
  - Chemical or thermal burns.
  - Foreign body in the larynx that cannot be removed expeditiously.
  - Post-extubation glottic edema.

Contraindications

- When the airway can be maintained by other more secure means.
- Complete obstruction to the normal egress of air due to the presence of glottic lesion, significant interarytenoid scarring, laryngospasm.
- Decreased cheat wall compliance.
- Advanced chronic obstructive pulmonary disease (COPD) with prolonged exhalation phase.
- Presence of pulmonary bullae.
- Subcutaneous emphysema in the neck.
- Damage to the larynx, cricoid cartilage, or trachea preclude successful oxygenation and ventilation via a transtracheal catheter
  - tracheal rupture.
  - tracheal dehiscence with distal displacement.
- Inability to align the axis of the direct laryngoscope with the long axis of the trachea (when used from above the vocal cords).
- Local infection.
- Local infiltration of tumor.

Relative Contraindications

However, in most instances, the benefit of establishing an airway will outweigh the risk of performing needle cricothyroidotomy in these circumstances:

- Anatomic distortion increases the risk of airway complications.
- Neck swelling that obscures the normal anatomical landmarks
- Anatomic anomalies or distortion of the larynx and trachea.
- Bleeding diathesis.

Complications

- Inadequate oxygenation and ventilation.
- Drying out the mucosa of the respiratory tract.
- Gastric distention and rupture.
- Regurgitation.
- Pneumomediastinum.
- Pneumothorax.
- Subcutaneous emphysema.
- Death.

Precautions

One should always use a longer expiratory time (e.g., I:E ratio of 1:3–1:5), the lowest oxygen pressure and flow rate that allows for chest rise, and as large a catheter as possible. If there is diminished chest fall with expiration, we should rule out the presence of pneumothorax or pulmonary barotrauma.

4.2.8.4 Apneic Oxygenation

Hypoxemia is not uncommonly encountered during endotracheal intubation of critically ill patients. This may predispose to the development of cardiac arrest, neurological injuries, or even death. In order to prevent rapid desaturation following induction of anesthesia, anesthesiologist have always resorted to a short period of preoxygenation. It has been shown that by providing preoxygenation, one may be able to delay the onset of hypoxemia. Normally during apnea, it has been shown that there is a net diffusion of about 250 ml/min of oxygen from the alveoli into the blood stream. Due to the buffering action of the red blood cells (RBCs) and the blood, only 10–20 ml of CO_2 is replaced into the alveoli, thus producing a net deficit in the volume and a negative alveolar pressure. This results in entrainment of air from the air passages as the apneic time continues. By providing continuous oxygen at the level of the pharynx, one may be able to delay the onset of hypoxemia [70–72].

4.2.8.5 High Flow Nasal Cannula

Conventionally, oxygen is delivered by nasal prongs, face, and nasal masks with or without a reservoir. Their maximum flow is limited by the breathing pattern, maximum flow rates, and the difficulty in heating and humidification of the inspired air. Most of these devices are associated with entrainment of the room air to meet the requirements of the peak inspiratory flow. The effective oxygen saturation provided by these conventional methods may not be able to meet the requirements of a patient in acute respiratory failure.

Administration of a high flow humidified and heated oxygen (often with flow rates as high as 70 L/min) has been shown to prevent entrainment of air from the surrounding, reduce the dead space, and generate some positive airway pressure by providing some resistance to expiration due to the high flow rates. Recent studies have suggested that it is not inferior to conventional noninvasive ventilator support and oxygen therapy in patients admitted to the intensive care unit (ICU) [73].

Active humidification has been shown to improve muco-ciliary function, [74] facilitate clearance of airway secretions, and prevent hyper-response symptoms. As an added benefit, they can potentially reduce the respiratory rate and increase patient comfort and overall satisfaction. Thus, they may have a role in management of patients with respiratory failure due to infections, asthma, and COPD. It has also been used safely in the neonatal period for respiratory support. Commercially available systems ensure that the inspired gas is heated to 37 °C and humidified by adding 44 mg H_2O/L [75].

There are no significant complications associated with the use of high flow nasal cannula.

4.2.9 Endobronchial Intubation

4.2.9.1 Double Lumen Endobronchial Tubes

Indication

- Isolation of lungs to prevent contamination or drowning from blood emanating from the contralateral lung.
- Facilitate ventilation and/or limit ventilation-perfusion mismatch
  - Bronchopleural fistula.
  - Bronchopleural cutaneous fistula.
  - Unilateral disruption of the main bronchus or major bronchi.
  - Giant unilateral lung cyst or bulla.
  - Whole lung lavage.
  - Differences in compliance between the 2 lungs.
- Facilitate surgical exposure
  - Thoracic aortic aneurysm.
  - Pneumonectomy.
  - Thoracoscopy.
  - Upper lobectomy.

Relative Indications

- To facilitate surgical exposure:
  - Lung resections involving the middle and lower lobes.
  - Segmental lung resections.
  - Esophageal resection.
  - Procedures on the thoracic spine.

- Lung trauma.
- Pulmonary edema after cardiopulmonary bypass.
- Preferential ventilation of 1 lung due to presence of unilateral lung disease.

Advantages

- Allows independent ventilation of each lung.
- Allows both sides to be ventilated if required with different modes or different ventilator setting.
- Allows for better surgical exposure.
- Better seal and less likelihood of displacement once properly positioned.

Disadvantages

- Larger size
  - Difficulty in patients with complex anatomy or distorted anatomy.
  - Rigid, hence more possibility for iatrogenic trauma to the airway.
  - Uncomfortable for patient being weaned from the ventilator.
- Not ideal for pulmonary toilet as lumen is not very wide.
- Not ideal for weaning the patient from the ventilator.
- Will need a smaller bronchoscope for visualization of the segments of the lung.

Contraindication

- Large tumor or external mass distorting the anatomy.

4.2.9.2 Procedure

Choosing the Correct Size

- It is challenging to precisely choose the correct double lumen tube (DLT) in a patient. If one chooses an inappropriate sized tube, there is a higher likelihood of tracheal trauma and failure to ventilate the lungs or failure to adequately separate the lungs [76].
- An intentional use of a smaller tube has not always proved to be helpful as it will require higher endobronchial cuff volumes and pressures that can damage the bronchus [77].
- Too large a size can cause iatrogenic trauma and can cause rupture of the bronchus.
- The ideal size should result in a near-complete seal of the bronchial lumen without inflation of the cuff.
- In general, women need a smaller size DLT as compared to men [76].
- In most instances, a 37, 39, or 41-F DLT is selected for men and a 28, 35, or 37-F DLT is selected for women.
- Direct tracheal measurement can be used to predict the size of tube to be selected [76].

Choosing the Correct Side

- There are 2 types of DLT, right- and left-sided, depending on the orientation of the bronchial arm at the distal end of the tube.
- As the DLT has 2 lumens, either tube can be used to ventilate either lung and this is dictated by which lumen is clamped.
- As the placement of a right-sided tube is technically more challenging, it is more often that we select a left-sided tube.
- This is due to the takeoff of the right upper lobe bronchus that arises from a variable distance and in a variable direction from the carina in different people, mostly very close to the origin of the right main bronchus. A malpositioned right-sided tube would not allow ventilation or drainage of the right upper lobe bronchus, resulting in collapse and or consolidation of the right upper lobe. The Rusch DLT addresses this issue by having a larger and more elongated Murphy eye compared to the Mallinckrodt DLT. Thus, the left-sided DLT is most commonly used, but in surgery for a left pneumonectomy for a tumor involving or very near the carina, it may be preferable to use a right-sided tube. An alternate technique is to use a left-sided tube and just withdraw it when the surgeon is ready to close the bronchus.

The tubes are bulky, rigid, and can be awkward to place in some individuals. They are a challenge to place in a patient with a known difficult airway. As the surgery proceeds, they tend to become softer. They can thus get dislodged from their position on movement of the patient or on manipulation around the mediastinum by the surgeon. Hence, there is a need to check the position of the tube and ensure that the tracheal lumen is above the carina, the bronchial lumen is in the correct bronchus, and that its cuff has not herniated into the trachea. With a right-sided tube, one needs to ensure that the takeoff of the right upper lobe is not occluded.

Placement

A double lumen tube can be placed with or without the help of a fiberoptic bronchoscope:

- Check the tube to ensure that both the lumen are patent and the cuffs are competent. Assemble the tube-breathing circuit connecting apparatus. Induce anesthesia and administer the neuromuscular blocking agent.

- Expose the vocal cords using a laryngoscope.
- Insert the endotracheal tube with bronchial concave curve facing anteriorly.
- After you pass the vocal cords, rotate the tube 90° (toward the side corresponding to the type of the DLT used) and advance the tube in the direction of the bronchus till some resistance is felt.
- Do not force the tube should you meet any resistance.
- Inflate the tracheal cuff and check that you can hear breath sounds on both sides of the chest.
- It is always better to confirm proper placement with bronchoscopy (auscultation is unreliable).
  - Pass the bronchoscope through the tracheal lumen
    - Look for the radio-opaque line encircling the bronchial lumen and if present, ensure that it is above the level of the carina.
    - For a left-sided tube with the endobronchial portion in the left main bronchus
      - The bronchial cuff should be just visible ~ 5 mm below the carina.
      - The cuff should not herniate above the carina.
  - Now pass the bronchoscope through the endobronchial lumen
    - For a left-sided tube
      Identify origins of the left upper and lower lobe bronchi.
    - For a right-sided tube
      The right upper lobe should be identified by the presence of its 3 lobar branches.
  - If you have not properly seated the DLT, guide the bronchoscopy into the side that you want and advance the DLT over it to sit correctly.
- Next confirm that you can ventilate and isolate the lungs.

You can also use a stylet or a bougie to help you guide the DLT into a proper position.

Complications

- Tracheal laceration.
- Bleeding.
- Rupture.
- Malposition, obstruction, and increased airway pressure.
- Herniation of the bronchial cuff.
- Failure of lung isolation.
- Obstruction of the right upper lobar bronchus (more common with right-sided tubes or aberrant origin of the right upper lobe bronchus).
- Vocal cord injury and postoperative hoarseness of voice.

4.2.9.3 Bronchial Blockers (Integral to Endotracheal Tube or Separate)

Another technique for lung isolation is the use of bronchial blockers. These can be in the form of a single lumen tube with integrated bronchial blocker or use of a single lumen tube with an external blocker. Some of the commonly used tubes include:

- Arndt blocker.
- Univent tube.
- Coopdech blocker.
- Wire-guided endobronchial blockers.
- EZ Blocker.

Indications

- Lung isolation in patients with a difficult airway.
- Lung isolation in a patient with airway abnormalities that preclude the use of a double lumen tube.
- Patients with a tracheostomy or stoma.
- Patients with small airway anatomy.
- Patients in whom during the course of surgery need a lung isolation due to airway or lung disruption (e.g., fistula), edema, bleeding, etc..
- As a selective distal bronchial blocker when the patient's medical condition does not permit complete lung isolation.
- Patients who need a nasotracheal intubation.

Disadvantages as Compared to a Double Lumen Tube

- Slow lung deflation following isolation.
- Slow lung inflation.
- Inability to maintain toilet or suctioning out secretions.
- Displacement of the blocker during positioning.
- Higher incidence of mucosal ischemia and damage due to low-volume high-pressure cuffs.
- Difficulty in management of desaturation
  - Inability to administer continuous positive airway pressure (CPAP).
  - Cumbersome to deflate and reinflate in case it becomes necessary.

Complications

- Loss of lung isolation.
- Obstruction to ventilation due to slipping of balloon into the trachea.
- Mucosal ischemia and damage.

Placement and Positioning Considerations

They need a fiberoptic scope to guide their placement and position check after any movement or repositioning.

4.2.10 Intubation and Tube Change Adjuncts

4.2.10.1 Bougies

The bougie has proved to be a very useful device to facilitate intubation when confronted with suboptimal visualization of the larynx following a direct laryngoscopy. With the bougie placed in the lumen of the trachea, an endotracheal tube can be railroaded over the bougie by Seldinger technique, thus securing the patient's airway.

It is moderately flexible and can be bent into a form that would follow the shape of the oropharynx. It is available in different sizes and lengths and in an adult, a 15F, 60–70 cm is usually selected. The tip of the bougie is angled anteriorly to about 30°. This allows it to enter a very anteriorly placed larynx.

Uses

1. Anterior larynx with difficulty in navigating the oropharynx.
2. Tube exchanger to an endotracheal tube and a tracheostomy tube.

Technique

- The tip of the bougie is either passed into the trachea under direct visualization or blindly hugging the curvature of the epiglottis.
- As the tip of the bougie glides over the tracheal rings, we feel the "clicks" and this helps us confirm the correct placement.
- The bougie should be then passed distally and it might turn into the left or right bronchus.
- Do not force the bougie should you meet with resistance as it could potentially perforate through the back of the trachea.
- Now mount an endotracheal tube onto the bougie and railroad it down into the trachea.
- It may be prudent to visualize the placement of the endotracheal tube into the trachea before removing the laryngoscope. The advantages include
  - Preventing the bougie from getting dislodged into the esophagus.
  - Preventing the bougie from further advancement into the airway producing trauma.
  - Early identification of disruption of the ETT cuff by sharp tooth.
- The disadvantage is the added bulk in the oral cavity that might preclude advancement of the tube.
- Always check proper placement prior to initiating ventilation.

Risks and Complications

- Perforation of trachea or bronchus.
- Perforation of esophagus.
- Injury to larynx.
- Pneumothorax/pneumomediastinum.

4.2.10.2 Jet Stylets (Tube Exchange Catheter)

The jet stylet was first introduced in 1987 to help maintain control of the difficult airway [78, 79]. They usually measure about 65 cm in length and are made of radio-opaque material to facilitate placement. It is often used for jet ventilation but with a regular adapter, it can be connected to a standard anesthesia circuitry as well. It is semirigid to allow for introduction even when visualization of the larynx may be difficult. There are usually multiple distal side ports to prevent a catheter from whipping during jet ventilation. They are usually marked to facilitate accurate placement in the airway.

Uses

- Exchanging the endotracheal tube in the difficult airway.
- For providing jet ventilation during a direct laryngoscopy prior to intubating a patient [79].
- As a first intermediate step in extubation of the difficult airway.
- As a tube exchanger tool for both an endotracheal tube or tracheotomy tube in a patient with a precarious airway.
- As a means of providing ventilation following extubation.
- To assess vocal cord mobility postoperatively while still maintaining the possibility of re-securing the airway.

4.2.11 Endotracheal Tube Types

4.2.11.1 Tube Material (Polyvinyl Chloride, Silicone, Laser-Resistant, Silver Impregnated, Other)

Most disposable endotracheal tubes available today are made of polyvinyl chloride (PVC). Under special circumstances, tubes made of silicone rubber, latex, or stainless steel are also used. Tubes vary from 2 to 10.5 mm in internal diameter.

Reusable red rubber tubes were used initially but as they are opaque and tend to crack with repeated use, they fell out of favor. They are more heat resistant as compared to the PVC tubes.

PVC tubes are relatively stiff and retain a memory and come preshaped. Usually, phthalates are added to the PVC to soften it, but there are concerns that they may be released with prolonged use and cause cancer. Because they are relatively stiff, the tubes can potentially navigate mild obstruction, but, if care is not taken during placement of the tube, they can damage the friable mucous lining of the trachea. When the PVC tubes are left in the body for a long time, they can soften due to the oropharyngeal temperature and thus may kink or obstruct the airflow.

Silicone tubes are nonporous, least allergenic, and do not deteriorate with prolonged use. They are softer than the PVC tubes and do not retain a memory. Due to their pliability, a stylet may have to be used to stiffen the catheter during intubation. They are the safest material and conform to the tracheal lumen. Their cost limits their usefulness.

4.2.11.2 Laser-Resistant Tubes

- Red rubber tubes work well with CO_2 lasers and KTP lasers—commercially available from Sheridian.
- Silicone-based tubes can be wrapped with aluminum and work well with CO_2 and KTP lasers. The cuff is pre-dyed with methylene blue and is available commercially from Xomed Laser shield II.
- Stainless steel spiral ETTs work well with CO_2 and KTP lasers. A tube with a double cuff design, which would allow for inflation of the second cuff should the laser damage the first, is available from Mallinckrodt Laser Flex.
- Soft white rubber tubes wrapped in copper foil work with Argon, Nd/YAG, and CO_2 lasers. A double cuff design is also commercially available.

4.2.11.3 Cuff Design (High Versu Low Volume/Pressure, Cuffed Versu Uncuffed, Cuff Shape)

Endotracheal tubes may be cuffed or uncuffed. Uncuffed endotracheal tubes are usually used in infants and small children as the lumen size would not allow the placement of a cuffed ETT. They are available in different sizes and lengths.

Cuffed endotracheal tubes come with either a high-pressure low-volume cuff or a low-pressure high-volume cuff.

4.2.11.4 High-Pressure Low-Volume Versus Low-Pressure High-Volume Cuffs

See ◉ Table 4.3 for differences between a high-pressure low-volume and a low-pressure high-volume cuff.

4.2.11.5 Specific Tube Types (Wire-Reinforced, Nasal and Oral RAE, Microlaryngeal, Supraglottic Secretion Suctioning, Other)

ETT may also be reinforced and these are usually used in head and neck and neuroanesthesia as well in long cases. They are usually made of silicone and need a stylet for intubation.

The oral and nasal RAE tubes are PVC tubes and are used in ENT procedures; they have the added advantage that they are preformed to facilitate getting them out of the way of the surgical procedure. The oral RAE is usually directed downward to tape to the chin while the nasal is directed to the forehead of the patient. They are marked to indicate the depth to which they have been placed in the trachea.

4.2.12 ASA Difficult Airway Algorithm

The American Society of Anesthesiologists (ASA) in line with their concern for and leadership in the patient safety movement in the US and the world issued the updated 2022 ASA Difficult Airway Practice Guidelines in 2022 [41] that addressed some of the shortcomings of the prior guidelines from 2012 due to changing practice parameters and new concepts in airway management. It is based on the available evidence, and when evidence is lacking, expert opinion including survey results from airway management experts from around the world and ASA members as well as collaborating medical societies. The reader is encouraged to review the entire article, however, we herein highlight some of the important concepts included in this 2022 update.

The practice guidelines address both anticipated and unanticipated clinical difficult airway scenarios. It encompasses difficult mask ventilation, visualization, placement

Table 4.3 Differences between high-pressure low-volume and low-pressure high-volume cuffs

High-pressure low-volume	Low-pressure high-volume
Mostly seen with silicone tubes	Mostly seen with PVC tubes
When deflated, the balloon rests flush with the ETT	When deflated, the balloon appears crimpled around the end of the ETT
When deflated, it does not obstruct view of the glottis during intubation	As it is more bulky, it might obstruct view when the mouth is narrow
Area of contact with the trachea is small	Area of contact with trachea is large
More commonly associated with tracheitis, pressure necrosis, stricture, rupture of the trachea	Less common but can occur with overinflation of the cuff
May impinge into the lumen of the tube if high pressure is used to obtain a seal	Not common

PVC polyvinyl chloride, *ETT* endotracheal tube

and securing both a supraglottic and endotracheal intubation, ventilation and avoidance of hypoxia, surgical airway issues, extubation challenges and better planning for the future. It also addresses the need for a robust follow-up following a difficult airway encounter and patient education to prevent an unanticipated DA scenario.

The highlight is the inclusion of both an adult and pediatric difficult airway algorithm. The new ASA 2022 pediatric difficult airway algorithm and the accompanying infographics are a welcome addition to the very popular "ASA DA algorithm." It follows almost the same principles regarding managing adult patient in terms of airway evaluation, and management, albeit with a focus on the concept of functional versu physiologic airway obstruction reminding clinicians of the need to monitor the patient's depth of anesthesia and muscle relaxation during the process of managing the difficult airway.

The decision making tool is a new feature in the present update that should be examined very carefully. It includes the consideration for awake airway management in patients with high risk for aspiration, and/or those who cannot tolerate a brief apneic episode.

The emphasis has been not only on the identification of patients with difficult airways but also on facilitating first attempt success, improving patient safety during airway management, and minimizing or avoiding adverse events that can have a devastating effect on the patient. These guidelines are applicable in all scenarios including planned diagnostic, elective and emergent anesthesia procedures in both an operating room and NORA locations.

Another important highlight is the realization of human factors that can not only affect our choices of the technique that we choose but also significantly affect the outcome for our patients.

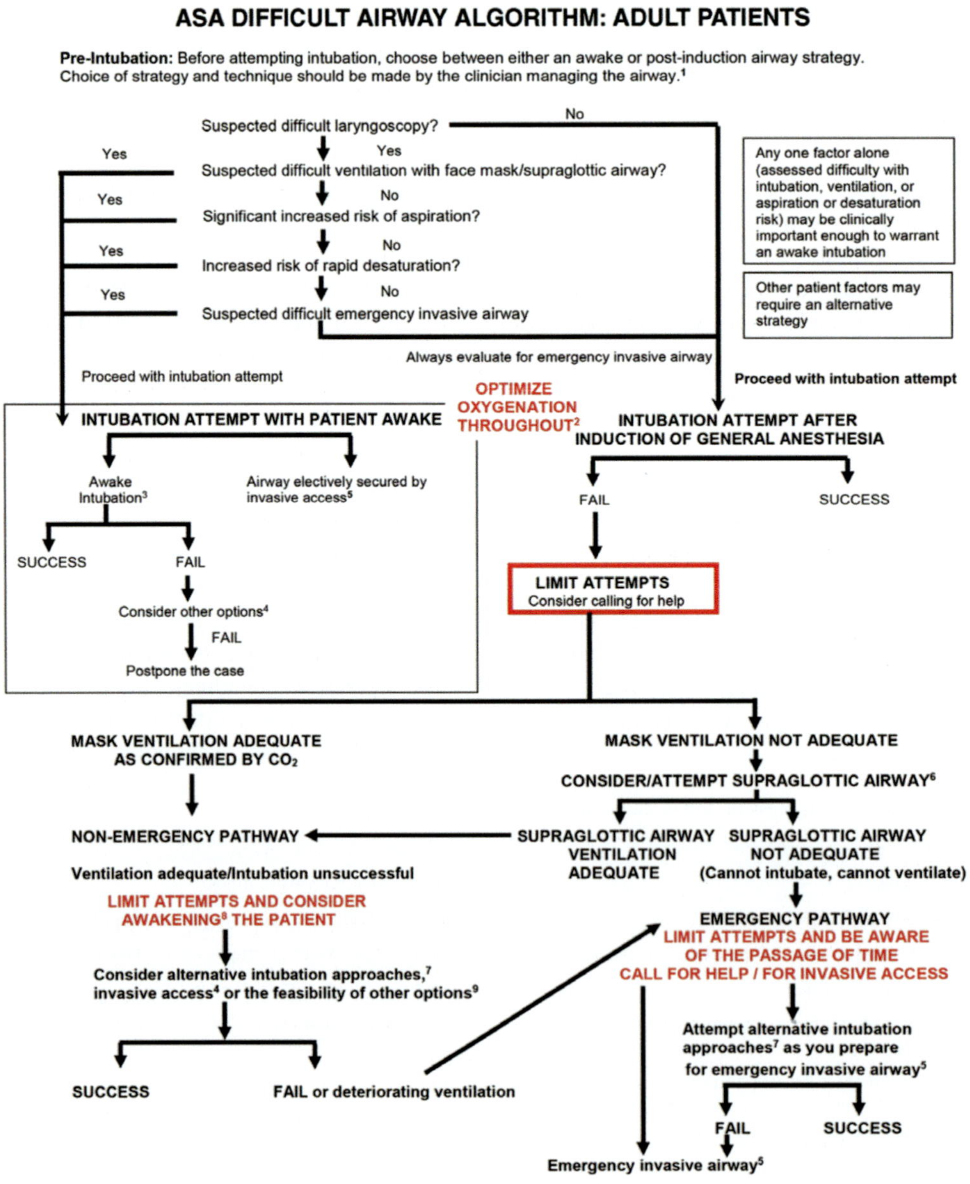

Difficult airway algorithm: Adult patients. [41] [1]The airway manager's choice of airway strategy and techniques should be based on their previous experience; available resources, including equipment, availability, and competency of help; and the context in which airway management will occur. [2]Low- or high-flow nasal cannula, head elevated position throughout procedure. Noninvasive ventilation during pre-oxygenation. [3]Awake intubation techniques include flexible bronchoscope, videolaryngoscopy, direct laryngoscopy, combined techniques, and retrograde wire-aided intubation. [4]Other options include, but are not limited to, alternative awake technique, awake elective invasive airway, alternative anesthetic techniques, induction of anesthesia (if unstable or cannot be postponed) with preparations for emergency invasive airway, and postponing the case without attempting the above options. [5]Invasive airway techniques include surgical cricothyrotomy, needle cricothyrotomy with a pressure-regulated device, large-bore cannula cricothyrotomy, or surgical tracheostomy. Elective invasive airway techniques include the above and retrograde wire-guided intubation and percutaneous tracheostomy. Also consider rigid bronchoscopy and ECMO. [6]Consideration of size, design, positioning, and first versus second-generation supraglottic airways may improve the ability to ventilate. [7]Alternative difficult intubation approaches include but are not limited to video-assisted laryngoscopy, alternative laryngoscope blades, combined techniques, intubating supraglottic airway (with or without flexible bronchoscopic guidance), flexible bronchoscopy, introducer, and lighted stylet or lightwand. Adjuncts that may be employed during intubation attempts include tracheal tube introducers, rigid stylets, intubating stylets, or tube changers and external laryngeal manipulation. [8]Includes postponing the case or postponing the intubation and returning with appropriate resources (e.g., personnel, equipment, patient preparation, awake intubation). [9]Other options include, but are not limited to, proceeding with procedure utilizing face mask or supraglottic airway ventilation. Pursuit of these options usually implies that ventilation will not be problematic.

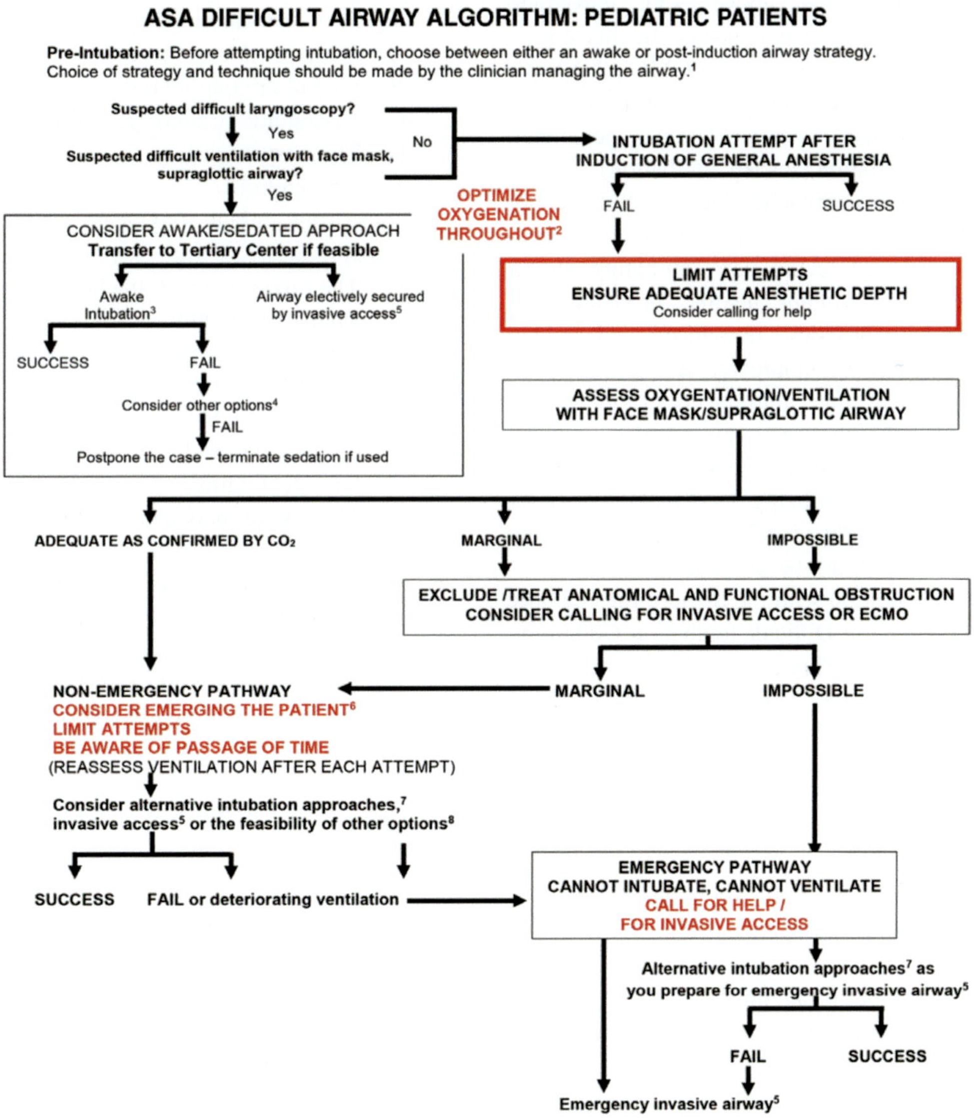

g. 2. Difficult airway algorithm: Pediatric patients. [41] [1]The airway manager's assessment and choice of techniques should be based on their previous experience; available resources, including equipment, availability, and competency of help; and the context in which airway management will occur. [2]Low- or high-flow nasal cannula, head elevated position throughout procedure. Noninvasive ventilation during preoxygenation. [3]Awake intubation techniques include flexible bronchoscope, videolaryngoscopy, direct laryngoscopy, combined techniques, and retrograde wire-aided intubation. [4]Other options include, but are not limited to, alternative awake technique, awake elective invasive airway, alternative anesthetic techniques, induction of anesthesia (if unstable or cannot be postponed) with preparations for emergency invasive airway, or postponing the case without attempting the above options. [5]Invasive airway techniques include surgical cricothyroidotomy, needle cricothyroidotomy if age-appropriate with a pressure-regulated device, large-bore cannula cricothyroidotomy, or surgical tracheostomy. Elective invasive airway techniques include the above and retrograde wire-guided intubation and percutaneous tracheostomy. Also consider rigid bronchoscopy and ECMO. [6]Includes postponing the case or postponing the intubation and returning with appropriate resources (e.g., personnel, equipment, patient preparation, awake intubation). [7]Alternative difficult intubation approaches include, but are not limited to, video-assisted laryngoscopy, alternative laryngoscope blades, combined techniques, intubating supraglottic airway (with or without flexible bronchoscopic guidance), flexible bronchoscopy, introducer, and lighted stylet. Adjuncts that may be employed during intubation attempts include tracheal tube introducers, rigid stylets, intubating stylets, or tube changers and external laryngeal manipulation. [8]Other options include, but are not limited to, proceeding with procedure utilizing face mask or supraglottic airway ventilation. Pursuit of these options usually implies that ventilation will not be problematic.

Developed in collaboration with the Society for Pediatric Anesthesia and the Pediatric Difficult Intubation Collaborative: John E. Fiadjoe, M.D., Thomas Engelhardt, M.D., Ph. D., F.R.C.A., Nicola Disma, M.D., Narasimhan Jagannathan, M.D., M.B.A., Britta S. von Ungern-Sternberg, M. D., Ph.D., D.E.A.A., F.A.N.Z.C.A., and Pete G. Kovatsis, M.D., F.A.A.P.

Updated highlights

In addition to the changes as alluded to above, some of the other important considerations include:

- Emphasis on the number of attempts.
- Emphasis on the passage of time: earlier invasive airway.
- Emphasis on provision of O_2 throughout the management of the difficult airway, including extubation.
- New list of suggested contents of standard anesthetizing location.

4.2.13 Questions and Answers

Questions (Choose the Most Appropriate Answer)

1. The muscles that serve as elevators of the larynx include all of the following except:
   A. Thyrohyoid
   B. Stylohyoid
   C. Sternothyroid
   D. Digastric
   E. Stylopharyngeus
2. All the intrinsic laryngeal muscles, except the cricothyroid muscle, are supplied by the recurrent laryngeal nerve. The latter is supplied by the external branch of the superior laryngeal nerve.
   A. Posterior cricoarytenoid
   B. Lateral cricoarytenoid
   C. Arytenoids (transverse and oblique)
   D. Thyroarytenoid
   E. Cricothyroid
3. Comparing infant (<1 year) and adult (>8 year) airways:
   A. The angle between trachea and right bronchus is smaller in infants.
   B. The narrowest position of the airway is glottis in infants and cricoid cartilage in adults.
   C. Only adults have a prominent protrusion of the corniculate and cuneiform tubercles into the laryngeal aditus.
   D. The angle between trachea and left bronchus remains unchanged.
4. Independent risk factors for difficult mask ventilation include all of the following, EXCEPT
   A. Sleep apnea
   B. Limited mandibular protrusion
   C. Body mass index < 21 kg/m2
   D. Facial hair
   E. Age > 55 years
5. The test that is the best indicator of a difficult intubation in a patient is:
   A. Obesity
   B. Mallampati score
   C. Neck circumference
   D. History of OSA
   E. History of snoring

6. A patient with bilateral superior laryngeal nerve palsy will present with
   A. Inspiratory stridor
   B. Expiratory stridor
   C. Complete airway obstruction
   D. Hoarseness of voice
   E. It will not affect the function of the vocal cords as it has no motor fibers
7. You have decided to undertake a cricothrotomy in a 40-year-old patient who cannot be intubated and cannot be ventilated. What is the largest size of tracheostomy tube that can be inserted through the cricothyroid membrane?
   A. Size 7.0
   B. Size 6.0.
   C. Size 5.0.
   D. Size 4.0.
   E. Size 3.0
8. Contraindications for transtracheal jet ventilation include all of the following except:
   A. Complete obstruction to the normal egress of air
   B. Increased cheat wall compliance
   C. Presence of pulmonary bullae
   D. Subcutaneous emphysema in the neck
   E. Local infiltration of tumor
9. Indications for the use of a double lumen endotracheal tube include all except
   A. Bronchopleural fistula
   B. Disruption of the main or major bronchi
   C. Prevent contamination of the lung from the contralateral side
   D. Esophageal surgery
   E. Lung lavage
10. Advantages of a bronchial blocker as compared to a double lumen tube include:
    A. Minimal displacement of the blocker once positioned
    B. Useful in patients with a tracheostomy stoma
    C. Rapid lung deflation following isolation
    D. Ease in clearing secretions from the isolated lung
    E. Lower incidence of mucosal ischemia and damaged

Answers

1. **C**. The sternothyroid is a part of the infrahyoid group of muscles and acts as a depressor of the larynx. All the other muscles are elevators.
2. **E**. The larynx is supplied by the recurrent laryngeal nerves and the internal and external branches of the superior laryngeal nerves. All the intrinsic muscles of the larynx except the cricothyroid muscle are supplied by the recurrent laryngeal nerve. The external branch of the superior laryngeal nerve supplies motor innervation to the cricothyroid muscle.
3. **D**. The angle between the trachea and the left bronchus is the same in infants as compared to adults. It usually measures about 45°. The right main stem bronchus tends to become shallower as the child ages.
4. **C**. Risk factors for difficult mask ventilation include older age greater than 55 years, body mass index greater than 30 kg/m^2, facial hair, limited mandibular protrusion, abnormal neck anatomy, sleep apnea, and a history of snoring.
5. **C**. The neck circumference was identified as a better predictor of difficult intubation in obese patients rather than the degree of obesity nor the presence of OSA.
6. **D**. The superior laryngeal nerve innervates the tensor of the vocal cord and its damage can lead to change in voice. The hoarseness might improve with time due to compensation from the other side. The cords may appear wavy on endoscopy. With total bilateral paralysis of the superior laryngeal nerves, the vocal cords are relaxed, abducted, and appear wavy (cadaveric position). On administration of muscle relaxants, a similar picture may be seen.
7. **B**. Size 6.0. The cricothyroid membrane's width varies between 22 and 33 mm in adults and the height between 9 and 10 mm. Hence, it would be difficult to pass a tracheostomy tube that measures greater the 9 mm (outer diameter). The outer diameter of a size 6 tracheostomy tube measures 8.3 mm. Therefore, size 6.0 is the largest tracheostomy tube that can be used for a surgical cricothyroidotomy in adult.
8. **B**. Decreased chest wall compliance is a contraindication.
9. **D**. Indications for a double lumen tube include:
   - 5 Isolation of lungs to prevent contamination from the contralateral lung
   - 5 Facilitate ventilation and/or limit ventilation-perfusion mismatch
   - 5 Facilitate surgical exposure
     - 5 Thoracic aortic aneurysm
     - 5 Pneumonectomy
     - 5 Thoracoscopy
     - 5 Upper lobectomy

     Relative indications include:
   - 5 To facilitate surgical exposure
     - 5 Lung resections involving the middle and lower lobes
     - 5 Segmental lung resections
     - 5 Esophageal resection
     - 5 Procedures on the thoracic spine

– 5 Lung trauma
– 5 Pulmonary edema after cardiopulmonary bypass
– 5 Preferential ventilation of 1 lung due to presence of unilateral lung disease

10. **B**. Disadvantages as compared to a double lumen tube:
    – 5 Slow lung deflation following isolation
    – 5 Slow lung inflation
    – 5 Inability to maintain toilet or suctioning out secretions
    – 5 Displacement of the blocker during positioning
    – 5 Higher incidence of mucosal ischemia and damage due to low-volume high-pressure cuffs
    – 5 Difficulty in management of desaturation
    – 5 Inability to administer CPAP
    – 5 Cumbersome to deflate and reinflate in case it becomes necessary.

They are indicated in patients with a tracheostomy tube in whom a double lumen tube cannot be placed in position.

References

1. Dalal PG, Murray D, Messner AH, Feng A, McAllister J, Molter D. Pediatric laryngeal dimensions: an age-based analysis. Anesth Analg. 2009;108(5):1475–9.
2. Masters IB, Ware RS, Zimmerman PV, Lovell B, Wootton R, Francis PV, et al. Airway sizes and proportions in children quantified by a video-bronchoscopic technique. BMC Pulm Med. 2006;6:5.
3. Boon JM, Abrahams PH, Meiring JH, Welch T. Cricothyroidotomy: a clinical anatomy review. Clin Anat. 2004;17(6):478–86.
4. Aslani A, Ng SC, Hurley M, McCarthy KF, McNicholas M, McCaul CL. Accuracy of identification of the cricothyroid membrane in female subjects using palpation: an observational study. Anesth Analg. 2012;114(5):987–92.
5. Bair AE, Chima R. The inaccuracy of using landmark techniques for cricothyroid membrane identification: a comparison of three techniques. Acad Emerg Med. 2015;22(8):908–14.
6. Elliott DS, Baker PA, Scott MR, Birch CW, Thompson JM. Accuracy of surface landmark identification for cannula cricothyroidotomy. Anaesthesia. 2010;65(9):889–94.
7. You-Ten KE, Desai D, Postonogova T, Siddiqui N. Accuracy of conventional digital palpation and ultrasound of the cricothyroid membrane in obese women in labour. Anaesthesia. 2015;70 (11):1230–4.
8. Mallampati SR, Gatt SP, Gugino LD, Desai SP, Waraksa B, Freiberger D, et al. A clinical sign to predict difficult tracheal intubation: a prospective study. Can Anaesth Soc J. 1985;32 (4):429–34.
9. Healy DW, LaHart EJ, Peoples EE, Jewell ES, Bettendorf RJ Jr, Ramachandran SK, et al. A comparison of the mallampati evaluation in neutral or extended cervical spine positions: a retrospective observational study of >80 000 patients. Br J Anaesth. 2016;116(5):690–8. https://doi.org/10.1093/bja/aew056; Br J Anaesth. 2016;117(Suppl 1):i103.
10. Samsoon GL, Young JR. Difficult tracheal intubation: a retrospective study. Anaesthesia. 1987;42(5):487–90.
11. Khan ZH. Airway assessment: a critical appraisal. In: Khan HZ, editor. Airway management. Cham: Springer International Publishing; 2014. p. 15–32.
12. Lewis M, Keramati S, Benumof JL, Berry CC. What is the best way to determine oropharyngeal classification and mandibular space length to predict difficult laryngoscopy? Anesthesiology. 1994;81(1):69–75.
13. Khan ZH, Khorasani AM, Yekaninejad MS. Mallampati Airway assessment test in upright and supine positions with and without noisy exhalation in the prediction of difficult mask ventilation. Intern Med. 2013;3:122. https://doi.org/10.4172/2165-8048.1000122.
14. Tremblay MH, Williams S, Robitaille A, Drolet P. Poor visualization during direct laryngoscopy and high upper lip bite test score are predictors of difficult intubation with the glidescope videolaryngoscope. Anesth Analg. 2008;106(5):1495–500. Table of contents.
15. Khan ZHMD, Kashfi AMD, Ebrahimkhani EMD. A comparison of the upper lip bite test (a simple new technique) with modified mallampati classification in predicting difficulty in endotracheal intubation: a prospective blinded study. Anesth Analg. 2003;96 (2):595–9.
16. Eberhart LHJMD, Arndt CMD, Cierpka TMD, Schwanekamp JMD, Wulf HMD, Putzke CMD. The reliability and validity of the upper lip bite test compared with the mallampati classification to predict difficult laryngoscopy: an external prospective evaluation. Anesth Analg. 2005;101(1):284–9.
17. Khan ZH, Mohammadi M, Rasouli MR, Farrokhnia F, Khan RH. The diagnostic value of the upper lip bite test combined with sternomental distance, thyromental distance, and interincisor distance for prediction of easy laryngoscopy and intubation: a prospective study. Anesth Analg. 2009;109(3):822–4.
18. Brodsky JB, Lemmens HJ, Brock-Utne JG, Vierra M, Saidman LJ. Morbid obesity and tracheal intubation. Anesth Analg. 2002;94(3):732–6. Table of contents.
19. Gonzalez H, Minville V, Delanoue K, Mazerolles M, Concina D, Fourcade O. The importance of increased neck circumference to intubation difficulties in obese patients. Anesth Analg. 2008;106 (4):1132–6. Table of contents.
20. Schmitt HJ, Kirmse M, Radespiel-Troger M. Ratio of patient's height to thyromental distance improves prediction of difficult laryngoscopy. Anaesth Intensive Care. 2002;30(6):763–5.
21. Butler PJ, Dhara SS. Prediction of difficult laryngoscopy: an assessment of the thyromental distance and mallampati predictive tests. Anaesth Intensive Care. 1992;20(2):139–42.
22. Etezadi F, Ahangari A, Shokri H, Najafi A, Khajavi MR, Daghigh M, et al. Thyromental height: a new clinical test for prediction of difficult laryngoscopy. Anesth Analg. 2013;117 (6):1347–51.
23. Cass NM, James NR, Lines V. Difficult direct laryngoscopy complicating intubation for anaesthesia. Br Med J. 1956;1 (4965):488–9.
24. White A, Kander PL. Anatomical factors in difficult direct laryngoscopy. Br J Anaesth. 1975;47(4):468–74.
25. Chou HC, Wu TL. Mandibulohyoid distance in difficult laryngoscopy. Br J Anaesth. 1993;71(3):335–9.
26. Munster T, Hoffmann M, Schlaffer S, Ihmsen H, Schmitt H, Tzabazis A. Anatomical location of the vocal cords in relation to cervical vertebrae: a new predictor of difficult laryngoscopy? Eur J Anaesthesiol. 2016;33(4):257–62.
27. Suzuki N, Isono S, Ishikawa T, Kitamura Y, Takai Y, Nishino T. Submandible angle in nonobese patients with difficult tracheal intubation. Anesthesiology. 2007;106(5):916–23.
28. Connor CW, Segal S. Accurate classification of difficult intubation by computerized facial analysis. Anesth Analg. 2011;112(1): 84–93.

29. Wilson ME, Spiegelhalter D, Robertson JA, Lesser P. Predicting difficult intubation. Br J Anaesth. 1988;61(2):211–6.
30. Krage R, van Rijn C, van Groeningen D, Loer SA, Schwarte LA, Schober P. Cormack-lehane classification revisited. Br J Anaesth [Research Support, Non-US Gov't Validation Studies]. 2010;105 (2):220–7.
31. Cook TM. A new practical classification of laryngeal view. Anaesthesia. 2000;55(3):274–9.
32. Levitan RM, Ochroch EA, Kush S, Shofer FS, Hollander JE. Assessment of airway visualization: validation of the percentage of glottic opening (pogo) scale. Acad Emerg Med. 1998;5(9):919–23.
33. Adnet F, Borron SW, Racine SX, Clemessy JL, Fournier JL, Plaisance P, et al. The intubation difficulty scale (ids): proposal and evaluation of a new score characterizing the complexity of endotracheal intubation. Anesthesiology [Comparative Study]. 1997;87(6):1290–7.
34. Lavi R, Segal D, Ziser A. Predicting difficult airways using the intubation difficulty scale: a study comparing obese and non-obese patients. J Clin Anesth. 2009;21(4):264–7.
35. Benumof and Hagberg's airway management. 3rd ed; Copyright: © Saunders 2013 Published: 24th September 2012: eBook ISBN: 9781455738106; Chapter 20 Retrograde intubation techniques. Antonio Sanchez. p. 412–29.
36. Li J, Murphy-Lavoie H, Bugas C, Martinez J, Preston C. Complications of emergency intubation with and without paralysis. Am J Emerg Med. 1999;17(2):141–3.
37. Schmidt UH, Kumwilaisak K, Bittner E, George E, Hess D. Effects of supervision by attending anesthesiologists on complications of emergency tracheal intubation. Anesthesiology. 2008;109(6):973–7.
38. Rosenstock C, Hansen EG, Kristensen MS, Rasmussen LS, Skak C, Ostergaard D. Qualitative analysis of unanticipated difficult airway management. Acta Anaesthesiol Scand. 2006;50 (3):290–7.
39. Richardson MG, Litman RS. Ventilation before paralysis: crossing the rubicon, slowly. Anesthesiology. 2012;117(3):456–8.
40. Calder I, Yentis SM. Could 'safe practice' be compromising safe practice? Should anaesthetists have to demonstrate that face mask ventilation is possible before giving a neuromuscular blocker? Anaesthesia. 2008;63(2):113–5.
41. Apfelbaum, J.L., Hagberg CA, Connis RT, Abdelmalak BB, Agarkar M, Dutton RP, Fiadjoe JE, Greif R, Klock PA, Jr., Mercier D, Myatra SN, O'Sullivan EP, Rosenblatt WH , Sorbello M, Avery, 2022 American society of anesthesiologists practice guidelines for management of the difficult airway. Anesthesiology. 2022;136(1):31–81.
42. Kheterpal S, Han R, Tremper KK, Shanks A, Tait AR, O'Reilly M, et al. Incidence and predictors of difficult and impossible mask ventilation. Anesthesiology. 2006;105(5):885–91.
43. Kopman AF, Klewicka MM, Neuman GG. An alternate method for estimating the dose-response relationships of neuromuscular blocking drugs. Anesth Analg. 2000;90(5):1191–7.
44. Smith CE, Donati F, Bevan DR. Dose-response curves for succinylcholine: single versus cumulative techniques. Anesthesiology. 1988;69(3):338–42.
45. Chestnut RJ, Healy TE, Harper NJ, Faragher EB. Suxamethonium–the relation between dose and response. Anaesthesia. 1989;44(1):14–8.
46. Donati F. Neuromuscular blocking drugs for the new millennium: current practice, future trends–comparative pharmacology of neuromuscular blocking drugs. Anesth Analg. 2000;90(5 Suppl): S2-6.
47. Jaradi H, Tay KH, Delilkan AE. Shortening the onset time of atracurium for rapid tracheal intubation. Med J Malaysia. 1989;44 (2):143–6.
48. Hung OR, Stewart RD. Lightwand intubation: I—a new lightwand device. Can J Anaesth. 1995;42(9):820–5.
49. Hung OR, Pytka S, Morris I, Murphy M, Launcelott G, Stevens S, et al. Clinical trial of a new lightwand device (trachlight) to intubate the trachea. Anesthesiology. 1995;83(3):509–14.
50. Hung OR, Pytka S, Morris I, Murphy M, Stewart RD. Lightwand intubation: Ii—clinical trial of a new lightwand for tracheal intubation in patients with difficult airways. Can J Anaesth. 1995;42(9):826–30.
51. Ellis DG, Jakymec A, Kaplan RM, Stewart RD, Freeman JA, Bleyaert A, et al. Guided orotracheal intubation in the operating room using a lighted stylet: a comparison with direct laryngoscopic technique. Anesthesiology. 1986;64(6):823–6.
52. Bannister FB, Macbeth RG. Direct laryngoscopy and tracheal intubation. Lancet. 1944;250(2):651–4.
53. Miller L. Choosing a laryngoscope blade: straight versu curved. Can J Anaesth. 2003;50(10):1079–80.
54. Benumof and Hagberg's airway management. 3rd ed; Copyright: © Saunders 2013 Published: 24th September 2012: eBook ISBN: 9781455738106; Chapter 24 Upper airway retraction: new and old laryngoscope blades Richard M Levitan, Carin A Hagberg. p. 508–35.
55. Negri de Sousa AC, Levy CE, Freitas MI. Laryngoscope blades and handles as sources of cross-infection: an integrative review. J Hosp Infect [Review]. 2013;83(4):269–75.
56. Asai T. Videolaryngoscopes: do they truly have roles in difficult airways? Anesthesiology [Comment Editorial]. 2012;116(3):515–7.
57. Brown CA 3rd, Bair AE, Pallin DJ, Laurin EG, Walls RM. National emergency airway registry I. Improved glottic exposure with the video macintosh laryngoscope in adult emergency department tracheal intubations. Ann Emerg Med. 2010;56 (2):83–8.
58. Piepho T, Fortmueller K, Heid FM, Schmidtmann I, Werner C, Noppens RR. Performance of the c-mac video laryngoscope in patients after a limited glottic view using macintosh laryngoscopy. Anaesthesia. 2011;66(12):1101–5.
59. Griesdale DE, Liu D, McKinney J, Choi PT. Glidescope(r) video-laryngoscopy versus direct laryngoscopy for endotracheal intubation: a systematic review and meta-analysis. Can J Anaesth. 2012;59(1):41–52.
60. Karalapillai D, Darvall J, Mandeville J, Ellard L, Graham J, Weinberg L. A review of video laryngoscopes relevant to the intensive care unit. Indian J Crit Care Med. 2014;18(7):442–52.
61. Kleine-Brueggeney M, Greif R, Schoettker P, Savoldelli GL, Nabecker S, Theiler LG. Evaluation of six videolaryngoscopes in 720 patients with a simulated difficult airway: a multicentre randomized controlled trial. Br J Anaesth. 2016;116(5):670–9.
62. Heuer JF, Heitmann S, Crozier TA, Bleckmann A, Quintel M, Russo SG. A comparison between the glidescope(r) classic and glidescope(r) direct video laryngoscopes and direct laryngoscopy for nasotracheal intubation. J Clin Anesth. 2016;33:330–6.
63. Vincent RD Jr, Wimberly MP, Brockwell RC, Magnuson JS. Soft palate perforation during orotracheal intubation facilitated by the glidescope videolaryngoscope. J Clin Anesth. 2007;19(8):619–21.
64. Manickam BP, Adhikary SD. Re: soft palate perforation during orotracheal intubation facilitated by the glidescope videolaryngoscope. J Clin Anesth. 2008;20(5):401–2; Author reply 403.
65. Benumof and Hagberg's airway management. 3rd ed; Copyright: © Saunders 2013 Published: 24th September 2012: eBook ISBN: 9781455738106; Chapter 30 Percutaneous dilational cricothyrotomy and tracheostomy David Cattano, Laura, F Cavallone: p. 613–39.
66. Freeman BD, Isabella K, Lin N, Buchman TG. A meta-analysis of prospective trials comparing percutaneous and surgical tracheostomy in critically ill patients. Chest. 2000;118(5):1412–8.

67. Friedman Y, Fildes J, Mizock B, Samuel J, Patel S, Appavu S, et al. Comparison of percutaneous and surgical tracheostomies. Chest. 1996;110(2):480–5.
68. Silvester W, Goldsmith D, Uchino S, Bellomo R, Knight S, Seevanayagam S, et al. Percutaneous versus surgical tracheostomy: a randomized controlled study with long-term follow-up. Crit Care Med. 2006;34(8):2145–52.
69. Freeman BD, Isabella K, Cobb JP, Boyle WA 3rd, Schmieg RE Jr, Kolleff MH, et al. A prospective, randomized study comparing percutaneous with surgical tracheostomy in critically ill patients. Crit Care Med. 2001;29(5):926–30.
70. Teller LE, Alexander CM, Frumin MJ, Gross JB. Pharyngeal insufflation of oxygen prevents arterial desaturation during apnea. Anesthesiology. 1988;69(6):980–2.
71. Wimalasena Y, Burns B, Reid C, Ware S, Habig K. Apneic oxygenation was associated with decreased desaturation rates during rapid sequence intubation by an australian helicopter emergency medicine service. Ann Emerg Med. 2015;65(4):371–6.
72. Jen Heng Pek HMK, Wong E. Improving apnoeic oxygenation use for rapid sequence intubation in an emergency department. Trends Anaesthesia Crit Care. 2017;13:25–31.
73. Nedel WL, Deutschendorf C, Moraes Rodrigues Filho E. High-flow nasal cannula in critically ill subjects with or at risk for respiratory failure: a systematic review and meta-analysis. Respir Care. 2017;62(1):123–32.
74. Williams R, Rankin N, Smith T, Galler D, Seakins P. Relationship between the humidity and temperature of inspired gas and the function of the airway mucosa. Crit Care Med. 1996;24(11):1920–9.
75. Parke RL, McGuinness SP, Eccleston ML. A preliminary randomized controlled trial to assess effectiveness of nasal high-flow oxygen in intensive care patients. Respir Care. 2011;56(3):265–70.
76. Brodsky JB, Macario A, Mark JB. Tracheal diameter predicts double-lumen tube size: a method for selecting left double-lumen tubes. Anesth Analg. 1996;82(4):861–4.
77. Slinger P. Choosing the appropriate double-lumen tube: a glimmer of science comes to a dark art. J Cardiothorac Vasc Anesth. 1995;9 (2):117–8.
78. Bedger RC Jr, Chang JL. A jet-stylet endotracheal catheter for difficult airway management. Anesthesiology. 1987;66(2):221–3.
79. Mandell-Brown MK, Bedger R, Chang JL, Johnson JT. Jet stylet catheter for airway management. Laryngoscope. 1987;97(9):1104–5.

Part II
Pharmacology

Contents

Pharmacology: General Concepts

5

Aaron Hawke and Kamal Maheshwari

Abstract

Medicine is intimately associated with a thorough understanding of clinical pharmacology. Many drugs have been discovered by observing natural materials—for example, plants—and their effects on animals. The physical effect of a drug, either positive or negative, can be observed without the knowledge of its mechanism of action. Modern drug discovery takes a different approach. Starting with a hypothesis that a certain protein is implicated in a disease, small molecules are screened for targeting the protein for the therapeutic effect; these are ultimately tested for a desired effect in basic science and clinical trials. The study of the interaction of the drug with the physiology of the body is the basis of clinical pharmacology. Pharmacokinetics describes the journey of the drug in the body whereas pharmacodynamics focuses on the physiological effects of the drug. Pharmacogenomics evaluate the role of genetics in drug response.

Keywords

Pharmacology • Anatomy • Pharmacokinetics • Absorption • Distribution • Metabolism • Excretion • Pharmacodynamics • Dose response • Potency • Efficacy • Therapeutic window • Drug interactions • Pharmacogenomics • Genetics

Key Points

- The role of the biological membrane includes encasing the aqueous compartment of the cell from its surroundings and housing membrane-bound proteins. It also plays an important role in signal transduction pathways. Transporter-membrane proteins control the influx of essential nutrients and ions and the efflux of cellular waste, environmental toxins, drugs, and other xenobiotics.
- Nervous tissues are composed of specialized cells called neurons whose major function is to receive, integrate, and transmit information to other cells. Signals are propagated electrically along the axon of the neuron, which terminates on the next cell at the synapse.
- The contractile apparatus of muscle tissues are made of thick filaments containing mainly myosin and thin filaments containing mainly actin arranged into an intercrossing array called sarcomeres. Contraction is due to the cyclic interaction between the two myofilaments coupled with the hydrolysis of adenosine triphosphate (ATP).
- Most drugs are weak acids or bases and exist in equilibrium between the ionized and non-ionized forms in the body, which in turn depends on the drug pKa. Non-ionized forms are usually more lipid soluble and diffuse readily across the cell membrane to their target site.
- Absorption of a drug depends on the route of administration, the physical characteristic of the drug, the dose, and the site of absorption. Bioavailability is the fraction of the administered drug that is present in the systemic circulation.
- Well-perfused organs receiving a high fraction of the cardiac output receive comparatively higher amounts of the drug early after drug administration. These vessel-rich tissue groups reach equilibrium quickly relative to blood concentration. Less well-perfused groups such as muscle,

A. Hawke
Anesthesiology Residency Program, Cleveland Clinic Foundation, Anesthesia Institute, Cleveland, OH, USA
e-mail: hawkea2@ccf.org

K. Maheshwari (✉)
Departments of General Anesthesiology and Outcomes Research, Cleveland Clinic Foundation, Anesthesia Institute, Cleveland, OH, USA
e-mail: mahesk@ccf.org

M. Argalious et al. (eds.), *Basic Sciences in Anesthesia*,
https://doi.org/10.1007/978-3-031-60203-0_5

fat, and skin may require hours before the drug reaches equilibrium with the blood concentration.
- Volume of distribution is the theoretical volume that the drug has distributed in the body. It can be calculated by dividing the bolus dose by the measured blood concentration after a defined period of time.
- Important parameters of the dose response curve are the EC 50 (concentration of the drug that achieves 50% of the maximum response) and Emax (maximum value of the body's response to the drug).
- Several metabolic enzymes were found to be due to monogenic phenotypic variations and thereby can be referenced according to their phenotype traits such as fast vs. slow metabolizer.

5.1 Introduction

Medicine is intimately associated with a thorough understanding of clinical pharmacology. Many drugs have been discovered by observing natural materials—for example, plants—and their effects on animals. The physical effect of a drug, either positive or negative, can be observed without the knowledge of its mechanism of action. Modern drug discovery takes a different approach. Starting with a hypothesis that a certain protein is implicated in a disease, small molecules are screened for targeting the protein for the therapeutic effect; these are ultimately tested for a desired effect in basic science and clinical trials. The study of the interaction of the drug with the physiology of the body is the basis of clinical pharmacology [1, 2].

5.2 General Concepts

We need to understand following basic anatomy and physiology concepts at the cellular level where most drugs exert their effects [3–5].

5.2.1 Lipid Bilayer and Membrane

Biological cells are surrounded by a lipid bilayer usually composed of an amphiphilic phospholipid bilayer with hydrophilic phospholipid head and hydrophobic fatty acid tail [6, 7]. The role of the biological membrane includes encasing the aqueous compartment of the cell from its surroundings, housing membrane-bound proteins, as well as playing an important role in signal transduction pathways. Movement of polar compounds (drugs) across the membrane requires transport proteins (◉ Fig. 5.1). Some transport proteins merely facilitate passive diffusion down a concentration gradient, while others transport chemicals against an electrochemical gradient, requiring metabolic energy.

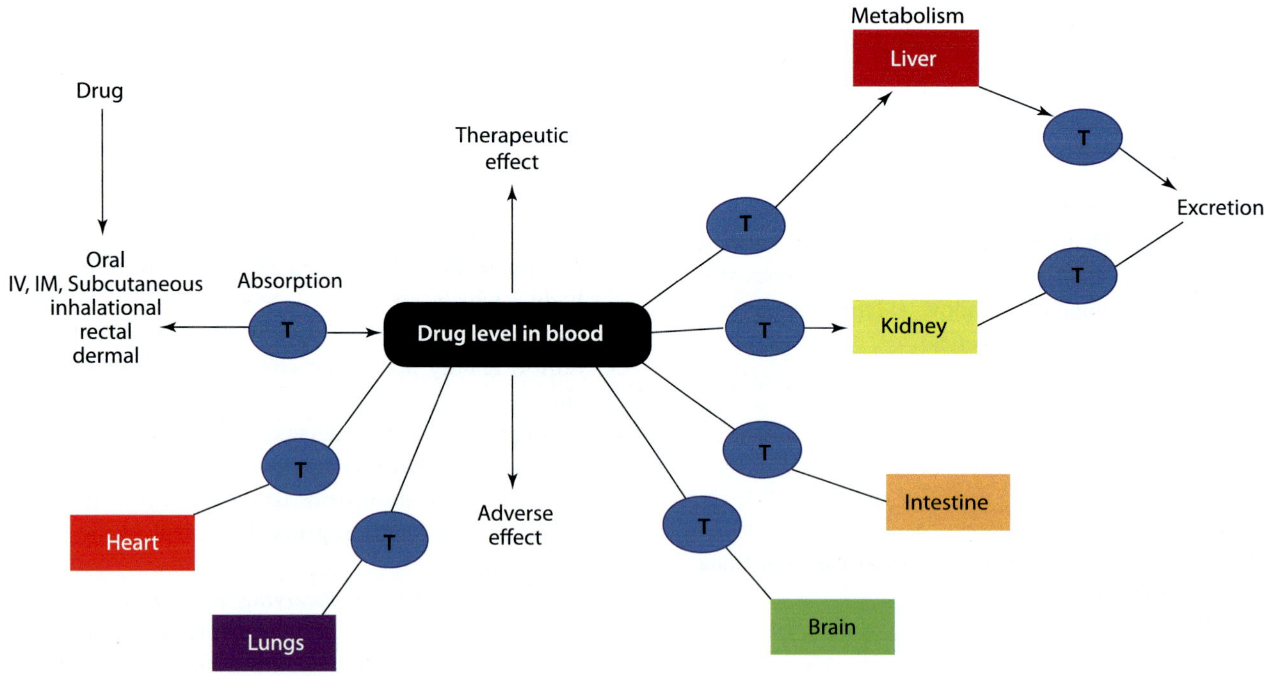

Fig. 5.1 Roles of membrane transporters in pharmacokinetic pathways. Membrane transporters (T) play important roles in pharmacokinetic pathways (drug absorption, distribution, metabolism, and excretion), thereby setting systemic drug levels. Drug levels often drive therapeutic and adverse drug effects

5.2.2 Nervous Tissue

There are three major nervous systems in the body: the central nervous system, the peripheral nervous system, and autonomic nervous system. Nervous tissues are composed of specialized cells called neurons whose major function is to receive, integrate, and transmit information to other cells. Signals are propagated electrically along the axon of the neuron, which terminates on the next cell at the synapse. Like other cells in the body, the membrane potential of neurons is primarily due to the function of Na+/K+ ATPase.

The resting membrane potential (normally − 60 to − 90 mV in unstimulated neurons) is determined by Na+ /K + ATPase and the membrane permeability. Na+/K+ ATPase actively pumps Na+out of the cell in exchange for K+. The cell membrane is practically impermeable to Na+ but K + leak channels that allow the transport of K+out of the cell until an equilibrium is reached between the balance of electrochemical gradient. In addition, neurons are highly specialized cells that are able to use rapid changes in membrane potential in order to generate electrical signals, mainly action potentials. This is accomplished by ligand-gated or voltage-gated ion channels that allow the passage of Na+, K+, Ca2+, and Cl− in response to electrical or chemical stimuli.

5.2.3 Muscle Tissue

Muscle tissues are composed of cells that are able to contract and shorten with the supply of ATP. Classic teaching divides muscle tissues into skeletal, cardiac, and smooth muscles. The contractile apparatus of muscle tissues are made of thick filaments containing mainly myosin and thin filaments containing mainly actin arranged into an intercrossing array called sarcomeres. Contraction is due to the cyclic interaction between the two myofilaments coupled with the hydrolysis of ATP. The shortening of the sarcomere is made possible by the relative movement of the myosin head along the actin filament.

Specialized synapses called neuromuscular junctions couple motor nerve impulses to muscle contractions by the action of Ca2+ ion on the troponin regulatory complex. Nerve impulses arriving at the junction cause the depolarization of myofilament resulting in the release of Ca2+ ion stored in sarcoplasmic reticulum. Binding of Ca2+ to troponin allows the cross-bridge formation between the myosin and actin filaments. Relaxation occurs when Ca2+ is pumped back into the sarcoplasmic reticulum.

5.2.4 Lipid Solubility

The lipid solubility can be defined as the relative partition of the substance between oil and water. The tissue distribution of the drug is determined by the partition of the drug between the blood and various tissues. The higher the lipid solubility of the substance, the easier it crosses the membrane bilayer to reach the target tissue. Most drugs are weak acids or bases and exist in equilibrium between the ionized and non-ionized forms in the body, which in turn depends on the drug pKa. pKa is the pH at which the amount of the substance in non-ionized form equals that of the ionized form. Non-ionized forms are usually more lipid soluble and diffuse readily across the cell membrane to their target site.

5.2.4.1 Ionization

Most drugs exist in both non-ionized and ionized forms in the body. The non-ionized (uncharged) form crosses the membrane easier compared to the ionized form. Flux across the membrane bilayer depends on the pKa of the drug and the pH gradient across the membrane.

5.2.4.2 Ion Trapping

Ion trapping is the accumulation of a drug across the membrane due to the pKa of the drug and the difference in pH across the membrane. For example, local anesthetics are weak bases; they are able to cross the placental membrane in the non-ionized or basic forms. Once crossing the placenta, the increased acidity of the fetal circulation favors the ionization of the local anesthetic into the acidic form. The ionized (acidic) form of the drug does not easily cross the placental membrane back to the maternal circulation, resulting in the "trapping" of local anesthetic in the fetus.

5.2.5 Water Solubility

The absorption, distribution, and elimination of a drug depends on its relative water solubility. Water-soluble substances do not readily diffuse through the membrane bilayer and require the facilitation of specific membrane transporter proteins. Oral absorption favors the non-ionized and more lipid-soluble form of the drug, while excretory organs favor the elimination of more polar compounds.

5.2.6 Transporter: Membrane Proteins

Transporter-membrane proteins control the influx of essential nutrients and ions and the efflux of cellular waste, environmental toxins, drugs, and other xenobiotics. The functions of membrane transporters may be facilitated (equilibrate, not requiring energy) or active (requiring energy). The active transport is of two types. Primary active transport is driven by ATP hydrolysis or electron transfer reaction. Secondary active transport is driven by coupled flow of two distinct solutes, in which one solute flows down its electrochemical gradient while pulling the other up against its gradient.

5.3 Pharmacokinetics

Pharmacokinetics are essentially what the body does to the drug. All drugs, as foreign substances, go through the processes of absorption, distribution, metabolism, and elimination in the body. The route of administration can influence this multi-step process.

5.3.1 Absorption

Absorption is the process by which the drug moves from the site of administration to the blood stream. Absorption depends on the route of administration, the physical characteristic of the drug, the dose, and the site of absorption. Bioavailability is the fraction of the administered drug that is present in the systemic circulation.

5.3.1.1 Route of Administration

Drugs can be administered via various routes: oral, sublingual, inhalational, rectal, transdermal, transmucosal, subcutaneous, intramuscular, and intravenous. Oral administration is most common and is cheap, easy, and relatively safe. The absorption from the gastrointestinal (GI) tract is determined by surface area, blood flow, and the concentration and the physical characteristic of the drug. Non-ionized (uncharged) forms of the drug are more readily absorbed than ionized (charged) forms. Most absorption occurs in the smaller intestine compared to the stomach due to the extremely large surface area provided by the villi and the longer transit duration. Accordingly, factors that accelerate gastric emptying will speed the rate of drug absorption while factors that delay gastric emptying will slow the rate of drug absorption.

Drugs follow the venous drainage of the stomach and small intestine and are delivered to the liver via the portal system. Therefore, bioavailability of orally administered drugs is limited to the first-pass hepatic metabolism. On the other hand, sublingual and transmucosal drug administration bypass the first-pass metabolism because veins of mouth and esophagus drain directly into the inferior vena cava. Around 50% of rectally administered drugs will bypass the liver, potentially increasing the bioavailability compared to orally administered drugs. However, rectal administration of a drug could be erratic and incomplete. In addition, many drugs cause irritation to mucosal membrane.

Transdermal absorption depends on the surface area, blood flow to the skin, and the lipid solubility of the drug because the dermis layer is essentially a lipid barrier. The epidermis allows passage of most substances easily. Thus, increased absorption through damaged skin, such as from burns, could result in toxicity. Similarly, inflammation increases cutaneous blood flow and also increases transdermal absorption of drugs. Examples of transdermal absorption of drugs include fentanyl and scopolamine patches.

The parental route of administration includes subcutaneous, intramuscular, intravenous, and intra-arterial. Subcutaneous and intramuscular absorption depend on the passive diffusion from the drug depot to the plasma. The rate is limited by the blood flow and the relative solubility of the drug in the interstitial fluid. Bioavailability of intravenous administration is rapid and complete by bypassing the process of absorption. The dose of the drug can be titrated to the response of the patient, for example, during the induction of anesthesia. The effect of the drug from intravenous administration must be monitored as toxicity often occurs with high plasma concentration attained in a short duration of time. Other than rare intra-arterial administration, all parental administration of drugs is subject to first-pass metabolism of the lung. The lung provides temporary storage for a number of substances, filters the particulate substance, and serves as a site of elimination for volatile agents.

5.3.1.2 Dosage

The drug dosage is based on patient characteristics and the route of administration. In pediatric patients, drugs are dosed by the total body weight. In adults, especially with the increasing prevalence of obesity, it is sometimes difficult to find the optimal dosage of a drug and drugs need to be titrated to effect.

Lean body weight (LBW) is calculated according to height and weight, while ideal body weight (IBW) is calculated only according to height [7, 8]:

For men: LBW = (0.32810 * Weight) + (0.33929 * Height) – 29.5336

IBW = 50 kg + 2.3 * (height over 60 in.) [7]

For women: LBW = (0.29569 * Weight) + (0.41813 * Height) – 43.2933

IBW = 45.5 kg + 2.3 * (height over 60 in.) [7]

Obese individuals have an increased total body weight and lean body weight. The ratio of lean body weight to total body weight, however, decreases as total body weight increases. Dosing drugs according to total body weight risks over dosing, while dosing drugs according to lean body weight risks under dosing [9]. A highly lipophilic or hydrophilic compound needs adjustment in particular due to the change in volume of distribution. However, most anesthetic drugs can be dosed by lean body weight, except for highly water-soluble drugs such as neuromuscular blockers, where dosing according to ideal body weight might be more appropriate. Drugs such as succinylcholine should be dosed according to total body weight.

5.3.1.3 First-Pass Metabolism

The venous drainage of the gastrointestinal system first passes the liver through the portal vein system before accessing the systemic venous system. Drugs administered by the oral route are all subjected to this first-pass hepatic metabolism, thereby decreasing their bioavailability in the systemic circulation.

5.3.2 Distribution

Once a drug is absorbed into the systemic circulation, it is distributed throughout the different tissues of the body depending on the cardiac output, regional blood flow, capillary permeability, and tissue volume. Well-perfused organs receiving a high fraction of the cardiac output (brain, heart, kidney, liver) receive a disproportionate amount of the drug early after drug administration. These vessel-rich tissue groups reach equilibrium quickly. Less well-perfused groups such as muscle, fat, and skin may require hours before equilibration with the blood concentration. Therefore, they have the potential of serving as a large reservoir for the drug after prolonged infusion. Tissue distribution of the drug depends on the partition between the blood and the specific tissue.

5.3.2.1 First-Order Kinetics

The clearance of the drug refers to the unit plasma that is completely clear of the drug per unit of time. Most drug clearance follow a first-order kinetics in which a constant fraction of the drug is eliminated from the body per unit of time. There is an exponential increase in metabolism with increase in the dose to maintain constant fraction metabolism (◉ Fig. 5.2a).

5.3.2.2 Zero-Order Kinetics

When the elimination mechanism of the drug becomes saturated, clearance kinetics approaches zero order, whereby a constant amount of drug is cleared per unit time. Examples of drugs that undergo zero-order kinetics include ethanol, salicylate, and phenytoin. The enzymes involved in the metabolic process are quickly saturated; thus, a constant amount of drug is eliminated regardless of the plasma concentration (◉ Fig. 5.2b).

5.3.2.3 Compartment Model

Volume of distribution is the theoretical volume that the drug has distributed in the body. It can be calculated by dividing the bolus dose by the measured blood concentration after a defined period of time. Most drugs in anesthesia can be modeled by a two-compartment model: a central compartment containing the blood and ultra-rapid equilibrating tissue such as the lung and a peripheral compartment containing other tissues. Some drugs are better modeled by a three-compartment model: (1) central, (2) rapid equilibrating peripheral (vessel-rich tissue groups), and (3) a

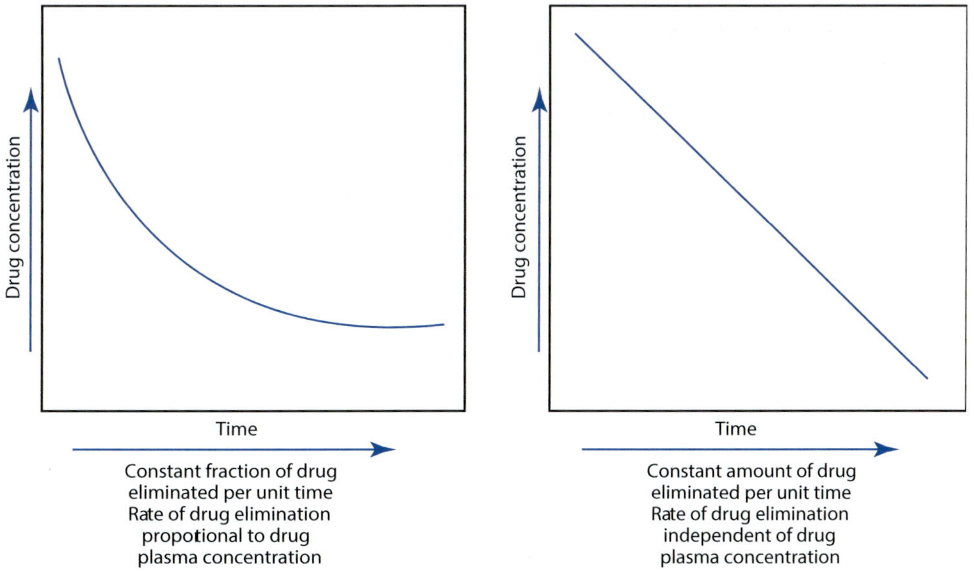

Fig. 5.2 **a** First and **b** zero kinetics of drug clearance

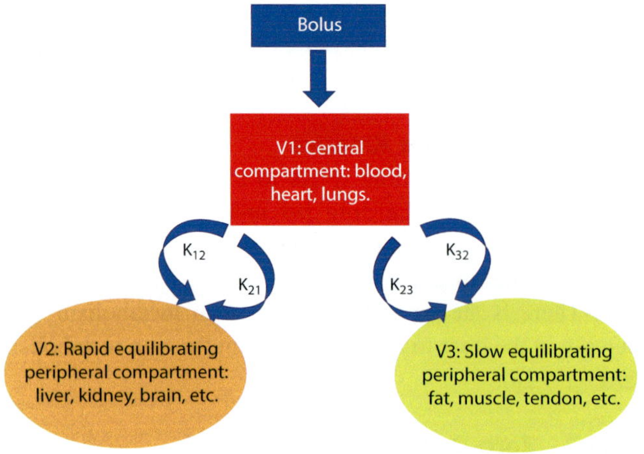

Fig. 5.3 Three-compartment model: central compartment, rapid equilibrating peripheral compartment (vessel rich), and slow equilibrating compartment (vessel poor). Two-compartment model: central compartment, peripheral compartment

slow equilibrating peripheral (vessel-poor tissue groups) (◉ Fig. 5.3). When modeled by two compartments, the course of the bolused drug first goes through a distribution phase in which the plasma concentration rapidly decreases due to the diffusion of the drug to the peripheral compartment, followed by the much slower elimination phase, which consists of metabolism and excretion.

5.3.2.4 Half-Life

The elimination half-life is the time required for the plasma drug concentration to fall by 50% [10]. Since many drugs used in anesthesia are best modeled using a multi-compartment model, there will be multiple elimination half-lives. Therefore, the half-life of the drug will be context dependent (discussed later). The clinical effect of the drug cannot be easily predicted using the terminal half-life.

5.3.2.5 Protein Binding

Many drugs in the systemic circulation are bound by plasma proteins. Albumin is chiefly responsible for binding acidic drugs while α(alpha)1-acid glycoprotein binds basic drugs. Bound and unbound drug molecules exist in almost instant equilibrium in the plasma and tissues. Distribution of drug molecules obey the law of mass action. If the free drug concentration gradient favors that of the tissue, the drug moves from plasma to the tissue. If a drug is not bound in the plasma but highly bound in the tissue, the free drug will move from the plasma to the tissue. On the other hand, if the drug is highly bound in the plasma but the binding site in the tissue is limited, the drug will stay in the plasma. Conditions that decrease plasma binding protein such as kidney failure, liver disease, chronic congestive heart failure, infection, and malignancies will decrease the relative solubility of the drug in the blood, thereby increasing tissue uptake.

5.3.2.6 Difference Between Bolus and Infusion Administration

Emergence is rapid after a bolus injection of a drug mainly due to the process of distribution to the peripheral compartment in a matter of minutes. After a prolonged infusion of a drug, tissue concentrations of the drug are in equilibrium with plasma; the redistribution process then delays the emergence after removal of drug infusion due to the drug returning to the plasma from the tissue reservoir.

5.3.2.7 Context Sensitive Half-Life

This refers to the time required for a 50% decrease in plasma concentration after a pseudo-state infusion (◉ Fig. 5.4). For many drugs, half-life depends on the length of the infusion; i.e., context.

5.3.3 Metabolism

Metabolism is the process in which the drug is altered in the body. Enzymes responsible for the majority of the drug biotransformation are located in the liver. Other tissues that play a role in drug metabolism include the gastrointestinal tract, the kidney, and the lung.

5.3.3.1 Phase I

Phase I metabolism deals with functionalization reactions, or the addition or exposure of functional groups to a compound by way of oxidation, reduction, or hydrolysis. This process generally results in a more reactive compound. Oxidation refers to the loss of electrons, loss of hydrogen, or gain of an oxygen atom, thereby increasing the chemical's oxidation state. Reduction refers to the gain of electrons, gain of hydrogen, or loss of oxygen atom, thereby decreasing the chemical's oxidation state. Hydrolysis refers

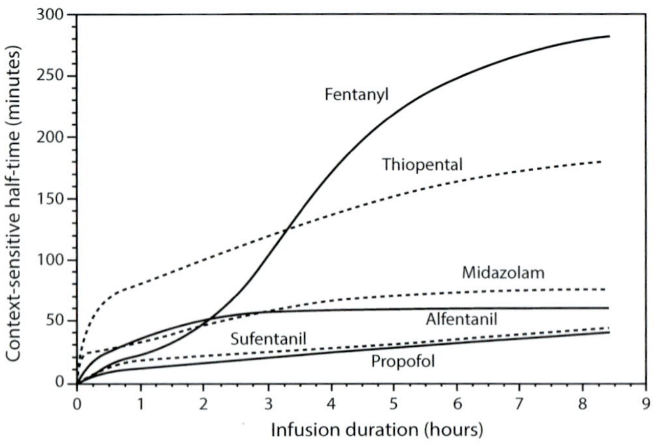

Fig. 5.4 Context sensitive half-life of common anesthetic agents (Reprinted with permission from Glass [10])

to the breaking of a covalent bond using a molecule of water. The majority of reactions that occur during phase I metabolism are oxidation reactions carried out by microsomal enzymes in the endoplasmic reticulum of hepatocytes, which constitute the cytochrome P450 system. Various isoforms are responsible for the metabolism of specific drugs. Drugs may also affect the function of specific P450 enzymes and can act as either inducers, which speed up the rate of metabolism of other drugs metabolized by that particular isoform, or inhibitors of the enzyme, which leads to a decreased rate of metabolism of other drugs. When certain substrates of a particular isoform are co-administered, drug–drug interactions may occur.

5.3.3.2 Phase II

Usually biosynthetic or conjugation reactions lead to the formation of a covalent bond between the parent drug compound or the phase I metabolite with endogenous polar groups such as glucuronic acid, sulfate, glutathione, amino acid, or acetate and thereby increase the water solubility of the compound resulting in rapid elimination in the urine or feces.

5.3.4 Excretion

About 25–50% of drugs are eliminated unchanged in the body; the rest undergo some process of metabolism. Opposite from absorption that favors lipophilic substances, the process of elimination favors polar compounds.

5.3.4.1 Renal Clearance

Renal clearance is the most important process by which drugs are eliminated from the body. Three important processes involved are glomerular filtration, active tubular secretion, and passive tubular reabsorption. Glomerular filtration of the drug to tubular fluid depends on the glomerular filtration rate (GFR) and amount of protein binding as only the free drug molecules are filtered. The apical cell membrane in the proximal tubule hosts transporters that actively secrete conjugated drug metabolites to the tubular fluid. The majority of tubular reabsorption is through diffusion of the non-ionized form of the drug metabolites and therefore depends on the pH gradient between the tubular urine and the plasma.

5.3.4.2 Hepatic Clearance

Hepatic clearance and biliary excretion depend on the transporter proteins on the canalicular membrane of hepatocytes. Drugs and metabolites are excreted into the gastrointestinal tract to be eliminated with feces. Enterohepatic recycling may occur as the drug metabolite is reabsorbed into the systemic circulation by the intestine. Such a process can increase the toxicity of the drug if it is not eliminated by other means.

5.4 Pharmacodynamics

Pharmacodynamics is defined as the action of the drug on the body. Major concepts include potency, efficacy, and therapeutic window.

5.4.1 Dose–Response Curves

As the body is exposed to increasing amounts of the drug, as more drugs are available to exert an effect on the specific receptors, the response of the body to the drug similarly increases, usually up to a maximum value. The typical relationship between the dose and response can be easily demonstrated graphically by plotting dose or exposure as the independent variable and the response or effect as the dependent variable. This is the fundamental concept of the receptor pharmacology. Two important parameters of the dose–response curve are the EC50 (concentration of the drug that achieves 50% of the maximum response) and Emax (maximum value of body's response to the drug) (◉ Fig. 5.5).

5.4.2 Potency

Potency is the amount of drug required to achieve a certain response in the body. A small quantity of a highly potent drug will be required to achieve the maximum response compared to a low potency drug. Highly potent drugs have low EC50 on the dose–response curve while non-potent drugs will have high EC50.

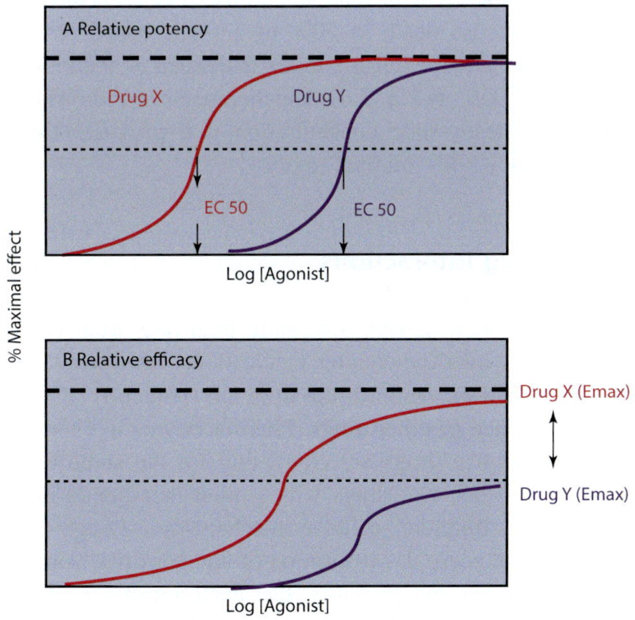

Fig. 5.5 Difference between drug potency and efficacy

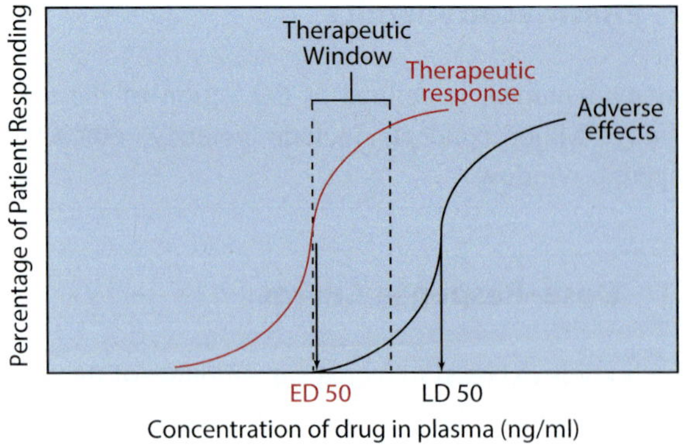

Fig. 5.6 Therapeutic response, toxicity, and therapeutic window

5.4.3 Efficacy

Efficacy refers to the capacity of the drug to generate the therapeutic effect regardless of the amount required. Drugs with high efficacy have a high Emax and generate greater response in the body while drugs with low efficacy have low Emax. For non-efficacious drugs, Emax will equal E0.

5.4.4 Therapeutic Window

The response to a particular drug has great inter-individual variability. Clinical trial data of efficacy and toxicity of all drugs must be taken into account for the variability of the pharmacodynamic response in the population. The median effective dose (ED50) is the dose of the drug required to produce a specified effect in 50% of the population based on clinical trial data. The median lethal dose (LD50) is the dose required to cause death in 50% of animals based on pre-clinical data. The therapeutic index is defined as the ratio of LD50 and ED50 (◉ Fig. 5.6). The therapeutic window is the theoretical steady-state concentration that provides therapeutic efficacy with minimal toxicity.

5.4.5 Drug Interactions

Patients are often treated with more than one drug, herbal substance, or over-the-counter medications. As a result, the absorption and excretion of the drug are frequently affected by the presence of other drugs. Pharmacodynamics interaction occurs when drugs are competing for the same target receptor, or when two drugs with similar therapeutic effect act through different cellular mechanisms. Drugs may increase or decrease the absorption of another drug from the intestinal lumen by changing the gastrointestinal pH or altering other aspects of the environment. Different drugs are often competing for the same plasma protein for binding; thereby, one drug can alter the free concentration of the other drug increasing its potency. A drug can frequently influence the metabolism of another drug by competing for the same liver metabolic enzyme or inducing the expression of the metabolic enzyme.

When two drugs are taken together, the result could be additive in which the net effect is the sum of individual drug effects ($1 + 1 = 2$). Thiazide and beta-blockers have additive antihypertensive effects. On the other hand, the result of the two drugs could be synergistic in which the net effect is greater than expected from the sum of the individual drug effects ($1 + 1 > 2$). An example is the synergistic antimicrobial effect when combining β(beta) lactam antibiotics and aminoglycosides. Potentiation refers to one drug with little effect on its own but able to increase the effect of other drugs ($1 + 0 > 2$). An example is the levodopa and carbidopa combination in treatment of Parkinson's disease. Lastly, two drugs could show an antagonism effect in which one drug inhibits the effect of another ($1 + 1 < 1$), such as concomitant administration of warfarin and high vitamin K food.

5.5 Special Populations

Response of the body to the drug has great individual variability, and it varies with the age, sex, race, and different disease states.

5.5.1 Elderly

Aging produces both pharmacokinetic and pharmacodynamic changes. Muscle mass progressively decreases with aging along with an increase in body fat content resulting in decreased total body water. This reduces the volume of distribution of water-soluble drugs while increasing the volume of distribution of lipid-soluble drugs. Renal function decreases with age resulting in the decline of the kidney's ability to excrete drugs. Liver mass and blood flow decrease with age; thus, the rate of biotransformation of certain drugs also declines. Phase I metabolism in particular declines with age, whereas phase II metabolism is relatively preserved. Distribution and elimination are also affected by protein binding. Albumin typically decreases with age while α(alpha)1-acidic glycoprotein increases.

5.5.2 Pregnancy

Pregnancy induces major physiological changes in females including increased cardiac output, increased oxygen consumption, increased tidal volume, respiratory rate, increased blood volume, vasodilatation, and increased GFR. The minimal alveolar concentration is significantly decreased as much as 40% during pregnancy for all general inhalational anesthetic agents and returns to normal on the third day after delivery. This change is likely to be partially due to the increase in progesterone level and level of endogenous opioids. Pregnancy also increases the sensitivity to local anesthetics such that the doses requirement during epidural anesthesia decreases by as much as 30%. This is mediated by hormonal change, decrease in alpha 1-acidic glycoprotein that binds basic local anesthetics resulting in an increase in unbound fraction, as well as the engorgement of epidural venous plexus as a result of the increase in blood volume and the obstruction of the inferior vena cava (IVC) as a result of the enlarging uterus during pregnancy.

5.5.3 Pediatrics

Neonates and infants have different physiological characteristics compared to adults. The cardiac output of an infant is heart rate dependent due to a relatively non-compliant left ventricle. Infants have increased heart rate, respiratory rate, metabolic rate, and increased total body water content. Thus, the volume of distribution of water-soluble drugs increases. Pediatric patients have decreased plasma protein available for drug binding. An increased amount of free drug increases the potency and reduces the dose required. Neonates and infants have decreased GFR, immature hepatic enzyme system, low hepatic blood flow, and renal tubular function. These factors impair the ability of the body to metabolize and excrete many drugs.

5.5.4 Obesity

The obese individual has a larger circulating blood volume, cardiac output, and modified regional tissue perfusion, leading to changes in absorption, distribution, metabolism, and elimination of drugs. Dosing drugs based on lean body weight is the optimal choice for water-soluble drugs including non-depolarizing neuromuscular blockers, most intravenous opioids, and anesthetics whereas for lipid-soluble drugs, the volume of distribution is increased and therefore requires dosing based on total body weight. But there are exception to these general rules, and we should follow drug-specific guidelines. For example, remifentanil should be dosed based on lean body weight. Propofol is dosed based on lean body weight when given as a bolus, but should be dosed based on total body weight when given as an infusion. Succinylcholine is dosed based on total body weight, as obese individuals have an increased extracellular fluid compartment and higher levels of butyrylcholinesterase, both of which are determinants of its duration of action. Also, the elimination half-life of lipid-soluble drugs is increased secondary to accumulation in the fat stores. Obese patients with otherwise normal renal function have an increased GFR and increased clearance of drugs that undergo renal excretion.

In addition to the above pharmacokinetics considerations, alterations in the pharmacodynamics profile of drugs must be taken into consideration. Obese patients suffer from impaired respiratory function with higher incidences of OSA and fat deposits in the pharyngeal tissue, putting them at risk for airway obstruction and adverse respiratory events when opioids and other sedating medications are administered. It is important to titrate these medications carefully with close monitoring for therapeutic effect.

5.6 Pharmacogenomics

Pharmacogenomics is the study of the genetic variation in humans that results in different responses to drugs. It is now understood that the individual's response to a drug involves a complex interplay between the genetic makeup and the environment.

Genetic polymorphism is the variation in the DNA sequence that occurs at a locus. The most common genetic polymorphism in humans is single-nucleotide polymorphism (SNP), which are single-nucleotide substitutions occurring at frequencies > 1% in the population. Substitution in the coding region could result in a change in amino acid and change the structure, stability, and substrate affinity of the protein. SNPs in a non-coding region could result in changes in promoter, intron, or regulatory region that results in differences in transcription factor binding, expression, or splicing of the gene. All those mechanisms are implicated in common pharmacogenetic polymorphisms. A genetic variability that encodes the determinants of the pharmacokinetics of the drug, especially the metabolic enzymes and transporters, greatly affects its therapeutic effect and toxicity. Several metabolic enzymes were found to be due to monogenic phenotypic variations and thereby can be referenced according to their phenotype traits, such as fast vs. slow metabolizer. Codeine is a prodrug and metabolized to morphine in the liver by cytochrome P450 enzyme CYP2D6. Multiple alleles exist for the gene coding CYP2D6 enzyme. Ultra-rapid metabolizers are at risk for adverse effects from morphine such as respiratory depression, while slow metabolizers experience limited analgesic effects. Genes that encode the target receptor of the drug have important roles. While some genetic variabilities are implicated in a disease process, others' more subtle variabilities may confer a difference in drug response.

5.7 Conclusion

As technology in biomedical research advances, an increasing number of drugs targeting new and old cellular processes are introduced in clinical practice. A thorough understanding of the pharmacokinetic (absorption, distribution, metabolism, and elimination) and pharmacodynamic (site of target, affinity, and selectivity) properties of a drug is a must for its appropriate use in research and clinical practice.

5.8 Questions and Answers

Questions (Choose the Most Appropriate Answer)

1. In normal cellular physiology, there is:
   A. high intracellular sodium concentration
   B. high intracellular potassium concentration
   C. high intracellular sodium and potassium concentration
   D. high extracellular sodium and potassium concentration
   E. high cytoplasmic calcium concentration
2. Relaxation of muscle is achieved by:
   A. hydrolysis of ATP by myosin head
   B. cross bridge formation of myosin head with actin filament
   C. entry of calcium ion into the cytoplasm
   D. binding of calcium ion to troponin
   E. pumping of calcium into the sarcoplasmic reticulum
3. A drug that is a weak acid with a pKa of 6.5 in an environment with pH of 5.5 will exist mainly in (1) acid form, (2) base form, (3) ionized form, (4) nonionized form:
   A. 1
   B. 2
   C. 1 and 3
   D. 1 and 4
   E. 2 and 3
4. After oral administration of the drug, absorption is the greatest in
   A. the esophagus because it bypasses the portal venous system
   B. the stomach because the acidic environment favors absorption of nonionized form
   C. the stomach because of the slower transit time
   D. the small intestine because of the basic environment favors absorption of nonionized form
   E. the small intestine because of the abundance of surface area and blood vessels
5. After one intravenous bolus, which of the following organs would receive the drug slowest?
   A. muscle
   B. fat
   C. liver
   D. kidney
   E. heart
6. Emergence from a single bolus of medication mainly depends on:
   A. hepatic metabolism
   B. renal metabolism
   C. renal clearance
   D. redistribution from vessel rich to vessel poor tissue groups
   E. redistribution from vessel poor to vessel rich tissue groups
7. Which of the following routes of administration has the highest hepatic first pass effect:
   A. oral
   B. sublingual
   C. rectal
   D. transdermal
   E. buccal
8. Which of the following routes of administration bypasses the first pass metabolism of the lung:
   A. transdermal
   B. rectal
   C. oral
   D. intravenous
   E. intra-arterial
9. In patients with hepatic failure, which of the following is incorrect?
   A. increased volume of distribution of water soluble drugs
   B. decreased possibility of tissue toxicity
   C. decreased plasma protein binding
   D. decreased hepatic metabolism
   E. decreased hepatic first pass effect
10. The main rationale for using sodium bicarbonate to treat aspirin overdose is:
    A. to neutralize the salicylic acid in blood and thereby keeping a normal plasma pH
    B. to facilitate the binding of salicylic acid to plasma proteins
    C. to alkalinize the urine thereby favoring the ionized form of salicylic acid in the urine
    D. to alkalinize the urine thereby preventing the acidic form of salicylic acid from entering back into the plasma
    E. to promote the reduction of salicylic acid by creating a favorable basic chemical environment

11. EC50 mainly reflects a drug's:
    A. efficacy
    B. potency
    C. tolerance
    D. safety
    E. rate of elimination
12. A competitive antagonist would shift the dose response curve:
    A. to the left
    B. to the right
    C. upward
    D. downward
    E. down and to the right
13. Partial agonist, compared to full agonist, would shift the dose response curve:
    A. to the left
    B. to the right
    C. upward
    D. downward
    E. downward and to the right
14. Compared to healthy adults, pregnant women have:
    A. increased cardiac output
    B. increased glomerular filtration rate (GFR)
    C. increased minimal alveolar concentration
    D. A and B
    E. A, B and C
15. Compared to healthy adults, pediatric population has:
    A. increased volume of distribution for water soluble drugs per weight
    B. increased renal clearance of water soluble drugs per weight
    C. increased plasma protein binding of water soluble drugs
    D. A and B
    E. A, B, and C
16. An otherwise healthy 5-year-old patient receives a standard pediatric dose of tramadol after a moderately painful procedure. The patient is later found to be apneic in the recovery area. What is the most likely explanation for this occurrence?
    A. increased oral bioavailability in the pediatric population
    B. decreased activity of the CYPD26 enzyme
    C. the patient is an ultra-rapid metabolizer of tramadol
    D. poor renal clearance of active metabolites

Answers

1. **B**. In normal cellular physiology, there is high intracellular potassium concentration. The resting membrane potential (normally − 60 to − 90 mV in unstimulated neurons) is determined by Na+/K+ATPase and the membrane permeability. Na+/K+ATPase actively pumps Na+out of the cell in exchange for K+. And the cell membrane is practically impermeable to Na+, but K +leak channels allows the transport of K+out of the cell until an equilibrium is reached between the balance of electrochemical gradient.
2. **E**. Specialized synapses called neuromuscular junctions couple motor nerve impulses to muscle contractions by the action of Ca2+ion on the troponin regulatory complex. Nerve impulses arriving at the junction cause the depolarization of myofilament resulting in the release of Ca2+ion stored in sarcoplasmic reticulum. Binding of Ca2+to troponin allows the cross-bridge formation between the myosin and actin filaments. Relaxation occurs when Ca2+is pumped back into the sarcoplasmic reticulum.
3. **D**. A drug that is a weak acid with a pKa of 6.5 in an environment with pH of 5.5 will exist mainly in acid and non-ionized forms.
4. **E**. After oral administration of a drug, absorption is the greatest in the small intestine because of the abundance of surface area and blood vessels.
5. **B**. Well-perfused organs receiving a high fraction of the cardiac output receive comparatively higher amounts of the drug early after drug administration. These vessel-rich tissue groups reach equilibrium quickly relative to blood concentration. Less well-perfused groups such as muscle, fat, and skin may require hours before the drug reaches equilibrium with the blood concentration.
6. **D**. Emergence from a single bolus of medication mainly depends on redistribution from vessel-rich to vessel-poor tissue groups. Emergence is rapid after bolus injection of drug mainly due to the process of distribution to the peripheral compartment in a matter of minutes. In comparison, after a prolonged infusion of a drug, tissue concentrations of the drug are in equilibrium with plasma; the redistribution process then delays the emergence after removal of drug infusion due to the drug returning to the plasma from the tissue reservoir.
7. **A**. Drugs follow the venous drainage of the stomach and small intestine and are delivered to the liver via the portal system. Therefore, bioavailability of orally

administered drugs is limited to the first-pass hepatic metabolism.

On the other hand, sublingual and transmucosal drug administration bypass the first-pass metabolism because veins of mouth and esophagus drain directly into the inferior vena cava. Around 50% of rectally administered drugs will bypass the liver, potentially increasing the bioavailability compared to orally administered drugs.

8. **E**. Other than rare intra-arterial administration, all parental administration of drugs is subject to first-pass metabolism of the lung. The lung provides temporary storage for a number of substances, filters the particulate substance, and serves as a site of elimination for volatile agents.
9. **B**. In patients with hepatic failure, there is no decreased possibility of tissue toxicity. Conditions that decrease plasma binding protein such as kidney failure, liver disease, chronic congestive heart failure, infection, and malignancies will decrease the relative solubility of the drug in the blood, thereby increasing tissue uptake.
10. **C**. The main rationale for using sodium bicarbonate to treat aspirin overdose is to alkalinize the urine, thereby favoring the ionized form of salicylic acid in the urine.
11. **B**. EC50 is the concentration of the drug that achieves 50% of the maximum response and mainly reflects a drug's potency. Potency is the amount of drug required to achieve a certain response in the body. A less amount of highly potent drug will be required to achieve the maximum response compared to drugs of low potency.
12. **B**. A competitive antagonist would shift the dose–response curve to the right. Highly potent drugs have low EC50 on the dose–response curve while non-potent drugs will have high EC50.
13. **D**. A partial agonist, compared to a full agonist, would shift the dose–response curve downward.
14. **D**. Pregnancy induces major physiological changes in females including increased cardiac output and increased GFR, as well as increased oxygen consumption, increased tidal volume, respiratory rate, increased blood volume, and vasodilatation.
15. **A**. Neonates and infants have different physiological characteristics compared to adults. The cardiac output of an infant is heart rate dependent due to a relatively non-compliant left ventricle. Infants have increased heart rate, respiratory rate, metabolic rate, and increased total body water content. Thus, the volume of distribution of water-soluble drugs increase. Pediatric patients have decreased plasma protein available for drug binding. An increased amount of free drug increases the potency and reduces the dose required. Neonates and infants have decreased GFR, immature hepatic enzyme system, low hepatic blood flow, and renal tubular function. These factors impair the ability of the body to metabolize and excrete many drugs.
16. **C**. Tramadol and codeine are two prodrugs that undergo metabolism by the cytochrome P450 enzyme CYP2D6 in the liver to become the active metabolites *O*-desmethyltramadol and morphine, respectively. Certain individuals have genetic polymorphisms of this enzyme and may be either fast or slow metabolizers of these drugs. Fast, or ultra-rapid, metabolizers are at risk for overdose as high concentrations of the active metabolites are produced and accumulate even in the presence of normal renal clearance.

References

1. Brunton L, Chabner B, Knollman B, editors. Goodman and Gilman's: the pharmacological basis of therapeutics. 13th ed. New York: McGraw-Hill Education; 2017.
2. Butterworth JF, Mackey DC, Wasnick JD. Morgan & Mikhail's clinical anesthesiology. 6th ed. New York: McGraw-Hill Education; 2018.
3. McPhee SJ, Hammer GD. Pathophysiology of disease: an introduction to clinical medicine. 8th ed. New York: McGraw-Hill Education; 2018.
4. Rhoades RA, Bell DR. Medical physiology: principles for clinical medicine. 5th ed. Philadelphia: Wolter Kluwer: Lippincott Williams & Wilkins; 2017.
5. Nelson DL, Cox MM. Lehninger principles of biochemistry. 8th ed. New York: W.H. Freeman and Company; 2021.
6. Phospholipid. Encyclopædia Britannica. Encyclopædia Britannica Online. Encyclopædia. Britannica Inc. 2015. http://www.britannica.com/science/phospholipid?oasmId=114973. Accessed 18 Apr 2022.
7. Devine BJ. Gentamicin therapy. Drug Intell Clin Pharm. 1974;8:650–5.
8. Hume R. Prediction of lean body mass from height and weight. J Clin Pathol. 1966;19(4):389–91.
9. Ingrade J, Lemmens HJM. Dose adjustment of anaesthetics in the morbidly obese. Br J Anaesth. 2010;105(S1):i16-23.
10. Glass PS. Half-time or half-life: what matters for recovery from intravenous anesthesia. Anesthesiology. 2010;112(5):1266–9.

Pharmacology of Non-opioid Intravenous Anesthetics

6

Mohamed Abdalla

Abstract

The progress in surgery would have been impossible if not coupled with progress and development of anesthetic techniques. The introduction and development of new sedative hypnotics is the corner stone in this progress. Barbiturates once were the most commonly used induction agents for general anesthesia but now are replaced with propofol. Nowadays, propofol is widely utilized in the operating rooms as a hypnotic for induction of general anesthesia, maintenance of general anesthesia in total intravenous anesthetic technique (TIVA), sedative during surgery and invasive procedures. In intensive care units (ICU), propofol complemented opioids and benzodiazepines for sedation. Ketamine is of great benefit in induction of general anesthesia in asthmatic patients, and utilizing ketamine for its analgesic properties has been revived. Etomidate is unmatched in its lack of hemodynamic depressant effects, rendering it the most appropriate agent to induce general anesthesia in patients with hemodynamic instability. Dexmedetomidine although not used as a general anesthesia induction agent but is a valuable sedative in the ICU and for procedures were respiratory depression is not tolerated with the added value of decreasing the anesthetic requirements. It is a never stopping effort in progress to provide us with sedative-hypnotics that lack the side effects of the currently available ones.

Keywords

Sedative • Hypnotics • Intravenous (IV) induction agents • Barbiturates • Benzodiazepines • Remimazolam • Ketamine • Etomidate • Etomidate analog • Propofol • Propofol derivatives • Dexmedetomidine

Key Points

1. The action of most intravenous (IV) anesthesia induction agents is through their interaction with $GABA_A$ receptors with the exception of ketamine.
2. Barbiturates, once the most commonly used IV general anesthesia induction agents (especially thiopental), are replaced now by propofol. Methohexital still has its place in anesthesia for electroconvulsive therapy (ECT) and short procedures as cardioversions. In 2010, thiopental ceased to be offered in the USA.
3. Etomidate is the drug of choice for induction of hemodynamically unstable patients due to its lacking of any cardiovascular depressant effect. Concerns about its adrenocortical suppression, especially in critically ill ventilated patients, stimulated the research for future analogs.
4. Ketamine has a dual effect: a direct depressant effect and an indirect effect that usually takes the upper hand resulting in sympathetic outflow, except in patients with exhausted sympathetic nervous system where the depressant effect is unmasked. Still ketamine is a valuable induction agent in asthmatic patients. The value of ketamine analgesic effect in opioid-sparing anesthetic techniques has been revived in the recent years.
5. The most commonly used benzodiazepines in the anesthetic practice nowadays are: midazolam, diazepam, and lorazepam. Midazolam is unique in its pharmacology due to changes in its imidazole ring rendering it more lipid soluble in physiologic pH.

M. Abdalla (✉)
Department of Anesthesiology, University Hospitals of Cleveland, Cleveland, OH, USA
e-mail: mohamed.abdalla2@uhhospitals.org

Case Western Reserve University, Cleveland, OH, USA

M. Argalious et al. (eds.), *Basic Sciences in Anesthesia*,
https://doi.org/10.1007/978-3-031-60203-0_6

6. Remimazolam the novel short-acting IV benzodiazepines shows high affinity for the $GABA_A$ receptor benzodiazepine site of action. It has a rapid onset and offset of sedation compared to midazolam and a unique structure that makes it a substrate to tissue esterases predicting its short duration of action.
7. Propofol, the most commonly used drug to induce general anesthesia, is widely used for sedation during surgery/procedures and in the intensive care unit (ICU). Propofol infusion syndrome (PRIS) is a serious fatal side effect of its prolonged used. Unexplained acidosis and elevated triglycerides during its usage may be a clue for PRIS.
8. Dexmedetomidine (an α [alpha] 2 receptor agonist), although not an IV general anesthesia induction agent, is a valuable sedative with anesthetic/analgesic-sparing effect and minimal effect on respiration.

6.1 Introduction

The introduction of intravenous sedative-hypnotics was a revolution in the practice of anesthesia, and a cornerstone was set in the armamentarium of the anesthetic pharmacology. Sodium thiopental was introduced by John Lundy and Ralph Waters in 1934, followed by the clinical use of benzodiazepines in 1960. Ketamine became available in 1969, etomidate in 1972, and propofol in 1983. In 1999, dexmedetomidine was approved by the US Food and Drug Administration (FDA) as a valuable addition.

Although sedative-hypnotics belong to different pharmacological drug groups and they might work on different receptors, they share a common pharmacological effect: sedation and hypnosis. The wide use of sedative-hypnotics for intravenous induction and maintenance of anesthesia as well as sedation highlights the importance of their pharmacology.

The ideal intravenous anesthetic:

- Water soluble and stable with long shelf-life
- Not painful when injected intravenously.
- Safe if injected intra-arterially and not an irritant if injected subcutaneously.
- Rapid onset of action.
- Rapid recovery.
- Analgesic effect.
- No excitatory phenomena (involuntary movement, coughing) on induction.
- Does not show emergence phenomena.
- Does not cause nausea and vomiting.
- Lacks histamine release and allergic reactions.
- No or minimal cardiorespiratory side effects.
- Safe in porphyria.
- Does not cause adrenocortical suppression.

Up until our present time, we do not have such an ideal intravenous sedative-hypnotic.

6.2 Barbiturates

Before the introduction of propofol, barbiturates were the most commonly used anesthetic induction agents.

6.2.1 Chemical Properties

Barbituric acid is the parent compound for barbiturates (◉ Fig. 6.1). Modification of the barbituric acid ring produces drugs of different pharmacological actions. Only two drugs of the barbiturates family are used in the current anesthetic practice: The first is a thiobarbiturate-thiopental sodium (substitution of a sulfur atom at C2 position), and the second is an oxybarbiturate-methohexital (substitution of oxygen at C2 position) (◉ Table 6.1).

Both sodium thiopental (◉ Fig. 6.2) and methohexital (◉ Fig. 6.3) are supplied for clinical use as a racemic mixture, prepared as sodium salts. Thiopental is no longer available in the United States, but it is still available in Europe and other parts of the world.

They are supplied as powder that is reconstituted with sterile water or normal saline. The powder is mixed with 6% anhydrous sodium carbonate to increase the water solubility.

The recommended solution is 2.5% for sodium thiopental and 1% for methohexital. These solutions are alkaline: pH 10.5 for sodium thiopental and 11 for methohexital. They can precipitate if mixed with acidic drugs such as rocuronium, atracurium, and vecuronium. It is recommended to flush the intravenous line before the addition of an acidic drug.

Barbituric Acid Ring

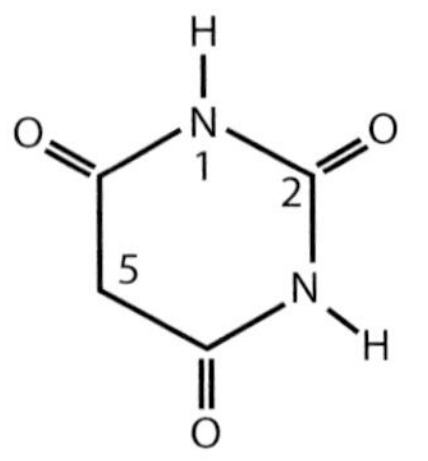

Fig. 6.1 Barbituric acid ring (Reprinted with permission, Cleveland Clinic Center for Medical Art & Photography © 2016. All Rights Reserved)

Table 6.1 Structure activity relationship

	Substitution	Effect
Position 5	Aryl or alkyl group	Hypnotic and sedative effect
Position 5	Phenyl group	Anticonvulsant effect
Position 2	Sulfur	Rapid onset of action (thiopental)
Position 1	Methyl or ethyl group	Rapid onset of action (methohexital)

Sodium thiopental prepared under a sterile hood remains sterile and chemically stable for 6 days at room temperature and longer if refrigerated. A reliable potency of prepared methohexital exists 6 weeks after preparation at room temperature and its pH (10–11) inhibits any bacterial contamination.

6.2.2 Mechanism of Action

Gamma amino butyric acid (GABA) is the most abundant inhibitory neurotransmitter in the central nervous system (CNS).

$GABA_A$ receptors (◉ Fig. 6.4) are believed to mediate the hypnotic effect of most intravenous anesthetics as well as depression of the spinal cord reflexes and amnesia.

$GABA_A$ is a pentameric transmembrane glycoprotein receptor. It is a ligand-gated ion channel; when activated, transmembrane chloride conductance increases, hyperpolarizing the postsynaptic cell membrane, and inhibits the function of the postsynaptic neurone.

Barbiturates act through modulating the action of $GABA_A$ receptors increasing the sensitivity to GABA. In high concentrations, barbiturates act as a direct agonist on $GABA_A$ receptors. On the $GABA_A$ receptor, barbiturates bind to a specific site on the B subunit.

It is believed that barbiturates inhibit neuronal nicotinic cholinergic receptors where thiopental acts as a competitive inhibitor. The clinical value of this action is unclear.

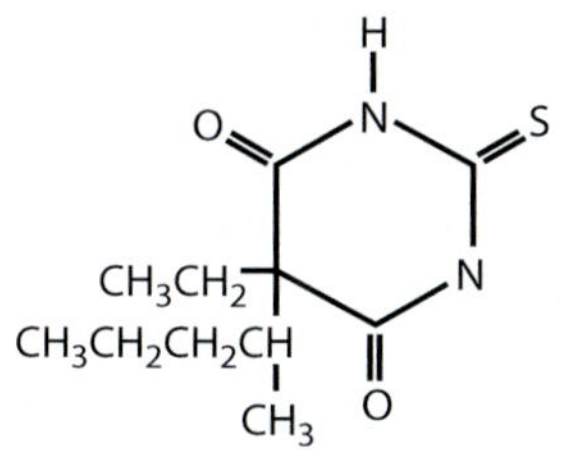

Fig. 6.2 Thiopental (Reprinted with permission, Cleveland Clinic Center for Medical Art & Photography © 2016. All Rights Reserved)

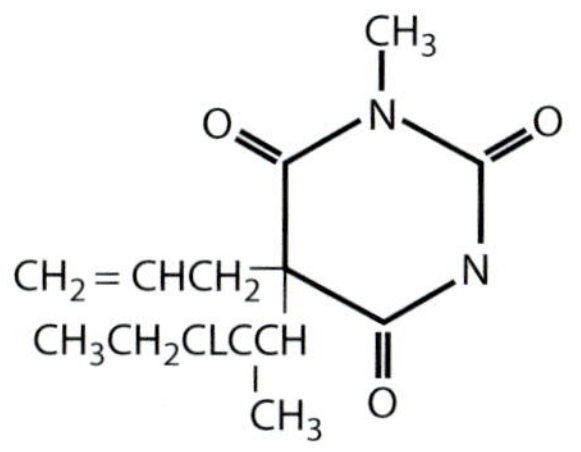

Fig. 6.3 Methohexital (Reprinted with permission, Cleveland Clinic Center for Medical Art & Photography © 2016. All Rights Reserved)

6.2.3 Pharmacokinetics of Barbiturates

Thiopental is alkaline, pH 10.5, but once it enters the circulation, it is buffered to the physiologic pH. It is highly lipid soluble, and this is the reason for its rapid onset of action that is within one circulation time. It is highly bound to albumin 75–90%. Protein binging is affected by the concentration of plasma proteins, displacement by other drugs, and changes in the blood pH where alkalemia decreases the protein binding. Hypoalbuminemia necessitates decreasing the induction dose and consequently the pharmacologically active free drug.

Redistribution out of the CNS is the main mechanism for termination of the anesthetic effect after injection of a single bolus dose. It takes 3–4 redistribution half-lives for termination of effect. The redistribution half-life (t1/2α[alpha]) is 2–4 min. Termination of the pharmacological effect is prolonged when the drug is given in repeated doses or as an infusion.

Subsequent metabolism and elimination is much slower with a half-life (t1/2β[beta]) of > 10 h. Thiopental is metabolized mainly in the liver. Thiopental undergoes ring desulfuration to pentobarbital that is an active metabolite with a longer duration of action and represents around 3.5% of the given dose, but this percent can increase with high doses.

Both pentobarbital and thiopental undergo oxidation to pharmacologically inactive metabolites. Oxidation is the most important pathway for thiopental metabolism. Hydroxylation also takes place to inactive metabolites. Thiopental inactive metabolites are excreted in urine.

Elderly patients show a slower rate of distribution, which warrants adjusting the dose of thiopental. Conversely,

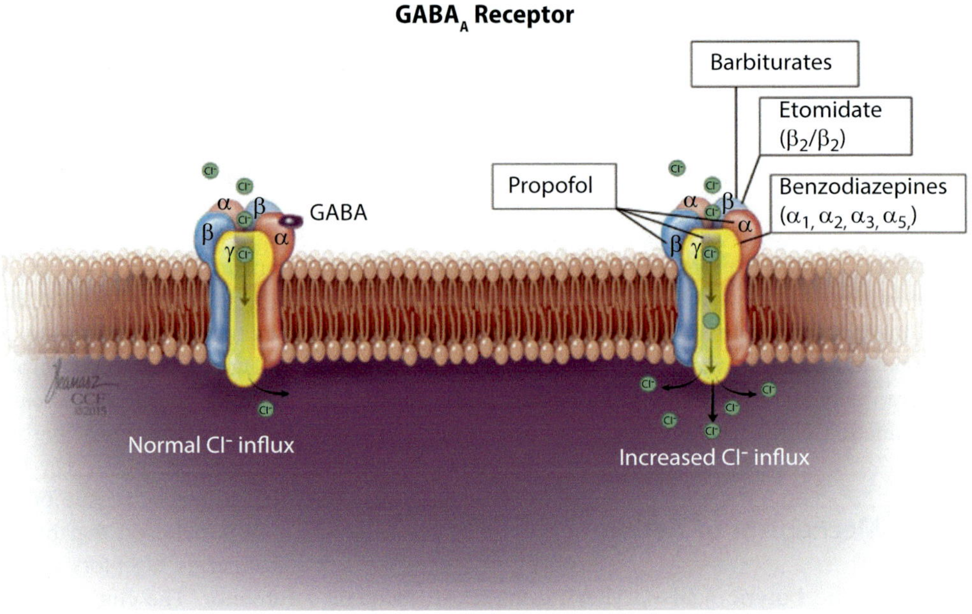

Fig. 6.4 GABA$_A$ receptor (Reprinted with permission, Cleveland Clinic Center for Medical Art & Photography © 2016. All Rights Reserved)

recovery time after large or repeated doses is faster in infants than adults due to accelerated elimination. Patients with poor cardiovascular reserve show an exaggerated response to the hypotensive effect of thiopental.

Zero-order kinetics (a constant fraction of the drug regardless of the total dose of the drug) describes the metabolism of thiopental after repeated doses or continuous infusion. Chronic administration of barbiturates or other drugs that induce the oxidative microsomal enzymes enhances the metabolism of barbiturates.

Methohexital is metabolized by the liver to inactive hydroxylated metabolites. It has a faster clearance than thiopental and accumulates less after prolonged infusions, and this can be explained by the hepatic extraction ratio of methohexital (0.5), which means that the liver extracts 50% of the drug reaching it while the hepatic extraction ratio for thiopental is 0.15.

6.2.4 Pharmacodynamics of Barbiturates

6.2.4.1 Cardiovascular System

Barbiturates cause direct myocardial depression and peripheral vasodilatation that is more pronounced on the capacitance vessels. They inhibit the medullary vasomotor center, which results in a decrease in the arterial blood pressure that is exaggerated with rapid injection, in hypovolemic patients, and the elderly. The depressive effect on the sympathetic nervous system is more than that on the parasympathetic, and this can result in bradycardia. In fact, tachycardia is more observed and attributed to the effect of hypotension on the baroreceptors.

The decrease in blood pressure with induction is more related to venodilatation than direct myocardial depression.

6.2.4.2 Central Nervous System

Barbiturates exert a dose-dependent, progressive depression of the central nervous system that involves the spinal reflexes. Thiopental suppresses the electroencephalogram (EEG) in a progressive fashion to burst suppression and electrical silence. Methohexital can increase the seizure activity in epileptic patients, which makes it suitable for induction of anesthesia in patients coming for electroconvulsive therapy (ECT). Thiopental is an excellent anticonvulsant; it terminates seizure activities fast, but status epilepticus might require repeated doses or continuous infusion.

Barbiturates decrease the cerebral metabolic oxygen consumption rate (CMRO2), the cerebral blood flow (CBF), cerebral blood volume (CBV), and intracranial pressure (ICP). They are potent cerebral vasoconstrictors and might have a protective effect against focal ischemia (inverse-steal phenomenon).

Thiopental lacks analgesic effect and even has an antanalgesic effect in sub-anesthetic doses.

6.2.4.3 Respiratory System

Barbiturates are respiratory depressants; they depress the medullary respiratory center and decrease the sensitivity to hypoxia and hypercapnia. The decrease in minute ventilation is mainly due to decrease in tidal volume.

Laryngeal spasm is noticed with barbiturates more than other sedative-hypnotics. Histamine release is described with thiopental, and the increase in bronchial smooth muscle tone might be attributed to it.

6.2.4.4 Hepato-Renal

There is no significant effect on the hepato-renal function with a single induction dose of barbiturates. Barbiturates are liver microsomal enzymes inducers and can increase the metabolism of other drugs.

6.2.4.5 Effect on Other Organs

Barbiturates have no direct neuromuscular junction effect but can decrease the skeletal muscle tone in high doses. During methohexital induction, muscle tremors, myoclonus, and hiccups are noticed.

Thiopental crosses the placenta and can depress the newborn and its activity, but it lacks a significant effect on the uterus.

Intraocular pressure decreases 25–40% with thiopental.

6.2.5 Uses of Barbiturates

- Induction of Anesthesia: A dose of 4–6 mg/kg of thiopental induces general anesthesia in 30 s, the dose is reduced in the elderly, patients with poor myocardial function and hypovolemia, and the rate of injection is slowed to avoid an exaggerated hypotensive response. In an obese patient, the dose should be calculated on the lean body weight. A dose of 1–1.5 mg/kg induces general anesthesia with methohexital, accompanied by mild pain. Barbiturates are not used in maintenance of anesthesia due to prolonged recovery. Barbiturates are used to induce barbiturate coma after neurological insults.
- Treatment of status epilepticus.
- Neuroprotection in elevated intracranial pressure and with focal ischemia.

6.2.6 Side Effects of Barbiturates

- Hypotension.
- Allergic reactions, true allergic reactions are rare but direct histamine release is noticed.
- Bronchospasm in asthmatic patients.
- Laryngeal spasm.
- Local irritation and tissue damage if injected in the subcutaneous tissues.
- Intra-arterial injection can precipitate acute ischemia because of the severe arterial spasm due to release of endogenous vasoconstrictors, precipitation of thiopental crystals, intimal damage, and thrombosis.
  On the occasion of intra-arterial injection, the catheter is left in place, a vasodilator (papaverine) is injected through the catheter, and a stellate ganglion block is used to promote vasodilatation and start heparin infusion.
- Barbiturates can precipitate acute porphyria in patients with intermittent or variegate porphyria due to aminolevulinic acid synthetase (ALA synthetase) induction with the accumulation of porphobilinogen during hemoglobin production. Acute attacks can be fatal. Patients present with severe abdominal pain, nausea, vomiting, and neurological abnormalities. For this reason, barbiturates are contraindicated in patients with porphyria.

Sodium thiopental production was interrupted in the United States in 2010, and due to controversy over its usage in lethal injections, the European import was halted.

6.3 Etomidate

Etomidate is a carboxylated imidazole intravenous sedative-hypnotic that is available as a single enantiomer, the R(+) isomer that is 10–20 times more potent as a hypnotic than the S(−) isomer. It is poorly soluble in water with moderate lipid solubility. It is prepared as a clear solution in 35% propylene glycol at a concentration of 2 mg/ml (Amidate in USA) or as a lipid emulsion containing medium-chain and long-chain triglycerides (Etomidate-Lipura in Germany).

It has a pH of 6.9, so the concern of precipitation with acidic drugs as rocuronium is nonexistent.

6.3.1 Mechanism of Action

Etomidate carries out its action through modulation of the $GABA_A$ receptors, acting as a positive allosteric modulator enhancing the effect of the inhibitory neurotransmitter GABA.

It shows high selectivity to the receptor with stereo-selectivity. It binds to receptors containing β (beta)2 and/or β(beta)3 subunits and less to receptors containing β(beta)1 subunits.

$Alpha_2$ adrenergic receptor activation is described, and it may contribute to its hemodynamic effects where activation of the vascular smooth muscle α(alpha)-2b receptors causes vasoconstriction and hypertension.

6.3.2 Pharmacokinetics

Etomidate is 75–77% bound to albumin. It is metabolized by ester hydrolysis to inactive carboxylic acid metabolite mainly in the liver by hepatic esterases. Excretion is mainly in urine and to a lesser extent in bile. Its elimination half-life is 1–5 h, and if given as a continuous infusion, its context-sensitive halftime is shorter than propofol. In elderly, renal failure and hepatic cirrhosis patients, smaller doses are required due to reduced protein binding and clearance.

6.3.3 Pharmacodynamics

6.3.3.1 Cardiovascular System

The superiority of etomidate among intravenous induction anesthetics arises from its stable hemodynamic profile preserving the cardiovascular stability. It shows minimal or no change in preload, heart rate, and myocardial contractility. It preserves the autonomic reflexes as baroreflex and shows no inhibition to the sympathetic tone. It does not cause hypotension due to its agonist effect on the vascular smooth muscle α(alpha)-2b receptors which causes vasoconstriction and hypertension.

6.3.3.2 Central Nervous System

Etomidate has a rapid onset of unconsciousness and a short duration of action (2–4 min after an induction dose). It decreases the CMRO2, decreasing CBF and the ICP. Etomidate maintains or even increases the cerebral perfusion pressure (CPP), and it is a potent cerebral vasoconstrictor.

When used for induction of general anesthesia in electroconvulsive therapy (ECT), the seizure activity is longer than that achieved with methohexital. It may increase the EEG activity in epileptogenic foci, but it still has an anticonvulsive effect.

Compared to propofol and barbiturates, it has less effect on the motor-evoked potentials.

6.3.3.3 Respiratory System

Etomidate has a minimal depressant effect on respiration, but this can be pronounced if combined with other respiratory depressants as opioids. The ventilatory depressant effect of etomidate is not exaggerated in chronic obstructive pulmonary disease (COPD).

6.3.3.4 Endocrine System

Etomidate is a potent inhibitor of cortisol and aldosterone synthesis, even more potent than its hypnotic effect. Adrenocortical suppression is dose dependent, and it is due to the inhibition of 11B-hydroxylase that catalyzes 11B-hydroxylation in cortisol synthesis and aldolase in aldosterone synthesis. It is believed that the imidazole structure is responsible for this adrenocortical suppression. A single induction dose of etomidate can inhibit the cortisol synthesis and the normal adrenocortical response up to 12 h. This can be prolonged more than 24 h after infusions. Prolonged infusion of etomidate in the critically ill ventilated patient has been shown to increase the mortality by twofold.

There is still controversy on the impact of the effect of etomidate single dose and using it in critically ill patients, especially those with hemodynamic instability where etomidate usage is attractive.

6.3.4 Uses of Etomidate

- The main usage for etomidate is for intravenous induction of anesthesia particularly in patients with compromised hemodynamics.
- 0.2–0.4 mg/kg for intravenous induction that needs to be modified in elderly patients with reduced protein binding.
- 6.5 mg/kg used for rectal induction of anesthesia.
- When used as an infusion; 5 mcg/kg/min for sedation and 10 mcg/kg/min for maintenance of anesthesia where its context sensitive halftime is shorter than propofol.

6.3.5 Side Effects of Etomidate

- Adrenocortical suppression (see earlier).
- Nausea and vomiting. It is reported to be 30–40% in propylene glycol preparation but the same incidence of nausea as propofol in the lipid emulsion preparation.
- Myoclonic activity and involuntary muscle movement (IMM) but not convulsions is commonly seen with etomidate induction that can be minimized by premedication with opioid, benzodiazepine, lidocaine, magnesium, or dexmedetomidine. The incidence in non-premedicated patients might reach 80%. It is hypothesized that this is due to depression of the inhibitory neuronal circuits earlier than the excitatory neuronal circuits and this disequilibrium can be attributed to the difference in local cerebral blood flow or difference in affinity.
- Pain on injection is more described if etomidate is injected in a small vein, especially with the propylene glycol preparation. This incidence of pain is less when preceded by lidocaine, injection in a big vein, or the lipid emulsion preparation is used. It is believed that this pain is due to activation of a member of the transient receptor potential (TRP) ion channel family, TRPA1. TRPA1 is a principle receptor in nociception and together with TRPV1 contributes to neurogenic inflammation and pain signaling. Etomidate and propofol evoke pain through activation and sensitization of TRPA1.
- Controversy exists about using etomidate in patients with porphyria and its safety. Some reports its safe usage, but it is an inducer for ALA synthetase.

6.3.6 The Future of Etomidate Analogs

The attractive pharmacological profile of etomidate with its cardiorespiratory stability effects stimulated the research for modifying its structure to avoid its side effects. The aim is to alter the design of etomidate to allow the ultra-rapid metabolism by non-specific esterases preventing it from binding to 11B-hydroxylase enzyme and reduce its adrenocortical suppression.

Cyclopropyl-methoxycarbonyl-metetomidate (CPMM) known as ABP-700 is under development and design to retain the favorable pharmacological properties of etomidate and diminish its adrenal suppression. It shows high hypnotic potency and a duration of action between etomidate and moc-etomidate. It is a 10 mg/ml solution with 10% sulfoether-B-cyclodextrine as a solvent. A dose of 0.25–0.35 mg/Kg is optimal to induce general anesthesia with a swift recovery after intravenous infusion regardless of the duration. IMM is still seen as with etomidate.

The methoxycarbonyl-etomidate (moc-etomidate) describes an analog that is rapidly metabolized by non-specific esterases. With a half-life of a few minutes, even when it suppresses the adrenocortical function, it would be for a much shorter duration than the parent drug. It shows a rapid onset of hypnosis and retains the hemodynamic stability profile of etomidate, but the ultrashort rapid metabolism causes ultra-rapid hypnotic recovery and large doses are needed to achieve adequate depth of anesthesia, and this leads to adrenocortical suppression.

Carboetomidate is another etomidate analogs. The imidazole ring of the parent drug that is responsible for the adrenocortical suppression is replaced by a pyrrole ring. This produces a drug that has the same hypnotic potency and cardiorespiratory effects of the parent drug but with less adrenal suppression and slower onset of hypnosis.

ET-26 hydrochloride is a novel analog in the preclinical stage. It shows a stable hemodynamic and anesthetic profile similar to etomidate and less adrenocortical suppression. In experimental animals sepsis model, it shows high survival rate compared to etomidate.

6.4 Ketamine

Ketamine is an arylcyclohexylamine related to phencyclidine (PCP) in its structure. It is prepared as ketamine hydrochloride that is water soluble and ten times more lipid soluble than thiopentone. The preparation available in the United States is a racemic mixture of its S(+) and R(−) isomers. Some countries in Europe and Latin America have the preparation that only contains the S(+) enantiomer that is 3–4 times more potent, has a shorter duration of action, and less emergence reactions.

6.4.1 Mechanism of Action

The pharmacological effect of ketamine compared to barbiturates, propofol, and benzodiazepines is through the interaction with different receptors in the CNS. It is widely known to be a non-competitive antagonist of the N-methyl-D-aspartate (NMDA) receptor, it has antagonist effect on the cholinergic muscarinic receptors, agonistic effect on the α (alpha) and β (beta) adrenergic receptors, agonist for the opioid receptor, and it enhances the dopaminergic activity.

The NMDA receptor complex is a cation-gated ion channel (mainly calcium and to a lesser extent potassium and sodium). When the receptor is activated by endogenous excitatory amino acid agonists (aspartic acid, glutamic acid, and glycine), the channel is opened, and the calcium influx increases causing depolarization of the membrane that plays an important role in the development of the sensory impulse at the cortical and subcortical levels.

Ketamine binds the phencyclidine (PCP) binding site within the ion channel in the open state preventing the influx of calcium and consequently preventing the membrane depolarization.

6.4.2 Pharmacokinetics of Ketamine

Ketamine is unique among intravenous induction agents in that it can be administered via different routes; it can be administered via intravenous, intramuscular, oral, nasal, and rectal route. It is water soluble, highly lipid soluble, 12% bound to plasma proteins with a pKa of 7.5.

Ketamine is rapidly absorbed; maximum plasma concentration is achieved in 5–15 min after intramuscular (IM) injection, 20 min after nasal, and 30 min after oral administration.

It undergoes extensive first-pass effect in the liver and intestines that is responsible for the low bioavailability of ketamine after oral and rectal administration (<30%).

It is the high lipid solubility and the low protein binding that allows ketamine to cross the blood brain barrier rapidly.

Termination of its pharmacological effect is through redistribution away from its CNS site of action. Redistribution half-life is 2.7 min.

Ketamine metabolism is mainly through N-demethylation to norketamine by hepatic cytochrome 450 enzymes. Norketamine is three-fourths the potency of the parent drug that undergoes hydroxylation, conjugation, and excretion mainly through the kidneys and to a lesser extent in feces. Ketamine elimination half-life is approximately 2 h. Oxidative metabolism of ketamine cyclohexanone ring is also described.

6.4.3 Pharmacodynamics of Ketamine

6.4.3.1 Cardiovascular System

Ketamine has a dual action, a direct cardiac depressing action that is seen in patients with exhausted catecholamines (critically ill and shocked patients), preventing the indirect effect of ketamine to take the upper hand. The indirect (predominant) effect is due to inhibiting the reuptake of circulating catecholamines causing tachycardia, hypertension, increase in contractility, increase in cardiac output, increase in systemic vascular resistance, and increase in the pulmonary artery pressure. These hemodynamic changes can cause an imbalance between myocardial oxygen supply and demand, precipitating myocardial ischemia.

6.4.3.2 Central Nervous System

Ketamine induces a state of dissociative anesthesia (dissociation between the thalamo-neocortical and limbic system), where patients seem awake, with opened eyes, a nystagmus gaze and phonating, but dissociated from the environment with variable degrees of hypertonus and muscle movements. The anesthetic state is accompanied by intense analgesia. On emergence, patients have alterations in their mood, dysphoria, floatation sensations, vivid dreams, and hallucinations.

Ketamine has unfavorable neurosurgical effects; it increases the CBF, CMRO2, and ICP, and its usage in head trauma or patients with space occupying lesions is not recommended.

On EEG, the wave patterns change from increase in frequency during light anesthesia to high-amplitude waves with increasing the depth of anesthesia. Electrical silence cannot be achieved with ketamine.

6.4.3.3 Respiratory System

Ketamine has minimal effect on the ventilatory drive, but transient apnea can be observed with bolus induction doses. It is a potent bronchial smooth muscle relaxant, a valuable induction agent in asthmatic patients.

Upper airway reflexes are preserved more than with other induction drugs. Ketamine effect on increasing salivation and preserving the upper airway reflexes can precipitate laryngospasm. An anti-sialagogue is recommended before the administration of ketamine.

6.4.3.4 Effect on Other Organs

Ketamine increases the skeletal muscle tone. Its effect on intraocular pressure and its usage for open eye injuries is controversial.

6.4.4 Uses of Ketamine

- Induction and maintenance of general anesthesia especially in asthmatic patients. Induction in hypovolemic/hypotensive patients, although this is replaced by etomidate. Ketamine's direct depressant effect can be unmasked in these patients who are at their maximum sympathetic discharge, and this can cause further hemodynamic compromise.
  For induction: 1-2 mg/kg IV (2-6 mg/kg for children), 8-10 mg/kg IM, 8–10 mg/kg rectally, and 1-2 mg/kg via intraosseous route.
  For maintenance: 25–100 mcg/kg/min can be used alone or with propofol for total intravenous anesthesia (TIVA).
- Analgesia: Ketamine is described to achieve analgesia that is comparable to opioids quantitatively and qualitatively but with less respiratory depression. For augmentation of incomplete peripheral nerve block or neuraxial blocks, for positioning orthopedics patients for peripheral nerve/neuraxial blocks, and for dressing change, ketamine can be used at a dose of 0.25–0.5 mg/kg.
  Ketamine analgesia can be used as an adjunct to general anesthesia, to decrease opioid tolerance and opioid-induced hyperalgesia at a dose of 3–5 mcg/kg/min.
  Administration of ketamine 0.5 mg/kg with induction of general anesthesia followed by 10mcg/kg/h reduces the intraoperative and postoperative requirement of opioids in opioid-dependent patients with chronic back pain undergoing spine surgery.
  There is evidence that ketamine can provide acute relief of chronic neuropathic pain presumably by inhibition of the NMDA receptor and possibly through central enhancement of descending inhibition and anti-inflammatory effects.
- Preoperative sedation for pediatrics 3–15 mg/kg orally alone or combined with midazolam but should be titrated to clinical effect. Intranasal dose of 0.25-4 mg/kg and IM dose of 4–5 mg/kg induce sedation. Intranasal sedation and analgesia is of particular importance when IV administration is difficult.
- Bronchodilator in patients with status asthmaticus as an adjunct to other bronchodilators.
- Antidepressant: Ketamine proved to be an effective treatment for major depression, suicidal behavior, and bipolar disorder. Its antidepressant effect is believed to be due to the action on the phencyclidine site on the NMDA receptor or the stimulation of the AMPA receptors. It showed a high response rate and rapid effect for treatment of resistant depression and suicidal ideation.

- Anti-inflammatory: Ketamine exerts both local and general anti-inflammatory effects, and it appears to be an immune-modulator promoting inflammatory homeostasis. As an antagonist to NMDA receptors, it can suppress T helper cell differentiation and subsequent in vitro cytokine production.
  S(+) ketamine 1-3 mg/kg bolus followed by 2-4 mg/kg/hr during elective coronary bypass surgery has been shown to provide anti-inflammatory effect during and after cardiopulmonary bypass.

6.4.5 Side Effects of Ketamine

- Emergence delirium with hallucinations and nightmares that can be minimized by the co-administration of benzodiazepines and minimizing the stimulation on emergence.
- Slow emergence with dysphoria and high incidence of nausea and vomiting.
- Increase salivation and airway secretions, necessitating premedication with an anticholinergic agent.
- Tachycardia and hypertension that might not be well tolerated in patients with ischemic heart disease.
- Increase in the ICP is of concern in patients with space occupying lesions.
- Involuntary movements.
- Nystagmus, diplopia, and pupillary dilatation.
- There is a concern that NMDA antagonists and GABA mimetic drugs can induce neuronal injury and death in the brain of juvenile rodents, but lack of solid information to date limits the ability to issue particular recommendations.

6.5 Benzodiazepines

The main IV benzodiazepines in the present anesthetic practice are diazepam, lorazepam, and midazolam. Remimazolam is the newest precious addition to our benzodiazepines armamentarium, approved for procedural sedation in the USA in 2020, China and Europe in 2021 and was approved for general anesthesia in Japan in 2020.

Diazepam is lipid soluble and together with lorazepam prepared in propylene glycol to render them water soluble, but this comes with pain on injection and the potential of glycol toxicity on prolonged infusions.

Diazepam is supplied as 0.5% solution in 40% propylene glycol, 10% alcohol, 5% sodium benzoate and benzoic acid added as buffers, and 1.5% benzyl alcohol added as a preservative. Its pH is 6.6 (6.2 to 6.9). Lorazepam is supplied as 0.4% solution in propylene glycol, 18% polyethylene glycol, and 2% benzyl alcohol.

Midazolam is unique in its structure (◉ Fig. 6.5); at the acidic pH, which is how it is supplied, it is water soluble with no pain or irritation on injection. At physiologic pH, it assumes a more lipid soluble form due to conformational changes in its imidazole ring.

6.6 Midazolam

Under physiologic pH, midazolam acquires its physiologically active lipophilic closed ring form.

6.6.1 Mechanism of Action

Benzodiazepines bind a specific site at the interface of α(alpha) and γ(gamma) subunits of those $GABA_A$ receptors that contain α(alpha)1,2,3, and 5 subunits. Benzodiazepines by potentiating the inhibitory effect of GABA increases the chloride conductance and consequently the neuronal membrane hyperpolarization. The nature of this modulatory effect of benzodiazepines on $GABA_A$ may explain their CNS ceiling effect.

In high doses, such as general anesthesia induction doses, benzodiazepines might inhibit adenosine reuptake as well.

The muscle relaxant effect of benzodiazepines might be related to their agonist effect on the spinal cord glycine receptors.

6.6.2 Pharmacokinetics of Benzodiazepines

Midazolam is not just unique in its structure that provides a benzodiazepine that is both water and lipid soluble, but also in the routes of administration. It can be administered by IV, IM, oral, intranasal, rectal, and sublingual routes. It is highly bound to plasma proteins mainly to albumin.

Lipid solubility accounts for the rapid onset of midazolam action, but it takes longer than other sedative-hypnotics to reach peak effect, around 10 min after IV dose. Consequently, repeated doses should be spaced to avoid oversedation.

Redistribution out of the CNS results in the termination of the drug effect, and then metabolism takes place. It is mainly metabolized in the liver by hepatic microsomal p450-3A4 enzyme system via hydroxylation to hydroxymidazolam. Hydroxymidazolam has half the potency of the parent drug, but it is rapidly conjugated to the inactive glucuronide metabolite that is excreted in urine.

Midazolam bioavailability is 83% after intranasal administration, which is higher than when given orally (15%) due to the extensive first-pass metabolism. Bioavailability after intramuscular administration is 90%. When

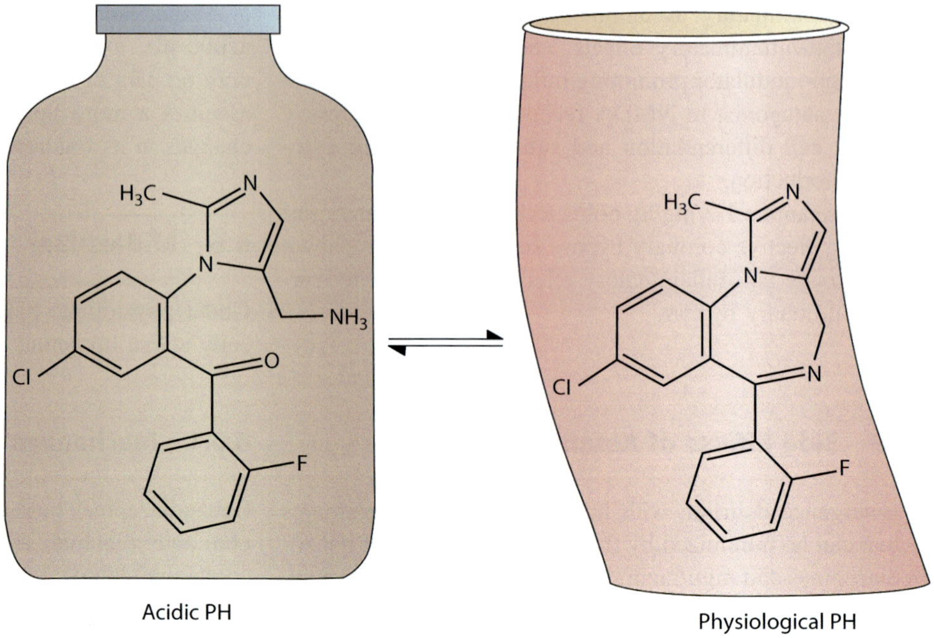

Fig. 6.5 Midazolam structural changes in acidic pH and physiologic pH (Reprinted with permission, Cleveland Clinic Center for Medical Art & Photography © 2016. All Rights Reserved)

given orally, midazolam shows onset of action in 10 min, peak in 20–30 min, and a duration of 45 min.

It is the shortest context-sensitive halftime compared to the other two benzodiazepines, which makes IV midazolam infusion attractive for sedation of mechanically ventilated patients in the intensive care unit (ICU).

Drugs known to inhibit p450-3A4 hepatic microsomal enzyme system—such as cimetidine, erythromycin, diltiazem, verapamil, ketoconazole, and itraconazole—can decrease the plasma clearance of midazolam and prolong its sedative effect.

Lorazepam differs from both midazolam and diazepam in its poor lipid and water solubility. It is highly bound to plasma proteins—approximately 90%. It can be administered via oral, IV, and IM routes. Its peak effect coincides with its peak serum level; 10 min after IV, 60 min after IM, and 90–120 min after oral administration with a bioavailability of 85% after an oral dose. Lorazepam is high protein binding and has poor lipid solubility, which may explain its relatively prolonged peak effect.

Lorazepam hepatic metabolism is not carried out by the microsomal p450 enzyme system but is conjugated to its inactive glucuronide metabolite and is excreted mainly in urine. For this reason, lorazepam metabolism is not affected in hepatic dysfunction like the other two benzodiazepines. Lorazepam's elimination half-life is 10–20 h.

Diazepam can be administered via oral, IV, and IM routes; the latter is not recommended due to its irritation (propylene glycol), pain, and erratic absorption. It is highly lipid soluble and highly protein bound, 96–99%. After IV administration, diazepam onset of action is twice as fast as midazolam but with a much longer duration of action. After IV dose, the onset of action is 1–5 min and peaks in effect in 15–60 min; after IM dose, it has an onset of action of 15–30 min and peak in effect in 30–60 min. When given via the oral route, diazepam has 100% bioavailability with a peak plasma level within 30–90 min.

In the liver, diazepam undergoes oxidative metabolism by demethylation, hydroxylation, as well as glucuronidation. It has several active metabolites (desmethyldiazepam, oxazepam, and temazepam), but the main active metabolite is desmethyldiazepam, which has an elimination half-life of 48–96 h, which is longer than the parent drug.

Oral contraceptive drugs can decrease the elimination of desmethyldiazepam while rifampin, phenytoin, and carbamazepine can enhance its metabolism.

6.6.3 Pharmacodynamics of Benzodiazepines

6.6.3.1 Cardiovascular System

Benzodiazepines cause venodilatation with decrease in venous return, causing a slight decrease in cardiac output and arterial blood pressure with slight increase in heart rate. A decrease in the arterial blood pressure is noticed in anxious hypertensive patients when given benzodiazepines.

6.6.3.2 Central Nervous System

Benzodiazepines cause a decrease in CMRO2 and CBF, but less than barbiturates, propofol, and etomidate. They have no significant effect on the ICP.

Benzodiazepines are potent anticonvulsants, but they have no neuroprotective effect and even in high doses cannot achieve burst suppression or isoelectric EEG.

They can induce anxiolysis and anterograde amnesia but not retrograde amnesia. Their muscle relaxant effect is believed to be through a central nervous system effect on the spinal cord. Tolerance has been described for their anticonvulsant and muscle relaxant effects.

6.6.3.3 Respiratory System

They decrease the ventilatory response to carbon dioxide in a dose-dependent fashion, and they decrease the hypoxic drive. This effect is pronounced in the elderly, COPD patients, and when combined with opioids. In induction doses, they can cause apnea.

6.6.4 Uses of Benzodiazepines

- For premedication, benzodiazepines are mainly used to relieve anxiety and tension before surgical procedures and to provide anterograde amnesia.
- For sedation during surgical procedures and for ventilated patients in the ICU where midazolam infusion plays an important role.
- For induction of general anesthesia, midazolam, and less commonly diazepam, can be used, but this has been replaced by other induction agents such as propofol and etomidate due to the delayed recovery with benzodiazepines.
- Diazepam is useful in relieving skeletal muscle spasms caused by local pathology or upper motor neurone disorders.
- Benzodiazepines are potent anticonvulsants, used for treating status epilepticus, especially diazepam and lorazepam. Midazolam is used for raising the threshold for convulsion in local anesthetic toxicity.

6.6.5 Side Effects

- Pain, local irritation, thrombophlebitis with diazepam injection that can be reduced by slow injection in a running IV fluid tubing. Erratic absorption on its IM administration.
- Can precipitate apnea in elderly patient with COPD and to be avoided in patients with hemodynamic instability.
- Benzodiazepines can cross the placenta and are avoided in pregnant ladies.
- Risk of precipitating porphyria in patients with acute intermittent porphyria, variegate porphyria, hereditary coproporphyria for the possibility of inducing ALA synthetase.
- They have the potential for drug abuse and dependence.
- Allergic reactions are rare with benzodiazepines.

6.6.6 Remimazolam

It is the newest addition to the benzodiazepines family, two salt forms have been developed: besylate and tosylate. Remimazolam shows high affinity for the $GABA_A$ receptor benzodiazepine site of action. It shows a rapid onset and offset of sedation compared to midazolam, and its effect is reversed by flumazenil. It is the unique structure of remimazolam with an added ester linkage that makes it a substrate to tissue esterases predicting its short duration of action.

It is known for its high clearance, small volume of distribution, a rapid onset and offset of sedation, and predictable effects over a wide dose range.

Remimazolam is highly bound in plasma (92%), very low bioavailability after oral administration (less than 2.2%) while its bioavailability after nasal administration is around 50%.

The breakdown of remimazolam is mainly via tissue esterases which differentiates it from other short-acting ester drugs that blood esterases play the predominant role in their metabolism. Carboxylesterase 1(CSE 1) is the major esterase responsible for remimazolam metabolism, and it is highly expressed in liver, gall bladder, and lungs. The carboxylic acid metabolite is 400 times weaker at $GABA_A$ receptor benzodiazepine site of action compared to the parent drug.

The context-sensitive halftime is largely insensitive to the duration of infusion, 6–11 min after 2 h of infusion.

Compared to propofol sedation, remimazolam sedation shows a lower incidence of hypotension, respiratory depression, and pain on injection while there is slightly higher incidence of nausea and vomiting.

Remimazolam shows a lower potential for drug interactions compared to midazolam, but flavonoids, fatty acids, and alcohol (known inhibitors for CSE 1) can prolong its duration of action.

6.7 Propofol

Propofol (2,6 diisopropylphenol) is an alkylated phenol that replaced thiopental sodium as the most commonly used drug for induction of general anesthesia. It made the concept of total intravenous anesthesia (TIVA) possible and widely applicable. Propofol induction is described as rapid, smooth induction with nearly no excitation phenomenon.

Propofol is highly lipid soluble but water insoluble, and for this reason, it is prepared as a 1% aqueous solution in an oil-in-water emulsion of soybean oil, glycerol, and purified egg phosphatide (from egg yolk lecithin). Since this medium is an inviting medium to microbial contamination, ethylenediaminetetraacetic acid (EDTA), metabisulfite, or benzyl alcohol is added as a bacteriostatic.

6.7.1 Mechanism of Action

Propofol exerts its hypnotic effect through enhancing the effect of GABA on $GABA_A$ receptors and directly activates the receptor. It is believed that propofol carries out its effect through interaction with α (alpha), β (beta), and γ(gamma) subunits of the receptor. It causes an inward directed chloride current that inhibits the neuronal depolarization by hyperpolarizing the postsynaptic membrane. It is a dose-dependent effect; at low concentration, propofol potentiates GABA-activated inward chloride current while at higher concentrations, it directly activates the channel opening.

6.7.2 Pharmacokinetics of Propofol

Propofol is highly protein bound (98%), predominantly to albumin. The pharmacologically active free portion of the drug is more available when the plasma protein concentration decreases.

Its extreme lipid solubility enables the drug to gain fast access to the CNS. The pharmacological effect of propofol is terminated by redistribution from the central compartment to the periphery with a redistribution half-life ($t1/2\alpha$[alpha]) of 1–2 min and the effect of an intravenous bolus fades in 8 min (approximately 4 half-lives).

Propofol has a context-sensitive halftime of < 40 min after 8 h infusion.

Metabolism is mainly through hepatic conjugation to the inactive glucuronide and sulfate metabolites (have no hypnotic activity) that are excreted in urine. Clearance of propofol is believed to have an extra hepatic component, mostly in the kidneys as its clearance exceeds the hepatic blood flow and it continues during anhepatic phase of liver transplantation.

Propofol is also excreted through exhalation; although extremely small amount, it correlates with the plasma concentration. Recently, a commercially available spectrometer is introduced to measure propofol concentration in exhaled air.

Neonates and elderly patients have a reduced clearance, but patients with cirrhosis and end-stage renal disease do not show reduced clearance.

6.7.3 Pharmacodynamics

6.7.3.1 Cardiovascular System

Propofol causes systemic hypotension through venous and arteriolar vasodilatation, decreasing the preload, systemic vascular resistance, and afterload. It might cause a slight myocardial depression as well. This hypotension is commonly not accompanied with increase in the heart rate due to attenuation of the baroreceptor reflex tachycardia that accompanies hypotension. Cases of severe bradycardia and sinus arrest have been reported.

The hemodynamic response lags behind the hypnotic effect of propofol.

It is believed that propofol exerts a dose-dependent cardioprotective effect that is less profound than sevoflurane. It attenuates ischemia–reperfusion myocardial injury by exerting free radical scavenging effects and decreases lipid peroxidase activity.

6.7.3.2 Central Nervous System

Propofol decreases CMRO2, causes cerebral vasoconstriction, decreases CBF, CBV, and ICP while maintaining the vascular responsiveness to carbon dioxide. The favorable effects of propofol on the cerebral physiology makes it the most ideal anesthetic for neurosurgery.

The hypotension that may accompany propofol administration can compromise the cerebral perfusion pressure (CPP).

It is believed that propofol has a neuroprotective effect, and it can induce burst suppression. The anticonvulsant effect of propofol is appreciated, and it can terminate resistant attacks of status epilepticus.

6.7.3.3 Respiratory System

Propofol is effective in suppressing the airway reflexes attenuating its responsiveness during manipulation. It facilitates the supraglottic airway devices placement. Endotracheal intubation without the need for neuromuscular blocking agents is feasible with propofol. Airway manipulation after propofol shows lower incidence of coughing and laryngospasm than other induction agents.

It interferes with ventilation in a dose-dependent manner by affecting the central chemoreceptor sensitivity, reducing the ventilatory response to hypercapnia and hypoxia. A dose-dependent decrease in the ventilatory drive is noticed with decrease in tidal volumes with propofol administration. Apnea is not uncommon with propofol induction. The bronchodilator effect of propofol may be due to attenuation of the vagally mediated bronchoconstriction.

Propofol potentiates hypoxic pulmonary vasoconstriction.

6.7.3.4 Effects on Other Organs

The antiemetic effect of propofol in sub-anesthetic doses is proven, but the exact mechanism is unclear. It has been demonstrated that propofol interacts with dopaminergic (D2) receptors in the chemoreceptor trigger zone, inhibits the limbic system, and consequently interacts with the cortical reflexes reaching the vomiting center. It inhibits 5-HT_3 receptors in the CNS in a dose-dependent non-competitive manner.

The antipruritic effect that it shows in cholestasis and after epidural morphine is another obscure mechanism.

It has no effect on the uterine tone, but it crosses the placenta. However, due to its clearance from the neonatal circulation, it has only minimal and short-lived clinical effects on unborn neonates.

6.7.4 Uses of Propofol

Propofol is only suitable for intravenous use.

- Induction and maintenance of general anesthesia.
  Induction dose: 2–2.5 mg/kg in adults.
  - 1–1.5 mg/kg in elderly patients.
  - 2.5–3.5 mg/kg for pediatrics.
  - Fentanyl significantly decreases the propofol required for loss of consciousness and suppression of responses to noxious stimuli.
    Following loss of verbal contact than checking the eye lash reflex with slow titrated administration might decrease the chance of hypotension.
    Maintenance dose: 100–200 mcg/kg/min for adults (lower doses with concomitant opioids administration).
  - 125–300 mcg/kg/min for pediatrics
- Sedation for procedures and surgeries done under monitored anesthesia care with or without regional blocks.
- Sedation of mechanically ventilated patients in the ICU where the level of sedation is assessed on a daily basis and reduction of the infusion rate as needed to avoid high plasma levels after prolonged infusions.
- Anticonvulsant that can terminate resistant attacks of status epilepticus.
  Antiemetic in sub-anesthetic doses.
  10 mg followed by an infusion of 1 mg/kg/h.
- Antipruritic.

6.7.5 Side Effects of Propofol

- Pain on injection, which is common on injecting propofol. This is believed to be due to direct and indirect irritation of the venous adventitia by free aqueous propofol through the interaction with TRPV1 and TRPA1 receptors. The free aqueous concentration of propofol is thought to be reduced when it is prepared in a solution containing more medium-chain triglycerides than intralipid.
  Several techniques are described to minimize it: injection in a large vein with a fast running carrier fluid and using lidocaine either prior to or mixed with propofol. It is found that keeping the lidocaine locally in the vein for 2 min by using a tourniquet is more efficient than mixing it. If lidocaine is to be premixed, limiting the dose to 20 mg is prudent due to reports on causing instability of the emulsion if more than 20 mg are used. Compared to thiopental, intra-arterial injection or subcutaneous extravasation is well tolerated with no sequelae.
- Myoclonic movements are noticed with propofol induction that might be mistaken for seizures.
- Bradycardia and possible asystole.
- Propofol infusion syndrome (PRIS): In genetically predisposed patients, propofol can interfere with the mitochondrial fatty acid oxidation and respiratory chain electron transfer, leading to accumulation of free fatty acids and failure to produce adenosine triphosphate (ATP). This is characterized by severe metabolic acidosis, hyperkalemia, hyperlipidemia, rhabdomyolysis, hepatomegaly, refractory bradycardia, and renal failure. It is noticed more in pediatrics and in patients receiving more than 4 mg/kg/h. Developing unexplained acidosis during propofol infusion should raise the concern about PRIS. Once diagnosed, propofol infusion should be stopped, and cardiorespiratory support even with ECMO (extracorporeal membrane oxygenation) support and hemodialysis provided to clear the acid load.
- On rare occasions pancreatitis.
- Allergic reactions to propofol are reported, but people who have egg allergy or soy bean allergy can receive propofol safely as the allergic reaction is usually to the protein component that is not in the drug emulsion.

6.7.6 Target-Controlled Infusions (TCI)

The goal when we administer drugs is to achieve and maintain therapeutic level according to the clinical need. A clear understanding of the pharmacokinetics and pharmacodynamics allows us to achieve this goal manually when we administer IV boluses and infusions as a dose/time.

Rather than setting a rate, the target-controlled infusion systems (TCI) through a well-understood pharmacokinetics principles, computers can calculate the infusion rate and boluses to achieve a user defined, predicted drug concentration in plasma or effect site, i.e., the brain.

TCI systems are used in more than 50 countries nowadays with drugs like propofol, fentanyl, sufentanil, remifentanil, and alfentanil.

As of this chapter's writing, TCI systems are not used in the USA due to disagreement on the pharmacokinetic model.

6.8 Propofol Derivatives

Efforts are attempted to overcome the disadvantage of propofol emulsion: risk of infection and pain on injection by modifying the emulsion formulation but unfortunately with limited success.

These attempts include decrease the oil content of the emulsion or use microemulsions with smaller droplets that those oil droplets in the current propofol emulsion.

Then another modification was attempted to increase the proportion of medium-chain triglycerides (MCTs) in the emulsion as they are more polar than the long-chain triglycerides (LCTs). Propofol-Lipuro is an example of the mixed MCT-LCT that has similar pharmacokinetics and pharmacodynamics as propofol but with less pain on injection. It has been used outside the USA since 1999. Modifying the emulsion by adding albumin was attempted as well.

Another approach was to work on nonemulsion formulations using alternatives to the oil emulsions as cyclodextrins and micelle formulation of propofol with no recent published data.

Propofol prodrugs and analogs have been developed to find an answer to the propofol formulation problem, where a water-soluble drug can be converted to propofol in vivo. Fospropofol disodium (Lusedra) has been approved by USA FDA. A methyl phosphate group substituted the hydroxyl on the propofol molecule first carbon. It requires alkaline phosphatase to cleave the molecule into the active propofol molecule. It is less painful on injection and has a slower onset and a longer duration of action compared to propofol but with greater perineal pain or paresthesia. Fospropofol was discontinued.

HX0507 and HX0969w are another water-soluble prodrugs of propofol under investigation.

6.9 Dexmedetomidine

Dexmedetomidine is a highly selective α (alpha)2 adrenergic receptor agonist chemically related to clonidine. It has unique effects of sedation that mimics normal sleep with easy transition from sleep to wakefulness, anxiolysis, decrease sympathetic tone, analgesia, and anesthetic-sparing effects with minimal respiratory depression. This provides the value of dexmedetomidine for sedation in the operating room and ICU.

6.9.1 Mechanism of Action

Dexmedetomidine is eight times more specific for α(alpha)2 adrenergic receptors than clonidine. The sedative hypnotic effect of dexmedetomidine is at the level of the brain stem locus ceruleus that modulates the state of wakefulness. The α(alpha)2 adrenergic receptors stimulation hyperpolarizes the noradrenergic neurones, suppressing the normal firing of the locus ceruleus, and inhibits the norepinephrine release and activity in the medullospinal pathway. This triggers a decrease in the histamine release resulting in hypnosis resembling normal sleep.

The interruption of the descending norepinephrine pathways that modulates nociception causes analgesia by interrupting the pain signaling.

At the spinal cord level, activation of the α(alpha)2 adrenergic receptors in the dorsal horn lamina II reduces the release of substance—p and glutamate, interrupting the nociceptive transmission.

Central postsynaptic α (alpha)2 receptors activation results in a sympatholytic effect that causes hypotension and bradycardia.

6.9.2 Pharmacokinetics

Dexmedetomidine follows zero-order kinetics (a constant amount of the drug is eliminated per hour). After IV administration, its onset of action is after 15 min and peak plasma concentration is reached 1 h after continuous IV infusion.

Dexmedetomidine can be administered via IV, IM, intranasal, oral, intrathecal, and buccal routes. It has a bioavailability of 65% and 81% after nasal and buccal administration, respectively. It shows a poor bioavailability (16%) after oral administration. Only the IV route is approved by the FDA.

It is 94% bound to albumin and α(alpha)-1 glycoprotein with a distribution half-life (t1/2α[alpha]) of 6 min and elimination half-life (t1/2β[beta]) of 2–2.5 h.

Dexmedetomidine is extensively metabolized in the liver through glucuronide conjugations and biotransformation by cytochrome p450 enzyme system to inactive metabolites that are excreted 95% in urine and 4% in feces.

6.9.3 Pharmacodynamics of Dexmedetomidine

6.9.3.1 Cardiovascular System

Dexmedetomidine has a biphasic effect when given by IV infusion. Initially, it causes hypertension and bradycardia that last for 10 min. Hypertension is caused by the stimulation of the peripheral vascular smooth muscles α(alpha)-2b adrenergic receptors and can be attenuated by slow IV infusion. This is followed by 10–20% decrease in the blood pressure due to the central sympatholytic effect that overrides the peripheral effect.

The baroreceptor reflex is well preserved during dexmedetomidine administration. There are reports on the cardioprotective effect of dexmedetomidine that warrants further studying.

6.9.3.2 Central Nervous System

Dexmedetomidine provides a unique sedative effect that resembles normal sleep. The analgesic effect is believed to be due to central as well as peripheral effect with a proven analgesics/anesthetic-sparing effect. Dexmedetomidine reduces CBF and decreases CMR, although there is still a debate on the reduction of CMR.

Animal studies showed that dexmedetomidine can decrease CBF despite raising the mean arterial pressure without reducing CMRO2. This might be due to stimulation of the postsynaptic α(alpha)2 receptors on the cerebral blood vessels causing vasoconstriction. There was no evidence that this effect in cerebral blood vessels could cause global ischemia. Despite the reported neuroprotective effects of dexmedetomidine in ischemic brain injury models, concerns were raised regarding its effect on CBF without altering CMRO2. It should be noted that α(alpha)2 agonists are more potent vasoconstrictors to cerebral venous more than arterial blood vessels.

At a low dose, dexmedetomidine decreased the ICP while at a higher dose had no effect on the ICP in rabbits.

Whether dexmedetomidine has a neuroprotective effect needs further studying.

6.9.3.3 Respiratory

Dexmedetomidine has a minimal effect on respiration, but in high doses, it can decrease the tidal volume. This effect makes dexmedetomidine attractive in patients who require sedation with minimal effect on their respiration, such as in awake craniotomies and for difficult airway awake intubation.

6.9.3.4 Effect on Other Organs

Dexmedetomidine decreases the intraocular pressure. It decreases the release of renin through its α(alpha)2 adrenoreceptor effect. It induces diuresis by inhibiting the release of antidiuretic hormone.

Dexmedetomidine has no muscle relaxing effect, but it reduces the requirement of rocuronium during sevoflurane anesthesia.

6.9.4 Uses

- Premedication for anxiolysis but lacks amnestic effect.
  Although the IV route is the only FDA-approved route, it is reported to be given via IM, buccal, and intranasal routes. A dose of intranasal dexmedetomidine 2.5 mcg/kg was found to be superior to 0.5 mg/kg oral midazolam in the pediatrics population.
- Sedation for mechanically ventilated patients in the ICU, where in the U.S. it is approved for IV infusion for 24 h.
- Sedation during regional blocks and surgical procedures where the benefit of cooperative sedation with minimal effect on ventilation is valued as in awake craniotomies and awake fiber-optic intubation where it provides the added benefit as anti-sialagogue.
  A loading dose of 1 mcg/kg over 10 min to be followed by 0.2–0.7 mcg/kg/h.
- Adjuvant to general anesthesia, blunting the sympathetic tone together with its opioid- and anesthetic-sparing effect.
- The use of dexmedetomidine as an adjunct to neuroaxial and peripheral nerve blocks is off label. Epidural dexmedetomidine showed synergism to local anesthetics, improving the quality and prolonging the motor and sensory block. It has a favorable effect on peripheral nerve blocks, reported to shorten the onset and prolong the duration of nerve blocks.
- Treatment of postoperative shivering: A single IV bolus dose of dexmedetomidine was found to shorten the duration of shivering by 15 min and a similar or better effect compared to meperidine.
- It decreases the emergence agitation in the pediatrics population.
- The anti-inflammatory benefits of dexmedetomidine is a new arena in research. It was found to decrease the serum or tissue inflammatory mediators as TNFα, IL-6, IL-1B, and C-reactive protein as well as the experimental evidence of reducing neuroinflammation.
- Dexmedetomidine may be beneficial as a new class of sleep-enhancing medication.
- It enhances the postoperative bowel recovery and relief of sore throat.

6.9.5 Side Effects

The main side effects of dexmedetomidine are due to its biphasic hemodynamic effect, with initial hypertension and bradycardia then hypotension. There are reports of severe bradycardia and even asystole with dexmedetomidine, but in the great majority of cases, this bradycardia does not need intervention. This can be avoided by administering the bolus doses as an infusion over 10 min or sometimes omitting the bolus dose. If it happens, usually IV fluids, ephedrine, or atropine can reverse the side effects.

6.10 Conclusion

The action of most IV anesthesia induction agents is through their interaction with $GABA_A$ receptors with the exception of ketamine.

Barbiturates, once the most commonly used IV general anesthesia induction agents (especially thiopental), are replaced now by propofol. Methohexital still has its place in anesthesia for ECT. In 2010, thiopental ceased to be offered in the USA.

Remimazolam the novel short-acting IV benzodiazepines shows high affinity for the $GABA_A$ receptor benzodiazepine site of action. It has a rapid onset and offset of sedation compared to midazolam and a unique structure that makes it a substrate to tissue esterases predicting its short duration of action.

Etomidate is the drug of choice for induction of hemodynamically unstable patients due to its lacking of any cardiovascular depressant effect. Concerns about its adrenocortical suppression, especially in critically ill ventilated patients, stimulated the research for future analogs.

Ketamine has a dual effect: a direct depressant effect and an indirect effect that usually takes the upper hand resulting in sympathetic outflow, except in patients with exhausted sympathetic nervous system where the depressant effect is unmasked. Still ketamine is a valuable induction agent in asthmatic patients.

The most commonly used benzodiazepines in the anesthetic practice nowadays are: midazolam, diazepam, and lorazepam. Midazolam is unique in its pharmacology due to changes in its imidazole ring rendering it more lipid soluble in physiologic pH.

Propofol, the most commonly used drug to induce general anesthesia, is widely used for sedation during surgery/procedures and in the ICU. Propofol infusion syndrome (PRIS) is a serious fatal side effect of its prolonged used. Unexplained acidosis and elevated triglycerides during its usage may be a clue for PRIS.

Dexmedetomidine (an α[alpha]2 receptor agonist), although not an IV general anesthesia induction agent, is a valuable sedative with anesthetic/analgesic-sparing effect with minimal effect on respiration.

6.11 Questions and Answers

Questions (Choose the Most Appropriate Answer)

1. Termination of Methohexital anesthetic induction effect is attributed to:
   A. Hepatic metabolism
   B. Renal excretion
   C. Destruction of the barbituric acid ring
   D. Redistribution
2. Drugs working on the $GABA_A$ receptor are:
   A. Ketamine
   B. Etomidate
   C. Dexmedetomidine
   D. All of the above
3. Precipitation in the IV tubing is noticed after atracurium is administered immediately and without flushing after:
   A. Etomidate
   B. Propofol
   C. Methohexital
   D. None of the above
4. Among the IV induction agents used for ECT, the maximum prolongation of the seizure activity is noticed with:
   A. Methohexital
   B. Ketamine
   C. Etomidate
   D. Propofol
5. Compared to propofol, etomidate has:
   A. Longer context-sensitive half-time
   B. Shorter context-sensitive half-time
   C. The same context-sensitive half-time
   D. Etomidate is context insensitive
6. Compared to thiopental, the lipid solubility of ketamine is:
   A. More than thiopental
   B. Less than thiopental
   C. The same as thiopental
   D. Ketamine does not show lipid solubility
7. When midazolam is given to a hypertensive patient on diltiazem, the sedative effect is expected to be:
   A. Shortened
   B. Prolonged
   C. No change in the sedative effect
   D. Weakens its sedative effect
8. The drug known for its metabolism via tissue esterase is:
   A. Midazolam

B. Remimazolam
C. Lorazepam
D. Diazepam

9. Propofol extrahepatic metabolism is carried out mainly in:
   A. Kidney
   B. Spleen
   C. Lungs
   D. RBCs
10. Dexmedetomidine can cause:
    A. Hypotension
    B. Hypertension
    C. Diuresis
    D. All of the above
    E. a and b

Answers

1. **D**. After an induction dose of methohexital, the termination of its pharmacological effect is due to redistribution from the CNS. Neither metabolism nor renal excretion play an important role unless the drug is given in repeated doses or by infusion for prolonged duration.
2. **B**. GABA is the most abundant inhibitory transmitter in the CNS. Etomidate, barbiturates, benzodiazepines, and propofol act on GABAA receptors either by modulation of its function or directly to induce general anesthesia or sedation. Ketamine works mainly as an antagonist to NMDA receptor, while dexmedetomidine acts on α(alpha)2 adrenoreceptor.
3. **C**. Methohexital is an alkaline drug, and when mixed with acidic drugs such as vecuronium, atracurium, rocuronium, it precipitates and this can occlude the IV tubing interrupting the anesthetic induction. It is recommended to flush the IV tubing with running IV fluids before adding an acidic drug after methohexital or thiopental.
4. **C**. It is found that when used for induction of general anesthesia for ECT, etomidate induces longer seizure activity than methohexital. Ketamine and propofol are less commonly used for ECT.
5. **B**. When etomidate is administered as an infusion (a practice that faded due to the adrenocortical suppression), it has a context-sensitive halftime that is shorter than propofol.
6. **A**. Ketamine is highly lipid soluble, eight times more than thiopental. It is its high lipid solubility and low protein binding that facilitates a rapid access to the CNS.
7. **B**. Midazolam is metabolized mainly by the hepatic microsomal p450-3A4 enzyme system. Drugs that inhibit P450-3A4 enzyme system as cimetidine, erythromycin, diltiazem, verapamil, ketoconazole, and itraconazole can decrease the plasma clearance of midazolam and prolong its sedative effect.
8. **B**. The breakdown of remimazolam is mainly via tissue esterases which differentiates it from other short-acting ester drugs that blood esterases play the predominant role in their metabolism.
9. **A**. Propofol clearance exceeds the hepatic blood flow, and its clearance continues in anhepatic phase. It is found that the kidneys are responsible for up to 30% of propofol clearance.
10. **E**. Dexmedetomidine as IV infusion has a biphasic effect, initially hypertension and bradycardia that last for 10 min due to stimulation of the peripheral vascular smooth muscles α(alpha)-2b adrenergic receptors causing hypertension and reflex bradycardia. This is followed by the central sympatholytic effect that takes the upper hand over the peripheral effect with decrease in the blood pressure by 10–20%.

Suggested Reading

1. Patel HH, Pearn ML, Patel PM, Roth DM. General anesthetics and therapeutic gases. In: Brunton LL, Hilal-Dandan R, Knollmann BC, editors. Goodman & Gilman's: the pharmacological basis of therapeutics, vol. 13e. McGraw Hill; 2017.
2. Sahinovic MM, Struys MMRF, Absalom AR. Clinical pharmacokinetics and pharmacodynamics of propofol. Clin Pharmacokinet. 2018;57(12):1539–58. https://doi.org/10.1007/s40262-018-0672-3.
3. Ingrande J, Lemmens HJ. Target-controlled infusion: not a one-sized-fits-all answer to drug administration. Anesth Analg. 2018;127(4):813–4. https://doi.org/10.1213/ANE.0000000000003461.
4. Valk BI, Struys MMRF. Etomidate and its analogs: a review of pharmacokinetics and pharmacodynamics. Clin Pharmacokinet. 2021;60(10):1253–69. https://doi.org/10.1007/s40262-021-01038-6.
5. Forman SA. Clinical and molecular pharmacology of etomidate. Anesthesiology. 2011;114(3):695–707.
6. Gao M, Rejaei D, Liu H. Ketamine use in current clinical practice. Acta Pharmacol Sin. 2016;37(7):865–72. https://doi.org/10.1038/aps.2016.5.
7. Sneyd JR, Gambus PL, Rigby-Jones AE. Current status of perioperative hypnotics, role of benzodiazepines, and the case for remimazolam: a narrative review. Br J Anaesth. 2021;127(1):41–55. https://doi.org/10.1016/j.bja.2021.03.028.
8. Sottas CE, Anderson BJ. Dexmedetomidine: the new all-in-one drug in paediatric anaesthesia? Curr Opin Anaesthesiol. 2017;30(4):441–51. https://doi.org/10.1097/ACO.0000000000000488. PMID: 28537937.
9. Mahmoud M, Mason KP. Dexmedetomidine: review, update, and future considerations of paediatric perioperative and periprocedural applications and limitations. Br J Anaesth. 2015;115(2):171–82.

Pharmacology of Opioids

7

Maria F. Ramirez, Siddhant Bhoir, and Juan P. Cata

Abstract

Opioids are the most effective analgesic used to manage acute and chronic pain. In general, the selection of opioids should be reserved for patients with acute moderate-to-severe postoperative pain or chronic malignant pain. It is anticipated that non-opioid therapy will not provide adequate treatment. When deciding which type of opioid is most appropriate for patients, one should consider the route of administration, pharmacokinetics/pharmacodynamics, patient's comorbidities, patient's individual needs, and most importantly, the clinical risk and benefits. For this, the fundamental understanding of the clinical pharmacology of opioids is paramount since opioids are associated with short- and long-term adverse events, including tolerance, addiction, and misuse. Opioid-based analgesia does not have a dose-related ceiling effect, but rather the severity of adverse events limits the escalation dose. Therefore, individual titration and combination with non-opioid analgesia should be considered to maximize the analgesic effect of opioids while reducing their adverse effects.

Keywords

Opioids • Pain management • Acute pain • Chronic pain • Opioid receptor

M. F. Ramirez · S. Bhoir · J. P. Cata (✉)
Department of Anesthesiology and Perioperative Medicine, MD Anderson Cancer Center, The University of Texas, Austin, TX, USA
e-mail: JCata@mdanderson.org

Anesthesiology and Surgical Oncology Research Group., Houston, TX, USA

7.1 Mechanism of Action

Opioids exert their effects by binding to specific proteins known as opioid receptors. Analgesia is achieved by opioids binding to three main receptors: mu (MOR), delta (DOR), and kappa (KOR) receptors [1] (Table 7.1). Each class of opioid receptor has subtypes, including MOR1, MOR2, and MOR3, KOR1, KOR2, and KOR3, DOR1, and DOR2. It is important to know that MOR forms and can function as heteromers with DOR (MOR-DOR) and KOR (MOR-KOR) [2].

MOR is a seven-transmembrane receptor that couples to intracellular G proteins. MOR receptors display an extracellular N-terminus and an intracellular C-terminus and are coupled with G_i/G_o proteins (Fig. 7.1). After binding a ligand, MOR activates the release of the inhibitory Gi protein, which causes adenylate cyclase inhibition, reducing cyclic 3′, 5′ adenosine monophosphate (cAMP) and reducing levels of protein kinase A activation [3]. The net result of activation of MORs in the reduction of intracellular cAMP, the opening of the voltage-sensitive K+ channels that allow K+ ions to flow out of the neuron, and ultimately hyperpolarization of cell membranes. Hyperpolarization of the cell membrane inhibits the neuron's action potential and the release of neurotransmitters [4].

The analgesic effect of MOR agonists is predominantly caused by the binding to the MOR1 subtype receptor. At the same time, their action on the MOR2 is responsible for most of the adverse effects related to opioids (i.e., respiratory depression, sedation, pruritus, prolactin release, dependence, anorexia, and sedation) [5]. Additionally, the interaction between the serotoninergic and dopaminergic with opioidergic systems also explains some of the analgesic effects of opioids [6, 7].

MOR receptors are expressed in the central nervous system and peripheral tissues of the body. In the central nervous system, MORs are distributed presynaptically in various regions, including the periaqueductal gray region of the brainstem, the thalamus, and the dorsal horn of the spinal

M. Argalious et al. (eds.), *Basic Sciences in Anesthesia*,
https://doi.org/10.1007/978-3-031-60203-0_7

Table 7.1 Opioid classification according to their action on opioid receptor

Full agonist	Partial agonist	Agonist–antagonist	Antagonist	
			Central	Peripheral
Alfentanil Codeine Fentanyl Hydrocodone Hydromorphone Methadone Morphine Remifentanil Sufentanil Oxycodone Oxymorphone Tramadol	Buprenorphine Dezocine	Nalbuphine Nalorphine Pentazocine	Naloxone Naltrexone	Alvimopan Methylnaltrexone Naloxegol Naldemedine

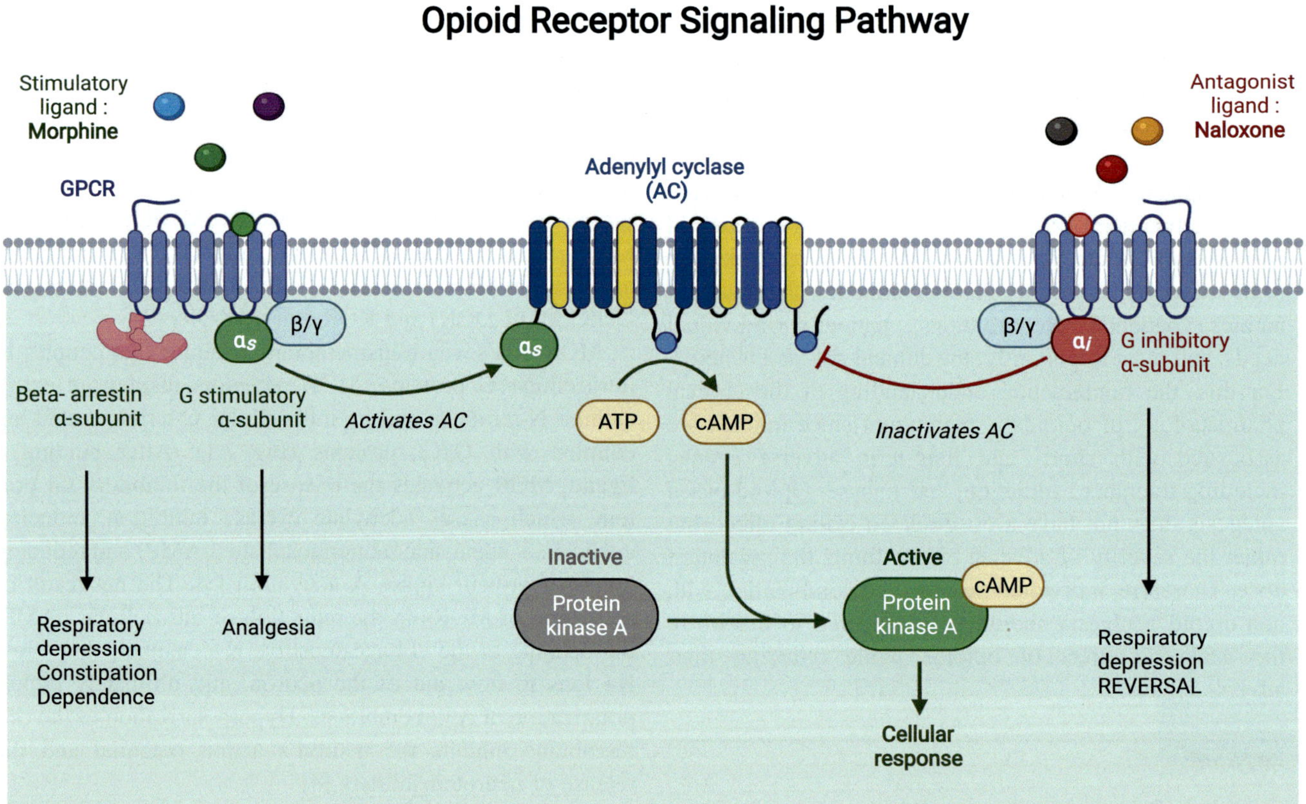

Fig. 7.1 Summary of opioid receptor signaling. Figure depicts opioid receptor signaling transduction. Like other G protein–coupled receptors, MOR signaling is mediated by adenylyl cyclase, the extracellular signal-regulated kinase pathway, and intracellular calcium and ion channels. The binding of agonist to the MOR leads to analgesia and respiratory. The binding of MOR antagonist leads to the reversal of the respiratory depression. Biased agonism acts of MOR to activate G protein signaling over β-arrestin 2 recruitment with less respiratory depression

cord [8, 9]. Activation of this receptor in neurons triggers a complex cascade of intracellular signals that lead to analgesia. MORs activation can promote inflammation, immunosuppression, and angiogenesis due to its activity in lymphocytes, macrophages, and cancer cells [10, 11].

Endogenous ligands of MOR include enkephalins, endorphin, dynorphin A, and nociceptins. Exogenous ligands include prescription drugs such as morphine, fentanyl, methadone, and oxycodone. All exogenous ligands can produce analgesia, tolerance, and physical or psychological dependence. They also cause unwanted gastrointestinal, cardiovascular, respiratory, and immunological adverse events. Interestingly, endogenous ligands can also mimic some of the exogenous opioid-related adverse effects [12]. Opioids that fully activate (i.e., morphine and oxycodone) are full agonists.

Table 7.2 Opioid pharmacokinetics

	Bioavailability % (oral dose)	Vd (L/kg)	Metabolism	Main metabolite	Excretion
Alfentanil	NA	0.4–10	Liver—CYP3A4	Noralfentanil	Urine (90%)
Codeine	60%	3–6	Liver—CYP3A4 and 2D6	Active—Morphine	Urine (70%)
Fentanyl	NA	3–5	Hydromorphone	None	Urine (75%)
Hydrocodone	25%	3.7–4.7	Liver—CYP2D6	Hydromorphone	Urine (25%)
Hydromorphone	25–50%	4	Liver—UGT	Unknown	Urine (75%)
Methadone	36–100%	1–8	Liver—CYP3A4, 2D6, 2B6, 2C19	None	Urine (<10%)
Morphine	30–40%	3–5	Liver—UGT	Inactive—M3G Active—M6G	Urine (90%)
Remifentanil	NA	0.2–0.3	Tissue esterases	Remifentanil acid	Urine
Sufentanil	NA	4.9–11.3	Liver—CYP3A4	None	Urine (90%)
Oxycodone	60–80%	2.6	Liver—CYP3A4 and 2D6	Active—Oxymorphone	Urine (19–64%)
Oxymorphone	10%	1.94–4.22	Liver—UGT	Active—6-OH	Urine (33–38%)
Tramadol	70%	2.6	Liver—CYP3A4 and 2D6	Active—M1	Urine (90%)

On the other hand, those opioids that occupy but do not activate the MOR are opioid antagonists (e.g., naltrexone and naloxone) [13]. Naloxone and naltrexone are also competitive antagonists at the kappa receptors. Partial agonist binds to the opioid receptor but produces a partial response independently of the amount of drug administered (buprenorphine) [14, 15]. It should be noted that buprenorphine is also an antagonist of KOR which makes it a commonly used drug to treat opioid abuse, induce detoxification, and as maintenance therapy. Agonists–antagonists can show a high affinity for MOR but exhibit little efficacy [16] (Table 7.2). Oliceridine is a biased agonist of MOR that has been recently approved for acute postoperative pain. It has been speculated that biased agonists such as oliceridine would produce potent analgesia while decreasing the risk of tolerance and other adverse effects (i.e., respiratory depression) associated with conventional full MOR agonists [17].

Most clinically available prescription opioids primarily produce their analgesic effects via binding to MOR [18]. The exogenous opioids can be classified into four chemical groups: the morphinan derivates (levorphanol and butorphanol), the benzomorphan derivates (pentazocine and pentazocine), the diphenylheptane derivates (methadone, and propoxyphene), and the phenylpiperidine derivates (pethidine, alfentanil, fentanyl, sufentanil, and remifentanil).

7.2 Pharmacokinetics and Pharmacodynamics

Absorption

Absorption is the transportation of the un-metabolized drug from the administration site to the body circulation. Multiple mechanisms of drug absorption have been described, including passive diffusion, facilitated passive diffusion, and active transport. Regardless of the route of administration, opioids need to cross the cell membranes to reach the systemic circulation. Most importantly, opioids must cross the blood–brain barrier to exert strong analgesic effects. Overall, opioids are well absorbed. However, multiple factors can affect drug opioid absorption, including molecular size, lipid solubility, degree of ionization, protein binding, and cell membrane properties [19]. In terms of solubility, high lipophilic opioids (i.e., fentanyl) cross the cell membrane rapidly and therefore are more efficiently absorbed when given transdermal or transmucosal.

Opioids are considered weak base molecules (pKa 6.5–8.7). In the stomach's acidic environment, opioids are highly ionized and poorly absorbed. In contrast, in an alkaline pH microenvironment such as the small intestine, the pH favors the creation of a unionized fraction of opioids and increases drug absorption [20]. Molecular size is another important determinant in the absorption of drugs; as the molecular weight decreases, the rate of the latter increases.

Distribution

Orally given opioids are absorbed in the gastric and duodenal mucosa and then transported to the systemic circulation via the portal venous system. Upon entering the systemic circulation, opioids are distributed throughout the body. In contrast, intravenous, intramuscular, sublingual, and subcutaneous administration allows for direct access to the systemic circulation providing more rapid onset of action. The distribution of opioids is uneven and is secondary to the differences in regional blood floods. The intravenous injection of morphine, hydromorphone, fentanyl, sufentanil, alfentanil, and remifentanil follows a three-compartment pharmacokinetic model [21]. The three-compartment model divides the body into a central compartment and two peripheral compartments. The central compartment represents the plasma and the tissue where the distribution of the drug is instantaneous. The peripheral compartment is composed of a rapidly equilibrating (organ and tissue highly perfused such as liver and brain) and a slowly equilibrating (organ and tissue scarcely perfused such as fat and muscle) compartment.

The volume of distribution (Vd) is defined as the hypothetical volume of plasma that would be necessary to dissolve the amount of drug needed to achieve the same concentration in the blood. Vd is affected by factors such as age or comorbidities and the fluid status of the patients. Vd may be increased by renal failure and liver failure and decreased in dehydration [22]. Furthermore, the Vd is usually larger in obese than non-obese patients. Opioids with a larger Vd are usually more lipophilic (i.e., fentanyl), not ionized with low protein binding, and therefore more likely to distribute faster across the blood–brain barrier. These opioids tend to have a quick onset and shorter duration of action in clinical practice and are more likely to cause adverse effects on the central nervous system. Sepsis, burns, and trauma are associated with larger Vd of most drugs, and opioids are not the exception. Thus, it has been suggested that the larger Vd leading to lower plasma therapeutic concentrations can explain the high requirements of drugs such as fentanyl in some of those conditions [23].

Metabolism and Excretion

Most opioids are subject to significant first-pass metabolism by the liver, and therefore, opioids are less potent orally than if delivered parenterally. Most opioids are metabolized by the liver in two phases to both active and inactive metabolites excreted in the bile and urine [24]. In phase I, opioids change their chemical structure to produce a more water-soluble and less active metabolite. This usually involves oxidation, reduction, or hydrolysis. In some instances, this process will transform an inactive prodrug into an active metabolic drug (e.g., codeine, hydrocodone, and tramadol). Phase II involves reactions that couple opioids with another polar molecule such as glucuronic acid, sulfate, or glycine in a process called conjugation (e.g., morphine). This process results in a water-soluble molecule that is inactive and easily excreted [25]. The major metabolic pathway for most opioids is oxidation except remifentanil, cleared by hydrolysis.

Most of the metabolic molecules produced during phases I and II are inactive or nontoxic. However, there are some important exceptions to consider. For instance, meperidine is metabolized to normeperidine, which is twice as neurotoxic as meperidine and has a longer half-life [26]. Morphine is metabolized to morphine-3-glucuronide (M3G) and morphine-6-glucuronide. The latter also binds to opioid receptors, and it is more potent than morphine [27]. While buprenorphine is not considered a prodrug, its major, N-dealkylated metabolite norbuprenorphine is a full agonist of MOR [28].

To exert a strong analgesic effect, opioids must cross the blood–brain barrier to reach the central nervous system. The blood–brain barrier plays a critical role by exerting bidirectional control over the passage of nutrients, electrolytes, and medication such as opioids. Several ATP-binding cassette (ABC) transporters are involved in transporting opioids and metabolites [29]. P-glycoprotein (ABCB1, MDR1) is the main co-transporter for opioids; however, also other co-transporter such as breast resistance protein (BCRP, ACBG2) and multidrug resistance-associated protein MRP4 (ABCC4), and MRP5(ABCC5) are involved to a lesser extent [30]. Additionally, the penetration of opioids into the blood–brain barrier depends on their solubility. Morphine has a low lipid-solubility molecule compared to drugs like fentanyl. Thus, the former takes a long time to cross the blood–brain barrier. Fentanyl and sufentanil, on the other hand, are lipophilic and cross the blood–brain barrier rapidly and therefore have a quick onset of action and a short duration of action [31].

The kidneys excrete most opioids except methadone which is excreted by the gastrointestinal tract through the bile acids.

7.3 Pharmacology of the Most Commonly Used Opioids

Morphine is one of the most widely used MOR agonists to treat acute and chronic pain. Morphine has poor liposolubility [32]. The usual dose of intravenous morphine is 2.5–10 mg. Morphine has a rapid distribution from the central compartment and an intermediate half-life. Morphine's half-life is 2–4 h after intravenous administration, intramuscular, subcutaneous, and oral administration. The oral-to-parenteral ratio for morphine is 3:1 [27]. **Hydromorphone** is structurally very similar to morphine. Hydromorphone also binds to the MOR and a lesser degree, to DOR. Hydromorphone can be administered orally, intravenously, and subcutaneously. The oral-to-parental administration ratio is 5:1. The onset of action after intravenous dosing varies between 5 and 20 min due to delayed penetration of the blood–brain barrier. Because it is more liposoluble than morphine, its onset of action is faster than morphine but slower than fentanyl [33]. **Fentanyl** has a 50–100-fold higher liposolubility than morphine. This property enables more accessible access to the central nervous system and more rapid onset of analgesia (within 1–2 min after administration) [34]. Fentanyl can be administrated intravenously, intramuscularly, transdermally, and intranasally. The duration of analgesic action intravenously is 30–40 min since serum levels decline rapidly from peak concentration due to redistribution and extensive tissue metabolism. The unique combination of high potency and short half-life allows the administration of multiple doses that can be titrated for a strong analgesic effect in the perioperative period [21]. **Alfentanil** is an agonist of MOR that has one-third to one-fourth of the potency of fentanyl. The preferred route of administration is intravenous. The high amount of non-ionized molecules of alfentanil results in a very short onset of action and a fast peak effect. Alfentanil is commonly used in the ambulatory perioperative setting [35]. **Sufentanil** is an analogue of fentanyl which is highly selective for MOR. It is 5–10 times more potent than fentanyl. It is also highly lipophilic and is rapidly distributed into the brain. Sufentanil can be given intravenously, intranasally, and epidurally, making it one of the preferred drugs in the perioperative setting. **Remifentanil** is an ultra-short-acting MOR agonist. The therapeutic potency of remifentanil is somewhat less than fentanyl but greater than alfentanil. Additionally, remifentanil has a rapid onset and offset therapeutic effect. The only route of administration is intravenous. Due to the rapid offset of analgesia, remifentanil can be associated with rebound pain [36]. **Meperidine** is a MOR and KOR agonist with local anesthetic properties. In terms of analgesic effect, meperidine lacks potency and has a short duration of action (2.5 h) compared to morphine [37]. In the United States, the use of meperidine has been significantly reduced as an analgesic drug. However, it remains a common choice for the treatment of postoperative shivering.

Oxycodone is an orally given MOR, DOR, and KOR agonist. Its potency equivalence to morphine is 1:2. The high oral bioavailability and short- (analgesia within 1 h) and long-acting [12 h] formulations of this drug facilitate the titration. Liver metabolites of oxycodone are also full agonists of MOR and include oxymorphone (potent agonist) and noroxycodone (weak agonist). Oxycodone and its metabolites are renally excreted [38]. **Hydrocodone** is also an orally given MOR agonist. This drug reaches maximum serum concentrations within 1 h; however, in single oral doses of the extended-release formulations hydrocodone formulations, blood concentration reaches the peak between 6 and 30 h. Hydrocodone is metabolized in the liver to norhydrocodone and hydromorphone (active drug). Patients can be grouped into extensive and poor metabolizers of hydrocodone. The latter may experience little or no analgesic effects after oral administration of the drug [39]. **Methadone** is an agonist of MOR, KOR, and DOR. It is also a non-competitive antagonist of the NMDA receptor. Methadone's half-life is 8–60 h. It is available in oral and intravenous formulations [40]. **Tramadol** is a weak opioid. The analgesic potency of tramadol is about 10% of morphine's potency, and its half-life is about 5–6 h. The mechanism of action of tramadol involves two enantiomers, both of which contribute to the analgesic effect differently. For instance, (+) –tramadol and metabolite (+)-O-desmethyl –tramadol are agonists of MOR, whereas (+) - tramadol inhibits serotonin reuptake and (-)- tramadol reduces noradrenaline reuptake [41]. Tramadol formulations include drops, oral, intramuscular, intravenous, and subcutaneous. **Buprenorphine** is a partial agonist of MOR with KOR antagonistic effects. Oral buprenorphine has an extensive first-pass effect and low bioavailability. However, its sublingual and transdermal bioavailability is high [28].

7.4 Opioid-Related Adverse Effects

Although opioids effectively treat moderate-to-severe acute and chronic pain, they are associated with clinically significant opioid-related adverse events (ORADEs). It is worth remembering that age, sex, race, body mass index, and patient's related comorbidities influence the development of ORADEs [42]. As an example, obese patients with obstructive sleep apnea have a higher risk of opioid-induced respiratory depression.

Gastrointestinal System

Nausea and vomiting are one of the most common ORADEs. Up to 25% of patients report nausea with chronic opioid treatment [42]. However, the incidence is even higher (80%) in surgical patients [43]. The mechanisms of opioid-induced nausea and emesis include central and direct stimulation of the chemoreceptor trigger zone in the area postrema located in the fourth ventricle and the reduction of gastrointestinal motility [44]. The DOR as well as interaction with other receptors such dopamine-2 (D2), histamine-1 (H1), 5-HT3 receptor, acetylcholine (ACh), tachykinin NK1 (NK-1), and cannabinoid receptor-1 (CB1) might also be involved in the pathophysiology of opioid-induced emesis [45]. Additionally, opioids impair esophageal peristalsis and slow gastric emptying, increasing the risk of acid reflux [46].

Opioids affect the gastrointestinal tract given the high density of opioid receptors in the esophagus, stomach, and small and large bowel [47]. Opioids decrease gastric emptying (gastroparesis), inhibit small bowel propulsion, and increase fluid reabsorption and the tone of the anal sphincter, which are the physiological bases of opioid-induced constipation [48]. Studies have reported that up to 20% of patients taking chronic opioids develop gastroparesis, an ORADE associated with a longer hospital stay, frequent hospitalization, and decreased work productivity [49]. Opioid-induced constipation is the most common side effect (40–60%) occurring with chronic opioid use. Opioid-induced constipation is defined as a change in bowel habits after the initiation of opioids. Roma IV criteria include: (1) hard stool in at least 25% of defecations, (2) straining of at least 25% of defecation, (3) less than three bowel movements per week, (4) a sensation of incomplete evacuation in at least 25% of defecation, and (5) use of maneuvers to facilitate the removal of stool from the rectum [50]. This common side effect is dose-dependent, and unfortunately, tolerance to constipation rarely develops [51]. However, genetic polymorphism of MOR may explain the inter-variability and severity of gastrointestinal side effects [52]. Opioid-induced constipation is a consequence of the action of MOR and DOR located in the submucosa and submucosa of the gastrointestinal tract [53]. However, in vivo and in vitro studies recently suggested that opioids might also interact with Toll-like receptor 4 and thus decrease gastrointestinal motility [54]. Furthermore, animal studies have demonstrated that the central actions of opioids might also affect gut motility [54].

Alvimopan, naloxegol, and methylnaltrexone are approved peripheral acting MOR antagonists for treating postoperative ileus after surgery or opioid-induced constipation [55].

Genitourinary System

Opioids can cause urinary retention. The incidence of this ORADE ranges from 0 to 8%. Opioid-induced urinary retention is caused by opioids acting on central and peripheral opioid receptors. Animal studies have shown that MOR and possibly DOR are the key mediators of this side effect [56]. After binding to MOR, opioids inhibit the parasympathetic fibers of the bladder peripherally and decrease the sensation of bladder fullness [57]. Additionally, the simultaneous stimulation of the sympathetic fibers in either the supraspinal or the spinal level increases the resistance of the outflow tract of the bladder and interferes with the function of the detrusor muscle. The potency and duration of these effects are correlated with the type of opioid, the dose, and the route of administration. Higher doses, long-acting opioids, and intrathecal administration are associated with the highest risk of presenting this side effect [58, 59].

Respiratory System

The incidence of opioid-induced respiratory depression varies between 0.01 and 7% [60, 61]. Opioids induce respiratory depression by activating MOR in the medullary pre-Bötzinger complex, parabrachial nucleus, and dorsal rostral pons [62]. Centrally, MOR activation decreases the frequency and regularity of the inspiratory rhythm [63], reduces the ventilator response to hypoxia and hypercapnia, and depresses the cough center in the medulla [64]. Activation of MOR mediates most of the effects of opioids on the respiratory system; however, DOR may also exert some inhibitory effects on respiration. KOR appears to be devoid of respiratory depressant activity [65, 66]. Opioid-induced respiratory depression depends on the degree of activation of the intracellular pathways [67]. Thus, it has been speculated that opioids biased toward the G-protein-dependent pathway (i.e., oliceridine) might retain analgesic effects but have fewer risks of respiratory depression [68]. Opioids also produce sedation and decrease the tone of the upper airway [69]. Peripherally, opioids acting on MOR and KOR inhibit voltage-gated Ca (2 +) influx in the carotid body (via G-protein pathway), reducing neurotransmitter release, which subsequently decreases the firing rate of the central neural system and eventually inhibits the acute hypoxic response [70].

Risk factors associated with respiratory depression include obstructive sleep apnea, obesity, the elderly, chronic pulmonary disease, cardiac disease, neurologic disease, renal failure, opioid dependence, patient-controlled analgesia, and concomitant use of sedatives [71]. Naloxone is an opioid antagonist and the first choice for life-threatening opioid-induced respiratory failure [72]. Side effects associated with the use of naloxone include pulmonary edema, cardiac arrhythmias, and hypertension secondary to the release of catecholamines (most likely in hemodynamically unstable patients).

Chest rigidity is an uncommon but severe side effect of opioids that can occur with administering supra-analgesic doses of potent MOR agonists such as alfentanil, fentanyl, sufentanil, and remifentanil. It presents a sudden onset of respiratory failure, hypercapnia, and worsening lung compliance. This side effect is dose-dependent and also observed after rapid intravenous injections, particularly in newborns or elderly patients. The exact mechanism of increased muscle tone after rapid infusion of opioids is not well known. However, animal studies indicate that this medical emergency is secondary to MOR activation. DOR and KOR receptors may attenuate this effect [73].

Cardiovascular System

Studies have shown that opioids have various effects on cardiovascular function. Overall, opioids reduce sympathetic tone and enhance the parasympathetic tone in a dose-dependent manner [74]. These effects are related to the stimulation of centrally located MOR, KOR, and DOR receptors and receptors located peripherally in the cardiac tissue [75, 76]. The function of opioids receptor in the heart includes the modulation of the heart rate (predominantly bradycardia), inotropic state (primarily depression), modulation of the vascular tone (vasodilation), and cellular adaptation to ischemic injury [77]. Thus, rapid opioid administration can result in bradycardia, vasodilation, hypotension, and syncope. Hypotension is mediated by MOR, while the cardioprotective effects of these medications seem to be related to KOR activation [76, 77]. Opioids have little impact on contractility when administered alone; however, when given in combination with other medication like intravenous anesthetics, they can decrease cardiac function. Morphine, hydromorphone, and meperidine can lead to histamine release and result in flushing, decreased vascular tone, and subsequently low blood pressure [78].

In vitro data suggest that all opioids can affect cardiac electrophysiology detrimentally. However, clinical data have shown that most opioids do not affect cardiac conductivity. Only methadone has shown clinical evidence of causing a deleterious effect on the electrophysiology of the heart [79]. Methadone has the highest risk of arrhythmia even at conventional doses due to its capacity to prolong the QT interval. The prolongation of the QT interval with subsequent torsades de point is attributed to its (R)-enantiomer due to a higher unbound fraction than the (S)-enantiomer [80]. The mechanism of QT prolongation is a block of cardiac delayed rectifier K (+) current (I(Kr)) [81]. Factors associated with a higher risk of QT prolongation and torsades de point include dose, electrolyte imbalances like hypokalemia, renal and hepatic failure, and concomitant use of other medications that prolong QT interval [82]. This adverse event has led to the issue of a black box warning on the use of methadone.

Some studies have suggested that opioids could protect cardiac tissue against ischemia–reperfusion injury. For instance, in rodent experimental studies, morphine diminishes neutrophil and endothelial activation in patients with acute myocardial infarction. Additionally, morphine increases the activity of neutrophil endopeptidase and metalloproteases necessary to mitigate the shedding of L-selecting and ICAM-1. This means that morphine attenuates the neutrophil–endothelium activation in patients with acute myocardial infarction [83]. Another mechanism involved in cardio-protection is activating the protein kinase-3 pathway, which enhances mitochondrial resistance to calcium overload [84].

Neurologic System

The ORADEs associated with the activity of opioids in the central nervous system can be classified into three different groups: The first group of side effects is related to a decreased level of arousal (sedation) and sleep disturbances. Overall, opioid administration is associated with progressive slowing in frequency and increased amplitude that results in delta waves. For instance, in clinical studies, low doses of sufentanil caused high-frequency beta activity and an increase in alpha activity. With increasing plasma concentration, further progressive slowing in electroencephalography frequency occurs [62, 85]. Sleep disturbances associated with the use of opioids include increased stage 2, decreased deep sleep (stages 3 and 4), inability to fall asleep, and reduced rapid eye movements (REM) [86].

The second group of side effects is associated with cognitive dysfunction and psychomotor impairment [87]. Patients with a history of cognitive disorders (i.e., Alzheimer's disease) have an increased risk of a sudden deterioration in their cognitive ability when opioids are administered. Opioid-induced cognitive dysfunction can reduce the attention span, cause disorientation, trigger agitation, and impair the quality of life [87, 88]. The third group of neurologic complications is those related to neurotoxicity (i.e., seizures) [89]. Seizures are more common with active metabolites of meperidine, codeine, and morphine. Typically, these side effects are dose-dependent and reversed by administering MOR antagonists [90].

Pruritus

The incidence of opioid-induced pruritus ranges between 30 and 100% [91]. This unwanted side effect is most likely to occur after intravenous, epidural, and intrathecal administration and appears to be dose-dependent. Parental opioids produce pruritus secondary to histamine release from mast cells, while neuraxial opioid administration produces pruritus secondary to neuronal disinhibition in the spinal cord dorsal horn [92]. In general, lipophilic opioids like fentanyl have a rapid onset and short duration of pruritus compared to less liposoluble opioids [93, 94]. The pharmacological treatment of opioid-induced pruritus includes antihistamines medication such as diphenhydramine. However, nalbuphine (opioid agonist–antagonist) is superior in treating pruritus when compared to antihistamines or naloxone [95].

7.5 Indications and Contraindications

The use of opioids has increased considerably over the past three decades, leading to the opioid crisis in the United States. Opioids are often prescribed for acute and chronic pain conditions, including postsurgical pain and palliative care. The prescription of opioids should be considered only when alleviating pain and improving functional capacity outweighs the risk of moderate-to-severe ORADEs. Current guidelines recommend opioid therapy for patients with moderate-to-severe pain, pain-related functional impairment, or diminished quality of life due to pain. When considering opioid treatment, the minimal dose and the shorter duration of therapy should be the goal.

In acute surgical pain, prescription opioids should be administered based on the type of surgery, patient's age and comorbidities, and pharmacokinetic and pharmacodynamics properties of each opioid. Fentanyl is one of the most commonly used opioids during surgery, given its potency, rapid initiation of action, short duration of action, and multiple routes of administration. Morphine and hydromorphone are widely given as single intravenous or epidural boluses. Hydrocodone and oxycodone are prescribed to manage moderate-to-severe postsurgical pain or ambulatory treatment of non-surgical injuries. However, an unnecessary increase in the prescription of both opioids has contributed to the so-called opioid epidemic. Although meperidine use for the treatment of acute and chronic pain has been discouraged, this opioid still plays a significant role in treating postoperative shivering. Opioids with serotoninergic activity like methadone, meperidine, buprenorphine, and tramadol can cause serotonin syndrome when used with other serotoninergic medications such as monoamine oxidase inhibitors.

Summary Questions (Choose the Most Appropriate Answer)

1- The primary mechanism of prescription opioid-induced analgesia is exerted by:
   a. **The mu-opioid receptor**
   b. The delta-opioid receptor
   c. The sigma-opioid receptor
   d. The kappa-opioid receptor
   The mu-opioid receptor is the main mechanism of action by which opioids cause analgesia

2- Opioid-related adverse effects are primarily mediated by:
   a. Mu-opioid receptor type 1
   b. **Mu-opioid receptor type 2**
   c. Serotoninergic receptors
   d. Dopaminergic receptor type 1
   The mu-opioid receptor type 2 is responsible for most of the adverse effects related to opioids (i.e., respiratory depression, sedation, pruritus, prolactin release, dependence, anorexia, and sedation).

3- The following opioid is considered a biased agonist of the mu-opioid receptor:
   a. Oxycodone
   b. Methadone
   c. Hydromorphone
   d. Oliceridine
   Oliceridine is a biased agonist of MOR that has been recently approved for acute postoperative pain.

4- Which route of administration should be considered to provide reliable and rapid-onset opioid-induced analgesia:
   a. Transdermal
   b. Oral
   c. **Intravenous**
   d. Rectal
   The intravenous route of administration provides reliable and rapid onset of analgesia and should be considered for the treatment of acute pain.

5- The liver is responsible for:
   a. Phase I metabolism
   b. Phase II metabolism
   c. Definite drug excretion
   d. **A and b**
   Most opioids undergo liver metabolism in 2 phases. In phase I, opioids change their chemical structure to produce a more water-soluble and less active metabolite. Phase II involves reactions that couple opioids with another polar molecule, such as glucuronic acid, sulfate, or glycine, in a process called conjugation.

6- Remifentanil is considered:
   a. A long-acting opioid
   b. A short-acting opioid
   c. An intermediate-acting opioid
   d. **An ultra-short-acting opioid**
   Remifentanil is the only ultra-short-acting opioid clinically available.

7- The longest-acting opioid – after single-dose intravenous administration – to treat acute pain is:
   a. **Methadone**
   b. Sufentanil
   c. Hydromorphone
   d. Fentanyl
   Methadone has a half-life between 8–60 h. it is available in oral and intravenous formulations.

8- Opioids:
   a. Increase gastric emptying
   b. Stimulate small bowel propulsion
   c. Decrease fluid reabsorption
   d. **None of the above**
   Opioids decrease gastric emptying (gastroparesis), inhibit small bowel propulsion, and increase fluid reabsorption and the tone of the anal sphincter, which are the physiological bases of opioid-induced constipation.

9- The following molecules are approved for opioid-induced constipation, except:
   a. Alvimopan
   b. Naloxegol
   c. **Oxymorphone**

d. Methylnaltrexone
Oxymorphone is a mu-opioid receptor agonist. alvimopan, naloxegol, and methylnaltrexone are peripheral antagonists of the mu-opioid receptor approved for the treatment of opioid-induced constipation.

10- A 55-year-old man is diagnosed with opioid-induced respiratory depression, which of the following can be administered for treatment:
  a. Alvimopan
  b. **Naloxone**
  c. Naloxegol
  d. Methylnaltrexone
  Naloxone is an opioid antagonist and the first choice for life-threatening opioid-induced respiratory failure.

References

1. Stein C. Opioid receptors. Annu Rev Med. 2016;67:433–51.
2. Fujita W, Gomes I, Devi LA. Revolution in GPCR signalling: opioid receptor heteromers as novel therapeutic targets: IUPHAR review 10. Br J Pharmacol. 2014;171(18):4155–76.
3. Christie MJ. Cellular neuroadaptations to chronic opioids: tolerance, withdrawal and addiction. Br J Pharmacol. 2008;154(2):384–96.
4. Al-Hasani R, Bruchas MR. Molecular mechanisms of opioid receptor-dependent signaling and behavior. Anesthesiology. 2011;115(6):1363–81.
5. Andoh T, Yageta Y, Konno M, Yamaguchi-Miyamoto T, Takahata H, Nojima H, et al. Evidence for separate involvement of different mu-opioid receptor subtypes in itch and analgesia induced by supraspinal action of opioids. J Pharmacol Sci. 2008;106(4):667–70.
6. Jolas T, Nestler EJ, Aghajanian GK. Chronic morphine increases GABA tone on serotonergic neurons of the dorsal raphe nucleus: association with an up-regulation of the cyclic AMP pathway. Neuroscience. 2000;95(2):433–43.
7. Juhasz JR, Hasbi A, Rashid AJ, So CH, George SR, O'Dowd BF. Mu-opioid receptor heterooligomer formation with the dopamine D1 receptor as directly visualized in living cells. Eur J Pharmacol. 2008;581(3):235–43.
8. Ben Hamida S, Boulos LJ, McNicholas M, Charbogne P, Kieffer BL. Mu opioid receptors in GABAergic neurons of the forebrain promote alcohol reward and drinking. Addict Biol. 2019;24(1):28–39.
9. Kline RHT, Wiley RG. Spinal mu-opioid receptor-expressing dorsal horn neurons: role in nociception and morphine antinociception. J Neurosci. 2008;28(4):904–13.
10. Eisenstein TK. The role of opioid receptors in immune system function. Front Immunol. 2019;10:2904.
11. Gorur A, Patino M, Takahashi H, Corrales G, Pickering CR, Gleber-Netto FO, et al. Mu-opioid receptor activation promotes in vitro and in vivo tumor growth in head and neck squamous cell carcinoma. Life Sci. 2021;278:119541.
12. Bodnar RJ. Endogenous opiates and behavior: 2012. Peptides. 2013;50:55–95.
13. Helm S, Trescot AM, Colson J, Sehgal N, Silverman S. Opioid antagonists, partial agonists, and agonists/antagonists: the role of office-based detoxification. Pain Physician. 2008;11(2):225–35.
14. Rosenblum A, Marsch LA, Joseph H, Portenoy RK. Opioids and the treatment of chronic pain: controversies, current status, and future directions. Exp Clin Psychopharmacol. 2008;16(5):405–16.
15. Pathan H, Williams J. Basic opioid pharmacology: an update. Br J Pain. 2012;6(1):11–6.
16. Hoskin PJ, Hanks GW. Opioid agonist-antagonist drugs in acute and chronic pain states. Drugs. 1991;41(3):326–44.
17. Stanczyk MA, Kandasamy R. Biased agonism: the quest for the analgesic holy grail. Pain Rep. 2018;3(3):e650.
18. Cox BM. A concise review of concepts in opioid pharmacology up to the discovery of endogenous opioids. Mol Pharmacol. 2020;98(4):392–400.
19. Overholser BR, Foster DR. Opioid pharmacokinetic drug-drug interactions. Am J Manag Care. 2011;17(Suppl 11):S276–87.
20. Del Vecchio G, Labuz D, Temp J, Seitz V, Kloner M, Negrete R, et al. PKA of opioid ligands as a discriminating factor for side effects. Sci Rep. 2019;9(1):19344.
21. Lotsch J. Pharmacokinetic-pharmacodynamic modeling of opioids. J Pain Symptom Manage. 2005;29(5 Suppl):S90-103.
22. Mansoor A, Mahabadi N. Volume of Distribution. StatPearls. Treasure Island (FL). 2022.
23. Han T, Harmatz JS, Greenblatt DJ, Martyn JAJ. Fentanyl clearance and volume of distribution are increased in patients with major burns. J Clin Pharmacol. 2007;47(6):674–80.
24. Smith HS. Opioid metabolism. Mayo Clin Proc. 2009;84(7):613–24.
25. DePriest AZ, Puet BL, Holt AC, Roberts A, Cone EJ. Metabolism and disposition of prescription opioids: a review. Forensic Sci Rev. 2015;27(2):115–45.
26. Danziger LH, Martin SJ, Blum RA. Central nervous system toxicity associated with meperidine use in hepatic disease. Pharmacotherapy. 1994;14(2):235–8.
27. Hasselstrom J, Sawe J. Morphine pharmacokinetics and metabolism in humans. Enterohepatic cycling and relative contribution of metabolites to active opioid concentrations. Clin Pharmacokinet. 1993;24(4):344–54.
28. Lutfy K, Cowan A. Buprenorphine: a unique drug with complex pharmacology. Curr Neuropharmacol. 2004;2(4):395–402.
29. Tournier N, Decleves X, Saubamea B, Scherrmann JM, Cisternino S. Opioid transport by ATP-binding cassette transporters at the blood-brain barrier: implications for neuropsychopharmacology. Curr Pharm Des. 2011;17(26):2829–42.
30. Uchida Y, Ohtsuki S, Katsukura Y, Ikeda C, Suzuki T, Kamiie J, et al. Quantitative targeted absolute proteomics of human blood-brain barrier transporters and receptors. J Neurochem. 2011;117(2):333–45.
31. McQuay HJ, Sullivan AF, Smallman K, Dickenson AH. Intrathecal opioids, potency and lipophilicity. Pain. 1989;36(1):111–5.
32. De Gregori S, De Gregori M, Ranzani GN, Allegri M, Minella C, Regazzi M. Morphine metabolism, transport and brain disposition. Metab Brain Dis. 2012;27(1):1–5.
33. Murray A, Hagen NA. Hydromorphone. J Pain Symptom Manage. 2005;29(5 Suppl):S57-66.
34. Playfor S, Jenkins I, Boyles C, Choonara I, Davies G, Haywood T, et al. Consensus guidelines on sedation and analgesia in critically ill children. Intensive Care Med. 2006;32(8):1125–36.
35. Scholz J, Steinfath M, Schulz M. Clinical pharmacokinetics of alfentanil, fentanyl and sufentanil. An update. Clin Pharmacokinet. 1996;31(4):275–92.
36. Egan TD. The clinical pharmacology of remifentanil: a brief review. J Anesth. 1998;12(4):195–204.

37. Pokela ML, Olkkola KT, Koivisto M, Ryhanen P. Pharmacokinetics and pharmacodynamics of intravenous meperidine in neonates and infants. Clin Pharmacol Ther. 1992;52(4):342–9.
38. Ordóñez Gallego A, González Barón M, Espinosa AE. Oxycodone: a pharmacological and clinical review. Clin Transl Oncol. 2007;9(5):298–307.
39. Cardia L, Calapai G, Quattrone D, Mondello C, Arcoraci V, Calapai F, et al. Preclinical and clinical pharmacology of hydrocodone for chronic pain: a mini review. Front Pharmacol. 2018;9.
40. Wolff K, Rostami-Hodjegan A, Hay AW, Raistrick D, Tucker G. Population-based pharmacokinetic approach for methadone monitoring of opiate addicts: potential clinical utility. Addiction. 2000;95(12):1771–83.
41. Grond S, Sablotzki A. Clinical pharmacology of tramadol. Clin Pharmacokinet. 2004;43(13):879–923.
42. Cepeda MS, Farrar JT, Baumgarten M, Boston R, Carr DB, Strom BL. Side effects of opioids during short-term administration: effect of age, gender, and race. Clin Pharmacol Ther. 2003;74 (2):102–12.
43. Yoo JH, Kim SI, Chung JW, Jun MR, Han YM, Kim YJ. Aprepitant in combination with palonosetron for the prevention of postoperative nausea and vomiting in female patients using intravenous patient-controlled analgesia. Korean J Anesthesiol. 2018;71(6):440–6.
44. Rung GW, Claybon L, Hord A, Patel C, Kallgren M, Koppel J, et al. Intravenous ondansetron for postsurgical opioid-induced nausea and vomiting. S3A-255 Study Group. Anesth Analg. 1997;84(4):832–8.
45. Smith HS, Smith JM, Seidner P. Opioid-induced nausea and vomiting. Ann Palliat Med. 2012;1(2):121–9.
46. Lacy BE. Effects of opioids on esophageal dysfunction. Gastroenterol Hepatol (N Y). 2016;12(5):323–5.
47. Holzer P. Opioid receptors in the gastrointestinal tract. Regul Pept. 2009;155(1–3):11–7.
48. Camilleri M, Lembo A, Katzka DA. Opioids in gastroenterology: treating adverse effects and creating therapeutic benefits. Clin Gastroenterol Hepatol. 2017;15(9):1338–49.
49. Jehangir A, Parkman HP. Chronic opioids in gastroparesis: relationship with gastrointestinal symptoms, healthcare utilization and employment. World J Gastroenterol. 2017;23(40):7310–20.
50. Aziz I, Whitehead WE, Palsson OS, Tornblom H, Simren M. An approach to the diagnosis and management of Rome IV functional disorders of chronic constipation. Expert Rev Gastroenterol Hepatol. 2020;14(1):39–46.
51. Nelson AD, Camilleri M. Chronic opioid induced constipation in patients with nonmalignant pain: challenges and opportunities. Therap Adv Gastroenterol. 2015;8(4):206–20.
52. Lang-Illievich K, Bornemann-Cimenti H. Opioid-induced constipation: a narrative review of therapeutic options in clinical management. Korean J Pain. 2019;32(2):69–78.
53. Farmer AD, Holt CB, Downes TJ, Ruggeri E, Del Vecchio S, De Giorgio R. Pathophysiology, diagnosis, and management of opioid-induced constipation. Lancet Gastroenterol Hepatol. 2018;3(3):203–12.
54. Farzi A, Halicka J, Mayerhofer R, Frohlich EE, Tatzl E, Holzer P. Toll-like receptor 4 contributes to the inhibitory effect of morphine on colonic motility in vitro and in vivo. Sci Rep. 2015;5:9499.
55. Rodriguez RW. Off-label uses of alvimopan and methylnaltrexone. Am J Health Syst Pharm. 2014;71(17):1450–5.
56. Dray A, Metsch R. Opioid receptor subtypes involved in the central inhibition of urinary bladder motility. Eur J Pharmacol. 1984;104(1–2):47–53.
57. Verhamme KM, Sturkenboom MC, Stricker BH, Bosch R. Drug-induced urinary retention: incidence, management and prevention. Drug Saf. 2008;31(5):373–88.
58. Kuipers PW, Kamphuis ET, van Venrooij GE, van Roy JP, Ionescu TI, Knape JT, et al. Intrathecal opioids and lower urinary tract function: a urodynamic evaluation. Anesthesiology. 2004;100 (6):1497–503.
59. Rawal N, Mollefors K, Axelsson K, Lingardh G, Widman B. An experimental study of urodynamic effects of epidural morphine and of naloxone reversal. Anesth Analg. 1983;62(7):641–7.
60. Cousins MJ, Mather LE. Intrathecal and epidural administration of opioids. Anesthesiology. 1984;61(3):276–310.
61. Shapiro A, Zohar E, Zaslansky R, Hoppenstein D, Shabat S, Fredman B. The frequency and timing of respiratory depression in 1524 postoperative patients treated with systemic or neuraxial morphine. J Clin Anesth. 2005;17(7):537–42.
62. Santiago TV, Edelman NH. Opioids and breathing. J Appl Physiol. 1985;59(6):1675–85.
63. Baertsch NA, Bush NE, Burgraff NJ, Ramirez JM. Dual mechanisms of opioid-induced respiratory depression in the inspiratory rhythm-generating network. Elife. 2021;10.
64. Bolser DC. Central mechanisms II: pharmacology of brainstem pathways. Handb Exp Pharmacol. 2009;187:203–17.
65. Dahan A, Sarton E, Teppema L, Olievier C, Nieuwenhuijs D, Matthes HW, et al. Anesthetic potency and influence of morphine and sevoflurane on respiration in mu-opioid receptor knockout mice. Anesthesiology. 2001;94(5):824–32.
66. Lonergan T, Goodchild AK, Christie MJ, Pilowsky PM. Presynaptic delta opioid receptors differentially modulate rhythm and pattern generation in the ventral respiratory group of the rat. Neuroscience. 2003;121(4):959–73.
67. Manglik A, Lin H, Aryal DK, McCorvy JD, Dengler D, Corder G, et al. Structure-based discovery of opioid analgesics with reduced side effects. Nature. 2016;537(7619):185–90.
68. Noble F, Marie N. Biased opioid ligands: revolution or evolution? Front Pain Res (Lausanne). 2021;2:722820.
69. Montandon G, Horner R. CrossTalk proposal: the preBotzinger complex is essential for the respiratory depression following systemic administration of opioid analgesics. J Physiol. 2014;592 (6):1159–62.
70. Ricker EM, Pye RL, Barr BL, Wyatt CN. Selective mu and kappa opioid agonists inhibit voltage-gated Ca2+ entry in isolated neonatal rat carotid body type I cells. Adv Exp Med Biol. 2015;860:49–54.
71. Gupta K, Prasad A, Nagappa M, Wong J, Abrahamyan L, Chung FF. Risk factors for opioid-induced respiratory depression and failure to rescue: a review. Curr Opin Anaesthesiol. 2018;31 (1):110–9.
72. Mueller SR, Walley AY, Calcaterra SL, Glanz JM, Binswanger IA. A review of opioid overdose prevention and naloxone prescribing: implications for translating community programming into clinical practice. Subst Abus. 2015;36(2):240–53.
73. Vankova ME, Weinger MB, Chen DY, Bronson JB, Motis V, Koob GF. Role of central mu, delta-1, and kappa-1 opioid receptors in opioid-induced muscle rigidity in the rat. Anesthesiology. 1996;85(3):574–83.
74. Goodarzi M, Narasimhan RR. The effect of large-dose intrathecal opioids on the autonomic nervous system. Anesth Analg. 2001;93 (2):456–9, 4th contents page.
75. Mousa SA, Shaqura M, Schaper J, Treskatsch S, Habazettl H, Schafer M, et al. Developmental expression of delta-opioid receptors during maturation of the parasympathetic, sympathetic, and sensory innervations of the neonatal heart: early targets for opioid regulation of autonomic control. J Comp Neurol. 2011;519 (5):957–71.

76. Bell SP, Sack MN, Patel A, Opie LH, Yellon DM. Delta opioid receptor stimulation mimics ischemic preconditioning in human heart muscle. J Am Coll Cardiol. 2000;36(7):2296–302.
77. Chen A, Ashburn MA. Cardiac effects of opioid therapy. Pain Med. 2015;16(Suppl 1):S27-31.
78. Ennis M, Schneider C, Nehring E, Lorenz W. Histamine release induced by opioid analgesics: a comparative study using porcine mast cells. Agents Actions. 1991;33(1–2):20–2.
79. Wedam EF, Haigney MC. The impact of opioids on cardiac electrophysiology. Curr Cardiol Rev. 2016;12(1):27–36.
80. Foster DJ, Somogyi AA, Dyer KR, White JM, Bochner F. Steady-state pharmacokinetics of (R)- and (S)-methadone in methadone maintenance patients. Br J Clin Pharmacol. 2000;50(5):427–40.
81. Katchman AN, McGroary KA, Kilborn MJ, Kornick CA, Manfredi PL, Woosley RL, et al. Influence of opioid agonists on cardiac human ether-a-go-go-related gene K(+) currents. J Pharmacol Exp Ther. 2002;303(2):688–94.
82. Vieweg WV, Hasnain M, Howland RH, Clausen T, Koneru JN, Kogut C, et al. Methadone, QTc interval prolongation and torsade de pointes: case reports offer the best understanding of this problem. Ther Adv Psychopharmacol. 2013;3(4):219–32.
83. Wang TL, Chang H, Hung CR, Tseng YZ. Attenuation of neutrophil and endothelial activation by intravenous morphine in patients with acute myocardial infarction. Am J Cardiol. 1997;80(12):1532–5.
84. Obame FN, Plin-Mercier C, Assaly R, Zini R, Dubois-Rande JL, Berdeaux A, et al. Cardioprotective effect of morphine and a blocker of glycogen synthase kinase 3 beta, SB216763 [3-(2,4-dichlorophenyl)-4(1-methyl-1H-indol-3-yl)-1H-pyrrole-2,5-dione], via inhibition of the mitochondrial permeability transition pore. J Pharmacol Exp Ther. 2008;326(1):252–8.
85. Scott JC, Cooke JE, Stanski DR. Electroencephalographic quantitation of opioid effect: comparative pharmacodynamics of fentanyl and sufentanil. Anesthesiology. 1991;74(1):34–42.
86. Robertson JA, Purple RJ, Cole P, Zaiwalla Z, Wulff K, Pattinson KT. Sleep disturbance in patients taking opioid medication for chronic back pain. Anaesthesia. 2016;71(11):1296–307.
87. Vella-Brincat J, Macleod AD. Adverse effects of opioids on the central nervous systems of palliative care patients. J Pain Palliat Care Pharmacother. 2007;21(1):15–25.
88. Chau DL, Walker V, Pai L, Cho LM. Opiates and elderly: use and side effects. Clin Interv Aging. 2008;3(2):273–8.
89. Gallagher R. Opioid-induced neurotoxicity. Can Fam Physician. 2007;53(3):426–7.
90. Wang JH, Rizak JD, Chen YM, Li L, Hu XT, Ma YY. Interactive effects of morphine and dopaminergic compounds on spatial working memory in rhesus monkeys. Neurosci Bull. 2013;29(1):37–46.
91. Kyriakides K, Hussain SK, Hobbs GJ. Management of opioid-induced pruritus: a role for 5-HT3 antagonists? Br J Anaesth. 1999;82(3):439–41.
92. Nguyen E, Lim G, Ross SE. Evaluation of therapies for peripheral and neuraxial opioid-induced pruritus based on molecular and cellular discoveries. Anesthesiology. 2021;135(2):350–65.
93. Wells J, Paech MJ, Evans SF. Intrathecal fentanyl-induced pruritus during labour: the effect of prophylactic ondansetron. Int J Obstet Anesth. 2004;13(1):35–9.
94. Kumar K, Singh SI. Neuraxial opioid-induced pruritus: an update. J Anaesthesiol Clin Pharmacol. 2013;29(3):303–7.
95. Jannuzzi RG. Nalbuphine for treatment of opioid-induced pruritus: a systematic review of literature. Clin J Pain. 2016;32(1):87–93.

Clinical Pharmacology of Drugs Acting at the Neuromuscular Junction

8

J. Ross Renew and Sorin J. Brull

Abstract

Since the first administration of d-tubocurarine in 1942 by Harold Griffith to facilitate muscle relaxation during an appendectomy, neuromuscular blocking agents (NMBAs) have been a class of medications utilized by anesthesiologists and intensivists to facilitate the performance of invasive and painful procedures. NMBAs are administered to improve the quality of intubating conditions and decrease the incidence of vocal cord injury during airway instrumentation. Furthermore, the use of NMBAs to relax major skeletal muscle groups during intra-cavitary operations significantly improves surgical conditions. The utility of NMBAs is not limited to the perioperative arena; they can be used to facilitate mechanical ventilation in patients with poor pulmonary compliance in the intensive care unit.

Keywords

Neuromuscular junction • Depolarizing neuromuscular blocking agent • Nondepolarizing neuromuscular blocking agent • Neuromuscular blockade monitoring • Residual neuromuscular blockade • Succinylcholine • Paralysis

Key Points

1. The vertebrate neuromuscular junction is the most studied synapse. Acetylcholine is released from the motor axon terminal, crosses the synaptic cleft, and binds to the recognition sites on the 2 α (alpha) subunits of postsynaptic nicotinic receptors. The generated action potential will result in excitation–contraction coupling.
2. Succinylcholine is an ultra-short-acting depolarizing neuromuscular blocking agent (NMBA). It produces the fastest, shortest, and most reliable neuromuscular blockade. Succinylcholine may result in postoperative myalgia, increases in plasma potassium levels that can reach pathologic levels under certain conditions, small increases in intracranial and intraocular pressure, and is one of the known triggers of malignant hyperthermia, while being one of the most common triggers of allergic reactions.
3. Atracurium is a benzylisoquinolinium compound of an intermediate duration of action; it contains 10 isomers and its metabolism occurs independently of renal and hepatic function by Hofmann degradation and plasma esterases hydrolysis. Doses used to facilitate rapid tracheal intubation may be associated with histamine release.
4. Cisatracurium, the *cis-cis* isomer of atracurium (a benzylisoquinolinium compound), is also metabolized by Hofmann degradation. The parent molecule does not undergo ester hydrolysis. Cisatracurium has an intermediate duration of action. There is virtually no histamine release when compared to its predecessor, atracurium.
5. Mivacurium, another benzylisoquinolinium compound, is a short-acting nondepolarizing NMBAA. It is metabolized by butyrylcholinesterases, similar to succinylcholine.
6. Pancuronium is a steroidal, long-acting NMBA that possesses vagolytic and sympathomimetic properties and yields active metabolites (3-OH pancuronium) that increase the incidence of residual neuromuscular blockade. In the modern era of rapid recovery protocols, its use has diminished significantly. The authors do not recommend its use.

J. Ross Renew · S. J. Brull (✉)
Department of Anesthesiology and Perioperative Medicine, Mayo Clinic College of Medicine and Science, Jacksonville, FL, USA
e-mail: Brull.Sorin@mayo.edu

J. Ross Renew
e-mail: renew.j@mayo.edu

M. Argalious et al. (eds.), *Basic Sciences in Anesthesia*,
https://doi.org/10.1007/978-3-031-60203-0_8

7. Vecuronium is a steroidal nondepolarizing NMBA with an intermediate duration of action. It is virtually devoid of hemodynamic effects. However, its degradation into active metabolites (3-OH vecuronium) precludes its use for prolonged periods in the intensive care unit.
8. Rocuronium is a steroidal nondepolarizing NMBA with an intermediate duration of action. At high doses (1.2 mg/kg or 4 × ED_{95}), it has an onset of action approaching that of succinylcholine.
9. The use of clinical signs, such as handgrip strength or sustained head lift, and subjective (visual and tactile) assessment obtained with a peripheral nerve stimulator are not reliable methods for determining recovery from neuromuscular blockade. Quantitative monitors—using acceleromyography, mechanomyography, or electromyography—are most reliable for excluding residual neuromuscular blockade.
10. Sugammadex is an encapsulating reversal agent, capable of rapidly antagonizing any level of rocuronium-induced neuromuscular blockade. Its use, however, does not preclude the need for monitoring the level of neuromuscular blockade, as the appropriate dose is dependent on the level of recovery at the time of its administration.

8.1 Background

Since the first administration of d-tubocurarine in 1942 by Harold Griffith to facilitate muscle relaxation during an appendectomy, neuromuscular blocking agents (NMBAs) have been a class of medications utilized by anesthesiologists and intensivists to facilitate the performance of invasive and painful procedures. NMBAs are administered to improve the quality of intubating conditions and decrease the incidence of vocal cord injury during airway instrumentation. Furthermore, the use of NMBAs to relax major skeletal muscle groups during intra-cavitary operations significantly improves surgical conditions. The utility of NMBAs is not limited to the perioperative arena; they can be used to facilitate mechanical ventilation in patients with poor pulmonary compliance in the intensive care unit.

Two major classes of NMBAs exist and are distinguished by the manner in which these medications interact with the neuromuscular junction (NMJ) to produce skeletal muscle relaxation. **Depolarizing** drugs act as acetylcholine receptor agonists at the postsynaptic nicotinic receptor. **Nondepolarizing** drugs act as competitive antagonists, as they compete with acetylcholine for the binding sites on the nicotinic acetylcholine receptors at the neuromuscular junction. Nondepolarizing NMBAs can be further subdivided into 2 categories, based on their molecular structures. Aminosteroidal and benzylisoquinolinium (tetrahydroisoquinolines) compounds have distinct structural characteristics that result in substantial differences in the pharmacological profiles of these compounds.

Despite nearly 75 years of experience, studies continue to demonstrate the potential deleterious side effects associated with the use of these medications. In 1954, Beecher and Todd demonstrated a six-fold increase in mortality in patients receiving curare compared with those who had not received curare. Such hazards persist today as the incidence of residual neuromuscular blockade may be as high as 40% of patients in the post-anesthesia care unit (PACU), a complication that leads to increases in pulmonary aspiration events, airway obstruction, attenuation of the hypoxic ventilatory response, and subjective reports of unpleasant weakness-related symptoms. Furthermore, the use of NMBAs has been repeatedly implicated in unintended awareness during surgery when paralyzed patients have inadequate level of anesthesia. Such findings suggest that many clinicians may have an incomplete understanding of the pharmacology of NMBAs, their interactions at the neuromuscular junction, and of the existing techniques available to monitor the level of neuromuscular blockade after NMBA administration.

8.2 The Neuromuscular Junction

The corticospinal tracts course in the ventral horns of the spinal cord and contain axons and cell bodies of motor neurons. The axons from this tract exit the spinal cord anteriorly via the ventral roots as they course to their destination skeletal muscle groups. The motor unit is the functional contractile unit and is composed of a single myelinated alpha motor neuron and all muscle fibers that receive innervation from this single neuron. A large motor nerve innervates more muscle fibers than a smaller motor nerve does. In general, small motor nerve units innervate the fatigue-resistant "slow" muscle fibers, whereas large motor units innervate the "fast" muscle fibers. Muscles contain a varying mixture of motor units depending on their function. The neuromuscular junction (NMJ) is composed of the presynaptic motor neuron terminal, the postsynaptic muscle surface, and a synaptic cleft (gap) that contains the enzyme acetylcholinesterase. The entire NMJ is capped by terminal Schwann cells.

When an electrical signal courses along the motor nerve to the presynaptic end, depolarization of the neuron occurs at the nerve terminal that opens voltage-gated calcium channels, allowing intracellular calcium concentration to increase, and the subsequent release of acetylcholine (ACh) via exocytosis into the synaptic cleft (◉ Fig. 8.1). ACh then traverses this cleft to reach the postsynaptic junction, where

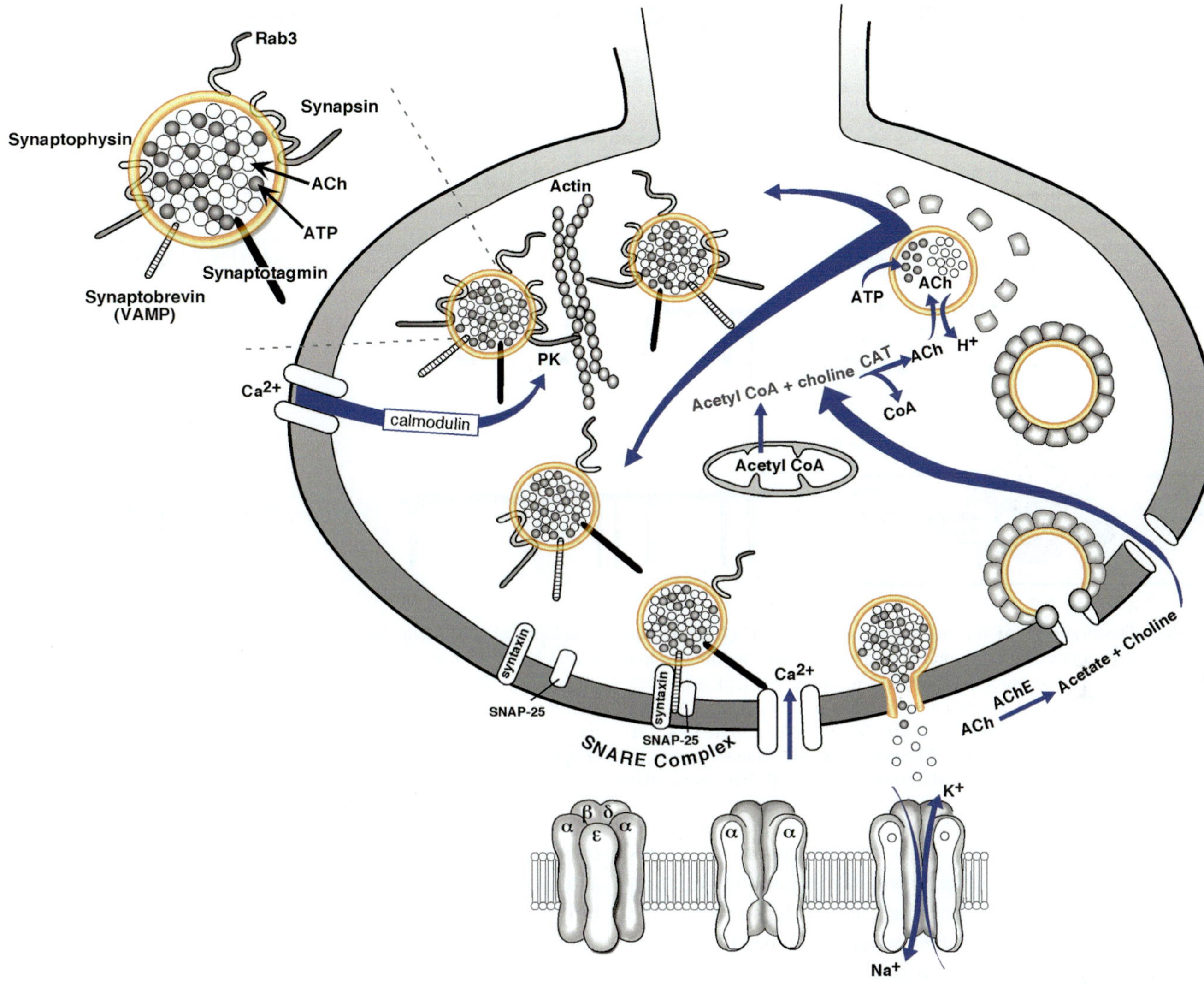

Fig. 8.1 The synaptic vesicle exocytosis–endocytosis cycle. After an action potential and Ca^{2+} influx, phosphorylation of synapsin is activated by calcium-calmodulin activated protein kinases I and II. This results in the mobilization of synaptic vesicles (SVs) from the cytomatrix toward the plasma membrane. The formation of the SNARE complex is an essential step for the docking process. After fusion of SVs with the presynaptic plasma membrane, acetylcholine (ACh) is released into the synaptic cleft. Some of the released acetylcholine molecules bind to the nicotinic acetylcholine receptors (nAChRs) on the postsynaptic membrane, while the rest is rapidly hydrolyzed by the acetylcholinesterase (AChE) present in the synaptic cleft into choline and acetate. Choline is recycled in the terminal by a high-affinity uptake system, making it available for the resynthesis of acetylcholine. Exocytosis is followed by endocytosis in a process dependent on the formation of a clathrin coat and of action of dynamin. After recovering of SV membrane, the coated vesicle uncoats, and another cycle starts again. See text for details. Acetyl CoA: acetylcoenzyme A; CAT: choline acetyltransferase; PK: protein kinase (Reproduced with permission from Naguib et al. [2])

it binds with nicotinic ACh receptors (nAChRs). Approximately 50% of the released acetylcholine is hydrolyzed during the time of diffusion across the synaptic cleft before reaching nAChRs. These nAChRs are concentrated on the folds of the postsynaptic muscle junction, also known as the motor endplate, with more than 90% of all such receptors located at this junction in adults. When managing patients with electrolyte abnormalities, it is important to remember that hypocalcemia and hypermagnesemia antagonize this release of ACh from the presynaptic motor neuron, leading to a decreased muscle response. In adult skeletal muscle, the postsynaptic nicotinic receptor consists of 5 protein subunits, 2 α (alpha) components and single β (beta), δ (delta), and ε (epsilon) subunits (◉ Fig. 8.2).

Once both binding sites on the α (alpha) subunits are bound by 2 ACh molecules or other agonist, a conformational change occurs that opens the ion channel, allowing for the entrance of sodium and calcium and the exit of potassium. The subsequent end-plate potential, when combined with enough other ACh-receptor interactions, depolarizes

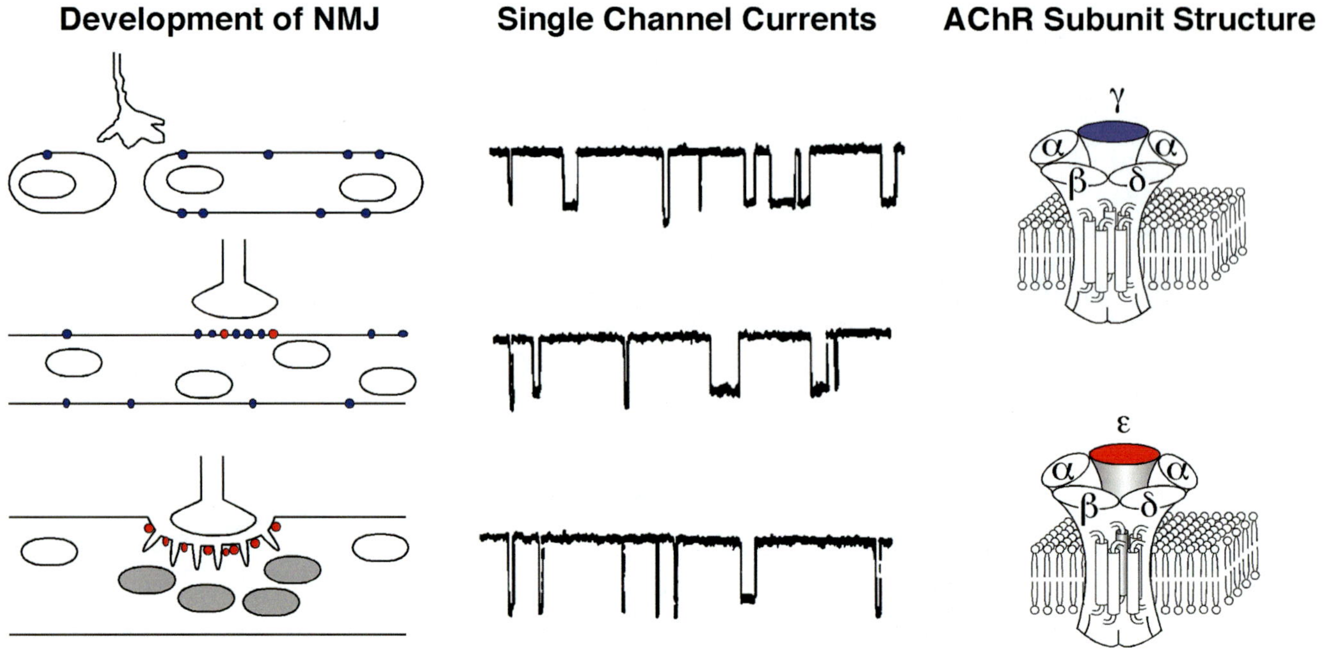

Fig. 8.2 Development of the neuromuscular junction. (*Left*) Motor neuron growth cones contact myotubes as they fuse from myoblasts and express mostly fetal nicotinic acetylcholine receptors (nAChRs; marked in *blue*) in their surface membranes. In adult muscle, adult nAChRs (marked in *red*) predominate and are largely concentrated at the neuromuscular junction. (*Center*) Records of AChR channel openings from muscle membranes at different stages of neuromuscular development. Fetal (*top*) and adult nAChRs (*bottom*) are activated by acetylcholine to form ion channels of different conductance and gating properties. (*Right*) Subunit composition of fetal and adult AChR subtypes. Fetal and adult AChR subtypes are characterized by the presence of a γ (gamma) and ε (epsilon) subunit, respectively (Reproduced with permission from Naguib et al. [2])

post-junctional membrane. This depolarization activates voltage-gated sodium channels, which mediate the initiation and propagation of action potentials across the surface of the muscle membrane and into the transverse tubules (T tubules) resulting in the upstroke of the action potential. There are 2 types of calcium channels: the dihydropyridine receptor (DHPR) in the transverse (T) tubules and the ryanodine receptor (RyR1) in the sarcoplasmic reticulum. DHPR-RyR1 interaction releases large amounts of calcium from the sarcoplasmic reticulum, causing muscle contraction. This process is known as excitation–contraction coupling. Repolarization of the muscle membrane is initiated by the closing of the sodium channels and by the opening of potassium ion channel that conducts an outward potassium current. Binding of ACh to only 1 α (alpha) subunit will not result in ion channel opening, current flow through these channels, or membrane depolarization. This scenario may occur in the presence of a nondepolarizing NMBA. Acetylcholine, succinylcholine, and nondepolarizing NMBAs have high affinity for the binding sites on the nAChRs.

Fetal nicotinic ACh receptors have a similar pentameric complex (◉ Fig. 8.2), although they contain a δ (delta) rather than an ε (epsilon) subunit; this accounts for its decreased cation conductance and subsequent longer opening time. Clinically, this translates to ACh causing brief activation of these receptors and a reduction in the probability of the channel opening and causing a muscle contraction. This trait makes such fetal receptors resistant to nondepolarizing NMBA and more sensitive to succinylcholine. Furthermore, these receptors increase in denervated states via upregulation, when they extend beyond the NMJ (extrajunctional receptors) throughout the muscle membrane. Such upregulation leaves patients vulnerable to exaggerated potassium plasma increases (from intracellular stores) when succinylcholine is administered.

8.3 Depolarizing Neuromuscular Blocking Agents

8.3.1 Succinylcholine

Succinylcholine is the only depolarizing NMBA in clinical use. This compound, also called suxamethonium, is composed of 2 ACh molecules adjoined through an acetate methyl group. This structure accounts for this medication's clinical effects. Succinylcholine produces the fastest, shortest, and most reliable neuromuscular blockade. This is accomplished by activating the postsynaptic ACh nicotinic

Table 8.1 Pharmacokinetic and pharmacodynamic properties of the depolarizing neuromuscular blocking agent succinylcholine

	Succinylcholine
Class	Depolarizing
Duration	Ultra-short acting
Potency—ED_{95} (mg/kg)	0.25–0.30
Intubating dose (mg/kg)	1.0–1.5
Onset time (min)	1.0–1.5
Clinical duration (min)	7–12
Recovery index (RI_{25-75}) (min)	2–4
Volume of distribution (L/kg)	0.04
Clearance (mL/kg/min)	35
Elimination half-life (min) Normal organ function Renal impairment Hepatic impairment	< 1 < 1 < 1
Maintenance dose (mg/kg)	N/A
Infusion dose (mcg/kg/min)	Titrate to ST muscle response
Elimination route/metabolism	Butyrylcholinesterase
Active metabolites	No active metabolites
Side effects	Myalgia; bradycardia/asystole in children or with repeated dosing; dual (phase II) block; anaphylaxis
Contraindications (other than specific allergy)	High serum K^+; MH; muscular dystrophy; children; receptor upregulation (e.g., patients with neurologic deficiencies, prolonged immobility, etc.); butyrylcholinesterase deficiency (see text for more details)
Comments	Fastest onset, most reliable NMBA for rapid tracheal intubation

Recovery index (RI_{25-75}) is the time required for the recovery of the first twitch from 25 to 75% of control twitch height. ED_{95}: effective dose that produces 95% depression of twitch height. The intubating dose for succinylcholine is ~ 3 × ED_{95} dose. NMBA: neuromuscular blocking drug; K^+: potassium; MH: malignant hyperthermia

receptor. Once bound to both binding sites on the α (alpha) subunits of the nicotinic ACh receptors, hyperpolarization occurs and flaccid paralysis then ensues as the membrane desensitizes. The clinical presentation of fasciculations noted after succinylcholine administration is variable (in location and severity) among patients. It appears that antidromic conduction of action potentials can lead to the activation of unparalyzed parts of the motor unit, resulting in fasciculations.

After an intravenous (IV) bolus of 1–1.5 mg/kg (3–5 × ED_{95}; ED_{95} is the dose that results in 95% depression of baseline twitch height), peripheral muscles become flaccid in 1–2 min, and remain so for 10–12 min. Such a large dose is required as nearly 90% of this compound is hydrolyzed by butyrylcholinesterase (also known as plasma cholinesterase or pseudocholinesterase) in the plasma prior to reaching the NMJ. Despite peripheral muscle paralysis, patients may be able to resume spontaneous breathing as soon as 5 min after administration, as central muscle groups (such as the diaphragm) recover before peripheral muscle groups. As very low concentrations of butyrylcholinesterase exist at the synaptic cleft, the termination of the effect of succinylcholine is determined primarily by its ability to diffuse into plasma (based on its concentration gradient) and the activity of butyrylcholinesterase for its hydrolysis (◉ Table 8.1).

While succinylcholine has many characteristics that make it ideal for facilitating endotracheal intubation, clinicians must be familiar with its ample side effect profile. Most patients experience muscle fasciculation after administration, a clinical sign that foreshadows the ensuing flaccid paralysis, which occurs approximately 1 min after offset of fasciculations. Myalgias are fairly common after succinylcholine exposure, with about half of patients reporting this side effect. While an intuitive causal relationship between uncomfortable-appearing fasciculations and myalgia seems plausible, large-scale reviews have never established such a link. Nonetheless, small "defasciculating" doses of nondepolarizing NMBAs or "self-taming" doses of succinylcholine have been used in an effort to decrease the fasciculations and postoperative myalgia. Such techniques may attenuate myalgia, but have not been found to reliably prevent these side effects; alternatively, such pretreatment

Table 8.2 Relationship between dibucaine number and duration of succinylcholine or mivacurium neuromuscular block

Type of butyrylcholinesterase	Genotype	Incidence	Dibucaine number[a]	Response to succinylcholine or mivacurium
Homozygous typical	$E_1^uE_1^u$	Normal	70–80	Normal
Heterozygous atypical	$E_1^uE_1^a$	1/480	50–60	Lengthened by 50–100%
Homozygous atypical	$E_1^aE_1^a$	1/3200	20–30	Prolonged to 4–8 h

[a] The dibucaine number indicates the percentage of enzyme inhibited

may expose patients to risks associated with partial paralysis, such as pulmonary aspiration. Non-steroidal anti-inflammatory drugs (NSAIDs) remain the only evidence-based treatment for succinylcholine-induced postoperative myalgias.

Again, owing to its similar structure to ACh, succinylcholine can produce bradycardia and even asystole, particularly in children or after repeated doses. In pediatrics, co-administration with atropine is a common practice to maintain the heart rate and subsequently, cardiac output, in the pediatric patients who have fixed stroke volumes.

Succinylcholine causes a reliable increase in the plasma potassium level (0.5 mEq/L) in otherwise healthy patients. This side effect has little clinical importance unless patients have preexisting hyperkalemia. Renal failure patients are no more susceptible to an exaggerated response to succinylcholine than are those with normal renal function. Alternatively, an exaggerated potassium increase that may lead to cardiac arrhythmia and even arrest can occur in patients with conditions associated with upregulation of extra junctional nicotinic nAChRs. As previously mentioned, such upregulation occurs in chronic denervated states, seen in patients with neuromuscular disease, massive trauma, sepsis, prolonged immobility or burns.

Succinylcholine is also associated with increases in intragastric pressure; however, proportional increases in the lower esophageal sphincter tone negate the potential risk of regurgitation. Transient increases in intraocular pressure also occur (up to 15 mm Hg) by unclear mechanisms. While this small increase in pressure must be considered and avoided in patients with preexisting high intraocular pressure, inadequate anesthesia, coughing, and ventilator dyssynchrony produce much greater increases in intraocular pressure. Co-administration with lidocaine or sufentanil can be used to attenuate succinylcholine-induced increases in intracranial pressure. Small increases in intracranial pressure also occur after succinylcholine administration; however, inadequate anesthesia during laryngoscopy with a subsequent hypertensive response is much more likely to elevate intracranial pressure.

The United States Food and Drug Administration (FDA) has issued a "black box" warning for succinylcholine in pediatrics, as these patients may have an undiagnosed myotonia or muscle dystrophy. Succinylcholine may trigger rhabdomyolysis and a fatal hyperkalemic state in these patients. Furthermore, succinylcholine is contraindicated in patients with malignant hyperthermia, a risk that is significantly increased when volatile anesthetics are used. Masseter muscle spasm is another complication that is specific to succinylcholine administration and may be associated with malignant hyperthermia.

The use of succinylcholine is also contraindicated in patients with butyrylcholinesterase deficiency (◉ Table 8.2). The heterozygous deficient state is present in approximately 1 in 480 patients, while the homozygous version may be present in 1 in 3,200 individuals. These patients require a much longer time to recover from succinylcholine administration and may require unanticipated postoperative mechanical ventilation and sedation/amnesia as they recover.

8.4 Nondepolarizing Neuromuscular Blocking Agents

Nondepolarizing NMBAs act as competitive antagonists by binding to the α (alpha) subunits of the nicotinic acetylcholine receptor. NMBAs have been classically categorized either based on their duration of action (long-, intermediate-, and short-acting agents) or based on their structure (steroids or benzylisoquinolinium) (◉ Tables 8.3 and ◉ 8.4). Nondepolarizing NMBAs are positively charged, relatively large molecules. In general, a dose of 2–3 × ED_{95} is used to facilitate tracheal intubation while a dose of 10% of the ED_{95} is used to maintain neuromuscular blockade (◉ Fig. 8.3).

8.4.1 Benzylisoquinolinium Compounds

Atracurium is a bis-benzylisoquinolinium compound that is mixture of 10 isomers. The ED_{95} is 0.2 mg/kg, with an intubating dose of 0.5 mg/kg that yields suitable laryngoscopy conditions after 2.5–4.0 min. This intermediate-duration nondepolarizing NMBA lasts 30–45 min after administration of an intubating dose. Atracurium is metabolized through 2 distinct pathways that are almost completely independent of renal and hepatic function: a nonenzymatic degradation (called Hofmann elimination) and hydrolysis by nonspecific plasma esterases. Hofmann

Table 8.3 Pharmacokinetic and pharmacodynamic properties of benzylisoquinolinium nondepolarizing neuromuscular blocking agents

	Mivacurium	Atracurium	Cisatracurium
Duration	Short	Intermediate	Intermediate
Potency—ED_{95} (mg/kg)	0.08	0.25	0.05
Intubation dose (mg/kg)	0.2	0.5	0.15–0.20
Onset time (min)	3–4	3–5	4–7
Clinical duration (min)	15–20	30–45	35–50
*Recovery index (RI_{25-75}) (min)	7–9	10–15	12–15
Volume of distribution (L/kg)	~ 0.2 for the 3 isomers	~0.15	~0.16
Clearance (mL/kg/min)	30–45	5.3–6.6	5.7
Elimination half-life (min) Normal organ function Renal impairment Hepatic impairment	2–2.5 3–4 3–6	21 21 21	23–30 Mild increase 23–30
Maintenance dose (mg/kg)	0.1	0.1	0.01
Infusion dose (mcg/kg/min)	5–8	10–20	1–3
Elimination route	Plasma cholinesterase (70% of succinylcholine rate)	Renal 10%; Hofmann elimination 30%; ester hydrolysis 60%	Hofmann elimination. No ester hydrolysis of the parent molecule
Active metabolites	No active metabolites	No active metabolites. Laudanosine and acrylates metabolite	No active metabolites. Laudanosine and monoquaternary acrylate metabolite
Side effects	Histamine release	Histamine release	
Contraindications (other than specific allergy)	Butyrylcholinesterase deficiency	Hemodynamically unstable patients due to histamine release	None
Comments	Composed of 3 isomers (*cis-trans, trans-trans and cis-cis*). Reversal by cholinesterase inhibitors; edrophonium for antagonism more effective during deep block	It is composed of 10 isomers. Organ-independent elimination	Cisatracurium is the *cis–cis* isomer of atracurium, accounting for 50% in terms of neuromuscular blocking activity of atracurium. It is approximately 4 times as potent as atracurium but does not cause histamine release. Minimal plasma laudanosine and acrylate levels

The data are averages obtained from published literature, assuming there is no potentiation from other co-administered drugs (such as volatile inhalational anesthetics), and the effects are measured at the adductor pollicis muscle. Other factors, such as muscle temperature, mode of evoked response monitoring, type/site of muscle monitoring, etc., will affect the data. ED_{95}: effective dose that produces 95% depression of twitch height. The intubating dose for nondepolarizing neuromuscular blocking drugs is traditionally 2 × ED_{95} dose. Recovery index (RI_{25-75}) is the time required for the recovery of the first twitch from 25 to 75% of control twitch height. This requires the use of a quantitative monitor and stabilization and calibration of the baseline twitch response before the administration of neuromuscular blocking drugs

Table 8.4 Pharmacokinetic and pharmacodynamic properties of aminosteroid nondepolarizing neuromuscular blocking agents

	Vecuronium	Rocuronium	Pancuronium
Duration	Intermediate	Intermediate	Long
Potency—ED_{95} (mg/kg)	0.05	0.3	0.07
Intubating dose (mg/kg)	0.1	0.6	0.1
Onset time (min)	3–4	1.5–3	3–5
Clinical duration (min)	25–50	30–70	60–120
Recovery index (RI_{25-75}) (min)	10–25	8–13	30–45
Volume of distribution (L/kg)	0.4	0.3–0.7	0.2–0.3
Clearance (mL/kg/min)	5	10	1.8
Elimination half-life (min) Normal organ function Renal impairment Hepatic impairment	65–75 Mild increase Significant increase	100–250 100–300 120–400	90–160 Increased x2 Increased x2
Maintenance dose (mg/kg)	0.01	0.1	0.02
Infusion dose (mcg/kg/min)	1–2	5–12	20–40 (not recommended)
Elimination route	Renal 10–50%; Hepatic 30–50%	Hepatic 90%; Renal 10%	Renal 40–70%; Hepatic 20%
Active metabolites	3-desacetyl-vecuronium	17-desacetyl-rocuronium (minimal)	3-OH-pancuronium; 17-OH-pancuronium
Side effects	Vagal blockade with large doses	Minimal	Vagal block (tachycardia), catecholamine release
Contraindications (other than specific allergy)	None	None	Short surgical procedures (< 60 min); not recommended for continuous infusion
Comments	In patients in the ICU who have renal failure, 3-desacetylvecuronium can accumulate and produce prolonged neuromuscular blockade; elimination half-life halved in late pregnancy; 3-desacetyl metabolite has 60% of the parent compound potency	Rocuronium is approximately 6–10 times less potent than pancuronium and vecuronium, respectively. Elimination half-life prolonged in ICU patient; 17-desacetyl metabolite has 20% activity	Significant accumulation, prone to residual block (3-OH metabolite has 50% activity of pancuronium); total clearance is delayed, and the duration of action is significantly lengthened by severe disorders of renal or hepatic function

The data are averages obtained from published literature, assuming there is no potentiation from other co-administered drugs (such as volatile inhalational anesthetics), and the effects are measured at the adductor pollicis muscle. Other factors, such as muscle temperature, mode of evoked response monitoring, type/site of muscle monitoring, etc., will affect the data. ED_{95}: effective dose that produces 95% depression of twitch height. The intubating dose for nondepolarizing neuromuscular blocking drugs is traditionally 2xED_{95} dose. Recovery index (RI_{25-75}) is the time required for the recovery of the first twitch from 25% to 75% of control twitch height. This requires the use of a quantitative monitor and stabilization and calibration of the baseline twitch response before the administration of neuromuscular blocking drugs. ICU: intensive care unit

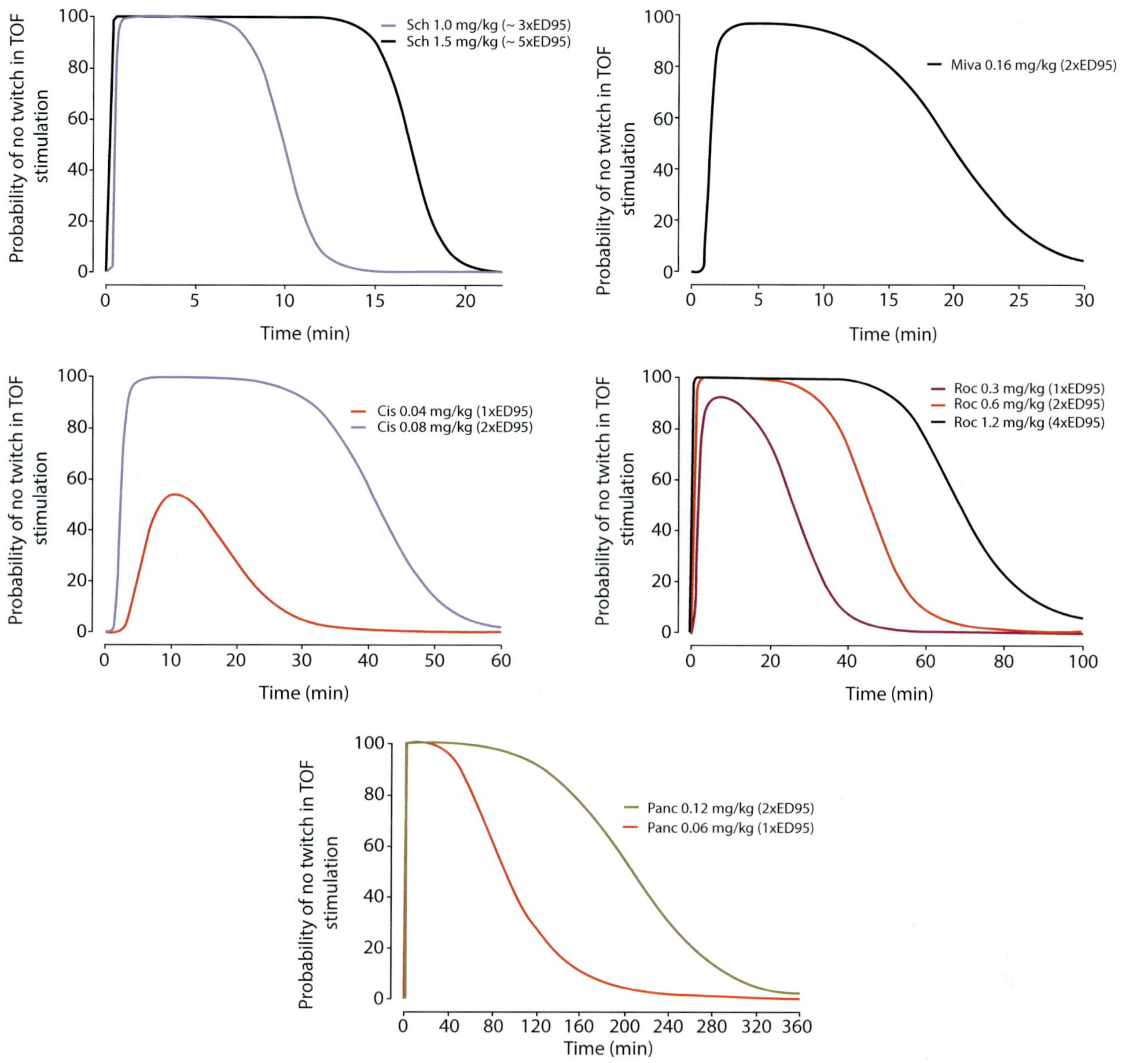

Fig. 8.3 Probability of no-twitch response to train-of-four (TOF) stimulation over time resulting from administration of different ED_{95} (the dose that results in 95% depression of twitch height) doses of different neuromuscular blocking drugs. Sch: succinylcholine; Miv: mivacurium; Cis: cisatracurium; Roc: rocuronium; Panc: pancuronium

elimination is a pH- and temperature-dependent reaction in which higher pH and temperature favor elimination. Atracurium is relatively stable at pH 3.0 and 4 °C and becomes unstable when injected into the bloodstream. Doses exceeding 0.5 mg/kg are associated with histamine release that can result in flushing, tachycardia, and hypotension. One breakdown product from Hofmann elimination, laudanosine, has been implicated in a theoretical risk of increased central nervous system excitability; however, at clinically relevant doses, such complications have not been reported.

Cisatracurium is the *cis*-isomer of atracurium and represents about 15% of the marketed atracurium mixture by weight, but accounts for more than 50% in terms of potency or neuromuscular blocking activity. It is approximately 4 times more potent than atracurium with an ED_{95} of 0.05 mg/kg and, unlike atracurium, it does not cause histamine release in the clinical dose range. The administration of 2 × ED_{95} of cisatracurium provides intubating conditions in about 3–5 min. Like atracurium, it is broken down by Hofmann elimination, but there is no ester hydrolysis of the parent molecule. Its organ-independent elimination pathway, combined with its hemodynamic stability and lack of associated histamine release make this NMBA ideal for use in the intensive care unit (ICU). The incidence of anaphylaxis from both cisatracurium and atracurium is lower than that of rocuronium and succinylcholine.

Mivacurium was developed in an effort to combine the safety profile of nondepolarizing NMBA with the rapid onset and short duration of action of depolarizing drugs. Its structure is similar to that of atracurium, save for an additional methylated phenolic group. It consists of 3 stereoisomers, with the trans-trans and *cis*-trans isomers accounting for the majority of its neuromuscular blocking activity. Like succinylcholine, it is metabolized by butyrylcholinesterases (with 75% efficiency) and therefore has a slightly longer duration of action (15–20 min). Like succinylcholine, mivacurium should not be used in patients with butyrylcholinesterase deficiency. With an ED_{95} of 0.08 mg/kg, 3–4 times this dose is needed for achieving intubating conditions reliably. Such doses, however, may result in significant histamine release and ideal intubating conditions are still not achieved for 2 min or longer. These limitations have prevented its widespread use in the USA, although efforts are currently being made to re-introduce this agent to the market.

8.4.2 Aminosteroidal Compounds

Pancuronium is a long-acting nondepolarizing NMBA with several clinical features of interest. It possesses vagolytic effects, as well as direct sympathomimetic stimulation as it blocks the reuptake of norepinephrine. The ED_{95} is 0.07 mg/kg, and a dose of 0.1 mg/kg will provide intubating conditions within 3–4 min. Recovery from such a dose, defined as time from injection until recovery of twitch height to 25% of control (clinical duration), takes nearly 90 min. This prolonged duration of action is at least partially due to the accumulation of an active metabolite, 3-OH pancuronium, following pancuronium's hepatic metabolism. The majority of pancuronium (85%) is eliminated renally, with the remainder being excreted by the liver. Given its prolonged effect and the concern for postoperative residual paralysis and associated morbidity, many clinicians elect to use other NMBAs for inducing neuromuscular blockade in their patients.

Vecuronium is an intermediate-acting nondepolarizing NMBA that produces paralysis with minimal hemodynamic effects. Its ED_{95} is 0.05 mg/kg, and an intubating dose ($2 \times ED_{95}$) results in adequate conditions within 3 min. Such a dose results in a 45–90 min recovery time. Specific to vecuronium are its various metabolites, one of which (3-OH vecuronium) has 60% potency relative to the parent compound. Like pancuronium, such metabolites are generated from hepatic metabolism and vecuronium is eliminated mostly (60%) through biliary excretion, with the remainder being excreted renally. These features preclude its safe use in the intensive care unit where repeated doses can lead to accumulation of its metabolites and prolonged duration of action, leading to critical illness polyneuromyopathy (CIPM).

Rocuronium is also an intermediate-acting nondepolarizing NMBA that can be used for rapid sequence induction and intubation, as its onset of action time approaches that of succinylcholine when a dose of 1.2 mg/kg ($4 \times ED_{95}$) is used. Its ED_{95} is 0.3 mg/kg, and the duration of recovery from an intubating dose is similar to that of vecuronium. Also, like vecuronium, it has a stable hemodynamic profile with no associated release of histamine. Rocuronium does not generate clinically relevant metabolites. While spontaneous recovery from a rapid sequence induction and intubating dose is much longer for rocuronium than for succinylcholine, the availability of sugammadex has allowed for a greater safety profile when using rocuronium. The incidence of anaphylaxis from any neuromuscular blocker is as high as 1 in 6500 administrations in some countries, and rocuronium (and succinylcholine) have the highest incidence of NMBA-induced anaphylaxis. Rocuronium is excreted unchanged through both biliary ($\sim$ 70%) and renal ($\sim$ 30%) mechanisms.

8.5 Drug Interactions

8.5.1 Mechanisms of Drug Interactions

Pharmacokinetic interactions are interactions in which one drug alters the rate or amount of absorption, distribution, metabolism, or excretion of another drug (or any combination of these processes). Pharmacodynamic interactions occur when the dose–response relationship of a drug is altered by the co-administration of a second drug. These interactions are generally described as being synergistic, antagonistic, or additive.

The interaction between succinylcholine and NMBAs depends on the order of administration and the doses used. Administration of small doses of different nondepolarizing NMBAs before succinylcholine to prevent fasciculations has an antagonistic effect on development of the subsequent depolarizing block produced by succinylcholine. Therefore, it is recommended that the dose of succinylcholine be increased after the administration of a defasciculating dose of a nondepolarizing NMBA. In contrast, the administration of succinylcholine before nondepolarizing NMBAs appears to potentiate the effects of these NMBAs.

In an era of polypharmacy, anesthesiologists must be aware of the various drug interactions that may occur with

NMBA use. For instance, inhalational anesthetics potentiate neuromuscular blockade, likely by affecting post-junctional receptors. This response depends not only on the type of such volatile anesthetics (desflurane > sevoflurane > isoflurane), but also the concentration and duration of exposure. Local anesthetics are another commonly utilized class of medications that interact with NMBAs. These drugs have the potential to prolong the duration of action of both depolarizing and nondepolarizing NMBAs. Certain antibiotics, such as streptomycin and neomycin, have been found to prolong the response to nondepolarizing NMBA as well, although newer antibiotics have not been implicated. Magnesium, a medication commonly used when treating obstetric patients with eclampsia, prolongs the normal response to neuromuscular blockade by preventing the release of acetylcholine from the presynaptic terminal. Similarly, patients receiving chronic lithium can have a prolonged response to both depolarizing and nondepolarizing NMBA as this medication inhibits presynaptic neuromuscular transmission and postsynaptic muscle contraction.

Antiepileptic drugs have a significant impact on the response to NMBA administration. Patients taking antiepileptic drugs chronically have a relative resistance to aminosteroidal nondepolarizing NMBAs and may require more frequent dosing during maintenance of neuromuscular blockade. However, acute administration of antiepileptic drugs is associated with a prolonged response to NMBA.

8.6 Reversal Drugs (Nondepolarizing NMBA Antagonists)

Traditionally, reversal of neuromuscular blockade has been achieved through the administration of acetylcholinesterase inhibitors. These medications inhibit the breakdown of ACh, causing an increase in ACh relative to nondepolarizing NMBA at the nicotinic ACh receptor. By more effectively competing with NMBAs for nAChR binding sites, ACh results in the generation of normal transmission and subsequent muscle contraction. Three acetylcholinesterase inhibitors are available today: edrophonium, neostigmine, and pyridostigmine. The latter of these medications has the longest onset of action, longest duration of action, and possesses central effects as its tertiary amine structure allows it to cross the blood-brain barrier. Pyridostigmine is not utilized in the operating arena; rather, it is utilized to treat weakness associated with myasthenia gravis.

Neostigmine is currently the most frequently used acetylcholinesterase inhibitor. As with all acetylcholinesterase inhibitors, neostigmine has significant parasympathomimetic effects as ACh interacts with cholinergic receptors throughout the body. For instance, these agents cause a pronounced bradycardia and other bradyarrhythmias as well as bronchoconstriction through muscarinic receptor activation. In order to mitigate these effects, anti-muscarinic agents are co-administered with acetylcholinesterase inhibitors. Glycopyrrolate is typically administered with neostigmine, and atropine is administered with edrophonium, as these pairings reflect similar onset times between the 2 classes of medications. The dose of neostigmine must be guided by the level of neuromuscular blockade: acetylcholinesterase inhibitors are ineffective at reversing deep levels of neuromuscular blockade when train-of-four (TOF) count is zero and only post-tetanic twitches are present. At the other extreme, administration of neostigmine once recovery is almost complete may have the paradoxical effect of inducing muscle weakness. Therefore, reversal with neostigmine should occur at moderate-to-shallow levels of neuromuscular blockade (TOF count of 2–4 with muscle fatigue or fade).

In addition to considering the depth of neuromuscular blockade, several other factors must be considered when utilizing acetylcholinesterase inhibitors for reversing NMBA-induced paralysis. As previously discussed, neuromuscular blockade can be potentiated by a variety of factors such as volatile anesthetics, aminoglycoside antibiotics, hypercarbia, acidosis, hypothermia, hypocalcemia, or hypermagnesemia. The type of nondepolarizing NMBA also affects recovery from neostigmine reversal, as recovery from long-acting agents such as pancuronium is prolonged when compared to recovery from intermediate-acting NMBA. The elderly population also has slower recovery following neostigmine reversal. Such confounding factors, combined with the fact that patients respond in a heterogeneous manner to both NMBA and pharmacologic reversal with acetylcholinesterases, may partly explain the high incidence of residual neuromuscular blockade, particularly when quantitative monitoring is not employed by clinicians.

Edrophonium is an acetylcholinesterase inhibitor with a faster peak onset of action time than neostigmine: 1–2 min versus 7–11 min, respectively. As a result of ionic bonds that it forms with the acetylcholinesterase enzyme, rather than the stronger covalent bonds of neostigmine, edrophonium has less affinity for this enzyme and therefore should only be used to antagonize shallow levels of blockade. The typical antagonist dose is 0.5–1.0 mg/kg. Given its fast onset time, atropine is co-administered with edrophonium. As of 2018, edrophonium is no longer available in the United States.

8.7 Selective Relaxant Binding Agents

Sugammadex is a modified gamma-cyclodextrin compound composed of an 8-membered ring with a central cavity that encapsulates aminosteroidal NMBAs. This modification entails: (1) the addition of 8 side chains to extend the cavity of gamma-cyclodextrin in order to better accommodate the 4 hydrophobic steroidal rings of rocuronium; and (2) the inclusion of negatively charged carboxyl groups at the end of the side chains in order to enhance electrostatic binding to the positively charged quaternary nitrogen of rocuronium. Sugammadex exerts its effect by forming very tight complexes at a 1:1 ratio with steroidal NMBAs (rocuronium/pipecuronium > vecuronium > > pancuronium). Sugammadex has little to no affinity for binding to benzylisoquinolinium neuromuscular blockers or to succinylcholine. The intravenous administration of sugammadex rapidly binds all available unbound (free) plasma rocuronium molecules, creating a concentration gradient that favors the movement of steroidal NMBA molecules from the NMJ back into the plasma. This removal of NMBA from the NMJ results in a fast recovery of neuromuscular function, as ACh no longer has to compete with the aminosteroidal NMBD for the receptor sites. The sugammadex-steroidal NMBA moiety is excreted in the urine. Sugammadex, therefore, acts as a binding agent and has no effect on acetylcholinesterase or any receptor system in the body. Such antagonism is devoid of the various side effects associated with acetylcholinesterase inhibition.

At doses of 2 mg/kg, sugammadex reverses rocuronium and vecuronium when the TOF count is at least 2 in about 3 min. A dose of 4 mg/kg is recommended for antagonism of deeper levels of blockade (such as when only post-tetanic twitches are present). A dose of 16 mg/kg can be used to rapidly and emergently reverse the effects of 1.2 mg/kg rocuronium during a failed rapid sequence induction scenario. This dose of sugammadex restores muscle function faster than the spontaneous recovery from succinylcholine administration (◉ Fig. 8.4). However, pharmacologic intervention with sugammadex should not be relied upon to rescue patients in the setting of "cannot intubate, cannot

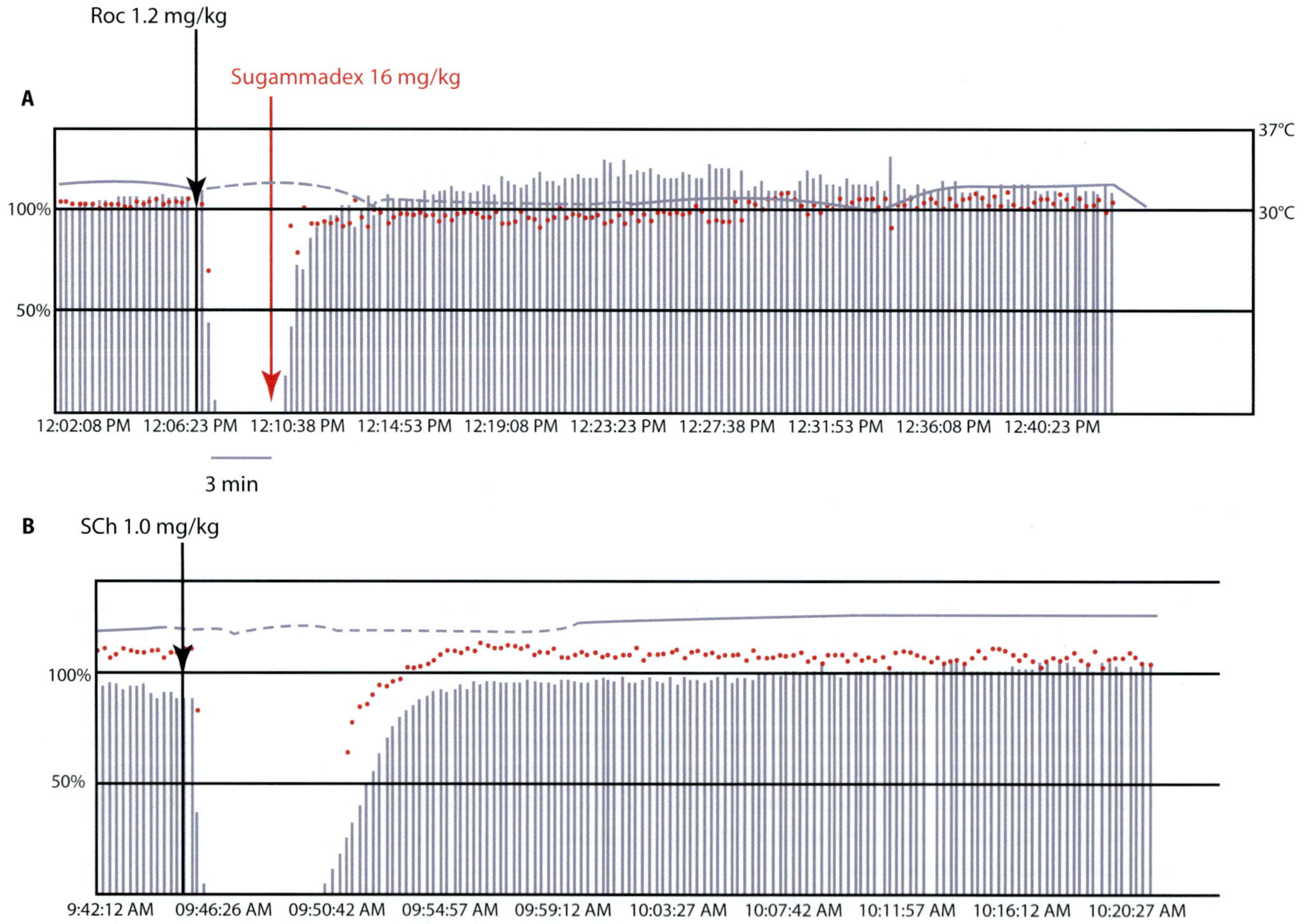

Fig. 8.4 *Panel A* shows the recovery of the twitch height and train-of-four (TOF) ratio after administration of 1.2 mg/kg rocuronium followed 3 min later by 16 mg/kg sugammadex, both given IV. Recovery to a first twitch height (T1) of 90% and a TOF ratio of 0.94 occurred 110 s later. The onset–offset time with this sequence (i.e., the time from the end of the injection of rocuronium to a T1 recovery to 90%) was 4 min 47 s. *Panel B* shows the effects of administering 1.0 mg/kg succinylcholine (SCh) with spontaneous recovery to a T1 of 90% occurring after 9 min and 23 s (Reproduced with permission from Naguib et al. [3])

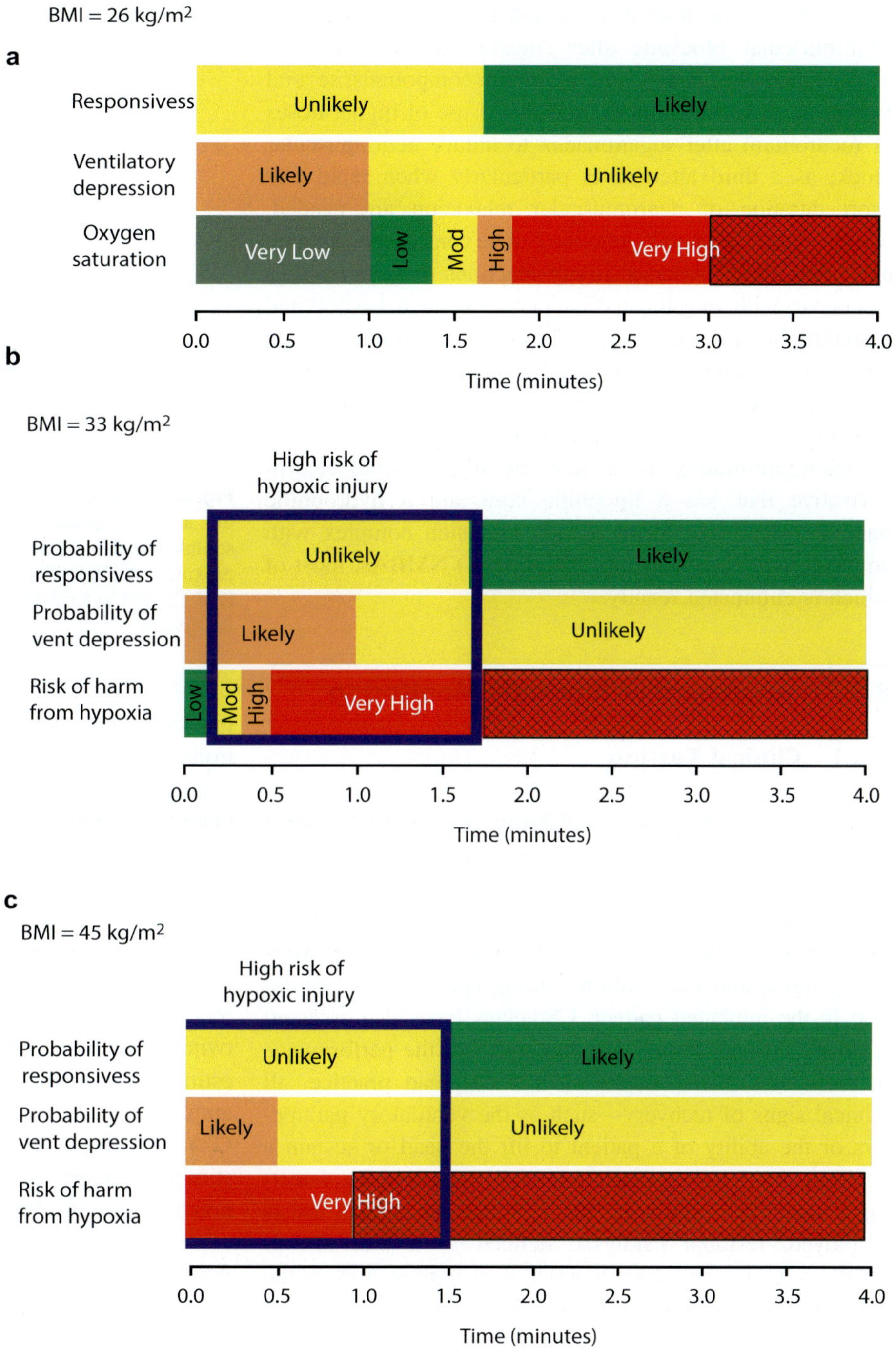

Fig. 8.5 Comparison of responsiveness, intolerable ventilatory depression, and hypoxia to estimate periods of *high risk of hypoxic injury* after induction with failure to ventilate or secure the airway. For discussion purposes, the duration of effects presented in this table are presented as the time from reversal of rocuronium neuromuscular blockade with sugammadex (*vertical pink line* in **c**) until selected endpoints in drug effects. See methods for criteria used to estimate a high risk of hypoxic injury. **a** and **b** present the definitions of the scales used to characterize the probability of effects. Time segments that met criteria are identified with a *blue rectangle*. The *blue rectangle* for the BMI of 45 kg/m^2 is truncated at time = 0 min because criteria were met for a high risk of injury 1.5 min before reversal with sugammadex (Reproduced with permission from Naguib et al. [4])

ventilate" (CICV) crisis (◉ Fig. 8.5). Following induction of anesthesia, rescue reversal of 1.2 mg/kg rocuronium with 16 mg/kg sugammadex in the setting of CICV may still not result in reliable, immediate return of spontaneous ventilation. In a simulation study, it was reported that, in obese and morbidly obese patients, even after adequate preoxygenation, neuromuscular reversal may not be sufficiently rapid to prevent significant hemoglobin desaturation. The clinical management of CICV should primarily focus on restoration of airway patency, oxygenation, and ventilation consistent with the American Society of Anesthesiologist's *Practice Guidelines for Management of the Difficult Airway* [1].

There are several patient factors that must be considered when utilizing this reversal agent. First, this drug binds oral contraceptive medications and patients receiving this medication should be advised to utilize alternative birth control means for the week succeeding its administration. As previously stated, sugammadex is cleared renally, but it can also be removed via high-flux hemodialysis. Reestablishing neuromuscular blockade after sugammadex reversal can involve the use of benzylisoquinolinium compounds; several studies have documented the successful use of higher doses of rocuronium after sugammadex to induce neuromuscular block; as a third alternative, particularly when rapid and short duration of neuromuscular relaxation are needed, administration of succinylcholine can be considered. As with any medication, hypersensitivity reactions to sugammadex can occur, with an estimated incidence between 1:3,500 and 1:20,000. Such reactions typically occur within the first 4-5 min after sugammadex administration, and the subsequent cardiovascular collapse has been successfully treated with epinephrine and volume resuscitation.

Adamgammadex is a new modified γ-cyclodextrin derivative that has a lipophilic core and a hydrophilic outer envelope that forms a tight inclusion complex with aminosteroidal (vecuronium, rocuronium) NMBAs, most of which is eliminated renally.

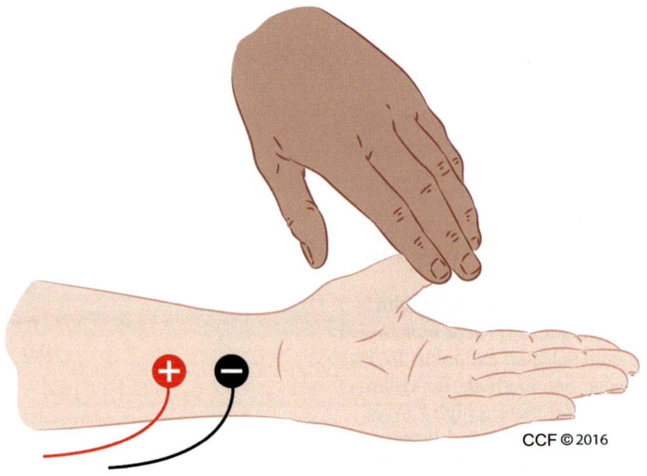

Fig. 8.6 Subjective (tactile) evaluation of neuromuscular responses at the adductor pollicis (thumb) muscle in response to ulnar nerve stimulation. Note that the *black* (*negative*) electrode is distal to the proximal, *red* (*positive*) electrode (Reprinted with permission, Cleveland Clinic Center for Medical Art & Photography ©2016. All Rights Reserved)

8.8 Neuromuscular Blockade Monitoring

8.8.1 Clinical Testing

Prior to the widespread availability of peripheral nerve stimulators and quantitative neuromuscular blockade monitors, clinicians relied on various clinical signs and tests to assess adequate recovery from neuromuscular blockade. Such tests include assessing vital capacity, negative inspiratory force, and tidal volume during spontaneous ventilation in the intubated patient. Clinicians have also assessed recovery through testing grip strength and the performance of a 5-s head lift. Despite such widespread practice, all clinical signs of recovery—such as the ventilatory parameters or the ability of a patient to lift the head or sustain a handgrip for 5 s—are inaccurate and insensitive for detecting residual neuromuscular block. Whatever clinical test is employed, residual paralysis, defined as a train-of-four (TOF, or T_4/T_1) ratio less than 0.9, is as high as 40% in the recovery room when objective monitoring is not used to guide the timing of tracheal extubation. Residual postoperative paralysis has numerous associated complications such as upper airway obstruction, aspiration, atelectasis, and hypoxemia. When such patients require unplanned re-intubation and intensive care unit admission, mortality increases significantly.

8.8.2 Subjective Evaluation

The use of a peripheral nerve stimulator (PNS) allows for the subjective evaluation of the level of neuromuscular blockade. This technique utilizes stimulating surface electrodes placed on the skin overlying a superficial motor nerve that innervates the muscle of interest. The negative (typically black) electrode is placed distally to the positive (typically red) electrode (◉ Figs. 8.6 and 8.7). Subjective assessment consists of evaluating and comparing the strength of sequential evoked muscle responses.

Peripheral nerve stimulators have been used clinically for more than 6 decades and typically involve delivering a train-of-four stimulation pattern in which 4 successive single twitch stimuli are delivered at 2 Hz. The degree of fade is estimated by evaluating the TOF ratio, which compares the amplitude of the fourth twitch (T_4) to that of the first twitch (T_1). In addition to evaluating recovery, performing a TOF stimulus pattern allows for assessment of the degree of nondepolarizing NMBA-induced paralysis, as the TOF count correlates with the percent of postsynaptic nicotinic Ach receptors occupied by nondepolarizing NMBA. Presence of 1 of 4 twitches (TOF count = 1) correlates with more than 95% of such receptors being blocked. Presence of two twitches (TOF count = 2) correlates with 85–90% occupancy. Presence of 3 twitches (TOF Count = 3) corresponds with 80–85% receptor occupancy. Presence of all 4 twitches after TOF stimulation suggests that 70–75% of receptors are blocked. Subjective evaluation of TOF stimulation with the use of a PNS requires the observer to determine the number of twitches and the strength of the first response in the train and compare it to the fourth evoked response by tactile or visual means. The major limitation of evaluating the TOF ratio subjectively is that once TOF ratio approaches 0.40, most clinicians cannot detect the presence

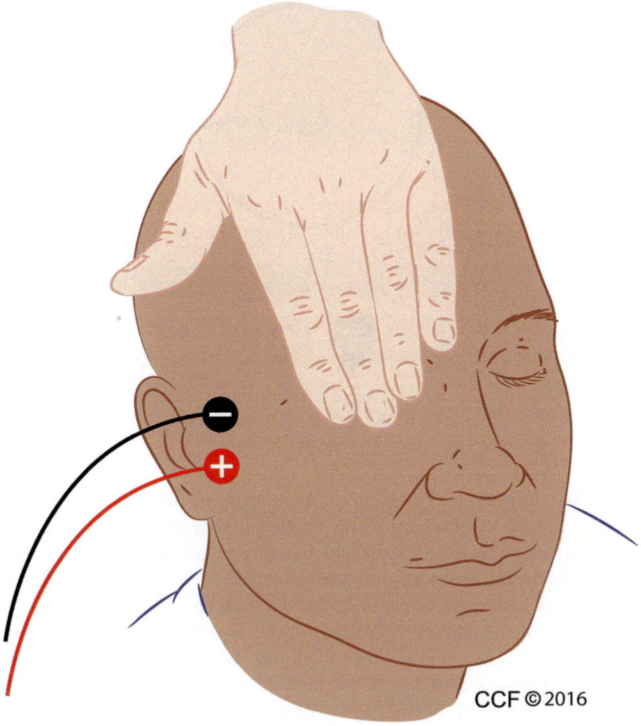

Fig. 8.7 Subjective (tactile) evaluation of neuromuscular responses at the orbicularis oculi (eye) muscle in response to facial nerve stimulation. Note the *negative* (*black*) electrode is placed distally (Reprinted with permission, Cleveland Clinic Center for Medical Art & Photography ©2016. All Rights Reserved)

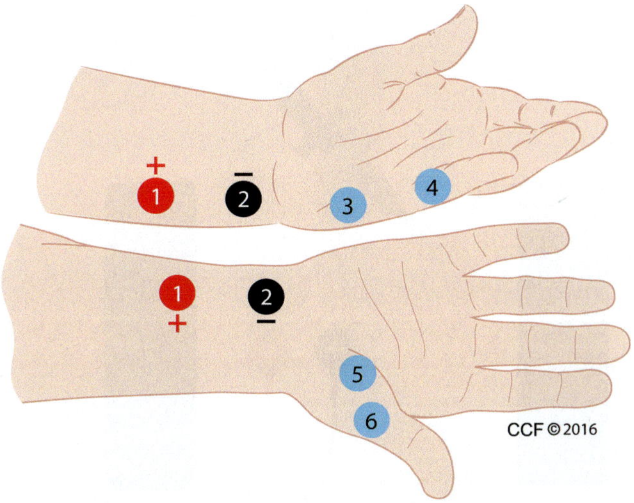

Fig. 8.8 Placement of the stimulating electrodes (*1* and *2*) along the ulnar nerve; and of the recording electrodes for monitoring the abductor digiti minimi (*3* and *4*) or the adductor pollicis (*5* and *6*) muscles by electromyography (Reprinted with permission, Cleveland Clinic Center for Medical Art & Photography ©2016. All Rights Reserved)

of fade. This failure underscores that subjective assessment is unreliable at determining recovery from neuromuscular blockade and exposes patients to the avoidable risks associated with residual neuromuscular weakness. The authors strongly recommend the use of objective (quantitative) monitoring.

8.8.3 Objective Evaluation

Objective evaluation involves the quantification of the TOF ratio through the measurement of electrical or mechanical response to nerve stimulation. There are numerous modalities that have been employed to provide such measurements, and the most clinically relevant techniques will be discussed.

Electromyography (EMG) is the oldest form of neuromuscular monitoring; it measures the electrical potential generated by myocytes upon activation (◉ Fig. 8.8). Active (recording) electrodes are placed over the muscle body (either intramuscular or at the surface), while a neutral electrode is placed at a remote site, usually near the muscle insertion site. EMG signals are subject to electrical interference, direct muscle stimulation, and hypothermia, although to a less extent than other techniques. It should be noted that this modality is inherently different from other techniques in that there is no muscle movement being analyzed; rather, EMG electrodes measure electrical activity (muscle action potential, MAP) in the muscle as a result of presynaptic nerve depolarization. EMG measures neuromuscular transmission and receptor activity and is therefore the most accurate technique of measuring neuromuscular transmission. EMG also has a significant clinical advantage because it does not require the unimpeded movement of the monitored muscle (thumb) that is needed for acceleromyography and kinemyography (see below). Therefore, the monitored arm can be tucked under surgical drapes without affecting EMG recordings.

Mechanomyography (MMG) measures the force created by muscle contraction in response to electrical stimuli applied to peripheral nerves (◉ Fig. 8.9). It is regarded as the historic gold standard of neuromuscular blockade monitoring, and a mechanomyographic adductor pollicis muscle (APM) TOF ratio of 0.9 or more is widely accepted as the threshold for exclusion of residual paralysis. However, its use in clinical settings is limited by the labor-intensive setup that includes the need for a large rigid support for the arm as well as pre-relaxant calibration and maintenance of a constant 200–300 gm preload (tension). MMG is primarily used for research purposes, as investigators compare new monitoring techniques to MMG.

Acceleromyography (AMG) is based on Newton's second law (force = mass X acceleration) and utilizes a piezoelectric transducer attached to a muscle (◉ Fig. 8.10). Upon stimulation of the nerve and contraction of the muscle, the

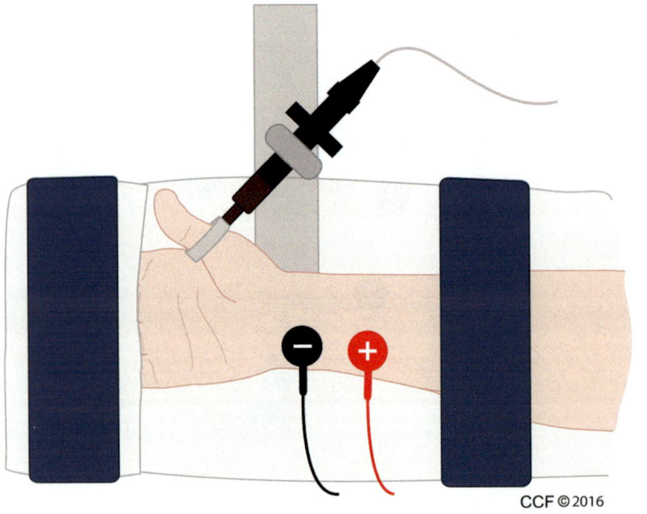

Fig. 8.9 Apparatus for objective monitoring of the adductor pollicis (*thumb*) muscle using mechanomyography. A force transducer ring is attached to the thumb, and the fingers are secured to prevent movement during nerve stimulation. Ulnar nerve stimulation (note that the negative electrode is distal to the positive electrode) will result in contraction of the adductor pollicis muscle, and the force of contraction is measured by the force transducer. The results are displayed on an interfaced screen (Reprinted with permission, Cleveland Clinic Center for Medical Art & Photography ©2016. All Rights Reserved)

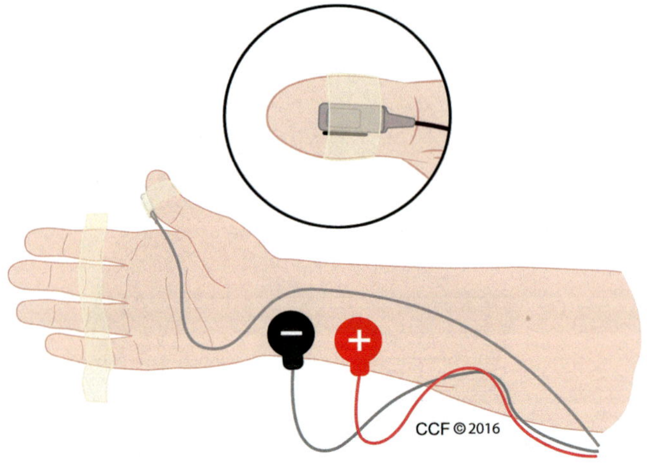

Fig. 8.10 Apparatus for objective monitoring of the adductor pollicis (*thumb*) muscle contraction using acceleromyography. An accelerometer is attached to the thumb, and the fingers are secured to prevent movement during nerve stimulation. Ulnar nerve stimulation (note that the negative electrode is distal to the positive electrode) will result in contraction of the adductor pollicis muscle, and the thumb acceleration is measured. The results are displayed on the monitor's screen (Reprinted with permission, Cleveland Clinic Center for Medical Art & Photography ©2016. All Rights Reserved)

force of the contraction is determined by measuring the acceleration of the piezoelectric crystal. As this technique relies on the free movement of the thumb and requires access to the hand for monitoring, surgical positioning may limit its clinical use. Additionally, TOF ratios at recovery should be put into the context of baseline values (normalization) when using AMG as this monitoring modality is associated with the reverse fade phenomenon in which baseline TOF ratios significantly exceed 1.0. For instance, if a patient has a baseline TOF ratio of 1.2 prior to NMBA administration, the patient should reach a normalized TOF ratio of 1.08 (1.2 X 0.9) prior to extubation in an effort to reduce the risk of complications from residual weakness. Nonetheless, multiple large-scale trials have demonstrated that the use of this quantitative monitor will decrease the incidence of postoperative paralysis as compared with the use of subjective assessment.

Kinemyographic (KMG) devices are based on the quantification of the degree of bending of a piezoelectric ceramic-wafer film sensor induced by muscle (thumb) contraction (◉ Fig. 8.11). When the sensor is bent and exposed to motion, it generates an electrical signal that is proportional to the magnitude of bending; the results are then analyzed. Commercially available devices are integrated into anesthesia workstations. However, the resulting measurements have been shown not to correlate with the MMG gold standard, limiting its clinical usefulness.

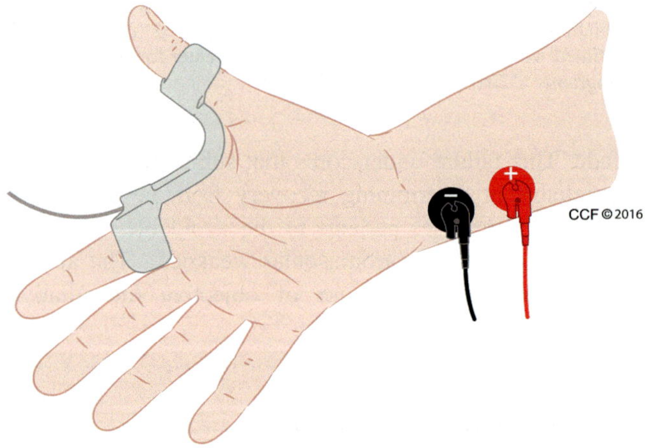

Fig. 8.11 Apparatus for objective monitoring of the adductor pollicis (*thumb*) muscle contraction using kinemyography. A mechanosensor (*metallic strip*) is placed in the groove between the thumb and index finger; ulnar nerve stimulation produces adductor pollicis muscle contraction that bends the strip, generating a current, which is proportional to the strength of muscle contraction. The results are displayed on the monitor's screen (Reprinted with permission, Cleveland Clinic Center for Medical Art & Photography ©2016. All Rights Reserved)

8.8.4 Clinical Considerations

The blockade produced by depolarizing and nondepolarizing NMBAs are distinct and can be distinguished by their response to peripheral nerve stimulation. Succinylcholine-induced (depolarizing) block is characterized by the absence

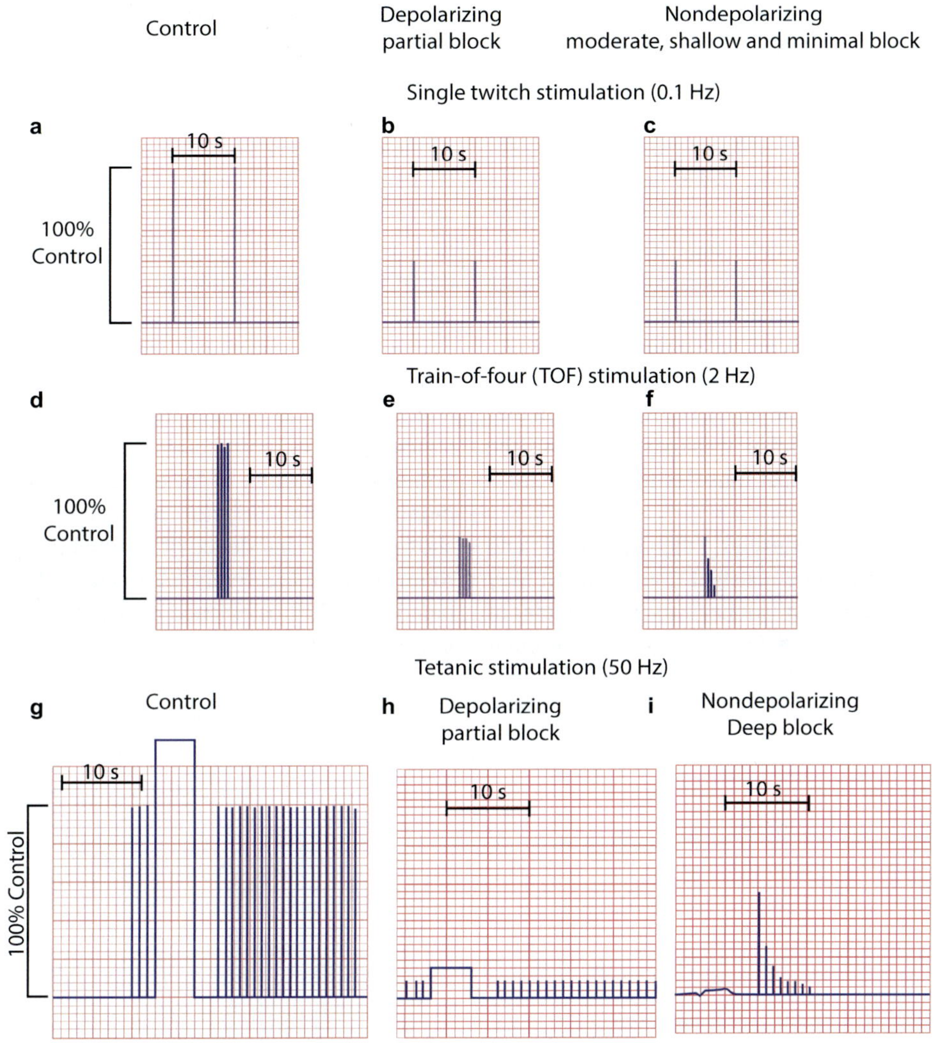

Fig. 8.12 Depiction of muscle contractions in response to single twitch (ST) stimuli delivered at a frequency of 0.1 Hz during normal conduction (Control, **a**); partial depolarizing block **b**; and moderate, shallow or minimal nondepolarizing block **c**. Note the lack of fade between the first ST and subsequent ST evoked responses during both depolarizing and nondepolarizing block when stimuli are delivered at this slow, 0.1 Hz frequency. **Train-of-four (TOF) stimulation.** Train-of-four (*TOF*) pattern in the absence of neuromuscular block (**d**, Control). The TOF ratio (TOFR) is calculated as the ratio between the fourth twitch of the TOF sequence (*T4*) and the first (*T1*). In the unblocked muscle, the TOF ratio is 1.0. During a partial depolarizing block **e**, there is minimal, if any, fade such that the TOF ratio remains close to 1.0. TOF fade is noted during moderate, shallow or minimal nondepolarizing block **f**. **Tetanic stimulation and post-tetanic count (PTC). g** In the unblocked muscle, the mechanical response to a 50 Hz tetanic stimulation is characterized by a sustained contraction with virtually no fade in tetanic response or post-tetanic potentiation of twitch response. During partial depolarizing block **h**, there is a reduction in the amplitude of tetanic stimulation but there is no tetanic fade or post-tetanic potentiation **i**. Application of tetanus during deep block resulted in a faint contraction for 5 s, and post-tetanic potentiation that results in 8 progressively weaker contractions (PTC = 8). Note that when measuring the PTC one always uses 1 Hz stimulation (Reprinted with permission, Cleveland Clinic Center for Medical Art & Photography ©2016. All Rights Reserved)

of both significant fade (to train-of-four or tetanic stimulation) and post-tetanic potentiation in response to nerve stimulation. The block produced by nondepolarizing NMBAs is characterized by fade after repeated stimulation as well as the ability to cause post-tetanic potentiation in which a 5-s tetanic stimulation produces an amplified subsequent response to stimulation. This tetanic stimulus mobilizes pre-junctional calcium, allows for the positive feedback on presynaptic acetylcholine receptors, and previously unavailable acetylcholine is manufactured and released into the synaptic cleft, producing a transiently exaggerated response. It should be noted that succinylcholine can produce fade or post-tetanic potentiation when used in large doses (>10 × ED_{95}), after prolonged exposure (>30 min), or in patients with butyrylcholinesterase deficiency (◉ Fig. 8.12).

Different muscle groups respond differently to the neuromuscular blocking effects of NMBAs. Vessel-rich, large, central muscle groups, such as the diaphragm, are initially more susceptible to NMBA effects than peripheral muscle groups, because the blood flow to these muscles is greater than to peripheral muscles. Thus, these central muscles become paralyzed before peripheral muscles following administration of NMBAs; however, they also recover faster. Understanding this relationship is essential to monitoring the level of neuromuscular blockade, regardless of which muscles are being monitored. Whether subjective or objective techniques are being used, monitoring the adductor pollicis muscle in response to ulnar nerve stimulation has been advocated to exclude residual weakness, because the adductor pollicis is one of the last muscles to recover from NMBA-induced paralysis.

Compared to peripheral muscles, the laryngeal and diaphragmatic muscles are more resistant (even though they may become partially blocked sooner) to the effects of neuromuscular blocking drugs (◉ Fig. 8.13). Neuromuscular blockade develops faster, it is less profound, lasts a shorter time, and recovers faster at the laryngeal and diaphragm muscles compared to the adductor pollicis muscle. The diaphragm and larynx have greater total blood flow than the adductor pollicis muscle, resulting in faster delivery of NMBA to these muscles. Conversely, washout of NMBA also occurs faster at the central muscles, so recovery occurs here before it does peripherally. Stimulation of the facial nerve will evoke contraction of the orbicularis oculi muscle (the eyelid) as well as the corrugator supercilii muscle (the eyebrow). The corrugator supercilii muscles have the same time course of paralysis and recovery as the laryngeal adductor muscles, while the orbicularis oculi muscles time course follows peripheral muscles such as the adductor pollicis. Monitoring of facial muscles is a poor substitute for monitoring the adductor pollicis muscle. A recent report showed a 52% incidence of residual paralysis in the recovery room using subjectively assessed eyebrow responses, compared with 22% incidence of residual paralysis during hand muscle monitoring.

	Muscle X	Adductor Pollicis
EC_{50} (μg/ml)	3.00	1.18
Keo	0.36	0.18
Hill coefficient	4.00	4.50

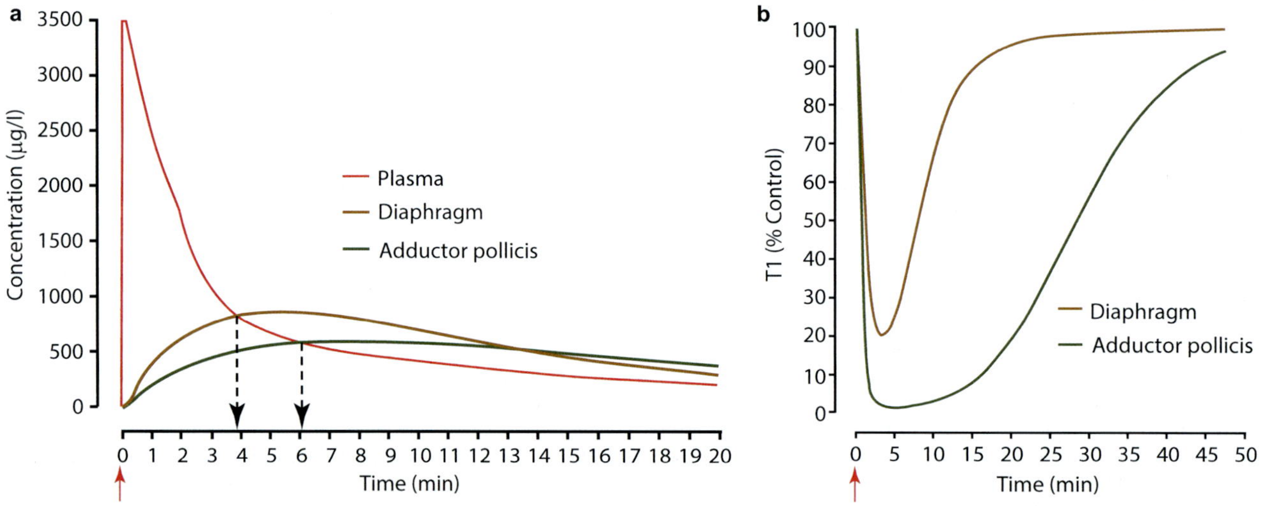

Fig. 8.13 Recovery characteristics of different muscles. Neuromuscular blockade develops faster, lasts a shorter time, and recovers faster at the laryngeal and diaphragmatic muscles than the adductor pollicis muscle although the laryngeal and diaphragmatic muscles are more resistant to neuromuscular blocking drugs. This figure depicts a computer simulation based on published models. Concentrations (*panel A*) and effect (*panel B*) over time for a 0.45 mg/kg rocuronium intravenous bolus. The ED_{95} of rocuronium at the adductor pollicis from this model is 0.33 mg/kg. Rocuronium 0.45 mg/kg is given as a bolus at time zero. Muscle X represents a muscle (such as the diaphragm, the laryngeal adductors, or corrugator supercilii muscle), which is less sensitive to the effects of nondepolarizing relaxants than the adductor pollicis muscle but has greater blood flow. *Panel A* presents the predicted rocuronium plasma and effect site concentrations at the adductor pollicis muscle and muscle X. Note that that concentration of rocuronium reaches higher levels at a faster rate in muscle X than in the adductor pollicis muscle. *Panel B* presents the predicted T1% as a percentage of control at muscle X and the adductor pollicis muscle. The EC_{50} represents the effect site concentration at which there is a 50% probability of effect. The k_{eo} represents the micro-rate constant for drug leaving the effect site compartment. The Hill coefficient represents the slope of the effect site concentration versus effect curve (not shown). In this example, the concentration of rocuronium producing 50% block (EC_{50}) of muscle X is 2.5 times that of the adductor pollicis muscle, but the half-life of transport between the plasma and effect compartment ($t_{½}k_{e0}$) of muscle X is only half as long. The rapid equilibration between plasma concentrations of rocuronium and muscle X results in the more rapid onset of blockade at muscle X than at the adductor pollicis muscle. The greater EC_{50} at muscle X explains the faster recovery of this muscle from neuromuscular block (faster rocuronium washout) than at the adductor pollicis muscle (Reproduced with permission from Naguib and Kopman)

8.9 Questions and Answers

Questions (Choose the most Appropriate Answer)

1. Atracurium is metabolized through mechanisms that are similar to all of the following **except**:
   A. Esmolol
   B. Chloroprocaine
   C. Remifentanil
   D. Oseltamivir
   E. Cisatracurium
2. Following a rapid sequence dose of rocuronium for a 100-kg patient, if you decide to reverse the block with sugammadex after 5 min, which of the following doses is appropriate:
   A. 100 mg
   B. 200 mg
   C. 400 mg
   D. 1600 mg
   E. 2000 mg
3. Which of the following clinical conditions can cause a prolonged response to nondepolarizing neuromuscular blockade:
   A. Propofol as the primary anesthetic
   B. Patient receiving chronic calcium channel blocker treatment for hypertension
   C. Patients with a contraction alkalosis from diuretic use
   D. A pregnant patient with eclamptic seizures being treated with intravenous magnesium
   E. All of the above can prolong the response to nondepolarizing neuromuscular blockade
4. Full recovery from neuromuscular blockade is defined as:
   A. A sustained 5-s head lift
   B. Presence of all 4 twitches elicited from a peripheral nerve stimulator with electrodes along the facial nerve
   C. Tidal volumes greater than 8 cc/kg on a spontaneous ventilation mode in an intubated patient
   D. A train-of-four (TOF) ratio greater than or equal to 0.9 as determined by a quantitative monitoring device of the adductor pollicis muscle
   E. All of the above represent definitive means of establishing complete reversal and recovery from neuromuscular blockade
5. Neostigmine-induced reversal of neuromuscular blockade can be delayed by which of the following conditions:
   A. Presence of a deep level of neuromuscular block
   B. Vecuronium block in elderly patients
   C. Patients whose primary anesthetic was sevoflurane
   D. Patients who received pancuronium
   E. All of the factors can prolong neostigmine reversal
6. Following a bolus dose of rocuronium, the order of muscle groups that will become paralyzed is:
   A. Diaphragm → orbicularis oculi
   B. Corrugator supercilii → laryngeal adductors
   C. Adductor pollicis → laryngeal adductors
   D. Flexor hallucis brevis → diaphragm
   E. Orbicularis oculi → corrugator supercilii
7. Upregulation of extrajunctional nicotinic receptors occurs in all of the following states **except:**
   A. After burns that cover more than 50% of total body surface area
   B. Within the first hours following a cervical neck fracture severing the spinal cord
   C. A septic shock patient who has been intubated, sedated, and receiving mechanical ventilation for 3 weeks
   D. An ICU patient with severe acute respiratory distress syndrome (ARDS) receiving a cisatracurium infusion for the past week
   E. A patient who experienced a stroke and subsequent hemiplegia several years ago
8. Succinylcholine administration is associated with:
   A. Rare instances of postoperative myalgias (<5%)
   B. Increasing intragastric pressure that significantly increases the risk of aspiration
   C. A transient decrease in intraocular pressure
   D. An exaggerated hyperkalemic response in patients with end stage renal disease
   E. The potential for triggering malignant hyperthermia
9. Mivacurium is metabolized through a mechanism similar to:
   A. Atracurium
   B. Succinylcholine
   C. Pancuronium
   D. Rocuronium
   E. Vecuronium
10. Sugammadex reversal is associated with which of the following:
    A. Rapid reversal of neuromuscular blockade from cisatracurium administration
    B. A clinically relevant increase in bleeding
    C. A cessation of the need to utilize quantitative monitors to determine the depth of neuromuscular blockade
    D. A disruption in the effectiveness of oral contraceptives
    E. Rapid reversal of succinylcholine-induced neuromuscular blockade

Answers

1. **B**. In addition to the Hofmann reaction, atracurium is metabolized by nonspecific plasma esterases, as is esmolol, remifentanil, and oseltamivir. Chloroprocaine is metabolized by butyrylcholinesterase.
2. **D**. The dose of sugammadex to reverse profound levels of neuromuscular blockade immediately after a rapid sequence dose of rocuronium is 16 mg/kg. This translates to a dose of 1600 mg in a 100 kg patient. Deep neuromuscular blockade with 1–2 post-tetanic twitches present can be reversed with a sugammadex dose of 4 mg/kg. Lighter levels of blockade, with at least 2 of 4 twitches present after a train-of-four stimulation can be reversed with sugammadex at a dose of 2 mg/kg.
3. **D**. The parturient receiving a magnesium infusion may have hypermagnesemia, a condition that prolongs the normal response to neuromuscular blockade by preventing the release of acetylcholine from the presynaptic junction. Inhalational anesthetics, rather than intravenous agents such as propofol, can also prolong neuromuscular blockade. While hypocalcemia prolongs neuromuscular blockade by similar mechanisms as hypercalcemia, patients on chronic calcium channel blockers do not have a clinically significant prolonged response to neuromuscular blockade. Acidosis, rather than alkalosis, also prolongs the response to neuromuscular blocking drugs.
4. **D**. The gold standard for determining recovery from neuromuscular blockade is a train-of-four ratio ≥ 0.9 as determined by monitoring the adductor pollicis muscle response via mechanomyography. Clinical tests such as assessing tidal volumes, negative inspiratory force, and sustained head lift do not reliably exclude residual paralysis. Furthermore, 4 of 4 twitches observed after train-of-four stimulation of the facial nerve can still be present despite up to ~30% of nicotinic receptors being blocked and such a response does not exclude residual paralysis.
5. **E**. Reversal with neostigmine is dependent on a number of variables and should not occur when patients have deep levels of neuromuscular blockade (e.g., when only post-tetanic twitches are present). The response can be prolonged in the elderly, in patients who received inhalational anesthetics, and following administration of long-acting NMBAs such as pancuronium.
6. **A**. Central muscles receive a higher proportion of blood flow and are more susceptible to the relaxant effects of NMBA than peripheral muscles. After administration of NMBA, the central muscles, such as the diaphragm and laryngeal adductors, are affected first. These muscles are also the first to recover. The response of corrugator supercilli muscle is similar to that of the laryngeal adductors while the orbicularis oculi mirrors the adductor pollicis muscle response.
7. **B**. Upregulation of extrajunctional nicotinic receptors occurs in a variety of settings, such as following major burns, in the intensive care unit after chronic debility from illnesses such as sepsis, after long-term NMB infusion, and in patients with history of stroke with resultant weakness. In the case of acute paralysis from recent (within hours) spinal cord transection, upregulation has not occurred yet.
8. **E**. The incidence of postoperative myalgias from succinylcholine is high (~50%). While administration of this agent is associated with increased intragastric pressure, the lower esophageal sphincter tone also increases, negating any potential increase in risk of aspiration. In fact, succinylcholine is commonly the drug of choice when aspiration is a concern given its reliably fast onset. While succinylcholine increases plasma potassium levels (~0.5 mEq), an exaggerated response is not noted in patients with end-stage renal disease. These patients commonly have preoperative hyperkalemia, but potassium levels increase similarly to that of the general population. Succinylcholine is a potent trigger for malignant hyperthermia, particularly when combined with inhalational anesthetics.
9. **B**. Mivacurium is metabolized through butyrylcholinesterase, just as succinylcholine (and chloroprocaine). Atracurium undergoes Hofmann reaction degradation and metabolism through plasma esterases. Pancuronium, rocuronium, and vecuronium are eliminated via the liver and kidney.
10. **D**. Sugammadex cannot reverse neuromuscular blockade from cisatracurium. It has been reported that within the first 60 min of sugammadex reversal, prothrombin time increases by 3% and activated partial thromboplastin time increases by 5.5%, but no increase in bleeding has been reported with use of sugammadex. The dose of sugammadex depends on the level of neuromuscular blockade and thus the need for quantitative monitoring to determine such. It does not reverse succinylcholine. Sugammadex binds oral contraceptives and is equivalent to missing 1 dose of such medications. Patients on these agents should be advised to utilize alternative forms of birth control up to 2 weeks afterward.

Acknowledgements The authors would like to acknowledge the late Mohammed Naguib for his contributions to the previous version of this chapter as well as his tremendous efforts to the overall body of literature on the topic. His work advanced our understanding of the neuromuscular junction, demonstrated the impact neuromuscular blocking drugs can have on patient safety, and developed techniques to reduce associated complications.

References

1. Apfelbaum JL, Hagberg CA, Caplan RA, Connis RT, Abdelmalak BB, Agarkar M, Dutton RP. American society of anesthesiologists practice guidelines for management of the difficult airway. Anesthesiology. 2022;136:31–81.
2. Naguib M, Flood P, McArdle JJ, Brenner HR. Advances in neurobiology of the neuromuscular junction: implications for the anesthesiologist. Anesthesiology. 2002;96:202–31.
3. Puhringer FK, Rex C, Sielenkamper AW, Claudius C, Larsen PB, Prins ME, et al. Reversal of profound, high-dose rocuronium induced neuromuscular blockade by sugammadex at two different time points: an international, multicenter, randomized, dose-finding, safety assessor-blinded, phase II trial. Anesthesiology. 2008;109:188–97.
4. Naguib M, Kopman AF. Low-dose rocuronium and tracheal intubation. Middle East J Anesthesiol. 2003;17:193–204.

Pharmacology of Local and Neuraxial Anesthetics

9

Sree Kolli and Adeeb Oweidat

Abstract

Local anesthetics are the pharmacologic cornerstone of regional anesthesia producing reversible and complete blockade of neuronal transmission when applied near the axons. Development of local anesthetics, since the 1950s, has focused on amide local anesthetics. Ester local anesthetics exhibit several limitations including instability when in solution, short shelf life, degradation when exposed to high temperatures, and an increased propensity to cause allergic reactions. Local anesthetics are widely used to prevent or treat acute pain; to treat inflammatory, cancer, and chronic pain; and for diagnostic and prognostic purposes. Nociceptive pain, as well as neuropathic pain, is targeted with this group of drugs. Any part of the nervous system, from the periphery to the brain, may be where local anesthetics act to produce a desired anesthetic or analgesic effect. This chapter describes the basic chemical structure of local anesthetics and gives an overview of pharmacologic properties of the different drugs. Clinical use, advantages, and side effects are compared, and local anesthetic toxicity is described.

Keywords

Local anesthetics • Pharmacokinetics • Metabolism • Pharmacodynamics properties • Individual local anesthetics • Side effects • Systemic toxicity of local anesthetics • Neuraxial LA

Key Points

1. Local anesthetics (LAs) cause reversible conduction blockade of nerve impulse transmission by inhibiting the sodium channels.
2. Local anesthetics bind to the interior portion of the sodium channel to inhibit and hence has to diffuse into the nerve membrane to block impulse conduction.
3. Local anesthetics are weak bases and pKa generally correlates with the speed of onset of action of most amide LA drugs; the closer the pKa to the body pH, the faster the onset.
4. Potency correlates with lipid solubility while duration of action is related to protein binding.
5. The rate of systemic absorption is proportionate to the vascularity of the site of injection: intravenous > tracheal > intercostal > caudal > paracervical > epidural > brachial plexus > sciatic > subcutaneous.
6. Ester local anesthetics are predominantly metabolized by pseudocholinesterase, while amide local anesthetics are metabolized by microsomal enzymes in the liver.
7. Addition of vasoconstrictors such as epinephrine can prolong the duration of action and limit toxic side effects of local anesthetics.
8. Systemic toxicity of local anesthetics is due to excess plasma concentration of the unbound drug that depends on the total dose, absorption, metabolism, and elimination.
9. Unintentional intravascular injection of bupivacaine can cause severe cardiotoxic reactions while with other local anesthetics central nervous system signs of toxicity usually precede cardiovascular manifestations.
10. ABC (Airway, Breathing, and Circulation) is the mainstay of treatment in local anesthetic toxicity. Lipid emulsion has been shown to significantly improve the outcomes.

S. Kolli (✉)
Department of MultiSpeciality Anesthesiology, Cleveland Clinic, Cleveland, OH, USA
e-mail: kollis@ccf.org

A. Oweidat
Department of Anesthesiology, University of Iowa, Iowa, USA

M. Argalious et al. (eds.), *Basic Sciences in Anesthesia*,
https://doi.org/10.1007/978-3-031-60203-0_9

9.1 Nerve Conduction

Local anesthetics (LAs) interrupt the nerve conduction by binding to specific receptor sites on the sodium (Na+) channels in nerves and block the movement of ions through these pores and cause reversible conduction blockade of impulses along central and peripheral nerve pathways. Both the chemical and pharmacologic properties of individual LA drugs determine their clinical properties.

Nerve conduction involves the propagation of an electrical signal generated by the rapid movement of small amounts of several ions (Na+ and potassium K+) across a nerve cell membrane. The ionic gradient for Na+ (high extracellularly and low intracellularly) and K+ (high intracellularly and low extracellularly) is maintained by a Na+-K + pump mechanism within the nerve.

The sodium channel "voltage-gated" protein structures consist of the large sodium-conducting pore (alpha-subunit) and varying numbers of adjacent smaller beta subunits. Those channels penetrate the full depth of the membrane bilayer and are in communication with both the extracellular surface and the axoplasm (interior) of the nerve.

The large polypeptide that forms the alpha-subunit is further divided into 4 subunits (DI-IV). The alpha-subunit that allows ion conduction and binds to local anesthetics is called the H subunit [1]. In the resting state, the nerve membrane is more permeable to K+ ions than to Na+ ions, resulting in the continuous leakage of K+ ions out of the interior of the nerve cell. This leakage of cations, in turn, creates a negatively charged interior relative to the exterior, resulting in an electric potential of 60–70 mV across the nerve membrane.

Sodium channels exist in activated-open, inactivated-closed, and rested-closed states during various phases of the action potential. When the threshold potential is achieved, an action potential results, with a sudden increase in the permeability of the nerve membrane to Na+ ions and a resultant rapid influx of positively charged Na+ ions leads to depolarization (◉ Fig. 9.1a, b). Repolarization takes place when sodium permeability decreases and K+ permeability increases, resulting in an efflux of K+ from within the cell and restoration of the electrical balance [4].

LAs prevent the generation and conduction of nerve impulses by selectively binding to the α(alpha) subunit of the Na+ channel in inactivated-closed states, stabilizing these channels in this configuration and preventing the influx of Na+ into the cell, halting the transmission of the advancing wave of depolarization down the length of the nerve, and preventing their change to the rested-closed and activated-open states in response to nerve impulses.

It is speculated that local anesthetics bind to specific sites located on the inner portion of sodium channels as well as obstructing sodium channels near their external openings. A resting nerve is less sensitive to an LA than a nerve that is repeatedly stimulated. A repeated depolarization and a more positive membrane potential increases the chance that an LA molecule will provide a greater degree of transmission block.

The minimum concentration of local anesthetic necessary to produce conduction blockade of nerve impulses is termed the Cm. Larger nerve fibers require higher concentrations of local anesthetic for production of conduction blockade. An increased tissue pH or high frequency of nerve stimulation decreases Cm.

9.2 Pharmacokinetics

The pKa (the pH at which 50% of the drug is ionized and 50% is present as base) of the LA is related to pH and the concentrations of the cationic and base forms.

Local anesthetics are weak bases; their pK values are slightly above physiologic pH. When injected into the human body, less than half of the LA exists in a lipid-soluble and nonionized form at physiologic pH.

Acidosis, if present due to tissue infection, increases the ionized fraction of drug. This is consistent with the poor quality of local anesthesia that often results when a local anesthetic is injected into an acidic infected area.

Local anesthetics with pKs nearest to physiologic pH have the most rapid onset of action, reflecting the presence of an optimal ratio of ionized to nonionized drug fraction. The pKa generally correlates with the speed of onset of action of most amide LA drugs; the closer the pKa to the body pH, the faster the onset. The coexistence of the 2 forms of the drug—the charged cation and the uncharged base—is important because drug penetration of the nerve membrane by the LA requires the base (un-ionized) form to pass through the nerve lipid membrane [5].

9.2.1 Chemical Structure

Local anesthetic molecules are comprised of 3 basic building blocks: a hydrophobic aromatic ring, a hydrophilic tertiary amine, and an intermediate chain connecting the two. The chemical connection between the intermediate chain and the aromatic ring divides local anesthetics into "esters" and "amides," depending on whether the hydrocarbon chain is joined to the benzene-derived moiety by an ester or an amide linkage (◉ Fig. 9.2). The type of linkage is important as it determines how local anesthetics are metabolized. Moreover, this chemical differentiation is clinically relevant because the amides are more stable and have less risk of allergic reaction than the esters.

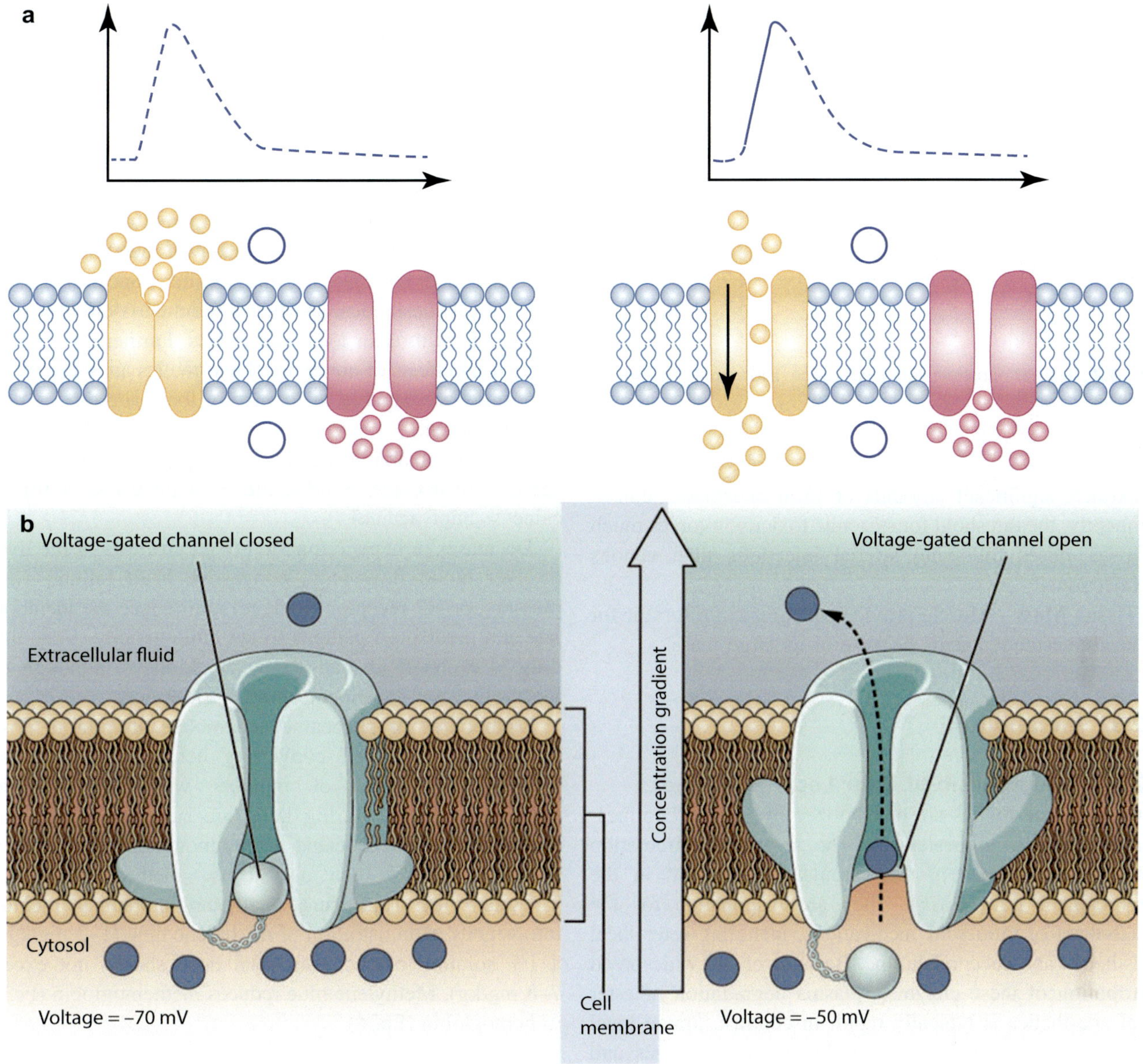

Fig. 9.1 **a**, **b** Sodium and potassium channel function and ion movements during nerve depolarization (**a** Reprinted with permission from Mulroy and Bernards [2]; **b** Reprinted under Creative Commons Attribution 4.0 International License from OpenStax [3]. Download for free at ► http://cnx.org/content/col11496/latest/)

9.2.2 Absorption and Distribution

The ultimate plasma concentration of a local anesthetic is determined by the rate of tissue distribution and the rate of clearance of the drug. Factors that affect the absorption and later redistribution are the following:

- **Lipid Solubility**—After distribution to highly perfused tissues, the local anesthetic is redistributed to less-well-perfused tissues, including skeletal muscles and fat. Ultimately, the local anesthetic is eliminated from the plasma by metabolism and excretion.
- **Tissue/Blood Partition Coefficient**—Strong plasma protein binding tends to retain anesthetic in the blood, whereas high lipid solubility facilitates tissue uptake.
- Patient-related factors are important such as age, cardiovascular status, and hepatic function. Protein binding parallels lipid solubility of the local anesthetic and is inversely related to the plasma concentration of drug.
- **Tissue Perfusion**—The highly perfused organs (brain, lung, liver, kidney, and heart) are responsible for the initial rapid uptake (α[alpha] phase), which is followed by a slower redistribution (β[beta] phase) to moderately perfused tissues (muscle and gut). In particular, the lung

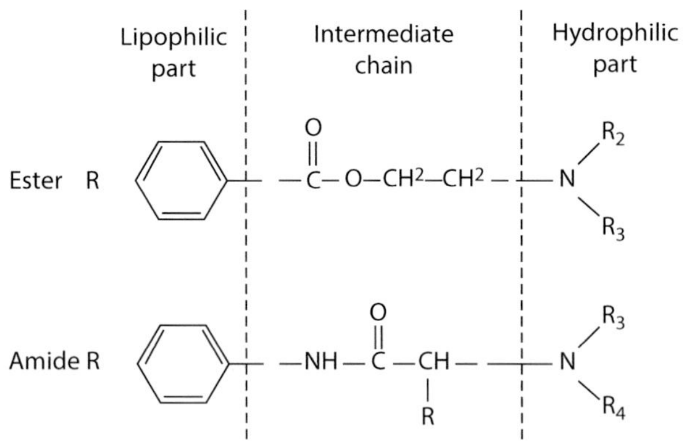

Fig. 9.2 Typical structure of local ester and amide anesthetic molecules

extracts significant amounts of local anesthetic; consequently, the threshold for systemic toxicity involves much lower doses following arterial injections than venous injections.

- **Tissue Mass**—Muscle provides the greatest reservoir for local anesthetic agents because of its large mass.

9.2.3 Metabolism

9.2.3.1 Metabolism of Ester Local Anesthetics

Ester local anesthetics are metabolized by plasma cholinesterases (pseudocholinesterase). The liver and circulation form these enzymes in the vascular system and in the cerebrospinal fluid (CSF). They are responsible for the metabolism of numerous medications, including ester local anesthetics and succinylcholine. Because of the widespread distribution of these enzymes, plasma degradation of ester local anesthetics is typically rapid. In contrast, amide local anesthetics undergo degradations by hepatic enzymes and typically have a longer serum half-life.

Ester hydrolysis is very rapid, and the water-soluble metabolites are excreted in the urine. Procaine and benzocaine are metabolized to p-aminobenzoic acid (PABA), which has been associated with allergic reactions.

Patients with genetically abnormal pseudocholinesterase are at increased risk for toxic side effects, as metabolism is slower. Cerebrospinal fluid lacks esterase enzymes, so the termination of action of intrathecally injected ester local anesthetics (e.g., tetracaine) depends on their absorption into the bloodstream. In contrast to other ester anesthetics, cocaine is partially metabolized (N-methylation and ester hydrolysis) in the liver and partially excreted unchanged in the urine.

9.2.3.2 Metabolism of Amide Local Anesthetics

Amide local anesthetics undergo varying rates of metabolism by microsomal enzymes located in the liver. The first step is conversion of the amide base to aminocarboxylic acid and a cyclic aniline derivative. Complete metabolism usually involves another steps, such as hydroxylation of the aniline moiety and N-dealkylation of the aminocarboxylic acid.

Prilocaine undergoes the most rapid metabolism; lidocaine and mepivacaine are intermediate; and etidocaine, bupivacaine, and ropivacaine undergo the slowest metabolism.

The metabolism of amide LA compared with that of ester is more complex and slower. This slower metabolism means that sustained increases of the plasma concentrations of amide local anesthetics, and thus systemic toxicity, are more likely than with ester local anesthetics. Furthermore, cumulative drug effects of amide local anesthetics are more likely. The lungs are capable of extracting local anesthetics from the circulation.

The rate of amide metabolism depends on the specific agent (prilocaine > lidocaine > mepivacaine > ropivacaine > bupivacaine).

Decreases in hepatic function (e.g., cirrhosis of the liver) or liver blood flow (e.g., congestive heart failure, vasopressors, or H2-receptor blockers) will reduce the metabolic rate and predispose patients to systemic toxicity. Very little drug is excreted unchanged by the kidneys, although the metabolites are dependent on renal clearance.

Metabolites of prilocaine accumulate after large doses of drug (>10 mg/kg), converting hemoglobin to methemoglobin. Neonates of mothers who have received prilocaine epidural during labor are susceptible to methemoglobinemia. Benzocaine, a common ingredient in local anesthetic sprays, can also cause methemoglobinemia. Treatment of significant methemoglobinemia includes intravenous administration of methylene blue (1–2 mg/kg of a 1% solution over 5 min; total dose should not exceed 7–8 mg/kg). Methylene blue reduces methemoglobin (Fe^{3+}) to hemoglobin (Fe^{2+}).

9.2.4 Site of Injection

The rate of systemic absorption is proportionate to the vascularity of the site of injection: intravenous > tracheal > intercostal > caudal > paracervical > epidural > brachial plexus > sciatic > subcutaneous.

9.2.5 Presence of Vasoconstrictors

The addition of epinephrine—or less commonly phenylephrine—causes vasoconstriction at the site of administration. The consequent decreased absorption increases neuronal uptake, enhances the quality of analgesia, prolongs the duration of action, and limits toxic side effects. The effects of vasoconstrictors are more pronounced with shorter-acting agents. For example, the addition of epinephrine to lidocaine usually extends the duration of anesthesia by at least 50%, but epinephrine has little or no significant effect when added to bupivacaine, whose long duration of action is due to a high degree of protein binding. Epinephrine can also augment and prolong analgesia through activation of α(alpha) 2-adrenergic receptors.

9.2.6 Placental Transfer

Plasma protein binding influences the rate and degree of diffusion of local anesthetics across the placenta. Bupivacaine, which is highly protein bound, has an umbilical vein–maternal arterial concentration ratio of about 0.32.

Ester local anesthetics are not available to cross the placenta significantly because of their rapid hydrolysis. Fetal acidosis can result in accumulation of local anesthetic in the fetus (ion trapping). While fetuses have less protein, the plasma concentration of drugs is nearly equal to that of their mothers. Fetal pH is slightly lower than maternal (7.32–7.38), thus most un-ionized drugs are "ion trapped" to a degree, even in a healthy fetus. In the presence of fetal acidosis, local anesthetics cross the placenta and become ionized in higher proportion than at normal pH.

Chloroprocaine has the least placental transfer because it is rapidly broken down by plasma cholinesterase in the maternal circulation.

9.2.7 Pharmacodynamic Properties

- **Potency** is the minimal concentration required to produce neural blockade. Lipophilicity correlates with potency.
- **Phasic (Rate-Dependent) Block –** The faster a nerve is stimulated, the lower the concentration of local anesthetic is needed to produce a blockade.
- **Nerve/Axon Exposed –** Myelinated axons: Myelin consists of Schwann cell plasma membranes wrapped around axons. There are gaps, called nodes of Ranvier; myelination results in much faster conduction velocities. Local anesthetics can gain access only at the nodes of Ranvier.
- Unmyelinated axons: The concentration of local anesthetic required to block conduction of unmyelinated axons decreases with increasing length of nerve exposed to the local anesthetic. Unmyelinated axons (C fibers) are in vitro the most resistant to local anesthetic blockade, followed by large (A fibers) and small (B fibers) myelinated axons. Intermediate-size myelinated axons (A d, A g fibers) are the easiest axons to block in vitro.
- **PKa** is the pH, where half of the drug is ionized (positively charged) and half is nonionized (base). The nonionized form penetrates the nerve membrane, while the ionized form binds to proteins on the intracellular side of the sodium channel.
- The percentage of each form present in a solution or in the tissue depends on the pH of the solution or tissue. Local anesthetics are weak bases (pKa = 7.6–9.0) that are commercially prepared as an acidic solution, typically at pH 4–5.
- **Hydrophobicity** correlates with potency and to the duration of action. The more hydrophobic the drug, the more potent it is. Hydrophobicity is determined by adding local anesthetic to a recipient containing 2 immiscible liquids, such as aqueous buffer and a hydrophobic lipid. The resultant ratio of the concentrations is called the "distribution (partition coefficient)." The charged form is more hydrophilic than the uncharged form. Hydrophobicity facilitates penetration of the neuronal cell membrane.
- **Protein Binding –** Duration of action correlates with the degree of protein binding (typically to albumin and alpha-1-acid-gylcoprotein). In general, more hydrophobic drugs have higher protein binding.

Short-acting local anesthetics have a fast onset of action, while long-duration local anesthetics have a slower onset. Only the free (protein unbound) local anesthetic fraction can induce toxicity. When serum proteins are saturated, any additional local anesthetics causes toxicity (patients show rapid progression to toxicity). Binding to plasma proteins is pH-dependent; binding decreases during acidosis due to the decrease of available binding sites.

9.3 Individual Local Anesthetics

The following is a summary of common local anesthetics used in clinical practice and their applications (◉ Table 9.1).

9.3.1 Ester Local Anesthetics

9.3.1.1 Cocaine

The clinically desired action of cocaine is local vasoconstriction due to inhibition of norepinephrine reuptake. However, its toxicity and the potential for abuse have precluded its clinical use. Topical mucous membrane applications of cocaine (4% solution) result in rapid anesthesia and vasoconstriction. At excessive doses, vasoconstrictive properties lead to hypertension, coronary ischemia, and arrhythmias.

Cocaine is metabolized in the liver to active metabolites. The half-life is 45 min. The maximum recommended dose of cocaine is 200 mg.

Table 9.1 Properties of local anesthetics

Anesthetic	Lipid solubility	Protein binding (%)	pKa (Unionized fraction pH 7.4) (%)	Molecular weight	Potency	Speed of onset	Duration of action	UV/MV ratio
Chloroprocaine	0.14	~ 0	8.7 (5)	271	Low	Very rapid	Short	~ 0
Procaine	0.02	6	8.9 (3)	236	Low	Rapid	Short	N/A
Lidocaine	2.9	64	7.7 (35)	234	Medium	Rapid	Medium	0.5–0.7
Mepivacaine	0.8	78	7.6 (39)	246	Medium	Medium	Medium	0.7–0.8
Bupivacaine	8.2	96	8.1 (15)	288	High	Slow	Long	0.2–0.4
Ropivacaine	8.0	92–94	8.1 (15)	274	High	Slow	Long	0.2

Reprinted with permission from Datta et al. [6]

Lipid solubility Heptanol or octanol/buffer partition ratio, *UV/MV ratio* ratio of concentration in umbilical vein to maternal vein, total concentration, not free drug concentration, is shown in the table, *N/A* not available

9.3.1.2 Procaine

Procaine is characterized by low potency, slow onset, and short duration of action. Its use now is confined to infiltration anesthesia (0.25–1.0%) and short-duration (30–45 min) spinal anesthesia (50–100 mg). Procaine is ineffective when used topically and for epidural anesthesia. It is not recommended for peripheral block since it has a very slow onset time paired with a short-acting time. Procaine is metabolized in the plasma by the cholinesterase; its elimination half-life is approximately 8 min.

9.3.1.3 2-Chloroprocaine

It is the most rapidly metabolized LA. The principal uses are in obstetrics and ambulatory anesthesia. It is frequently chosen for urgent forceps or cesarean deliveries for epidural anesthesia. In the 2–3% concentrations, chloroprocaine is rapidly metabolized by plasma cholinesterase, and with duration of action between 30 and 60 min, it is a good drug for outpatient procedures. Since serum half-life is approximately 40 s, fetal accumulation and systemic toxicity are unlikely. The preservative-free solution should be used for central neuraxial blocks because of the concern of neurotoxicity. Chloroprocaine has been previously associated with muscle spasms, but it is believed to be due to calcium chelation by the preservative EDTA. The current preparations are preservative-free.

9.3.1.4 Tetracaine

Tetracaine is the longest-acting ester local anesthetic. It is more potent and has a longer duration of action than procaine or 2-chloroprocaine. Tetracaine is more slowly metabolized and it is more toxic. Currently, it is used in spinal anesthesia when a drug of long duration is needed, as well as in various topical anesthetic preparations. It is used rarely for peripheral nerve blocks. It is less chemically stable compared to lidocaine and bupivacaine. This instability may result in an occasional failed spinal anesthetic due to degradation of the local anesthetic during storage.

9.3.1.5 Benzocaine

Benzocaine has a low pKa (3.5), it only exists in the uncharged form at physiological pH, and it is hardly soluble in aqueous solutions. Therefore, it is exclusively used as a topical spray. Methemoglobinemia is observed more frequently when benzocaine is used.

9.3.2 Amide Local Anesthetics

9.3.2.1 Lidocaine

Lidocaine is the most widely used local anesthetic. It combines significant potency, fast onset, intermediate duration, good tissue penetration, and minimal cardiac toxicity.

Lidocaine is widely used for infiltration (1–2%), intravenous regional anesthesia (0.5%), peripheral nerve blocks (1 and 1.5%), topical airway (4%), spinal anesthesia (0.2–5%), and epidural anesthesia (2%). It produces moderate vasodilation. The allergic potency is very low. Lidocaine 5% has been implicated in the occurrence of cauda equina syndrome with the use of small-diameter microcatheters for continuous spinal anesthesia. Single-shot spinal anesthesia can be associated with transient neurologic syndrome (TNS), the etiology of which is uncertain. Hepatic disease or decreases in hepatic blood flow, which may occur during anesthesia, can decrease the rate of metabolism of lidocaine. Maternal clearance of lidocaine is prolonged in the presence of pregnancy-induced hypertension, and repeated administration of lidocaine can result in higher plasma concentrations than in normotensive parturients.

9.3.2.2 Mepivacaine

Mepivacaine offers slightly longer duration and better tissue penetration than lidocaine. Chemically, it is a cyclic tertiary amine like bupivacaine. It is used primarily for intermediate-duration blocks. It has a mild vasoconstricting effect. Mepivacaine is not used anymore in obstetric epidural anesthesia since it is poorly metabolized in the fetus.

9.3.2.3 Prilocaine

Prilocaine was withdrawn from use in the USA following cases of methemoglobinemia. Prilocaine is metabolized to nitro- and orthotoluidine, which can oxidize hemoglobin to methemoglobin. It is used commercially in topical eutectic mixture of local anesthetics (EMLA) cream, as well as in proprietary mixtures of local anesthetics specifically for airway anesthesia.

9.3.2.4 Etidocaine

Etidocaine is a derivate of lidocaine, more hydrophilic, and rarely used in practice. Its onset is similar to lidocaine, but its high protein binding is similar to bupivacaine, as are its duration of action and cardiac toxicity.

9.3.2.5 Bupivacaine

The first long-acting amide local anesthetic, bupivacaine, is more hydrophobic than mepivacaine and lidocaine, and highly protein bound, which is consistent with long duration and potential for cardiotoxicity. Bupivacaine is used in an array of applications, including infiltration (0.25%), peripheral nerve blocks (0.375–0.5%), spinal (0.5 and 0.75%), and epidural (0.5 and 0.75%) anesthesia. Because of systemic toxicity, it is not used for intravenous (IV) regional anesthesia. Bupivacaine is more slowly absorbed into plasma than lidocaine and produces plasma peak concentrations that are approximately 40% lower.

9.3.2.6 Levobupivacaine

Levobupivacaine is the levorotatory enantiomer of bupivacaine. It is approximately 35% less cardiotoxic compared to racemic bupivacaine. Levobupivacaine is used in the same concentrations, doses, and applications as racemic bupivacaine.

9.3.2.7 Ropivacaine

Because only a very small fraction of ropivacaine is excreted unchanged in the urine (about 1%) when the liver is functioning normally, dosage adjustments based on renal function do not seem necessary. Overall, clearance of ropivacaine is higher than that determined for bupivacaine, and its elimination half-time is shorter. The higher clearance of ropivacaine may offer an advantage over bupivacaine in terms of systemic toxicity. The lipid solubility of ropivacaine is intermediate between lidocaine and bupivacaine.

Ropivacaine was specifically designed to minimize cardiotoxicity. At higher concentration, its potency is equivalent to that of bupivacaine. At lower concentration, ropivacaine was shown to be 40% less potent than bupivacaine. Ropivacaine appears to be approximately 40% less cardiotoxic as compared to bupivacaine. Ropivacaine produces vasoconstriction, so there is little advantage of adding epinephrine to prolong the block.

9.3.2.8 Dibucaine

Dibucaine is metabolized in the liver and is the most slowly eliminated of all the amide derivatives. It inhibits pseudocholinesterase and is used to detect genetically abnormal enzyme.

9.3.2.9 Liposome-Based Local Anesthetic Carriers

Liposomes are microscopic spheres containing an aqueous core and surrounded by bilayer phospholipid vesicles that allows it to encapsulate different compounds such as LAs. The polar core of the liposphere allows lipophilic molecules to become encapsulated [7]. It can trap drugs in the aqueous or lipid form and that enables it to carry both hydrophilic and hydrophobic drugs. The benefit of encapsulating LA in liposomes is controlled delivery by slow drug release to prolong duration of action. They are non-toxic and biodegradable [8]. The most commonly used liposome-based local anesthetic carrier in clinical practice is liposomal bupivacaine. It is FDA-approved for use as surgical site infiltration, thoracoabdominal plane blocks, and interscalene block. Liposomal bupivacaine reliably produced plasma levels of bupivacaine up to 72 hours after infiltration [9]. Clinical duration of action lasts around 24 hours [10].

Liposomal bupivacaine is packaged in a 10ml or 20ml vial at 1.3% concentration. It is recommended not to use more than 266mg (one vial). Approximately 3% of the LA in liposomal bupivacaine is present in the free form. It has two peaks in plasma concentration following tissue infiltration. The first Tmax occurs within the first hour, followed by a second Tmax within 12 hours (See Fig. 9.3) [11, 12].

9.3.3 Additives

- **Sodium bicarbonate** can be added to local anesthetic solutions to raise the pH, thereby increasing the nonionized form, enabling it to penetrate the nerve membranes more readily. Thus, the speed of onset is increased. It also prolongs the duration and intensity of the block. Bicarbonate reduces the pain of injection (injection pain is associated with a low pH and cold solution). The recommended dose is 1 ml of 8.4% sodium bicarbonate per 10 ml of local anesthetic. There is little advantage in adding it to bupivacaine or ropivacaine. The practice of mixing sodium bicarbonate with local anesthetics is rarely used.
- **Epinephrine** causes vasoconstriction. This reduces the local anesthetic absorption and results in prolonging the block duration and reducing toxicity. These effects vary significantly among different types of LAs and individual nerve blocks. For example, because lidocaine is a natural vasodilator, the effect is pronounced for those blocks compared with blocks using ropivacaine, which has its

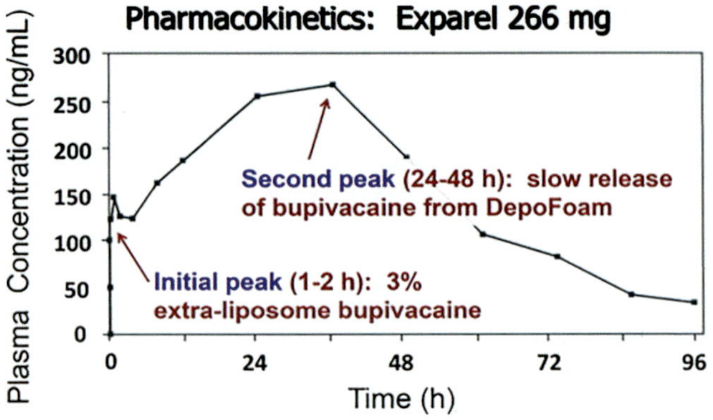

Fig. 9.3 Pharmacokinetics of a single 266-mg dose of Exparel infiltrated directly into tissue

own slight vasoconstricting effect. Epinephrine does not significantly prolong the duration of bupivacaine or ropivacaine but it does slow the absorption of these agents and thus reduces peak plasma levels. This reduces the toxicity risk of these 2 local anesthetics. Epinephrine also serves as a marker of intravenous injection of local anesthetic [13].

- **Clonidine** is a centrally acting selective partial alpha-2 adrenoreceptors agonist. Clonidine has widespread effects on the nervous system. It acts on the brain to cause sedation and has analgesic effects on the central and peripheral nervous systems. It prolongs and intensifies blocks when added to local anesthetics. Preservative-free clonidine, administered into the epidural or subarachnoid space (150–450 μ[mu]g), produces dose-dependent analgesia and, unlike opioids, does not produce depression of ventilation, pruritus, nausea, or vomiting. Adding clonidine 75–100 micrograms can extend the duration of peripheral blocks by 50–100%. Side effects—notably sedation, orthostatic hypotension, and fainting—should be considered when using clonidine. The latter 2 effects, in particular, can interfere with mobilization postoperatively.
- **Hyaluronidase** is used to break down connective tissue in the extracellular matrix, thereby increasing drug dispersion through tissue. It is used in peribulbar block (sub-Tenon's block).
- **Opioids**—The injection of opioids into the epidural or subarachnoid space to manage acute or chronic pain is based on the knowledge that opioid receptors are present in the substantia gelatinosa of the spinal cord. When added to short-duration local anesthetics used for spinal anesthesia, short-acting opioids (fentanyl and sufentanil) prolong and intensify sensory block without prolonging motor block. However, post-anesthesia nausea and vomiting (PONV), and itching can be a problem. When added to intrathecal local anesthetics, the peak plasma concentrations for sufentanil occur between 20 and 30 min and are greater than what is necessary for postoperative analgesia. This explains the many reports of "early" respiratory depression in mothers and fetal heart rate abnormalities in infants when sufentanil is added to intrathecal local anesthetics for labor analgesia or cesarean delivery. However, in peripheral nerves, similar receptors are absent or the effects of opiates are negligibly weak. For this reason, opiates do not have a significant clinical role in peripheral nerve blockade.

9.4 Combinations of Local Anesthetics

LAs can be combined to produce a rapid onset (chloroprocaine) and prolonged duration (bupivacaine) of action. Clinical trials have yielded mixed results. Clinically there are few advantages to this technique. Nevertheless, placement of chloroprocaine in the epidural space may decrease the efficacy of subsequent epidural bupivacaine-induced analgesia during labor. It is speculated that the low pH of the chloroprocaine solution could decrease the nonionized pharmacologically active fraction of bupivacaine. Tachyphylaxis to the local anesthetic mixture could also reflect local acidosis due to the low pH of the bathing solution. For these reasons, adjustment of the pH of the chloroprocaine solution with the addition of 1 mL of 8.4% sodium bicarbonate added to 30 mL of chloroprocaine solution just before placement into the epidural space may improve the efficacy of the chloroprocaine–bupivacaine combination. It should be noted that when mixing local anesthetics, the risk of toxicity remains. LA toxicity of combinations of drugs is additive rather than synergistic.

Evidence for and against adding short and long-acting LA's for onset time:

An ideal LA for a peripheral nerve block should have rapid onset of action, with a long duration, and have low side effects. Since there are still no ideal agents, we try to achieve an ideal mixture by compounding different local anesthetics.

Substantial controversy exists regarding pros and cons of various mixtures of LA, and there is little evidence to guide clinical practice. Most studies show conflicting results.

Before the use of US, one RCT compared bupivacaine 0.5% alone with mixture of chloroprocaine 3% and bupivacaine 0.5% for axillary brachial plexus blocks. There was 50% decrease in onset time with addition of chloroprocaine [14].

In 2009, a double-blinded RCT involving equal volume mixtures of bupivacaine 0.5% or ropivacaine 0.75% with lidocaine 2% versus long-acting agents alone for both femoral and sciatic nerve blocks in patients undergoing lower-extremity surgery reported significantly shorter latency by 33% to 50% with mixtures containing lidocaine. Another study by Lawal & Adetunji looked at the effects of mixing lidocaine and bupivacaine for spinal anesthesia in cats. The onset time was no faster when adding lidocaine to bupivacaine compared with lidocaine alone or bupivacaine alone. So mixing lidocaine did not achieve the goal of improving onset time. Further, the duration in the lidocaine/bupivacaine mixture was shorter than in the bupivacaine group alone. So mixing lidocaine with bupivacaine actually resulted in a shorter duration than bupivacaine alone [15].

However, in 2011, another RCT study for US-guided interscalene block, a combination of mepivacaine 1.5% and bupivacaine 0.5% results in a block onset similar to either local anesthetic alone but with significantly shorter duration of action than the block with bupivacaine 0.5% alone [16]. However, the volume used was 30 ml which could account for the lack of difference in onset time.

In 2013, a study comparing saline, lidocaine, lidocaine/bupivacaine, and bupivacaine blocks for the metacarpi of rams and then did sensory testing. Duration in the lidocaine/bupivacaine group was shorter than the bupivacaine group, and the time to onset was not different.

A study comparing lidocaine, lidocaine/bupivacaine, low-dose bupivacaine, and high-dose bupivacaine. The onset time was no better for lidocaine or lidocaine/bupivacaine compared with high-dose bupivacaine, and the duration was longer in the high-dose bupivacaine group. Another group compared 40 mL of bupivacaine 0.5% and 40 mL of mepivacaine 1.5% with a same volume combination of each LA for US infraclavicular block. The onset time was equivalent for the mepivacaine and mixed group and longer for the bupivacaine group [17].

9.5 Side Effects

9.5.1 Allergic Reactions

True allergy (type I or IgE mediated) to local anesthetics is rare, estimated at less than 1% of all adverse reactions to local anesthetics.

Ester LAs produce metabolites related to para-aminobenzoic acid (PABA) that are more likely than amide local anesthetics to evoke an allergic reaction. Allergy to amide local anesthetics is exceedingly rare. An allergic reaction after the use of a local anesthetic may be due to methylparaben (in multidose vials), which can elicit allergy in patients allergic to PABA or similar substances used as preservatives in commercial preparations of ester and amide local anesthetics. These preservatives are structurally similar to para-aminobenzoic acid. PABA is frequently used in the pharmaceutical and cosmetic industries. As a result, an allergic reaction may reflect prior stimulation of antibody production by the preservative and not a reaction to the local anesthetic.

Hypotension associated with syncope or tachycardia when an epinephrine-containing local anesthetic solution is administered suggests an accidental intravascular injection of drug. Use of an intradermal test requires injection of preservative-free preparations of local anesthetic solutions to eliminate the possibility that the allergic reaction was caused by the preservative. There is no cross-allergy between esters and amides.

9.5.2 Chondrolysis After Intrarticular Continuous Infusion of Local Anesthetics

The US Food and Drug Administration (FDA) issued a warning about the use of continuous intra-articular infusion of local anesthetics. Chondrolysis was diagnosed a median of 8.5 months after the infusion and in 97% of the cases involved the shoulder joint. The local anesthetics bupivacaine, chloroprocaine, lidocaine, mepivacaine, procaine, ropivacaine with or without epinephrine were used for 48–72 h.

9.5.3 Systemic Toxicity of Local Anesthetics

Systemic toxicity of a local anesthetic is due to an excess plasma concentration of the drug. Accidental direct intravascular injection of local anesthetic solutions during performance of peripheral nerve block anesthesia or epidural anesthesia is the most common mechanism for production of excess plasma concentrations of local anesthetics.

Systemic toxicity in association is estimated to result in seizures in 1–4 per 1,000 patient exposures to local anesthetics, with bupivacaine being the drug most likely to be associated with this adverse response.

The capacity of a local anesthetic to produce systemic toxicity is directly related to the plasma level of unbound drug, which depends on:

1. Total dose
2. Absorption
3. Metabolism and elimination.

Central nervous system (CNS) signs of toxicity usually precede cardiovascular (CV) manifestations.

The absorption of local anesthetics from different sites is from highest to lowest: endotracheal > intercostal > caudal > epidural > plexus blocks > sciatic/femoral > subcutaneous infiltration.

Peak blood levels may also be affected by the rate of biotransformation and elimination, for the actively metabolized drugs such as 2-chloroprocaine, which has a plasma half-life of about 45–60 s. For amide local anesthetics, such as lidocaine, peak plasma levels after regional anesthesia primarily result from absorption and usually occur within 1 h.

9.5.4 Central Nervous System Toxicity

Toxic plasma levels are usually produced by inadvertent intravascular injection. Symptoms tend to be biphasic with initial excitatory symptoms followed by depression. These symptoms may include numbness of the tongue, light-headedness, tinnitus, restlessness, tachycardia, and convulsions followed then by unconsciousness, respiratory arrest, and cardiac manifestations. The initial manifestations of CNS excitation culminating in seizures are the result of local anesthetic inhibitory effect on gamma-aminobutyric acid(GABA)-related pathways, which is followed by effects both on GABA and N-methyl-D-aspartate (NMDA) receptors leading to an overall depression of the CNS.

The onset of seizures may reflect selective depression of inhibitory cortical neurons by local anesthetics, leaving excitatory pathways unopposed. Plasma concentrations of local anesthetics producing signs of central nervous system toxicity depend on the specific drug involved.

Lidocaine, mepivacaine, and prilocaine demonstrate effects on the CNS at plasma concentrations of 5–10 μ(mu) g/mL. The typical plasma concentration of bupivacaine associated with seizures is 4.5–5.5 μ(mu)g/mL. The threshold plasma concentration at which CNS toxicity occurs may be related more to the rate of increase of the serum concentration than to the total amount of drug injected. There is an inverse relationship between the PaCO2 and seizure thresholds of local anesthetics. Increases in the serum potassium concentration can facilitate depolarization and thus markedly increase local anesthetic toxicity. Conversely, hypokalemia, by creating hyperpolarization, can greatly decrease local anesthetic toxicity.

9.5.5 Cardiovascular System Toxicity

Cardiovascular (CV) system toxicity usually follows the CNS effect with the exception of bupivacaine, which can produce cardiac toxicity at subconvulsant concentrations. The incidence of CV toxicity with local anesthetics is higher in pregnancy due to higher proportion of unbound fraction, increased under conditions of hypoxia and acidosis. The hypotension reflects both decreased systemic vascular resistance and cardiac output. Part of the cardiac toxicity that results from high plasma concentrations of local anesthetics occurs because these drugs block cardiac sodium channels. Excessive plasma concentrations of lidocaine slow conduction of cardiac impulses through the heart, manifesting as prolongation of the P-R interval and QRS complex and reentry ventricular cardiac dysrhythmias on the electrocardiogram (ECG).

For a patient using propranolol, CVS toxicity occurred at plasma bupivacaine concentrations of 2–3 μ(mu)g/ml. Propranolol reduces the hepatic blood flow and thus the clearance of bupivacaine, which can lead to toxic concentrations of bupivacaine. This suggests that caution must be taken in the use of bupivacaine in patients who are on antidysrhythmic drugs or other cardiac medications known to depress impulse propagation. Epinephrine and phenylephrine may increase bupivacaine cardiotoxicity. The cardiac toxicity of bupivacaine in animals is enhanced by arterial hypoxemia, acidosis, or hypercarbia.

Both bupivacaine and lidocaine block cardiac sodium ion channels during systole, whereas during diastole, highly lipid-soluble bupivacaine dissociates off these channels at a slow rate compared with lidocaine. The R enantiomer of bupivacaine is more toxic than the S enantiomer. In animals, levobupivacaine compared with bupivacaine was associated with a lower incidence of ventricular cardiac dysrhythmias, and successful resuscitation. Ropivacaine is a pure S enantiomer that is less lipid soluble and less cardiotoxic than bupivacaine but more cardiotoxic than lidocaine. Tachycardia can enhance frequency-dependent blockade of cardiac sodium channels by bupivacaine.

9.5.6 Maximum Dose

The recommended maximum recommended doses (◉Table 9.2) are extrapolated from animal data and do not necessarily apply to the clinical practice. The peak plasma levels do not correlate with patient size or body weight in adults. Experts argue that the safe doses should be block specific and related to patient's age (e.g., higher epidural spread in the elderly), organ dysfunction (especially for repeated doses), and whether the patient is pregnant (◉ Table 9.3).

Table 9.2 Suggested maximum doses of local anesthetics

Drug (per 70 kg patient)	Concentration (%)	Volume (cc)	Suggested maximum dose (mg)
Lidocaine	1–2	30–50	500
Mepivacaine	1–1.5	30–50	500
Prilocaine	1–2	30–50	600
Bupivacaine	0.25–0.5	30–50	225
Levobupivacaine	0.25–0.5	30–50	225
Ropivacaine	0.2–0.5	30–50	250

Reprinted with permission from Patel and Sadoughi [18]

Table 9.3 Recommended concentrations of anesthetics for pregnant patients

Drug (per 70 kg patient)	Concentration (%)	Volume (cc)
Procaine	10.0	1–2
Lidocaine	1.5, 5.0	1–2
Mepivacaine	4	1–2
Tetracaine	0.25–1.0	1–4
	0.25	2–6
	1.0	1–2
Bupivacaine	0.5	3–4
	0.75	2–3
Levobupivacaine	0.5	3–4
	0.75	2–3
Ropivacaine	0.5	3–4
	0.75	2–3

Reprinted with permission from Patel and Sadoughi [8]

9.5.7 Prevention of Local Anesthetic Systemic Toxicity

As recognized in the American Society of Regional Anesthesia and Pain Medicine (ASRA) 2010 guidelines:

- Use the lowest clinically effective dose of local anesthetic.
- Inject the local anesthetic incrementally in volumes of 3–5 mL, pausing for 15–30 s.
- Aspirate before injection.
- Use epinephrine as an intravascular marker.

9.5.8 Treatment of Local Anesthetic Systemic Toxicity

When local anesthetic-induced seizures occur, hypoxia, hypercarbia, and acidosis develop rapidly. ABC (Airway, Breathing, and Circulation) is the mainstay of treatment.

If seizures interfere with ventilation, benzodiazepines, small-dose propofol or thiopental can be used. The use of succinylcholine effectively facilitates ventilation and, by abolishing muscular activity, decreases the severity of acidosis. However, neuronal seizure activity is not inhibited, and therefore, cerebral metabolism and oxygen requirements remain increased. The 2010 ASRA guidelines for local anesthetic systemic toxicity (LAST) treatment specifically recommends avoiding vasopressin, based on an animal study. Amiodarone should be favored over lidocaine to treat arrhythmias.

9.5.9 Lipid Emulsion

The most likely mechanism of action of lipid emulsion, according to Groban and Butterworth (2003), is that "the lipid is serving to more rapidly remove LA molecules from whatever binding site serves to produce the cardiovascular depression" [19]. It is recommended to store lipid emulsion in all sites where local anesthetics are used.

Propofol has the same vehicle as Intralipid® or other lipid emulsion solutions, but only half the concentration (10%). Using propofol to treat local anesthetic toxicity will not provide enough lipids, and its active ingredient will produce cardiac depression. Therefore, propofol is not indicated to treat local anesthetic-induced cardiac toxicity.

The administration of local anesthetics should be stopped immediately. Prompt and effective airway management can prevent hypoxia and acidosis.

For seizures, promptly administer a benzodiazepine, small doses of propofol, lipid emulsion. If seizures persist, small doses of succinylcholine should be considered to minimize acidosis and hypoxemia.

If cardiac arrest occurs follow Advanced Cardiovascular Life Support (ACLS) guidelines with the following modifications [20]:

- The use of small initial doses(10–100 mcg boluses) of epinephrine.
- Vasopressin is not recommended.
- Avoid calcium channel blockers and beta-blockers.
- In ventricular arrhythmias prefer Amiodarone.
- Treatment of ventricular arrhythmias with local anesthetics (lidocaine, procainamide) is not recommended.

- Use lipid emulsion at first signs of LAST after airway management.
- Give a bolus of 20% lipid emulsion 1.5 mL/kg (lean body mass).
- Followed by 0.25 mL/kg/min infusion for at least 10 min after circulatory stability. If circulatory stability is not attained consider re-bolusing and increasing your infusion to 0.5 mL/kg/min.
- Approximately 10 mL/kg of lipid emulsion in 30 min is recommended as the upper limit for initial dosing. Failure to respond to lipid emulsion and vasopressor therapy should prompt institution of cardiopulmonary bypass (CPB).

In short, treatment of seizures includes ventilation of the patient's lungs with oxygen because arterial hypoxemia and metabolic acidosis occur within seconds. Hyperventilation is to decrease the delivery of local anesthetic to the brain. IV administration of a benzodiazepine such as midazolam or diazepam is effective in suppressing local anesthetic-induced seizures. Early use of lipid emulsion for the treatment of local anesthetic toxicity is becoming standard of care, acknowledging that a prolonged effort may be needed to increase the chance of resuscitation [21, 22].

9.5.10 Neurotoxicity

9.5.10.1 Transient Neurologic Symptoms

The etiology of transient neurologic symptoms (TNS) is unclear, but some have speculated that this syndrome represents a form of neurotoxicity.

TNS manifests as moderate to severe pain in the lower back, buttocks, and posterior thighs that appear within 6–36 h after complete recovery from uneventful single-shot spinal anesthesia.

The incidence of transient neurologic symptoms is greatest following the intrathecal injection of lidocaine (as high as 30%). Initial reports of transient neurologic symptoms involved spinal anesthesia produced by hyperbaric 5% lidocaine. Several risk factors (lidocaine, lithotomy position, outpatient status, arthroscopic knee surgery, and obesity) for developing TNS have been identified. Decreasing spinal lidocaine concentrations does not alter the incidence of transient neurologic symptoms. The risk of TNS associated with bupivacaine, tetracaine, mepivacaine, prilocaine, or procaine is significantly less than with lidocaine.

Sensory and motor neurologic examination is normal, and relief of pain with trigger point injections and nonsteroidal anti-inflammatory drugs (NSAIDs) suggests a musculoskeletal component. Full recovery from transient neurologic symptoms usually occurs within 1–7 days [23, 24].

9.5.11 Direct Nerve Injury from Local Anesthetic

Toxicity can result from either local anesthetics themselves or from additives, preservatives, antiseptics, or the pH of the formulations. The mechanism of local anesthetic-induced neurotoxicity is multifactorial.

Direct nerve injury is evident when isolated nerves are exposed to high concentration of local anesthetics, particularly lidocaine and tetracaine. Hyperbaric 5% lidocaine and tetracaine have been associated with cauda equina syndrome after continuous spinal anesthesia. In these cases, spinal microcatheters were used to administer supernormal doses (up to 300 mg) of hyperbaric 5% lidocaine. Because spinal microcatheters (25–32 gauge) greatly limit the speed of drug administration, badly distributed local anesthetics presumably pool near the catheter tip.

9.5.12 Myotoxicity

Skeletal muscle toxicity is a rare side effect of local anesthetic. Intramuscular injections result in reversible myonecrosis. The extent of muscle damage is dose-dependent. The extent of such damage depends on pharmacological properties of each local anesthetic, dose injected, and site of injection. Interactions with the Ca 2+ metabolism seem to be a key pathway and explain most damage; also, changes in the mitochondrial metabolism. First reports of muscular dysfunction were related to retrobulbar injection of local anesthetics. Bupivacaine seems to be the most toxic local anesthetic.

9.5.13 Anterior Spinal Artery Syndrome

Anterior spinal artery syndrome consists of lower-extremity paresis with a variable sensory deficit. Thrombosis or spasm of the anterior spinal artery as well as effects of hypotension or vasoconstrictor drugs is possible.

9.5.14 Methemoglobinemia

Methemoglobinemia is a rare but potentially life-threatening complication that may follow the administration of certain drugs or chemicals that cause oxidation of hemoglobin to methemoglobin more rapidly than methemoglobin is reduced to hemoglobin. Known oxidant substances include topical local anesthetics (prilocaine, benzocaine, lidocaine), nitroglycerin, phenytoin, and sulfonamides.

9.5.15 Drug Interactions

Local anesthetics potentiate the effects of non-depolarizing muscle relaxants. Succinylcholine and ester local anesthetics are metabolized by pseudocholinesterases. Simultaneous administration may potentiate the effect of each other. Propranolol decreases hepatic blood flow and amide local anesthetic clearance.

9.6 Epidural Anesthesia

Local anesthetic can produce epidural anesthesia by 2 presumed mechanisms. First, local anesthetic diffuses across the dura to act on nerve roots and the spinal cord. Second, local anesthetic also diffuses into the paravertebral area through the intervertebral foramina, producing multiple paravertebral nerve blocks. Lidocaine is commonly used for epidural anesthesia because of its good diffusion capabilities through tissues.

Bupivacaine and ropivacaine at similar concentrations (0.5–0.75%) produce similar prolonged sensory anesthesia (ropivacaine has a greater tendency to block A-delta and C fibers) when used for epidural anesthesia, but the motor anesthesia produced by ropivacaine is less intense and of shorter duration. Ropivacaine and bupivacaine both provide excellent labor analgesia with no significant differences between the 2 drugs in the incidence of measured obstetric outcomes.

Local anesthetics cross the placenta and may produce detectable, although not necessarily adverse, effects on the fetus for 24–48 h. Use of a more lipid-soluble and protein-bound local anesthetic such as bupivacaine may limit passage across the placenta to the fetus.

The large dose required for producing epidural anesthesia leads to systemic absorption of the local anesthetic. For example, peak plasma concentrations of lidocaine are 3–4 μ(mu)g/mL after placement of 400 mg into the epidural space. Addition of epinephrine to the local anesthetic solution may decrease systemic absorption of the local anesthetic by approximately one-third. Addition of opioids to local anesthetic solutions placed results in synergistic analgesia.

9.7 Spinal Anesthesia

The principal site of action is the preganglionic fibers as they leave the spinal cord in the anterior rami. The total dose of local anesthetic administered for spinal anesthesia is more important than the concentration of drug or the volume of the solution injected.

- **Bupivacaine** produces greater motor block than tetracaine.
- **Ropivacaine**, 3 mL of 0.5 or 0.75%, produces sensory anesthesia, although complete motor blockade was present in only about 50% of patients receiving the lower dose. Ropivacaine is an acceptable local anesthetic to produce spinal anesthesia for cesarean delivery, and its decreased lower-extremity blockade compared with bupivacaine may be a desirable feature.
- **Levobupivacaine** has equivalent clinical efficacy to bupivacaine for spinal anesthesia.
- **Chloroprocaine** was not recommended for placement in the subarachnoid space because of potential neurotoxicity.
- **Addition of glucose** to local anesthetic solutions increases the specific gravity of local anesthetic solutions above that of cerebrospinal fluid (hyperbaric).
- **Addition of distilled water** lowers the specific gravity of local anesthetic solutions below that of cerebrospinal fluid (hypobaric).

9.8 Questions and Answers

Questions (Choose the most Appropriate Answer)

1. Injection of local anesthetics into which of the following sites is MOST likely to result in the highest peak plasma concentration?
   A. Caudal
   B. Epidural
   C. Intercostal
   D. Brachial plexus
2. Which local anesthetic undergoes the LEAST hepatic clearance?
   A. Chloroprocaine
   B. Bupivacaine
   C. Etidocaine
   D. Prilocaine
   E. Lidocaine
3. The primary determinant of local anesthetic potency is
   A. pKa
   B. Molecular weight
   C. Lipid solubility
   D. Concentration
   E. Protein binding
   F. Patient position
4. The common element thought to be present in every case of cauda equina syndrome after continuous spinal anesthesia is
   A. Use of microcatheter
   B. Maldistribution of local anesthetic
   C. Administration of lidocaine
   D. Addition of epinephrine
   E. Hyperbaricity

5. According to a recent study regarding hemodynamic instability due to bupivacaine toxicity, which of the following statements about initial treatment is MOST likely true?
   A. Higher doses of lipid emulsion (4 mL/kg vs. 2 mL/kg) resulted in lower mortality.
   B. Rapid lipid emulsion administration resulted in increased risk for side effects.
   C. Normalization of hemodynamic variables occurred more rapidly when epinephrine was given before lipid emulsion.
   D. Epinephrine produced fewer rhythm disturbances compared to lipid emulsion.
6. The maximum dose of lidocaine containing 1:200,000 epinephrine that can be administered to a 70-kg patient for regional anesthesia (other than spinal anesthesia) is:
   A. 50 mg
   B. 100 mg
   C. 200 mg
   D. 500 mg
   E. 1000 mg
7. Injection of which of the following local anesthetics in a preservative-free solution is MOST likely to cause an allergic reaction?
   A. Bupivacaine
   B. Ropivacaine
   C. Chloroprocaine
   D. Prilocaine
8. After receiving an uneventful 45 mg, 5% hyperbaric lidocaine spinal anesthetic for an outpatient hysteroscopy, a patient calls on postoperative day 1 to complain of severe burning in her buttocks and posterior thighs. Which statement about this patient's condition is MOST likely true?
   A. This is a dose-dependent phenomenon.
   B. The patient should be treated with nonsteroidal anti-inflammatory agents.
   C. A neurology consult should be obtained for suspected cauda equina syndrome.
   D. Use of a lower concentration of lidocaine would have reduced the risk
9. In a patient with known history of allergy to chloroprocaine, injection of which of the following local anesthetics in a preservative-free solution is MOST likely to be safe?
   A. Benzocaine
   B. Tetracaine
   C. Bupivacaine
   D. Procaine
10. Which statement about methemoglobinemia in association with ester local anesthetics is MOST likely false?
   A. Methemoglobinemia is common and easily treatable complication.
   B. Methemoglobinemia is easily treated by the administration of methylene blue.
   C. Blood normally contains approximately 1% methemoglobin levels.
   D. Methemoglobin is incapable of oxygen transport.
   E. Neonates may be at greater risk because of more readily oxidized fetal hemoglobin.
11. What term best describes the mechanism of action of local anesthetics for spinal anesthesia?
   A. The level of motor anesthesia is 2 segments above sensory anesthesia.
   B. The principal site of action is the postganglionic fibers.
   C. Sympathetic denervation extends 2 spinal segments cephalad to the level of sensory anesthesia.
   D. Cerebrospinal fluid contains significant amounts of cholinesterase enzyme.
12. Mixing of lidocaine 2% with bupivacaine 0.5% in brachial plexus blocks results in the following?
   A. Prolonged duration of action
   B. Increased latency time
   C. No change in duration of action or onset time
   D. Faster onset time
   E. Decreased duration of action with no effect on onset time
13. What are important properties of Liposomal Bupivacaine?
   A. It is safe to mix with different types of LAs.
   B. It is FDA approved for use in Interscalene block, Tap blocks, and local infiltration
   C. If used alone, it can achieve adequate analgesia
   D. It has clinical effect lasting 72 hours
   E. It is less cardiotoxic than Ropivacaine

Answers

1. **C**. Intercostal. The rate of systemic absorption is proportionate to the vascularity of the site of injection: intravenous > tracheal > intercostal > caudal > paracervical > epidural > brachial plexus > sciatic > subcutaneous.
2. **A**. Chloroprocaine is an ester. Esters are metabolized by pseudocholinesterase. Ester hydrolysis is very rapid, and the water-soluble metabolites are excreted in the urine.
3. **C**. Lipid solubility:
   - The potency of local anesthetics is directly related to their lipid solubility.
   - In general, the speed of onset of action of local anesthetics is related to the pKa of the drug.

- Drugs with lower pKa values have a higher amount of non-ionized molecules at physiologic pH and penetrate the lipid portion of nerves faster (an exception is chloroprocaine, which has a fast onset of action that may be related to the higher concentration of drug used).
- The amount of protein binding seems related to the duration of action of local anesthetics (more protein binding has longer duration of action)

4. **B**. Maldistribution of local anesthetic. Direct nerve injury is evident when isolated nerves are exposed to high concentration of local anesthetics, particularly lidocaine and tetracaine.
   Hyperbaric 5% lidocaine and tetracaine have been associated with cauda equina syndrome after continuous spinal anesthesia. In these cases, spinal microcatheters were used to administer supernormal doses (up to 300 mg) of hyperbaric 5% lidocaine. Because spinal microcatheters (25–32 gauge) greatly limit the speed of drug administration, badly distributed local anesthetics presumably pooled near the catheter tip.
5. **C**. Normalization of hemodynamic variables occurred more rapidly when epinephrine was given before lipid emulsion.
6. **D**. 500 mg. Maximal allowable dose:
   - Lidocaine 5 mg/Kg
   - Lidocaine with epinephrine 7 mg/Kg
   - Ropivacaine/Levobupivacaine/Bupivacaine 3 mg/Kg
   - Addition of epinephrine to ropivacaine does not result in increase in the maximum allowable dose.
   - Care should be exercised not to exceed the maximum dose.
   - Toxicities of local anesthetics are not independent, but additive. A solution containing 50% of the toxic dose of local anesthetic A, and 50% of the toxic dose of local anesthetic B, will have the same implications as 100% of the toxic dose of either local anesthetic alone.
7. **C**. Chloroprocaine:
   - Ester LA have a higher incidence (chloroprocaine, procaine, tetracaine)
   - There metabolism to a compound similar to PABA, which associated with allergic reaction
   - The esters include procaine, chloroprocaine, and tetracaine (all have 1 letter “i” in the name).
   - The amides are lidocaine, mepivacaine, prilocaine, bupivacaine, levobupivacaine, etidocaine, and ropivacaine (all have 2 “i”s in the name).
   - The esters undergo plasma clearance by cholinesterases and have relatively short half-lives, whereas the amides undergo hepatic clearance and have longer half-lives.
8. **B**. The patient should be treated with non-steroidal anti-inflammatory agents. Lidocaine-associated TNS is neither dose-dependent nor concentration (0.5–5%)-dependent, and lidocaine-associated TNS appears to occur at a similar rate regardless of the preparation (hyperbaric, isobaric) as it is diluted with cerebrospinal fluid.
   The rate does vary with the type of surgery being performed and is highest after outpatient gynecologic procedures performed in the lithotomy position. Patients undergoing surgery in the lithotomy position have a risk rate of 30–36%, while those undergoing surgery in the supine position have a risk rate of 4–8%. Transient and self-limiting, it can be very uncomfortable for patients, and prior to instituting therapy, it is important to seek other symptoms that might suggest other etiology.
   Treatment: Opioids, NSAIDS, muscle relaxants, and symptomatic therapy (e.g., heating pads). NSAIDs have been the most successful therapy.
9. **C**. Bupivacaine. Cross-sensitivity between local anesthetics reflects the common metabolite para-aminobenzoic acid (PABA). A similar cross-sensitivity, however, does not exist between classes of local anesthetics. Therefore, a patient with a known allergy to an ester local anesthetic can receive an amide local anesthetic without an increased risk of an allergic reaction. Likewise, an ester local anesthetic can be administered to a patient with a known allergy to an amide local anesthetic. It is important that the “safe” local anesthetic be preservative-free.
10. **A**. Methemoglobinemia is common and easily treatable complication.
    Methemoglobinemia is a rare but potentially life-threatening complication (decreased oxygen-carrying capacity) that may follow the administration of certain drugs or chemicals that cause oxidation of hemoglobin to methemoglobin more rapidly than methemoglobin is reduced to hemoglobin. Known oxidant substances include topical local anesthetics (prilocaine, benzocaine, lidocaine), nitroglycerin, phenytoin, and sulfonamides. Neonates may be at greater risk because of more readily oxidized fetal hemoglobin.
    Normal hemoglobin contains an iron molecule in the reduced or ferrous form (Fe^{2+}), the only form suitable for oxygen transport by hemoglobin. When hemoglobin is oxidized, the iron molecule is converted into the ferric state (Fe^{3+}) or methemoglobin. Because red blood cells are continuously exposed to various oxidant stresses, blood normally contains approximately 1% methemoglobin levels. Prilocaine and benzocaine can oxidize the ferrous form of the

hemoglobin to the ferric form, creating methemoglobin. It is more frequently seen with nitrates such as nitroglycerin.

Depending on the degree, methemoglobinemia can lead to tissue hypoxia. The oxyHb curve shifts to the left (P50 <27 mm Hg). MetHb has a larger absorbance than Hb and oxyHb at 940 nm, but simulates Hb at 660 nm. In the presence of high MetHb concentrations, the SaO2 falsely approaches 85%, independent of the actual arterial oxygenation. Central cyanosis usually occurs when methemoglobin concentrations exceed 15%. The presence of methemoglobinemia is suggested by a difference between the calculated and measured arterial oxygen saturation. The diagnosis is confirmed by qualitative measurements of methemoglobin by cooximetry and clinical suspicion.

Methemoglobinemia is easily treated by the administration of methylene blue (1–2 mg/kg of a 1% solution over 5 min) or less successfully with ascorbic acid (2 mg/kg).

11. C. Sympathetic denervation extends 2 spinal segments cephalad to the level of sensory anesthesia. The principal site of action is the preganglionic fibers as they leave the spinal cord in the anterior rami. Because preganglionic sympathetic nervous system fibers are blocked by concentrations of local anesthetics that are insufficient to affect sensory or motor fibers, the level of sympathetic nervous system denervation during spinal anesthesia extends approximately 2 spinal segments cephalad to the level of sensory anesthesia. For the same reasons, the level of motor anesthesia averages 2 segments below sensory anesthesia.

    Cerebrospinal fluid does not contain significant amounts of cholinesterase enzyme; therefore, the duration of action of ester local anesthetics as well as amides placed in the subarachnoid space depends on systemic absorption of the drug.
12. E. Most studies on mixing shorter-acting LA (chloroprocaine, mepivacaine, Lidocaine) with a long-acting LA (bupivacaine, Ropivacaine) for upper and lower-extremity surgeries failed to show a faster onset time. However, the duration of action with mixing LA did decrease. There is still not much evidence to support the mixing of LA to achieve an ideal LA that has rapid onset, longer duration of action, and lower toxicity.
13. B. Liposomal bupivacaine is FDA-approved for use as surgical site infiltration, thoracoabdominal plane blocks, and interscalene block. Liposomal bupivacaine reliably produced plasma levels of bupivacaine up to 72 hours after infiltration. Clinical duration of action last around 24 hours. It is should not be mixed with different local anesthetics as this can make the molecule unstable and cause excess secretion of content from the vesicles. It encapsulates bupivacaine so can still cause cardiotoxicity.

References

1. Lee-Son S, Wang GK, Concus A, Crill E, Strichartz G. Stereoselective inhibition of neuronal sodium channels by local anesthetics. Evidence for two sites of action? Anesthesiology. 1992;77(2):324–35.
2. Mulroy MF, Bernards CM. A practical approach to regional anesthesia. 4th ed. Philadelphia: Wolters Kluwer/Lippincott Williams & Wilkins; 2009.
3. Creative Commons Attribution 4.0 International License from OpenStax. Anatomy & physiology. Houston: OpenStax, Rice University; 2016.
4. Butterworth JFT, Strichartz GR. Molecular mechanisms of local anesthesia: a review. Anesthesiology. 1990;72(4):711–34.
5. Tetzlaff JE. Clinical pharmacology of local anesthetics. Boston: Butterworth-Heinemann; 2000.
6. Datta S, Kodali BS, Segal S. Ch 2. Local anesthetic pharmacology. In: Obstetric anesthesia handbook, 5th ed. New York: Springer; 2010.
7. Samad A, et al. Liposomal drug delivery systems: an update review. Curr Drug Deliv. 2007;4(4):297–305.
8. Kulkarni PR, et al. Liposomes: a novel drug delivery system. Int J Curr Pharm Res. 2011;3(2):10–8.
9. *Marcaine (Bupivacaine HCl)* [US prescribing information]. Hospira Inc.; 2009.
10. Exparel (Bupivacaine Liposome Extended-Release Injectable Suspension)[prescribing information]. Pacira Pharmaceuticals Inc.; 2011.
11. Langford RM, et al. A single administration of depobupivacaine intraoperatively results in prolonged detectable plasma bupivacaine and analgesia in patients undergoing inguinal hernia repair. In: Presented at 62nd Postgraduate Assembly in Anesthesiology, December 12–16, 2008, New York, Poster 9088.
12. Ilfeld BM. Liposomal bupivacaine: its role in regional anesthesia and postoperative analgesia. Adv Anesth. 2014;32(1):133–47.
13. Mossetti V, Vicchio N, Ivani G. Local anesthetics and adjuvants in pediatric regional anesthesia. Curr Drug Targets. 2012;13(7):952–60.
14. Cunningham NL, Kaplan JA. A rapid-onset, long-acting regional anesthetic technique. Anesthesiology. 1974;41:509–11.
15. Cuvillon P, Nouvellon E, Ripart J, et al. A comparison of the pharmacodynamics and pharmacokinetics of bupivacaine, ropivacaine (with epinephrine) and their equal volume mixtures with lidocaine used for femoral and sciatic nerve blocks: a double-blind randomized study. Anesth Analg. 2009;108:641–9.
16. Gadsden J, Hadzic A, Gandhi K, et al. The effect of mixing 1.5% mepivacaine and 0.5% bupivacaine on duration of analgesia and latency of block onset in ultrasound-guided interscalene block. Anesth Analg. 2011;112(2):471-476. https://doi.org/10.1213/ANE.0b013e3182042f7f
17. Laur JJ, Bayman EO, Foldes PJ, Rosenquist RW: Triple-blind randomized clinical trial of time until sensory change using 1.5% mepivacaine with epinephrine, 0.5% bupivacaine, or an equal mixture of both for infraclavicular block. Reg Anesth Pain Med 2012;37:28–33.

18. Patel N, Sadoughi A. Ch 11. Pharmacology of local anesthetics. In: Kaye AD, editor. Essentials of pharmacology for anesthesia, pain medicine, and critical care. New York: Springer; 2015.
19. Groban L, Butterworth J. Lipid reversal of bupivacaine toxicity: has the silver bullet been identified? Reg Anesth Pain Med. 2003;28(3):167–9.
20. Neal JM, Bernards CM, Butterworth JF, Di Gregorio G, Drasner K, Hejtmanek MR, et al. ASRA practice advisory on local anesthetic toxicity. Special Article Reg Anesth Pain Med. 2010;35:152–61.
21. Di Gregorio G, Schwartz D, Ripper R, Kelly K, Feinstein DL, Minshall RD, et al. Lipid emulsion is superior to vasopressin in a rodent model of resuscitation from toxin-induced cardiac arrest. Crit Care Med. 2009;37:993–9.
22. Neal JM, Mulroy MF, Weinberg GL. American Society of Regional Anesthesia and Pain Medicine checklist for managing local anesthetic systemic toxicity: 2012 version. Reg Anesth Pain Med. 2012;37(1):16–8.
23. Silvanto M, Tarkkila P, Makela ML, Rosenberg PH. The influence of ambulation time on the incidence of transient neurologic symptoms after lidocaine spinal anesthesia. Anesth Analg. 2004;98 (3):642–6.
24. Faccenda KA, Finucane BT. Complications of regional anaesthesia incidence and prevention. Drug Saf. 2001;24:413–42.

10 Pharmacology of Inhaled Anesthetics

Elizabeth Demers Lavelle and Swamy Kurra

Abstract

Inhalational agents are chemical compounds that produce general anesthesia and are delivered via inhalation. They are used in anesthesia primarily to produce a loss of consciousness, but may have other lesser effects such as muscle relaxation and analgesia. Nitrous oxide is the only currently used inorganic inhalational agent. Volatile anesthetics, including halothane, methoxyflurane, enflurane, isoflurane, desflurane, and sevoflurane, exert their effects at multiple sites throughout the central nervous system. Each agent has its own specific chemical structure that leads to different solubilities, potencies, biotransformation, and side effects of each drug. The modern volatile inhalational agents of fluorinated ethers including isoflurane, sevoflurane, and desflurane were introduced in the 1980s. The modern volatile agents mainly resist metabolism and make organ toxicity unlikely. As research continues, the noble gas, xenon, has a potential for future development.

Keywords

Inhalational anesthetics • Nitrous oxide • Halothane • Isoflurane • Desflurane • Sevoflurane • Meyer–Overton hypothesis • MAC • Blood:gas partition coefficient • Compound A

Key Points

1. Inhalational agents are chemical compounds that possess general anesthetic properties and can be administered via inhalation. The contemporary agents available for clinical use include nitrous oxide and the volatile agents: halothane, isoflurane, desflurane, and sevoflurane.
2. Currently, the mechanics of inhaled volatile anesthetics are believed to occur through a combined effect by prolongation of inhibitory effects ($GABA_A$ and glycine receptors) and inhibition of excitatory effects. This has minimized the belief in the Meyer and Overton theory that proposed the lipid membrane was the primary site of anesthetic action.
3. Volatile anesthetics decrease mean arterial pressure in a dose-dependent manner, which varies with the type of agent used. All volatile agents depress ventilation and blunt responses to changes in $PaCO_2$.
4. The minimum alveolar concentration (MAC) of an inhaled anesthetic is the alveolar concentration at which 50% of patients will not show a motor response to a standardized surgical incision.
5. Inhalational anesthetics undergo biotransformation to many different degrees and locations depending primarily on their lipophilicity and clinical stability. The major organs involved in biotransformation, the liver and kidneys, are exposed to the highest metabolite concentrations; and therefore, are the primary sites of toxicity
6. The single most important factor in determining the speed of induction and recovery for inhalational agents is the blood:gas coefficient, which expresses the agent's distribution between the blood and gas at the same partial pressure. The higher the agent's solubility in the blood, the slower its induction rate.

The original version of this chapter was revised. The abbreviation "MAP mean arterial pressure" was additionally present in the footnote of Table 10.2. This has now been removed. The correction to this chapter can be found at https://doi.org/10.1007/978-3-319-62067-1_39

E. D. Lavelle (✉) · S. Kurra
Department of Anesthesiology, SUNY Upstate Medical University, Syracuse, NY, USA
e-mail: Bethdemers@yahoo.com

M. Argalious et al. (eds.), *Basic Sciences in Anesthesia*,
https://doi.org/10.1007/978-3-031-60203-0_10

10.1 Introduction

Inhalational agents are used in anesthesia primarily to produce a loss of consciousness, but may have other effects such as muscle relaxation and analgesia. Inhalational anesthetics have been in use since the 1840s, when agents such as ether, chloroform, and nitrous oxide were introduced. Due to safety issues, the search for better inhalational agents was begun and fluorinated ethers and hydrocarbons were introduced. Halothane was introduced into clinical practice in 1956 and revolutionized anesthetic practices. However, secondary to its arrhythmogenic effects with epinephrine and possible postoperative liver failure, alternative agents were developed to minimize negative effects. Enflurane, a methyl ether derivative, was not arrhythmogenic or hepatotoxic, but had side effects including lowering the seizure threshold. With further research, the modern inhalational agents of fluorinated ethers including isoflurane, sevoflurane, and desflurane were introduced by the 1980s. These drugs resist metabolism and make organ toxicity unlikely. As research continues, the noble gas, xenon, has a potential for future development. These agents have improved safety and reliability.

10.2 Physical and Chemical Properties of Inhaled Anesthetics

10.2.1 Nitrous Oxide

Nitrous oxide (◉ Fig. 10.1) is a low-molecular weight inorganic gas that is odorless and colorless. Although it is non-explosive, it does support combustion [1]. Because of its low potency and poor blood solubility (◉ Table 10.1), it is commonly administered in conjunction with volatile anesthetics or narcotics to produce general anesthesia. Nitrous oxide has the lowest potency of the inhalational agents, with a minimum alveolar concentration (MAC) value of 104%, which is clinically not achievable and thus cannot provide general anesthesia when administered solely. Nitrous oxide is a gas at room temperature, but can be stored as a liquid under pressure as its critical temperature lies above room temperature. Although it does have amnestic and analgesic properties, it does not provide muscle relaxation as other inhalational agents do. Controversy exists over the role of nitrous oxide in postoperative nausea and vomiting (PONV), which may occur through activation of the chemoreceptor trigger zone and vomiting center in the medulla [4].

10.2.2 Halothane

Halothane is a halogenated alkane (◉ Fig. 10.1) that remains a clear liquid at room temperature. Carbon-fluoride bonds make it non-flammable and non-explosive. It is well tolerated for inhalational inductions with a notable sweet, non-pungent odor. It has a high potency and intermediate solubility, which allows for an intermediate onset and recovery from anesthesia (◉ Table 10.1). Thymol must be added to halothane which also must be stored in amber bottles to prevent spontaneous oxidative decomposition [5, 6].

10.2.3 Enflurane

Enflurane is a halogenated ether (◉ Fig. 10.1) with an ethereal odor that remains a liquid at room temperature. It has an intermediate solubility and high potency allowing for intermediate onset and recovery times from anesthesia (◉ Table 10.1). Enflurane is oxidized in the liver and can produce nephrotoxic fluoride ions [7, 8].

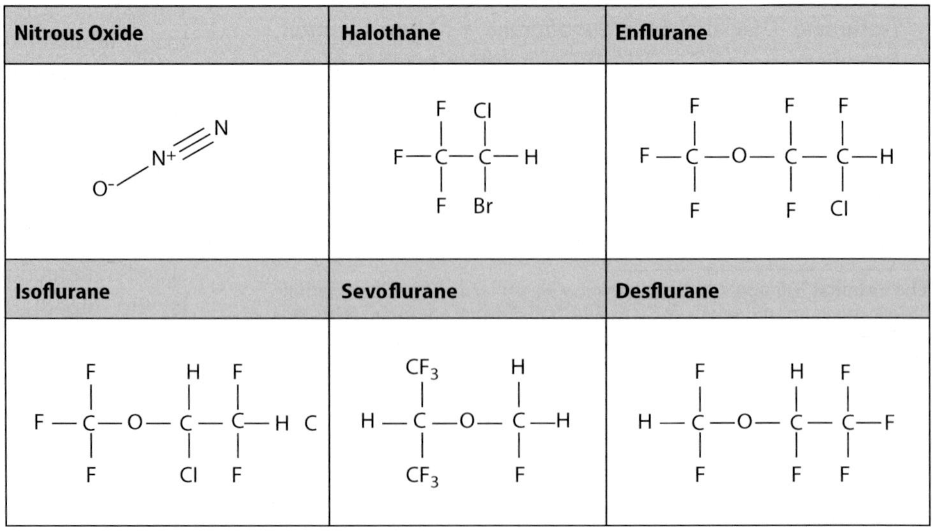

Fig. 10.1 Molecular structure of inhalational anesthetics

Table 10.1 Physical and chemical properties of inhaled anesthetics

	Nitrous Oxide	Halothane	Methoxyflurane	Enflurane	Isoflurane	Desflurane	Sevoflurane
Molecular weight	44	197	165	184	184	200	168
Boiling point (°C)	−89	51	105	57	48	23	59
Blood:gas coefficient @ 37 °C	0.47	2.5	12	1.9	1.4	0.45	0.65
Oil: gas coefficient @ 37 °C	1.3	197	950	99	97	19	53
Vapor pressure (mmHG @ 20 °C)	Gas	244	22.5	172	240	669	170
MAC % (30–55 year old at 1 atm)	104	0.75	0.2	1.63	1.17	6.0	2.0
Stable in soda lime	Yes	No	Yes	Yes	Yes	Yes	No

Sources Bovill [2] and Yasuda et al. [3]

10.2.4 Isoflurane

Isoflurane is a fluorinated methyl ethyl ether (◉ Fig. 10.1) that is a non-flammable liquid at room temperature. Although it is an isomer of enflurane, it has different physiochemical properties and different manufacturing methods. Like enflurane and halothane, it has an intermediate solubility and high potency allowing for intermediate onset and recovery times from anesthesia (◉ Table 10.1). It has a pungent ethereal odor [8].

10.2.5 Sevoflurane

Sevoflurane is a fluorinated methyl isopropyl ether (◉ Fig. 10.1). It has a potency similar to enflurane. However, it has a significantly lower solubility in blood (◉ Table 10.1). This property allows for a rapid increase in alveolar concentration and a rapid on and offset of anesthesia. Combined with its non-pungent odor, these attributes make sevoflurane an ideal inhalational induction agent. Its vapor pressures allow for the use of a conventional vaporizer. Sevoflurane is susceptible to metabolism, with 3–5% undergoing biodegradation. Unlike other volatile agents, sevoflurane is not metabolized to acyl halide intermediates (as with halothane, enflurane, isoflurane, and desflurane), which can potentially cause hepatotoxicity or cross-sensitivity between drugs.

10.2.6 Desflurane

Desflurane is also a fluorinated methyl ethyl ether (◉ Fig. 10.1) that differs from isoflurane only by a substitution of a fluoride for the chlorine atom. The "minor change" of fluorination increases the vapor pressure, enhances molecular stability, and decreases the potency of the drug [9]. Because of its vapor pressure (◉ Table 10.1), desflurane will boil at room temperature at high altitudes. This requires a vaporizer (Tec 6, GE Healthcare, Chicago, IL) designed specifically to handle this inhalational agent. The vaporizer is heated to 39°C and pressurized to 2 atm. No fresh gas flows through the vaporizer pump; rather pure desflurane vapor joins the fresh gas flows before exiting the vaporizer [10]. Low solubility and potency allow for a rapid on and offset of anesthesia. Its lower blood:gas solubility creates precise control and the ability for more rapid recovery times from anesthesia [8]. Desflurane has a pungent odor, which limits its utility for inhalational inductions.

10.2.7 Xenon

Xenon is a noble gas found in the atmosphere; and was recognized as an anesthetic in 1951. It has a MAC value of 71% and can be combined with oxygen to deliver anesthesia. The blood:gas partition coefficient is 0.12, which results in rapid onset and recovery. Xenon depresses postsympathetic excitatory transmission through N-methyl-D-aspartate (NMDA) receptor blocks. There are minimal cardiovascular side effects, even in the setting of severely limited myocardial reserve. Xenon affects anesthetic-induced preconditioning of the heart and brain against ischemic damage in the same way as volatile agents. Xenon may have neuroprotective action, but it may be offset by an increase in cerebral blood flow. It is a non-irritant to the airway for easy induction. Although a mild respiratory depressant, it decreases respiratory rate and increases tidal volume, in contrast to the volatile agents. Xenon has a high relative density, which causes an increase in pulmonary resistance. Caution is advised in patients who have severe chronic obstructive pulmonary disease (COPD) or in premature infants. It is not metabolized in the liver or kidneys, and it does not trigger malignant hyperpyrexia. Xenon is also a potent intraoperative analgesic, attenuating responses to surgical stimuli to a greater extent than sevoflurane.

Xenon anesthesia provides more stable intraoperative blood pressure, lower heart rate, and faster recovery from anesthesia than volatile agents. However, it is associated with higher postoperative nausea and vomiting. The main limitations for wider use are lack of studies, need for hyperbaric conditions, impracticality in surgery, and inefficiency of conventional anesthesia equipment. These limitations make xenon cost prohibitive.

10.3 Mechanism of Action

The exact mechanism of action for volatile anesthetics is complex and still unknown. Currently, the mechanics of inhaled volatile anesthetics is believed to occur through a combined effect by prolongation of inhibitory effects ($GABA_A$ and glycine receptors) and inhibition of excitatory effects (nicotinic acetylcholine and glutamate receptors). Typical anesthetic agents produce anesthesia, amnesia, analgesia, and immobilization.

Initially, Meyer and Overton proposed a lipid theory and believed the lipid membrane was the primary site of anesthetic action by correlating inhaled anesthetics potency with their solubility in lipids. They observed a strong correlation between the potency of inhalational anesthetics and their solubility in oil, theorizing they had a non-specific lipid membrane mechanism of action [11]. Later, researchers demonstrated that proteins may also be the site of action for inhaled anesthetics [12, 13]. Additional research on the mechanism of action for inhaled anesthetics explained ligand-gated ion channels proteins are mostly likely the targets of inhaled anesthetics [14].

Electrical activity in human cells is generated through influx and efflux of ions (mostly Na+, Ca2+, Cl−, and K+) through a variety of ion channels. Some receptor-mediated ion channels are targets of inhaled anesthetics at clinical anesthetic concentrations, such as serotonin receptors, $GABA_A$ receptors, glycine receptors, and NMDA or AMPA (α[alpha]-amino-3-hydroxy-5-methyl-4-isoxazolepropionic acid) receptors (glutamate neurotransmitter) [15–18].

$GABA_A$-related anesthetic action is common for all volatile anesthetics due to its abundancy in the brain. Normal physiologic function of $GABA_A$ and glycine receptors (Cl− ion channels) is to inhibit the excitation of postsynaptic neurons. At effective clinical concentrations, volatile anesthetics enhance the $GABA_A$ receptor-mediated activity by increasing its sensitivity to gamma-aminobutyric acid (GABA) and the sensitized receptors prolong the inhibition of excitatory neurons. Gaseous anesthetics, such as nitrous oxide, have a minimal effect on GABA-related mechanisms [19–23]. Normally K+ channels maintain a polarized state of neurons and are targeted sites for isoflurane. Isoflurane activates the K+ channel and leads to a decrease of neuronal excitation [24].

Inhibition of excitatory neurotransmission can be achieved either by inhibition of a neurotransmitter release from presynaptic nerve endings or a postsynaptic receptor blockade. Halothane and isoflurane at clinical concentrations inhibit the NMDA receptor (Na+ ion channel) associated excitation by postsynaptic blockades or decreasing presynaptic glutamate release. The volatile anesthetics also can inhibit the presynaptic release of an excitatory neurotransmitter by blocking presynaptic voltage-gated Na+ channels at clinical concentrations [25]. Excitatory postsynaptic nicotinic acetylcholine receptors and NMDA-sensitive glutamate channels are inhibited by gaseous anesthetics to inhibit the excitation of excitatory neurons [26].

The mechanism of action for immobilization and amnesia occurs at distinct sites. Studies have proven that immobilization to surgical stimulus can be achieved at the spinal cord level without brain involvement. Immobility to surgical stimuli occurs by inhibiting ascending transmission of pain stimuli to the brain from the spinal cord. At the spinal cord level, volatile anesthetics prolong the inhibitory effects of glycine receptors and inhibit the postsynaptic excitatory effects of NMDA and AMPA receptors [27–29]. Amnesia can be induced without immobilization at lower clinical concentrations. Specific loci in the brain are responsible for this amnesic effect. Inhaled anesthetics act on nicotinic acetylcholine receptors in the brain and impair the memory process leading to amnesia [30–33].

GABA receptors function differently between the growing brain in children and the brain in adults. In the growing brain, GABA receptors function as stimulators, and in the adult brain they act as inhibitors; therefore, a neurotoxic effect from anesthetics can be seen in the growing brain. In contrast to its inhibitory action in the adult brain, GABA receptors act as an excitatory neurotransmitter in the growing brain of the child. These GABA receptors generate action potentials directly opening voltage-dependent calcium channels and increase the calcium concentration in the brain. This increase in intracellular calcium can lead to apoptosis. In addition, the mitochondrion appears to be the mediator between anesthesia-induced increased calcium levels and cell apoptosis, leading to mitochondrial damage. Every year, millions of children are treated with anesthetic agents. There is evidence that suggests that exposure to anesthetics may be neurotoxic to the developing brain and lead to long-term neurological effects.

Lithium protects against anesthesia-induced developmental neuroapoptosis along with melatonin. Coadministration of hydrogen gas acts as part of the carrier gas mixture and may suppress neuronal apoptosis. Therefore, there may not be a safe anesthetic, but only safe anesthetic concentrations and exposure durations.

Table 10.2 Systemic effects of inhaled anesthetics

	Nitrous Oxide	Halothane	Methoxyflurane	Enflurane	Isoflurane	Desflurane	Sevoflurane
Cardiovascular	↔	↓	↓	↓	↓	↓	↓
HR	↔	↓	↑	↑	↑	↑[b]	↔
SVR	↔	↔	↔	↓	↓	↓	↓
CO	↑[a]	↓	↓	↓	↔	↔	↓
Myocardial contractility	↔	↓	↔	↓	↔	↔	↔
Respiratory	↓	↓	↓	↓	↓	↓	↓
TV	↑	↑	↑	↑	↑	↑	↑
RR	↔	↑	↑	↑	↑	↑	↑
$PaCO_2$	↑	↔	↔	↔	↔	↔	↔
PVR	↓	↓↓	↓	↓	↓	Irritant	↓
Airway resistance							
Cerebral	↑	↑↑	↑	↑	↑	↑	↑
Blood flow	↑	↑	↑	↑	↑	↑	↑
ICP	↑	↑[a]	↓	↓	↓	↓	↓
$CMRO_2$	↓	↓	↓	↑	↓	↓	↓/↑
Seizures							
Non-depolarizing blockade	↑	↑	↑	↑	↑	↑	↑
Renal	↓	↓	↓	↓	↓	↓	↓
Blood flow	↓	↓	↓	↓	↓	Unknown	Unknown
GFR	↓	↓	↓	↓	↓	Unknown	Unknown
Urine							
Hepatic	↓	↓	↓	↓	↓	↓	↓
Blood flow							

Abbreviations: HR heart rate, *SVR* systemic vascular resistance, *CO* cardiac output, *TV* tidal volume, *RR* respiratory rate, $PaCO_2$ partial pressure of carbon dioxide, *PVR* pulmonary vascular resistance, *ICP* intracranial pressure, $CMRO_2$ cerebral metabolic rate of oxygen, *GFR* glomerular filtration rate

[a] Minimal

[b] With rapid change in inhaled concentration

10.4 Systemic Effects of Inhaled Anesthetics

Inhaled anesthetics have several effects on systemic organs. Anesthetics effects on the central nervous system, cardiovascular system, pulmonary function, neuromuscular junction, renal and liver function, and hematology and immune systems have been described in sub-sections and are summarized in ◉ Table 10.2.

10.4.1 Effects on Central Nervous System

The changes in an electroencephalogram (EEG) are noticed after the induction of inhaled anesthetics. At lower clinical concentrations (low MAC), the volatile anesthetics and gaseous anesthetics produce high frequency and low amplitude (Beta waves) waves in the EEG, and are transformed to low frequency and high amplitude waves (Delta waves) at clinical anesthetic concentrations [33]. Some volatile anesthetics, such as isoflurane and desflurane at 1.5–2 MAC anesthetic concentration, cause electrical silence in the EEG [34].

Enflurane has the tendency to induce convulsions (seizures) to decreased $PaCO_2$, MAC >2, and repetitive auditory stimuli [35]. Isoflurane has anti-convulsive properties, and desflurane does not produce seizures [36, 37]. There are case reports that support that sevoflurane can produce seizure activity [38, 39].

Typically, cerebral blood flow is autoregulated and depends on the cerebral oxygen consumption ($CMRO_2$), and $PaCO_2$. All inhaled anesthetics increase cerebral blood flow in a dose-dependent manner despite a decrease in cerebral oxygen consumption. Inhalation agents also partially preserve the autoregulation of CBF to changes in $PaCO_2$. Desflurane and isoflurane preserve the responsiveness of CBF to changes in $PaCO_2$ [40]. Cerebral metabolic oxygen requirements are dose-dependent and are decreased with volatile anesthetics [41]. Increased intracranial pressure is seen with halothane use due to significant increases in cerebral blood flow compared to other inhaled anesthetics [42].

Preconditioning and postconditioning is a mechanism for inhaled anesthetics for neuroprotective effects. Inhalational anesthetics provide neuroprotective effects against brain ischemia by pre-, pro- and post-conditionings. Preconditioning is a process where a relatively small amount of inhalational agent is administered prior to the ischemic insult. Postconditioning is applied after the cerebral ischemic event has developed. Many studies have confirmed the protection of pre- and post-conditioning of inhalational anesthetics in their neuroprotection against cerebral ischemia. Sevoflurane preconditioning and early postconditioning reduced both cerebral infract size and neurological defect score at 24 h of reperfusion. Pretreatment with sevoflurane or its early administration at reperfusion provided neuroprotection via mitoKATP in a rat model for focal cerebral ischemia.

Although sevoflurane and isoflurane are similar in their systemic effects, they appear to differ in cerebral circulation. Sevoflurane can maintain cerebral autoregulation up to 1.5 MAC, whereas isoflurane results in loss of autoregulation. Thus, cerebral autroregulation is better preserved during 1.5 MAC sevoflurane than isoflurane and is a better neuroanesthetic agent.

10.4.2 Effects on Cardiovascular System

Volatile anesthetics decrease mean arterial pressure in a dose-dependent manner, which varies with the type of agent used. At clinical anesthetic concentration, halothane decreases the mean arterial pressure by decreasing myocardial contractility and cardiac output; however, isoflurane, sevoflurane, and desflurane decrease systemic vascular resistance. Enflurane decreases both systemic vascular resistance and cardiac output. The change in heart rate is variable with type of agent used and the type of pharmacological agent administrated during surgery. The decrease in heart rate is observed with halothane use due to suppression of the carotid sinus to changes in systemic blood pressure and rate of sinus node depolarization. At anesthetic concentrations, the heart rate is increased with desflurane, enflurane, sevoflurane (>1 MAC), and isoflurane use [41, 43]. Nitrous oxide has very little effect in mean arterial pressure and heart rate changes [44, 45]. Significant decrease in cardiac output is noticed with halothane and enflurane, and sevoflurane can decrease cardiac output at MAC between 1 and 1.5. Sevoflurane can prolong the QT interval and should be cautiously used in patients with prolonged QT interval syndrome or patients susceptible to QT interval changes [46]. Volatile agents can induce arrhythmias. Halothane and isoflurane sensitize the heart to epinephrine, compared to desflurane and sevoflurane, and cause cardiac arrhythmias [47, 48]. Coronary steal syndrome, wherein normally responsive coronary arterioles are dilated “stealing” blood from vessels supplying ischemic zones, may be associated with isoflurane [49]. Isoflurane is known to be a potent coronary artery vasodilator. Isoflurane-induced coronary artery vasodilatation can lead to redistribution of coronary blood flow away from diseased areas, which have decreased ability to vasodilate. Thereby, blood is redistributed in greater amounts to areas with normally responsive coronary arteries. However, most clinical studies failed to prove a higher incident of myocardial ischemia due to isoflurane. Sevoflurane and desflurane do not cause coronary steal syndrome.

10.4.3 Effects on Respiration

All volatile agents depress ventilation and blunt responses to changes in $PaCO_2$. Volatile agents cause rapid, shallow breathing. There is a reduction in the tidal volumes and minute ventilation. The increase in respiratory rate does not adequately compensate for the amount of tidal volume decrease and hence causes an increase in $PaCO_2$.

Volatile agents reduce minute ventilation by reducing tidal volumes. Reduced tidal volume causes a slight increase in $PaCO_2$. The agents minimally suppress the responsiveness to increased $PaCO_2$ (hypercapnia) from decreased tidal volume at central medullary respiratory centers [50, 51]. Nitrous oxide has very little effect in ventilation depression, bronchial muscle tone, and in hypoxic drive [52]. Increases in respiratory rate are associated with all volatile anesthetics. Halothane, isoflurane, and sevoflurane decrease airway resistance in COPD and asthmatic patients [53]. Due to low airway irritant effects, nitrous oxide, halothane, and sevoflurane can be used for induction of anesthesia. Isoflurane and desflurane can irritate the airways during induction with MAC greater than 1.5 and 1, respectively, but have little or no effect during the maintenance of anesthesia. Desflurane is a pungent gas that can cause airway irritability during induction, manifested as breath-holding, salivation, coughing, and possibly laryngospasm. Small doses of opioid administration and humidification help to reduce irritant properties [54–56].

10.4.4 Effects on Neuromuscular Junction

Volatile anesthetics enhance the effects of neuromuscular blocking drugs by inhibiting nicotinic acetylcholine receptors [57]. Volatile anesthetics produce dose-dependent muscle relaxation, whereas nitrous oxide can cause skeletal muscle rigidity (>1 MAC) [44]. One potential complication of volatile agents is malignant hyperthermia (MH). Succinylcholine administration with a volatile agent potentiates a patient susceptible to MH. Malignant hyperthermia can occur even without succinylcholine administration in genetically susceptible patients [58–60]. Halothane has a higher tendency to produce MH than other volatile agents. MH can appear hours after uneventful anesthesia with desflurane [61] and sevoflurane [62, 63]. Nitrous oxide does not manifest this complication [11].

10.4.5 Effects on Renal Function

Volatile agents have little effect on renal physiology. The decrease in renal blood flow that is clinically observed is a product of their glomerular filtration rate, and urine output is systemic vascular effects. There is no direct effect of inhalational agents on renal blood flow. Inorganic fluorides and metabolites, such as compound A, produced from the metabolism of volatile anesthetics can be nephrotoxic; and these effects are further discussed in the next section (Biotransformation and Toxicity of Inhaled Anesthetics).

10.4.6 Effects on Hepatic Function

All inhaled anesthetics reduce the hepatic blood flow. Severe hepatic injury following volatile anesthetics administration is very rare, with a ratio of 1:10,000,000 [64]. Anesthetics agents interfere with hepatic metabolism of other pharmacological agents that are administrated during the anesthesia [65, 66]. Hepatotoxicity can occur with inhaled anesthetics due to inadequate hepatic oxygenation from reduced hepatic blood flow. Hepatotoxicity incidences are higher with halothane induction compared with other inhaled anesthetics. These effects are further discussed in the next section (Biotransformation and Toxicity of Inhaled Anesthetics).

10.4.7 Effects on Hematologic and Immune Systems

Prolonged exposure to nitrous oxide can interfere with bone marrow function. Nitrous oxide affects DNA synthesis by inhibiting vitamin B_{12} dependent enzymes (methionine synthetase) [67, 68]. Megaloblastic changes are noticed in patients who receive nitrous oxide for a duration of 24 h. Agranulocytosis occurs in patients with 4 days or longer exposure to nitrous oxide. Volatile anesthetics have an immunosuppressive effect on both innate immunity (neutrophils, NK cells, and macrophages) and cell-mediated immunity (T-cells and B-cells), and are dose-dependent. Volatile agents impair neutrophil, macrophage, dendritic, and T-cell function. The suppressive action on immunity is from a combined exposure of the patient to surgery and anesthesia. Surgery releases stress hormones (catecholamines and corticosteroids) [69]. Inhaled anesthetics inhibit the actions of polymorphonuclear cells such as chemotaxis and phagocytosis. Sevoflurane and isoflurane can induce dose-dependent apoptosis in lymphocytes. Isoflurane and sevoflurane also reduce the expression of adhesion molecules on lymphocytes and macrophages, and thus, decrease the recruitment and accumulation of immune cells at inflammatory sites [70].

10.5 Biotransformation and Toxicity of Inhaled Anesthetics

Inhalational anesthetics undergo biotransformation to many different degrees and locations depending primarily on their lipophilicity and clinical stability. The major organs involved in biotransformation, the liver and kidneys, are exposed to the highest metabolite concentrations, and therefore, are the primary sites of toxicity (see ◉ Table 10.3).

10.5.1 Nitrous Oxide

Nitrous oxide undergoes very little biotransformation (0.004%) and is almost solely eliminated by exhalation during emergence [8]. Anaerobic bacteria in the gastrointestinal (GI) tract are responsible for the minimal amount of metabolism. Nitrous oxide irreversibly oxidizes the cobalt atom in vitamin B_{12}, including methionine synthetase and thymidylate synthetase. These enzymes are responsible for myelin formation and DNA synthesis; and thus, nitrous oxide has been questioned to cause bone marrow suppression and neurologic deficiencies in prolonged usage.

10.5.2 Halothane

The liver is the primary site of biotransformation and metabolism for most drugs, particularly lipophilic drugs such as halothane [73, 74]. Approximately 25% of administered halothane is oxidized by an isoenzyme of P450 (CYP2E1) into its principal metabolite trifluoroacetic acid (TFA), as well as lesser amounts of bromide and chloride [75]. The TFA metabolites react with tissue proteins to form trifluoroacetylated protein adducts. Clinical exposure to halothane results in two distinct types of hepatitis [76–78]. Type I hepatotoxicity is benign and self-limiting and occurs in 25–30% of patients receiving halothane. Symptoms include transient nausea, fever, and serum transaminase levels. "Halothane hepatitis," or type II hepatotoxicity, has been reported in 1:5000 to 1:35,000 cases of halothane administration. This immune-mediated reaction is believed to result from the trifluoroacetylated protein adducts in the liver. Clinical symptoms of halothane hepatitis include fever, eosinophilia, and jaundice. Laboratory findings include elevated serum alanine and aspartate transferase and elevated bilirubin. Patients also have a positive IgG against TFA.

Table 10.3 Biotransformation and toxicity of inhaled anesthetics

	Nitrous Oxide	Halothane	Methoxyflurane	Enflurane	Isoflurane	Desflurane	Sevoflurane
Tissue metabolism (%)	0.004	25	70	2.5	0.2	0.02	5
Oxidating enzymes	Anaerobic bacteria in gastrointestinal tract	CYP2E1, CYP2A6	CYP2E1, CYP1A2, CYP2C9/10, CYP2D6	CYP2E1	CYP2E1	CYP2E1	CYP2E1
Principal metabolite	Inactivation of methionine synthetase	TFA, bromine, chloride	Oxalic acid, free fluoride	TFA, small fluoride level rise	TFA, small fluoride level rise	TFA (fluoride levels unchanged from pre-anesthetic levels)	Fluoride
Trifluoroacetylated hepatocellular protein degree of modification	None	++++++	None	++	+	+	None
CO_2 stability	Yes	CO from desiccated carbon dioxide absorbent	CO from desiccated carbon dioxide absorbent	CO from desiccated carbon dioxide absorbent	CO from desiccated carbon dioxide absorbent	CO from desiccated carbon dioxide absorbent	Compound A from desiccated carbon dioxide absorbent, heat production
Possibly toxicities	DNA synthesis, Bone marrow suppression, Vitamin B12 deficiency	**Hepatic** (1:20,000 fulminant hepatitis)	**Renal**, hepatic	Hepatic (1:300,000 fulminant hepatitis)	Hepatic (rare fulminant hepatitis)	Hepatic (rare fulminant hepatitis)	Hepatic (few case reports fulminant hepatitis)

Sources Yasuda et al.[71, 72]
Abbreviations TFA trifluoroacetic acid, *CO_2* carbon dioxide, *CO* carbon monoxide

Severe cases are associated with centrilobular necrosis that may lead to fulminant liver failure with a mortality rate of 50% [79]. Higher rates of halothane hepatitis are found in patients exposed to multiple halothane anesthetics in a short period of time, obese patients, patients >50 years old, female patients, and patients with a history of postanesthetic fever or jaundice.

10.5.3 Methoxyflurane

As the most lipophilic inhaled anesthetic, methoxyflurane undergoes the most biotransformation at an estimated 70% of the drug administered [80]. Only a small amount of the drug, taken into body tissue, is exhaled and respiratory clearance from muscle and fat can extend over a period of several days. Methoxyflurane is metabolized in both the kidneys and the liver, and inorganic fluoride (F-) is produced during its metabolism in clinically significant quantities [81, 82]. Many studies have demonstrated direct links between methoxyflurane dosages, metabolism, and fluoride production. Inorganic fluoride likely causes renal injury with a nephrotoxic threshold of 50 μ(mu)mol/L [83]. Methoxyflurane, the first modern halogenated ether anesthetic, is no longer in clinical use because it is now known to produce polyuric renal insufficiency. More recent anesthetics have been cautiously studied for their renal impairment and fluoride production abilities [84].

10.5.4 Isoflurane

The minimal metabolism (0.2%) of isoflurane results in extremely low rates of hepatic or renal impairment. TFA is the primary metabolite, but serum fluoride levels have not been shown to cause renal dysfunction [85].

10.5.5 Desflurane

Desflurane undergoes extremely low metabolism rates in humans (0.02%); and thus, the serum and urine fluoride levels are essentially unchanged from pre-anesthetic levels. More than the other volatile agents (desflurane > enflurane > isoflurane), desflurane is susceptible to degradation in dessicated carbon dioxide absorbancy to carbon monoxide, when water content falls below 1.4% for soda lime and 5% for baralyme. This carbon monoxide can lead to increased levels of blood carboxyhemoglobin [86–88].

10.5.6 Sevoflurane

Inorganic fluoride ions in plasma concentrations greater than enflurane and hexafluoroisopropanol are produced during the metabolism of sevoflurane in humans. The overall rate of sevoflurane metabolism is more than 10 times that of isoflurane (5%), clinically producing higher serum fluoride levels. Despite this, clinical studies have demonstrated no clinical nephrotoxicity with sevoflurane administration, even with peak concentrations of 50 μ(mu)mol/L. Production of fluoride ions of sevoflurane is mainly in the liver and, therefore, has minimal effect on the kidney function. The liver metabolizes 2–5% of the sevoflurane. Typical fluoride levels after 2–3 MAC hours are 20–30 μ(mu)mol/L [89]. Because of sevoflurane's low blood:gas solubility and rapid elimination, fluoride concentrations fall quickly and renal toxicity is not clinically present. In the presence of a strong alkali, such as those in carbon dioxide absorbents, sevoflurane has been shown to degrade to compounds toxic to animals, particularly compound A (fluoromethyl-1, 1-difluro-1(trimethyl) vinyl-ether) [90–92]. Larger amounts of compound A are produced with lower gas flows, increased respiratory temperatures, high sevoflurane concentrations, anesthetics of long duration, and dessicated soda lime. Amsorb® (Armstrong Ltd., Coleraine, Northern Ireland) is a newer absorbent that does not contain strong base and does not form CO or compound A in vitro. It is clinically recommended to maintain fresh gas flows greater than 2 L/min to limit possible compound A production. Despite proven nephrotoxicity in rats, no postoperative renal impairment or injury has been seen in humans. This difference may be secondary to the lower β(beta)-lyase activity in humans [93]. Degradation of sevoflurane to hydrogen fluoride in the presence of metal and environmental impurities can also occur. Hydrogen fluoride can cause respiratory mucosal burns. Degradation is inhibited through the addition of water in manufacturing and packaging in plastic containers [89]. The US Food and Drug Administration (FDA) recommends the use of sevoflurane with fresh gas flow rates at least 1 L/min for exposure up to 1 h and at least 2 L/min for exposures greater than 1 h.

10.5.7 Possible Neurotoxicity of Inhaled Anesthetics

The possibility of neurotoxic effects of inhaled and other general anesthetics does exist in patients of extreme ages [94, 95]. The greatest concern is the use of general anesthetics in the youngest patients, where rapid brain development is occurring. Widespread neuronal apoptosis in 7-day-old rats after exposure to midazolam, isoflurane, and nitrous oxide caused lasting deficits in behavior, learning, and memory centers [96, 97]. Continued research has demonstrated, in non-human species including primates, sensitive periods of early brain development when anesthetics can accelerate apoptosis [98]. Clinical studies in humans have demonstrated mixed results. Although a possible association with multiple anesthetic exposure and impaired neurocognitive development was demonstrated in one study, others have found no cognitive outcome differences [99–101]. Ongoing clinical trials will provide more information on this important issue, and additional information is available at smarttots.org.

10.6 Minimum Alveolar Concentration and Its Affecting Factors

Minimal alveolar concentration of an inhaled anesthetic is defined as the alveolar concentration at which 50% of the patients are immobile to a standard surgical incision at 1 atmospheric pressure [61, 102]. The immobility is achieved in 99% of patients with 1.3 MAC. This is the state where somatic responses are lost. The potency of the anesthetics is measured by MAC. Anesthetics with higher MAC have a lower potency (e.g., N_2O) and vice versa. As the MAC of nitrous oxide exceeds 100%, it cannot be used alone to provide general anesthesia. It is typically combined in a 70% concentration with 30% oxygen and in concert with more potent agents. The MAC values are additive when used in combinations. The MACs of different inhalational anesthetics are summarized in ◉ Table 10.1. Numerous factors are involved in affecting MAC values, and they are described in ◉ Table 10.4 [103, 104].

"MAC-awake" is defined as the concentration at which response to the vertebral commands are lost in 50% of the patients. This is the state where amnesia occurs. Amnesia is observed before the immobility occurs. The MAC-awake values are significantly lower than the MAC values.

Many studies have demonstrated an age-related MAC value for the volatile agents. MAC is highest at 6 months of age, after which it begins to decline. After age 40, MAC declines ~6% per decade such that by 80 years of age, MAC is about 0.75 that of a 40-year-old.

10.7 Trace Concentrations, Operating Room Pollution, and Personnel Hazards

Health-care workers, surgeons, and anesthesiologists in operating theaters or anesthetizing locations are at risk of exposure to trace concentrations of anesthetics. Spontaneous abortions and congenital defects were observed in rats that were exposed to nitrous oxide for longer times [105, 106]. Even in humans, potential occupational associated risks are noticed after prolonged exposure to nitrous

Table 10.4 Factors affecting minimum alveolar concentrations (MAC)

Factors decreasing MAC requirements	Factors increasing MAC requirements
Decreased catecholamine levels in CNS	Increased catecholamine levels in CNS
Hyponatremia	Hypernatremia
Hypothermia	Hyperthermia
Older age (elderly)	Infants (greatest MAC at 6 months)
Acute alcohol intoxication	Chronic alcohol usage
Anemia (hematocrit <10%)	Red hair (20% increase)
Hypercarbia ($PaCO_2$ >95 mmHg)	Hyperthyroidism
Hypoxia (PaO_2 <40 mmHg)	
Pregnancy (decreased by 30% at 8 weeks)	
Drugs	Drugs
Opioids	Cocaine
Ketamine	Ephedrine
Benzodiazepines	MAO inhibitors
Clonidine, dexmedetomidine, methyldopa	Amphetamine (acute)
Local anesthetics	
Lithium	
Amphetamines (chronic)	

CNS central nervous system, *$PaCO_2$* partial pressure of carbon dioxide, *PaO_2* partial pressure of oxygen, *MAO* monoamine oxidase

oxide. Spontaneous abortions and decreases in fertility occurred in female workers who were exposed to nitrous oxide in the absence of scavenging systems during nitrous oxide administration [107, 108]. Halogenated agents in vitro are embryolethal and produced teratogenic effects in animals [109–111]. In humans, halogenated agents can cause spontaneous abortions and there is some evidence they might produce congenital defects in the offspring of exposed pregnant women [111–113]. Appropriate safety measures, such as scavenging systems and proper ventilation systems, must be taken in hospital operating rooms and anesthetizing locations to prevent occupational-related hazards, especially in females.

Nitrous oxide enhances the greenhouse effect just as carbon dioxide does, but is 300 times more potent, accounting for 6% of the heating effect and causing ozone depletion. In addition, inhaled anesthetics also contribute to global climate change. Isoflurane, sevoflurane, and desflurane undergo very little in vivo metabolism in clinical use, and upon exhalation these agents remain in a form that may pollute the environment. Whenever N_2O or a volatile anesthetic is administered, a continuous flow fresh air ventilation system or scavenger must be used to prevent waste gas accumulation (WGA). Health-care facilities are accountable for ensuring that all anesthesia equipment, including the scavenging system, is properly maintained to promote a safe and healthy environment.

10.8 Comparative Pharmacokinetics of Inhaled Anesthetics

The pharmacokinetics of inhaled anesthetics describes their uptake from the alveoli into the systemic circulation, distribution in the body, and primary elimination by the lungs or liver metabolism. Although the mechanism of action of these agents remains hypothetical, their therapeutic effect ultimately depends on their tissue concentration in the central nervous system. The goal of delivering the inhaled anesthetic is to obtain an optimal brain partial pressure (P_{br}) of the anesthetic. The alveolar partial pressure (P_A), in equilibrium, mirrors the P_{br} and is used as an index of anesthetic depth. The pharmacokinetics can be influenced by aging and increases in body fat [114].

10.8.1 Uptake and Partial Pressure Equilibrium

There are many steps involved between the administration of the inhaled anesthetic from a vaporizer and its distribution into the central nervous system (see ◉ Fig. 10.2).

A series of partial pressure gradients drives the forward movement and systemic absorption of the gas. The principal objective is to achieve equal partial pressures on both sides of each single barrier in the gas flow.

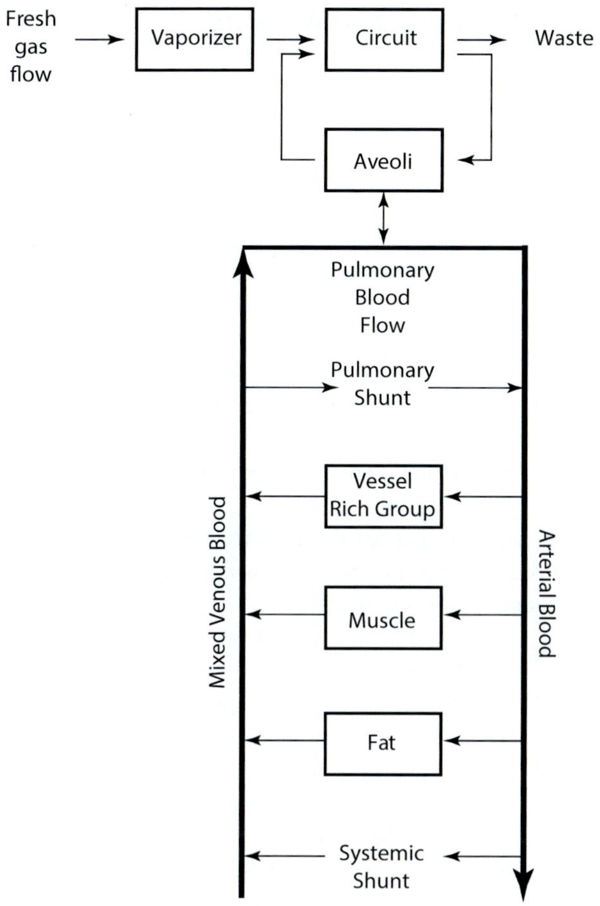

Fig. 10.2 Uptake and distribution of inhaled anesthetics in the body (Adapted from Miller and Pardo [115])

***P_A* (alveolar partial pressure)** ↔ *P_a* (arterial partial pressure) ↔ *P_{br}* (brain partial pressure):

The alveolar partial pressure is dependent on the inspired pressure, ventilation, and breathing system components. This gradient begins with the inspiratory concentration of the gas leaving the anesthesia machine. This content depends on the concentration set by the vaporizer as well as the fresh gas flow, the volume of the breathing circuit, and the possible absorption of the gas by the circuit. Increasing ventilation promotes the input of anesthetics to offset the tissue uptake. The effect is a more rapid rate of increased in the P_A [116].

The second component in the uptake of inhaled anesthetics is the alveolar gas concentration that is achieved in lung tissues during anesthesia. As the agent is taken up in the pulmonary blood stream during induction, the alveolar tissue concentrations remain less than in inspired concentrations. When the blood uptake of the agent is greater, its rate of rise in the alveolar gas is slower. Increasing the inspired concentration of an agent not only increases its alveolar concentration, but also its rate of rise (F_A/ F_I). This phenomenon is known as the concentration effect. The alveolar partial pressure of an agent is important because it determines the partial pressure of the anesthetic in the blood and ultimately in the brain. Hence, the partial pressure in the brain is directly proportional to its brain tissue concentration and therefore its clinical effect.

The impact of a right-to-left shunt on the rate of increase in the P_a depends on the solubility of the anesthetic. A right-to-left shunt slows the rate of increase of the P_a of a poorly soluble anesthetic more than that of a soluble anesthetic. It appears unlikely that a right-to-left shunt alone will alter the speed of induction of anesthesia significantly. Left-to-right shunts result in delivery to the lungs of blood containing a higher partial pressure of anesthetic than that present in blood that has passed through tissues. As a result, left-to-right shunts offset the dilutional effects of a right-to-left shunt on the P_a.

P_A (alveolar partial pressure) ↔ ***P_a* (arterial partial pressure)** ↔ *P_{br}* (brain partial pressure):

The uptake of the inhaled anesthetics from the alveoli into the pulmonary capillary blood depends on its solubility in body tissue (the partition coefficients), the cardiac output, and the alveolar-venous partial pressure difference [3, 117]. A slower rate of induction occurs if there is a greater uptake of the agent and a greater difference between the inspired and alveolar concentrations. The blood:gas partition coefficient is the single most important factor in determining the speed of induction and recovery (◉ Table 10.5). A partition coefficient is a property of a chemical that describes its relative distribution at equilibrium given the same temperature, pressure, and volume. For anesthetics, the blood:gas coefficient is an important measure describing an inhalational agent's distribution between the blood and gas at the same partial pressure. A higher blood:gas coefficient correlates with higher blood solubility and thus a slower induction rate. A lower blood:gas coefficient transiently corresponds with a faster induction rate; for instance, nitrous, desflurane,

Table 10.5 Partition coefficients of inhaled anesthetics

Partition coefficient @ 37 ° C	Nitrous oxide	Halothane	Methoxyflurane	Enflurane	Isoflurane	Desflurane	Sevoflurane
Blood: gas	0.47	2.5	12	1.9	1.4	0.45	0.65
Brain: blood	1.1	2.9	2	1.5	2.6	1.3	1.7
Fat: blood	2.3	60	49	36	45	27	48

and sevoflurane have faster induction rates than isoflurane and halothane (see ◉ Table 10.5). The second-gas effect states that a high volume of uptake of one gas will accelerate the rate of increase of the P_A of a simultaneously administered second gas. For instance, a high uptake of nitrous oxide will accelerate the uptake of a second gas, such as a volatile anesthetic [118, 119].

The cardiac output, in the absence of pulmonary shunting, directly affects the uptake of the inhaled agent into the blood stream. As the cardiac output increases, a more rapid uptake will occur, which causes the rate of rise in the P_A to slow and the induction rate to decrease. Insoluble anesthetics display less effect from the cardiac output since little is taken up in the alveolar blood flow.

The final factor in determining the alveolar blood anesthetic uptake is the alveolar to venous partial pressure difference. A larger gradient slows the rise in P_A. These factors are determined by the tissue uptake of the anesthetic, primarily in vessel-rich groups that receive 75% of the cardiac output. The vessel-rich groups—including the brain, heart, and kidneys—equilibrate rapidly with the P_a. In approximately 3 time constants, 75% of the returning venous blood has the same partial pressure as the P_A.

P_A (alveolar partial pressure) ↔ P_a (arterial partial pressure) ↔ $\boldsymbol{P_{br}}$ **(brain partial pressure)**:

The anesthetic partial pressure in the brain is the final component, and the clinically significant end result of drug administration. It is affected by the blood:brain partition coefficient, the cerebral blood flow, and the arterial to venous partial pressure difference (◉ Table 10.4).

10.8.2 Elimination

Recovery from anesthesia is represented as the lowering of the anesthetic concentration in the brain tissue. A majority of modern anesthetic elimination is through exhalation; however, a small percentage is elimination in biotransformation or transcutaneous loss. The most important route of elimination is through ventilation and the alveolus. As such, many of the same factors that determine induction speed account for the speed of recovery: elimination of rebreathing, high fresh gas flows, low circuit absorption, decreased agent solubility, high cerebral blood flow, and increased ventilation [71, 72]. The main difference in recovery from anesthetics is that, in recovery, different tissues in the body have different partial pressures of the inhaled anesthetic. Therefore, recovery is not as controllable as induction [120]. Because nitrous oxide is eliminated so quickly, it can dilute alveolar oxygen and carbon dioxide, causing diffusion hypoxia. Clinically, this hypoxia is avoided by administering 100% oxygen for 5–10 min after discontinuing nitrous oxide [121].

10.9 Questions and Answers

Questions (Choose the Most Appropriate Answer)

1. The rate of uptake of an anesthetic gas from the lungs and hence the rate of induction with an inhalational anesthetic:
   A. Increases when a premedication has been administered prior to induction
   B. Is proportional to the solubility of the inhalational agent in the blood
   C. Is increased if tidal volumes are decreased
   D. Is dependent only on the MAC of the inhalational agent
   E. Correlates with the vapor pressure of the inhalational agent
2. A pediatric patient presents for an inhalational induction. The reason desflurane is not the most appropriate agent in this scenario is:
   A. Desflurane has a low blood:gas partition coefficient
   B. Desflurane has a high vapor pressure
   C. Desflurane may produce hepatitis postoperatively
   D. Desflurane may produce airway irritability
   E. Desflurane cannot attain adequate potency due to its higher MAC value
3. The anesthetic agent that should be avoided in patients with a history of seizure activity is:
   A. Halothane
   B. Isoflurane
   C. Desflurane
   D. Enflurane
   E. All of the above
4. While administering only an inhalational agent, you notice that the cardiac output of your patient has decreased. The agent that you are most likely using is:
   A. Halothane
   B. Isoflurane
   C. Desflurane
   D. Nitrous Oxide
   E. Sevoflurane
5. The recommended fresh gas flows when using sevoflurane is 2 L/min because:
   A. Sevoflurane biodegrades into peak concentrations of 50 μ(mu)mol/L of fluoride, which may cause nephrotoxicity.
   B. Metal degrades sevoflurane into hydrogen fluoride.
   C. Alkali, such as soda lime, can degrade sevoflurane compound A.
   D. Nitrous oxide remaining in the circuit can cause degradation of sevoflurane.

E. Sevoflurane is less pungent to airways with higher gas flows.

6. A patient presents to the operating room for a knee arthroscopy. She is a 65-year-old woman with obesity. Postoperatively, she develops fever, eosinophilia, jaundice, and elevated serum transaminase levels. Which is the most likely inhalational agent he received during his case?
   A. Halothane
   B. Isoflurane
   C. Desflurane
   D. Nitrous Oxide
   E. Sevoflurane
7. A patient undergoes a 25-h anesthetic for hand reconstruction after a crush injury with sevoflurane, nitrous oxide, fentanyl, and rocuronium. He is observed on postoperative day one to have megaloblastic anemia. What is the most likely source?:
   A. Sevoflurane
   B. Nitrous Oxide
   C. Fentanyl
   D. Inadequate Ventilation
   E. Rocuronium
8. The anesthetic agent that most can produce regional myocardial ischemia during tachycardia due to a preferential dilation of the normal coronary arteries is:
   A. Halothane
   B. Isoflurane
   C. Desflurane
   D. Nitrous Oxide
   E. Sevoflurane
9. The resting $PaCO_2$ is elevated in patients undergoing a general anesthetic with volatile agents primarily because:
   A. The respiratory rate is decreased.
   B. Central ventilator depression occurs.
   C. Bronchodilation causes an elevated $PaCO_2$.
   D. The patient becomes apneic.
   E. The tidal volumes are decreased.
10. Metabolism plays an important role in the emergence from anesthesia with which of the following agents:
   A. Halothane
   B. Methoxyflurane
   C. Desflurane
   D. Nitrous Oxide
   E. None of the above

Answers

1. **B**. Inhalational agents with high solubility in the blood are taken up very rapidly from the alveoli. This rapid uptake lowers their partial pressure in the lung and increases the latency for induction of anesthesia. Therefore, the higher the agent's solubility in the blood, the slower its induction rate. A low blood solubility of an agent is desirable as induction and recovery times are faster.
2. **D**. Desflurane is a pungent gas that can cause airway irritability during induction, manifested as breath-holding, salivation, coughing, and possibly laryngospasm. Although its low blood:gas partition coefficient would allow for a rapid induction, this agent is not well suited for pediatric inductions due to its airway irritability.
3. **D**. Enflurane has the tendency to induce convulsions (seizures) to decreased $PaCO_2$, MAC >2, and repetitive auditory stimuli. Isoflurane has anti-convulsive properties, and desflurane does not produce seizures. There are case reports that support sevoflurane can produce seizure activity.
4. **A**. At clinical anesthetic concentration, halothane decreases the mean arterial pressure by decreasing myocardial contractility and cardiac output; however, isoflurane, sevoflurane, and desflurane decrease systemic vascular resistance. Nitrous oxide increases cardiac output due to a mild increase in sympathetic tone.
5. **C**. Alkali, such as soda lime, can degrade sevoflurane into another proven nephritic product in animal models, compound A. Larger amounts of compound A are produced with lower gas flows, increased respiratory temperatures, high sevoflurane concentrations, anesthetics of long duration, and dessicated soda lime. It is clinically recommended to maintain fresh gas flows greater than 2 L/min to limit possible compound A production. Despite proven nephrotoxicity in rats, it has never shown postoperative renal impairment to indicate injury or toxicity in humans.
6. **A**. "Halothane hepatitis," or type II hepatotoxicity, has been reported in 1:5000 to 1:35,000 cases of halothane administration. This immune-mediated reaction is believed to result from the trifluoroacetylated protein adducts in the liver. Clinical symptoms of halothane hepatitis include fever, eosinophilia, and jaundice. Severe cases are associated with centrilobular necrosis that may lead to fulminant liver failure with a mortality rate of 50%.
7. **B**. Nitrous oxide irreversibly oxidizes the cobalt atom in vitamin B_{12}, including methionine synthetase and thymidylate synthetase. These enzymes are responsible for myelin formation and DNA synthesis; and thus, nitrous oxide has been questioned to cause bone marrow suppression. Megaloblastic changes are noticed in patients who receive nitrous oxide for duration of over 24 h.
8. **B**. Coronary steal syndrome may be associated with isoflurane. Sevoflurane and desflurane do not cause coronary steal syndrome. When the perfusion pressure

of a coronary artery is reduced, only the vessels that are capable of dilation can effectively compensate. Atherosclerotic coronary vessels cannot effectively dilate and blood is diverted further from these areas to those with the dilation, "stealing" the blood and causing ischemia.

9. **E**. Volatile agents cause rapid, shallow breathing. There is a reduction in the tidal volumes and minute ventilation. The increase in respiratory rate does not compensate for the amount of tidal volume decrease and hence causes an increase in $PaCO_2$.
10. **B**. As the most lipophilic inhaled anesthetic, methoxyflurane undergoes the most biotransformation at an estimated 70% of the drug administered. Only a small amount of the drug, taken into body tissue, is exhaled and respiratory clearance from muscle and fat can extend over a period of several days. Methoxyflurane is metabolized in both the kidneys and the liver and inorganic fluoride (F-) is produced during its metabolism in clinically significant quantities.

References

1. Neuman GG, Sidebotham G, Negoianu E, et al. Laparoscopy explosion hazards with nitrous oxide. Anesthesiology. 1993;78(5):875–9.
2. Bovill JG. Inhalation anaesthesia from dietyl ether to xenon. Handb Exp Pharmacol. 2008;182:121–42.
3. Yasuda N, Targ AG, Eiger EI 2nd. Solubility of I-653, sevoflurane, isoflurane, and halothane in human tissues. Anesth Analg. 1989;69(3):370–3.
4. Fernandez-Guisasola J, Gomez-Arnau JI, Cabrera Y, et al. Association between nitrous oxide and the incidence of postoperative nausea and vomiting in adults: a systematic review and meta-analysis. Anaesthesia. 2010;65(4):378–87.
5. Gmehling J, Onken U, Schulte HW. Vapor-liquid equilibria for the binary systems diethyl ether-halothane (1,1,1-trifluoro-2-bromo-2-chloroethane), halothane-methanol, and diethyl ether-methanol. J Chem Eng Data. 1980;25(1):29–32.
6. Stachnik J. Inhaled anesthetic agents. Am J Health Syst Pharm. 2006;63(7):623–34.
7. Cousins MJ, Greenstein LR, Hitt BA, Mazze RI. Metabolism and renal effects of enflurane in man. Anesthesiology. 1976;44(1):44–53.
8. Eger EI 2nd. Characteristics of anesthetic agents used for induction and maintenance of general anesthesia. Am J Health Syst Pharm. 2004;61(Suppl 4):S3–10.
9. Eger EI 2nd. Desflurane animal and human pharmacology: aspects of kinetics, safety, and MAC. Anesth Analg. 1992;75(4 Suppl):S3–7. discussion S8-9.
10. Andrews JJ, Johnston RV Jr. The new Tec 6 desflurane vaporizer. Anesth Analg. 1993;76(6):1338–41.
11. Eger EI 2nd. The pharmacology of inhaled anesthetics. J Crit Care. 2005;24(2):89–100
12. Franks NP, Lieb WR. Where do general anaesthetics act? Nature. 1978;274(5669):339–42.
13. Franks NP, Lieb WR. Do general anaesthetics act by competitive binding to specific receptors? Nature. 1984;310(5978):599–601.
14. Sonner JM, Antognini JF, Dutton RC, et al. Inhaled anesthetics and immobility: mechanisms, mysteries, and minimum alveolar anesthetic concentration. Anesth Analg. 2003;97(3):718–40.
15. Narahashi T, Aistrup GL, Lindstrom JM, et al. Ion channel modulation as the basis for general anesthesia. Toxicol Lett. 1998;100–101:185–91.
16. Frazer MJ, Lynch C 3rd. Halothane and isoflurane effects on Ca2 + fluxes of isolated myocardial sarcoplasmic reticulum. Anesthesiology. 1992;77(2):316–23.
17. Franks NP, Lieb WR. Which molecular targets are most relevant to general anaesthesia? Toxicol Lett. 1998;100–101:1–8.
18. Franks NP, Lieb WR. Molecular and cellular mechanisms of general anaesthesia. Nature. 1994;367(6464):607–14.
19. Jones MV, Harrison NL. Effects of volatile anesthetics on the kinetics of inhibitory postsynaptic currents in cultured rat hippocampal neurons. J Neurophysiol. 1993;70(4):1339–49.
20. cZimmerman SA, Jones MV, Harrison NL. Potentiation of gamma-aminobutyric acidA receptor Cl- current correlates with in vivo anesthetic potency. J Pharmacol Exp Ther. 1994;270(3):987–91.
21. Yamakura T, Harris RA. Effects of gaseous anesthetics nitrous oxide and xenon on ligand-gated ion channels. Comparison with isoflurane and ethanol. Anesthesiology. 2000;93(4):1095–101.
22. Mennerick S, Jetovic-Todorovic V, Todorovic SM, et al. Effect of nitrous oxide on excitatory and inhibitory synaptic transmission in hippocampal cultures. J Neurosci. 1998;18(23):9716–26.
23. Gyulai FE, Mintun MA, Firestone LLFE. Dose-dependent enhancement of in vivo GABA(A)-benzodiazepine receptor binding by isoflurane. Anesthesiology. 2001;95(3):585–93.
24. Patel AJ, Honore E, Lesage F, et al. Inhalational anesthetics activate two-pore-domain background K+ channels. Nat Neurosci. 1999;2(5):422–6.
25. Hemmings HC Jr. Sodium channels and the synaptic mechanisms of inhaled anaesthetics. Br J Anaesth. 2009;103(1):61–9.
26. Nishikawa K, MacIver MB. Excitatory synaptic transmission mediated by NMDA receptors is more sensitive to isoflurane than are non-NMDA receptor-mediated responses. Anesthesiology. 2000;92(1):228–36.
27. Kendig JJ. In vitro networks: subcortical mechanisms of anaesthetic action. Br J Anaesth. 2002;89(1):91–101.
28. Daniels S, Roberts RJ. Post-synaptic inhibitory mechanisms of anaesthesia; glycine receptors. Toxicol Lett. 1998;100–101:71–6.
29. Cheng G, Kendig JJ. Enflurane directly depresses glutamate AMPA and NMDA currents in mouse spinal cord motor neurons independent of actions on GABAA or glycine receptors. Anesthesiology. 2000;93(4):1075–84.
30. Flood P, Ramirez-Latorre J, Role L. Alpha 4 beta 2 neuronal nicotinic acetylcholine receptors in the central nervous system are inhibited by isoflurane and propofol, but alpha 7-type nicotinic acetylcholine receptors are unaffected. Anesthesiology. 1997;86(4):859–65.
31. Raines DE, Claycomb RJ, Forman SA. Nonhalogenated anesthetic alkanes and perhalogenated nonimmobilizing alkanes inhibit alpha(4)beta(2) neuronal nicotinic acetylcholine receptors. Anesth Analg. 2002;95(3):573–7.
32. Cordero-Erausquin M, Marubio LM, Klink R, Changeux JP. Nicotinic receptor function: new perspectives from knockout mice. Trends Pharmacol Sci. 2000;21(6):211–7.
33. Campagna JA, Miller KW, Forman SA, Mechanisms JA. Of actions of inhaled anesthetics. N Engl J Med. 2003;348(21):2110–24.

34. Eger EI 2nd, Stevens WC, Cromwell TH. The electroencephalogram in man anesthetized with forane. Anesthesiology. 1971;35 (5):504–8.
35. Oshima EE, Urabe N, Shingu K, Mori K. Anticonvulsant actions of enflurane on epilepsy models in cats. Anesthesiology. 1985;63 (1):29–40.
36. Koblin DD, Eger EI 2nd, Johnson BH, et al. Are Convulsant Gases Also Anesthetics? Anesth Analg. 1981;60(7):464–70.
37. Neigh JL, Garman JK, Harp JR. The electroencephalographic pattern during anesthesia with ethrane: effects of depth of anesthesia, $PaCo_2$, and nitrous oxide. Anesthesiology. 1971;35(5):482–7.
38. Oda Y, Toriyama S, Tanaka K, et al. The effect of dexmedetomidine on electrocorticography in patients with temporal lobe epilepsy under sevoflurane anesthesia. Anesth Analg. 2007;105 (5):1272–7.
39. Kaisti KK, Jaaskelainen SK, Rinne JO, et al. Epileptiform discharges during 2 MAC sevoflurane anesthesia in two healthy volunteers. Anesthesiology. 1999;91(6):1952–5.
40. Mielck F, Stephen H, Buhre W, et al. Effects of 1 MAC desflurane on cerebral metabolism, blood flow and carbon dioxide reactivity in humans. Br J Anaesth. 1998;81(2):155–60.
41. Torri G. Inhalation anesthetics: a review. Minerva Anestesiol. 2010;76(3):215–28.
42. Adams RW, Gronert GA, Smith TM, Michenfekder JD. Halothane, hypocapnia and cerebrospinal fluid pressure in neurosurgery. In: Brock M, Deitz, editors. Intracranial pressure. New York: Springer; 1972. p. 320–5.
43. McKay RE, Sonner J, McKay WR. Inhaled anesthetics. In: Stoelting RK, Miller RD, editors. Basics in anesthesia. 5th ed. Phildelphia: Churchill Livingstone Elsevier; 2007. p. 77–96
44. Hornbein TF, Eger EI 2nd, Winter PM, et al. The minimum alveolar concentration of nitrous oxide in man. Anesth Analg. 1982;61(7):553–6.
45. Eger EI. Isoflurane (Forane®): A compendium and reference. Madison, Wisconsin: Ohio Medical Products; 1981.
46. Khan KS, Hayes I, Buggy DJ. Pharmacology of anaesthetic agents II: inhalation anaesthetic agents. Contin Educ Anaesth Crit Care Pain. 2014;14(3):106–11.
47. Moore MA, Weiskopf RB, Eger EI 2nd, et al. Arrhythmogenic doses of epinephrine are similar during desflurane or isoflurane anesthesia in humans. Anesthesiology. 1993;79(5):943–7.
48. Navarro R, Weiskopf RB, Moore MA, et al. Humans anesthetized with sevoflurane or isoflurane have similar arrhythmic response to epinephrine. Anesthesiology. 1994;80(3):545–9.
49. Sakai EM, Connolly LA, Klauck JA. Inhalation anesthesiology and volatile liquid anesthetics: focus on isoflurane, desflurane, and sevoflurane. Pharmacotherapy. 2005;25(12):1773–88.
50. Doi M, Ikeda K. Respiratory effects of sevoflurane. Anesth Analg. 1987;66(3):241–4.
51. Lockhart SH, Rampil IJ, Yasuda N, et al. Depression of ventilation by desflurane in humans. Anesthesiology. 1991;74(3):484–8.
52. Lam AM, Clement JL, Chung DC, Knill RL. Respiratory effects of nitrous oxide during enflurane anesthesia in humans. Anesthesiology. 1982;56(4):298–303.
53. Goff MJ, Shahbaz R, Arain SR, et al. Absence of bronchodilation during desflurane anesthesia: a comparison to sevoflurane and thiopental. Anesthesiology. 2000;93(2):404–8.
54. Jones RM, Cashman JN, Mant TG. Clinical impressions and cardiorespiratory effects of a new fluorinated inhalation anaesthetic, desflurane (I–653), in volunteers. Br J Anaesth. 1990;64 (1):11–5.
55. Kong CF, Chew ST, Ip-Yam PC. Intravenous opioids reduce airway irritation during induction of anaesthesia with desflurane in adults. Br J Anaesth. 2000;85(3):364–7.
56. Wilkes AR, Hall JE, Wright E, Grundler S. The effect of humidification and smoking habit on the incidence of adverse airway events during deepening of anaesthesia with desflurane. Anaesthesia. 2000;55(7):685–9.
57. Vitez TS, Miller RD, Eger EI 2nd, et al. Comparison in vitro of isoflurane and halothane potentiation of d- tubocurarine and succinylcholine meeting abstractss. Anesthesiology. 1974;41 (1):53–6.
58. Papadimos TJ, Almasri M, Padgett JC, Rush JEA. Suspected case of delayed onset malignant hyperthermia with desflurane anesthesia. Anesth Analg. 2004;98(2):548–9.
59. Ducart A, Adnet P, Renaud B, et al. Malignant hyperthermia during sevoflurane administration. Anesth Analg. 1995;80(3): 609–11.
60. Ochiai R, Toyoda Y, Takeda J, et al. Possible association of malignant hyperthermia with sevoflurane anesthesia. Anesth Analg. 1992;74(4):616–8.
61. Merkel G, Eger EI 2nd. A comparative study of halothane and halopropane anesthesia including method for determining equipotency. Anesthesiology. 1963:346–57.
62. Hoenemann CW, Halene-Holtgraeve TB, Booke M, et al. Delayed onset of malignant hyperthermia in desflurane anesthesia. Anesth Analg. 2003;96(1):165–7.
63. Gillmeister I, Schummer C, Hommann M, Schummer W. Delayed onset of malignant hyperthermia crisis during a living donor liver transplantation caused by sevoflurane. Article in German. Anaesthesiol Intensivmed Notfallmed Schmerzther. 2004;39(3):153–6.
64. Eger EI 2nd, Eisenkraft JB, Weiskopf. The pharmacology of inhaled anesthetics. San Francisco (CA). Not in PubMed. 2002
65. Whelan E, Wood AJ, Koshakji R, et al. Halothane inhibition of propranolol metabolism is stereoselective. Anesthesiology. 1989;71(4):561–4.
66. Reilly CS, Wood AJ, Koshakji R, Wood M. The effect of halothane on drug disposition: contribution of changes in intrinsic drug metabolizing capacity and hepatic blood flow. Anesthesiology. 1985;63(1):70–6.
67. Eger EI 2nd, Lasiter MJ, Winegar R, et al. Compound A induces sister chromatid exchanges in Chinese hamster ovary cells. Anesthesiology. 1997;86(4):918–22.
68. Flippo TS, Holder WD Jr. Neurologic degeneration associated with nitrous oxide anesthesia in patients with vitamin B12 deficiency. Arch Surg. 1993;128(12):1391–5.
69. Stevenson G, Hall SC, Rudnick S, et al. The effect of anesthetic agents on the human immune response. Anesthesiology. 1990;72 (3):542–52.
70. Stollings LM, Jia LJ, Tang P, et al. Immune modulation by volatile anesthetics. Anesthesiology. 2016;125(2):399–411.
71. Yasuda N, Lockhart S, Eger EI 2nd, et al. Kinetics of desflurane, isoflurane, and halothane in humans. Anesthesiology. 1991;74 (3):489–98.
72. Yasuda N, Lockhart S, Eger EI 2nd, et al. Comparison of kinetic of sevoflurane and isoflurane in humans. Anesth Analg. 1991;72 (3):316–24.
73. Krishna DR, Klotz U. Extraheptatic metabolism of drugs in humans. Clin Pharmacokinet. 1994;26(2):144–60.
74. Eiger EI 2nd. Partition coefficients of I-653 in human blood, saline, and olive oil. Anesth Analg. 1987;66(10):971–3.

75. Spracklin DK, Thummel KE, Kharasch ED. Human reductive halothane metabolism in vitro is catalyzed by cytochrome P450 2A6 and 3A 4. Drug Metab Dispos. 1996;24(9):976–83.
76. Summary of the national halothane study. Possible association between halothane anesthesia and postoperative hepatic necrosis. JAMA. 1966;197(10):775–88.
77. Gut J, Christen U, Huwyler J. Mechanisms of halothane toxicity: novel insights. Pharmacol Ther. 1993;58(2):133–55.
78. Ray DC, Drummond GB. Halothane hepatitis. Br J Anesth. 1991;67(1):84–99.
79. Kenna JG. Immunoallergic drug-induced hepatitis: lessons from halothane. J Hepatol. 1997;26(Suppl 1):5–12.
80. Yoshimura N, Holaday DA, Fiserova-Bergerova V. Metabolism of methoxyflurane in man. Anesthesiology. 1976;44(5):372–9.
81. Vandam LD. Report on methoxyflurane. Anesthesiology. 1966;27(5):534–5.
82. Crandell WB, Pappas SG, MacDonald A. Nephrotoxicity associated with methoxyflurane anesthesia. Anesthesiology. 1966;27 (5):591–607.
83. Cousins MJ, Mazze RI. Methoxyflurane nephrotoxicity: a study of dose response in man. JAMA. 1973;225(13):1611–6.
84. Mazze RI. Methoxyflurane revisited: tale of an anesthetic from cradle to grave. Anesthesiology. 2006;105(4):843–6.
85. Kharasch ED, Thummel KE. Identification of cytochrome P450 2E1 as the predominant enzyme catalysing human liver microsomal defluorination of sevoflurane, isoflurane, and methoxyflurane. Anesthesiology. 1993;79(4):795–807.
86. Koblin DD. Characteristics and implications of desflurane metabolism and toxicity. Anesth Analg. 1992;75(4 Suppl):S10–6.
87. Baxter PJ, Garton K, Kharasch ED. Mechanistic aspects of carbon monoxide formation from volatile anesthetics. Anesthesiology. 1998;89(4):929–41.
88. Wissing H, Kuhn I, Warnken U, Dudziak R. Carbon monoxide production from desflurane, enflurane, halothane, isoflurane, and sevoflurance with dry soda lime. Anesthesiology. 2001;95 (5):1205–12.
89. Kharasch ED. Biotransformation of sevoflurane. Anesth Analg. 1995;81(6 Suppl):S27-38.
90. Anders MW. Formation and toxicity of anesthetic degradation products. Annu Rev Pharmacol Toxicol. 2005;45:147–76.
91. Iyer RA, Anders MW. Cysteine conjugate beta-lyase-dependent biotransformation of the cysteine Sconjugates of the sevoflurane degradation product compound A in humans, nonhuman primate, and rat kidney cytosol and mitochondria. Anesesthesiology. 1996;85(6):1454–61.
92. Kharasch ED. Sevoflurane and the kidney: a current perspective. Anesth Clin North Am Annu Anesthetic Pharmacol. 1996;1:205–22.
93. Kharasch ED, Schroeder JI, Sheffels P, Liggitt HD. Influence of sevoflurane on the metabolism and renal effects of compound A in rats. Anesthesiology. 2005;103(6):1183–8.
94. Rappaport B, Mellon RD, Simone A, Woodcock J. Defining safe use of anesthesia in children. N Engl J Med. 2011;364(15):1387–90.
95. Hudson AE, Hemmings HC Jr. Are anaesthetics toxic to the brain? Br J Anaesth. 2011;107(1):30–7.
96. Jevtovic-Todorovic V, Hartman RE, Izumi Y, et al. Early exposure to common anesthetic agents causes widespread neurodegeneration in the developing rat brain and persistent learning deficits. J Neurosci. 2003;23(3):876–82.
97. Loepke AW, Soriano SG. An assessment of the effects of general anesthetics on developing brain structure and neurocognitive function. Anesth Analg. 2008;106(6):1681–707.
98. Zou X, Liu F, Zhang X, et al. Inhalation anesthetic-induced neuronal damage in the developing rhesus monkey. Neurotoxicol Teratol. 2011;33(5):592–7.
99. Wilder RT, Flick RP, Sprung J, et al. Early exposure to anesthesia and learning disabilities in a populationbased cohort. Anesthesiology. 2009;110(4):796–804.
100. Hansen TG, Pedersen JK, Henneberg SW, et al. Academic performance in adolescence after inguinal hernia repair in infancy: a nationwide cohort study. Anesthesiology. 2011;114 (5):1076–85.
101. Sun LS, Li G, DiMaggio CJ, et al. Feasibility and pilot study of the Pediatric Anesthesia NeuroDevelopment Assessment (PANDA) project. J Neurosurg Anesthesiol. 2012;24(4):382–8.
102. Eger EI 2nd. Age, minimum alveolar anesthetic concentration, and minimum alveolar anesthetic concentration-awake. Anesth Analg. 2001;93(4):947–53.
103. Hall RI, Sullivan JA. Does cardiopulmonary bypass alter enflurane requirements for anesthesia? Anesthesiology. 1990;73 (2):249–55.
104. Al Q, Eger EI 2nd, Tinker JH. Determination and applications of MAC. Anesthesiology. 1980;53(4):315–34.
105. Vieira E, Cleaton-Jones P, Auston JC, et al. Effects of low concentrations of nitrous oxide on rat fetuses. Anesth Analg. 1980;59(3):175–7.
106. Fink B, Shepard T, Blandau R. Teratogenic activity of nitrous oxide. Nature. 1967;214(5084):146–8.
107. Rowland AS, Baird DD, Weinberg CR, et al. Reduced fertility among women employed as dental assistants exposed to high levels of nitrous oxide. N Engl J Med. 1992;327(14):993–7.
108. Rowland AS, Baird DD, Shore DL, et al. Nitrous oxide and spontaneous abortion in female dental assistants. Am J Epidemiol. 1995;141(6):531–8.
109. Basford AB, Fink BR. The teratogenicity of halothane in the rat. Anesthesiology. 1968;29(6):1167–73.
110. Wharton RS, Wilson AI, Mazze RI, et al. Fetal morphology in mice exposed to halothane. Anesthesiology. 1979;51(6):532–7.
111. Corbett TH, Cornell RG, Endres JL, Lieding K. Birth defects among children of nurse-anesthetists. Anesthesiology. 1974;41 (4):341–4.
112. Occupational disease among operating room personnel: a national study. Report of an Ad Hoc Committee on the Effect of Trace Anesthetics on the Health of Operating Room Personnel, American Society of Anesthesiologists. Anesthesiology. 1974;41(4):321–40.
113. Pharoah PO, Aberman E, Doyle P, Chamberlain G. Outcome of pregnancy among women in anaesthetic practice. Lancet. 1977;309(8001):34–6.
114. Strum DP, Eger EI 2nd, Unadkat JD, et al. Age affects the pharmacokinetics of inhaled anesthetics in humans. Anesth Analg. 1991;73(3):310–8.
115. Miller RD, Pardo MC, editors. Basics of anesthesia. 8th ed. Philadelphia: Saunders; 2015.
116. Eger EI 2nd. The effect of inspired concentration on the rate of rise of alveolar concentration. Anesthesiology. 1963;24:153–7.
117. Eger EI 2nd. Desflurane (Suprane): A compendium and reference. Anaquest: Nutley, NJ; 1993.
118. Stoelting RK, Eger EI 2nd. An additional explanation for the second gas effect: a concentrating effect. Anesthesiology. 1969;30(3):273–7.
119. Epstein RM, Rackow H, Salanitre E, Wolf GL. Influence of the concentration effect on the uptake of anesthetic mixtures: the second gas effect. Anesthesiology. 1964;25:364–71.

120. Carpenter RI, Eger EI 2nd, Johnson BH, et al. Pharmacokinetics of inhaled anesthetics in humans: measurements during and after the simultaneous administration of enflurane, halothane, isoflurane, methoxyflurane, and nitrous oxide. Anesth Analg. 1986;65(6):575–82.
121. Fink BR. Diffusion anoxia. Anesthesiology. 1955;16(4):511–9.

Cardiovascular Anatomy and Pharmacology 11

Maria Bauer

Abstract

Patients in the perioperative period often receive agents that affect hemodynamic variables such as heart rhythm and rate, blood pressure, or cardiac output. This chapter reviews cardiovascular anatomy, the effects of medications on the cardiovascular system, and the current guidelines.

Keywords

Cardiac anatomy • Cardiovascular pharmacology • Electrophysiology • Antiarrhythmic agents • Pulmonary hypertension

Key Points

The major determinants of myocardial O_2 *supply* are coronary blood flow and arterial O_2 content. Coronary blood flow is determined by the patency of the coronaries, coronary perfusion pressure, and coronary vascular resistance.

The major determinants of myocardial O_2 *demand* are heart rate, inotropic state, and wall tension (which is the function of intracavitary pressure, radius and wall thickness, preload and afterload).

Critical O_2 delivery is the point at which the extraction ratio is maximized, and any further incongruence between demand and supply will lead to tissue hypoxia.

In the perioperative setting, the continuation of long-standing beta-blocker therapy is recommended.

Beta-blockers should not be started on the day of surgery in beta-blocker-naïve patients.

Patients with coronary artery disease undergoing surgical coronary revascularization should be administered a beta-blocker before surgery.

Although recent perioperative guidelines suggested continuing angiotensin-converting enzyme (ACE) inhibitors/angiotensin receptor blockers (ARBs) before non-cardiac surgery, adverse circulatory effects during anesthesia in patients chronically treated with ACE inhibitors/ARBs have led to the recommendation that these drugs be discontinued 24 h before surgery.

Epinephrine inhibits uterine contractions, especially during the second stage of labor.

11.1 Part 1: Cardiac Anatomy

11.1.1 Development and Anatomy of the Heart

The heart is a conical hollow muscular organ located between the lungs in the mid-mediastinal portion of the thorax, suspended in the pericardial sac. As a dual pump, it maintains unidirectional blood flow to the body and the lungs by its rhythmical torsion and untwisting throughout the series of cardiac cycles. Its receiving chambers (the left and right atrium, composed of two myocardial layers) and its pumping chambers (the left and right ventricle, composed of three layers of myocardium building up the two separate vortices each ventricle) are structurally separated by their respective interchamber septa corresponding with the long axis of the heart and are electrically isolated by the left and right fibrous rings comprising the fibrous cardiac skeleton in the short axis of the heart, perpendicular to the long axis [1].

A Brief Review of Cardiogenesis

The development of the cardiovascular system begins on day 17 of gestation, when mesoderm-derived blood islands, consisting of endothelial cells and hemoblasts, begin to form. These blood islands coalesce to form a pair of endothelial heart tubes, which on day 21 fuse into a single

M. Bauer (✉)
Department of Anesthesiology and Critical Care Medicine, The Johns Hopkins Hospital, Baltimore, MD, USA
e-mail: MABAUER@augusta.edu

M. Argalious et al. (eds.), *Basic Sciences in Anesthesia*,
https://doi.org/10.1007/978-3-031-60203-0_11

primitive heart tube with a cranial inflow (arterial) and a caudal outflow (venous) end. This primitive heart tube is divided into five regions: truncus arteriosus, bulbus cordis, primitive ventricle, primitive atrium, and sinus venosus. Initial contractions occur on days 21–22, and unidirectional circulation is established by week 4. From weeks 4–7, folding and septation of the heart and the great vessels take place, critical to the development of the four chambers and the normal embryonic vascular circuit. In the developed heart, the atrial chambers lie cephalad and to the right of their corresponding ventricles, and the right-sided chambers lie anterior to their corresponding left-sided chambers. The atrial and ventricular septation is summarized later.

11.1.2 Review of the Gross Anatomy of the Heart

11.1.2.1 Fibrous Skeleton

The fibrous skeleton of the heart is a framework of four dense collagen rings around the atrioventricular (AV) and semilunar valves, as well as the left and right fibrous trigones (also known as the central fibrous body), and the membranous portion of the interatrial and interventricular septum. Its main component is the central fibrous body, where the leaflets of all four cardiac valves converge. The fibrous skeleton reinforces the ostia of the valves and prevents the annuli from overdistension by resisting forces of pressure developing through the cardiac cycle. It provides attachment for the valvular leaflets and cusps, as well as for some of the musculature of the atrial and ventricular wall. It is electrically impermeable, only allowing electrical propagation from the atrioventricular node across the right fibrous trigone to the bundle of His. Chronic degenerative changes and calcium deposition into the collagen skeleton result in delayed conduction and depolarization, arrhythmias, the rigidity of the valvular ostia, restricted leaflet opening, or leaflet malcoaptation.

11.1.2.2 Interatrial Septum

The interatrial septum is a blade-shaped wall between the left and right atrium. Its development begins during the fifth gestational week with the septum primum growing from the posterior wall of the primary atrium toward the endocardial cushion, formed within the atrioventricular canal. With the incomplete fusion of the septum primum and the endocardial cushion, a progressively diminishing space above the endocardial cushion, the ostium (also known as foramen) primum remains. During this process, small coalescing perforations in the upper portion of the septum primum create the ostium (or foramen) secundum. Concurrently, a second septum, the septum secundum begins to form to the *right* of the septum primum, growing from the anterior wall, and partially covering the foramen primum. Its growth stops at the seventh week of gestation, leaving a gap known as the foramen ovale. This is essential in reducing pulmonary blood flow through the inactive fetal lungs.

The foramen ovale is continuous with the ostium secundum and is covered by the septum secundum on its *left* side. As a result of normal adaptive changes in the neonatal circulation, the decreasing pulmonary vascular resistance (PVR) and the resultant reversal of interatrial pressure gradient result in the permanent functional closure of the foramen ovale. In one-third of the population, incomplete fusion between the septum primum and the septum secundum results in a residual flap valve and a probe patent foramen ovale (PFO).

Excessive apoptosis within the septum primum, or incomplete development of the septum secundum results in an atrial septal defect (ASD), the most common congenital heart defect to manifest in adulthood:

There are four types of ASD, the most common being the secundum type ASD, accounting for 80–90% of all ASDs. The secundum type ASD is located centrally, it is larger than a PFO, and it is commonly associated with mitral valve prolapse.

The primum type ASD is less common, it represents 2–3% of ASDs. It is located in the lower portion of the interatrial septum, and it is associated with endocardial cushion defects, AV-valve abnormalities, or ventricular septal defects such as in Down syndrome.

The sinus venosus ASD represents 2–10% of ASDs. It is associated with abnormal pulmonary venous return.

The fourth type, the coronary sinus ASD or unroofed coronary sinus is the least common. It results from incomplete septation between the inferior portion of the left atrium and the coronary sinus and is commonly associated with a persistent left superior vena cava.

ASDs often remain clinically silent with preserved normal left atrial size; however, long-standing left-to-right shunting and resultant dilatation of the right-sided chambers along with persistent pulmonary hypertension may reverse the direction of the shunt, resulting in hypoxemia and Eisenmenger physiology.

11.1.2.3 Interventricular Septum

The interventricular septum (IVS) separates the left and right ventricles from one another. Under physiologic pressure and filling conditions, its convexity is bowing into the right ventricle. Its margins are marked externally by the anterior and posterior interventricular grooves. The upper, posterior part of the interventricular septum is thin and constitutes the membranous interventricular septum. The greater, anterior portion is the muscular interventricular septum.

During cardiogenesis, along with the atrial septation, concurrent ventricular septation is also taking place. With the development of the endocardial cushions and the atrioventricular separation, there is tissue growth between the left and the right sides of the developing atrioventricular canal. This is the muscular portion of the interventricular septum, growing from the inferior portion of the ventricle toward the endocardial cushion. As the muscular IVS reaches the endocardial cushion, a small interventricular foramen remains. This is closed by tissue growth from the endocardial cushion, connective tissue from the muscular IVS, as well as tissue from the septation of the truncus pulmonalis and the conus arteriosus. Inadequate contribution from either component results in different types of ventricular septal defects.

11.1.3 Chambers and Valves of the Right Heart

11.1.3.1 Right Atrium

The right atrium is the cardiac chamber receiving the systemic and cardiac venous return via the superior and inferior vena cava (SVC and IVC) and the coronary sinus. It is divided into three components.

The venous component receives deoxygenated blood from the SVC and the IVC. At the inferior cavoatrial junction lies the Eustachian valve, important before birth in directing blood from the IVC to the left atrium across the foramen ovale. A network of fine filamentous strands, the Chiari network, may be seen in this region. The variably sized Eustachian valve and Chiari network are normal variants within the right atrium.

The second component is the vestibule, which converges into the leaflets of the tricuspid valve, and the third is the appendage (also known as the auricle). The right atrial appendage has a wide junction with both the vestibule and the venous component. The vestibuloauricular junction is identified by the terminal groove, the external marking of the prominent terminal crest on the internal surface. A consistent feature of the right atrial anatomy is the extension of the auricular pectinate muscles beyond the appendage to the atrioventricular junction.

The sinus node, a cluster of specialized myocardial cells capable of spontaneous electrical impulse generation, lies at the superior cavoatrial junction at the terminal groove. It is supplied by the nodal artery, arising from the right coronary artery in 55% of cases, or the proximal left circumflex artery in the remaining 45%. The atrioventricular node is embedded into the floor of the right atrium, near the opening of the coronary sinus. Preserving blood flow to the sinus node and other conductive tissues is key to avoiding arrhythmias and other conduction abnormalities.

11.1.3.2 Tricuspid Valve

The tricuspid valve is located nearly vertically behind the aortic valve. With a valve area of 4–6 cm^2, it is the largest of the four valves in the heart. Its annular plane is saddle-shaped and is apically displaced relative to that of the mitral valve. A displacement index greater than 8 mm/m^2 (body surface area) suggests the presence of Ebstein's anomaly. Its three leaflets are the septal, anterior, and posterior tricuspid valve leaflets, attached by their chordae tendineae to the right ventricular papillary muscles (true chords), or, not uncommonly, directly to the septum (false chords). The subvalvular apparatus of the tricuspid valve is variable. Most commonly, the chordae tendineae originate from two or three papillary muscles, the anterior being the most prominent; the posterior, which is usually less prominent and may have several subdivisions; and the septal, which is the least prominent or may be entirely absent.

11.1.3.3 Right Ventricle

The right ventricle is the most anterior of the four chambers of the heart, located immediately behind the sternum. Its geometry is complex: The right ventricle is crescent-shaped when viewed in the short axis, and triangular when viewed longitudinally. Current guidelines identify its walls as the anterior, inferior, and lateral free walls. Medially, the right ventricle shares the septum with its left-sided counterpart. For purposes of functional quantification, these walls are further divided into basal, mid, and apical segments.

Anatomically and functionally, the right ventricle is composed of three portions: the smooth muscular right ventricular inflow tract, the apical trabecular, and the right ventricular outflow tract. The inlet portion encircles the tricuspid valve. The trabecular portion of the right ventricle extends into the apical region. The wall of the ventricle is thin here, making it vulnerable to perforation by catheters and electrodes.

The most prominent of the trabeculas is the septomarginal trabecula. It carries part of the right bundle branch of the conduction system. It was once wrongly thought to prevent the right ventricle from overdistention, hence the name "moderator band." The septomarginal trabecula originates from the base of the septum, and it divides into an anterior limb that supports the pulmonic valve cusps, and a posterior limb, from which the medial papillary muscle arises. Its main mass extends from the base of the septum to the apex and divides into smaller muscle ridges. Two of these are particularly prominent, one giving rise to the anterior papillary muscle, and the other crossing the right ventricular cavity as the moderator band.

The outlet portion consists of the circumferential muscular infundibulum that supports the pulmonic valve, which is the only one of the cardiac valves with no single ring-like annulus. It is supplied by the conus branch of the right coronary artery.

11.1.3.4 Pulmonic Valve

The pulmonic valve separates the right ventricular outflow tract from the pulmonary artery. It is located anteriorly and to the left of the aortic valve. It is a semilunar valve formed by three cusps, labeled anterior (non-septal), left, and right, each with a fibrous nodule at the midpoint of their free edges. The leaflets coapt via their crescent-shaped surfaces. The cusps of the pulmonic valve are formed by endocardial folds that are supported by internal dense collagenous plates as well as elastic connective tissue, continuous with the fibrous skeleton of the heart. They are thinner than the cusps of the aortic valve and, lacking fibrous continuity with the septal leaflet of the tricuspid valve, are supported only by a prominent ridge of the posterior subpulmonary infundibular musculature. This is the supraventricular crest that separates the pulmonic and tricuspid valves from one another and supports the semilunar attachments of the pulmonic valve. Surgical incisions made through this crest may run toward the interventricular septum and jeopardize the right coronary artery.

11.1.4 Chambers and Valves of the Left Heart

11.1.4.1 Left Atrium

Oxygen-rich blood returning from the lungs via the four pulmonary veins is received first by the left atrium. The left atrium has three basic components: first, the largest, smooth-walled pulmonary venous component; second, the vestibule; and third, the left atrial appendage. The wall of the vestibule is continuous with both the venous component and the posterior (mural) leaflet of the mitral valve, and may affect normal valvular function when left atrial dilation is present. Pectinate muscles are confined almost exclusively to the appendage in the left atrium. The flap valve of the fossa ovalis is found on the left atrial side of the interatrial septum.

Recurrent, symptomatic, drug-refractory atrial fibrillation most often originates from the pulmonary veins or their pulmonary venous ostia. Circumferential or segmental ablation of potential triggers is considered effective means to control refractory atrial fibrillation, as scar forming is thought to prevent the propagation of abnormal signals to the rest of the atrial musculature. The ablation and mapping catheters are inserted via the femoral or jugular veins and are placed through separate transseptal punctures. Most often, radiofrequency energy is used to make ablation lesions around the pulmonary vein ostia. In the presence of a left atrial appendage thrombus, or inability to anticoagulate in the 30-day peri- and post-procedural period, pulmonary vein isolation for atrial fibrillation ablation is contraindicated. A rare, frequently disabling, sometimes fatal complication of the procedure is an *atrio-esophageal fistula* resulting from thermal damage. Other potential complications are cardiac tamponade, arrhythmias or atrioventricular block, embolic events, valvular complications, or peripheral vascular damage.

11.1.4.2 Mitral Valve

The bileaflet mitral valve is located between the left atrium and left ventricle, embedded into the saddle-shaped mitral valve annulus. It serves as a unidirectional valve directing blood from the atrium toward the ventricle by passively opening during diastole and closing in systole, as determined by the pressure gradient between the chambers.

The mitral valve apparatus consists of the left atrial wall, the annulus, the anterior leaflet attached to the aortic root, the posterior leaflet attached to the left atrial myocardium, the chordae tendineae attached to the ventricular side of the mitral valve leaflets, and the anteromedial and posterolateral papillary muscles.

The anterior leaflet of the mitral valve is wide. It occupies about one-third of the annular circumference and forms the anterior portion of the left ventricular outflow tract. In contrast with the posterior leaflet, its free edge has no indentations. The posterior (mural) leaflet is narrower, it occupies about two-thirds of the annular circumference, and it is further divided into three scallops by two clefts. Because the posterior aspect of the mitral valve annulus contains little fibrous tissue, the posterior leaflet, especially the middle scallop, is more prone to prolapse than the anterior. The circumflex artery courses near the left half of the posterior leaflet, whereas the right half is in close proximity to the coronary sinus and the arterial branch supplying the AV node.

The mitral valve leaflets are supported by a dense collagen annulus. The most vulnerable portion of the mitral valve annulus is its aspect continuous with the right fibrous trigone, due to the proximity of the atrioventricular node and the penetrating bundle of His.

The muscular components of the mitral valve apparatus are the anteromedial and posterolateral papillary muscles. The anteromedial papillary muscle is more prominent and is supplied by the left coronary system. The posteromedial papillary muscle is smaller and is supplied by the right coronary artery. The mitral valve closes with the of the papillary muscles and opens when they relax. Papillary rupture, as a result of ischemia, will result in acute mitral regurgitation. Because the anterolateral papillary muscle is supplied by both the left anterior descending (LAD) artery and the left circumflex artery, its ischemic dysfunction is relatively uncommon. In about 60–65% of individuals, the posteromedial papillary muscle was found to be perfused by a single vessel, most commonly by the right coronary artery.

11.1.4.3 Left Ventricle

The left ventricle (LV) is the largest and thickest chamber of the heart. It receives oxygenated blood from the left atrium during diastole, to transfer it to the body across the aortic valve during systole. Relative to the right ventricle, it is located laterally and posteriorly. Its superior, widest aspect is termed the base, leaning upward and toward the right shoulder, opposing its apex, pointing down and to the left. By consensus, its four walls are termed septal, and the free anterior, inferior, and lateral walls. For purposes of functional quantification, these are further divided into basal, mid, and apical segments.

Morphologically, the left ventricle also has an inlet, a fine trabecular, and an outlet component. The inlet portion extends from the mitral valve annulus to the origins of the papillary muscles and contains the mitral valve apparatus. In contrast to the coarsely trabeculated right ventricle, the left ventricular free wall is finely trabeculated. The trabeculation extends to the apex, where, due to the progressively decreasing number of myocardial fibers, the wall thickness is thin. The left ventricle outflow tract differs from that of the right ventricle, and in that it is anatomically and functionally contiguous with the inlet via the aortic-mitral continuity. The left ventricular outflow tract supports the aortic valve, and its septal portion, in contrast with the primarily muscular right ventricular infundibulum, includes the membranous interventricular septum. The left bundle branch of the conduction system courses posteriorly to the membranous septum between the right and non-coronary cusps of the aortic valve.

The interventricular septum is formed by subendocardial myocardial fibers of both the left and the right ventricle, intermingled with circumferentially arranged fibers derived from the left ventricle. For this reason, in a normally functioning heart, the septum thickens toward the left ventricle during systole. During contraction, the high left ventricular pressure along with the septum provides a "splint" against which the right ventricle is able to shorten, thereby contributing to the emptying of the right ventricle (systolic ventricular interdependence). Under pathologic conditions, for example, during acute right ventricular volume or pressure overload, or due to conduction abnormalities or pacemaker activation, the septum may appear flat, or move paradoxically toward the right ventricle during systole. Blood flow to the anterior two-thirds of the septum is supplied by the septal perforators of the left anterior descending artery. The posterior one-third is supplied by the distal branches of the right coronary artery.

The two papillary muscles of the left ventricle arise from the anterolateral and posteromedial portions of the left ventricular free wall. Their arrangement ensures parallel alignment of the chordae tendineae with the LV axis during systole, allowing for complete leaflet coaptation and closure of the mitral valve in the normally functioning heart.

All three coronary branches contribute to the blood supply of the left ventricle, and acute ischemic events therefore predictably manifest as regional wall motion abnormalities based on the coronary distribution. The left anterior descending artery and its branches, the septal perforators, and the diagonals perfuse the anterior wall, the anterior two-thirds of the septum, and the apex. The obtuse marginal branches of the left circumflex artery supply the lateral wall. The right coronary artery perfuses the medial portions of the inferior wall, as well as the posterior one-third of the interventricular septum. Anastomotic connections between the left and the right coronary system allow for preserved myocardial perfusion distal to a significant obstruction or total coronary occlusion.

11.1.4.4 Aortic Valve

The aortic valve is part of the aortic root consisting of the annulus, the aortic valve cusps, the sinuses of Valsalva, the junction between the sinuses and the proximal ascending aorta (the sinotubular junction), and the proximal ascending aorta. It is located at the left ventricular outlet, separating the aorta and the ventricle. Owing to its central location, it is the only valve in the heart that is related to all four chambers and each of the valves. As a trileaflet semilunar valve, it consists of three cusps: the left and right coronary cusps giving rise to their respective coronary arteries, as well as the non-coronary cusp, which faces the interatrial septum. The right coronary cusp is the most anterior and is adjacent to the right ventricular outflow tract. The left coronary cusp is located posteriorly relative to the other two. Histologically, its cusps are composed of dense collagenous plates, which are in continuity with the fibrous skeleton of the heart, covered by the endocardium. Each cusp has its attachment to the aorta and the left ventricle. Immediately behind the cusps, the wall of the proximal ascending aorta bulges outward to form the aortic sinuses of Valsalva. The function of these sinuses is to prevent coronary ostial occlusion by creating eddy currents of blood flow during rapid ejection. As with the pulmonic valve, each cusp has a fibrous nodule at the midpoint of their free edges, forming the nodule of Arantius. The leaflets coapt via their crescent-shaped surfaces. Incomplete coaptation of the valve leaflets during diastole results in aortic regurgitation, whereas limited systolic leaflet excursion due to excessive leaflet thickening resulting from degenerative or rheumatic disease process suggests the presence of aortic stenosis. The severity of aortic stenosis can be assessed by various methods. *A peak transaortic velocity of greater than 4 m/second, a peak transaortic gradient of at least 70 mm Hg, and a mean gradient of at least 40–50 mm Hg, as well as* *an aortic valve area of less than*1 cm^2 *are consistent with severe aortic stenosis.*

Coronary Circulation

The first pair of arteries branching off the proximal ascending aorta are the left and right coronaries, originating from their respective sinus of Valsalva in the aortic root. While there is some variability in their point of origin and their distribution, the right coronary artery (RCA) almost always supplies the right ventricle (RV), whereas the left coronary artery (LCA) supplies the anterior and lateral wall of the left ventricle (LV), as well as the anterior portion of the interventricular septum. Blood supply to the remainder of the left ventricle is determined by the coronary dominance. This refers to the artery that supplies the posterior descending artery (PDA) and the posterior lateral branch (PLB). Right dominance (when the right coronary artery gives off the PDA and the PLB) occurs in 80–90% of normal individuals. Left dominance (the PDA and the PLB originating from the left circumflex artery) is slightly more common in men than in women. If the PDA is supplied by the RCA and the PLB branches off the left circumflex artery, the system is codominant.

11.1.4.5 The Left Coronary System

The left coronary artery arises from the left coronary sinus as the left main stem, which then bifurcates into two segments: the left anterior descending (LAD) and the circumflex (LCx) artery. The relatively short left main stem courses between the left atrial appendage and the pulmonary trunk before giving off the LAD and the LCx, and, in 15–30% of cases the variant coronary ramus intermedius, the branch supplying the anterior aspect of the heart.

The left anterior descending artery traverses the anterior interventricular groove and perfuses the anterior wall via the diagonal branches, as well as the anterior two-thirds of the interventricular septum via its septal perforators coursing along the anterolateral wall, and a small portion of the anterior wall of the right ventricle, adjacent to the interventricular groove, via the right ventricular branches.

The circumflex artery courses in the left atrioventricular groove. Its primary branches are the obtuse marginals, supplying the lateral aspect of the left ventricle, including the posteromedial papillary muscle. In 10 to 15% of individuals, it gives off the posterior descending artery (left dominance). Further branches of the left circumflex artery supply the left atrium, and, in 45% of the cases, the sinus node. A left dominant coronary system also supplies the atrioventricular node.

11.1.4.6 The Right Coronary System

The right coronary artery emerges from the right sinus of Valsalva and is carried by the right atrioventricular groove. In about half of the cases, it gives off the conus branch that supplies the right ventricular outflow tract. The RCA perfuses the anterior free wall of the right ventricle via its acute marginal branches, the sinus node via the nodal artery in 55% of individuals, and the atrioventricular node in patients with right-dominant coronary circulation. It bifurcates into the posterior descending artery and the posterolateral branch at the posterior interventricular groove. The posterior descending artery gives off the posterior septal perforators that supply the posterior one-third of the interventricular septum. The posterolateral branch supplies the inferoposterior wall of the left ventricle along with the acute marginal branches of the RCA and/or the circumflex artery. The Kugel's artery is an anastomotic branch between the RCA and the LCx that may give off a branch that supplies collateral circulation to the atrioventricular node.

11.1.4.7 The Coronary Veins

Of the cardiac veins, the great cardiac vein courses in the anterior interventricular groove upward from the apex, alongside the LAD. It drains into the coronary sinus. The middle cardiac vein courses in the inferior interventricular groove, upward from the apex, accompanying the PDA.

The coronary sinus courses in the posterior atrioventricular groove, alongside the left circumflex artery. It receives the great cardiac vein proximally and the middle cardiac vein distally, and drains into the right atrium. Its orifice is guarded by the Thebesian valve.

The anterior right ventricular veins course on the anterior surface of the right ventricle, where they may drain directly into the right atrium, or coalesce to form the small cardiac vein. The small coronary vein runs posteriorly through the right AV groove.

The Thebesian veins are small veins draining directly into the cardiac chambers, primarily into the right atrium and the right ventricle.

11.2 Part 2: Cardiovascular Pharmacology

11.2.1 Overview of Subcellular Mechanisms: Ion Channels and Receptors

Patients in the perioperative period often receive agents that affect hemodynamic variables such as heart rhythm and rate, blood pressure, or cardiac output. The effect of these agents is governed predominantly by transmembrane ion fluxes. Drugs used for rhythm and rate control act by modulating Na^+, K^+, and Ca^{2+} currents. Intracellular calcium is a key mediator in coupling electrical excitation to mechanical contraction and is an important determinant of the contractile state of the myocardium. The vascular tone of resistance vessels is regulated by ion fluxes via different types of K^+, Ca^{2+}, and Cl^- channels [2].

Much of human physiology (for example, responses to stimuli by hormones, neurotransmitters, ions, or photons) is regulated by GTP binding (G) protein-linked signal transduction. G-proteins serve as points of communication between the extracellular and intracellular environment.

Adrenergic receptors are membrane-spanning molecules coupled to adenylate cyclase via a G-protein located on the inner membrane of the cell. Their activation ultimately leads to the modulation of downstream effectors. G-proteins consist of 3 (α, β, and γ) subunits. The binding of an agonist to the adrenergic receptor replaces guanosine diphosphate (GDP) with guanosine triphosphate (GTP). This causes the α-subunit of the G-protein to break free from the β-γ complex, and to act as a primary messenger. In beta receptors, the α-subunit stimulates adenylate cyclase and triggers cyclic adenosine monophosphate (cAMP) production, which, as a second messenger in the process of signal transduction, activates its target kinases that phosphorylate regulator proteins and ultimately increase intracellular calcium levels.

Pure alpha-adrenergic agonists also increase intracellular calcium levels by stimulating phospholipase C, an enzyme that catalyzes the hydrolysis of phosphatidyl inositol to diacylglycerol and inositol triphosphate. Inositol triphosphate stimulates the release of calcium from the sarcoplasmic reticulum, and both molecules act as myofilamental calcium sensitizers [3].

11.2.2 Review of Electrophysiology and the Anatomy of the Cardiac Conduction System

Under physiologic conditions, electrical impulse generation, conduction, and propagation occur in specialized excitatory and conductive tissues within the myocardium and are driven by a sequence of ion fluxes through sarcolemmal ion channels. The pacemaker of the normal cardiac muscle is the sinoatrial (SA) node, located in the right atrium, below and lateral to the ostium of the superior vena cava, supplied by the nodal branch of the right coronary artery (RCA). Its intrinsic rate (60–100 beats per minute) is determined by the resting transmembrane potential, the threshold potential, and the rate of phase 4 spontaneous diastolic depolarization. The SA node has the steepest slope of phase 4 depolarization. For this reason, its intrinsic rate is the highest; therefore, this is the dominant, primary pacemaker of the heart.

Rhythmical, automatic impulses generated by the sinus node spread directly to the right atrium via its own non-contractile sinus fibers that fuse with excitable and contractile atrial fibers, as well as anteriorly to the left atrium via the Bachmann's bundle. The electrical impulse from the right atrium propagates via three other internodal tracts, including the posterior (Thorel's) and median (Wenkebach's) pathways to the atrioventricular (AV) node. The AV node, supplied by the AV-nodal branch of the distal RCA and the septal perforators of the left anterior descending (LAD) coronary artery, and located in the right atrial side of the interatrial septum behind the tricuspid valve and superior to the coronary sinus, delays impulses from the atria by approximately 70–100 ms before allowing them to pass to the bundle of His. These slow conduction velocities allow the atria to empty before a ventricular contraction begins. The AV node is the primary regulator of ventricular rate in atrial fibrillation and flutter. Its intrinsic rate is 40–60 beats per minute, and it is considered a latent intrinsic pacemaker.

The bundle of His is located just above the interventricular septum (IVS) and is supplied by the septal perforators of the LAD, as well as the posterior descending artery. As a latent pacemaker, its intrinsic rate is 20–40 beats per minute. From the bundle of His, impulses rapidly travel down the bundle branches on either side of the membranous portion of the interventricular septum, to depolarize the left (left bundle branch, LBB, which also depolarizes the IVS) and the right (right bundle branch, RBB) ventricles. The left bundle branch further divides into the anterior and posterior fascicles. Both bundles terminate in the Purkinje fibers that penetrate the ventricular myocardium, initiating its contraction from the endocardium toward the epicardium. An organized sequence of impulse generation and conduction is required for the cardiomyocytes to synchronously contract, and, by coordinated chamber contraction, to maintain cardiac output.

Understanding normal cardiac electrophysiology is the foundation for understanding the basic principles of disease mechanisms and antiarrhythmic pharmacotherapy. The following is a brief review.

11.2.2.1 Cardiac Action Potential

In the normal resting myocardium, the transmembrane potential is determined primarily by potassium conductance and is maintained by the Na^+/K^+ ATPase. The resting transmembrane potential is stable around − 90 mV (the intracellular compartment being more negative relative to the outside of the cell), approaching the potassium equilibrium potential.

Phase 0

An action potential is triggered by either the cardiac pacemaker cells or by the surrounding cardiomyocytes. This results in a transient increase in Na^+ conductance, which in turn initiates an increase in Na^+-influx through fast sodium channels. When the threshold potential is reached at around − 70 mV, a large enough number of sodium channels have been opened to generate a self-sustaining sodium influx. Above − 40 mV, long-opening (L-type) Ca^{2+} channels open with resultant Ca^{2+} influx down its concentration gradient. At around 0 mV, fast Na^+-channels start to close. This is phase 0 (early rapid depolarization), peaking at + 20 mV (Na^+-equilibrium potential).

Phase 1

The increase in Na^+-conductance is inactivated. This, with the outward movement of K^+ via transient K^+ channels, results in a brief period of initial repolarization. The transmembrane potential returns from slightly positive to approximately 0 mV. This is phase 1.

Phase 2

Following the initial repolarization, a constant Ca^{2+} influx via slow (L-type, "long-opening") Ca^{2+} channels, and an increase in K^+ conductance via delayed rectifiers maintain the membrane potential just below 0 mV. The electrical countercurrents are balanced. This is phase 2, the plateau. The phase between the initiation of the upstroke and the end of the plateau is the absolute refractory period, during which the cell is unable to be depolarized regardless of the strength of the stimulus, and corresponds with the phase between the beginning of the QRS complex and the beginning of the T-wave on the electrocardiogram (ECG).

Phase 3

The next phase of the cardiac action potential is rapid repolarization. Ca^{2+} conductance via the L-channels is inactivated, but the K^+ channels remain open. Potassium is rapidly shifted out of the cell, and the transmembrane potential rapidly approaches the K^+ equilibrium. This is phase 3. The phase between the initiation of the upstroke and the transition between phases 2 and 3 is the relative refractory period, during which the cell may be able to be depolarized to allow for a non-propagated stimulus. This corresponds with the early upstroke of the T-wave. During phase 3, the cell is able to be depolarized by supranormal stimuli (relative refractory period), resulting in an action potential. This corresponds with the dome of the T-wave on the ECG. Membrane hyperpolarization at the end of this phase results in a hyperexcitable period, during which even weak stimuli can trigger an action potential. This brief phase corresponds with the downward slope of the T-wave.

Phase 4

During phase 4, Na^+ and Ca^{2+} channels are closed. There is a constant outflow of potassium ions through inward rectifier channels. This is the resting phase in the contractile cells or spontaneous diastolic depolarization in the cardiac pacemaker cells.

11.2.2.2 Pacemaker Cells

Pacemaker cells are found primarily in the dominant and subsidiary rhythm generators (SA node, AV node, His-Purkinje system) of the heart. However, impulses may originate from other sites; for example, cells at the coronary sinus, atrioventricular valves, or cells at the crista terminalis. Abnormally, impulses may originate from around the pulmonary veins. These cells are different from contractile cardiomyocytes in that they share the characteristic to generate spontaneous cardiac action potentials. They exhibit automaticity, have an unstable membrane potential, and have no rapid depolarization phase.

Automaticity means that pacemaker cells are capable of initiating their own action potential without external stimulus. These cells undergo a spontaneous diastolic depolarization, and action potential is triggered when threshold potential is reached.

Pacemaker cells undergo spontaneous diastolic depolarization during phase 4 (as opposed to the resting phase during phase 4 in contractile cells) and have no rapid depolarization phase. These cells have fewer inward K rectifier channels than contractile myocytes do, and their transmembrane potential is never lower than − 60 mV. Therefore, the fast Na^+-channels that need − 90 mV to get activated are permanently inactivated in these cells.

Multiple ion currents are responsible for the generation of spontaneous action potentials. The synergy of three different currents— (1) the decay of the K^+ efflux; (2) an inward depolarizing "funny" mixed Na^+-K^+ inward current, activated by membrane hyperpolarization, and playing a major role in the spontaneous depolarization of the sinoatrial node; and (3) an inward Ca^{2+} current in the late phase of the spontaneous diastolic depolarization—determines the rate and shape of action potentials in cardiac pacemaker cells. Physiologically, the dominant pacemaker is the sinoatrial node. When its rate drops below the intrinsic rate of a latent, non-dominant pacemaker—for example, as a result of parasympathetic stimulation or SA-nodal disease—the removal of the sinus overdrive leads to the "escape-activation" of these non-dominant centers. Junctional rhythm may also occur when the AV junctional pacemaker rate exceeds and suppresses the sinoatrial rate.

11.2.2.3 Mechanisms of Cardiac Dysrhythmias

Cardiac arrhythmias are commonly defined as abnormalities of the normal sequence of impulse generation and propagation within the myocardium. While benign arrhythmias—for example, premature atrial contractions, isolated premature ventricular contractions, or atrial fibrillation in the absence of structural heart disease—are very common, malignant ventricular arrhythmias (monomorphic or polymorphic ventricular tachycardia [VT], ventricular fibrillation) accounted for an estimated 180,000–250,000 sudden cardiac deaths in the United States.

Underlying provoking factors are, for example, arterial hypoxemia, acidosis or alkalosis, electrolyte abnormalities, ischemia, increased sympathetic activity, atrial or ventricular dilation, or arrhythmogenic drugs. In some cases, correction of these factors is sufficient to suppress ectopic cardiac beats. However, when this alone does not control cardiac arrhythmias, and/or hemodynamic compromise ensues, or the presence of a disturbance increases the risk of a life-threatening arrhythmia, administration of antiarrhythmic agents may be warranted.

The main mechanisms of cardiac dysrhythmias have been identified as:

Focal activity due to abnormal impulse generation

This results from:

Enhancement or reduction of normal automaticity (such as in sinus tachycardia and sinus bradycardia, accelerated junctional rhythm).

Enhanced abnormal automaticity of the Purkinje fibers, atrial or ventricular myocytes; i.e., cells that do not normally display automaticity (for example, atrial tachycardia or accelerated idioventricular rhythm. Purkinje fibers are catecholamine sensitive, and their activation can be augmented by increased sympathetic tone, for example during myocardial ischemia).

Triggered activity. This occurs when early after-depolarizations and delayed after-depolarizations initiate spontaneous multiple depolarizations, such as in torsades de pointes, or ventricular arrhythmias in the setting of digitalis toxicity.

Abnormal conduction

Delayed conduction (such as in atrioventricular blocks), or re-entrant mechanisms (for example, SA-nodal re-entry, atrial flutter, AV-nodal re-entry tachycardia, or ventricular tachycardia). Re-entrant tachycardias can be generated by three different mechanisms: reflection, circus movement re-entry, and phase 2 re-entry. Circus movement re-entry due to an anatomical or functional block is a major mechanism and the most commonly described. For a re-entrant circuit to occur, two roughly parallel conductive pathways must be connected with conductive tissue, capable of forming an electrical circuit. One of these pathways must have a refractory period substantially longer than that of the other pathway (pathway A). Finally, the pathway with the shorter refractory period (alternate pathway, pathway B) must conduct impulses more slowly than pathway A. Once an extra impulse (for example, premature contraction) encounters these two separate pathways of conduction when pathway A is unable to be depolarized due to being in the refractory period but pathway B is capable of depolarization, the impulse will be conducted via pathway B. The signal then travels to the distal end of pathway A to reconnect with it if it is no longer refractory, then it is conducted retrograde to the site where it reconnects with pathway B. Pathway B has a shorter refractory period, and therefore, it recovers faster: The impulse will travel into pathway B where it will re-enter that portion of the circuit, completing the loop. Micro-re-entry occurs with ventricular tachycardia from conduction around scar tissue such as in myocardial infarction (MI). Macro-re-entry occurs via conduction through concealed accessory pathways, such as in Wolff–Parkinson–White syndrome.

Antiarrhythmic Agents: Classification and Mechanism of Action

Pharmacologic management of arrhythmias is warranted when treatment of the underlying causes does not break the arrhythmia, the arrhythmia results in hemodynamic compromise, or it increases the risk of the development of a life-threatening arrhythmia. The most widely used classification system of antiarrhythmic drugs was proposed by Vaughan Williams. This system classifies the antiarrhythmic agents based on their ability to abolish an arrhythmia by blocking specific ion currents during the action potential.

Ion-specific channels exist in three different stages. During the upstroke phase (phase 0) of the action potential, the channels are in the activated state. During the plateau phase of repolarization (phase 2), the inactivated state occurs. During the effective refractory period, channels are unresponsive to new or continued stimulus. Ion channels are closed during the resting phase (phase 4).

The effects on the action potential and the effective refractory period of the cardiac action potential determine the clinical effect of antiarrhythmic drugs. Drugs blocking inward sodium ion flow will slow conduction and result in suppression of the maximum upstroke velocity of the cardiac action potential. Potassium channel blockers prolong repolarization by prolonging the duration QTc prolongation. L and T-type calcium channels are present in the myocardium and are targets of calcium channel blockers.

Classification

Class I

Class I antiarrhythmic drugs are fast Na-channel inhibitors. Fast sodium channels are blocked during phase 0 (upstroke), and phase 4 depolarization of the action potential with resultant decreases in the amplitude and rate of the action potential and conduction velocity.

Class IA

For example, quinidine, procainamide, and disopyramide. These drugs lengthen both the action potential and the effective refractory period reflecting sodium channel inhibition and lengthening of repolarization reflecting potassium channel blockade. These drugs are considered membrane stabilizers in the treatment of atrial, AV-nodal, and ventricular arrhythmias. They may prolong the QRS and QT intervals.

Quinidine—Quinidine has mild parasympatholytic and alpha-blocking effects and decreases systemic vascular resistance (SVR).

Procainamide—Procainamide is used to suppress premature atrial and ventricular contractions and to prevent precipitation of atrial fibrillation or flutter. It increases refractoriness and can prevent accessory pathway re-entry tachycardias. High serum levels may cause direct myocardial depression and bradycardia requiring temporary pacing or administration of beta-agonists. Procainamide and its active metabolite N-acetyl-procainamide may induce QT-prolongation and torsades de pointes. Long-term therapy may cause lupus-like symptoms.

Disopyramide—Disopyramide has a vagolytic effect that is dose-dependent and reversible by pyridostigmine. It depresses myocardial contractility and increases SVR, and may thus precipitate or exacerbate congestive heart failure.

Class IB

Class IB drugs are less powerful Na-channel blockers, for example, lidocaine, tocainide, and mexiletine. They shorten action potential duration and refractory period in normal ventricular myocytes. Class II drugs have minimal effect on inotropy or SVR. In the ischemic tissue, lidocaine may block adenosine triphosphate-dependent channels, preventing ischemic-mediated shortening of ventricular depolarization. Lidocaine depresses the slope of phase 4 depolarization in Purkinje fibers and increases the fibrillation threshold in ventricular myocytes. Signs of toxicity are frequent with concentrations above 9 mcg/ml.

Class IC

Class IC drugs are potent sodium channel blockers, indicated for the treatment of ventricular arrhythmias, for example, flecainide and propafenone. They markedly decrease the rate of phase 0 depolarization and speed of conduction. They have little effect on the duration of the action potential and the effective refractory period in ventricular muscular cells but do shorten the duration of the action potentials in the Purkinje fibers. This inhomogeneity on the rate of cardiac repolarization plus the slowing of cardiac conduction may contribute to the pro-dysrhythmic effects of these drugs, particularly in patients with a history of myocardial infarction, left ventricular dysfunction, or previous sustained ventricular tachycardia. Class IC drugs, especially flecainide, significantly depress inotropy and prolong the PR and QT intervals.

Class II

Class II drugs are beta-adrenergic receptor blockers. Beta-adrenergic receptor antagonists decrease the rate of spontaneous phase 4 depolarization, important in the suppression of ventricular arrhythmias during ischemia and reperfusion. They are effective in the treatment of adrenergically mediated disease states, in which increased phase 4 depolarization, enhanced conduction velocity, and a shorter refractory period all contribute to increased automaticity. Beta-blockers decrease the rate of V_{max} of the action potential, by prolonging its duration as well as the effective refractory period. Drug-induced slowing of the heart rate with resulting decreases in myocardial oxygen requirements is desirable in patients with coronary artery disease. Beta-blockers slow the sinus rate, prolong AV-nodal conduction, and enhance refractoriness. They prolong the PR interval on the ECG. Esmolol is used to convert atrial fibrillation with rapid ventricular response to normal sinus rhythm, or to maintain a slow ventricular rate. It also predictably reverses the fibrillation threshold-lowering effects of catecholamines.

Class III

Class III drugs are potassium channel blockers; for example, amiodarone, bretylium, and sotalol. These drugs prolong cardiac repolarization, action potential duration, and the effective refractory period possibly by interference with sodium and calcium exchange. These effects are beneficial in preventing cardiac dysrhythmias by decreasing the proportion of the cardiac cycle during which myocardial cells are excitable and susceptible to a triggering event. Re-entrant tachycardias may be suppressed if the action potential duration becomes longer than the cycle length of the tachycardia circuit.

Amiodarone—In addition to class III effects, amiodarone exhibits class I Na^+-channel blocking, class II beta-blocking, and class IV Ca^{2+}-channel blocking properties. It prolongs repolarization and cardiac action potential; it produces negative chronotropy in nodal tissues. As a Ca^{2+} and K^+-channel blocker, it slows SA-nodal conduction speed and prolongs the refractory period. It is an α- and β-receptor antagonist with potent vasodilating and myocardial depressant potential. It may produce sinus bradycardia or heart block, necessitating the administration of positive chronotropes or the initiation of temporary pacing. Long-term side effects include pulmonary fibrosis, corneal microdeposits, liver cirrhosis, hyperthyroidism, or hypothyroidism.

Sotalol—Sotalol is a mixture of isomers that possess similar class III effects, used for the treatment of atrial fibrillation or atrial flutter, as well as to treat ventricular arrhythmias. The L isomer of sotalol acts as a beta-antagonist, whereas the D isomer may increase mortality in patients with ventricular dysfunction and recent myocardial infarction. Sotalol lacks intrinsic sympathomimetic activity or membrane-stabilizing properties. The lower incidence of dysrhythmia effects seen with amiodarone and racemic sotalol may be related to the beneficial class II effects.

Bretylium is no longer available in the United States for clinical use.

Class IV

Calcium Channel Blockers These agents act by inhibiting inward slow inward calcium currents that may contribute to the development of ventricular arrhythmias. These drugs are useful in the treatment of idiopathic ventricular tachycardias. Calcium channel blockers prolong neuromuscular blockade.

Prodysrhythmic Effects

Prodysrhythmia effects of antiarrhythmic agents describe bradydysrhythmias or tachydysrhythmias that represent new dysrhythmias associated with chronic antidysrhythmic drug treatment. Types of dysrhythmias include torsades de pointes, incessant VT, and wide complex ventricular rhythm.

Torsades de pointes (polymorphic VT) is the most common dysrhythmia and is triggered by early after-depolarizations in a setting of a delayed depolarization and increased duration of refractoriness manifesting as prolonged QT_c interval on the ECG. Class IA (especially quinidine) and class III drugs prolong QT_c by potassium channel blockade and provide the setting for torsades de pointes. Drug-induced torsades is often associated with bradycardia because the QT_c interval is longer at slower heart rates. Exacerbating factors such as hypokalemia, hypomagnesemia, poor LV function, and concomitant administration of other QT-prolonging drugs are important predisposing factors in the development of torsades de pointes.

Incessant ventricular tachycardia may be precipitated by cardiac antidysrhythmic drugs that slow the conduction of cardiac impulses (class IA and class IC) sufficiently to create a continuous ventricular re-entry circuit. Incessant ventricular tachycardia is more likely to occur with high doses of class IC drugs and in patients with prior history of sustained ventricular tachycardia and poor LV function. Ventricular tachycardia due to this mechanism is generally slower because of the drug effect but may be resistant to drugs or electrical therapy.

Wide complex ventricular rhythm is usually associated with class IC drugs in the setting of structural heart disease with excessive plasma concentrations or abrupt changes in the dose. A wide complex rhythm is thought to reflect a re-entrant tachycardia and easily degenerates to ventricular fibrillation.

11.2.2.4 Antianginal Drugs: Coronary Vasodilators and Cardioinhibitory Drugs

Under normal physiologic conditions, oxygen delivery (DO_2, the amount of oxygen delivered to the cells) is adequate to meet cellular oxygen demand (VO_2, the amount of oxygen extracted from arterial blood) and maintain aerobic metabolism. The ratio of oxygen consumption to the oxygen available to tissues is the oxygen extraction ratio, which varies for different organs. During periods of increased workload and increased cellular demand, and/or decreased supply, aerobic metabolism can still be maintained independently of blood flow by increasing O_2 extraction. Critical O_2 delivery is the point at which the extraction ratio is maximized, and any further incongruence between demand and supply will lead to tissue hypoxia and subsequent activation of anaerobic metabolic pathways. When myocardial oxygen consumption exceeds the reserve in coronary blood supply to meet a given O_2 demand, ischemia is precipitated. The heart's high, 60–70% O_2 extraction ratio (compared to 25–30% for the rest of the body) can make it susceptible to even short periods of ischemia.

The major determinants of myocardial O_2 *supply* are coronary blood flow and arterial O_2 content. Coronary blood flow is further determined by the patency of the coronaries, coronary perfusion pressure, and coronary vascular resistance. The three major determinants of myocardial O_2 *demand* are heart rate, inotropic state, and wall tension (which is the function of intracavitary pressure, radius, and wall thickness, as well as preload and afterload). Antianginal pharmacotherapy is indicated when the supply/demand imbalance results in ischemia. In accordance with the 2014 American College of Cardiology/American Heart Association (ACC/AHA) Guideline for the Management of Patients with Non-ST-Elevation Acute Coronary Syndromes, standard medical therapy includes the use of beta-blockers, nitroglycerin, calcium channel blockers, analgesics, and cholesterol management. This section will focus on role of nitroglycerin, beta-blockers, and calcium channel blockers in the management of angina pectoris [4, 5].

Coronary Vasodilators

Nitroglycerin

Nitroglycerin (NTG) is an endothelium-independent smooth muscle relaxant that acts predominantly on venous capacitance vessels and large epicardial coronary arteries, maximizing blood flow to the subendocardial areas. Peripheral vasodilatory effects are prominent even at low doses and are not dose-dependent, whereas dilation of peripheral conductance and resistance vessels occur at higher doses, and further increases in dose result in more pronounced vasodilation. Nitroglycerin reduces myocardial O_2 demand and increases oxygen supply by reducing preload and decreasing ventricular dimension and wall tension, dilating normal and atherosclerotic coronary arteries, and enhancing collateral circulation. The degree to which coronaries are able to dilate is dependent on their baseline vascular tone. Nitroglycerin produces a dose-dependent systemic and pulmonary arterial vasodilatory effect and predictably decreases cardiac filling pressures. Its use is indicated for the initial treatment of nearly all types of myocardial ischemia, as well as for managing hypertension and heart failure. The elimination half-life of nitroglycerin is approximately 1.5 min.

Mechanism of Action

NTG enters the smooth muscle cells and generates nitric oxide through a glutathione-dependent pathway, which stimulates cyclic GMP production and causes peripheral vasodilation via a sequence of protein phosphorylation and dephosphorylation within the smooth muscle. Nitric oxide production via guanylate cyclase stimulation and cGMP production is a sulfhydryl (SH)-group-dependent process. Depletion of SH-groups by prolonged exposure leads to dose- and duration-dependent tolerance, which may manifest within the first 24 h of treatment. Restoring SH supplies with reducing agents (for example, N-acetylcysteine) does not reliably reverse nitrate tolerance, and therefore, a drug-free interval of 12–24 h is recommended to maintain drug efficacy. Rebound myocardial ischemia may occur during drug-free intervals.

Common Clinical Use

Nitroglycerin is available in intravenous (IV), sublingual, or topical formulations. A typical IV dose to treat acute ischemia is 50–10 mcg. For a continuous infusion, the dose range is 0.1–7 mcg/kg/min.

Adverse Effects

Nitroglycerin at low doses causes predominantly splanchnic venodilation that results in venous pooling, decreased cardiac filling, and decreased biventricular end-diastolic volume and pressure. Excessive decreases in diastolic blood pressure may decrease coronary blood flow and trigger reflex tachycardia and increased contractility mediated by the baroreceptor reflex. The combination of decreased coronary blood flow and increased myocardial O_2 demand may provoke angina pectoris. With the administration of intravenous phenylephrine, adequate coronary perfusion pressure can be maintained.

In the lungs, nitroglycerin inhibits hypoxic pulmonary vasoconstriction and worsens hypoxia and gas exchange. It has been shown to have platelet-inhibitory effects, the clinical significance of which has not been elucidated.

Although an uncommon complication of nitroglycerin therapy, the nitrite metabolite of NTG is capable of oxidizing the ferrous (Fe^{2+}) ion in the hemoglobin into the ferric (Fe^{3+}) state, producing methemoglobin. Ferric (oxidated) iron is unable to carry O_2 effectively, and in sufficiently high concentrations (> 40%), it can impair tissue oxygenation. The treatment of methemoglobinemia is methylene blue, to facilitate the conversion of methemoglobin to hemoglobin. High doses of NTG are more likely to produce methemoglobinemia in patients with hepatic dysfunction.

The 2014 ACC/AHA guidelines recommend that nitrates should not be administered to patients with non-ST-elevation-acute coronary syndrome (ACS) who recently received a phosphodiesterase inhibitor (class III, level of evidence: B). Nitrates should not be administered to patients with signs of hypovolemia or hypotension, and it should be used with caution in patients with right ventricular infarction.

Cardioinhibitory Drugs

Beta-Adrenergic Blockers

As discussed in the previous section, beta-blockers are class II antiarrhythmics with a multitude of favorable properties utilized in the treatment of cardiac ischemia. Their negative inotropic, negative chronotropic, and antihypertensive properties allow for a reduction in O_2 consumption and an increase in blood supply during diastole. Beta-blockers slow spontaneous diastolic depolarization and shorten the duration of cardiac action potentials. The ventricular fibrillation threshold is increased. Beta-blockers reduce myocardial infarct size. In the absence of contraindications (cardiogenic shock, decompensated heart failure, severe sinus bradycardia, second- or third-degree atrioventricular block, or active bronchospasm), beta-blockers should be administered early in the treatment of myocardial ischemia. While early administration has not been shown to improve short-term survival, beta-blockers decrease re-infarction and the frequency of ventricular dysrhythmias, and their use has been associated with mortality benefits after myocardial infarction. Perioperative beta-blockers should be continued in patients already taking them, according to class 1 indications for perioperative beta-blockade from the 2014 ACC/AHA recommendations; patients at high perioperative risk for adverse cardiac events should be started on beta-blockers preoperatively, and continued up to 30 days postoperatively. In these patients, it is reasonable to titrate beta-blockers to heart rate and blood pressure.

Mechanism of Action

Beta-blockers are competitive, reversible inhibitors of beta-adrenergic receptors. Beta-adrenergic receptors are G-protein coupled receptors. Stimulation by their agonists activates adenylate cyclase to produce cyclic AMP. Cyclic AMP, in turn, activates protein kinase pathways with subsequent phosphorylation of L-type calcium channels and troponin C, the net effect being enhanced inotropy, positive chronotropy, and dromotropy. These responses are all blunted by receptor occupancy by beta-antagonists.

Propranolol—Propranolol is a non-selective β-1 and β-2 receptor blocker with no alpha-receptor activity. As the most soluble beta-blocker, its use is associated with the highest frequency of central nervous system side effects. It is well absorbed when taken by mouth. For a comparable effect, higher oral than intravenous doses are required due to its very high (90%) hepatic first-pass metabolism. Its active metabolite does not add to the primary clinical effect due to its short half-life. Propranolol decreases cardiac output by decreasing the heart rate and reducing myocardial contractility, effects that are especially prominent in sympathetically driven disease states. Owing to its β-2 receptor antagonism, propranolol may increase systemic vascular and coronary vascular resistance. Increased airway resistance may be evoked by propranolol in asthmatic patients. Renal and hepatic blood flow is reduced with the administration of propranolol.

Metoprolol—Metoprolol was the first β-1 selective receptor antagonist used in clinical practice to prevent increased chronotropy and inotropy in response to sympathetic stimulation. Its receptor selectivity is dose related. Metoprolol is lipid-soluble, it diffuses more readily into ischemic regions than hydrophilic drugs. Fifty percent of the drug administered is metabolized during first-pass hepatic metabolism. At the intravenous dose of 0.2 mg/kg, the maximum beta-receptor blockade is achieved.

Esmolol—Esmolol is a short-acting cardioselective agent metabolized rapidly by red blood cell esterases. It is primarily a β-1 blocking agent, producing significant decreases in heart rate and contractility. It lacks the ability to block peripheral vascular β-2 receptors; therefore, decrease in blood pressure and cardiac index is more pronounced due to unopposed peripheral vasodilation. Esmolol has been safely used in patients with reactive airway disease.

Sotalol—Sotalol is a class III antiarrhythmic agent with both β-receptor and K^+-channel antagonistic effects. A relatively recent Cochrane database review found significant reductions in the incidence of postoperative atrial fibrillation in the cardiac surgical population. Despite the conclusions of this review, the use of sotalol in the post-cardiac surgical population remains limited, owing to sotalol's undesired side effects, such as hypotension, bradycardia, QT-prolongation, and inducing torsade-type ventricular arrhythmias.

Calcium Channel Blockers

Calcium channel blockers (CCBs) comprise a diverse group of agents that selectively inhibit calcium influx into myocardial and vascular smooth muscle cells. *Dihydropyridines* (such as nifedipine, nicardipine, nimodipine, amlodipine, felodipine, and isradipine) exert their effect on the peripheral arteriolar beds (nimodipine favors cerebral vessels) and produce marked peripheral vasodilation with little direct effect on heart rate, AV conduction, and inotropy. They may elicit reflex sympathetic activation via the baroreceptor reflex. *Non-dihydropyridines* (phenylalkylamines, for example, verapamil; and benzothiazepines, for example, diltiazem), on the other hand, block AV-nodal calcium channels and have significant negative inotropic, chronotropic, and dromotropic effects. Their main anti-ischemic effects are due to their ability to reduce myocardial O_2 consumption by depressing contractility, decreasing heart rate and systemic afterload, and increasing O_2 supply by coronary and collateral vasodilation. Calcium channel blockers are preferred in vasospastic (variant) angina, as beta-blockers may provoke or aggravate ischemia in some patients. All calcium channel blockers are effective in the treatment and prevention of coronary vasospasm. They may reduce re-infarctions and long-term events in hypertensive patients with acute myocardial infarction.

Calcium Channels

Calcium channels display selectivity to calcium ions and are present among others in myocardial, smooth muscle, skeletal muscle, and neural tissues, as well as in membranes of subcellular organelles, such as the mitochondria or the sarcoplasmic reticulum. Calcium channel blockers bind to voltage-gated transient (T), long (L) type channels in the myocardium and smooth muscle, or to neural (N) type channels, rendering them inactive. T-type calcium channels are activated at low voltages, play a major role in phase 0 depolarization, and are not affected by calcium channel blockers. L-type channels are activated at higher voltages, playing a role in the phase 2 plateau of the cardiac action potential. These are the Ca^{2+} channels that are able to be blocked by calcium antagonists.

11.2.3 Dihydropyridines: Smooth-Muscle-Selective Vasodilators

Dihydropyridines prevent calcium entry into the vascular smooth muscle cell by *extracellular modulation* of the L-type channels. The primary target of dihydropyridines is the peripheral arteriolar bed except for nimodipine, which favors cerebral vessels. Reflex tachycardia may be elicited with their use. Examples include nifedipine, nicardipine, nimodipine, amlodipine, and felodipine. The predominant action of these agents is decreasing systemic, coronary, and cerebrovascular vasomotor tone. Dihydropyridine calcium channel blockers, with the exception of the primarily antianginal nifedipine, will be discussed later.

Nifedipine—Nifedipine was the first dihydropyridine calcium channel blocker in clinical use for its coronary and peripheral vasodilator properties. It has greater coronary and peripheral vasodilatory properties than verapamil with negligible effects on venous capacitance vessels. It has little or no effect on cardiac impulse generation and on SA- and AV-nodal conduction. Peripheral vasodilation and the resultant decrease of systemic blood pressure activate baroreceptors, leading to reflex sympathetic nervous system activity manifesting as tachycardia. In the absence of concomitant beta-receptor blockade, it may increase the risk of myocardial infarction or recurrent angina. Excessive peripheral vasodilation can be antagonized with phenylephrine. It may be combined with beta-blockers without increasing the risk of AV-block. Nifedipine is used in angina pectoris due to coronary artery vasospasm. No IV preparation is available due to its extreme instability when exposed to light. Its abrupt discontinuation has been associated with coronary artery vasospasm.

11.2.4 Non-Dihydropyridines: Antiarrhythmics

11.2.4.1 Phenylalkilamines

Phenylalkilamines bind to the *intracellular portion* of the L-type calcium channel when it is in the open state, and occlude the channel.

Verapamil—Verapamil is a synthetic derivative of papaverine. It is supplied as a racemic mixture, in which the D isomer lacks Ca^{2+}-channel blocking properties and acts as a fast Na^{+}-channel blocker, accounting for local anesthetic effects, and the L isomer is specific for slow Ca^{2+} channels. The predominance of this action accounts for the classification of this drug as a calcium channel blocker. Verapamil decreases the heart rate by depressing sinoatrial and AV-nodal activity (hence, its utility in the treatment of supraventricular arrhythmias), lowers systemic blood pressure due to myocardial depression and peripheral vasodilation, and produces moderate coronary artery dilation (preferred in essential hypertension and vasospastic angina). Its negative inotropy is more pronounced in patients who already have a depressed left ventricular function; therefore, verapamil should be avoided in symptomatic heart failure, severe bradycardia, sinus node dysfunction, and AV-nodal block. These effects of verapamil may be enhanced with concomitant β(beta)-blockade. In the presence of drug-induced heart block, isoproterenol may be useful to increase heart rate. Verapamil may also precipitate dysrhythmias in patients with Wolff–Parkinson–White (WPW) syndrome, and has proven effective in the treatment of hypertrophic cardiomyopathy with or without left ventricular outflow tract (LVOT) obstruction. Verapamil may be useful in the treatment of premature labor, as well as fetal and maternal tachydysrhythmias. It may decrease uterine blood flow and should be administered with caution to parturients with impaired uteroplacental perfusion.

11.2.4.2 Benzothiazepines

Benzothiazepines block L-type channels via a mechanism that is not well understood. Diltiazem may act on the Na^{+}/K^{+} pump, decreasing the amount of intracellular Na^{+} available for exchange with extracellular calcium, and it may inhibit the calcium-calmodulin binding.

Diltiazem—Diltiazem, like verapamil, blocks the calcium channels at the AV node. It is considered the first-line treatment for supraventricular tachydysrhythmias. It may also be used for the control of chronic essential hypertension. Diltiazem has minimal cardio-depressant effects and is unlikely to interact with β-blockers to decrease contractility.

11.2.4.3 Inotropes and Vasopressors

Adrenergic Receptors

Alpha- and beta-adrenergic receptors are G-protein-coupled receptors present on various types of cells: pre-and post-synaptic sympathetic nerve terminals; as well as cardiac, skeletal, or smooth muscle cells; hepatocytes; pancreatic islets (beta cells); adipose tissue; platelets; and the renal juxtaglomerular apparatus. They bind endogenous and synthetic catecholamines. There are two discrete types of adrenergic receptors, each with several subtypes: alpha and beta.

Alpha receptors are predominant in the peripheral and pulmonary vasculature. They have two subtypes, α-1 and α-2.

The α-1 subtype is G_q-protein-coupled, expressed by smooth muscle, adipose tissue, the liver, sweat glands, and the kidneys. G_q-protein-coupled receptors activate the phospholipase C (PLC) pathway: PLC cleaves phosphatidylinositol 4,5-bisphosphate (PIP_2) into diacylglycerol (DAG) and inositol triphosphate (IP_3). IP_3 in turn interacts with intracellular calcium stores and increases the intracellular calcium content. DAG activates protein kinase C, which further modulates ion channels. Stimulation of the α-1 receptor results primarily in vascular smooth muscle contraction. Other effects include contraction of the pregnant uterus, contraction of urogenital smooth muscle (bladder neck, prostate), bronchoconstriction, mydriasis, glycogenolysis and gluconeogenesis, secretion from sweat glands, and renal sodium reabsorption.

Alpha-2 receptors are G_i-coupled receptors expressed by central presynaptic nerve terminals. G_i-proteins inhibit the production of cAMP from ATP, reduce Ca^{2+} permeability, and increase K^+ permeability. Presynaptic neuronal α_2 agonists cause inhibition of acetylcholine as well as norepinephrine release by negative feedback from norepinephrine present in the synaptic cleft. Stimulation of central presynaptic α_2 receptors inhibits sympathetic nervous system output and causes sedation. Peripheral α_2 receptor stimulation causes decreased insulin secretion from pancreatic beta cells, inhibition of lipolysis, platelet aggregation, and vascular smooth muscle contraction.

Beta-1 adrenergic receptors are found on the sinus node, AV node, and myocardium. These are G_s-protein coupled receptors and are expressed predominantly in the cardiac pacemaker cells, myocardium, salivary glands, as well as eccrine and apocrine sweat glands. Their stimulation activates adenylate cyclase, increasing intracellular cAMP-synthesis. cAMP as a second messenger activates intracellular signaling pathways that result in increased Ca^{2+} levels during systole. Calcium binds to troponin C, facilitates actin-myosin cross-bridge formation, and increases sarcomere contraction. This translates into a faster heart rate, increased myocardial excitability, increased conductivity, and more forceful contractions.

Beta-2 receptors are located on the smooth muscle of the bronchial tree, some coronary vessels, skeletal muscle arteries, the gastrointestinal tract, and the urinary bladder. Stimulation of a β_2 receptor may activate 2 G-proteins that regulate adenylate cyclase differently: the excitatory G_s and the inhibitory G_i-proteins. Stimulation of the Gi protein results in decreased smooth muscle tone.

11.2.4.4 Adrenergic Receptor Agonists

Epinephrine

Epinephrine is an endogenous catecholamine produced by the adrenal medulla. It is a potent direct α_1-, α_2-, β_1-, and β_2-adrenergic agonist. In all dose ranges, it has strong positive inotropic effects. Peripheral vascular resistance varies according to the dominant effect of the receptors activated: at low doses ($\beta > \alpha$), SVR is usually decreased. At moderate doses (β comparable to α), SVR may remain unchanged. At high doses ($\alpha > \beta$), SVR is increased. It increases myocardial oxygen consumption.

1. **Hemodynamic Effects**

Preload: increased due to α_1-effect on capacitance vessels.

Contractility: augmented due to β_1-effect on the myocardium; its lusitropic effects account for an enhanced rate of relaxation.

Lusitropy: As a β_1-agonist, epinephrine enhances early diastolic filling by accelerating relaxation, augmenting filling, and reducing end-systolic ventricular size.

Afterload: dose-dependent effect. Pulmonary hypertension may occur.

Heart rate: tachycardia due to β_1-effect, increased excitability and conduction, increased risk of arrhythmias.

Cardiac output: augmented.

Common Clinical Use: first-line agent in the treatment of asystole or cardiac arrest due to ventricular fibrillation; cardiogenic shock when administered with a vasodilator (for example, nicardipine or milrinone); low cardiac output after separation from cardiopulmonary bypass; drug of choice in anaphylaxis and anaphylactoid reactions; severe asthma due to its β_2 effects. It is not currently recommended as first-line pressor in the management of sepsis.

Administration: (1) By central intravenous line via controlled infusion device. Peripheral extravasation may cause skin necrosis; (2) via an endotracheal tube (ETT); (3) subcutaneously for mild allergic reactions or bronchospasm.

Adverse Effects: hypertension, tachycardia, arrhythmias, and decreased peripheral perfusion (kidney function, urine output, and extremity perfusion should be monitored).

Warnings and Contraindications: There are no contraindications to the use of epinephrine in a life-threatening medical emergency. Contraindications include narrow-angle glaucoma, labor, and thyrotoxicosis. Epinephrine should be used with caution in patients with the following conditions: severe coronary artery disease, angina pectoris, irritable myocardium, diabetes, cerebrovascular insufficiency, thyroid disease, and pregnancy. Rapid administration, for example, in cardiac arrest, may cause devastating cerebrovascular hemorrhage. Clostridium gas gangrene has been reported after intramuscular injection for anaphylaxis, injection into the buttock should therefore be avoided. Hypovolemia should be corrected before administration. End-organ ischemia (myocardial, renal) may result from prolonged administration at high infusion rates. Epinephrine inhibits uterine contractions, especially during the second stage of labor.

Norepinephrine

Norepinephrine (NE) is an endogenous catecholamine produced by the adrenal medulla and sympathetic neurons, which stimulates both alpha- and beta-adrenergic receptors, and acts as both a hormone and the primary post-synaptic sympathetic neurotransmitter. Its pharmacologic effects are predominant on peripheral α_1 receptors, resulting in vasoconstriction of both resistance *and* capacitance vessels. In most dose ranges, norepinephrine increases mean systemic and pulmonary arterial blood pressure. In low dose ranges, its less potent β_1 effects—translating into increased heart rate, positive inotropy, and a mild increase in cardiac output—become noticeable. Norepinephrine does not have significant β_2 effects.

2. **Hemodynamic Effects**

Preload: NE recruits cardiac preload reserve and reduces preload dependency in patients with septic shock.

Contractility: augmented.

Lusitropy: As a β_1-agonist, norepinephrine enhances early diastolic filling by accelerating relaxation, augmenting filling, and reducing end-systolic ventricular size.

Afterload: increased SVR and PVR. Increased systolic, diastolic, and mean arterial pressure.

Heart rate (HR): varies, depending on blood pressure. Positive chronotropy is usually offset by a reflexive increase in vagal tone in response to increased blood pressure. Heart rate may increase if hypotension persists.

Cardiac output: increased or unchanged (depending on HR).

Common Clinical Use: peripheral vasoconstrictor. Agent of choice in septic shock and other states where the normal sympathetic tone is lost. Short-term hemodynamic support in non-hypovolemic shock.

Administration: via central venous line, typical starting dose 0.03 mcg/kg/min via controlled infusion device.

Adverse Effects: Peripheral vasoconstriction reduces peripheral organ perfusion and risks ischemia. May precipitate arrhythmias or coronary vasospasm. May worsen pulmonary hypertension.

Warnings and Contraindications: contraindicated as sole therapy in hypovolemic patients.

Dopamine

Dopamine is an endogenous catecholamine, a precursor to epinephrine and norepinephrine, found in the adrenal medulla and peripheral nerve terminals. It has effects on alpha, beta, and dopaminergic (DA) receptors. At the lowest doses (1–3 mcg/kg/min), its dopaminergic effects are dominant, resulting in the dilation of the cerebrovascular, renal, and mesenteric vascular beds. In low-to-moderate dose ranges, its β_1-adrenergic effects are predominant, resulting in increased heart rate, increased contractility, and increased cardiac output. At high doses (greater than 10–20 mcg/kg/min), its α_1-agonist effects predominate: high-dose dopamine increases SVR and PVR, and decreases peripheral perfusion. It is an effective mixed inotrope and vasoconstrictor; however, it is not recommended as first-line therapy in the treatment of septic shock due to the side effects associated with its use. Dopamine has positive chronotropic effects in all dose ranges, and in higher dose ranges, it may induce arrhythmias due to increased excitability and conduction. It does not have significant β_2 effects. Dopamine causes less increase in O_2 consumption than isoproterenol.

3. **Hemodynamic Effects:** Direct agonist on α_1, β_1, β_2, and DA-receptors. Indirectly, it increases norepinephrine levels by its conversion into norepinephrine and by inducing norepinephrine release from storage sites. In low doses, it redistributes blood flow from skeletal muscle to the kidneys and mesentery.

Preload: Dopamine increases venous return.

Contractility: augmented.

Lusitropy: As a β_1-agonist, dopamine enhances early diastolic filling by accelerating relaxation, augmenting filling, and reducing end-systolic ventricular size.

Afterload: increases SVR and PVR. Dopamine usually widens pulse pressure by increasing systolic, and to a much less extent, diastolic pressure. At low doses, dopamine produces renal and mesenteric vasodilation. At high infusion rates, renal perfusion is decreased.

Heart rate: increased,

Cardiac output: augmented,

Common Clinical Use: treatment of hypotension due to low SVR or cardiac output. It may be the first choice for temporizing hypotension until the intravascular volume is restored. Current evidence discourages its use to treat kidney insufficiency or failure as it provides no mortality benefit or risk reduction.

Administration: IV only, preferably via central venous line via controlled infusion device, typical dose range 1–20 mcg/kg/min,

Adverse Effects: Dopamine increases myocardial work without compensatory coronary vasodilation, and increases the size of myocardial ischemia; increases the risk of arrhythmia.

Warnings and Contraindications: In patients with prior history of occlusive peripheral vascular disease, dopamine may elicit peripheral circulatory insufficiency. Monoamine oxidase (MAO) inhibitors may potentiate and prolong the effects of dopamine. Extravasation may result in skin necrosis. Contraindications to dopamine use include hypersensitivity to dopamine, uncorrected tachyarrhythmias, ventricular fibrillation, uncorrected hypovolemic shock, and pheochromocytoma.

Dobutamine

Dobutamine is a synthetic derivative of dopamine that does not affect endogenous norepinephrine release. It is a racemic mixture of enantiomers of (−) dobutamine with a vasoconstrictor (α_1-agonist), and (+) dopamine with vasodilator (α_1-antagonist) properties. It is a myocardial β_1-agonist with a predominant positive inotropic effect. Its β_2 and α_1 effects are limited, and it completely lacks α_2 effects. In the heart, it augments myocardial contractility and O_2 consumption and increases cardiac output by increasing heart rate and stroke volume. Increased myocardial work is compensated by increased coronary blood flow. On all systemic vascular beds and pulmonary blood vessels, it acts as a vasodilator and may cause hypotension. This is primarily mediated by its mild β_2 effects, which are partially unopposed by dobutamine's α_1 effects.

4. **Hemodynamic Effects**:

Preload: Dobutamine decreases venous resistance and mean systemic filling pressure. Left ventricular end-diastolic pressure is decreased.

Contractility: augmented.

Lusitropy: Dobutamine increases early peak diastolic filling rate in normal-weight patients, and this increase is linearly related to the increased heart rate. In obese patients, the correlation between heart rate and diastolic filling rate is lost as the rate of relaxation is significantly lower, suggesting that baseline relaxation reserve is impaired in obesity, and this impaired diastolic function is not resolved during stress.

Afterload: decreased SVR and PVR. SVR may increase in the presence of β-adrenergic blockade.

Heart rate: increased.

Cardiac output: augmented.

Common Clinical Use: short-term inotropic support in low cardiac output states, especially in right ventricular failure, afterload reduction in left and/or right systolic heart failure (pulmonary congestion, cardiogenic shock; drug of choice in right heart failure), and stress echocardiography. May be combined with dopamine to augment preload, contractility, and systemic vascular resistance.

Administration: IV or IO, central venous administration is preferred via a controlled infusion device. Typical dose range: 0.5–20 mcg/kg/min.

Common Side Effects: dose-dependent tachycardia and arrhythmias (less likely to induce tachycardia at therapeutic doses than dopamine or isoproterenol), angina pectoris, exaggerated hypertension (especially in patients with pre-existing hypertension), hypokalemia.

Warnings and Contraindications: Contraindications to the use of dobutamine include hypersensitivity to dobutamine, dynamic left ventricular outflow tract obstruction such as in idiopathic hypertrophic subaortic stenosis/hypertrophic obstructive cardiomyopathy, pre-existing tachydysrhythmias or hypertension, and acute coronary syndrome with ventricular irritability. Contraindicated as sole therapy in severely hypovolemic patients: Hypovolemia should be corrected before administration. May provoke atrial fibrillation with rapid ventricular response in patients with pre-existing atrial fibrillation.

Dopexamine

Dopexamine is a synthetic dobutamine-analog with positive inotropy, positive chronotropy, and peripheral vasodilator action, as well as minimal alpha-receptor activity. It is a potent agonist of DA1-receptors (and thus decreases renovascular resistance). It is indicated for the treatment of low cardiac output states. It is widely used in Europe, but it is not approved by the Food and Drug Administration (FDA) in the United States.

Ephedrine

Ephedrine is an alkaloid derivative with sympathomimetic effects. It has mild direct agonist on α_1-, β_1-, and β_2-receptors, and leads to indirect norepinephrine release from the neurons. It is an easily titratable pressor and inotrope with a short duration of action that does not reduce placental blood flow and is therefore safe to administer in pregnancy.

5. **Hemodynamic Effects**

Preload: increased due to β_1 effects on venous capacitance vessels.

Contractility: increased.

Lusitropy: likely enhances early diastolic filling by reducing end-systolic ventricular size.

Afterload: increased.

Heart rate: increased.

Cardiac output: increased.

Common Clinical Use: correction of drug-induced hypotension and bradycardia under general anesthesia, or drug-induced sympathectomy with resultant relative hypovolemia and low SVR after placement of a neuraxial block. May be used to temporize blood pressure in hypovolemia until the intravascular volume is restored.

Administration: may be administered as an IV bolus via a peripheral vein. Typical dose: 5–10 mg titrated to target blood pressure. May be administered intramuscularly, subcutaneously, or by mouth.

Adverse Effects: Its efficacy diminishes with the depletion of endogenous norepinephrine. The use of ephedrine increases the risk of malignant hypertension when used with cocaine or MAO inhibitors. Tachyphylaxis may develop with repeated doses.

Warnings/Contraindication: hypersensitivity to ephedrine. Overdose may manifest as convulsions, mydriasis, pulmonary edema, visual disturbances, pyrexia, hypertension, and tachycardia.

Phenylephrine

Phenylephrine is a synthetic non-catecholamine with nearly selective post-synaptic α_1 and minimal β effects. Due to its vasoconstrictor effects on resistance vessels, it is widely used for the treatment of intraoperative drug-induced hypotension. Its vasoconstrictor potency is less than that of epinephrine and norepinephrine. It is a direct α-agonist with a short duration of action. It raises both systemic and pulmonary vascular resistance. Phenylephrine constricts coronary blood vessels and augments coronary blood flow. It constricts cerebral and renal vessels but does not compromise blood flow to these organs. Phenylephrine may reduce renal, skeletal muscle, mesenteric, and skin blood supply. Myocardial O_2 requirement is usually unchanged unless hypertension is present. Vagally mediated reflex bradycardia commonly occurs as a response to increased vascular resistance and usually responds well to atropine; this response can be blocked by atropine. Its effects on cardiac output appear to be determined by preload dependency.

6. **Hemodynamic Effects**

Preload: Direct α_1-stimulation decreases venous capacitance and minimally increases venous return.

Contractility: no direct effect.

Lusitropy: unchanged.

Afterload: increased SVR and PVR.

Heart rate: unchanged or reflex bradycardia due to the aortic baroreceptor reflex. Phenylephrine is the adrenergic agonist least likely to elicit tachycardia.

Cardiac output: unchanged in preload-independent patients, or decreased in preload-dependent patients.

Common Clinical Use: low SVR states, iatrogenic hypotension, non-hypovolemic shock, treatment of hypotension on patients with coronary artery disease, aortic stenosis, tetralogy of Fallot to counteract right-to-left shunting, or idiopathic hypertrophic subaortic stenosis. Although not harmful, phenylephrine is not the drug of choice in septic shock due to its decreased potency relative to norepinephrine.

Administration: IV, may be administered peripherally via the vein of the antecubital fossa via a controlled infusion device; intramuscular (IM), subcutaneous (SC), or intranasal.

Adverse Effects: hypertension, reflex bradycardia, pulmonary edema, and metabolic acidosis. An increased SVR may decrease stroke volume, subsequently decreasing the cardiac output.

Warnings and Contraindications: Contraindications to the use of phenylephrine include hypersensitivity to phenylephrine or sulfites, severe coronary disease, severe hypertension, ventricular tachycardia, and close-angle glaucoma. Rarely, it may provoke a spasm of a coronary artery or a coronary bypass graft.

Isoproterenol

Isoproterenol is a pure direct β_1- and β_2-receptor agonist. It increases cardiac output by 1.) increasing heart rate, augmenting myocardial contractility, and 2.) afterload reduction. When inhaled, β_2-receptors mediate its bronchodilator effects.

7. **Hemodynamic Effects**

Preload: increased.

Contractility: augmented.

Lusitropy: enhances early diastolic filling by reducing end-systolic ventricular size.

Afterload: reduced SVR and PVR.

Heart rate: increased.

Cardiac output: increased due to increased heart rate and reduced afterload.

Common Clinical Use: bradycardia not responding to atropine in the absence of a temporary pacemaker. Treatment of low cardiac output in cases when increased inotropy and chronotropy is needed; for example, in the denervated heart, in pediatric patients with fixed stroke volume, or in ventricular aneurysm resection. Treatment of pulmonary hypertension. Status asthmaticus (continuous cardiac monitoring is required). β-blocker overdose. Heart block.

Administration: PO or IV: safe to administer via peripheral veins.

Adverse Effects: tachycardia, arrhythmias, hypokalemia, dyspnea, pulmonary edema, and angina pectoris.

Warnings and Contraindications: Isoproterenol is contraindicated in digitalis intoxication, angina, and pre-existing ventricular arrhythmias. Not to be used for asystolic arrest. Isoproterenol may increase the size of myocardial infarction and may cause transient hyperglycemia.

11.3 Non-Adrenergic Vasoconstrictors

11.3.1 Vasopressin

Vasopressin is a naturally occurring antidiuretic nonapeptide synthesized as a pro-hormone primarily in the supraoptic, and secondarily in the paraventricular nuclei of the posterior hypothalamus. After binding to carrier protein neurophysin, it is transported via the supraoptic hypophyseal tract to the posterior hypophysis, where it is stored and released into the circulation when plasma osmolality is higher than physiologic, or when profound hypovolemia is present. Normal plasma concentrations are less than 4 pg/ml. The half-life of endogenous vasopressin is 10–35 min, and it is metabolized via renal and hepatic pathways. Due to trypsin activity in the gastrointestinal tract, it must be administered parenterally or intranasally. In concentrations higher than required for its antidiuretic effect, it acts as a non-adrenergic vasoconstrictor on peripheral vascular beds. It completely lacks beta-adrenergic effects; therefore, it produces less tachycardia compared to adrenergic agonists. In severe shock states, or in conditions where refractory vasoplegia is present, a deficiency in vasopressin levels may necessitate restoration of its physiologic concentration by administration of low-dose exogenous vasopressin.

The effects of vasopressin are mediated by a family of G-protein-coupled vasopressin receptors. V_{1a} and V_{1b} are G_q-protein-linked, whereas V_2 is G_s-protein-linked receptors.

V_{1a} is located primarily on the vascular smooth muscle of the systemic, coronary, splanchnic, and renal vessel bed, mediating pressor response by increasing peripheral vascular resistance. Intra-arterial infusion of vasopressin constricts all major celiac artery branches except the hepatic artery. A less well-appreciated aspect is vasopressin's pulmonary vasodilatory effect by inducing constitutive endothelial nitric oxide synthase and increasing nitric oxide production. Vasopressin's vasodilatory effects are mediated by endothelial oxytocin receptors. V_{1a} is also expressed in diverse tissues such as hepatic, central neuronal, and myometrial tissues, as well as platelets. V_{1a} receptors are G_q-protein linked, activate phospholipase C, and ultimately increase intracellular calcium, leading to vasoconstriction. V_{1b} receptors activate adrenocorticotropic hormone (ACTH) release from the anterior pituitary gland.

V_2 receptors are located primarily in the distal tubules and collecting ducts of the kidneys, and play a role in the homeostatic regulation of plasma volume and preservation of serum osmolality. These receptors are Gs-protein-linked and activate adenylate cyclase to ultimately increase intracellular cAMP levels. This in turn leads to the mobilization of aquaporin two channels and their insertion into the luminal surface of the collection tubules and the subsequent increase of water reabsorption. V_2 receptors are also expressed in endothelial cells, where they are involved in the release of von Willebrand factor (VWF) and factor VIII (F VIII). VWF protects F VIII from breakdown and plays an important role in binding platelets to the site of bleeding.

1. **Hemodynamic Effects:** adrenergic-independent direct peripheral vasoconstriction via V_{1a} receptors without affecting chronotropy or inotropy. Redistributes blood to the coronaries and the cerebral vasculature without a β_1-induced increase in myocardial O_2 consumption.

Preload: Vasopressin increases blood volume and venous return via constriction of capacitance vessels.

Contractility: unchanged.

Lusitropy: unchanged.

Afterload: increased SVR; elevated systolic and diastolic pressures.

Heart rate: unchanged.

Cardiac output: unchanged or decreased due to increased SVR.

Common Clinical Uses: The 2015 AHA guidelines no longer recommend the use of vasopressin during advanced cardiac life support, and vasopressin has been removed from the adult cardiac arrest algorithm. Vasopressin is still recommended for the treatment of vasoplegia refractory to maximal catecholamine replacement such as in septic shock, vasoplegic syndrome after separation from cardiopulmonary bypass, residual ACE inhibitor, or ARB effect under general anesthesia.

Administration: in vasoplegic states: second-line agent, typical dose 0.02–0.04 units/minute via controlled infusion device.

Side Effects: pallor, angina pectoris, bronchoconstriction, abdominal cramping, nausea, vomiting, uterine contractions, decreased platelet count, and lactic acidosis.

Warnings and Contraindications: Treatment is contraindicated in patients with hypersensitivity to vasopressin. In patients with coronary artery disease, peripheral vascular disease, heart failure, angina pectoris, migraine, and renal failure, vasopressin should be used with caution.

11.4 Phosphodiesterase-3 Enzyme Inhibitors

11.4.1 Milrinone

Milrinone is a non-catecholamine and non-glycoside inodilator with potent positive inotropic and vasodilator properties. It acts as a competitive inhibitor of phosphodiesterase-3 (PDE-3) in the cardiac and vascular smooth muscle cells, independently of β-adrenergic mechanisms. PDE-3 is an enzyme that hydrolyzes intracellular cAMP into its inactive metabolite. Inhibition of the cAMP breakdown allows for the cAMP levels to remain elevated. This in turn increases the Ca^{2+} influx into the myocardium and increases Ca^{2+} efflux from the vascular smooth muscle, an effect translating into increased inotropy in the heart, and vasodilation of the peripheral arteries and veins. In the myocardium, milrinone augments contractility, facilitates diastolic relaxation, enhances automaticity, and shortens AV-nodal conduction time. Afterload reduction in the peripheral vessels usually has little effect on chronotropy. Overall, milrinone improves myocardial contractility, cardiac output, and ejection fraction. Myocardial O_2 consumption is unchanged or slightly increased.

1. **Hemodynamic Effects**

Preload: decreased.

Contractility: augmented.

Lusitropy: augmented.

Afterload: decreased SVR and PVR. Milrinone is primarily an afterload reducer.

Heart rate: no direct effect; may induce supraventricular and ventricular arrhythmias or increase ventricular response rate in atrial fibrillation or flutter.

Cardiac output: increased.

Common Clinical Uses: short-term treatment of low cardiac output syndrome, especially when the pulmonary capillary wedge pressure/left ventricular end-diastolic pressure is elevated; may be considered as first-line therapy in decompensated congestive heart failure and evidence of pulmonary hypertension; depressed right ventricular function. Retains hemodynamic effects in the presence of beta-blockade.

Administration: by mouth, or through a central vein. When administered intravenously, milrinone should be administered with a loading dose (50 mcg/kg) over 10 min followed by slow continuous infusion by central intravenous line via a controlled infusion device. The typical maintenance rate is 0.375–0.75 mcg/kg/minute. In renal impairment, the maintenance dose should be reduced.

Adverse Effects: ventricular arrhythmias, supraventricular arrhythmia, hypotension, angina, rarely hypokalemia, bronchospasm, elevated liver enzymes, and thrombocytopathy.

Warnings and Contraindications: hypersensitivity to milrinone or inamrinone. Hemodynamics should be closely monitored. Liver function should be monitored during treatment with milrinone. Milrinone should be used with caution in patients with atrial fibrillation or flutter, due to positive dromotropy. It precipitates furosemide when administered in the same intravenous line.

Inamrinone

Inamrinone (formerly, amrinone; a selective competitive PDE-3 inhibitor) is another example of β-independent, non-catecholamine non-glycoside inotropes. It is a potent inodilator; its mechanism of action is similar to that of milrinone. It decreases preload and afterload and enhances cardiac output. Generally, if any, there is little change in the myocardial O_2 consumption; the decreased ventricular wall tension and end-diastolic left ventricular pressure offset the increased M_{VO2} resulting from the increased cardiac output. This agent is losing popularity to milrinone due to milrinone's less pronounced effect on platelet function.

2. **Hemodynamic Effects**

Preload: decreased. Inamrinone is primarily a preload reducer.

Contractility: augmented.

Lusitropy: augmented.

Afterload: decreased. Mean arterial pressure (MAP) may or may not change, as the decrease in SVR and PVR may be offset by an augmented cardiac output.

Heart rate: little or no change. At high doses, milrinone may potentiate atrial or ventricular arrhythmias.

Cardiac output: increased.

Common Clinical Uses: severe decompensated congestive heart failure refractory to conventional therapy with diuretics, vasodilators, and inotropic agents. Effective in the presence of β(beta)-adrenergic blockade.

Administration: central IV infusion via a controlled infusion device. The typical loading dose is 0.75–1.5 mg/kg, and maintenance rate is 5–20 mcg/kg/minute. Incompatible with furosemide.

Adverse Effects: arrhythmia (low risk), thrombocytopenia/thrombocytopathy, hypotension, and hepatotoxicity with chronic administration.

Warnings and Contraindications: hypersensitivity to inamrinone, milrinone, or bisulfite preservatives. Inamrinone should be used with caution in patients with recent myocardial infarction, hypotension, severe aortic or pulmonic stenosis, or renal impairment. Inamrinone is not dialyzable.

Levosimendan

Levosimendan is a PDE-3 inhibitor that acts as an intracellular calcium-sensitizer to troponin C. It improves contractility in a calcium-dependent manner by binding to cardiac troponin C and stabilizing its calcium-induced conformational changes, and has vasodilatory effects by opening ATP-sensitive potassium (K_{ATP}) channels of the vascular smooth muscle. K_{ATP} channels close as intracellular ATP concentration increases, their selective blockade results in arteriolar vasoconstriction. Activation of K_{ATP} channels may also account for its antistunning effects without increasing intracellular calcium concentrations or energy consumption in the myocardium. The effects of levosimendan are greatest during systole when intracellular calcium levels are the highest, and diminish along with the decreasing intracellular calcium availability during diastole. Levosimendan acts independently of cAMP and has been used in beta-blocked patients. It does not increase myocardial oxygen consumption. It does not impair the baseline diastolic function and is tolerated without arrhythmogenicity. It is a systemic and coronary vasodilator used for the treatment of acute decompensated congestive heart failure. The Levosimendan Infusion versus Dobutamine (LIDO) study demonstrated a significant survival benefit of levosimendan over dobutamine, and smaller studies described its benefits for pulmonary hypertension complicated by right ventricular failure. It is not FDA-approved for clinical use in the United States.

Papaverine

Papaverine is a non-specific phosphodiesterase inhibitor, derived from opium; however, as a benzyl-isoquinoline, it is structurally and functionally unrelated to opioid alkaloids. It is used by surgeons to treat and prevent spasms of the internal mammary artery during cardiac surgery.

Antihypertensive Agents

Hypertension is a major risk factor for cardiovascular morbidity and mortality. Essential hypertension accounts for the vast majority of adult cases. Based on recommendations of the Seventh Report of the Joint National Committee on Prevention, Detection, Evaluation, and Treatment of High Blood Pressure (JNC-7), the classification of blood pressure (BP) for adults have been as follows:

Normal: Systolic lower than 120 mm Hg, diastolic lower than 80 mm Hg

Prehypertension: Systolic 120–139 mm Hg, diastolic 80–89 mm Hg

Stage 1: Systolic 140–159 mm Hg, diastolic 90–99 mm Hg

Stage 2: Systolic 160 mm Hg or greater, diastolic 100 mm Hg or greater.

Antihypertensive pharmacotherapy is indicated when lifestyle modifications (weight loss; smoking cessation; limiting alcohol consumption; reducing dietary saturated fat and sodium intake; maintaining adequate dietary calcium, magnesium, and potassium intake; engaging in moderate-intensity aerobic exercise for 30 min on most days) fail to achieve adequate blood pressure control. The updated eighth report of the JNC recommends treating to 150/90 mm Hg in patients over age 60 years; for everybody else, the goal BP is 140/90.

Diuretics, beta-blockers, angiotensin-converting enzyme (ACE) inhibitors/angiotensin receptor blockers (ARBs), calcium channel blockers (CCBs), and aldosterone antagonists are the mainstays of pharmacologic management of essential hypertension. Specific antihypertensive classes target specific end-organ damage, hence the difference in drug combinations when coexisting risk factors are taken into consideration:

Heart failure: diuretics, beta-blockers, ACE inhibitors/ARBs, and aldosterone antagonists

Post-myocardial infarction: beta-blockers, ACE inhibitors, and aldosterone antagonists

High coronary disease risk: diuretics, beta-blockers, ACE inhibitors, and CCBs

Diabetes: Diuretics, beta-blockers, ACE inhibitors/ARBs, and CCBs

Chronic kidney disease: ACE inhibitors/ARBs

Recurrent stroke prevention: diuretics and ACE inhibitors

This section will focus on drugs used in the management of systemic hypertension, pulmonary hypertension, and heart failure.

Management of Systemic Hypertension

The primary determinants of blood pressure are cardiac output and peripheral vascular resistance. Cardiac output is maintained by heart rate and stroke volume. Stroke volume is determined by preload, contractility, and afterload, as well as the left ventricular and vascular compartmental size. Modulation of these factors by controlling input from vasoactive hormones, neurotransmitters, and local endothelium-derived factors will bring about a change in blood pressure: peripheral resistance is decreased by peripheral α-1 blockers, central α-2 agonists, angiotensin-converting enzyme inhibitors, angiotensin receptor blockers, calcium channel blockers, diuretics, or direct vasodilators. Heart rate is modulated by beta-blockers, calcium channel blockers, or the novel agent ivabradine. Stroke volume is reduced by preload-reducer diuretics and venodilators, negative inotropy of calcium channel blockers, or afterload-reducing agents.

Peripheral α_1 Receptor Blockers

Labetalol—Labetalol is a non-selective beta-blocker with selective α_1 receptor blocking properties. The potency of β-blockade is approximately sevenfold greater than α_1 blockade. Its partial β_2 agonism promotes peripheral vasodilation. Labetalol can be considered a peripheral vasodilator not triggering reflex tachycardia. In a dose-related fashion, it decreases heart rate and peripheral vascular resistance, leaving the stroke volume and cardiac output unchanged. After oral administration, labetalol is completely absorbed. Its significant first-pass metabolism produces inactive metabolites.

Phentolamine—Phentolamine is a reversible non-selective competitive antagonist at the adrenergic α_1 and α_2 receptors, as well as at serotonin receptors. Its main action is arterial vasodilation with minimal venodilation. SVR and PVR is therefore decreased. Heart rate and contractility drastically increase due to both the baroreceptor reflex and phentolamine's direct effect on central presynaptic α_2 receptors, allowing for increased norepinephrine release and decreased reuptake. This results in unopposed β effects that may provoke arrhythmias and myocardial ischemia, and respond well to β-blockers. In patients pre-treated with phentolamine, administration of epinephrine may result in hypotension due to unopposed β_2 effects. Phentolamine is a gastrointestinal stimulant, may lower blood glucose, and causes histamine release. It is used for the diagnosis of pheochromocytoma (a drop in SBP > 35 mm Hg and DBP > 25 mm Hg is diagnostic for pheochromocytoma), management of hypertensive episodes associated with the resection of pheochromocytoma, as well as local treatment of skin necrosis associated with norepinephrine extravasation.

Phenoxybenzamine—Phenoxybenzamine is a non-selective, non-competitive adrenergic α_1- and α_2-antagonist at postganglionic synapses in smooth muscle and exocrine glands. Its main action is arterial vasodilation with minimal venodilation. It decreases SVR and PVR. Heart rate and contractility are increased due to both the baroreceptor reflex and phentolamine's direct effect on central presynaptic α_2 receptors, allowing for increased norepinephrine release and decreased reuptake. This results in unopposed β effects that may provoke arrhythmias and myocardial ischemia, and respond well to β-blockers. Phenoxybenzamine is available in PO form only. It is used for the treatment of pheochromocytoma; it is started 10–14 days preoperatively to allow for the expansion of blood volume. To avoid unopposed alpha-stimulation and life-threatening hypertensive episodes, β-blockers are not introduced until after adequate alpha-blockade. Due to its side effects—for example, orthostatic hypotension and tachycardia—especially after administering the initial dose, its dose should be increased slowly. Alpha- and beta-blockers should be continued until the morning of surgery.

Prazosin, Doxazosin, Terazosin, and Tamsulosin—Prazosin, doxazosin, terazosin and tamsulosin are selective α_1-antagonists. Their main cardiovascular action is decreasing SVR and PVR with only minimal increases in heart rate. Prazosin acts on arteries and veins. Prazosin and doxazosin are indicated for the treatment of chronic hypertension. Terazosin blocks vascular α_{1B}, as well as α_{1A} receptors in the prostate and bladder neck. It is used for the treatment of benign prostate hypertrophy (BPH) and hypertension. Tamsulosin is a selective α_{1A} receptor blocker used for symptomatic BPH and to help with the passage of kidney stones. Orthostatic hypotension with syncope may occur with the use of peripheral α-blockers, especially after the first dose.

Tolazoline—Tolazoline is a non-selective competitive α-adrenoceptor antagonist, structurally similar to phentolamine. It acts as a sympathomimetic and also stimulates muscarinergic ACh-receptors and causes histamine release. It decreases systemic and pulmonary vascular resistance. It markedly increases heart rate and may provoke arrhythmias due to its sympathomimetic effects and the reflex sympathetic activation associated with its use. Although it is used to treat persistent pulmonary hypertension in neonates, it is not a selective pulmonary vasodilator and may worsen the SVR/PVR ratio when fixed pulmonary hypertension is present.

Central α_2 Receptor Agonists

Central α_2 receptor agonists reduce sympathetic outflow by stimulating bulbar α_2 activity and reducing peripheral norepinephrine release without eliciting reflex tachycardia and increased contractility. These agents potentiate the effects of anesthetics and may substantially reduce anesthetic and narcotic requirements. Central α_2 receptor agonists may exacerbate depression and are contraindicated for the management of hypertension in patients treated with monoamine oxidase inhibitors.

Clonidine—Clonidine is a centrally acting α-agonist with near selectivity on α_2-receptors (220:1 α_2 to α_1 effect). As a partial agonist–antagonist, it elicits a submaximal response on central pre-and post-junctional α_2-receptors while blocking the effects of other agonists. It is a coronary vasodilator and acts as a sympatholytic—a property utilized to manage withdrawal symptoms in opioid and alcohol addicts. Clonidine effectively reduces SVR, PVR, and renal vascular resistance. Its half-life is 12 h.

Clonidine blocks pain signal transmission in the brain. It may potentiate opioid effects on the central nervous system and has local anesthetic properties. When administered epidurally, it produces dose-dependent analgesia not reversed by opioid antagonists—an effect utilized in the treatment of cancer pain. It doubles the duration of intermediate-duration local anesthetics when used as an adjunct to peripheral nerve blocks. Due to the risk of hypotension and bradycardia, epidural clonidine is not recommended in the perioperative, obstetric, and postpartum settings. It causes sedation in a dose-dependent manner. Due to a lack of adequate data, it should not be administered above the C4 dermatome.

Clonidine should not be discontinued abruptly, as rebound hypertension is frequently triggered. Its immediate-release oral formulations should be discontinued within 4 h before surgery and resumed as soon as possible in the early postoperative period.

Methyldopa—Methyldopa is a centrally acting antihypertensive. Its mechanism of action is not fully elucidated. Its antihypertensive effects are most likely due to its metabolism to α-methyl-norepinephrine, which stimulates central inhibitory α-receptors and lowers blood pressure by false neurotransmission and possibly by reducing plasma renin activity. It has no direct effect on cardiac and renal function. Reversible thrombocytopenia and leukopenia, hemolytic anemia, a positive Coombs test, and liver dysfunction including fatal liver necrosis have been reported with the use of methyldopa. Despite these adverse effects, methyldopa is still commonly used for the treatment of pregnancy-induced hypertension due to the lack of adverse effects of long-term treatment on the fetus.

Guanabenz—Guanabenz is an oral antihypertensive active on central α_2-receptors. Its action is mediated by bulbar α_2 activation, leading to attenuated sympathetic outflow at the level of the brain stem. It effectively controls blood pressure without significant effects on renal function. It frequently causes sedation; therefore, additive sedative effects should be considered when used with other centrally acting depressants. Its abrupt discontinuation may rarely result in an increased production of endogenous catecholamines and subsequent rebound hypertension. In patients with coexisting liver and kidney disease, careful monitoring of blood pressure is recommended.

Guanfacine—Guanfacine is a selective oral central post-synaptic α_{2A}-receptor agonist with a duration of action longer than that of clonidine. It reduces sympathetic outflow with a resultant decrease in heart rate and vasomotor tone. Guanfacine preferentially binds post-synaptic α_{2A}-receptors in the prefrontal cortex and modulates behavioral responses. Its immediate-release form is used for the management of hypertension, whereas its extended-release form is used for the treatment of attention-deficit hyperactivity disorder as monotherapy or as an adjunct to central nervous system stimulants. Its dose should be reduced with concomitant use with CYP3A4 inhibitors, and slowly increased with the use of CYP3A4 inducers.

Dexmedetomidine—Dexmedetomidine is a selective central α_{2A} and peripheral α_{2B}-agonist with sedative and anesthetic properties. Centrally, it reduces sympathetic outflow and inhibits norepinephrine release at regular doses. At high doses, it activates peripheral α_{2B} receptors with resultant vasoconstriction, increased SVR, PVR, pulmonary artery occlusion pressure, and central venous pressure. Its use is indicated for procedural sedation for awake fiberoptic intubation, as well as sedation of intubated and mechanically ventilated patients in the intensive care unit. Its initial loading dose is 1 mcg/kg over 10 min, followed by a maintenance rate of 0.2–0.7 mcg/kg/hour, administered via a controlled infusion device, and titrated to effect. No dose adjustments are required in patients with severe renal impairment. In patients with severe hepatic impairment, dose reduction is recommended. It may cause episodes of hypotension, bradycardia, or sinus arrest. These adverse effects are enhanced in the presence of beta-blockers and antihypertensive agents, as well as in patients with advanced age, diabetes mellitus, pre-existing heart block, bradycardia, hypovolemia, or depressed ventricular function. Limited information is available regarding its use in pregnancy. Dexmedetomidine is expected to cross the placenta.

Perioperative Management

Perioperative continuation of α_2 agonists is not recommended for the prevention of major adverse cardiac events.

Angiotensin Converting Enzyme Inhibitors

When the circulating blood volume is low and renal perfusion is reduced (the afferent glomerular arteriolar pressure is decreased), the renal juxtaglomerular apparatus converts proenzyme prorenin into renin, which is then released into circulation. Upon entering the circulation, renin cleaves a decapeptide from plasma protein angiotensinogen to produce angiotensin I, a precursor to the potent vasoconstrictor angiotensin II. Angiotensin II (AT-II) is the primary vasoactive hormone of the renin-angiotensin system. It is generated from angiotensin I by the proteolytic action of the angiotensin-converting enzyme (ACE). It also stimulates aldosterone secretion by the adrenal cortex [6, 7].

AT-II is therefore a potent vasoconstrictor of arteries and veins. It is responsible for increased aldosterone secretion and sympathetic nervous system stimulation. Angiotensin II normally binds to the AT1 receptor which ultimately leads to the increased release of calcium from the sarcoplasmic reticulum to produce vasoconstriction. Besides its effects on vasomotor tone, AT-II also mediates alveolar permeability and lung injury: excessive ACE inhibition is related to worse lung injury, an important consideration in the management of critically ill patients. Decreased generation of angiotensin II (for example, by inhibition of ACE) results in decreased vasoconstrictive effects, usually without eliciting reflex tachycardia or an increase in cardiac output. In addition, decreased concentrations of plasma aldosterone result in decreased sodium and water retention. ACE inhibitors block the AT-I to AT-II conversion, as well as the breakdown of bradykinin, an endogenous vasodilator substance, which contributes to the antihypertensive effects of these drugs. ACE inhibitors reduce the activation of low-density lipoprotein (LDL) receptors and decrease the concentrations of LDL cholesterol. If the concentration of LDL is already sufficiently low, ACE inhibitors may no longer be effective in reducing the rate of cardiovascular events.

ACE inhibitors can be classified according to the structural element that interacts with the zinc ion of the enzyme, as well as the form in which the drug is administered (prodrug or active). Administration of ACE inhibitors (for example, benazepril, fosinopril, ramipril, or quinapril) as prodrugs increases the bioavailability prior to their hepatic metabolism to the active drug. Enalapril is the prodrug of the active ACE inhibitor enalaprilat, and its conversion may be altered in patients with hepatic dysfunction. Captopril, enalaprilat, and lisinopril are not prodrugs. The major difference among the clinically used ACE inhibitors is in the duration of action.

In the absence of contraindications, ACE inhibitors and angiotensin receptor blockers are recommended in patients with systolic heart failure to reduce morbidity and mortality. They may be preferred in hypertensive patients with chronic kidney disease and/or diabetes mellitus. Unless contraindicated, ACE inhibitors are prescribed together with a beta-blocker. Contraindications to the use of ACE inhibitors are prior life-threatening reactions (angioedema) and known or planned pregnancy. Caution should be used in the presence of low baseline blood pressure, elevated levels of serum potassium, increased serum creatinine, or bilateral renal artery stenosis.

Side Effects

Common side effects are cough, upper respiratory congestion, rhinorrhea, and allergic-like symptoms. It is speculated that these airway responses reflect potentiation of the effects of kinins due to drug-induced inhibition of peptidyl-dipeptidase activity and subsequent breakdown of bradykinin. If respiratory depression develops, prompt injection of epinephrine is advised. Angioedema is a potentially life-threatening complication of treatment with ACE inhibitors. Decreases in glomerular filtration rate may occur. For this reason, ACE inhibitors are used with caution in patients with pre-existing renal dysfunction and are not recommended for patients with renal artery stenosis. Hyperkalemia is possible due to decreased production of aldosterone. The risk of hyperkalemia is greatest in patients with recognized risk factors (congestive heart failure with renal insufficiency). Measurement of plasma concentrations of potassium may be indicated in treated patients. ACE inhibitors are to be avoided in pregnancy due to their potential to induce oligohydramnios, other fetal developmental abnormalities, or fetal demise.

Perioperative Management

Although previous perioperative guidelines have suggested continuing ACE inhibitors/ARBs before non-cardiac surgery, adverse circulatory effects during anesthesia have been recognized in patients chronically treated with ACE inhibitors/ARBs, leading to the recommendation that these drugs be discontinued 24 h before anesthesia and major, low-risk, urgent, or emergent surgery. While not affecting major postoperative outcomes such as major adverse cardiac events or death, prolonged hypotension has been observed in patients undergoing general anesthesia for minor surgery in whom ACE inhibitor therapy was maintained until the morning of surgery. Surgical procedures with major fluid shifts have also been associated with hypotension in patients treated with ACE inhibitors [8].

Treatment with ACE inhibitors does not increase the incidence of hypotension after the induction of anesthesia in patients with infarction-induced myocardial dysfunction. Exaggerated hypotension attributed to continued ACE inhibitor therapy has been responsive to crystalloid fluid infusion and/or administration of sympathomimetics such as ephedrine or phenylephrine. If hypotension is refractory to treatment, treatment with vasopressin is usually effective. ACE inhibitors may increase insulin sensitivity and hypoglycemia, which is a concern when these drugs are administered to patients with diabetes mellitus.

Captopril—Captopril is an oral vasodilator that inhibits the formation of angiotensin II in the lung. The subsequent decrease in plasma AT-II levels leads to decreased arterial and venous vasomotor tone, generally without eliciting tachyphylaxis or reflex hemodynamic changes.

In common with all ACE inhibitors, captopril reduces preload and afterload on the heart. It promotes renal excretion of sodium and water, reducing the circulating blood volume. Treatment with captopril is associated with survival benefits after myocardial infarction, congestive heart failure, or hypertension. Captopril may delay the development of renal disease in patients with diabetes mellitus, and counteracts ventricular remodeling after myocardial infarction.

Also, in common with all ACE inhibitors, captopril may reversibly reduce kidney perfusion and decrease kidney function. Patients with bilateral renal artery stenosis are at risk for kidney failure. Due to suppressed aldosterone activity, hyperkalemia may occur. A common side effect is chronic non-productive cough, secondary to the inhibition of the breakdown of bradykinin. Angioedema, a life-threatening condition potentially causing airway obstruction, is a rare adverse effect.

Enalapril and Enalaprilat—Enalapril is an oral ACE inhibitor used for the treatment of hypertension and congestive heart failure. The therapeutic and side effects of enalapril are very similar to those of captopril. As an inactive prodrug, it first must undergo hepatic metabolism into its active form, enalaprilat.

Enalaprilat is an intravenous ACE inhibitor, used primarily to treat severe hypertension. Its therapeutic and side effects are similar to those of captopril. It has a duration of action longer than nitrates, eliminating the need for continuous infusion. Enalaprilat decreases peripheral vascular resistance without eliciting reflex tachycardia, an increase in cardiac output, and myocardial oxygen consumption.

Lisinopril and Ramipril—Lisinopril and ramipril are oral ACE inhibitors—prodrugs used for the treatment of hypertension. They must first undergo hepatic metabolism into their active form. Their therapeutic and side effect profile is very similar to that of captopril. In renal insufficiency, dose adjustment is required.

Fosinopril—Fosinopril is an oral ACE inhibitor used for the treatment of hypertension. It must be converted into an active metabolite in the liver and the gastrointestinal tract. It is eliminated by biliary excretion, and therefore, unlike other ACE inhibitors, it does not need dose adjustment in patients with kidney insufficiency.

Perindopril, Trandolapril, and Moexipril—Perindopril, trandolapril, and moexipril are oral ACE inhibitors used for the management of left ventricular dysfunction after myocardial infarction, as well as the treatment of hypertension. These prodrugs must be hydrolyzed in the liver into their active metabolites. Their action and side effect profile is similar to that of captopril.

Angiotensin II Receptor Blockers

Angiotensin II levels may increase and maintain elevated blood pressure despite adequate treatment with ACE inhibitors, due to AT-II production via non-ACE-dependent pathways. Angiotensin II receptor blockers produce antihypertensive effects by blocking the vasoconstrictive actions of AT-II without affecting ACE activity. Because these drugs do not inhibit ACE, they do not cause an increase in bradykinin, which contributes to some of the side effects, for example, dry cough and angioedema, of ACE inhibitors. Their effects and indications (hypertension, post-myocardial infarction, and heart failure, prevention of renal insufficiency in diabetics) are similar to angiotensin-converting enzyme inhibitors.

ARBs are preload- and afterload-reducers, they down-regulate sympathetic activity by blocking the AT-II effect on peripheral norepinephrine release and reuptake, they act as diuretics and natriuretics by blocking aldosterone secretion, and counteract cardiac remodeling associated with hypertension, heart failure, and myocardial infarction. ARBs may be preferred to ACE inhibitors in hypertensive patients with heart failure, ischemic heart disease, and/or post-myocardial infarction. Angiotensin receptor blockers are generally well tolerated with a low incidence of side effects and drug interactions. In common with ACE inhibitors, ARBs are contraindicated in pregnancy.

In the presence of bilateral renal artery stenosis, AT-II constricts the efferent glomerular arteriole more than the afferent arteriole, allowing for adequate glomerular capillary pressure and filtration. ACE inhibitors and ARBs eliminate this effect of AT-II. In the presence of at least one unaffected kidney, sufficient filtration can still be maintained even after AT-1 receptors are blocked; however, when a solitary kidney or bilateral renal artery stenosis is present, kidney function may worsen.

Losartan—Losartan is an oral ARB indicated for the treatment of hypertension and lowering fatal and non-fatal cardiac and cerebrovascular events, especially when left ventricular hypertrophy is present. Both losartan and its first metabolite are active and effectively antagonize AT-II action on the AT-1 receptor. Volume and salt deficit should be corrected before treatment with losartan. In the presence of liver and kidney disease, or in patients whose kidney function depends on the activity of the renin–angiotensin–aldosterone system, dosage adjustment, withholding, or discontinuation may be required, and periodic monitoring of kidney function and potassium is necessary. It is contraindicated in pregnancy.

Valsartan—Valsartan is an ARB used as monotherapy or in combination with amlodipine and/or hydrochlorothiazide for the initial management of hypertension and heart failure with reduced ejection fraction. It conveys morbidity and mortality benefit in clinically stable patients with symptomatic heart failure or left ventricular dysfunction after MI. Valsartan may be given as part of the standard post-MI regimen, along with aspirin, beta-blockers, statins, and thrombolytics. It is contraindicated in pregnancy.

Irbesartan—Irbesartan is an oral ARB. Its indications, therapeutic, and side effect profile is similar to that of losartan and valsartan.

Olmesartan, Candesartan, Telmisartan, and Eprosartan—Olmesartan and candesartan are taken as prodrugs and which are metabolized into their active form during their absorption from the gastrointestinal tract. Candesartan is the only ARB depending on its metabolism for clinical effect.

Dose adjustment is required in the presence of kidney disease.

Olmesartan, telmisartan, and eprosartan do not require dose adjustment in the presence of mild to moderate kidney disease.

Beta Receptor Blockers

Beta-blockers have been shown to reduce mortality after myocardial infarction, congestive heart failure, hypertension, and chronic angina. The properties of these antiarrhythmic agents have been discussed previously. This section will briefly review the role of beta-blockers in the treatment of hypertension and congestive heart failure [9].

Beta adrenoceptor antagonists blunt the effect of sympathetic stimulation on the cardiovascular system. The magnitude of this effect depends on the density of receptors at the effector sites, and the availability and relative concentration of both the agonist catecholamines and the antagonist receptor blockers. Beta-blockers inhibit myocardial and peripheral vascular β_1-receptors to reduce heart rate, contractility, and myocardial O_2 consumption. By decreasing heart rate, beta-blockers increase diastolic filling time and improve O_2 and substrate delivery to the left ventricle. By decreasing contractility, beta-blockers reduce left ventricular ejection velocity and decrease shear forces on the aorta in the presence of dissection, and reduce dynamic ventricular outflow tract obstruction; for example, in hypertrophic obstructive cardiomyopathy or the tetralogy of Fallot. SVR may increase due to the inhibition of β_2 vasodilation; beta-blockers should therefore be used with caution in patients with peripheral vascular disease. Beta-blockers are generally not preferred as a first-line agent for the initial management of hypertension but may be considered as add-on therapy in patients who do not respond adequately to treatment with other drug classes. They can precipitate congestive heart failure, especially when used with other myocardial depressants; for example, calcium channel blockers. Abrupt perioperative discontinuation of beta-blocker therapy may produce rebound tachycardia and hypertension.

Traditionally, beta-receptor antagonists are classified on the basis of their relative selectivity for β_1- and β_2-receptors, the presence or absence of intrinsic agonistic (sympathomimetic) activity, and their pharmacokinetic features.

Cardioselectivity

The first generation of beta-blockers (propranolol) non-selectively blocked both β_1- and β_2-receptors. Second-generation cardioselective beta-blockers have a greater affinity for β_1- than for β_2-adrenoceptors and are less likely to produce undesired side effects (bronchoconstriction, increased SVR). β_1-selectivity is dose-dependent; therefore, caution should be exercised when administering a beta-blocker to a patient with reactive airway disease.

Examples of cardioselective beta-blockers are metoprolol, atenolol, bisoprolol, esmolol, betaxolol, and acebutolol.

Examples of non-selective beta-blockers are labetalol, carvedilol, nadolol, timolol, sotalol, and propranolol. Timolol eye drops can produce systemic beta-blockade.

Labetalol—Labetalol is a long-acting non-selective beta-receptor blocker with selective α_1-receptor blocking properties. Its α_1 to β-receptor blocking ratio is 1:3 when administered by mouth, and 1:7 when administered intravenously. It produces dose-related vasodilation without eliciting reflex tachycardia. Labetalol decreases blood pressure and systemic vascular resistance. Heart rate may slightly increase; stroke volume and cardiac output remain unchanged. Due to its long duration of action, it is usually not preferred for intraoperative minute-to-minute control of hemodynamic variables.

Carvedilol—Carvedilol is a non-selective beta-adrenergic blocking agent with selective activity on peripheral alpha_1 receptors. It is used for the management of hypertension, either as monotherapy or in combination with other agents. Carvedilol has demonstrated survival benefits and is now also part of the standard treatment regimen for clinically stable patients who have survived the acute phase of MI and have a left ventricular ejection fraction of less than 40%. In hypertensive patients with left ventricular dysfunction (those who depend on beta-adrenergic stimulation in order to maintain cardiovascular compensation), the usual (lower) heart failure dosage applies (instead of that for hypertension). Contraindications to the use of carvedilol include high-degree atrioventricular block, bronchial asthma or other reactive airway diseases, cardiogenic shock, decompensated congestive heart failure (CHF) requiring inotropes, severe liver dysfunction, and a history of severe hypersensitivity reactions. Abrupt discontinuation of carvedilol may precipitate cardiac ischemia or malignant ventricular arrhythmias, as well as thyroid storm in patients with thyrotoxicosis.

Intrinsic Sympathomimetic Activity

Certain beta-blockers may act as a competitive partial agonist–antagonist on peripheral β-receptors, and elicit a submaximal response at maximal occupancy. This phenomenon is referred to as intrinsic sympathomimetic activity or ISA. These agents will prevent a beta-agonist from binding to its receptor and will decrease blood pressure and systemic vascular resistance while resulting in less resting bradycardia and maintaining resting cardiac output than is observed with beta-blockers without ISA. Long-term treatment with agents with ISA results in a decrease in blood pressure due to decreased vascular resistance, rather than decreased cardiac output. These agents may be useful in patients who are unable to tolerate excessive bradycardia resulting from treatment with beta-blockers. Agents with ISA have not been shown to be beneficial after myocardial infarction and are not included in standard post-MI treatment regimens. They are less effective than other beta-blockers in the treatment of angina and tachycardia.

Examples of beta-blockers with ISA are pindolol and acebutolol.

Perioperative Management

Perioperative cardiac complications are not uncommon, with 2% of patients suffering major cardiac complications, and 8% showing evidence of significant myocardial injury. According to the 2014 ACC/AHA Perioperative Clinical Practice Guideline, a continuation of long-standing beta-blocker therapy is recommended. Beta-blockers should not be started on the day of surgery in beta-blocker-naïve patients. In patients with intermediate or high perioperative risk, or in patients with at least 3 Revised Cardiac Risk Index (RCRI) risk factors, it may be reasonable to initiate beta-blocker therapy at least 24 h prior to surgery. It may also be reasonable to initiate perioperative beta-blocker therapy long enough in advance to assess safety and tolerability; however, it is uncertain whether starting beta-blockers benefits those with long-term indications, but no other RCRI risk factors. In the perioperative setting, beta-blockers have been confirmed to reduce the incidence of postoperative atrial fibrillation when started before or immediately after surgery. Initiation of beta-blocker therapy prior to surgery is currently reserved for patients with significant coronary artery disease undergoing surgical coronary revascularization.

Calcium Channel Blockers: Dihydropyridines

Calcium channel blockers have a multifaceted profile of therapeutic effects. Calcium channel blockers are used primarily as anti-ischemic agents for the treatment and prevention of stable angina pectoris. Common to all calcium channel blockers, but to a different extent in each class, they act as peripheral vasodilators without eliciting reflex tachycardia, induce coronary vasodilation, they are negative inotropes, and have electrophysiologic depressant properties. The non-dihydropyridine diltiazem and verapamil are used for rate control in acute cardiac ischemia when beta-blockers are contraindicated. Most importantly, calcium channel blockers are first-line agents as potent coronary vasodilators in the treatment of Prinzmetal (variant, vasospastic) angina.

As discussed previously, dihydropyridines act on the peripheral arteriolar beds and produce marked peripheral vasodilation with a direct and indirect effect on heart rate, AV conduction, and inotropy. Examples are the rapid-acting antianginal nifedipine, the long-acting vasodilator nicardipine, the highly lipid-soluble nimodipine (favoring cerebral vessels), amlodipine, felodipine, or isradipine.

Nifedipine—Nifedipine is primarily indicated in the management of Prinzmetal angina. Only its extended-release formulations are recommended for the treatment of hypertension, as well as the management of Raynaud's disease. Conventional (immediate-release) formulations are contraindicated in the management of acute myocardial infarction due to their negative inotropy and reflex sympathetic activation.

Nicardipine—Nicardipine is a highly potent peripheral vasodilator that inhibits calcium influx into the myocardium and vascular smooth muscle. Nicardipine has no effects on the SA node and AV node. It produces clinically insignificant negative inotropy and may be combined with a beta-blocker for the treatment of angina. This drug has the greatest vasodilating effects of all the CCBs, with vasodilation being particularly prominent in the coronary arteries. Because of all the antianginal drugs dihydropyridines produce the greatest peripheral vasodilation, either nifedipine or nicardipine may be useful in patients who have residual hypertension despite the adequate beta-adrenergic blockade. Nicardipine produces a dose-related decrease in both systolic and diastolic blood pressure. Nicardipine is frequently used as a tocolytic. When administered, it binds to the inside of the myometrial L-channels causing them to remain closed and inhibiting uterine contractions. Pulmonary edema has been reported when nicardipine was used as a tocolytic. Its use is contraindicated in patients with severe aortic stenosis: A decrease in diastolic pressure may worsen myocardial oxygen balance.

Nimodipine—Nimodipine is a highly lipid-soluble analog of nifedipine. This high degree of lipid solubility facilitates its penetration into the central nervous system, where it blocks the influx of extracellular calcium necessary for the contraction of large cerebral arteries. This is especially valuable during the treatment and prevention of cerebral vasospasm after subarachnoid hemorrhage. Nimodipine has a minimal negative inotropic effect on the myocardium.

Amlodipine—Amlodipine is a dihydropyridine calcium antagonist only available in oral form, with minimal cardio-depressant effects. Its anti-ischemic effects are comparable to beta-blockers in patients with acute coronary syndrome. The combination of amlodipine and a beta-blocker is more effective in the treatment of myocardial ischemia than either drug alone. Its actions are resembling those of nifedipine. It is used primarily for the oral treatment of hypertension.

Felodipine—Felodipine is primarily a peripheral vasodilator with no clinically significant negative inotropy. Its actions are resembling those of nifedipine. It is used for the oral treatment of hypertension.

Isradipine—Isradipine is a peripheral vasodilator with no clinically significant negative inotropy. Its actions are resembling those of nifedipine. It is used for the oral treatment of hypertension.

Direct Vasodilators: Hydralazine, Nitroglycerine, and Nitroprusside

Hydralazine—Hydralazine is a direct systemic arteriolar vasodilator, with minimal venodilator (preload and postural) effects. Its mechanism of action is not fully understood. It appears to interfere with calcium movements within the cell that initiate and maintain the contractile state. Hydralazine decreases systemic blood pressure (systolic less than diastolic). Hydralazine may produce reflex sympathetic nervous system stimulation: It increases renin and AT-II activity, which leads to aldosterone stimulation and sodium reabsorption; tachycardia and increased myocardial contractility results in an increase in cardiac output, and may provoke angina. Patients with coronary artery disease should be monitored for myocardial ischemia. The use of hydralazine to treat pulmonary hypertension is not recommended since the associated systemic vasodilation may result in systemic hypotension. Hydralazine has a relatively slow onset of action with a peak effect occurring by 20 min. With chronic PO use, a lupus-like reaction may occur.

Nitroglycerine—Nitroglycerine is a direct coronary vasodilator with greater effects on the venous than on the arterial system. Its mechanism of action and effects are described in a previous section.

Nitroprusside—Sodium nitroprusside (SNP) is a direct-acting, non-selective vasodilator. It is indicated for rapid correction of hypertensive emergencies. It produces vasodilation by directly increasing intracellular nitric oxide levels; its effects on arteries and veins are balanced. Nitroprusside lacks effect on non-vascular smooth muscle and the myocardium; however, reflex tachycardia and increased inotropy may occur, making it an undesirable drug of choice for the treatment of aortic dissection, where shear forces should be minimized. Its immediate onset of action and short duration allows for IV infusion and precise titration of dosage.

As nitroprusside interacts with oxyhemoglobin ($HbFe^{2+}$), it dissociates immediately and forms methemoglobin ($HbFe^{3+}$) while releasing nitric oxide (NO) and the highly toxic free cyanide ions. In contrast to organic nitrates (for example, nitroglycerin), nitroprusside does not require the presence of sulfhydryl compounds to generate NO, instead it spontaneously produces them and therefore acts as a prodrug. Nitric oxide is the active mediator in the vasodilating effects of SNP: It activates the guanylate cyclase present in vascular smooth muscle and increases cGMP, which in turn decreases Ca^{2+} entry into the cell and intracellular Ca^{2+} concentration.

Nitroprusside's degradation products are rapidly cleared via non-enzymatic pathways. Each SNP molecule releases five cyanide ions. Cyanide ions undergo sulfurilation by the hepatic and kidney enzyme rhodanase (also known as thiosulfate sulfurtransferase, indicating that thiosulfate must be available for the transsulfuration to take place) to form thiocyanate, and are excreted in the urine. The availability of thiosulfate is the rate-limiting step in cyanide detoxification. Excess cyanide ions immediately react with methemoglobin to form cyanmethemoglobin. When sulfur donors and methemoglobin are exhausted, unscavenged free cyanide radicals may accumulate and bind to tissue cytochrome oxidase, to inhibit mitochondrial oxidative phosphorylation. This leads to tissue hypoxia despite adequate levels of available oxygen.

The most common adverse effect of SNP is hypotension and dysrhythmias. Tachyphylaxis may occur, requiring adjustments in dosage for the necessary effect. Thiocyanate toxicity is infrequent and presents with nausea, abdominal pain, hyperreflexia, tinnitus, seizures, and changes in mental status. Thiocyanate clearance can be facilitated by dialysis. Rarely, cyanide toxicity ensues.

Signs and symptoms of cyanide toxicity are hypertension (secondary to tachyphylaxis), arrhythmias, ST-segment changes, altered mental status, seizures, coma, elevated mixed venous pO2 (due to inhibition of cellular O_2 utilization), increasing the base deficit, and metabolic acidosis. No cyanosis is seen; SpO_2 remains high.

Treatment includes immediate discontinuation of nitroprusside, mechanical ventilation with 100% oxygen, and correction of acidosis with bicarbonate. Mild toxicity (stable hemodynamics with discontinuation of SNP, base deficit less than 10) can be treated with thiosulfate (150 mg/kg IV bolus over 15 min). Severe toxicity (worsening hemodynamics even after discontinuation of SNP, base deficit greater than 10) is treated with 3% sodium nitrite (4–6 mg/kg over 5 min). Sodium nitrite converts oxyhemoglobin to methemoglobin, which competes with cytochrome oxidase for the cyanide ions. Hydroxocobalamin is an alternative to thiosulfate or sodium nitrite. It binds cyanide to form cyanocobalamin, which acts as a non-toxic reservoir and is excreted by the kidneys.

Ganglionic Blockade: Trimethaphan

Trimethaphan dilates peripheral arteries by blocking cholinergic transmission on nicotinergic autonomic ganglia by binding to the post-synaptic ACh-receptor. It is a short-acting competitive acetylcholine antagonist with both sympatholytic and parasympatholytic effects. It causes vasodilation and tachycardia. Common side effects are mydriasis, urinary retention, and ileus. Its use is very limited; it has been used for inducing controlled hypotension during surgery, reduction of blood pressure during hypertensive emergencies (for example, in patients with a dissecting aortic aneurysm), or for the emergency treatment of pulmonary edema.

Considerations for Treatment of Pulmonary Hypertension

Pulmonary hypertension—sustained elevated pressure within the pulmonary artery—is a heterogenous and frequently progressive disorder of the pulmonary vasculature that ultimately leads to increased pulmonary vascular resistance, right heart failure, and death, due to constrained pulmonary blood flow and vascular remodeling of the resistance arteries. Multiple pathways of pathogenesis have been implicated in the development of pulmonary arterial hypertension; excessive cell proliferation, reduced apoptosis, endothelial dysfunction, and an imbalance of the vasoconstrictor/vasodilator milieu appearing to be the predominant cause. Based on the etiology, the World Health Organization (WHO) classifies pulmonary hypertension into five groups:

1. Idiopathic pulmonary arterial hypertension, familial arterial hypertension, and pulmonary arterial hypertension associated with connective tissue disorders, portal hypertension, human immunodeficiency virus (HIV) infection, congenital left-to-right shunt, or venous or capillary involvement
2. Pulmonary arterial hypertension with left heart disease
3. Pulmonary arterial hypertension associated with hypoxia and/or lung disease
4. Pulmonary arterial hypertension caused by chronic thrombotic and/or embolic disease4
5. Pulmonary arterial hypertension due to miscellaneous causes

Treatment is geared toward symptomatic relief, enhancement of functional capacity, improvement of quality of life, slowing disease progression, and prolongation of survival. Basic management strategies involve lifestyle modifications including physical activity appropriate to functional capacity, oxygen supplementation when chronic hypoxemia develops, diuresis for right ventricular preload reduction, avoidance of pregnancy, and oral anticoagulant therapy to decrease the risk of venous thromboembolism. The optimal management of pulmonary hypertension is always individualized.

Calcium Channel Blockers

Based on the American College of Cardiology Foundation (ACCF)/AHA 2009 Expert Consensus Document on Pulmonary Hypertension, vasodilator testing (administration of a pulmonary vasodilator to assess pulmonary vascular reactivity) should be performed in patients with idiopathic pulmonary arterial hypertension, and chronic responders should be considered for long-term treatment with calcium channel blockers. Commonly used agents are long-acting nifedipine, diltiazem, or amlodipine. Verapamil should be avoided [10].

Endothelin-Receptor Antagonists

Endothelin-1 (ET-1) is a proinflammatory mediator—a direct vasoconstrictor that stimulates pulmonary vascular smooth muscle cell proliferation and induces fibrosis. Its effects are mediated through the ET_A receptors that mediate vasoconstriction and smooth muscle proliferation, and the ET_B receptors that induce the production of nitric oxide and prostacyclin, and mediate ET-1 clearance. Clearance of ET-1 is diminished in pulmonary hypertension.

Bosentan—Bosentan is an orally active dual ET_A and ET_B antagonist. It is approved for the treatment of WHO group 1 pulmonary hypertension to slow clinical deterioration and enhance functional capacity in patients who are not candidates for treatment with calcium channel blockers.

The use of bosentan increases the risk of severe hepatic injury, liver cirrhosis, and liver failure. Liver function should be monitored monthly while taking bosentan. Bosentan may cause serious birth defects. Pregnancy should be ruled out prior to initiation of treatment and monthly thereafter. It should be avoided in patients with elevated transaminases and is contraindicated in pregnancy. Angioedema, fluid retention, and possible dose-related decreases in hemoglobin and hematocrit have been reported.

Prostaglandin Analogues

Prostacyclin (prostaglandin I_2, PGI_2, PGX) and thromboxane A_2 are the main metabolites of arachinoid acid with opposing effects on the vascular smooth muscle. Thromboxane A_2 induces vasoconstriction and promotes platelet activation, whereas PGI_2 is a vasodilator with platelet inhibitor effects. In pulmonary arterial hypertension, their physiologic balance is shifted toward thromboxane A_2. This promotes smooth muscle cell proliferation, vasoconstriction, and thrombogenesis. The activity of prostacyclin synthase is decreased in pulmonary hypertension, leading to low levels of the vasodilator and antiproliferative PGI_2. Restoring the balance between vasodilating and vasoconstricting factors, including the administration of prostacyclin analogs, is a mainstay of the medical management of pulmonary hypertension.

Epoprostenol—PGI_2-analog epoprostenol is used for the long-term treatment of idiopathic pulmonary hypertension, and pulmonary hypertension associated with scleroderma spectrum diseases. It improves functional class, exercise tolerance, and hemodynamics. Its two main pharmacologic actions are (1) direct pulmonary and systemic vasodilation, and (2) platelet inhibition. It is an afterload reducer for both the left and the right ventricle. It produces dose-related decreases in pulmonary vascular resistance; it increases stroke volume and cardiac output.

Epoprostenol is usually administered as a continuous infusion into a central vein. Dosing must be individualized; however, the optimal dose range for long-term therapy is believed to be 25–40 ng/kg/minute, when used as monotherapy. Alternatively, it may be delivered as an inhaled aerosol, for example for the treatment of acute right ventricular failure in the intraoperative or early postoperative setting. Common side effects are headache, flushing, nausea, diarrhea, and musculoskeletal pain. Contraindications to its chronic use include congestive heart failure due to severe left ventricular systolic dysfunction, pulmonary edema during initial treatment, or known hypersensitivity to epoprostenol or structurally related agents. Abrupt withdrawal or sudden dose adjustments should be avoided. Its use should be limited to centers experienced with its administration and with systematic follow-up with patients.

Iloprost—Iloprost is a stable prostacyclin analog delivered as an inhaled aerosol to patients with idiopathic pulmonary hypertension, pulmonary hypertension associated with scleroderma spectrum diseases or appetite suppressants, or pulmonary hypertension related to chronic thromboembolic disease. In the acute setting, iloprost decreases pulmonary vascular resistance; with long-term use, in addition to its pulmonary vasodilator effects it suppresses pulmonary vascular smooth vessel proliferation.

Iloprost is delivered as an inhaled aerosol. It is approved for functional class III and IV to relieve symptoms, enhance exercise tolerance, and diminish disease progression. Its adverse effects are similar to those of epoprostenol. Its use should be avoided in pre-existing hypotension. It may induce bronchospasm in patients with reactive airway disease. Caution should be used with its administration in the presence of increased risk of bleeding, anticoagulation, or other bleeding disorders. Abrupt withdrawal or sudden dose adjustments should be avoided. The use of iloprost should be limited to centers experienced with its administration and with systematic follow-up with patients.

Treprostinil—Treprostinil is a stable prostacyclin analog that can be taken by mouth, administered into a central vein, or subcutaneously (preferred). Its main actions are pulmonary arterial vasodilation and inhibition of platelet aggregation. It is approved to decrease exercise-related symptoms and diminish clinical deterioration.

Treprostinil may induce symptomatic hypotension. It may increase the risk of bleeding. There appears to be an increased risk of Gram-negative bloodstream infections, especially in patients receiving intravenous treatment via a chronic indwelling catheter. Its side effects are similar to those of epoprostenol. Abrupt withdrawal or sudden dose adjustments should be avoided. Its use should be limited to centers experienced with its administration and with systematic follow-up with patients.

Phosphodiesterase-5 Inhibitors

Phosphodiesterase-5 (PDE-5) is the intracellular enzyme responsible for degrading cyclic nucleotide monophosphates. It limits signal transduction by cAMP and cGMP—second messengers implicated in pathogenetic pathways leading to pulmonary hypertension. cGMP is involved in mechanisms of pulmonary vasodilation; its rapid hydrolysis by PDE-5 significantly limits its effect on vasomotor tone.

Sildenafil—Sildenafil is a PDE-5 inhibitor initially indicated for the treatment of erectile dysfunction. It enhances the effect of nitric oxide in the corpus cavernosum and the pulmonary arterial smooth muscle. It is approved for the treatment of WHO group 1 pulmonary hypertension to improve functional capacity and delay disease progression; its unlabeled indication is the treatment of pulmonary hypertension after recent left ventricular assist device placement.

Common side effects associated with the use of sildenafil are headache, flushing, dyspepsia, epistaxis, and disturbances of color discrimination. It may potentiate the effects of antihypertensive agents. The use of sildenafil for pulmonary hypertension should be avoided with strong CYP3A4 inhibitors. The use of sildenafil is contraindicated with the concurrent use of organic nitrates and guanylate cyclase stimulant riociguat.

Tadalafil—Tadalafil is a longer-acting PDE-5 inhibitor approved for the treatment of erectile dysfunction, benign prostate hypertrophy, and WHO group 1 pulmonary hypertension in patients who are not candidates for treatment with calcium channel blockers. Its mechanism of action is similar to that of sildenafil. It is taken by mouth as a once-daily dose. It may be considered for combination therapy with a prostacyclin analog or ET-1 receptor antagonist.

Its side effects are similar to those of sildenafil. It may potentiate the effects of antihypertensive agents.

Its use is not recommended in patients with recent myocardial infarction or stroke within 6 months; uncontrolled arrhythmias, hypotension, uncontrolled hypertension, heart failure, or unstable angina. It should be avoided when severe aortic stenosis or dynamic left ventricular outflow tract obstruction is present. Concomitant use of organic nitrates is contraindicated.

Nitric Oxide

Nitric oxide (NO) is a potent, endothelium-derived, cGMP-dependent direct vasodilator generated from the terminal guanidine nitrogen of L-arginine. It is produced by three isoforms of nitric oxide synthase (NOS) in response to hypoxia, pulsatile flow, and flow-induced sheer stress on the arterial wall. It exists in the gaseous form and is administered as an inhalational agent. Once inhaled, it diffuses to target cells and activates guanylate cyclase to increase cGMP production: an increased cGMP concentration subsequently leads to vasorelaxation. NO diffuses across the pulmonary capillary endothelium into the circulation. Once in circulation, it avidly binds to the iron of heme-based proteins; it is rapidly inactivated by hemoglobin.

In pulmonary arterial hypertension, decreased NOS3 activity is present, resulting in decreased NO-induced pulmonary vasodilation. The use of nitric oxide is favored in the treatment of pulmonary hypertension for its selective pulmonary vasodilator and antiproliferative effects. It vasodilates the well-ventilated areas and improves V/Q matching. It inhibits platelet activation, aggregation, and adhesion. It is synergistic with PGI2, allowing the endothelium to maintain its antithrombotic properties.

Nitric oxide is used to treat persistent pulmonary hypertension in the newborn. As with inhaled prostaglandin analogs, it does not appear to improve clinical outcomes in acute respiratory distress syndrome (ARDS).

Drug Therapy for Heart Failure

Heart failure is a constellation of clinical symptoms (primarily fatigue and dyspnea) secondary to impaired left ventricular systolic (reduced ejection fraction) or diastolic (preserved ejection fraction) function, and/or elevated intracardiac pressures. The 2013 AHA/ACC guidelines classify the syndrome by its evolution from asymptomatic preclinical stages to progression to advanced structural heart disease and symptomatology at rest, refractory to maximal medical management. These guidelines also complement the widely accepted functional classification of symptomatic heart failure by the New York Heart Association (NYHA I-IV) [11].

Chronic heart failure is a condition characterized by vasoconstriction, volume overload, and neurohormonal activation. The goal of its pharmacologic management is to reduce vascular tone, reduce sympathetic activation, and improve cardiac function. Conventional treatment options include angiotensin-converting enzyme inhibitors, angiotensin II receptor blockers, aldosterone antagonists, beta-blockers, and the combination of isosorbide dinitrate and hydralazine and diuretics. Novel approaches are now the use of ivabradine and angiotensin receptor-neprilysin inhibitor/ARB combinations.

Nesiritide

Nesiritide is a recombinant human B-type natriuretic peptide with vasodilatory properties. It binds to vascular endothelial and smooth muscle A- and B-type natriuretic peptide receptors. It increases cGMP levels. cGMP serves as a second messenger to produce arterial and venous dilation. Much like endogenous natriuretic peptides, it suppresses the sympathetic nervous system, the renin–angiotensin–aldosterone system, and endothelin. Based on the results of initial trials and the observed reduction of pulmonary capillary wedge pressure and symptomatic relief, it was first approved for the treatment of patients with acute decompensated heart failure; however, the Acute Study of Clinical Effectiveness of Nesiritide in Decompensated Heart Failure (ASCEND-HF) demonstrated that nesiritide did not convey advantage over standard treatment of acute decompensated heart failure [12].

Ivabradine

Ivabradine is a novel sinoatrial modulator used for the treatment of chronic stable angina pectoris and heart failure with an ejection fraction lower than 35% inadequately controlled by beta-blockers, in patients with native sinus rhythm. It reduces the heart rate by inhibiting the cardiac pacemaker inward "funny" current in the sinoatrial node, which, unlike beta-blockers or calcium channel blockers, produces selective heart rate control without affecting ventricular repolarization or myocardial contractility. It may prove beneficial for the treatment of heart failure with reduced ejection fraction. It is contraindicated in sick sinus syndrome, as well as concomitant use of CYP3A4 inhibitors; for example, azole antifungals, macrolides, and protease inhibitor antiretrovirals. It is contraindicated with the concomitant use of verapamil or diltiazem.

Angiotensin Receptor-Neprilysin Inhibitors (ARNI)

Sacubitril/Valsartan

ARNI combinations have been shown to convey mortality benefits in patients with chronic heart failure, a condition in which neurohormonal activation, volume overload, and vasoconstriction play important roles. Natriuretic peptides are potent vasodilators with natriuretic properties. They reduce sympathetic tone and inhibit the renin–angiotensin–aldosterone (RAAS) axis. Neprilysin is an endopeptidase that degrades vasoactive and natriuretic peptides. Sacubitril is a neprilysin inhibitor; therefore, it increases the concentration of natriuretic peptides. Its combination with a RAAS-inhibitor angiotensin receptor blocker conveys cardiovascular and renal protection. The PARADIGM-HF (Prospective Comparison of ARNI with ACEI to Determine Impact on Global Mortality and Morbidity in Heart Failure) trial demonstrated a significant reduction in cardiovascular and all-cause mortality, as well as heart failure-related hospital readmissions in patients with Class II-IV heart failure and reduced ejection fraction when treated with sacubitril/valsartan compared to enalapril alone. It should be avoided in pregnancy, and it should not be administered concomitantly with ACE inhibitors.

The updated 2016 ACC/AHA/Heart Failure Society of America (HFSA) Guidelines for Management of Heart Failure include the addition of ivabradine and sacubitril/valsartan to the list of treatment options for patients with heart failure and reduced ejection fraction.

Digitalis

Digitalis is a cardiac glycoside that selectively and reversibly inhibits the integral membrane protein Na^+/K^+ ATPase ion transport system: the Na^+/K^+ ATPase maintains gradients for Na^+ and K^+ that determine myocardial excitability and action potential. Digoxin is the only commercially available digitalis preparation available in the United States. It binds on the external alpha subunit, increases intracellular Na^+ concentration, decreases Ca^{2+} efflux, and augments inotropy by releasing calcium from the sarcoplasmic reticulum into the cytoplasm, making more calcium available to generate contraction. Digoxin makes resting potential less negative with a resultant increase in myocardial excitability. M_{VO2} is decreased due to its effects on wall tension, preload, and afterload.

Electrophysiologic Effects

1. Inhibits Na efflux during phase 0
2. Shortens the duration of phase 2. This results in a decreased duration of the action potential.
3. Decreases the slope of phase 3 depolarization. This results in digoxin's characteristic effect on the ST segment of the EKG.
4. Increases the slope of phase 4 repolarization. This leads to increased automaticity and ectopic beats.
5. Shortens AV conduction time. Shortens the refractory period in the atria and the ventricles.

ECG Changes

1. Increases the PR interval due to delayed AV conduction.
2. Characteristic scaphoid ST-segment depression due to decreased slope of phase 3 depolarization.
3. Flat or inverse T-waves. The diminished amplitude or negative deflection does not correlate with serum levels.
4. Shortens QT interval. This leads to more rapid ventricular repolarization. This is independent of parasympathetic activity.

Hemodynamic Effects

1. Preload: decreased
2. Contractility: augmented, ejection fraction increased
3. Lusitropy: increased
4. Afterload: decreased
5. Heart rate: Digoxin reduces ventricular response rate in atrial fibrillation or flutter. It sensitizes arterial baroreceptors in the carotid sinus, and increases parasympathetic activity by activating the vagal nuclei and the ganglion nodosum with resultant decreases in SA node activity, prolonged effective refractory period and AV conduction time, resulting in slowed heart rate. Digoxin may trigger any type of arrhythmia.
6. Cardiac output: increased.

Common Clinical Uses

Treatment of supraventricular tachyarrhythmias, ventricular rate control for atrial fibrillation with a rapid ventricular response. It has been used for the treatment of paroxysmal supraventricular tachycardia due to AV-nodal re-entry or AV-re-entry. Historically, it is used for the treatment of symptomatic heart failure associated with left ventricular dysfunction. Treatment may be initiated in patients who have not yet responded to the conventional treatment regimen with an ACE inhibitor or a beta-blocker. Digoxin does not provide overall mortality benefits, but alleviates symptoms and decreases heart failure-related hospital admissions. Digoxin does not appear to have a significant effect on disease progression in asymptomatic individuals.

Administration

PO or IV. Assuming normal renal function, the loading dose for an adult is typically 0.25–0.5 mg increments IV or IM for a total of 1–1.25 mg. The maintenance dose is 0.125–0.250 mg/day, based on serum levels and clinical effects.

Adverse Effects

Dizziness, mental disturbances, diarrhea, nausea, vomiting, cardiac dysrhythmias, heart block, and visual disturbances.

Warnings and Contraindications

Administration of digoxin is not recommended for asymptomatic (NYHA class I) patients. Digoxin is contraindicated when dynamic LVOT obstruction is present and in pre-excitation arrhythmias. Caution should be used with the concomitant use of beta-blockers, calcium channel blockers, or calcium. Digoxin has a very low therapeutic index with a nonlinear dose response. The dose should be reduced in hypokalemia, hypothyroidism, extensive myocardial or renal damage, and geriatric patients.

Digitalis Toxicity

Due to its very narrow therapeutic range, increased latency of onset, and long duration of action, careful dosage determination is essential to avoid digitalis toxicity. In addition to drug pharmacokinetics and pharmacodynamics, patient characteristics—for example, age, cardiac and renal functional status, other medical comorbidities, and pharmacotherapy—should be considered. Doses should be individualized. Digoxin toxicity has a relatively high mortality rate.

Therapeutic digoxin levels fall between 0.5 and 2.5 ng/ml. Levels lower than 0.5 ng/ml are non-toxic. Levels higher than 3 ng/ml are definitely toxic. Infants and children appear to be more tolerant of higher digoxin levels without manifesting signs and symptoms of toxicity.

Signs of toxicity include extracardiac (primarily central nervous system and gastrointestinal) and cardiac effects. Extracardiac manifestations are similar in both acute and chronic intoxication.

In pediatric patients, drowsiness, nausea, and vomiting are common signs of early toxicity and may present before or after the manifestation of cardiotoxicity. In neonates and infants, sinus bradycardia is a premonitory sign of digitalis cardiotoxicity.

In adults, early gastrointestinal effects include nausea, vomiting, and anorexia. These may present before or after the manifestation of cardiotoxicity. Central nervous system effects include headache, drowsiness, generalized weakness, visual disturbances (color vision is commonly affected), disorientation, confusion, delusions, hallucinations, delirium, or amnesia. Cardiovascular toxicity may develop in the absence or presence of other signs and symptoms of toxicity, and includes new arrhythmias, especially those that exhibit features of increased automaticity and AV-block, premature atrial and ventricular beats, and malignant ventricular arrhythmias.

Acute toxicity is usually associated with hyperkalemia, whereas chronic toxicity is associated with hypokalemia or normokalemia.

Factors that predispose to toxicity are electrolyte derangements such as hypokalemia, hypomagnesemia, or hypercalcemia, diuretic use, alkalosis or acidosis, impaired kidney function, hyperventilation, hypocapnia, arterial hypoxemia, treatment with quinidine, and decreased muscle mass. Hypokalemia increases myocardial binding of glycosides; binding of cardiac glycosides to the Na^+/K^+ ATPase enzyme complex is inhibited by elevated potassium levels.

Treatment of Digitalis Toxicity

Immediate discontinuation of digoxin, correction of predisposing factors, treatment of cardiac dysrhythmias (phenytoin, amiodarone, and beta-blockers), and temporary pacing. Supplemental K decreases the binding of digitalis to myocardial tissue. Digoxin Fab is a special digoxin-binding antidote that prevents and reverses toxic effects and enhances elimination; as there is no comparable alternative treatment, it should be promptly administered to patients with digitalis toxicity.

11.5 Questions and Answers

Questions (Choose the Most Appropriate Answer)

1. You are taking care of a patient undergoing mitral annular valvuloplasty for severe mitral regurgitation. Shortly after separation from cardiopulmonary bypass, ST-segment elevations are noted in lead V5 with reciprocal ST-segment depression in lead II. The hypokinetic region of the left ventricle most likely reflects compromised flow through which coronary artery?

    Left anterior descending artery
    Left circumflex artery
    Left main stem
    Right coronary artery

2. Common ECG findings of hypercalcemia are:
   A. Slightly prolonged PR interval, shallow or biphasic T-waves, prominent U-waves, ST-segment depression
   B. Wide or flat P wave, prolonged PR interval, wide QRS, prolonged QT, peaked T-waves, ventricular fibrillation
   C. Prolonged QT_c (lengthened ST segment), third-degree AV-block, torsades de pointes, ventricular tachycardia
   D. Short PR or QT interval (shortened ST segment), flattened T-wave, Osborn-waves
3. For a chronic beta-blocker user patient with a recent history of percutaneous myocardial revascularization with a bare metal stent 10 days prior to his non-emergent non-cardiac surgery, the recommended course of action is:
   A. Continue beta-blockers and proceed to surgery in 10 days.
   B. Wait at least 30 days after bare metal stent placement before undergoing non-emergent non-cardiac surgery, and continue beta-blockers in the perioperative period.
   C. Wait at least 365 days after bare metal stent placement, and hold beta-blockers preoperatively.
   D. Start clonidine for perioperative cardiac risk reduction.
4. Through what mechanisms does propofol affect blood pressure?
   A. Propofol decreases systemic vascular resistance and directly depresses the myocardium in the absence of significant cardiovascular disease.
   B. At standard induction doses, propofol maintains baseline mean arterial pressure by augmenting inotropy in response to vasodilation.
   C. At high doses, propofol maintains baseline cardiac output by proportionally increasing the heart rate for a given decrease in SVR and mean arterial pressure.
   D. Propofol does not affect systemic vascular resistance or cardiac output.
5. Through what mechanisms does ketamine change blood pressure?
   A. Ketamine enhances cardiac output by directly stimulating the sympathetic nervous system; it causes tachycardia and acts as a vasoconstrictor by increasing peripheral arteriolar resistance.
   B. Ketamine augments myocardial contractility in patients with depleted sympathetic reserves.
   C. In patients with adequate myocardial and catecholamine reserve, ketamine decreases baseline mean arterial pressure as a result of vasodilation and myocardial depression.
   D. Ketamine does not have significant cardiovascular effects at standard induction doses.
6. Which statement about the hemodynamic effects of etomidate is correct?
   A. Etomidate causes significant cardiorespiratory depression in the presence of cardiac and pulmonary disease.
   B. Etomidate causes significant cardiorespiratory depression in the absence of cardiac and pulmonary disease.
   C. Etomidate may cause a small increase in heart rate and cardiac output, and may decrease systemic vascular resistance and mean arterial pressure regardless of pre-existing cardiopulmonary reserves.
   D. Etomidate does not have any cardiovascular effects.
7. An 82-year-old patient presents for laparoscopic cholecystectomy. His medical history is significant for severe aortic stenosis with an estimated orifice area of 1 cm^2. The goals of induction are:
   A. Ensure full preload to maintain adequate left ventricular end diastolic pressure and forward stroke volume, maintain normal sinus rhythm, avoid extremes of heart rate, maintain adequate coronary perfusion by avoiding any significant drop in cardiac output or systemic vascular resistance.
   B. Decrease afterload to promote forward flow.
   C. Allow the heart rate to increase above 90 beats per minute to raise aortic diastolic pressure.
   D. Minimize IV hydration to avoid volume overload.
8. The preferred agent to treat drug-induced hypotension in the patient from question 7 is
   A. Ephedrine
   B. Phenylephrine
   C. Epinephrine
   D. Norepinephrine
9. In patients with an intact circulation, rapid infusion of intravenous amiodarone leads to
   A. Rapid restoration of native sinus rhythm and hemodynamic stability
   B. Shortened refractory period
   C. Hypotension and bradycardia
   D. Increased speed of conduction in the sinoatrial node
10. Which of the following statements about the cardiovascular effects of norepinephrine is correct?
    A. The primary effect of norepinephrine is direct β(-beta)$_2$-agonism.
    B. Norepinephrine increases cardiac output to a greater extent than phenylephrine.

C. Norepinephrine augments renal and mesenteric blood flow.
D. The arrhythmogenicity of norepinephrine is significantly greater than that of epinephrine, dobutamine, dopamine or isoproterenol.

Answers

1. **B**. Left circumflex artery. ST elevation in the septal (V1, V2) and anterior (V3, V4) leads reflect compromised flow across the left anterior descending artery. ST-changes in the high (I-aVL) and low (V5, V6) lateral leads reflect compromised flow through the left circumflex artery. The inferior wall (leads II, III, and aVF) is supplied by the right coronary artery in 80–90% of the cases, and by the left circumflex artery in the remaining 10%. A recognized immediate surgical complication of mitral valve surgery is left circumflex coronary injury, due to the proximity of the left circumflex artery to the mitral valve annulus: Any suture placed during mitral annuloplasty, or changes in the coronary caliper as a result of a posterior leaflet plication may result in compromised blood supply to the lateral wall of the left ventricle. ST-segment elevations in leads V1-V6, I, and aVL indicate an extensive anterior myocardial infarct, and would most likely result from compromised flow through the left main coronary artery.
2. **D**. Electrolyte abnormalities may cause ECG changes due to altered ion flux across the membrane resulting in altered transmembrane potentials. The cardiac effects of hypercalcemia (usually at levels greater than 15 mg/dL) are shortened PR or QT interval with or without widening of the QRS complex, flattened T-wave, or the Osborne-waves, typically seen in hypothermia. Treatment is hydration with normal saline to decrease plasma calcium levels by dilution, administration of non-thiazide diuretics, and avoidance of thiazides. Non-depolarizer muscle relaxant doses should be decreased in patients with hypercalcemia and muscle weakness. The cardiac effects of hyperkalemia are peaked T-waves at mildly elevated potassium levels (6–7 mEq/L), wide or flat P wave, prolonged PR interval, wide QRS, prolonged QT, ventricular fibrillation, and asystole at higher serum potassium levels (10–12 mEq/L). Treatment is: (1) temporary membrane stabilization with IV calcium (commonly administered dose: 500 mg $CaCl_2$ or 1 g Ca-gluconate), (2) inducing intracellular K + − shift by administering intravenous insulin and glucose (commonly administered dose: 25 to 50 g intravenous dextrose along with 5 to 10 units of insulin), and (3) promoting excretion (diuretics, hemodialysis, resins). Slightly prolonged PR interval, shallow or biphasic T-waves, prominent U-waves, and ST-segment depression reflects hypokalemia; whereas prolonged QT_c, third-degree AV-block, torsades de pointes or ventricular tachycardia may reflect hypocalcemia.
3. **B**. According to the most recent ACC/AHA guidelines, there is a Class I recommendation for continuing beta-blocker therapy in patients using beta-blockers chronically. It may be reasonable to start beta-blockers in patients with 3 or more RCRI risk factors; however, beta-blockers should not be started on the day of surgery. Alpha-2 agonists are not recommended for risk reduction of major adverse cardiac events. It is a Class I recommendation to wait at least 14 days after percutaneous myocardial revascularization with balloon coronary angioplasty, 30 days after bare metal stent placement, and 365 days after drug-eluting stent placement.
4. **A**. Propofol is a GABAergic agent. It causes central nervous system inhibition by decreasing the rate of dissociation of GABA from its receptor, and prolonging the GABA-mediated chloride influx into the cell, causing membrane hyperpolarization. Its induction dose for a normovolemic adult patient with normal cardiac function is 2–2.5 mg/kg. Propofol decreases mean arterial pressure by producing direct myocardial depression and decreasing SVR. It alters the baroreceptor reflex and causes a disproportionally small compensatory increase in heart rate relative to the decrease in blood pressure. It decreases the cerebral metabolic rate of oxygen consumption, cerebral blood flow, and ICP; however, at high doses, it may significantly decrease cerebral perfusion pressure. Propofol may trigger histamine release, and allergic reactions are therefore possible. It is not associated with an increased incidence of postoperative nausea and vomiting.
5. **A**. Ketamine is a phencyclidine derivative interacting with numerous receptors. Primarily, it acts as a glutamate antagonist at both NMDA and non-NMDA receptors; additionally, it is an opioid receptor agonist (opioid-sparing effects) and an M2 muscarinergic acetylcholine receptor antagonist (bronchodilation). It interacts with nicotinic and monoaminergic receptors, as well as with voltage-dependent Na^+- and L-type Ca^{2+} channels. Its actions on the NMDA receptors account for its psychomimetic, analgesic, and amnestic effects. The incidence of emergence delirium may be reduced by concomitant administration of a benzodiazepine and by minimizing external stimulation during emergence. Ketamine produces centrally mediated sympathetic activation: It increases plasma epinephrine levels, heart rate, and mean arterial pressure. It is the only anesthetic that increases peripheral arteriolar tone. In

catecholamine-depleted patients, or in those with limited inotropic reserve, its intrinsic cardio-depressant properties predominate and may cause hypotension. Absolute contraindications to the use of ketamine are hypersensitivity to ketamine or chemically related agents, significantly elevated blood pressure, stroke, intracranial hemorrhage, active delirium or psychosis, porphyria, pregnancy, and preeclampsia.

6. **C**. Etomidate is a lipid-soluble non-barbiturate hypnotic and anesthetic without analgesic effects. It is a carboxylated imidazole, structurally unrelated to other intravenous anesthetics. It is frequently used for rapid intravenous induction of anesthesia at standard doses of 0.2–0.3 mg/kg. Its short duration of action is subsequent to its rapid redistribution to peripheral compartments. Etomidate causes minimal cardiorespiratory depression even in the presence of cardiac and pulmonary disease. It may increase heart rate and cardiac output by 3% to 4% and may produce a 10–15% decrease in systemic vascular resistance and mean arterial pressure. It decreases cerebral blood flow, $CMRO_2$, and ICP. Even a single induction dose of etomidate suppresses cortisol production by inhibiting the activity of 11-β(beta)-hydroxylase. Etomidate causes pain on injection and it is associated with increased incidence of postoperative nausea and vomiting. There are no absolute contraindications to the use of etomidate as an induction agent.
7. **A**. Aortic stenosis, congenital or acquired, is the most common valvular disease in the United States. The most common etiologies are senile degeneration and congenital bicuspid aortic valve. Asymptomatic patients even with severe aortic stenosis carry a small risk of sudden cardiac death, whereas the occurrence of symptoms is ominous sign of poor outcome. The classic triad of symptomatic aortic stenosis is angina pectoris (life expectancy is about 5 years unless the aortic valve is replaced), syncope (average life expectancy: 3–4 years), and congestive heart failure (average life expectancy: 1–2 years). Treatment is surgical.
   As the severity of the stenosis progresses, a pressure gradient develops between the left ventricle and the aorta, causing the left ventricular wall tension to increase (fixed increase in LV afterload). This leads to a compensatory increase in wall thickness. According to the law of Laplace, the wall tension within a sphere filled to any given pressure depends on the thickness of the sphere: Pressure = (2 * wall thickness * wall tension)/radius. Consequently, at constant pressure, wall tension can be decreased by increasing the thickness of the sphere's wall: left ventricular wall tension = (LV pressure * radius)/2* LV wall thickness. Wall stress is a major determinant of myocardial O_2 demand. Concentric left ventricular hypertrophy with an increasing wall thickness but unchanged chamber size, therefore, reduces wall stress and O_2 demand. Chamber size, contractility, and stroke volume are usually preserved until late in the disease process.
   The increasing LV wall thickness will eventually lead to impaired left ventricular relaxation and decreased compliance, and eventually a fixed stroke volume. To maintain an adequate stroke volume, preload augmentation is necessary.
   A thick, non-compliant heart has an increased basal myocardial O2 consumption. In the hypertrophied left ventricle, capillary density does not adapt to the increased wall thickness, and any decrease in coronary perfusion pressure will compromise myocardial O2 supply. Maintenance of adequate afterload to ensure adequate systemic diastolic and coronary perfusion pressure is essential in preventing hypotension and the resultant risk of subendocardial ischemia.
   Extremes of heart rate are poorly tolerated in patients with hemodynamically significant aortic stenosis. Maintenance of normal rate and sinus rhythm is essential, as a non-compliant left ventricle is unable to augment stroke volume to maintain cardiac output during bradycardic episodes to restore cardiac output, and excessive tachycardia will reduce coronary perfusion during diastole. Atrial contraction contributes up to 30% to 40% of the left ventricular filling, maintenance of sinus rhythm is essential, and any supraventricular arrhythmias should be aggressively treated.
8. **B**. Patients with concentric LVH and hemodynamically significant aortic stenosis are unable to augment cardiac output in response to any sudden decrease in systemic vascular resistance. Administration of an α_1- adrenergic agent—for example, phenylephrine—improves coronary perfusion pressure without adding to the already existing fixed afterload, and increasing myocardial work. Concomitant venoconstriction increases venous return and augments preload. Reflex bradycardia may improve myocardial O_2 consumption. It is essential not to delay the treatment of hypotension, as the thick myocardium is at risk for ischemia, further worsening cardiac output, and coronary perfusion, leading to sudden death. Agents with the potential to increase heart rate or myocardial O2 consumption are not the first choices for the treatment of hypotension in this patient with severe aortic stenosis.
9. **C**. Amiodarone is a class III antiarrhythmic agent used for the treatment of atrial and ventricular arrhythmias. It is used during cardiac arrest to aid in the defibrillation of recurrent or refractory ventricular fibrillation. Amiodarone has Na^+, K^+, Ca^{2+} − channels, as well as alpha- and beta-adrenergic receptor blocker properties.

Its rate-dependent (rapid) administration may cause profound hypotension and bradycardia. Treatment is volume expansion, administration of vasoconstrictors and positive chronotropes, or temporary pacing.

10. **B**. Norepinephrine is an endogenous catecholamine with peripheral post-synaptic α_1- and β effects. Its peripheral α effects predominate over its myocardial β_1 effects. The effects of norepinephrine mediated by β_2-receptors are not clinically significant. Norepinephrine is a potent vasoconstrictor (MAP and SVR are increased) with mild positive inotropy. It does increase myocardial O2 requirements. Its β-induced positive chronotropy is counteracted by the reflex bradycardia resulting from the α-mediated increase in afterload. Norepinephrine does not significantly increase cardiac output; an effect different from that of phenylephrine (phenylephrine may decrease cardiac output). Norepinephrine is less likely to induce tachyarrhythmias than epinephrine, dobutamine, dopamine, or isoproterenol.

References

1. Mill MR, Anderson RH, Cohn LH (2012) Chapter 2. Surgical anatomy of the heart. In: Cohn LH, (eds.) Cardiac surgery in the adult. 4th ed. New York: McGraw-Hill;. ► http://accesssurgery.mhmedical/content.aspx? Bookid+476&sectioned=39679013.
2. Barash PG, Cullen BF, Stoelting RK, Cahalan MK, Stock MC (2009) (eds.) Chapters 10, 18, 41. In: Clinical anesthesia. 6th ed. Philadelphia: Lippincott Williams & Wilkins.
3. Butterworth JF. Chapter 2. Cardiovascular drugs. In: Gravlee GP, Martin ED, Hensley F, editors. A practical approach to cardiac anesthesia. Philadelphia: Lippincott Williams & Wilkins; 2013.
4. Fleischer LA, Fleischmann KE, Auerbach AD, et al. 2014 ACC/AHA guideline on perioperative cardiovascular evaluation and management of patients undergoing noncardiac surgery. A report of the American College of Cardiology/American Heart Association Task Force on Practice Guidelines. J Am Coll Cardiol. 2014;64(22):e77–137.
5. Kristensen SD, Knuuti J, Saraste A, et al. 2014 ESC/ESA Guidelines on non-cardiac surgery: cardiovascular assessment and management: the Joint Task Force on non-cardiac surgery: cardiovascular assessment and management of the European Society of Cardiology (ESC) and the European Society of Anaesthesiology (ESA). Eur Heart J. 2014;35(35):2383–431. https://doi.org/10.1093/eurheartj/ehu282.
6. Shiffermiller JF, Monson BJ, Vokoun CW, et al. Prospective randomized evaluation of preoperative angiotensin-converting enzyme inhibition (PREOP-ACEI). J Hosp Med. 2018;13 (10):661–7. https://doi.org/10.12788/jhm.3036.
7. Hollmann C, Fernandes NL, Biccard BM. A systematic review of outcomes associated with withholding or continuing angiotensin-converting enzyme inhibitors and angiotensin receptor blockers before noncardiac surgery XE "Noncardiac surgery." Anesth Analg. 2018;127(3):678–87. https://doi.org/10.1213/ANE.0000000000002837.
8. Roshanov PS, Rochwerg B, Patel A, et al. Withholding versus continuing angiotensin-converting enzyme inhibitors or angiotensin II receptor blockers before noncardiac surgery: an analysis of the vascular events in noncardiac surgery patIents cOhort evaluatioN prospective cohort. Anesthesiology. 2017;126:16–27.
9. Wijeysundera DN, Duncan D, Nkonde-Price C, Virani SS, Washam JB, Fleischmann KE, Fleisher LA. Perioperative XE "Perioperative" beta-blockade in noncardiac surgery: a systematic review for the 2014 ACC/AHA guideline on perioperative cardiovascular evaluation and management of patients undergoing noncardiac surgery: a report of the American College of Cardiology/American Heart Association Task Force on practice guidelines. Circulation. 2014;130:000–000.
10. McLaughlin VV, Archer SL, Badesch DB, et al. ACCF/AHA 2009 expert consensus document on pulmonary hypertension a report of the American College of Cardiology Foundation Task Force on Expert Consensus Documents and the American Heart Association developed in collaboration with the American College of Chest Physicians; American Thoracic Society, Inc.; and the Pulmonary Hypertension Association. J Am Coll Cardiol. 2009;53(17):1573–619.
11. Ponikowski P, Voors AA, Anker SD, et al. 2016 ESC guidelines for the diagnosis and treatment of acute and chronic heart failure. Eur Heart J. 2016;37(18):2129–200.
12. van Deursen V, Hernandez AF, Stebbins A, et al. Nesiritide, renal function, and associated outcomes during hospitalization for acute decompensated heart failure. Results from the acute study of clinical effectiveness of nesiritide and decompensated heart failure (ASCEND-HF). Circulation. 2014;130:958–65.

Respiratory Pharmacology 12

Ahmad Maher Adi

Abstract

The pathological triad of pulmonary disease consists of: bronchospasm, airway inflammation, and retained secretion. Respiratory pharmacology deals with agents used to treat this "pathological triad." Medications used to treat these conditions can be divided into different categories based on their mechanism of action. They include bronchodilators, anticholinergics, corticosteroids, mucolytics, decongestants, and biological drugs just to name a few. Research is currently focused on the persistent inflammation that characterizes chronic obstructive pulmonary disease (COPD) but no medications are currently available.

Keywords

Respiratory pharmacology • Pathological triad • Bronchodilators • Anti-inflammatory modifier drugs • Biological drugs

Key Points

- Medications used to manage the pulmonary "pathologic triad" include bronchodilators and anti-inflammatory medication. Bronchodilators include beta 2 adrenergic receptor agonists and cholinergic/muscarinic acetylcholine receptor antagonists. Anti-inflammatory medications include leukotriene modifier drugs, mast cell stabilizers, and immunoglobulin E blockers.
- Bronchodilators are essential in the treatment of airway disorders. They are a mainstay treatment for the management of chronic obstructive lung disease (COPD) and are critical in the symptomatic management of asthma.
- There is a uniform distribution of β (beta)-adrenoceptors on the alveolar wall with 2:1 ratio of β (beta) 1/β (beta) 2 receptors.
- β (beta) 2-adrenergic agonists should be used with caution in patients with hyperthyroidism and cardiovascular disease due to the potential for QT prolongation and arrhythmias.
- Airway tone is mainly controlled by parasympathetic nerves carried by the vagus nerve.
- There are 5 different subtypes of muscarinic acetylcholine receptors (M1-M5), which are expressed in almost every cell type of the airway and lung tissue, including airway and vascular smooth muscle, different glandular and surface epithelium cells, endothelial cells, and inflammatory cells.
- Steroids are considered first-line medications in the treatment of asthma. Using the inhaled rather than intravenous forms can reduce their side effects.
- Low-dose inhaled steroids in regular daily doses are highly effective in reducing asthma symptoms and reducing the risk of asthma-related exacerbations, hospitalization, and death.
- Headache is a common side effect in patients receiving leukotriene-modifying drugs.
- The use of biological drugs can reduce the requirements for steroids and improve quality of life in asthmatic patients with frequent asthma exacerbation. Its use is reserved for severe uncontrolled asthmatic patients despite best available therapy. Biological drugs are approved to treat patients with severe uncontrolled Asthma and are directed against mediators of Type 2 immunity.
- Combination therapy combines a medication from 2 or more classes. Combination therapy, by using a lower dose of medication from each class, can reduce systematic side effects.

A. M. Adi (✉)
Department of Cardiothoracic Anesthesiology and Critical Care, Cleveland Clinic, Cleveland, OH, USA
e-mail: adia@ccf.org

M. Argalious et al. (eds.), *Basic Sciences in Anesthesia*,
https://doi.org/10.1007/978-3-031-60203-0_12

12.1 Introduction

The pathological triad of pulmonary disease consists of: bronchospasm, airway inflammation, and retained secretion. Respiratory pharmacology deals with agents used to treat this "pathological triad." Medications used to treat these conditions can be divided into different categories based on their mechanism of action. They include bronchodilators, anticholinergics, corticosteroids, mucolytics, decongestants, and biological drugs just to name a few. Other agents used to treat pulmonary disease such as oxygen, antibiotics, local aesthetics, respiratory stimulants, and muscle relaxers are beyond the scope of this chapter.

12.2 Bronchodilators

Bronchodilators are essential in the treatment of airway disorders. They are the primary treatment for the management of chronic obstructive pulmonary disease (COPD) and are critical in the symptomatic management of asthma. Bronchodilators work through a direct relaxation effect on airway smooth muscle cells. Three major classes of bronchodilators exist at the present time: β (beta) 2-adrenoreceptor (AR) agonists, cholinergic receptor antagonists, and xanthines. This chapter will discuss the first 2 treatments, which can be used individually or in combination, as is currently preferred in order to minimize systemic effects. Fast- and short-acting agents are best used for acute symptom relief, whereas long-acting agents are best for maintenance therapy. Treatment adherence has been improved by new formulations that allow once-daily administration.

Understanding the neurological innervation of the airway is key to understanding how bronchodilators work. Airway tone is mainly controlled by parasympathetic nerves carried by the vagus nerve.

Postganglionic parasympathetic cholinergic and non-noradrenergic noncholinergic (NANC) fibers innervate airway smooth muscles (ASM), providing the dominant control of the muscle tone and airway caliber as well as airway glands and microvasculature.

There is no direct sympathetic innervation of ASM, but there is innervation of the airway vasculature.

Acetylcholine (ACh) is the classic neurotransmitter of the parasympathetic nervous system at both the ganglionic and neuroeffector junctions, which then activate the cholinergic/muscarinic receptors.

Five different subtypes of muscarinic receptors (mAChs) have been identified (M1-M5), and they are expressed in almost every cell type of the airway and lung tissue, including airway and vascular smooth muscle, different glandular and surface epithelium cells, endothelial cells, and inflammatory cells.

β (beta)-ARs are present in high concentrations in lung tissue and are divided into 3 types: β (beta) 1, β (beta) 2, and β (beta) 3. The majority of pulmonary β (beta)-ARs are of the β (beta) 2-AR subtype, localized in the ASM, epithelium, vascular smooth muscle, and submucosal glands. They are more prevalent in small airways than large airways but are also expressed on many inflammatory and immune cells, whereas (beta) 1-ARs are located in the gland and alveoli. There is a uniform distribution of β (beta)-ARs on the alveolar wall with a 2:1 ratio of β (beta) 1/β (beta) 2.

β(beta)2-ARs are coupled to Gs (part of the (protein-coupled receptors), where stimulation by B(beta)2-AR agonist activates the adenyl cyclase and increases cyclic adenosine monophosphate (cAMP) levels, which in turn increases protein kinase A (PKA), activity. This reduces the intracellular Calcium level and activates large conductance potassium channels leading to relaxation of airway smooth muscle.

12.3 β (beta)-Adrenergic Receptors Agonists

Ephedrine from the plant ephedra: equisetina was used for more than 2000 years for the short-term treatment of respiratory systems. The discovery of epinephrine and isoproterenol followed, but due to the fact that these drugs were non-selective alpha- and beta-adrenergic receptor agonists, they caused unwanted side effects and warranted the need of selective β (beta)-AR receptors agonist.

12.3.1 Short-Acting β (beta) 2-Adrenergic Receptors Agonists

Short-acting β(beta)2-AR agonists (SABA) can be divided into 2 groups dependent on the duration of action using conventional doses: (1) very short-acting, duration 1–2 h (isoproterenol and rimiterol); and short-acting, duration 3–6 h (fenoterol, albuterol, and terbutaline).

12.3.1.1 Albuterol

Albuterol has greater selectivity between (beta) 2 and B (beta) 1-AR than any other product previously available. It also has negligible a (alpha)-AR activity. It causes maximum bronchodilation but with minimal cardiovascular responses compared to isoproterenol. After inhalation, its maximum effect can be seen in 15 min. However, albuterol weakly binds to the receptor and quickly diffuses to the microcirculation, which accounts for the short action of duration (4–6 h), but it is the drug of choice to relieve symptoms of bronchospasm. It also can be used intravenously if the inhalation response is reduced or absent.

Levalbuterol ([R]-Albuterol), an isomer of albuterol, can be used instead of albuterol. It may reduce hospitalization, have fewer adverse effects, and provide similar bronchodilators effects at reduced dose, but recent studies have questioned these benefits.

12.3.1.2 Fenoterol

Fenoterol has a similar effect to albuterol, with β (beta) 2-AR selectivity and minimal α (alpha)-AR stimulation. The only difference is that it can exhibit a slightly longer duration of action. A 200 μg dose was required to produce a maximal response.

12.3.1.3 Terbutaline

Synthetic sympathomimetic amine has a greater specificity for β (beta) 2-AR. Due to its structure, with a dihydroxybenzene group at the β (beta)-carbon atom, it has a longer duration of action (4–6 h).

Terbutaline is administered by aerosol inhalation. When given parenterally, it loses much of its selectivity, and cardiovascular effects similar to isoproterenol are observed. Compared to epinephrine, subcutaneous terbutaline can induce more bronchodilation for a longer period of time but with more side effects.

Bambuterol is an oral terbutaline prodrug with prolonged duration of bronchodilator action.

12.3.2 Long-Acting (beta) 2-Adrenergic Receptor Agonists

Long-acting β (beta) 2-AR agonists (LABA) such as salmeterol and formoterol provide 12-h bronchodilation.

12.3.2.1 Salmeterol

Salmeterol binds specifically to the β(beta)2-AR via albuterol "head group"-the molecule of which is > 10,000 times more lipophilic than albuterol. The process of its diffusion to reach the active site of the (beta)2-AR is slow (=30 min) and accounts for the slow onset of action on the airway smooth muscle (ASM). Salmeterol does not induce desensitization or internalization of receptors, which may also contribute to its long therapeutic duration of action.

Studies have shown that salmeterol is a partial agonist, which may attenuate the effects of β(beta)2-AR agonist with greater efficacy, thus raising the possibility of pretreatment with this drug.

The onset of action is approximately 10 min. Maximal bronchodilation may take hours to achieve.

12.3.2.2 Formoterol

Due to its structural molecule, formoterol has greater affinity to the β(beta)2-AR and has the highest bronchoselectivity among the LABA.

Formeterol has a faster onset of action compared to salmeterol and has been shown in a concentration dependent to inhibit antigen-induced mediator release from human lung fragments.

Formolerol has the same effect of salmeterol at a lower dose (50 μg vs 12 μg).

12.3.3 Ultra-Long-Acting β(beta)2-Adrenergic Receptors Agonists

Ultra-long acting β(beta)2-ARs were developed to simplify the treatment to 1 dose daily so that patients can adhere to their treatment.

12.3.3.1 Indacaterol

Indacaterol is a highly lipophilic drug that is retained in the lipid rafts of the plasma membrane, an area particularly rich in B(beta) receptors. This means that these receptors are repeatedly stimulated by this drug and for a long period of time, achieving an effect that lasts 24 h. Indacaterol has high intrinsic activity, which explains the rapid onset of action within 5 min of administration. Mild cough is the only significant side effect, which may lead to discontinuation of the treatment.

Multiple studies have shown the superiority of daily dose indacaterol over formoterol, salmeterol, and tiotropium bromide in improving through forced expiratory volume 1 (FEV1). It also provides a significant health-related quality of life.

12.3.3.2 Olodaterol

Olodaterol is a potent β(beta)2 receptor agonist with high intrinsic activity. This ultra-LABA binds moderately to lipid rafts, although its dissociation half-life is about 18 h. It has a 2-stage profile of dissociation from β(beta)2 receptors. Its slow component has a dissociation half-life of 12 h. These 2 features explain the fact that the bronchodilator effect lasts 24 h.

12.3.3.3 Vilamterol

Vilamterol has greater intrinsic activity than salmeterol and appears to be more potent than indacaterol. All doses of vilamterol were associated with low incidence of treatment-related side effects.

12.3.3.4 Carmoterol

Carmoterol is over 100 times more selective for bronchial muscle than myocardial tissue. It displays a fast onset and long duration of action.

Carmoterol has better improvement of trough FEV1 than salmeterol, and it has no side effects.

12.3.4 Intravenous (beta)2-Adrenergic Receptors Agonists

12.3.4.1 Bedoradrine

Many patients with acute exacerbation of asthma are non-responders to inhaled §(beta)-adrenergic agonists. Intravenous bedoradrine is a highly selective β(beta)2-AR agonist. In a recent study to show the efficacy of bedoradrine, there was no significant difference in % FEV1 at 3 h between the bedoradrine compared to the placebo groups. The dyspnea scores were significantly improved for patients treated with bedoradrine [1–7].

12.3.5 Side Effects of β(beta)2-Adrenergic Receptors Agonists

Because of the widespread distribution of B(beta)2-AR, several side effects are noted when (beta)2-AR agonists are absorbed into the systemic circulation. The number of side effects is the greatest when (beta)2-AR is administered orally or parenterally.

Increased heart rate and palpitation are less common with the selective β(beta)2-AR agonists than the non-selective, but they can cause reflex tachycardia secondary to vasodilation. Some of these atrial and ventricular effects could be the result of β(beta)2-AR receptors that may be present in the atria and ventricles.

All agonists should be used with caution in patients with hyperthyroidism or cardiovascular disease.

(Arrhythmias, hypertension, QT-interval prolongation).

Transient mild decrease in partial pressure of oxygen in arterial blood could result from the administration of β(beta) 2-AR agonists despite concomitant bronchodilation. This could be attributed to pulmonary vasodilation and increased blood flow to poorly ventilated lung region, which causes a ventilation-perfusion mismatch.

In diabetics, β(beta)2-AR agonists should be used with caution because of the risk of ketoacidosis. β(beta)2-AR agonists stimulate liver glycogenolysis, which results in an increase in glucose blood level.

Hypokalemia is a risk secondary to stimulation of the Na +/K+ pump in skeletal muscle, which causes an extracellular shift of sodium in exchange for potassium, thereby lowering potassium plasma levels.

Selective (beta)2-AR agonists can cause fine tremors of skeletal muscles, particularly the hands.

β(beta)2-AR agonists can induce the mobilization of triglycerides resulting in elevated blood levels of fatty acids and glycerol.

Albuterol, terbutaline, and fenoterol can induce mild appetite suppression, headache, nausea, and sleep disturbances due to their ability to cross the blood–brain barrier.

12.4 Cholinergic/Muscarinic Acetylcholine Receptors Antagonists

Inhaled muscarinic acetylcholine receptors (mAchR) antagonists have been used for many years. The smoking of plant alkaloids was recommended in the seventeenth century for the treatment of asthma in India, and it was later introduced in the nineteenth century to Great Britain.

Atropa belladonna and *Datura stramonium* are rich in anticholinergic alkaloids, atropine, and stramonium. If dried and smoked, they relieve the symptoms of asthma.

Atropine is well absorbed into the systemic circulation and can cross the blood–brain barrier. It therefore has multiple unmanned side effects, but the modification of its chemical molecule lessens the amount of mucosal absorption and blood–brain barrier crossing.

12.4.1 Short-Acting Muscarinic Acetylcholine Receptors Antagonists

Short-acting mAchR agents have a duration of action of 6–8 h, but compared to SABAs they have a slower onset of action.

12.4.1.1 Atropine Methonitrate

Quaternary ammonium of atropine, a more potent bronchodilator, reaches its peak effect in 40–60 min and duration of action can last up to 6 h.

12.4.1.2 Ipratropium Bromide

Unlike atropine, ipratropium bromide has low lipid solubility, does not cross the blood–brain barrier, and is poorly absorbed by the mucosa or the gastrointestinal tract.

It is a non-selective antagonist of M1, M22, and M3 mChRs and starts acting within 15–30 min with peak concentration in 3 h. The duration of action is approximately 6 h when given as inhalation. It has little or no systemic side effects.

12.4.1.3 Oxitropium Bromide

Oxitropium bromide's base molecule is scopolamine. It has a longer duration of action than ipratropium, but peak bronchodilation may take 60–90 min. It has a slight clinical advantage over ipratropium, but at higher doses it causes tachycardia.

12.4.2 Long-Lasting Muscarinic Acetylcholine Receptors Antagonists

12.4.2.1 Tiotropium Bromide

Tiotropium bromide is a long-acting AChR antagonist (LAMA) with higher affinity to the mAChRs than ipratropium by (6- to 20-fold). It binds to all the M receptors but dissociates faster from the M2 receptors. Its long duration of action can be explained by the slow dissociation from M1-M3 mAChRs.

It has a very long half-life of approximately 35 h, which allows for once-daily dose. It is rapidly absorbed into the circulation with peak plasma concentration within 5 min followed by rapid fall within 1 h a steady state and a terminal half-life of 5–6 days. Peak onset occurs between 1 and 3 h with improvement in FEV1 for more than 24 h. Recently, tiotropium bromide has been shown to be more effective than salmeterol in preventing COPD exacerbation.

12.4.3 Novel Long-Acting Muscarinic Acetylcholine Receptors Antagonists

12.4.3.1 Glycopyrronium Bromide

Glycopyrronium bromide is a mAChR antagonist and has a fast onset that is sustained over 24 h.

Fifty micrograms of glycopyrronium bromide once daily produces immediate and significant improvement in exercise tolerance from day 1. It also improves inspiratory capacity and through FEV1. in patients with COPD.

12.4.3.2 Aclidinium Bromide

Aclidinium bromide exhibits M3/M2 selectivity. Its action is related to its inhibition of M3 receptors with resultant bronchodilation. The major route of metabolism of aclidinium bromide is hydrolysis, which occurs both chemically and enzymatically by esterases.

It has a faster onset and shorter duration of action than tiotropium bromide.

12.4.3.3 Umeclidinium Bromide

Umeclidinium bromide is a long-acting muscarinic antagonist (LAMA) that blocks action of acetylcholine at muscarinic receptors (M1-M5) in the bronchial airways (M3) by preventing increases in intracellular calcium concentration. This leads to relaxation of airway smooth muscle, improved lung function, and decreased mucous secretion. It dissociates slowly from M3 muscarinic receptors, extending its duration of action.

Primary metabolic routes for umeclidinium are oxidative (hydroxylation, O-dealkylation) followed by conjugation (e.g., glucuronidation) to inactive metabolite. It is mostly secreted in the feces.

12.4.3.4 Trospium

Trospium is currently used as a urinary antispasmodic drug, but when used as an inhaler it induces a fast onset of bronchodilation with an onset of 15 min and duration of 24 h.

12.4.4 Side Effects of Muscarinic Acetylcholine Receptors Antagonists

All of the mChR antagonists are very well tolerated because they are very poorly absorbed after inhalation.

If these agents contact the eye, they can cause papillary dilation and blurred vision. In patients with glaucoma, they can cause an acute angle-closure glaucoma.

In patients with prostatic hyperplasia, they should be used with caution, since the risk of further increase and acute urinary retention can follow.

Patients with moderate to severe renal impairment should be monitored under the treatment of tiotropium bromide because it is mainly excreted by the kidneys.

Bad breath or dry mouth is another side effect of the treatment, though usually well tolerated in the long-term treatment.

Paradoxical bronchoconstriction could occur with these drugs. One possible cause is the blockade of prejunctional M2 mChRs on airway cholinergic nerves, which normally inhibits the release of ACh.

Recent systemic reviews and meta-analyses showed that tiotropium bromide inhaler is associated with an increased risk of cardiovascular morbidity and mortality. A possible explanation is that new formulation and device may lead to greater systemic absorption.

12.5 Steroids

Corticosteroids are very useful when the common bronchodilators are less effective. Previously they were used as rescue medication, but presently they are considered a first-line medication for asthma.

Corticosteroids are primarily anti-inflammatory by reducing the numbers of inflammatory cells in the airway, such as eosinophils, T lymphocytes, mast cells, and dendritic cells. Corticosteroids inhibit the recruitment of inflammatory cells by reducing chemotaxis and adhesion, phagocytosis, and the production of inflammatory mediators such as cytokines and eicosanoids. Corticosteroids also increase the expression of 2-adrenergic receptors in the lung and prevent their down-regulation and uncoupling in response to 2 agonists.

The primary effects of corticosteroids are at the genetic level, activating transcription of anti-inflammatory genes while repressing pro-inflammatory genes. The steroid hormone is initially taken up by the target cell before binding to specific cytoplasmic receptor proteins. This "steroid-receptor complex" is then transported to the nucleus of the cell. There it binds to a specific acceptor site on the DNA molecule. Messenger RNA is then formed from the DNA. The messenger RNA is transported to the cytoplasm where it causes new protein synthesis along the ribosomes. The new protein then gives a cellular response to the steroid, promoting vasoconstriction in areas of inflammation and decreasing capillary permeability. This decreases edema fluid in the airway, which will decrease the wall thickness, increase lumen size, and decrease airway resistance. Steroids stabilize cell membranes resulting in a decrease in synthesis, storage, and release of histamine. This makes it useful in preventing allergic bronchospasm.

Steroids are administered orally, intravenously, or aerosolized for respiratory symptoms. Intravenous formulations include hydrocortisone or methylprednisolone. Oral choices are prednisone or prednisolone. Aerosolized steroids are beclomethasone dipropionate, flunisolide, triamcinolone acetone, and fluticasone. It may take 4–6 h to have a noticeable improvement in asthmatic symptoms.

Between 10 and 60% of inhaled corticosteroid (ICS) is deposited in the lung, where it is absorbed into the circulation and cleared by the liver. The remainder of the dose is deposited in the oropharynx and may cause local side effects.

Oral steroid undergoes absorption into the portal circulation and undergoes first-pass elimination.

- Hydrocortisone is administered parenterally and rarely aerosolized. The dose ranges from 300 to 2000 mg.
- Prednisone has 3–4 more inflammatory potency than hydrocortisone, ineffective when aerosolized.
- Prednisolone is a synthetic steroid, rarely aerosolized. Its half-life is 2–4 h and its duration of action can be up to 36 h.
- Methylprednisolone is 4–5 times more potent than prednisone. It has little effect on electrolyte balance. It is used for severe shock, persistent asthma, acute respiratory distress syndrome (ARDS), and aspiration pneumonia. Onset is fast, and its half-life is 78–188 min, with duration of action lasting up to 36 h.
- Dexamethasone—With 30 times the anti-inflammatory potency than hydrocortisone, it is as effective as an aerosolized steroid but does not potentiate the effect of B (beta) 2 agonists. It also may cause adrenal insufficiency.
- Triamcinolone—As a synthetic steroid, it may cause sodium and water diuresis. It has a similar potency to methylprednisolone. Its half-life is 3 h, and duration can last up to 48 h. Prolonged use can cause muscle weakness and depression.
- Beclomethasone Dipropionate—This is 100 times more potent that hydrocortisone. The major side effect is fungal infection of the oropharynx. The maximum adult daily dose is 840 mcg.
- Pediatric dosing is half of that.
- Flunisolide is several hundred times more potent than hydrocortisone. Maximum dose is 2 mg, and pediatric dosage is half that dose.
- Fluticasone—The highest recommended dose is 440 mcg daily, which may be doubled if the patient is taking oral steroids.

12.5.1 Side Effects of Steroid Treatment

Usually, side effects are more common with systemic steroids than with inhaled agents. These side effects can be improved with reducing the dosage or treatment duration, if possible.

Long-term use can be associated with weight gain, increase susceptibility to infection secondary to immunosuppression, osteoporosis, and growth retardation in kids.

Bone health is adversely affected in systemic steroid utilization, and it is related to daily use, prolonged duration of use, and high cumulative lifetime dose. This can be manifested as osteoporosis, osteoporotic fractures, and avascular osteonecrosis. These complications are seen with doses as low as 5–7.5 mg/day of prednisone.

Adrenal insufficiency is another side effect from systemic steroids. This risk seems minimal with inhaled steroidal agents. Morning cortisol level suppression does occur with inhaled steroids, but it is clinically not significant.

When a systemic steroid is prescribed in higher doses and for a prolonged period of time, it carries a risk for *Pseudomonas, Pneumocystis* infections, tuberculosis, and herpes zoster. This is all secondary to immunosuppression.

Inhaled steroids can cause deposition of the drug in the oropharynx, which in turn can increase the risk of fungal infection, such as oral candidiasis. Rinsing the mouth after taking the medication may reduce the incidence of fungal infection. Inhaled steroids may cause dysphonia.

The TORCH (Towards a Revolution in COPD Health) trial found an increased frequency of pneumonia among patients receiving inhaled steroids. Proper education of patients in the utilization of the inhaled steroid and washing of the mouth after use can reduce the side effects mentioned previously.

Patients also should be referred for routine ophthalmologic exams, as secondary glaucoma or cataracts may develop while on chronic use of systemic steroids. Routine checkups for cardiovascular side effects are also recommended to monitor for hypertension, hyperglycemia, and hyperlipidemia.

Bone density measurements should be done routinely in patients on chronic steroid therapy, and they should be encouraged to perform weight-bearing exercise and take calcium supplements with vitamin D.

Avoidance of nonsteroidal anti-inflammatory drugs (NSAIDs) is appropriate in patients receiving steroid therapy, due to increased risk of stomach ulcer and gastrointestinal bleeding.

Psychiatric symptoms should be monitored, if any, and they should be managed by reducing the dose or adding an additional treatment targeting the psychiatric symptoms.

12.6 Leukotriene Modifier Drugs

Leukotrienes are formed from arachidonic acid that is released from the cell-membrane phospholipid bilayer by phospholipase A2 (PLA2). The liberated arachidonic acid may then be metabolized by one of several pathways. The cyclooxygenase pathway, to generate prostaglandins, thromboxanes, and prostacyclin: or the 5-lipoxygenase pathways, generates the cysteinyl leukotrienes C4, D4, and E4. In humans, 5-lipoxygenase is present only in myeloid cells (i.e., monocytes, eosinophils, basophils, alveolar macrophages, and mast cells).

Leukotrienes can impair mucociliary clearance, enhance mucus secretion, chemotactically attract leukocytes to the airways, and cause edema by facilitating pulmonary vascular permeability. Inhaled leukotrienes C4 and D4 can cause airflow obstruction 1000 times more potently than histamine in normal subjects. In patients with asthma, the airways are 100 to 1000 times more sensitive to inhaled leukotrienes D4 and E4 than are the airways of normal subjects.

Two approaches have been developed to decrease the action of leukotrienes. One is by enzyme inhibition to block leukotriene synthesis, and the other is by blocking the binding of a leukotriene to its receptor.

Inhibitors of leukotriene synthesis block the formation of both the cysteinyl leukotrienes and leukotriene B4. These inhibitors can be grouped on their site of action into 2 groups. Inhibitors of 5-lipoxygenase prevent the formation of leukotriene A4, which is the unstable intermediate. Zileuton is a representative 5-lipoxygenase inhibitor.

Alternatively, leukotriene synthesis can be inhibited by blocking the action of the 5-lipoxygenase-activating protein. These agents are still under investigation.

Leukotriene modifiers also work as competitive antagonists of the leukotriene B4 receptor.

12.6.1 Zafirlukast

Zafirlukast (Accolate®) is a synthetic peptide leukotriene-receptor antagonist recommended for children 7 years of age and older. It is used for the management of mild, persistent asthma, a step-up therapy for moderate persistent asthma, treatment of exercise-induced asthma, and management of allergic rhinitis. It inhibits the binding of leukotrienes that are responsible for smooth muscle constriction and hyper-responsiveness after contact with an allergen challenge including exercise. The dose is 10 mg for 7–12 years old twice a day. For older patients, it is 20 mg BID.

Headache is the major side effect. Nausea, abdominal pain, diarrhea, rash, and elevated liver functions tests (LFTs) have occurred in clinical trials. Patients on warfarin treatment should be monitored closely because this drug may affect the warfarin level and increase prothrombin time.

12.6.2 Montelukast

Montelukast (Singulair®) is also a leukotriene-receptor antagonist. It is used for the long-term management of children with asthma over the age of 2 years. Montelukast is recommended as an alternative medication to inhaled corticosteroids or as adjunctive therapy for the treatment of mild and moderate persistent asthma.

The rapid onset, safety of the drug in children, ease of administration, once-daily dose, and chewable tablets are all advantages to using this drug. Headaches are the major side effect affecting 18–19% of patients. Cough, abdominal pain, and increased LFTs, diarrhea, and rash are other side effects of this drug.

12.6.3 Zileuton

Zileuton (Zyflo®) is a 5-lipoxygenase inhibitor. Zyflo is indicated for children greater than 12 years of age for the treatment of chronic asthma. Headaches are a side effect experienced by 25% of patients taking zileuton. Additional reported side effects include unspecified pain, dyspepsia, nausea, and abdominal pain. Increase in LFT is reported, so it is contraindicated in children with liver disease or elevated LFTs.

Leukotriene modifiers drugs are effective treatment against exercise-induced bronchospasm and aspirin-induced asthma. They are not recommended in acute exacerbations of asthma, but should be continued during acute episodes.

12.7 Mast Cell Stabilizer

Mast cell stabilizing drugs inhibit the release of allergic mediators from mast cells and are used clinically to prevent allergic reactions to common allergens.

Mast cells play a fundamental role in the occurrence and maintenance of allergic disease in response to substances that induce an allergic reaction.

This allergic reaction begins with the allergen interacting with immunoglobulin E (IgE) complex, expressed on the surface of the sensitized mast cell, through complex signaling cascade. It leads to calcium influx and release of preformed chemical mediators such as histamine from mast cells, which induces the production of cytokine and chemokines. The effect of these mediators on surrounding cells and tissues is responsible for the symptoms and the severity of an allergic reaction.

Mature mast cells are widely distributed throughout the body where they reside in vascularized tissue, including nerves, smooth muscle cells, mucus production glands, and hair follicles. They are also found in sites that are directly exposed to the environment including the skin, airway, and gastroenterology tract.

Mast cells are classified into 2 subtypes depending on their location: (1) connective tissue mast cells, which reside in tissue such as skin, small bowel submucosa, and peritoneal cavity; and (2) mucosal mast cells, which mature in mucosal tissue such as the intestine and in the airways.

An allergic reaction may be prevented or attenuated by interfering with certain signaling molecules within the signaling cascade of the mast cell. Agents that prevent mediator release from the mast cells are termed mast cell stabilizers. They can be natural, semisynthetic, and synthetic products.

12.7.1 Cromolyn Sodium

One of the earliest mast cell stabilizers, cromolyn sodium inhibits release of histamine, leukotrienes, and slow-reacting substance of anaphylaxis from mast cells by inhibiting degranulation following exposure to reactive antigens.

Peak onset is 15 min with duration of action of 6 h and half-life 80–90 min.

Multiple side effects have been reported, most of which are diarrhea, headache, angioedema, and neutropenia. Inhalation of cromolyn sodium has side effects including cough, nasal congestion, nausea, and wheezing.

12.7.2 Nedocromil Sodium

Nedocromil sodium has been shown to inhibit the activation of, and mediator release from, a variety of inflammatory cell types associated with asthma, including eosinophils, neutrophils, macrophages, mast cells, platelets, and monocytes. In humans, nedocromil sodium has been shown to inhibit acutely the bronchoconstriction response to several kinds of allergens.

At higher concentrations, nedocromil sodium showed more effective inhibition of histamine release from mast cells isolated from the lung, and tonsillar and adenoid tissues than cromolyn sodium.

Systemic absorption of nedocromil sodium administered as an inhaled aerosol is low.

Studies have shown that nedocromil sodium improved symptom control and pulmonary function when it was added to an as-needed inhaled beta 2-adrenergic bronchodilator regimen, and a beneficial effect could be detected within 2 weeks.

12.7.3 Ketotifen

Ketotifen is another mast cell stabilizer drug, but is currently not available in the United States.

The aforementioned drugs are used mainly as prophylaxis, and they cannot be used in the acute phase of any bronchoconstriction events.

12.8 Biological Drugs

In recent years, evidence suggests that bronchial asthma and other allergic conditions have become more common worldwide, in both developed and developing countries.

It is estimated that more than 50% of asthma is related to allergy and the majority of patients with severe asthma have allergic-atopic asthma. Immunoglobulin E(IgE) antibodies, allergen type 2 helper T cells derived cytokines and eosinophils, play a major role in the development of chronic airway disease, even in mild forms of the disease. This airway inflammation is the pathogenesis of bronchial asthma, which causes an increase in airway responsiveness to many trigger factors such as aeroallergens alone or in combination with other triggers such as air pollution and viruses.

There are two major types of asthma endotypes based on inflammatory pathway involved, high 2 type (T2-high) which include the allergic and nonallergic eosinophilic phenotypes and affect half of patients with asthma and type2 low (T2-low) driven by neutrophilic inflammation and oxidative stress and affect the other half of patients with asthma.

Corticosteroids have been the main treatment for asthmatic patients, suggested by the Global Initiative for Asthma (GINA), but there are asthmatic patients who continue to have severe symptoms with multiple regimen treatments. These patients have increased recurring hospitalizations and mortality within 1 year of initial hospitalization. These conditions also have high economic and social costs.

Biological drugs are approved to treat the patient with severe asthma and are directed against mediators of type 2 immunity. Current Biological drugs are for the treatment of severe asthma and are directed against T2-high inflammatory target.

Omalizumab

Is an anti-IgE monoclonal antibody that binds IgE at the same site where the antibody binds, resulting in the inhibition of IgE effector function. This means that in allergic subjects, omalizumab prevents the activation of cellular response and the occurrence of asthma symptoms.

Treatment with omalizumab reduces airway wall thickness in patients with severe persistent asthma treated with conventional treatment. The use of omalizumab also has resulted in decreased corticosteroid use and improved quality of life in asthmatic patients.

Omalizumab treatment is reserved for severe uncontrolled asthmatic patients despite best available therapy. Multiple studies have shown that adding omalizumab reduces asthma exacerbation, total emergency visits, hospitalizations, and steroid utilization, thus improving quality of life.

Omalizumab is very safe with few side effects. The most frequent side effects are nasopharyngitis and sinusitis. No data exist about patients with renal or hepatic dysfunction prior to starting omalizumab, thus caution should be used in administering this drug in these patients.

Mepolizumab

The first commercialized anti-IL-5mAB approved by the FDA for patients above the age of 6 with severe eosinophilic asthma that remains uncontrolled despite all other treatment. It targets circulating IL-5 required for eosinophil development and survival, prevents interactions with alpha-subunit of IL-5 of IL-5 receptor on the surface of eosinophils, thereby reducing asthma exacerbations, the use of oral steroid and improving lung function (FEV1).

Reslizumab

Is a monoclonal antibody directed against IL-5 similar to mepolizumab, approved for patients above 18 years with severe eosinophilic asthma, it demonstrated reduction in absolute eosinophilic count, a reduction in asthma exacerbation, and improvement in lung functions.

Benralizumab

It is humanized afucosylated mAB directed against IL-5Ralpha; the complex mAB/IL-5Ralpha promotes the apoptosis of eosinophils through antibody-dependent cell-mediated cytotoxicity involving natural killer cells which result in active peripheral eosinophil depletion.

It is approved for patients above 12 years old. Benralizumab significantly reduces asthma exacerbation rate and improves lung function (FEV1) while reducing blood eosinophil count.

Dupilumab

Fully humanized mAB directed against alpha chain of IL-4 receptor (IL4-R) is similar to IL13R, both of which play a role in type 2 inflammation in asthma, by stimulating goblet cell hyperplasia and modulating airway hyperresponsiveness and airway remodeling. It is approved for patients above 12 years old. It reduces asthma exacerbations, reduces steroid utilization, and improves lung function.

12.9 Combination Therapy

Combination therapy is used when airway symptoms are not controlled by maintenance monotherapy.

Moreover, combining 2 or more classes allows the use of lower doses to achieve the same result.

Combination therapy with a long-acting beta agonist (LABA) and inhaled corticosteroid (ICS) is an essential approach to patients with frequent exacerbation.

The combinations present in clinical use are:

1. Combining β (beta) 2-adrenergic receptors agonist and muscarinic acetylcholine receptor antagonists
2. Combining β (beta) 2-adrenergic receptor agonists and inhaled corticosteroid
3. Combining muscarinic acetylcholine receptor antagonists and inhaled corticosteroid

Repairing damaged lungs using regeneration therapy is ongoing research that might prove beneficial in treating COPD/IPF/ARDS/COVID patients.

Increasing evidence suggests that there is acceleration of normal lung aging in COPD, with accumulation of senescent cells in the lung that release an array of inflammatory proteins which leads to disease progression, several treatments that may target cellular senescence are in development.

12.10 Conclusion

Inhaled bronchodilators are the primary drugs for the management of COPD, and they are critical in the symptomatic management of asthma.

According to the guidelines for the management of COPD by the British National Institute for Health and Clinical Excellence (NICE), the treatment choice after initial SAMA or SABA bronchodilators for persistent breathlessness or exacerbations is determined by the level of post bronchodilator FEV1.

International guidelines on asthma management recommend the utilization of rapid onset inhaled β (beta) 2-AR agonists alone for symptom relief and pretreatment of exercise-induced asthma.

The field of obstructive lung disease treatment is currently undergoing major development in pharmacogenetic studies, which could target the use of specific medications in populations most likely to benefit.

Biological drugs are approved to treat the patients with severe asthma and are directed against mediators of type 2 immunity. There is two major type of asthma endotypes based on inflammatory pathway involved, high 2 type (T2-high) and type 2 low (T2-low).

12.11 Questions and Answers

Questions (Choose the Most Appropriate Answer)

1. Airway tone is mainly controlled by which of the following
   A. Parasympathetic nerves carried by the vagus nerve
   B. Parasympathetic nerves carried by the phrenic nerve
   C. Sympathetic nerves carried by the vagus nerve
   D. Sympathetic nerves carried by the phrenic nerve
2. How many subtypes of muscarinic receptors are present in the airways?
   A. 3
   B. 4
   C. 5
   D. 6
   E. 7
3. Levalbuterol has an advantage over albuterol in which category
   A. Duration
   B. Side effect
   C. Hospitalization
   D. All of the above
4. Side effects of B2 adrenergic receptors agonists include all of the following EXCEPT
   A. Tachycardia
   B. Transient increase in partial pressure of oxygen
   C. Risk of ketoacidosis in patients with diabetes mellitus
   D. Hypokalemia
   E. Fine tremor
5. Which of the following is a side effect of muscarinic acetylcholine receptors antagonists?
   A. Dry mouth
   B. Urinary retention
   C. Paradoxical bronchoconstriction
   D. Blurred vision
   E. All of the above

Answers

1. A. Airway tone is mainly controlled by parasympathetic nerves carried by the vagus nerve.
2. C. There are 5 subtypes of muscarinic receptors in the airways.
3. D. Levalbuterol may reduce hospitalization, have fewer adverse side effects, and provide similar bronchodilators effects at reduced dose compared to albuterol.
4. B. Transient mild decrease (rather than an increase) in partial pressure of oxygen in arterial blood could result from the administration of (beta) 2-AR agonists despite concomitant bronchodilation.
5. E. All are side effects:
   - Bad breath or dry mouth is a side effect, though usually well tolerated in long-term treatment.
   - In patients with prostatic hyperplasia, these agents should be used with caution, since the risk of further increase and acute urinary retention can follow.
   - Paradoxical bronchoconstriction could occur with these drugs. One possible cause is the blockade of prejunctional M2 mChRs on airway cholinergic nerves, which normally inhibits the release of ACh.
   - If these agents contact the eye, they can cause papillary dilation and blurred vision.

Suggested Reading

1. Calverley PM, Anderson JA, Celli B, Ferguson GT, Jenkins C, Jones PW, Yates JC, Vestbo J. Salmeterol and fluticasone propionate and survival in chronic obstructive pulmonary disease. N Engl J Med. 2007;356(8):775–89.
2. Cazzola M, Metersa MG, Calzetta L, Rogliani P. Pulmonary pharmacology—The emergence of new treatment in pulmonary medicine is finally providing real therapeutic perspectives. Curr Opin Pharmacol 2021;60:54–58
3. Cazzola M, Page CP, Calzetta L, Matera MG. Pharmacology XE "Pharmacology" and therapeutics of bronchodilators. Pharmacol Rev. 2012;64(3):450–504.
4. Expert Panel Working Group of the National Heart, Lung, and Blood Institute (NHLBI) Administered and Coordinated National Asthma Education and Prevention Program Coordinating Committee (NAEPPCC); Cloutier MM, Baptist AP, Blake KV, Brooks EG, Bryant-Stephens T, DiMango E, Dixon AE, Elward KS, Hartert T, Krishnan JA, Lemanske RF Jr, Ouellette DR, Pace WD, Schatz M, Skolnik NS, Stout JW, Teach SJ, Umscheid CA, Walsh CG. 2020 Focused updates to the Asthma Management guidelines: A report from the National Asthma Education and Prevention Program Coordinating Committee Expert Panel Working Group. J Allergy Clin Immunol. 2020 Dec;146(6):1217–270.
5. Montuschi P, Peters-Golden ML. Leukotriene modifiers for asthma treatment. Clin Exp Allergy. 2010;40(12):1732–41.
6. Pelaia G, Vatrella A, Maselli R. The potential of biologics for the treatment of asthma. Nat Rev Drug Discovery. 2012;11(12):958–72.
7. Fong WC, Azim A, Knight D, Mistry H, Freeman A, Felongco M, Kyyaly A, Harvey M, Dennison P, Zhang H, Howarth P. Real-world Omalizumab and Mepolizumab treated difficult asthma phenotypes and their clinical outcomes. Clin Exp Allergy. 2021;51 (8):1019–32.

Renal Pharmacology

13

Sekar S. Bhavani

Abstract

The term diuretic describes a drug that increases urinary solute and water excretion thus affecting the extracellular volume status of the individual. In addition, they alter the excretion of other cations such as K + , H + , Ca + + , and Mg + + and anions such as Cl − , HCO_3 − , and H_2PO_4 − , and uric acid. They thus have a significant effect on the body's electrolyte balance. The diuretic effect largely depends on the volume of the extracellular fluid. Chronic diuretic administration to a patient with a fixed sodium intake produces «diuretic braking,» also known as post diuretic sodium retention, which describes avid sodium retention occurring in response to rapid diuresis. Increasing the dose of diuretic to counter this can be detrimental in patients. When you fail to initiate an adequate response to a diuretic, you would need addition or substitution from a different class of diuretic in order to obtain a response.

Keywords

Diuretics • Classification of diuretics • Osmotic diuretics • Loop diuretics • Carbonic anhydrase inhibitors • Thiazides • Potassium-sparing diuretics • Dopaminergic agents

Key Points

1. The effect of a diuretic depends on the volume of the extracellular fluid.
2. Chronic diuretic administration to a patient with a fixed sodium intake initially causes a loss in total-body Na+ , but, with time, renal compensatory mechanisms balance the Na+ excretion to Na+ intake. This phenomenon is known as diuretic braking [1–3].
3. Diuretics may be detrimental and patients receiving higher doses have worse outcomes.
4. The failure to initiate an adequate response to a diuretic would need addition or substitution from a different class of diuretic in order to obtain a response [4].
5. Loop and thiazide diuretics increase the expression of the transporters they inhibit. This leads to decreased efficacy, and when the administration of diuretics is terminated, there may be a rapid increase in NaCl reabsorption.
6. The use of dopamine for potential renoprotective effects is not warranted, especially in light of several large-scale trials that have shown lack of benefit.

13.1 Part 1: Diuretics

13.1.1 What Are Diuretics?

The term diuretic describes a drug that increases urinary solute and water excretion thus affecting the extracellular volume status of the individual. Irrespective of their chemical class, most of the diuretics bring about their action by affecting the Na+ transport at one or more nephron segments resulting in natriuresis. Some produce kaliuresis (preferential loss of potassium) while others act as aquaretics (preferential loss of free water—antivasopressin-like action). In addition, diuretics alter the excretion of other cations such as K + , H + , Ca + + , and Mg + + and anions such as Cl − , HCO_3 − , and H_2PO_4 − , and uric acid. Thus, they have a significant effect on the body's electrolyte balance.

The time course of natriuresis is finite as renal compensatory mechanisms bring Na+ excretion in line with Na+ intake—a phenomenon known as "diuretic braking" [1, 3, 5].

S. S. Bhavani (✉)
Cleveland Clinic Lerner College of Medicine, Anesthesiology Institute, Cleveland Clinic, Cleveland, OH, USA
e-mail: sekarbhavani@gmail.com

M. Argalious et al. (eds.), *Basic Sciences in Anesthesia*,
https://doi.org/10.1007/978-3-031-60203-0_13

In addition, activation of the sympathetic nervous system, the renin–angiotensin–aldosterone axis, induction of renal cell hypertrophy, and increased expression of the transporter mechanisms that alter the renal hemodynamics facilitate this braking phenomenon.

13.1.2 Classification of Diuretics

1. Historically, the classification of diuretics can be based on the site of Primary Action
   a. Proximal-Osmotic Diuretics and Carbonic Anhydrase Inhibitors.
   b. Loop diuretics
   c. Distal tubules
   d. Potassium-sparing diuretics
2. Efficacy
   a. High-ceiling diuretics
   b. Moderate-ceiling diuretics
   c. Low-ceiling diuretics
3. Chemical nature
   a. Polysaccharides
   b. Sulfonamide and its derivatives
   c. Benzothiadiazine or its derivatives
   d. Steroid pyrazine carboxamides, pteridine derivative
4. Effect on K + excretion
   a. Potassium-sparing

13.1.3 Site of Action of the Diuretics

Diuretic class	Site of action
Proximal Tubules-Osmotic diuretics	Proximal tubule Thin descending limb of the loop of Henle
Proximal Tubules-Carbonic anhydrase inhibitors	Epithelial cells of the proximal convoluted tubules Modest effect along the distal nephron
Loop diuretics	Medullary ascending portion of the thick loop of Henle
Distal Convoluted Tubules-Thiazides	Distal convoluted tubule Some effect on the collecting ducts
Distal Convoluted Tubules-Potassium-sparing diuretics	Distal convoluted tubule Some effect on the collecting ducts
Collecting Tubules-Mineralocorticosteroid antagonists and Vasopressin receptor antagonists	Collecting tubules

13.2 Osmotic Diuretics

Osmotic diuretics are all small molecules. These agents are freely filtered at the glomerulus and are poorly reabsorbed. The osmotic diuretics exert their action by increasing the osmotic pressure and are effective only on the most permeable portions of the renal tubules: proximal tubule and the thin descending limb of the loop of Henle. Through osmotic effects, they also oppose the action of antidiuretic hormone (ADH) in the collecting tubule.

Normally, about 65–70% of the filtered sodium is passively absorbed in the proximal tubules. The presence of the osmotic diuretic interferes with the passive reabsorption of water. The reabsorption of sodium, however, continues normally in the thick ascending loop of Henle. The net effect is therefore only a mild natriuresis (10–25% net loss of $Na+$) [6].

Osmotic agents do not act directly on any of the Na transport pathways nor do they interact with any specific transport proteins or enzymes. The osmotic diuretics increase the excretion of sodium, potassium, calcium, magnesium, chloride, and bicarbonate.

The commonest agents considered in this class of diuretics include mannitol, urea, sorbitol, and glycerol. Hyperglycemia can also cause an osmotic diuresis. The prototypical osmotic diuretic is mannitol, which is an alcohol produced by the reduction of mannose.

13.2.1 Pharmacokinetics of Mannitol

Mannitol is poorly absorbed by the gastrointestinal (GI) tract. When administered orally, it causes osmotic diarrhea rather than diuresis. For its diuretic effects, therefore, it must be given intravenously. The usual dose is 0.25–1 g/kg. Following an IV infusion, it is slowly distributed into the extravascular compartment. Mannitol is not metabolized and is excreted unchanged by glomerular filtration within 30–60 min. About 10% is reabsorbed in the loop of Henle but a similar amount is metabolized by the liver[6].

13.2.2 Pharmacodynamics of Mannitol

Mannitol tends to mobilize the fluid from the extravascular compartment and expand the intravascular volume. It increases the renal blood flow by causing the release of renal prostaglandins that decrease the renal vascular resistance, increase the release of atrial natriuretic peptide (ANP), and net result is a decrease in the hematocrit and blood viscosity [6].

This increase in renal blood flow results in washout of the medullary tonicity that further decreases reabsorption of water from the tubules. It also acts as a free-radical scavenger and reduces the harmful effects of free radicals during ischemia–reperfusion injury. This latter property may have a protective effect following an ischemic insult to the kidneys by reducing the tubular endothelial swelling and maintaining tubular patency. Mannitol has no effect on the urinary pH.

13.2.3 Uses of Osmotic Diuretics

Osmotic diuretics are used for the following purposes [7]:

1. Reduction of raised intracranial pressure
   a. Mannitol is often administered to reduce intracranial pressure (ICP) following a closed head injury when the blood–brain barrier is still intact.
   b. There is some evidence that hypertonic saline is effective at reducing raised ICP resistant to mannitol and that it has a more favorable effect than mannitol on mortality after traumatic brain injury (TBI) [8].
   c. Preservation of perioperative renal function following:
      i. Major intra-abdominal surgery
      ii. Cardiac surgery
      iii. Aortic surgery
      iv. Renal transplantation
   d. Promotion of urinary excretion of toxic materials following:
      i. Rhabdomyolysis secondary to crush injuries and compartment syndrome
      ii. Jaundice
      iii. Incompatible blood transfusions
   e. Orally for bowel preparation before colorectal surgery, colonoscopy, and barium enemas.

13.2.4 Side Effects

Side effects include.

1. Fluid and electrolyte imbalance
   a. Rapid initial volume expansion resulting in increased risk of heart failure, pulmonary congestion
   b. Progressive loss of volume resulting in delayed hypovolemia and hypotension. In large doses, it can also cause renal failure because of intra-renal vasoconstriction and intravascular volume depletion
   c. Metabolic acidosis
   d. Hypernatremia and hypokalemia
2. Repeated administration may result in very high serum osmolality
3. Allergic reactions
4. Thrombophlebitis
5. Skin necrosis should accidental extravasation occur
6. Rebound increase in ICP

13.3 Carbonic Anhydrase Inhibitors

Carbonic anhydrase is present in many nephron sites, but the predominant location of this enzyme is the epithelial cells of the proximal convoluted tubules, where it catalyzes the dehydration of H_2CO_3 to CO_2 at the luminal membrane and rehydration of CO_2 to H_2CO_3 in the cytoplasm:

$$H^+ + HCO_2^- \leftrightarrow H_2CO_2 \leftrightarrow CO_2 + H^+$$

By blocking the carbonic anhydrase, these inhibitors decrease the reabsorption of NaHCO3 by 25–30% and cause diuresis. They have a weak natriuretic effect due to compensatory mechanisms that come into play following chronic administration [6].

The prototypical carbonic anhydrase inhibitor is acetazolamide.

13.3.1 Pharmacokinetics

The carbonic anhydrase inhibitors are well absorbed after oral administration. There is an increase in urine pH from HCO_3 − and diuresis is apparent within 30 min and maximal at 2 h. The effect persists for 12 h after a single dose. Excretion of the drug is by Glomerular filtration and tubular secretion in the proximal tubule S2 segment. Dosing must be reduced in renal insufficiency to prevent accumulation.

13.3.2 Uses of Carbonic Anhydrase Inhibitors

Carbonic anhydrase inhibitors are used for the following:

1. Glaucoma – The reduction of aqueous humor formation by carbonic anhydrase inhibitors decreases the intraocular pressure.
2. Urinary Alkalization – Uric acid and cysteine are relatively insoluble and may form stones in acidic urine. Alkalization of the urine can prevent their precipitation.
3. Metabolic Alkalosis: When the alkalosis is due to excessive use of diuretics, acetazolamide can be useful in correcting the alkalosis as well as producing a small additional diuresis for correction of volume overload.

4. Acute Mountain Sickness: By decreasing cerebral spinal fluid (CSF) formation and by decreasing the pH of the CSF and brain, acetazolamide can increase ventilation and diminish symptoms of mountain sickness. This is also useful in the treatment of sleep apnea.

   Miscellaneous:

5. Hypokalemic periodic paralysis
6. CSF leak
7. Severe hyperphosphatemia
8. As a short-term therapy in combination with other diuretics when patients develop resistance to the second agent.

13.3.3 Side Effects

Side effects include:

1. Hyperchloremic metabolic acidosis
2. Renal stones. There is a higher incidence of calcium and phosphate stones as they are insoluble in an alkaline pH.
3. Hypokalemia
4. Drowsiness and paresthesia
5. Hypersensitivity reactions (fever, rashes, bone marrow suppression, and interstitial nephritis)

13.3.4 Contraindications

Carbonic anhydrase inhibitors are contraindicated in patients with cirrhosis of liver as they may develop hyperammonemia and hepatic encephalopathy.

13.4 Loop Diuretics

Loop diuretics act selectively on the medullary ascending portion of the thick loop of Henle's and inhibit NaCl reabsorption. The decreased reabsorption of sodium chloride alters the tonicity of the normally hypertonic medullary interstitium and leads to a reduced urine-concentrating ability of the kidneys thus facilitating diuresis. Loop diuretics also lead to a loss of potassium and hydrogen ions.

The two drugs that were initially available were the sulfonamide derivative furosemide and the phenoxyacetic acid derivative ethacrynic acid. The prototypical agents of this class in common clinical use are the sulfonamide derivatives furosemide, bumetanide, and torasemide.

13.4.1 Pharmacokinetics

The loop diuretics are rapidly absorbed after oral administration. Absorption of orally administered loop diuretics is variable for each agent. It is about 10–50% with furosemide but is about 80–90% for torasemide and bumetanide. Because of this, changing from intravenous to oral dose will require a doubling of the furosemide dose but not that of bumetanide or torsemide doses.

Approximately 90–95% of loop diuretics are bound to plasma proteins and its volume of distribution is relatively low. This protein binding is essential for the delivery of furosemide to the kidney, the site for its action [9].

Loop diuretics have to be secreted into the luminal side of the proximal tubules in order to have an effect. Medications that compete for the same weak acid secretion (NSAIDs or probenecid) may interfere with their secretion and thus make it ineffective.

Thirty percent of the drug is metabolized and excreted via the gastrointestinal tract. It is primarily eliminated by the kidney by glomerular filtration and tubular secretion. Half-life varies from 1 to 3 h and depends on renal function and the dose has to be adjusted in patients with renal failure.

The diuresis lasts for 2–3 h following an oral dose of furosemide but lasts for about 4–6 h following use of torasemide.

13.4.2 Pharmacodynamics

Loop diuretics inhibit the luminal $Na^+/K^+/2Cl^-$ transporter in the thick ascending loop of Henle. They thus reduce the reabsorption of NaCl.

Loop diuretics increase the excretion of water, Na, K, Cl, phosphate, Mg, and Ca. In normal circumstances, this increased loss of calcium is counter-balanced by increased intestinal absorption and parathyroid hormone-induced renal reabsorption of $Ca2^+$ and hypocalcemia does not develop.

Loop diuretics have also been shown to increase synthesis of prostaglandins. This increases renal blood flow and decreases the peripheral vascular tone. The latter reduces pulmonary congestion and left ventricular filling pressures in the presence of heart failure.

13.4.3 Uses of Loop Diuretics

Loop diuretics are used in treatments for the following [6]:

1. Hyperkalemia
2. Acute pulmonary edema
3. Increased intracranial pressure: they can be used even in the presence of disrupted blood–brain barrier.

4. Acute renal failure
5. Edematous conditions
6. Congestive heart failure
7. Cirrhotic ascites
8. Nephrotic syndrome
9. Hypercalcemia
10. Hyponatremia
11. Toxicity due to ingestion of bromide, fluoride, and iodide.

13.4.4 Side Effects

Side effects include

1. Hyponatremia
2. Hypokalemic metabolic alkalosis
3. Hypomagnesemia
4. Hyperuricemia
5. Hypercalciuria, which can lead to mild hypocalcemia and secondary hyperparathyroidism
6. Hypercalcemia in volume-depleted patients with metastatic breast or squamous cell lung carcinoma
7. Dehydration
8. Ototoxicity: dose-related hearing loss that is usually reversible
9. Furosemide may increase the toxicity of aminoglycosides and cephalosporins.
10. Allergic reactions: skin rash, eosinophilia, and less often, interstitial nephritis. Allergic reactions are much less common with ethacrynic acid.
11. Direct toxic action resulting in interstitial nephritis

13.4.5 Contraindications

Furosemide, bumetanide, and torasemide may exhibit allergic cross-reactivity in patients who are sensitive to other sulfonamides, but this appears to be very rare.

Use with caution in patients with hepatic cirrhosis, borderline renal failure, or heart failure.

13.4.6 Furosemide

Furosemide can be administered orally (0.75–3 mg kg^{-1}) or intravenously (0.1–1 mg kg^{-1}). Absorption is variable after an oral dose and ranges from 15–50%. The peak effect is seen 60–90 min after an oral dose. Approximately 90% of the drug is bound to plasma proteins and its volume of distribution is relatively low.

About 30% of the elimination is via the GI tract while the rest is excreted unchanged by the kidneys by glomerular filtration and tubular secretion. The elimination half-life of furosemide is 60–90 min.

Furosemide increases renal artery blood flow if the intravascular fluid volume is maintained. It increases the blood flow to the inner cortex and medullary regions. This is mediated through release of prostaglandins.

Loop diuretics have a high-ceiling effect (i.e., increasing doses leads to increasing diuresis).

13.4.7 Ethacrinic Acid

Unlike other loop diuretics, ethacrynic acid does not have a sulfonamide group in its structure and so can be used even in patients with sulfa-allergies. The main site of action is limited to the ascending limb of the loop of Henle [10–12].

In addition, Ethacrynic acid causes venous dilation and thus can produce rapid pulmonary decongestion even before its onset of diuresis when used in patients with CCF. More recently, it has been used as a potential anticancer agent [13].

After oral intake, onset of action is usually within 30 min, peak effect occurs in 2 h and lasts for 6–8 h. After intravenous injection, onset is in 5 min, peaks in 30 min, and effect lasts for 2–4 h.

Most side effects of ethacrynic acid can be attributed to its effectiveness (volume depletion); however, it may cause metabolic alkalosis that is preventable by KCl replacement. Ethacrynic acid has ototoxic effect that occasionally results in temporally or permanent deafness [14].

13.4.8 Bumetanide

Bumetanide is used for managing various edematous conditions secondary to cardiac failure or hepatic or renal disease, including nephrotic syndrome. It may also be indicated for refractory edema resistant to other loop diuretics.

The mechanism of action and its effects are similar to those of furosemide. Bumetanide is absorbed completely after oral administration. Its rate of elimination is less dependent on renal function.

Onset of diuretic action occurs between 0 to 30 min following intravenous use and 30 to 60 min following oral administration. The peak of the drug's action occurs at 90 min after oral administration. The diuretic effect and the total duration of action last for 3 to 4 h. Bumetanide is primarily excreted in the urine (80% of dose; 50% unchanged) [15].

Ototoxicity may be slightly less frequent than with furosemide, but renal toxicity is more of a problem. Because it is more potent, smaller doses are required.

13.4.9 Torasemide

Torasemide (torsemide) is a high-ceiling loop diuretic which acts on the thick ascending limb of the loop of Henle to promote rapid and marked excretion of water, sodium, and chloride. Like furosemide (frusemide), its major site of action is from the luminal side of the cell. Torasemide is at least twice as potent as furosemide on a weight-for-weight basis, produces equivalent diuresis and natriuresis at lower urinary concentrations, and has a longer duration of action, allowing once-daily administration without the paradoxical antidiuresis seen with furosemide.

The bioavailability of oral torsemide is high (80%) even after oral administration, so the dose of oral and IV forms are the same. Food does not interfere with absorption of Torsemide. Diuresis lasts approximately 6–8 h [16].

Torsemide is well tolerated with adverse effects of a mild and include hypotension, electrolyte abnormalities, and photosensitivity. It is contraindicated in patients with sulfa allergy, anuria, and patients in hepatic coma.

13.4.10 Thiazides

The thiazide diuretics are chemically related to carbonic anhydrase inhibitors. These agents inhibit the NaCl, rather than $NaHCO_3$ transportation. They have their predominant site of action at the distal convoluted tubule and have some effect on the collecting ducts [17].

13.4.11 Pharmacokinetics

Thiazides can be administered orally. They are highly protein-bound like the loop diuretics. Also like the loop diuretics, they are secreted by the organic acid secretory system in the proximal tubule and compete with the secretion of uric acid by that system. Hence, this might result in hyperuricemia.

13.4.12 Pharmacodynamics

Thiazides inhibit NaCl reabsorption from the luminal side of epithelial cells in the distal convoluted tubules by blocking the Na^+/Cl^- transporter. They increase the excretion of Na, K, Cl, HCO_3, phosphate, and urate.

Thiazides actually enhance $Ca2^+$ reabsorption. This effect can be helpful in some patients to prevent calcium stones in patients with hypercalciuria.

13.4.13 Uses of Thiazide Diuretics

Thiazides are used to treat the following:

1. Hypertension
2. Heart failure
3. Nephrolithiasis due to idiopathic hypercalciuria
4. Nephrogenic diabetes insipidus
5. Cirrhotic ascites
6. Nephrotic syndrome
7. Presence of osteoporosis or hypoparathyroidism

13.4.14 Side Effects

Side effects of thiazides include:

8. Hypokalemic metabolic alkalosis
9. Hyperuricemia
10. Impaired Carbohydrate Tolerance—occurs at higher doses of hydrochlorothiazide (HCTZ) (> 50 mg/d) due to both impaired pancreatic release of insulin and diminished tissue utilization of glucose
11. Hyperlipidemia—5–15% increase in total serum cholesterol and low-density lipoproteins (LDLs).
12. Hyponatremia
13. Allergic Reactions—Being sulfonamides, they share cross-reactivity with other members of this chemical group. Serious allergic reactions—such as hemolytic anemia, thrombocytopenia, and acute necrotizing pancreatitis—are extremely rare.

13.4.15 Contraindications

Use with caution in patients with hepatic cirrhosis, borderline renal failure, or heart failure.

13.5 Potassium-Sparing Diuretics

Potassium-sparing diuretics act primarily along the aldosterone-sensitive distal nephron and prevent the secretion of potassium by antagonizing the effect of aldosterone. They are weak diuretics and are usually used in combination with thiazides or loop diuretics.

Potassium-sparing diuretics comprise three distinct groups:

A. Aldosterone antagonists (spironolactone)—Directly inhibit the mineralocorticoid receptor
B. Pteridines (triamterene)—Inhibit the Na^+ influx
C. Pyrazinoylguanidines (amiloride)—Inhibit the Na^+ influx

13.5.1 Uses of Potassium-Sparing Diuretics

Potassium-sparing diuretics are used for the following:

1. Hyperaldosteronism
2. Hypertension
3. Female hirsutism (spironolactone)
4. The Na^+ channel blockers can be used as adjuncts to other diuretics
5. Amiloride is used for the treatment of diabetes insipidus

13.5.2 Side Effects

Side effects include:

1. Acidosis
2. Hyperkalemia
3. Azotemia
4. Gynecomastia
5. Libido changes (spironolactone)
6. Nephrolithiasis (triamterene)

13.6 Sodium Glucose Cotransporter 2 Inhibitors

The Sodium Glucose Cotransporter 2 inhibitors block glucose reabsorption in the proximal tubule and thus increase the excretion of glucose in the urine (inducing an osmotic diuresis effect). Inhibiting this transporter will result in glucose excretion of 30–50% of the amount of glucose filtered. Three SGLT2 inhibitors (*Empagliflozin, canagliflozin, and dapagliflozin* are currently available.

13.6.1 Pharmacokinetics

The SGLT2 inhibitors are rapidly absorbed by the GI tract. The elimination half-life of dapagliflozin is 10–12 h and up to 70% of the given dose is excreted in the urine. The drugs are not recommended in patients with severe renal failure or advanced liver disease.

13.6.2 Clinical Indications and Adverse Reactions

1. Currently, the only indication for the use of these drugs is as third-line therapy for patients with diabetes mellitus or in patients to help relieve loop diuretic resistance and preserve renal function.
2. SGLT2 inhibitors may also be used as an adjunct to weight loss treatment.
3. There is a six-fold increased incidence of genital fungal infection in women and a slightly higher risk of urinary tract infections [18].

13.7 Aquaretics (Vasopressin Receptor Antagonists)

Vasopressin receptor antagonists promote the excretion of solute-free water, and thus are known as "aquaretics." Vasopressin mediates its effects by acting on the V2 receptors in the distal nephron and the collecting tubules. Arginine vasopressin (AVP) brings about its effects by triggering the cAMP, which in turn stimulates the expression of the aquaporin-2 channels on the luminal surface of the collecting tubules.

The US Food and Drug Administration (FDA) has only approved conivaptan, a combined V1a/V2-receptor antagonist, for clinical use in the United States. There are concerns about its interactions with other drugs metabolized by the CYP3A4 pathway [19, 20].

13.8 Adenosine A-1 Receptor Antagonists

Adenosine A-1 receptor antagonists prevent tubuloglomerular feedback by interfering with the activation of NHE3 in the proximal convoluted tubules and the adenosine-mediated enhancement of collecting tubule K^+ secretion.

Caffeine and theophylline are the prototypical agents. They exhibit a modest and nonspecific inhibition of these adenosine receptors and produce a mild diuretic effect.

13.9 Nesiritide and Neprilysin Inhibitors

13.9.1 Nesiritide

Nesiritide is the recombinant form of B-type natriuretic peptide, that is used in the treatment of acute decompensated congestive heart failure. It produces both a natriuresis and relaxation of smooth muscle by stimulating cGMP in the blood vessels, kidney, adrenal gland, and brain. When given intravenously, it produces peripheral vasodilation resulting in decrease in the left and right ventricular filling pressures and thus increases the stroke volume and cardiac output without any significant increase in heart rate. In addition, nesiritide lowers aldosterone, catecholamines, and endothelin-1 levels and this leads to an increased natriuresis and diuresis without effect on serum potassium or renal function [21].

13.9.2 NeprilysinInhibitors

Neprilysin inhibitors prevent the breakdown of natriuretic peptides, and therefore contribute to natriuresis. The combined use of an ARB and neprilysin inhibitor (LCZ696) has been shown to reduce rates of cardiovascular death and hospitalization for heart failure in patients with class II, III, or IV heart failure.233.

13.10 Part 2: Dopaminergic Drugs

13.10.1 Dopamine

Dopamine is an endogenous catecholamine with a broad range of activity on dopaminergic, beta-adrenergic, and alpha-adrenergic receptors [22]. "Low dose" dopamine (less than 3 mcg/kg/min) has long been thought to be useful as a renal protection agent due to its effect in producing renal vasodilation and producing natriuresis by blocking the tubular reabsorption of sodium [23].

The pharmacokinetics of dopamine varies between individuals by as much as tenfold to 75-fold and can also vary in the same individual [23]. Therefore, dosing the drug based on body weight may not reflect the true plasma concentration of the medication. Thus, what is considered as a "low dose dopamine" may in fact produce beta 1 or alpha stimulation resulting in unwanted tachycardia and hypertension [23].

The "renoprotective" effects have not been established in a large randomized controlled trial, and use of dopamine remains controversial [24–27]. The increase in cardiac output that may follow its use, however, may be beneficial in improving the renal perfusion and increasing the urine output.

13.10.2 Fenoldopam

Fenoldopam is a phenolated derivative of dopamine that has been shown to have some advantages over the latter. It is a selective dopaminergic-1 receptor agonist. Its effects are similar to dopamine and it induces a dose-dependent renal vasodilation, increase in renal blood flow (RBF), and natriuresis [22].

Being a selective D-1 effect, it lacks the beta- or alpha-adrenergic effects and hence has the potential to be safer and more effective as compared to dopamine as an effective renoprotective agent without inducing some of the adverse effects of dopamine, including tachycardia or vasoconstriction [28].

It can produce some hypotension and a reflex increase in the heart rate. It can be administered by a peripheral venous catheter.

A meta analysis has demonstrated its usefulness in reducing the risk of acute kidney disease [29].

13.11 Factors Affecting Diuretic Efficacy and Diuretic Resistance [30]

Following administration of a diuretic, the effect can be variable. This depends on:

1. The volume status of the individual.
   a. Inappropriate salt and fluid intake
   b. Incorrect diagnosis
2. Absorption from the gut following orally administration.
   a. Non compliance
   b. Inadequate dose
   c. Interference with food intake
3. Delivery of the drug to its effector site due to renovascular disease or humoral changes as seen in heart failure or cirrhosis.
4. Secretion of the drug into the lumen of the primary segment of the nephron at which it has its effect. Most diuretics, except the potassium-sparing diuretics, mediate their effect via the solute reabsorptive pumps that are located on the luminal surface of the nephron. Hence, these drugs have to be secreted into the lumen of the tubules in order to produce their effects.
5. Renal dysfunction
   a. AKI
   b. CKD
   c. Nephrotic syndrome
6. The secondary structural changes downsteam from its effort site due to Epithelial Hypertrophy and Hyperplasia or Nephron adaptation
7. Effect of the humoral and neuronal modulators
   a. Renin–Angiotensin–Aldosterone system
   b. Inhibition of PG synthesis by ANSAIDS-[31–34]

13.12 Diuretic Combinations

1. It is important to realize that continuing to increase the dose beyond the maximum therapeutic dose when we do not get an adequate response may not be the best option.
2. Adding another drug that acts on the same transport mechanism does not provide any added benefit and may even be associated with a higher incidence of complications, whereas, use of a combination of diuretics acting on a separate mechanism may be synergistic.
   a. A loop diuretic and a thiazide or thiazide-like drug act synergistically in both normal subjects and in patients with edema or renal insufficiency.
   b. Adding a loop diuretic or a thiazide with a potassium-sparing diuretic may not affect the natriuresis but will curtail the loss of K + and net acid. However, one must be cautious in adding a potassium-sparing agent in patients with renal failure because of the risk of hyperkalemia.

13.13 Questions and Answers

Questions (Choose the Most Appropriate Answer)

1. Which class of diuretics act predominantly on the proximal tubule?
   a. Carbonic anhydrase inhibitors
   b. Loop diuretics
   c. Potassium-sparing diuretics
   d. Thiazide diuretics
2. You are planning on short trip to the Andes while on vacation. A drug that is useful in preventing high-altitude sickness is:
   a. Acetazolamide
   b. Amiloride
   c. Demeclocycline
   d. Desmopressin
   e. Ethacrynic acid
3. A 50-year-old patient presents to the emergency department with mental status changes. An electrolyte panel is ordered and it shows serum Ca + + of 16.5 (normal = 8.5–10.5 mg/dL). Which of the following would be your first choice in the management of his severe hypercalcemia?
   a. Acetazolamide plus saline infusion
   b. Furosemide plus saline infuse
   c. HCTZ plus normal saline
   d. Mannitol plus hypertonic saline
4. You are seeing a patient with a history of traumatic head injury with signs suggestive of cerebral edema and herniation. The diuretic that would be most useful in acute management of this patient would be:
   a. Amiloride
   b. Ethacrynic Acid
   c. Furosemide
   d. Mannitol
5. You are seeing a patient with a history of hypertension for which he has been placed chronic therapy with Lasix (furosemide). What would be one of the complications of such a treatment protocol?
   a. Decreased urinary Ca + + excretion
   b. Elevation of pulmonary vascular pressure
   c. Metabolic acidosis
   d. Ototoxicity
6. A 40-year-old patient presents with a history of passing renal stones. A prior analysis of his stones suggested that they are calcium stones. What would be your first choice for a diuretic for this patient?
   a. Acetazolamide
   b. Furosemide
   c. Hydrochlorothiazide (HCTZ)
   d. Mannitol
7. A 60-year-old patient with long-standing heart failure has been on large doses of furosemide. His blood gas reveals the presence of metabolic alkalosis. Which of the following diuretics would have a positive impact on his treatment?
   a. Acetazolamide
   b. Digoxin
   c. Dobutamine
   d. Spironolactone
8. You see a patient who is complaining of gynecomastia following initiation of a water pill. He does not have his prescription with him. Which of the following diuretics has this effect?
   a. Hydrochlorothiazide (HCTZ)
   b. Furosemide
   c. Spironolactone
   d. Mannitol
9. Chlorothiazide produces its action by blocking the sodium and chloride co-transport at the
   a. Proximal convoluted tubule
   b. Loop of Henle
   c. Distal convoluted tubule
   d. Collecting ducts
10. Sodium bicarbonate is mostly reabsorbed at the
    a. Proximal tubule
    b. Loop of Henle
    c. Distal tubule
    d. Collecting tubule

Answers

1. A. Carbonic anhydrase inhibitors act predominantly on the proximal tubule.
2. A. By decreasing cerebral spinal fluid (CSF) formation and by decreasing the pH of the CSF and brain, acetazolamide can increase ventilation and diminish symptoms of high-altitude sickness.
3. B. Furosemide plus saline infuse.
4. D. Mannitol is often administered to reduce intracranial pressure (ICP) following a closed head injury when the blood–brain barrier is still intact.
5. D. Ototoxicity is a dose-related hearing loss that is usually reversible.
6. C. Hydrochlorothiazide (HCTZ). Thiazides actually enhance $Ca2+$ reabsorption. This effect can be helpful in some patients to prevent calcium stones in patients with hypercalciuria.
7. A. Acetazolamide. When the alkalosis is due to excessive use of diuretics, acetazolamide can be useful in correcting the alkalosis as well as producing a small additional diuresis for correction of volume overload.
8. C. Spironolactone. One of the side effects of potassium-sparing diuretics, such as spironolactone, is gynecomastia.
9. C. The thiazide diuretics have their predominant site of action at the distal convoluted tubule and have some effect on the collecting ducts.
10. A. Proximal tubule. Normally about 65–70% of the filtered sodium is passively absorbed in the proximal tubules.

References

1. Ellison DH. Diuretic resistance: physiology and therapeutics. Semin Nephrol. 1999;19(6):581–97.
2. Jardim SI, et al. A 2018 overview of diuretic resistance in heart failure. Rev Port Cardiol. 2018;37(11):935–45.
3. Felker GM, et al. Diuretic therapy for patients with heart failure: JACC State-of-the-art review. J Am Coll Cardiol. 2020;75 (10):1178–95.
4. Brater DC. Pharmacology of diuretics. Am J Med Sci. 2000;319 (1):38–50.
5. Imbs JL, Grima M, Stephan D. Diuretic resistance: mechanisms and therapeutic possibilities. Arch Mal Coeur Vaiss. 1998;91 (11):1383–8.
6. Ellison DH (2013) Physiology and pathophysiology of diuretic action, in Seldin and Giebisch's the kidney, 5*th Edition*, M.J.C.a. O.W.M. Edited by Robert J Alpern, (eds.) 2013, Academic Press. pp 1353–4
7. Shawkat H, Westwood M-M, Mortimer A. Mannitol: a review of its clinical uses. Contin Educ Anaesth CritAl Care & Pain. 2012;12 (2):82–5.
8. Wakai A, et al. Mannitol for acute traumatic brain injury. Cochrane Database Syst Rev. 2013;8:001049.
9. Inoue M, et al. Mechanism of furosemide resistance in analbuminemic rats and hypoalbuminemic patients. Kidney Int. 1987;32 (2):198–203.
10. Ricci Z, et al. Furosemide versus ethacrynic acid in pediatric patients undergoing cardiac surgery: a randomized controlled trial. Crit Care. 2015;19(1):2.
11. Cannon PJ, Kilcoyne MM. Ethacrynic acid and furosemide: renal pharmacology and clinical use. Prog Cardiovasc Dis. 1969;12 (1):99–118.
12. Krumlovsky FA, del Greco F. Diuretic agents Mechanisms of action and clinical uses. Postgrad Med. 1976;59(4):105–10.
13. Yu L, et al. Ethacrynic acid: a promising candidate for drug repurposing as an anticancer agent. Int J Mol Sci. 2023;24 (7):6712.
14. Molnar J, Somberg JC. The clinical pharmacology of ethacrynic acid. Am J Ther. 2009;16(1):86–92.
15. Flamenbaum W, Friedman R. Pharmacology, therapeutic efficacy, and adverse effects of bumetanide, a new "loop" diuretic. Pharmacotherapy. 1982;2(4):213–22.
16. Blose JS, Adams KF Jr, Patterson JH. Torsemide: a pyridine-sulfonylurea loop diuretic. Ann Pharmacother. 1995;29(4):396–402.
17. Akbari P, Khorasani-Zadeh A (2023) *Thiazide Diuretics*, in *StatPearls*. 2023: Treasure Island (FL) ineligible companies. Disclosure: Arshia Khorasani-Zadeh declares no relevant financial relationships with ineligible companies
18. Anders H-J, Davis JM, Thurau K. Nephron protection in diabetic kidney disease. N Engl J Med. 2016;375(21):2096–8.
19. Corry JJ, et al. Conivaptan for the reduction of cerebral edema in intracerebral hemorrhage: a safety and tolerability study. Clin Drug Investig. 2020;40(5):503–9.
20. Li-Ng M, Verbalis JG. Conivaptan: evidence supporting its therapeutic use in hyponatremia. Core Evid. 2010;4:83–92.
21. Elkayam U, et al. Nesiritide: a new drug for the treatment of decompensated heart failure. J Cardiovasc Pharmacol Ther. 2002;7 (3):181–94.
22. Diaz GC, Moitra V, Sladen RN. Hepatic and renal protection during cardiac surgery. Anesthesiol Clin. 2008;26(3):565–90.
23. Olsen NV, et al. *Dopamine*, *dobutamine*, and *dopexamine*. A comparison of renal effects in unanesthetized human volunteers. Anesthesiology. 1993;79(4):685–94.
24. Bellomo R, et al. Low-dose dopamine in patients with early renal dysfunction: a placebo-controlled randomised trial. Australian and New Zealand Intensive Care Society (ANZICS) Clinical Trials Group. Lancet. 2000;356(9248):2139–43.
25. Marik PE. Low-dose dopamine: a systematic review. Intensive Care Med. 2002;28(7):877–83.
26. McDonald RH Jr, et al. Effect of dopamine in man: augmentation of sodium excretion, glomerular filtration rate, and renal plasma flow. J Clin Invest. 1964;43(6):1116–24.
27. Carey RM, et al. Dopamine-1 and dopamine-2 mechanisms in the control of renal function. Am J Hypertens. 1990;3(6 Pt 2): 59S-63S.
28. Mathur VS, et al. The effects of fenoldopam, a selective dopamine receptor agonist, on systemic and renal hemodynamics in normotensive subjects. Crit Care Med. 1999;27(9):1832–7.
29. Landoni G, et al. Beneficial impact of fenoldopam in critically ill patients with or at risk for acute renal failure: a meta-analysis of randomized clinical trials. Am J Kidney Dis. 2007;49(1):56–68.
30. Cox ZL, Rao VS, Testani JM. Classic and novel mechanisms of diuretic resistance in cardiorenal syndrome. Kidney360. 2022;3 (5):954–67.

31. Kramer HJ, et al. Interaction of conventional and antikaliuretic diuretics with the renal prostaglandin system. Clin Sci. 1980;59 (1):67–70.
32. Tan SY, Mulrow PJ. Inhibition of the renin-aldosterone response to furosemide by indomethacin. J Clin Endocrinol Metab. 1977;45 (1):174–6.
33. Kirchner KA, et al. Mechanism of attenuated hydrochlorothiazide response during indomethacin administration. Kidney Int. 1987;31 (5):1097–103.
34. Favre L, et al. Interaction of diuretics and non-steroidal anti-inflammatory drugs in man. Clin Sci. 1983;64(4):407–15.

Pharmacology of Anticoagulants, Antithrombotics, and Antiplatelet Drugs

14

G. Burkhard Mackensen and Melanie Liu

Abstract

Anticoagulant therapies, which include antiplatelet and antithrombotic drugs, prevent and treat many cardiovascular disorders and are some of the most universally prescribed drugs. Rapid onset anticoagulant therapy is also required to perform a number of clinical procedures including percutaneous coronary interventions (PCI), structural heart interventions, cardiovascular surgery, and other surgeries, as well as dialysis. This therapy is also used as a treatment for a number of thrombotic diseases including acute coronary syndromes (myocardial infarction and unstable angina), deep vein thrombosis, and pulmonary embolism. The hematologic system involves a complex interaction of the vascular endothelium, platelets, and coagulation factors. As long as the fine-tuned interplay within the system is balanced, neither thrombus formation or bleeding and any associated consequences will take place. Perioperatively, hemostasis is often challenged but perturbations of the integrity of the vascular endothelium and subsequent platelet activation may result in acute clot formation in the arteries or veins, which ultimately manifests as arterial or venous thromboembolism. This is where anticoagulant drugs including antiplatelet therapies and antithrombotic agents are utilized to interfere with hemostasis. When selecting the most appropriate anticoagulant drug, thorough consideration of the efficacy to safety ratio is warranted. In addition, there are a number of pharmacological factors that affect a drug's success: the absorption rate, the overall metabolism, an active parent drug rather than a prodrug that needs to be metabolized, drug interactions, interpatient variability in anticoagulant effects (e.g., drug, environment, and genetic), onset of action, pharmacokinetics with a dose-dependent drug effect, elimination, and a direct target. The overarching goal over the last several years has been to develop antithrombotic, anticoagulant, and antiplatelet drugs that carry more favorable pharmacological properties (e.g., faster onset of action, fewer interactions, and less interpatient variability in their antithrombotic effects) thus reducing thrombotic events without generation of unacceptably high bleeding rates. Besides more original drugs such as unfractionated heparin (UFH), the antiplatelet agents aspirin and clopidogrel and the vitamin K antagonist warfarin, modern treatment options now include anticoagulants that directly target factor IIa (bivalirudin, argatroban, dabigatran) or Xa (rivaroxaban, apixaban, edoxaban) and the next-generation antiplatelet drugs prasugrel and ticagrelor. This chapter focuses on the pharmacological properties, monitoring, and strategies for reversal of the most commonly used anticoagulants, antithrombotics, and antiplatelet drugs.

Keywords

Anticoagulant • Antithrombotic • Antiplatelet • Pharmacology • Oral • Intravenous • Medications • Agents and therapies

Key Points

- The perioperative management of anticoagulation and the prevention of thrombosis and bleeding remain challenging and require a comprehensive understanding of the coagulation cascade and the pharmacology of anticoagulants, antithrombotics, and antiplatelet agents.
- The hematologic system involves a complex and balanced interaction of the vascular endothelium, platelets, and coagulation factors.

G. Burkhard Mackensen (✉) · M. Liu
Division of Cardiothoracic Anesthesiology,
Department of Anesthesiology and Pain Medicine,
University of Washington, 1959 N.E. Pacific St.,
Seattle, WA 98195, USA
e-mail: gbmac@uw.edu

M. Liu
e-mail: melanliu@uw.edu

M. Argalious et al. (eds.), *Basic Sciences in Anesthesia*,
https://doi.org/10.1007/978-3-031-60203-0_14

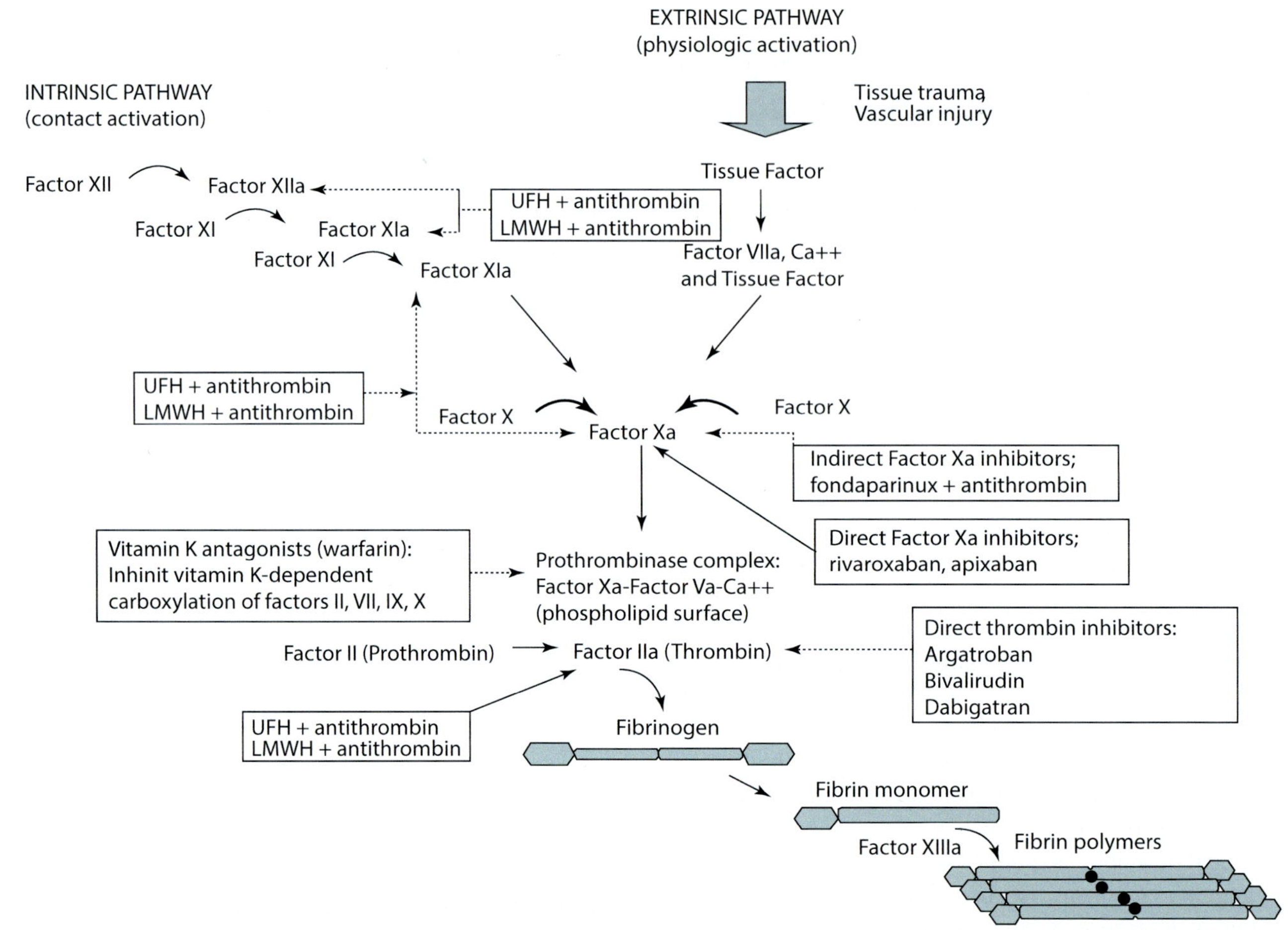

Fig. 14.1 Illustration of the coagulation cascade with its intrinsic (contact activation) and extrinsic (tissue factor) pathway. Each pathway generates a series of reactions in which inactive circulating enzymes and their co-factors are activated. The key elements of the extrinsic pathway involve the release of tissue factor from trauma or vascular injury. In the presence of calcium, tissue factor forms a complex with factor VIIa and cleaves clotting factors X and IX to their active forms. The intrinsic pathway is based on contact activation where factor IXa binds to factor VIIIa and forms intrinsic tenase, which activates factor X. The interaction of factor Xa with factor Va results in the formation of prothrombinase, which converts factor II to IIa (thrombin). Factor IIa further amplifies the coagulation system, converts soluble fibrinogen to insoluble fibrin, and also activates platelets. Anticoagulants are interacting at various stages with this coagulation system and interrupt the enzymatic reactions. With permission from Alquwaizani et al. [1]

- Anticoagulant therapy is required to perform a number of clinical procedures including percutaneous coronary and transcatheter interventions, cardiovascular surgeries, and other surgeries, as well as dialysis. This therapy is also used as a treatment for a number of thrombotic diseases including acute coronary syndromes (myocardial infarction and unstable angina), deep vein thrombosis, and pulmonary embolism.
- The ideal anticoagulant possesses a fast onset and offset of action, few drug interactions, and little interpatient variability in its anticoagulant effects.

Anticoagulant therapy is required to perform a number of clinical procedures including percutaneous coronary interventions (PCI), structural heart interventions, cardiovascular surgery, and other surgeries, as well as dialysis [1–4]. This therapy is also used as a treatment for a number of thrombotic diseases including acute coronary syndromes, deep vein thrombosis, and pulmonary embolism. The hematologic system involves a complex interaction of the vascular endothelium, platelets, and coagulation factors (Fig. 14.1: coagulation cascade). When selecting the most appropriate anticoagulant drug, thorough consideration of the efficacy to safety ratio is warranted. In addition, there are a number of pharmacological factors that affect a drug's success: the absorption rate, the overall metabolism, an active parent drug rather than a prodrug that needs to be metabolized, drug interactions, interpatient variability in anticoagulant effects (e.g., drug, environment, and genetic), onset of action, pharmacokinetics with a dose-dependent drug effect, elimination, and a direct target [1, 5]. The overarching goal over the last several years has been to develop antithrombotic, anticoagulant and antiplatelet drugs that carry more favorable pharmacological properties (e.g., faster onset of action, fewer interactions, and less interpatient variability in their antithrombotic effects) thus reducing thrombotic events without generation of unacceptably high bleeding rates [6]. Besides more original drugs such as unfractionated heparin (UFH), the antiplatelet agents aspirin and clopidogrel and the vitamin K antagonist warfarin, modern treatment options now include anticoagulants that directly target factor IIa (bivalirudin, argatroban, dabigatran) or Xa (rivaroxaban, apixaban, edoxaban) and the next-generation antiplatelet drugs prasugrel and ticagrelor [1, 4, 7–10].

14.1 Unfractionated Heparin, Low Molecular Weight Heparin and Fondaparinux

Unfractionated heparin (UFH) is the anticoagulant of choice in acute settings (such as cardiovascular procedures or surgery) while both UFH and low molecular weight heparin (LMWH) are preferred agents in acute thrombosis [1, 11, 12]. Heparin is an endogenously produced, linear polysaccharide that consists of repeating units of pyranosyluronic acid and glucosamine residues. Heparins contain an active pentasaccharide sequence that binds to the endogenous serin protease inhibitor antithrombin (AT), thus causing a conformational change of AT which results in accelerated AT binding and inactivation of coagulation factors XIIa, IXa, XIa, Xa, and thrombin. Neither UFH nor LMWH have significant intrinsic fibrinolytic activity and neither provides direct thrombolysis. Most important for the clinical effect of heparin is the accelerated inhibition of thrombin and factor Xa. Once a heparin molecule has formed a complex with AT, it can easily dissociate and bind to other AT molecules, thus providing a continuous anticoagulant effect. The active pentasaccharide sequence (e.g., high-affinity-material) responsible for catalyzing AT is more prevalent in the chains of UFH than LMWH, and only 30–50% of the UFH- and < 20% of the LMWH molecules contain the specific and active pentasaccharide sequence. Fondaparinux is a fully synthetic analog of the naturally occurring pentasaccharide found in heparins, which selectively and irreversibly binds to AT [1, 8, 13, 14]. This results in neutralization of factor Xa, which ultimately inhibits thrombin formation and thrombus development.

Unfractionated heparin is administered either intravenously (IV) or subcutaneously. As with other medications, intravenously administered UFH achieves therapeutic plasma concentrations and its clinical effect more quickly compared to subcutaneous administration. Owing to its low bioavailability, subcutaneous UFH needs to be dosed more generously (>30,000 U/day) to reach a clinically effect. Intravenously administered heparin can be effectively monitored and adjusted based on infusion rates. To monitor the antiocoagulant effect of UFH, the activated partial thromboplastin time (aPTT) or the anti-factor Xa essay (range 0.3–0.7 IU/mL) is being utilized [15].

The clearance of UFH from the systemic circulation is dose-dependent and follows two independent mechanisms. The initial clearance is rapid and depends on saturable binding of UFH to endothelial cells, macrophages, and local proteins where UFH undergoes depolymerization. The second phase depends on renal-mediated clearance, is non-saturable, and results in non-linear UFH pharmacokinetics with anticoagulation increasing disproportionally at high therapeutic doses. At clinically effective doses, UFH is primarily cleared via depolymerization. However, if clearance becomes dependent on the kidney function and especially if the renal function is impaired, prolonged administration of UFH results in a disproportionate increase in both the intensity and the duration of the anticoagulant effect. In patients with moderate (CrCl 30–50 mL/min) to severe renal dysfunction (CrCl < 30 mL/min), over-anticoagulation occurs once saturation of reticuloendothelial clearance is reached. Hospital-specific weight-based dosing nomograms are useful to streamline the administration of UFH and have been associated with shorter time to therapeutic UFH levels and no increase in bleeding events. Major complications of UFH therapy include bleeding and heparin-induced thrombocytopenia (HIT) [16–18]. Heparin-induced thrombocytopenia (HIT) is a prothrombotic disorder caused by antibodies to complexes of platelet factor 4 (PF4) and heparin. Diagnostic tests for HIT consist of the platelet count (decrease of > 50% from baseline), immunoassays, and functional assays. Immunoassays identify antibodies against heparin/platelet factor 4 (PF4) complexes and use an enzyme-linked immunosorbent assay (ELISA). Functional assays such as the serotonin release essay measure the platelet-activating capacity of PF4/heparin-antibody complexes. While functional assays have greater specificity than immunoassays, they are also time-consuming and not as widely available.

Intracranial, intraspinal, intraocular, mediastinal, or retroperitoneal bleeding is typically classified as major bleeding and usually results in hospitalization, transfusion, possible organ failure, and death [19–21]. Risk factors for major bleeding during anticoagulation with UFH include the intensity of the anticoagulant effect, increased age, female sex, history of gastrointestinal bleeding, concomitant use of other anticoagulants, and duration of therapy [1]. Patients receiving long-term heparin therapy are also at increased risk to suffer from osteoporosis and may be prone to vertebral fractures [22].

Perioperative anticoagulation management is procedure-dependent and informed by the patient's risk factors for bleeding and thrombosis. Evidence-based guidelines for the

Table 14.1 Pre- and postoperative recommendations for regional anesthesia in the patient receiving antithrombotic or thrombolytic therapy as recommended by the American Society of Regional Anesthesia and Pain Medicine Evidence-Based Guidelines (Third Edition) [35]

Preoperative
• Discontinue warfarin at least 5d before elective procedure
• Assess INR to 2d before surgery, if > 1.5, consider 1–2 mg of oral vitamin K
• Reversal for urgent surgery/procedure, consider 2.5–5 mg of oral or intravenous vitamin K; for immediate reversal, consider fresh-frozen plasma
• Patients at high risk for thromboembolism
o Bridge with therapeutic subcutaneous LMWH (preferred) or intravenous UFH
o Last dose of preoperative LMWH administered 24 h before surgery, administer half of the daily dose
o Intravenous heparin discontinued 4 h before surgery
• No bridging necessary for patients at low risk for thromboembolism
Postoperative
• Patients at low risk for thromboembolism
o Resume warfarin on postoperative day
• Patients at high risk for thromboembolism (who received preoperative bridging therapy)
o Minor surgical procedures – resume therapeutic LMWH 24 h postoperatively
o Major surgical procedures – resume therapeutic LMWH 48–72 h postoperatively or administer low-dose LMWH
• Assess bleeding risk and adequacy of hemostasis when considering timing of the resumption of LMWH or UFH therapy
Recommendations from Douketis et al. [12]
• Not all invasive procedures/surgeries require normalization of the INR

INR International normalized ratio, *LMWH* Low-molecular-weight heparain, *UFH* Unfractionated heparin

perioperative management of antithrombotic therapy contain specific recommendations. Bridging therapy is recommended in patients at moderate to high risk of thromboembolism (e.g., the prevention of thromboembolism outweighs the potential for increased surgical bleeding) [2]. For patients at low risk for thromboembolism, no bridging therapy is recommended. Preoperatively, UFH is routinely halted for 4 h prior to the surgical procedure, and the effect is monitored with a normalization of the aPTT. Postoperatively, therapeutic UFH is restarted after about 12 h but will be delayed if surgical bleeding continues. One key advantage of UFH anticoagulation is that its effect may be rapidly reversed with protamine. Each mg of protamine can neutralize 100 U of heparin. Importantly, protamine is associated with development of a number of adverse effects, ranging from life-threatening anaphylactic complications in 0.16% of patients to minor reactions associated with systemic hypotension in 13% of patients. Risk factors for adverse protamine reactions include fish allergy, vasectomy, and prior exposure to protamine (e.g., use of NPH insulin) [11, 23–25]. The incidence and severity of the reaction to protamine may depend on the rate of administration (maximum recommended administration rate is 5 mg/min). Patients with risk factors for adverse protamine reaction should be given protamine with a slow rate of administration under close monitoring. Pre-treatment with corticosteroids and antihistamines can be considered [19]. A history of prior anaphylaxis to protamine should prompt careful consideration for risks, benefits, and alternatives to heparin administration.

Evidence-based guidelines help to provide safe regional anesthesia in patients receiving antithrombotic or thrombolytic therapy [26]. As long as patients receive only low-dose UFH subcutaneously, there is no contraindication for neuraxial techniques. However, in the patient that is receiving intraoperative (and possibly high-dose) anticoagulation with UFH, therapy should be started at least one hour after the neuraxial needle placement. The removal of indwelling catheters such as epidural catheters should not be performed unless the UFH therapy has been halted for at least 2–4 h and not without demonstration of an effect on the coagulation (see Table 14.1).

Low molecular weight heparin or UFH is routinely administered as high-dose (therapeutic), intermediate dose, and low-dose (prophylactic). Prophylactic-dose LMWH is commonly prescribed to prevent venous thromboembolism (VTE) but is not sufficient in the prevention of arterial thromboembolism (e.g., stroke in atrial fibrillation). Due to the homogeneity of the polysaccharide chains, LMWHs have a superior pharmacodynamic and pharmacokinetic profile in comparison to UFHs. Other advantages of LMWH include the convenience of its fixed daily dosing regimens (once or twice), the fact that routine monitoring is not required and its track record of safety and efficacy in practice. The renal clearance for LMWH is dose-independent and the half-life is longer than for UFH (17–21 h). Anti-Xa testing is optional in high-risk patients (renal insufficiency, pregnancy, non-compliance) and its interpretation is product specific.

When administered subcutaneously, fondaparinux undergoes rapid and complete absorption, exhibits a half-life of 17–21 h, and is excreted primarily unchanged in the urine in patients with normal renal function. Similar to LMWH and UHF, fondaparinux has been proven to be safe and effective as treatment of DVT and pulmonary embolism (PE). When studied in clinical trials, fondaparinux demonstrates superior efficacy in reducing VTE in various orthopedic surgeries but its incidence of major bleeding is higher compared with LMWH. Of note, the timing of fondaparinux administration has been shown to be associated with its efficacy and outcomes and the incidence of major bleeding. Fondaparinux currently does not have Food and Drug Administration (FDA) approval for acute coronary syndromes.

Protamine only partially reverses the anti-Xa activity of LMWH and has no effect on the anti-Xa activity of fondaparinux. In the absence of specific reversal agents, recombinant factor VIIa has been used off-label for reversal of LMWH and fondaparinux in cases of severe bleeding not responsive to supportive measures; the safety and efficacy of this practice have not been well studied. Ciraparantag, a small synthetic cationic molecule currently being studied as a "universal" reversal agent, shows some promise as a reversal agent for LMWH and fondaparinux as well as the non-vitamin K oral anticoagulants.

14.2 Direct Thrombin Inhibitors (DTIs)

The direct thrombin inhibitors lepirudin and hirudin are naturally occurring anticoagulants derived from the salivary glands of the medicinal leech and have demonstrated efficacy in models of thrombosis [9, 22]. The synthetic analogs of hirudin, bivalirudin, and desirudin exert their anticoagulant activity by direct, selective, and reversible binding to the active catalytic site and the anion binding site of thrombin, which antagonizes the recognition and binding of fibrinogen at the anion binding exosite 1 of thrombin. Argatroban, which is derived from the amino acid arginine, is another smaller synthetic thrombin inhibitor, which also binds reversibly but non-covalently to an active thrombin site. The currently available DTIs vary significantly in regards to their pharmacologic profiles. Bivalirudin possesses a predictable, dose-dependent anticoagulant activity, has the shortest half-life, and, therefore, is the most suitable agent in the perioperative space. Patient specific factors (age, cardiovascular function, and hepatic or renal dysfunction) dictate the choice of DTIs. Comorbidities and organ dysfunction in critically ill patients typically dictate lower infusion rates. Standard monitoring of DTI administration follows the aPTT, with a goal of 1.5–2.5 times control (bivalirudin) and 1.5–3 times control (argatroban) while desirudin does not require routine monitoring. As an alternative to aPTT levels and because of inconsistencies in aPTT measurements, the plasma diluted thrombin time can be considered [27, 28]. While there is no direct reversal agent for these parenterally administered DTIs, their short and relatively predictable half-lives should allow for restoration of native coagulation function soon after cessation of therapy, until which point supportive measures should be maintained.

14.3 Oral Antiplatelet Treatments

Platelets are essential to hemostasis and to the development of a pathological thrombus. In a multifactorial process, initial disruption of the endothelium exposes platelets to the adhesive proteins of the subendothelial matrix. Interactions between the matrix proteins and platelet-receptor glycoproteins enable platelet adhesion and subsequent activation of intracellular signaling pathways that trigger the release of activators such as ADP, serotonin, adrenaline, thrombin, and thromboxane A2. Via G-protein-coupled receptors, these agonists potentiate each other's actions. Ultimately, the glycoprotein IIb/IIIa complexes on platelets bind to fibrinogen, a process that results in platelet aggregation and can culminate in thrombus formation (Fig. 14.2). In summary, there are multiple steps involved in the adhesion, activation, and aggregation of platelets and more recently developed antiplatelet drugs either target platelet-activating factors or associated receptors.

14.3.1 Aspirin

Aspirin (acetylsalicylic acid) is the most commonly prescribed antiplatelet drug for prevention of cardiovascular disorders [7, 29]. While low doses of aspirin selectively inhibit cyclooxygenase (COX)-1, resulting in its antiplatelet effects, higher doses of aspirin inhibit both COX-1 and COX-2 leading to anti-inflammatory and analgesic effects [30].

Aspirin prevents the access of arachidonic acid to its receptor and inhibits production of thromboxane A2 by acetylating a serine residue near the narrow catalytic site of the COX-1 channel.

Repeated low doses of aspirin result in permanent and irreversible thromboxane A2 inhibition throughout the 7–10 day lifetime of anucleated platelets. This is why aspirin can be administered once daily and still remains effective

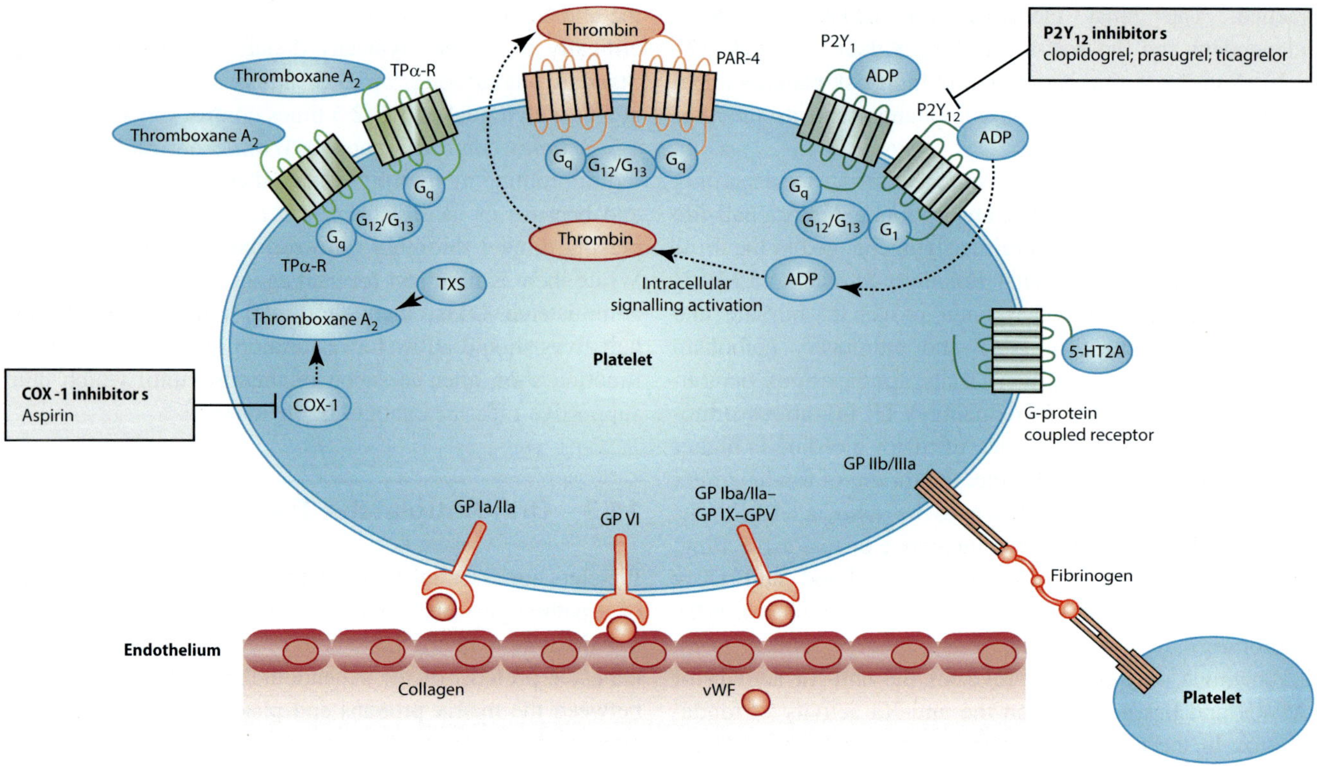

Fig. 14.2 Platelet pathways and commonly used oral antiplatelet treatments such as COX-1 inhibitors, $P2Y_{12}$ inhibitors, and others. Following the disruption of the endothelium, adhesive proteins of the subendothelial matrix (collagen and von Willebrand factor [vWF]) are being exposed. These proteins then interact with platelet-receptor glycoproteins (GP). Intracellular signaling activation results in the release of platelet activators such as ADP, adrenaline, serotonin, thrombin, and thromboxane A2. These agonists bind to G-protein-coupled receptors and further potentiate the process. Ultimately, GP IIb/IIIa binds to fibrinogen and results in platelet aggregation. 5-HT2A = serotonin receptor 2A. COX-1 = cyclooxygenase 1. PAR = protease-activated receptor. TP-R = thromboxane prostanoid receptor. TXS = thromboxane A2 synthase. G = G-protein. Dotted arrows show movement of molecules. Adapted from Franchi and Angiolillo, [4] by permission of Nature Reviews Cardiology [10]

despite its very short half-life (15–20 min). Of note, aspirin also exerts other relevant (indirect) properties such as the reduction of inflammatory cytokines, oxygen radicals, and growth factors relevant.

Absorption of aspirin is rapid and mediated by passive diffusion through gastrointestinal membranes. Single or repeated oral administration of aspirin results in systemic bioavailability of about 45–50% but the enteric-coated formulation has a much lower bioavailability. With regular aspirin, peak plasma concentrations of aspirin are reached within 30 min after ingestion but up to 4 h after ingestion of the enteric-coated formulation. In patients with acute coronary syndrome (ACS), rapid inhibition of thromboxane A2 can be achieved with a recommended dose of 150–325 mg of aspirin. There appears to be no evidence that patients with ACS benefit from higher versus lower doses of oral aspirin, but lower doses (81–100 mg) have been shown to result in relatively less bleeding than higher doses of aspirin. Alternatively, lower doses of aspirin can also be given intravenously.

The return of platelet function after aspirin administration is related to the natural turnover of platelets. Assuming a daily generation of 10–12% new platelets from megakaryocytes, near normal hemostasis can be seen within 2–3 days after the last aspirin dose in patients with a typical rate of platelet turnover. Variability in inhibition of platelet thromboxane A2 often termed as "aspirin resistance" can be seen in proinflammatory settings (such as in patients with ACS or diabetes) that promote a faster rate of platelet turnover and platelet hyper-reactivity [31].

14.3.2 P2Y12 Receptor Antagonists

Dual antiplatelet therapy with aspirin and a P2Y12 receptor antagonist such as clopidogrel is considered as standard treatment of patients with ACS and those undergoing coronary interventions with placement of intracoronary stents [4, 10, 32]. Although the first generation P2Y12 receptor antagonist ticlopidine proved to reduce the risk of stent

Table 14.2 Properties of oral $P2Y_{12}$ inhibitors

	Prasugel	Ticagrelor	Clopidogrel
Drug class	Thienopyrindine	Cyclopentyl-triazolopyrimidine	Thienopyrindine
P2Y12 receptor blockade	Irreversible	Reversible	Irreversible
Prodrug	Yes	No	Yes
Onset of action	30 min–4 h	30 min–4 h	2–8 h
Offset of action	7–10 days	3 – 5 days	7–10 days
Percentage of active metabolite	85%	90 – 100%	15%
Interactions with CYP-targeted drugs	No	CYP3A4 or CYP3A5	CYP2C19
Elimination	Urine (68%) Feces (27%)	Urine (~ 30%) Feces (~ 60%)	Urine (60%) Feces (40%)

CYP CYtochrome P450

thrombosis compared with standard treatments, it was soon replaced with clopidogrel, which had fewer hematological side effects. Common to all PSY12 receptor antagonists is that they either irreversibly (clopidogrel and prasugrel) or reversibly (ticagrelor) block the binding of adenosine diphosphate (ADP) to a specific platelet-receptor P2Y12, which consequently inhibits the activation of the glycoprotein (GP) IIb/IIIa complex and platelet aggregation. Improved understanding of the P2Y12 receptor and the pharmacology of antiplatelet drugs resulted in the production of prasugrel and ticagrelor. Compared to clopidogrel, both prasugrel and ticagrelor have faster onset of action and are associated with reduced interpatient variability in platelet inhibition (See Table 14.2). Although the reasons for the significant interpatient variability associated with clopidogrel are likely multifactorial, they include drug, environmental, and genetic interactions, in addition to clinical factors such as diabetes and obesity.

While the thienopyridines clopidogrel and prasugrel represent prodrugs that need biotransformation involving CYP450 to become active, they also irreversibly inhibit the P2Y12 receptor. After absorption, 85% of clopidogrel is hydrolyzed by esterases into an inactive carboxylic acid. By contrast, ticagrelor is the first clinically available oral cyclopentyltriazolopyrimidine, which represents an active drug with a simpler metabolism that leads to the formation of an active metabolite. As a consequence, ticagrelor results in faster inhibition of platelet function than the two other compounds. Unlike the thienopyridines, it reversibly binds to a separate site of the P2Y12 receptor and it inhibits G-protein activation and signaling without binding to the ADP-binding site.

For clopidogrel, the recommended loading dose is 600 mg and maintenance dose is 75 mg. The loading dose achieves an onset of antiplatelet action within 2 h and it is necessary because it takes 5–7 days to achieve a steady state inhibition of platelet function with maintenance dosing. The onset of prasugrel antiplatelet action is reported at 30 min after a loading dose of 60 mg for prasugrel (maintenance dose 10 mg). Both drugs have a similarly slow offset of action of 7–10 days. The recommended loading and maintenance doses of ticagrelor are 180 mg once and 90 mg twice per day. Ticagrelor's onset of action is reported at 30 min after dosing, its peak effect is observed after about 2 h and it appears to reach its steady state after 2–3 days.

Of note, the different mechanism of action of the P2Y12 receptor antagonists also affects the approach to treatment for patients who are bleeding. While circulating ticagrelor and its metabolite are likely to inhibit transfused platelets, studies have shown that the effects of aspirin and the thienopyridines can be offset with platelet transfusions.

14.4 Oral Anticoagulant Treatments

Since the concept of the coagulation cascade was initially introduced in 1964, there have been numerous revisions and refinements. The key elements of the so-called extrinsic pathway involve the release of tissue factor from trauma or vascular injury. In the presence of calcium, tissue factor forms a complex with factor VIIa and cleaves clotting factors X and IX to their active forms (factors Xa and IXa). The intrinsic pathway is based on contact activation where factor IXa binds to factor VIIIa and forms intrinsic tenase, which activates factor X. The interaction of factor Xa with factor Va results in the formation of prothrombinase, which converts factor II to IIa (thrombin). Factor IIa further amplifies the coagulation system, converts soluble fibrinogen to insoluble fibrin, and also activates platelets.

14.4.1 Vitamin K Antagonists

Vitamin K-dependent antagonists (VKAs) such as warfarin and phenprocoumon are synthetic analoges of the naturally occurring dicumarol [1, 10]. They produce their anticoagulant effect by inhibiting the vitamin K-dependent carboxylation of factors II, VII, IX, and X. Warfarin has a mean plasma half-life of 40 h and reaches its full anticoagulant effects 48–72 h after administration. Inactivation and metabolism of this drug occur via cytochrome P450 enzymes (CYP2C9, CYP1A2, and CYP3A4). However, dose and effects of warfarin have been shown to vary greatly among patients. Besides a number of patient-specific factors such as diet, drug interactions, and underlying disease states, there are genetic variations (polymorphisms) in the proteins CYP2C9 and VKORC1, which influence the primary metabolism and pharmacodynamics of warfarin and place patients at increased risk of bleeding. Based on this information, the FDA has recommended clinicians to consider a patient's genotype, before prescription of warfarin. In fact, despite more than 60 years of clinical experience with VKAs, bleeding complications with warfarin remain as one of the most significant causes of severe adverse drug events. To achieve a therapeutic international normalized ratio (INR), a wide dosing range of warfarin is often required and due to the narrow therapeutic index, frequent routine blood testing is required. Absolute contra-indications of VKAs include liver failure, history of intracranial hemorrhage, active bleeding, and dementia.

Withholding therapy alone in the absence of a reversal agent takes several days until an effect is seen. In patients with severe bleeding complications or patients who need emergency surgery, acute reversal of anticoagulant effects of warfarin is required. Vitamin K can be given orally or parenterally, but its efficacy depends on adequate hepatic synthetic function. Parenteral administration of vitamin K achieves correction of INR within 6–8 h, compared to after 24 h for oral administration. Vitamin K-dependent factors can be replenished through administration of fresh frozen plasma (FFP) or prothrombin complex concentrates (PCCs). Four-factor (4F) PCCs, which contain factors II, VII, IX, and X as well as proteins C and S, were developed and approved as a reversal agent for warfarin. While FFP was formerly the standard of care, a recent meta-analysis showed mortality benefit to using PCCs over FFP for reversal of VKA in major bleeding, as well as more rapid correction of INR and less volume overload. Current American College of Cardiology guidelines for reversal of VKA-associated bleeding recommend administration of vitamin K 5–10 mg IV over 30 min, along with 4F-PCCs. Dosing strategies for 4F-PCCs can be based on INR (25 units/kg for INR 2 to < 4, 35 units/kg for INR 4–6, 50 units/kg for INR > 6) or fixed dose (1500 units for intracranial hemorrhage, 1000 units for any other major bleed). If 4F-PCCs are unavailable, FFP can be administered at a dose of 10–15 ml/kg.

14.4.2 Non-VKA Anticoagulants

In light of the narrow therapeutic index of VKAs, their multiple interactions, and the need for (invasive) blood monitoring of patients, an intense search for new anticoagulants with more predictable pharmacological effects has resulted in the availability of numerous alternatives to warfarin [1, 20]. These non-VKA oral anticoagulants (NOACs), also known as direct-acting oral anticoagulants (DOACs), directly target factor IIa (dabigatran) or Xa (rivaroxaban, apixaban, and edoxaban). Compared to warfarin, NOACs have faster onset and offset of action and do not require routine blood tests. The comparatively short half-life of NOACs versus warfarin is advantageous when the unwanted side effect of bleeding is considered. Additionally, within the past decade, specific reversal agents for dabigatran and the factor Xa inhibitors have been developed and approved in the United States and Europe. As such, NOACs are increasingly used for the prevention and treatment of VTE and for stroke prevention in patients with non-valvular (i.e., not due to moderate-to-severe mitral stenosis or in the presence of a mechanical heart valve) atrial fibrillation. In fact, the most recent American College of Cardiology / American Heart Association guidelines now recommend the use of NOACs over warfarin for stroke prevention in patients with non-valvular atrial fibrillation, with the exception of patients with end-stage renal disease or on dialysis. This was based on the results of multiple randomized controlled trials showing at least noninferiority of NOACs compared to warfarin in stroke prevention, along with a superior safety profile of NOACs over warfarin with respect to bleeding risk.

Dabigatran selectively inhibits thrombin (factor IIa) similar to other already established injectable direct thrombin inhibitors (DTIs) such as recombinant hirudin, bivalirudine, and argatroban. Dabigatran contains a prodrug, has a half-life of 12–17 h, has by far the lowest bioavailability of present NOACs (3–7%), and is to 80% cleared by the kidneys. Therefore, renal function should be monitored regularly in patients taking dabigatran and most of the other NOACs. Given that renal clearance varies greatly amongst NOACs, every NOAC comes with specific dose adjustment recommendations based on renal function. Because NOACs have not been widely studied in patients with more severe disease or those on dialysis, they are generally avoided in patients on dialysis.

Rivaroxaban exhibits its anticoagulant effect by direct, selective, and reversible inhibition of factor Xa. Rivaroxaban does not contain a prodrug, has a half-life of 5–13 h, has the highest bioavailability of present NOACs (66% and ~ 100% with food) and is to 66% cleared by the kidneys. Similar to rivaroxaban, apixaban exhibits its anticoagulant effect by direct and reversible inhibition of factor Xa. Apixaban does not contain a prodrug, has a half-life of 9–14 h, has a bioavailability 50% and is to 27% cleared by the kidneys.

Although the NOACs have generally fewer interactions with other medications than warfarin, there are a number of contraindicated medications and some that make a dose-reduction of NOACs necessary. Currently, none of the NOACs are FDA-approved for patients with valvular disease. For instance, a randomized trial of dabigatran compared with warfarin in patients with mechanical heart valves demonstrated an increase in both bleeding and ischemic events among patients on dabigatran.

While routine monitoring of patients receiving NOACs is not required, there are circumstances in which measurements of the anticoagulant effect are reasonable. For factor Xa inhibitors, the prothrombin time (PT) can be used to make a qualitative assessment as it is prolonged in a dose-dependent manner, though it is not sufficiently sensitive to exclude therapeutic drug levels if normal. Anti-Xa activity assays provide the best measurement of therapeutic effect, especially when calibrated with drug-specific standards. In the case of dabigatran, therapeutic effect is best measured by dilute thrombin time and ecarin-based assays, though these tests are not widely available. Thrombin time is extremely sensitive to dabigatran, and a normal value essentially rules out therapeutic levels. While activated partial thromboplastin time (aPTT) can be prolonged in the presence of dabigatran, neither aPTT nor PT is sensitive enough to provide quantitative assessment of drug effect. Valid absolute and relative contra-indications of NOACs include the following: life failure, history of intracranial hemorrhage, active bleeding, renal failure (CrCl < 15 ml/min), and mechanical heart valves.

For bleeding complications in patients taking NOACs, supportive care measures should be instituted including discontinuation of anticoagulation, local hemostasis if possible, and volume resuscitation and/or blood transfusion as indicated [33, 34]. Activated charcoal can be given if NOAC has been recently ingested (within 2–4 h) in order to prevent drug absorption. If rapid reversal of anticoagulant effect is required, a number of reversal options are now available. Idarucizumab is approved in the United States and Europe for reversal of dabigatran in patients with severe or life-threatening bleeding or need for emergency surgery. It is a monoclonal antibody fragment with high affinity for dabigatran (350 times the affinity of thrombin, in fact) that is able to sequester and reverse the anticoagulant effect of dabigatran within minutes when given as a fixed dose of 5 g. Dabigatran can also be removed via hemodialysis. Andexanet alfa is currently approved in the United States for reversal of rivaroxaban and apixaban in patients with severe or life-threatening bleeding; studies on its use for reversal of other factor Xa inhibitors and for patients undergoing emergency surgery are ongoing. It is a recombinant human factor Xa protein that acts as a decoy for the drug, binding it with high affinity to allow native factor Xa to participate in the coagulation cascade. Its availability remains limited at the present time. In situations where these specific reversal agents are not available for use, 4F-PCCs may be used off-label in an attempt to "bypass" the factor Xa inhibitors by overloading the coagulation cascade with upstream factors. The evidence for use of 4F-PCCs is limited, and optimal dosing has not been established. Based on the available data, the most recent American College of Cardiology guidelines suggests an initial intravenous dose of 50 units/kg.

Questions

1. Which of the following anticoagulants contains the highest number of pentasaccharide sequences responsible for catalyzing antithrombin to inactivate several coagulation factors?

A) Coumadin
B) Unfractionated heparin (UFH)
C) Low molecular weight heparin (LMWH)
D) Desirudin

Correct answer: B

The active pentasaccharide sequence (e.g., high-affinity-material) responsible for catalyzing antithrombin is most prevalent in the chains of unfractionated heparin (UFH) than low molecular weight heparin (LMWH) and only 30–50% of the UFH- and <20% of the LMWH molecules contain the specific and active pentasaccharide sequence.

2. Which of the following four antiplatelet drugs represents an active drug, is orally available, and reversibly binds to a separate site of the P2Y12 receptor?

A) Clopidogrel
B) Prasugrel
C) Ticagrelor
D) Aspirin

Correct answer: C

Ticagrelor is the first clinically available oral cyclopentyltriazolopyrimidine. Ticagrelor is an active drug and results in faster inhibition of platelet function than clopidogrel and prasugrel. Unlike the thienopyridines, it reversibly binds to a separate site of the P2Y12 receptor and it inhibits G-protein activation and signaling without binding to the ADP-binding site. The thienopyridines clopidogrel and prasugrel represent prodrugs that need biotransformation involving CYP450 to become active and they irreversibly inhibit the P2Y12 receptor.

3. Which statement about the so-called extrinsic pathway of the coagulation cascade most accurately describes its key components?
A) Contact activation activates factor IXa that binds to factor VIIIa and forms intrinsic tenase, which then activates factor X.
B) In the presence of calcium, tissue factor forms a complex with factor VIIa and cleaves clotting factors X and IX to their active forms (factors Xa and IXa).
C) Factor IIa and factor Xa convert soluble fibrinogen to insoluble fibrin and also activate platelets.
D) The interaction of factor Xa with factor Va results in the formation of prothrombinase, which converts factor II to IIa.

Correct answer: B
The key elements of the so-called extrinsic pathway involve the release of tissue factor from trauma or vascular injury. In the presence of calcium, tissue factor forms a complex with factor VIIa and cleaves clotting factors X and IX to their active forms (factors Xa and IXa).

4. Which of the following patient scenarios would be best suited to receive a non-VKA oral anticoagulants (NOACs)?
A) Patient with persistent atrial fibrillation who will require frequent lung biopsies, necessitating discontinuation of anticoagulation
B) Patient with prior stroke and atrial fibrillation, and undergoing surgery with spinal anesthesia
C) Patient with prior stroke, atrial fibrillation, and mechanical heart valves, with labile international normalized ratio (INR)
D) Patient with paroxysmal atrial fibrillation and structurally normal heart, with labile INR

Correct answer: D
While NOACs have several attractive features, such as minimal interaction with medications and foods and no need for blood work to monitor the required dose, they also have several important limitations. Currently, none of the NOAC medications are FDA-approved for patients with valvular disease. For instance, a randomized trial of dabigatran compared with warfarin in patients with mechanical heart valves demonstrated an increase in both bleeding and ischemic events among patients on dabigatran. The only approved oral anticoagulant for patients with mechanical heart valves is warfarin. All three FDA-approved NOAC medications carry a black-box warning to avoid discontinuation in the absence of adequate alternative anticoagulation, owing to a risk for rebound hypercoagulability and stroke. In addition, they should not be used in patients receiving spinal anesthesia.

5. Which option describes the most appropriate combination of measures to reverse the anticoagulant effects of warfarin?
A) Acute reversal of the anticoagulant effects can be achieved with intravenous administration of Vitamin K alone.
B) Acute reversal of the anticoagulant effects of warfarin can be best achieved by administration of vitamin K and prothrombin complex concentrate (PCC).
C) Acute reversal of the anticoagulant effects of warfarin can be best achieved by administration of protamine.
D) Acute reversal of the anticoagulant effects of warfarin can be best achieved by administration of fresh frozen plasma (FFP).

Correct answer: B
Acute reversal of anticoagulant effects of warfarin (in patients with acute bleeding or in surgical patients) can best be achieved by administration of vitamin K and prothrombin complex concentrate (PCC). IV vitamin K achieves reversal of anticoagulant effect in 6-8 hours in patients with normal hepatic synthetic function, while PCC allows for immediate replacement of the vitamin K-dependent factors (II, VII, IX, and X and proteins C and S).

6. How many days after the last aspirin dose in patients with a typical rate of platelet turnover can you expect near normal hemostasis?
A) After 1 day
B) Within 4–5 days
C) Within 9–10 days
D) Within 2–3 days

Correct answer: D
The return of platelet function after aspirin administration is related to the natural turnover of platelets. Assuming a daily generation of 10–12% new platelets from megakaryocytes, near normal hemostasis can be seen within 2–3 days after the last aspirin dose in patients with a typical rate of platelet turnover.

7. Of the currently available direct thrombin inhibitors, which provides the most predictable, dose-dependent anticoagulant activity and has the shortest half-life making it the most suitable agent in the perioperative space?
A) Argatroban
B) Bivalirudin
C) Desirudin
D) Lepirudin

Correct answer: B

The currently available DTIs vary significantly in regard to their pharmacologic profiles. Bivalirudin possesses a predictable, dose-dependent anticoagulant activity, has the shortest half-life, and therefore is the most suitable agent in the perioperative space.

8. Which of the following statements in regard to the heparin-induced thrombocytopenia (HIT) are correct?
A) Heparin-induced thrombocytopenia (HIT) is a pro-thrombotic disorder caused by antibodies to complexes of platelet factor 4 (PF4) and heparin.
B) Functional HIT assays such as the serotonin release essay measure the platelet-activating capacity of PF4/heparin-antibody complexes.
C) All heparin administration should be immediately stopped if the diagnosis of HIT is made and an alternative anticoagulant should be started.
D) All of the above

Correct answer: D

All of the statements are correctly describing the pathophysiology, diagnosis, and treatment in cases of HIT.

9. From the list below, please select the anticoagulant or antiplatelet drug that has a direct antidote?
A) Edoxaban
B) Unfractionated heparin
C) Bivalirudin
D) All of the above

Correct answer: B

Unfractionated heparin is the only medication listed that may be rapidly reversed by an antidote. One mg of protamine can neutralize 100 U of heparin. Currently, specific antidotes to direct thrombin inhibitors (bivalirudin) are not available, and the reversal agent andexanet alfa is approved for the factor Xa inhibitors rivaroxaban and apixaban only.

10. Please select valid absolute and relative contra-indications of a non-VKA oral anticoagulants (NOACs) from the following:
A) History of intracranial hemorrhage
B) Renal failure (creatine clearance < 15 ml/min)
C) Mechanical heart valve
D) All of the above

Correct answer: D

Valid absolute and relative contra-indications of NOACs include the following: life failure, history of intracranial hemorrhage, active bleeding, renal failure (CrCl < 15 ml/min), and mechanical heart valves.

References

1. Alquwaizani M, Buckley L, Adams C, Fanikos J. Anticoagulants: A Review of the Pharmacology, Dosing, and Complications. Curr Emerg Hosp Med Rep. 2013;1(2):83–97.
2. Douketis JD, Berger PB, Dunn AS, Jaffer AK, Spyropoulos AC, Becker RC, et al. The perioperative management of antithrombotic therapy: American college of chest physicians evidence-based clinical practice guidelines (8th Edition). Chest. 2008;133 (6):299S-339S.
3. Eriksson BI, Lassen MR. Investigators PEiH-FSP Duration of prophylaxis against venous thromboembolism with fondaparinux after hip fracture surgery: a multicenter, randomized, placebo-controlled, double-blind study. Arch Intern Med. 2003;163(11): 1337–42.
4. Franchi F, Angiolillo DJ. Novel antiplatelet agents in acute coronary syndrome. Nat Rev Cardiol. 2015;12(1):30–47.
5. Hughes S, Szeki I, Nash MJ, Thachil J. Anticoagulation in chronic kidney disease patients-the practical aspects. Clin Kidney J. 2014; 7(5):442–9.
6. January CT, Wann LS, Calkins H, Chen LY, Cigarroa JE, Cleveland JC Jr, et al. 2019 AHA/ACC/HRS Focused Update of the 2014 AHA/ACC/HRS guideline for the management of patients with atrial fibrillation: a report of the american college of cardiology/American Heart association task force on clinical practice guidelines and the heart rhythm society in collaboration with the society of thoracic surgeons. Circulation. 2019;140(2): e125–51.
7. Awtry EH, Loscalzo J. Aspirin. Circulation. 2000;101(10):1206–18.
8. Buller HR, Davidson BL, Decousus H, Gallus A, Gent M, Piovella F, et al. Fondaparinux or enoxaparin for the initial treatment of symptomatic deep venous thrombosis: a randomized trial. Ann Intern Med. 2004;140(11):867–73.
9. Di Nisio M, Middeldorp S, Buller HR. Direct thrombin inhibitors. N Engl J Med. 2005;353(10):1028–40.
10. Mega JL, Simon T. Pharmacology of antithrombotic drugs: an assessment of oral antiplatelet and anticoagulant treatments. Lancet. 2015;386(9990):281–91.
11. Bussey HFJ. Heparin consensus group. Heparin overview and issues. Pharmacotherapy. 2004;24:103S-S107.

12. Weitz DS, Weitz JI. Update on heparin: what do we need to know? J Thromb Thrombolysis. 2010;29(2):199–207.
13. Buller HR, Davidson BL, Decousus H, Gallus A, Gent M, Piovella F, et al. Subcutaneous fondaparinux versus intravenous unfractionated heparin in the initial treatment of pulmonary embolism. N Engl J Med. 2003;349(18):1695–702.
14. Turpie AGGBK, Eriksson BI, et al. Fondaparinux vs enoxaparin for the prevention of venous thromboembolism in major orthopedic surgery. A meta-analysis of 4 randomized double-blind studies. Arch Intern Med. 2001;162:1833–40.
15. Lehman CMFE. Laboratory monitoring of heparin therapy: partial thromboplastin time or Anti-Xa assay? LabMedicine. 2009;40 (1):47.
16. Cuker A, Arepally GM, Chong BH, Cines DB, Greinacher A, Gruel Y, et al. American Society of Hematology 2018 guidelines for management of venous thromboembolism: heparin-induced thrombocytopenia. Blood Adv. 2018;2(22):3360–92.
17. Greinacher A, Potzsch B, Amiral J, Dummel V, Eichner A, Mueller-Eckhardt C. Heparin-associated thrombocytopenia: isolation of the antibody and characterization of a multimolecular PF4-heparin complex as the major antigen. Thromb Haemost. 1994;71(2):247–51.
18. Selleng K, Warkentin TE, Greinacher A. Heparin-induced thrombocytopenia in intensive care patients. Crit Care Med. 2007;35 (4):1165–76.
19. Kambam J, Meszaros R, Merrill W, Stewart J, Smith BE, Bender H. Prophylactic administration of histamine1 and histamine2 receptor blockers in the prevention of protamine-related haemodynamic effects. Can J Anaesth. 1990;37(4 Pt 1):420–2.
20. Milling TJ Jr, Ziebell CM. A review of oral anticoagulants, old and new, in major bleeding and the need for urgent surgery. Trends Cardiovasc Med. 2020;30(2):86–90.
21. Piran S, Schulman S. Treatment of bleeding complications in patients on anticoagulant therapy. Blood. 2019;133(5):425–35.
22. Garcia DA, Baglin TP, Weitz JI, Samama MM. American College of Chest P. parenteral anticoagulants: antithrombotic therapy and prevention of thrombosis, American college of chest physicians evidence-based clinical practice guidelines. Chest. 2012;141 (2):24S-43S.
23. Carr JA, Silverman N. The heparin-protamine interaction. A review J Cardiovasc Surg (Torino). 1999;40(5):659–66.
24. Levy JH, Zaidan JR, Faraj B. Prospective evaluation of risk of protamine reactions in patients with NPH insulin-dependent diabetes. Anesth Analg. 1986;65(7):739–42.
25. Porsche R, Brenner ZR. Allergy to protamine sulfate. Heart Lung. 1999;28(6):418–28.
26. Horlocker TT, Wedel DJ, Rowlingson JC, Enneking FK, Kopp SL, Benzon HT, et al. Regional anesthesia in the patient receiving antithrombotic or thrombolytic therapy: American Society of Regional Anesthesia and Pain Medicine Evidence-Based Guidelines (Third Edition). Reg Anesth Pain Med. 2010;35(1):64–101.
27. Love JE, Ferrell C, Chandler WL. Monitoring direct thrombin inhibitors with a plasma diluted thrombin time. Thromb Haemost. 2007;98(1):234–42.
28. Samuelson BT, Cuker A. Measurement and reversal of the direct oral anticoagulants. Blood Rev. 2017;31(1):77–84.
29. Gurbel PA, Myat A, Kubica J, Tantry US. State of the art: Oral antiplatelet therapy. JRSM Cardiovasc Dis. 2016;5:2048004016 652514.
30. Loll PJ, Picot D, Garavito RM. The structural basis of aspirin activity inferred from the crystal structure of inactivated prostaglandin H2 synthase. Nat Struct Biol. 1995;2(8):637–43.
31. Patrono C, Rocca B. Drug insight: aspirin resistance–fact or fashion? Nat Clin Pract Cardiovasc Med. 2007;4(1):42–50.
32. Investigators C-O, Mehta SR, Bassand JP, Chrolavicius S, Diaz R, Eikelboom JW, et al. Dose comparisons of clopidogrel and aspirin in acute coronary syndromes. N Engl J Med. 2010;363(10):930–42.
33. Kaide CG, Gulseth MP. Current Strategies for the Management of Bleeding Associated with Direct Oral Anticoagulants and a Review of Investigational Reversal Agents. J Emerg Med. 2020;58(2):217–33.
34. Schulman S, Beyth RJ, Kearon C, Levine MN. American College of Chest P. Hemorrhagic complications of anticoagulant and thrombolytic treatment: American College of chest physicians evidence-based clinical practice guidelines (8th Edition). Chest. 2008;133(6):257S-98S.
35. Horlocker TT, et al. Regional anesthesia in the patient receiving antithrombotic or thrombolytic therapy: American Society of Regional Anesthesia and Pain Medicine Evidence-Based Guidelines (Third Edition). Reg Anesth Pain Med. 2010;35(1):64–101.

Perioperative Intravenous Fluid Therapy

15

Marta Kelava and Maged Argalious

Abstract

The goal of this chapter is to provide an overview of two major types of resuscitation fluids: crystalloids and colloids. This includes a discussion of types of crystalloids and indications for the use of specific types of crystalloids. In addition, an overview of commonly used colloids (albumin and hetastarches) and their side effects is included. The concept of early goal-directed fluid therapy and the literature supporting its use is also presented. Finally, the difference between static and dynamic parameters of fluid responsiveness in both mechanically ventilated and spontaneously breathing patients is discussed. In a nutshell, the chapter reviews choice of fluid resuscitation type, amount of fluid that should be given, and mechanisms to assess adequacy of fluid resuscitation.

Keywords

Fluids • Crystalloids • Colloids • Albumin • Hetastarch • Goal-directed fluid therapy • Fluid responsiveness • Perioperative

Key Points

1. Total body water comprises around 60% of the lean body mass of an adult.
2. Osmolarity takes into account the total concentration of penetrating solutes and non-penetrating solutes, while tonicity takes into account the total concentration of non-penetrating solutes only.
3. Infusion of 0.9% NaCl is accompanied by a hyperchloremic metabolic acidosis, especially if large volumes are administered.
4. Balanced crystalloid solutions avoid the hyperchloremic metabolic acidosis caused by isotonic NaCl. In addition, they reduce antidiuretic hormone (ADH) secretion, thereby reducing the typical salt and water retention that occurs.
5. Hypotonic fluids should be avoided in cases of increased intracranial pressure and in cases of traumatic brain injury for fear of worsening of cerebral edema.
6. Glucose-containing solutions should be avoided in cases of traumatic brain injury for fear of worsening of neurologic outcome.
7. In large-scale prospective trials, the volume of crystalloid resuscitation to achieve prespecified resuscitation endpoints is around 1.5 to 2 times the colloid resuscitation volume, which is much less than the crystalloid to colloid resuscitation ratio (3:1) previously recommended.
8. In patients with sepsis, the use of hetastarches is associated with an increased incidence of acute kidney injury, the need for renal replacement therapy, and an increased mortality. The use of hetastarches should be avoided in patients with sepsis and in those with underlying kidney disease.
9. Goal-directed fluid therapy aims to achieve and maintain a specific goal: an optimum cardiac output that ensures adequate delivery of oxygen to the tissues, thereby avoiding tissue hypoperfusion and the

M. Kelava
Division of Cardiothoracic and Vascular Anesthesiology, Department of Anesthesiology, Integrated Hospital-Care Institute Cleveland Clinic, Cleveland, OH, USA
e-mail: kelavam@ccf.org

M. Argalious (✉)
Division of Multispecialty Anesthesiology, Department of Anesthesiology, Integrated Hospital Care Institute, Cleveland Clinic, Cleveland, OH, USA
e-mail: argalim@ccf.org

M. Argalious
Cleveland Clinic Lerner College of Medicine of Case Western Reserve University, Cleveland, OH, USA

M. Argalious et al. (eds.), *Basic Sciences in Anesthesia*,
https://doi.org/10.1007/978-3-031-60203-0_15

associated cascade of cellular changes that can ultimately result in organ dysfunction and failure.
10. Dynamic measures of fluid responsiveness are indices evaluating the response to a cyclic preload variation and provide better prediction of fluid responsiveness than static measures.

15.1 Body Fluid Compartments

Total body water comprises around 60% of the lean body mass of an adult. The intracellular fluid compartment accounts for two-thirds of the total body water, while the extracellular fluid accounts for the remaining one-third. The extracellular body water is distributed between the interstitial fluid and the plasma volume in a ratio of 3:1.

For a 70 kg patient, the following total body water composition is applied:

$$\text{Total body water} = 60\% \times 70\,\text{kg} = 42\,\text{L}$$
$$\text{Intracellular water volume} = 66\%\ \text{of} 42\,\text{L} = 28\,\text{L}$$
$$\text{Extracellular water volume} = 33\%\ \text{of}\ 42\,\text{L} = 14\,\text{L}$$
$$\text{Interstitial water volume} = 75\%\ \text{of} 14\,\text{L} = 10.5\,\text{L}$$
$$\text{Plasma(intravascular)water volume} = 25\%\ \text{of}\ 14\,\text{L} = 3.5\,\text{L}$$

Osmolarity refers to the concentration of osmotically active particles in a solution expressed in milliosmoles per liter (mOsm/L).

Normal plasma osmolarity $= 275$ to $295\ \text{mOsmol/L}$.

Plasma osmolarity is calculated based on the following osmotically active particles in plasma $=2[\text{Na}+] + \text{Glucose}/18 + \text{BUN}/2.8$.

15.1.1 Osmolarity Versus Tonicity

Both osmolarity and tonicity compare the solute concentrations of 2 solutions separated by a membrane.

Osmolarity takes into account the total concentration of penetrating solutes and non-penetrating solutes, while tonicity takes into account the total concentration of only non-penetrating solutes.

15.2 Crystalloids

Crystalloids are intravenous fluids containing electrolytes and/or dextrose dissolved in water. ◘ ◉ Table 15.1 lists the composition of commonly used intravenous crystalloid solutions.

15.2.1 NaCl 0.9%

Infusion of 0.9% NaCl is accompanied by a hyperchloremic metabolic acidosis, especially if large volumes are administered [1]. Its effects on the kidneys include renal vasoconstriction, reduced glomerular filtration rate (GFR), and a reduction in renal cortical perfusion. Observational trials showed that the use of isotonic normal saline could increase the incidence of acute kidney injury (AKI) and the requirement for renal replacement therapy, likely through a reduction in renal perfusion. Among patients receiving crystalloid fluid therapy in the ICU, the use of a buffered crystalloid compared with normal saline did not reduce the risk of acute kidney injury.

In a single-center alternating cohort trial of 8616 patients undergoing major noncardiac surgery (SOLAR trial), infusion of large volumes of normal saline versus lactated Ringer's solution showed comparable postoperative renal, respiratory, infectious, and hemorrhagic complications.

15.2.2 NaCl 3%

The use of hypertonic NaCl is limited to patients with increased intracranial pressure to reduce cerebral edema as well as for the treatment of hypo-osmolar hyponatremia. Its use as a volume expander has been considered in prehospital trauma with no demonstrable improvement in patient outcomes [2].

15.2.3 Balanced Crystalloid Solutions

Balanced crystalloid solutions including PlasmaLyte (isotonic) and Ringer's lactate, gluconate, and acetate (mildly hypotonic) have a lower sodium and chloride concentration as compared to isotonic NaCl. The reduced anion content is compensated for by the addition of buffers, such as lactate, gluconate, and acetate. Following administration, the buffer is metabolized to HCO_3^-. Balanced crystalloid solutions avoid the hyperchloremic metabolic acidosis caused by isotonic NaCl. In addition, they reduce antidiuretic hormone (ADH) secretion, thereby reducing the typical salt and water retention that occurs with isotonic NaCl administration and allow diuresis in response to intravascular fluid expansion [3]. While several meta-analyses failed to show a benefit of balanced crystalloids versus normal saline in reducing mortality, [4–6] randomized control trials in the critically ill patients (SMART trial) and in patients treated in an emergency department and subsequently hospitalized outside the intensive care unit showed a reduction in major adverse kidney events within 30 days [7, 8].

Table 15.1 Composition of commonly used crystalloid solutions

Solution	mOsm/L	Tonicity	pH	Na^{+a}	Cl^{-a}	K^{+a}	Ca^{2a}	Mg^{2a}	Glucose (g/L)	Lactate[a]	HCO_3^{-a}	Gluconate[a]	Acetate[a]
Lactated Ringer's (LR)[b]	273	Iso	6.5	130	109	4	3	–	–	28	–	–	–
PlasmaLyte A	294	Iso	7.4	140	98	5	–	3	–	–	–	23	27
PlasmaLyte —148	294	Iso	5.5	140	98	5	–	3	–	–	–	23	27
Normal Saline (NS)	308	Iso	5.0	154	154	–	–	–	–	–	–	–	–
5% dextrose (D5) in water	253	Hypo	–	–	–	–	–	–	50	–	–	–	–
D5 ¼ NS	355	Iso	4.0	38.5	38.5	–	–	–	50	–	–	–	–
D5 ½ NS	406	Hyper	4.3	77	77	–	–	–	50	–	–	–	–
D5 NS	586	Hyper	4.0	154	154	–	–	–	50	–	–	–	–
D5 LR	525	Hyper	5.0	130	109	4	2.7	–	50	28	–	–	–
½ NS	154	Hypo		77	77	–	–	–	–	–	–	–	–
3% Saline	1027	Hyper	5.0	513	513	–	–	–	–	–	–	–	–
5% Saline	1711	Hyper	5.0	856	856	–	–	–	–	–	–	–	–
7.5% $NaHCO_3$	1786	Hyper	–	893	–	–	–	–	–	–	893	23	27
Normasol	280	Iso	7.4	140	98	5	–	–	–	–	–	23	27

[a] Standard SI units: mEq/L
[b] Lactate Ringer's = Hartmann's solution = Compound Sodium Lactate

In patients receiving large amounts of crystalloids in the perioperative period and in patients with pre-existing kidney disease and those at risk for acute kidney injury, it is prudent to avoid hyperchloremic metabolic acidosis and its potential deleterious consequences on kidney-related outcomes by using balanced crystalloid solutions instead of normal saline.

15.2.4 Dextrose Solutions

Dextrose solutions are typically used for acute management of hypoglycemia (D50) and for maintenance of patients' nutritional requirements as part of parenteral nutrition. Dextrose solutions are not suitable for intravascular fluid expansion since water is able to move across fluid compartments and is not confined to the intravascular space. Glucose solutions can also be used in conjunction with insulin for management of hyperkalemia (by shifting K+ intracellular) as well as to reduce the occurrence of hypoglycemia in diabetic patients receiving insulin infusions.

15.2.5 Crystalloids to be Avoided in Certain Conditions and Disease States

- Acute and chronic kidney disease: Avoid large volumes of 0.9% NaCl.
- Hyperparathyroidism: Avoid Ca^{2+} containing solutions including Ringer's lactate
- Blood product transfusion: Avoid Ca^{2+} containing solutions to prevent clotting caused by interaction of Ca^{2+} with citrate. The small amounts of Ca^{2+} in Ringer's lactate make this a rare and hypothetical occurrence.
- Traumatic brain injury: Avoid hypotonic solutions for fear of worsening cerebral edema; avoid glucose containing solutions for fear of worsening of neurologic outcome.
- Liver Disease: Avoid hypotonic solutions that may exacerbate ascites/interstitial edema due to a reduced oncotic pressure.
- Hyperglycemia: Avoid glucose containing solutions to prevent worsening hyperglycemia.
- Increased Intracranial Pressure: Avoid hypotonic solutions for fear of worsening cerebral edema.

15.3 Colloids

Colloids are small, finely divided particles that remain dispersed in a liquid for a long time due to their small size (usually less than 1 mm) and electron charge. While these particles are too small to be seen by the optical microscope, they are too big to pass through a semipermeable membrane. These particles have negligible settling velocity because of their small mass and have a low gravitational force compared to surface frictional forces. Colloids can be classified into natural and synthetic colloids. Albumin is the typical example of natural colloids, while synthetic colloids include various hydroxyethyl starches, dextran, and gelatins [9].

15.3.1 Albumin

Human serum albumin is a 66.5-kDa, negatively charged, and elliptically shaped protein that contributes up to 80% of the intravascular oncotic pressure and serves as a transport protein in blood. Albumin 5–25% is a sterile liquid solution that contains variable concentrations of albumin (5–25%) in normal saline. Albumin is derived from large pools of human plasma, manufactured by cold ethanol fractionation followed by ultra- and diafiltration. The manufacturing also includes final container pasteurization and additional bulk pasteurization at 60 ± 0.5 °C for 10–11 h. The combination of fractionation and pasteurization virtually eliminates the risk of potential viral transmission.

The effective oncotic pressure of the 5% albumin solution approaches that of human plasma (around 25 mm Hg) while that of the 25% solution is approximately four to five times that of human plasma.

Albumin traverses the intravascular space, a phenomenon known as "transcapillary filtration," into the interstitial space via both passive filtration at areas with large gaps in the endothelium and active filtration via the receptor albondin. Albondin is an avid receptor for the transport of albumin into the interstitial space, but is lacking in certain tissue compartments, such as brain, resulting in low albumin levels in the cerebrospinal fluid. In experimental animal models, however, albumin has been shown to interact with the endothelial glycocalyx, thereby preserving the integrity of the endothelial surface layer and more effectively limiting fluid extravasation compared to crystalloids and other synthetic colloids.

While most studies report that albumin is safe but not significantly better than saline (0.9% NaCl) in reducing mortality, [10, 11] albumin has been shown to be beneficial for the following patient populations:

- Hypoalbuminemia and multiorgan dysfunction: Dubois and colleagues used intravenous albumin to correct hypoalbuminemia and used the Sequential Organ Failure Assessment (SOFA) score to evaluate for changes in organ dysfunction [12]. They concluded that the administration of albumin to critically ill hypoalbuminemic patients showed improved organ function especially in the central nervous system, the cardiovascular system, and the pulmonary system.
- Sepsis: A meta-analysis reported that the use of albumin-containing solutions for the resuscitation of patients with sepsis was associated with lower mortality.[13]
- Spontaneous bacterial peritonitis complicating cirrhosis.
- Children with severe malaria.

On the other hand, several studies reported an increase in mortality with the use of albumin in patients with traumatic brain injury. While the exact mechanism is not well understood, a disruption in the blood–brain barrier with leakage of albumin into the brain parenchyma causing rebound intracranial hypertension has been suggested.

15.3.2 Hydroxyethyl Starch

Hydroxyethyl starch (HES) is a synthetic colloid solution in which the molecular mass of at least 80% of polymers ranges between 10 thousand and 2 million Daltons (Da). Larger molecules are degraded enzymatically by amylase. HES is stored in the reticuloendothelial system for several hours and is believed to be renally excreted. HES is mixed in a salt solution so that its salt concentration resembles that in blood. HES has become one of the most frequently used colloidal plasma expanders worldwide, mainly due to its lower cost compared to albumin. Most HES preparations have oncotic pressures around 30 mm Hg, (hetastarch: 450/0.7, Voluven®: 130/0.4) with some preparations having much higher oncotic pressures of 55 mm Hg (pentastarch: 260/0.5).

HES is derived from amylopectin, a polysaccharide from maize, and is similar to glycogen. HES is prepared by hydrolysis, in vivo, by serum alpha-amylase and amylopectin hydroxyethylation. HES is excreted by the kidneys and the rate of decomposition of starch is based on the molar substitution and C2/C6 ratio. The higher the molar substitution and C2/C6 ratios, the slower the decomposition, ultimately leading to plasma accumulation [14–18].

15.3.2.1 Classification of HES

Various hetastarches can be classified according to their:

- In vitro molecular weight (MW): Increased MW = decreased degradation.
- Molar substitution (hydroxyethylation): the proportion of glucose units on the starch molecule that have been substituted by hydroxyethyl units. The higher molar substitution means a larger molecule; so the larger the molecule, the slower the degradation in the body.
- C2 to C6 ratio: the substitution of hydroxyethyl at the C2 or C6 location. Increased C2 substitution = decreased degradation, since a high C2/C6 ratio decreases the rate of hydrolysis by alpha-amylase.
- Concentration %: HES 6% means that there are 6 g of HES per each 100 ml of diluent.
- Diluent (also called carrier solution): typically, 0.9% NaCl or lactated Ringer's solution.

Three generations of hetastarches, based on their average molecular weights and their molar substitutions, have been introduced into clinical practice:

- First generation: also referred to as high molecular weight HES. Examples include hydroxyethyl starch HES 450/0.7, 550/0.7, and 670/0.75.
- Second generation: Medium molecular weight HES. The typical example is pentastarch 200/0.5, which is prepared as 10% in normal saline.
- Third generation: Low molecular weight HES (130/0.4). HES 130/0.4 is the latest generation of the commercially available HES solutions. It is characterized by a mean in vitro MW of 130,000 Da, a molar substitution (MS) of 0.4, and a C2/C6 ratio of about 9:1. HES 130/0.4 is one of the most frequently used resuscitation fluids worldwide [19].

15.3.2.2 Side Effects of HES

- Anaphylactoid reactions: All synthetic colloids are associated with a several-fold increased incidence of anaphylactoid reactions compared with albumin, with HES having the lowest risk of anaphylactoid reactions among the synthetic colloids.
- Coagulopathy and bleeding: HES 450/0.7 and 200/0.5 administration increased bleeding when used during cardiac surgery after which hetastarch received a warning label in the United States. HES 200/0.6 was associated with fatal bleeding in patients with intracranial hemorrhage. HES can produce dilutional effects like other volume expanders and decrease factor VIII and von Willebrand factor levels. HES can also reduce the accessibility of glycoprotein IIb/IIIa on the surface of platelets. All these effects on coagulation parameters can result in severe coagulopathy. In a retrospective propensity matched study of patients undergoing cardiac surgery, the use of low molecular weight HES (130/0.4) was associated with more coagulopathy and blood product transfusion when compared to the crystalloid group.
- Acute kidney injury and need for renal replacement therapy: HES is associated with renal tubular injury characterized by increased urinary excretion of alpha 1-microglobulin, Tamm–Horsfall protein, and the brush border enzyme acetyl-b glucosaminidase. A proinflammatory action on the kidney interstitium also has been described. The mechanism of renal failure may include reabsorption of the macromolecule into renal tubular cells leading to osmotic nephrotic lesions or renal plugging due to hyperviscous urine. HES 130/0.4 at doses more than 33 mL/kg was an independent risk factor for acute renal failure (ARF) in a large observational study of 2911 surgical intensive care unit (ICU) patients (adjusted OR, 1.85; CI, 1.01–3.41). In a multicenter parallel group blinded trial of septic patients randomized to either HES 130/0.4 or Ringer acetate, the HES group was more likely to require renal replacement therapy compared to the Ringer acetate group. In 7000 patients admitted to an ICU and randomly assigned to HES 130/0.4 versus normal saline, the use of HES resulted in a higher requirement for renal replacement therapy compared to the normal saline group. In a systematic review of 92 studies, including 23 randomized clinical trials, renal impairment was demonstrable after usage of HES solutions spanning the full spectrum of molecular weights and substitutions.
- Mortality: High doses of HES may be associated with higher mortality in patients at risk. In the VISEP trial (Efficacy of Volume Substitution and Insulin Therapy in Severe Sepsis), septic patients showed a trend toward increased 90-day mortality if they received 10% HES 200/0.5 compared with modified lactated Ringer's (41.0% vs. 33.9%, $P = 0.09$). This excess mortality seemed to be driven by patients who received HES in higher cumulative doses. In the Scandinavian Starch for Severe Sepsis/Septic Shock Trial: HES 130/0.4 versus Ringer's acetate solution in severe sepsis patients, patients with severe sepsis assigned to fluid resuscitation with HES 130/0.4 had an increased risk of death at day 90 and were more likely to require renal replacement therapy, as compared with those receiving Ringer's acetate. It is unclear how HES administration might impair survival, but tissue storage may have a role. Synthetic colloids are either broken down by serum amylase and excreted via the kidneys or temporarily absorbed into lysosomes of liver, kidney, lymph nodes, and other tissue. This phenomenon is dose-dependent and may be increased in the presence of renal failure. In patients with impaired renal function, frequent plasma replacement with HES resulted in an increase in plasma chitotriosidase activity, which is a marker of activated foamy macrophages. Massive colloidal tissue storage may impair ventilation and contribute to acute kidney injury, and higher cumulative doses may be responsible for extensive organ depositions with the appearance of a foamy macrophage syndrome. There is no evidence of an overall beneficial effect of HES in any subgroup of critically ill patients. On the other hand, the use of HES (including low molecular weight) shows clear signals of harm, including adverse effects on the kidneys, on hemostatic functions as well as a trend toward increased mortality. HES should therefore be avoided in patients with acute or chronic renal disease, coagulopathy, as well as in critically ill septic patients.

15.3.3 Dextrans

Dextrans are glucose polymers synthetized from sucrose medium by lactic acid bacteria *Leuconostoc mesenteroides*. Dextrans are available as 10% dextran 70 and 40 in normal saline. Dextran 70 is a volume expander, whereas dextran 40 is used to increase blood flow. Both dextrans have an oncotic pressure of 40 mm Hg, greater than that of plasma at 20 mm Hg. Dextran can be antigenic and can lead to anaphylactoid reactions, but the incidence of such severe reactions has been reduced dramatically from about 5% to 0.032% in the past 20 years. Dextrans can disable the crossmatch for blood by coating red blood cells and increasing the erythrocyte sedimentation rate. Dextrans are also considered as a cause of acute renal failure because their oncotic pressure is higher than plasma, reducing filtration pressure in the kidneys. Because of all the side effects, dextrans are rarely used as fluid expanders.

15.3.4 Gelatins

Gelatins are polypeptides produced by degradation of bovine collagen. Gelatins, like starches, impair platelet function and reduce von Willebrand and coagulation factor VIII: c. In patients with intracranial bleeding, 4% gelatin and 6% HES 200/0.5 increased blood transfusion requirements and inflammatory markers. Gelatin may also be associated with renal impairment in patients at risk. In patients with severe sepsis, both HES and gelatins in doses >33 mL/kg were associated with an increased incidence of renal failure. Due to allergic reactions and altered plasma viscosity, gelatins are not approved by the Food and Drug Administration (FDA) in the US.

15.4 Crystalloid Versus Colloid Resuscitation

In patients with burns, trauma, or following surgery, there is no evidence from randomized controlled trials and meta-analyses that resuscitation with colloids reduces the risk of death, compared to resuscitation with crystalloids. The use of the colloid HES in a critically ill patient may worsen renal outcomes, increase coagulopathy and the need for blood product transfusion, and may increase mortality. Since colloids are more expensive and do not confer a mortality benefit, there is little evidence to support their preferential use over crystalloids.

In large-scale prospective trials, the volume of crystalloid resuscitation to achieve prespecified resuscitation endpoints is around 1.5 to 2 times the colloid resuscitation volume, which is much less than the crystalloid to colloid resuscitation ratio (3:1) previously recommended. In the Saline versus Albumin Fluid Evaluation (SAFE) trial, the ratio of normal saline to 4% albumin resuscitation over the first 4 days was 1.4 to 1. Similarly, in the VISEP trial, the ratio of lactated Ringer's to HES over the first 4 days was 1.6. Recent publications in animal models point to the fact that the volume effects of crystalloid solutions have been underestimated.

Several randomized controlled trials also examined the effect of crystalloids vs. colloids on postoperative nausea and vomiting in noncardiac surgery, and a meta-analysis of available RCTs by Jong Lee and colleagues suggests no significant difference in this outcome, although sub-analysis suggested that colloids may be associated with less PONV in surgeries > 3 h [20]. There is little evidence to support the preferential use of colloids versus crystalloid for early goal-directed fluid therapy [21].

Accurately identifying and following resuscitation end points and the use of evidence-based methods for assessment of fluid responsiveness may be more important determinants of outcomes than the type of fluid used for resuscitation.

15.5 Perioperative Fluid Management

The classic and now outdated approach to fluid management in the perioperative period utilizes an empiric weight-based formula to estimate fluid requirements. The formula differentiates three types of fluid losses: preoperative fluid loss, maintenance requirements, and surgical fluid losses. This approach to fluid management is also known as the 4/2/1 rule and has been largely abandoned for a more goal-oriented approach.

- Preoperative fluid losses:
  The estimated fluid requirements follow the 4/2/1 rule: 4 cc/kg/h for the first 10 kg, 2 cc/kg/h for the second 10 kg, and 1 cc/kg/h for every kg above 20 kg.
  The hourly fluid requirements are then multiplied by the number of hours the patient remained NPO.
- Ongoing intraoperative maintenance requirements:
  using the same 4/2/1 rule as used to calculate preoperative maintenance requirements.
- Surgical fluid losses based on type of surgery:
  - Minimal tissue trauma (e.g., breast surgery): 2–4 cc/kg/h
  - Moderate tissue trauma (ventral hernia surgery): 4–6 cc/kg/h
  - Severe tissue trauma (e.g., laparotomy): 6–8 cc/kg/h

15.6 The Concept of Early Goal-Directed Fluid Therapy

Fluid overload through "liberal" fluid resuscitation regimens has been shown to negatively affect vascular barrier competence, increase cardiopulmonary complications, and prolong recovery of bowel function and hospital stay. Goal-directed fluid therapy aims to achieve and maintain a specific goal: an optimum cardiac output that ensures adequate delivery of oxygen to the tissues, thereby avoiding tissue hypoperfusion and the associated cascade of cellular changes that can ultimately result in organ dysfunction and failure.[22]

The concept of early goal-directed therapy was introduced by Rivers and colleagues, who randomized 263 patients presenting with severe sepsis to a protocol of early goal-direct fluid therapy (EGDT) or standard therapy during the initial 6 h of resuscitation.[23] In that study, The EGDT protocol used fluid therapy, blood transfusion, and vasoactive drug infusion to optimize tissue oxygen delivery, and EGDT was associated with a significant mortality benefit (30.5% for EGDT vs. 46.5% for standard, $P = 0.009$).

In several subsequent large-scale randomized multicenter trials of critically ill patients presenting to the hospital with early septic shock, EGDT did not reduce all-cause mortality at 90 days compared to standard care [24–26].

In the perioperative period, the use of goal-directed fluid therapy may avoid the deleterious effects of liberal fluid practices with their deleterious effects on pulmonary complications, delayed return of bowel function, and delayed hospital discharge. Conclusive data from randomized trials regarding the benefits of goal-directed fluid therapy in the perioperative period is lacking, and this represents an important research question for current and future clinical trials.

It is worthwhile mentioning that in patients with hypotension caused by penetrating trauma, delay in fluid resuscitation may improve outcome. The rationale behind delayed fluid resuscitation or "permissive hypotension" in these circumstances is that uncontrolled bleeding may have temporarily stopped due to hypotension, vasoconstriction, and in situ thrombus formation. Efforts to normalize circulating blood volume and hemodynamics prior to definitive surgical homeostasis may cause a paradoxical increase in blood loss.

15.7 Fluid Responsiveness: Static Versus Dynamic Parameters

Static markers of cardiac preload—especially central venous pressure or pulmonary artery occlusion pressure, but also left ventricular end-diastolic area and early/late diastolic wave ratio—do not identify fluid responders from nonresponders. These static markers, including those derived from echocardiography, can identify whether a cardiac chamber is full or empty and may help identify different mechanisms of shock states, but they do not reliably predict the hemodynamic response to a subsequent fluid bolus administration.

Dynamic markers are indices evaluating the response to a cyclic preload variation and provide better prediction of fluid responsiveness.

15.7.1 Actual Change in Preload: Fluid Challenge

The physiologic benefit of a fluid challenge is based on the Frank–Starling relationship, whereby an increase in cardiac preload results in an increased stroke volume and subsequently an increased cardiac output. This concept assumes that a patient's preload is on the steep portion of the Frank–Starling curve. However, it is the actual interaction among the three parameters—preload, stroke volume, and cardiac contractility—that determines fluid responsiveness (◉ Fig. 15.1).

15.7.2 Functional Change in Preload in Mechanically Ventilated Patients

Although inducing an actual change in cardiac preload can be simply and quickly accomplished by a fluid bolus, an alternative method to predicting volume responsiveness is to challenge the Frank–Starling curve by inducing a functional change in cardiac preload and monitoring the response in stroke volume, cardiac output, or their surrogates.

In mechanically ventilated patients, this functional change in preload is already occurring because of mechanical ventilation-induced changes in cardiac preload and can be monitored by observing the magnitude of change in hemodynamic signals in relation to cyclic changes in airway pressure. Arterial pressure rises during inspiration and falls during expiration because of changes in intrathoracic pressure secondary to positive pressure ventilation. In patients with preload reserve, mechanical ventilation will result in greater cyclic changes in the right ventricle and subsequently the left ventricle stroke volume and can therefore predict volume responsiveness.

Respiratory variations in hemodynamic signals do not predict volume responsiveness in spontaneously breathing patients, in patients with cardiac arrhythmias, and are inaccurate in patients with isolated right ventricle dysfunction or pulmonary hypertension.

Echocardiographic "dynamic" measures of fluid responsiveness, including inferior vena cava (IVC) and superior

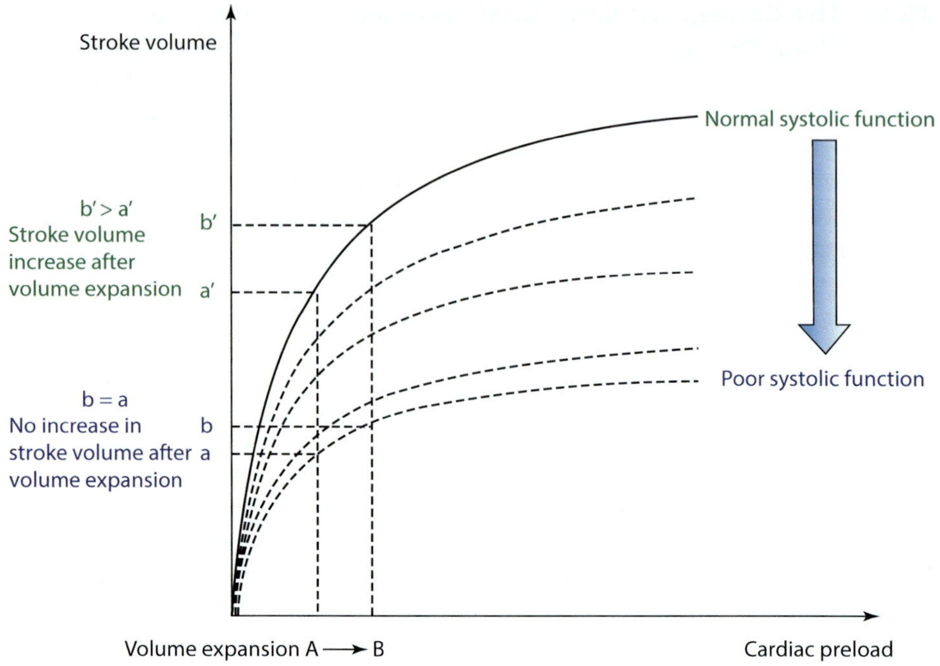

Fig. 15.1 Frank–Starling curve and its relationship to fluid responsiveness. A given value of cardiac preload can be associated with an increase in stroke volume in patients with good ventricular function, whereas the same value of preload will not be associated with an increase in stroke volume (no preload reserve) in patients with poor ventricular function

vena cava (SVC) collapsibility index and respiratory variations in left and right ventricle stroke volume, can also be used to predict the response to fluid loading in mechanically ventilated patients before an actual fluid bolus is given and are therefore important components of goal-directed fluid therapy.

15.7.3 Functional Change in Preload in Spontaneously Breathing Patients

In spontaneously breathing patients, the functional change in preload is accomplished by the passive leg-raising test [27]. It consists of lifting the legs passively 45° from the horizontal (supine) position (or tilting the bed to the same extent) and observing the change occurring in hemodynamic effects (change in stroke volume, cardiac output, or arterial pulse pressure) as a result of the gravitational transfer of blood from the lower extremities toward the intrathoracic compartment. This test has the advantage of being simple, reversible, and applicable in spontaneously breathing patients.

15.8 Questions and Answers

Questions (Choose the Most Appropriate Answer)

1. What percentage of total body water does the extracellular fluid compartment constitute?
   A. 25%
   B. 33%
   C. 50%
   D. 66%
2. Administration of 0.9% NaCl is associated with the following metabolic abnormality?
   A. Hypochloremic metabolic acidosis
   B. Hyperchloremic metabolic acidosis
   C. Hypochloremic metabolic alkalosis
   D. Hyperchloremic metabolic alkalosis
3. Which of the following crystalloids has the highest tonicity?
   A. NaCl 0.9%
   B. NaCl 0.45% in Dextrose 5%
   C. PlasmaLyte
   D. Lactated Ringer's
4. The use of albumin is not recommended in patients with:
   A. Spontaneous bacterial peritonitis
   B. Severe malaria
   C. Traumatic brain injury
   D. Sepsis
5. Which of the following hetastarch generations should be avoided in critically ill septic patients:
   A. First-generation hetastarches
   B. Second-generation hetastarches
   C. Third-generation hetastarches
   D. 1st, 2nd, and 3rd generation hetastarches
6. Static parameters of fluid responsiveness include all of the following except:
   A. Mechanical ventilation-induced changes in stroke volume

B. Central venous pressure
C. Pulmonary artery occlusion pressure
D. Left ventricle end-diastolic area

7. Which of the following is the most appropriate goal during goal-directed fluid therapy:
A. PAO2 (Alveolar oxygen tension)
B. Mean arterial pressure
C. Cardiac output
D. Central venous pressure

8. Which of the following fluids are associated with the highest incidence of anaphylactoid reactions:
A. PlasmaLyte
B. Hypertonic saline (3% NaCl)
C. Hetastarch 200/0.5
D. Albumin 5%

9. A high molar substitution on hetastarches is associated with
A. Slower degradation
B. Shorter half-life
C. Less anaphylactoid reactions
D. Less coagulopathy

10. Plasma osmolarity is calculated based on the following osmotically active particles except:
A. Blood urea nitrogen
B. Creatinine
C. Glucose
D. Sodium

Answers

1. **B**. In adults, the extracellular fluid constitutes 33% of total body water, while the intracellular fluid constitutes 66% of total body water.
2. **B**. Infusion of 0.9% NaCl is accompanied by a hyperchloremic metabolic acidosis, especially if large volumes are administered.
3. **B**. NaCl 0.45% in Dextrose 5% has the highest tonicity. Please see ◘ ◉ Table 15.1 for details.
4. **C**. Several studies reported an increase in mortality with the use of albumin in patients with traumatic brain injury. While the exact mechanism is not well understood, a disruption in the blood–brain barrier with leakage of albumin into the brain parenchyma causing rebound intracranial hypertension has been suggested.
5. **D**. All hetastarch preparations have been associated with an increased incidence of acute kidney injury and an increased mortality in critically ill septic patients and should therefore be avoided in this patient population.
6. **A**. Static markers of cardiac preload, especially central venous pressure or pulmonary artery occlusion pressure, but also left ventricular end-diastolic area, do not identify fluid responders from nonresponders. These static markers, especially those derived from echocardiography (left ventricle end-diastolic area), can identify whether a cardiac chamber is full or empty and may help identify different mechanisms of shock states, but do not reliably predict the hemodynamic response to a subsequent fluid bolus administration.
7. **C**. Goal-directed fluid therapy aims to achieve and maintain a specific goal: an optimum cardiac output that ensures adequate delivery of oxygen to the tissues, thereby avoiding tissue hypoperfusion and the associated cascade of cellular changes that can ultimately result in organ dysfunction and failure.
8. **C**. All synthetic colloids (hetastarch, gelatin, dextran) are associated with a several-fold increased incidence of anaphylactoid reactions compared with albumin, with HES having the lowest risk of anaphylactoid reactions among the synthetic colloids.

19. **A**. Molar substitution (hydroxyethylation) refers to the proportion of glucose units on the starch molecule that have been substituted by hydroxyethyl units. The higher molar substitution means a larger molecule; so the larger the molecule, the slower the degradation in the body.

10. **B**. Plasma osmolarity is calculated based on the following osmotically active particles in plasma = 2[Na +] + Glucose/18 + BUN/2.8.

References

1. Gheorghe C, Dadu R, Blot C, Barrantes F, Vazquez R, Berianu F, Feng Y, Feintzig I, Amoateng-Adjepong Y, Manthous CA. Hyperchloremic metabolic acidosis following resuscitation of shock. Chest J. 2010;138(6):1521–2.
2. Bulger EM, May S, Kerby JD, Emerson S, Stiell IG, Schreiber MA, Brasel KJ, Tisherman SA, Coimbra R, Rizoli S, Minei JP. Out-of-hospital hypertonic resuscitation after traumatic hypovolemic shock: a randomized, placebo controlled trial. Ann Surg. 2011;253(3):431.
3. Lorenzo M, Davis JW, Negin S, Kaups K, Parks S, Brubaker D, Tyroch A. Can Ringer's lactate be used safely with blood transfusions? Am J Surg. 1998;175(4):308–10.
4. Sohail et al. Perioperative administration of buffered versus non-buffered crystalloid intravenous fluid to improve outcomes following adult surgical procedures. Cochrane Database Syst Rev. 2017 9
5. Odor Peter M, et al Perioperative administration of buffered versus non-buffered crystalloid intravenous fluid to improve outcomes following adult surgical procedures: a Cochrane systematic review. Perioper Med 2018;7(1):1–3.
6. Kawano-Dourado L, et al Low-versus high-chloride content intravenous solutions for critically ill and perioperative adult patients: a systematic review and meta-analysis. Anesth Analg. 2018;126(2):513–21.
7. Semler MW, et al Balanced crystalloids versus saline in critically ill adults. N Engl J Med. 2018;378(9):829–39.

8. Self WH, et al Balanced crystalloids versus saline in noncritically ill adults. N Engl J Med. (2018);378(9):819–28.
9. Argalious MY. Colloid update. Curr Pharm Des. 2012;18(38): 6291–7.
10. Neel DR, McClave S, Martindale R. Hypoalbuminaemia in the perioperative period: clinical significance and management options. Best Pract Res Clin Anaesthesiol. 2011;25(3):395–400.
11. Finfer S, Bellomo R, Boyce N, French J, Myburgh J, Norton R, SAFE Study Investigators. A comparison of albumin and saline for fluid resuscitation in the intensive care unit. N Engl J Med. 2004;350(22):2247–56.
12. Dubois MJ, Orellana-Jimenez C, Melot C, De Backer D, Berre J, Leeman M, Brimioulle S, Appoloni O, Creteur J, Vincent JL. Albumin administration improves organ function in critically ill hypoalbuminemic patients: a prospective, randomized, controlled, pilot study. Crit Care Med. 2006;34(10):2536–40.
13. Delaney AP, Dan A, McCaffrey J, Finfer S. The role of albumin as a resuscitation fluid for patients with sepsis: a systematic review and meta-analysis. Crit Care Med. 2011;39(2):386–91.
14. Wilkes MM, Navickis RJ, Sibbald WJ. Albumin versus hydroxyethyl starch in cardiopulmonary bypass surgery: a meta-analysis of postoperative bleeding. Ann Thorac Surg. 2001;72(2):527–33.
15. Jonville-Béra AP, Autret-Leca E, Gruel Y. Acquired type I von Willebrand's disease associated with highly substituted hydroxyethyl starch. N Engl J Med. 2001;345(8):622–3.
16. Hans GA, Ledoux D, Roediger L, Hubert MB, Koch JN, Senard M. The effect of intraoperative 6% balanced hydroxyethyl starch (130/0.4) during cardiac surgery on transfusion requirements. J Cardiothorac Vasc Anesth. 2015;29(2):328–32.
17. Perner A, Haase N, Guttormsen AB, Tenhunen J, Klemenzson G, Åneman A, Madsen KR, Møller MH, Elkjær JM, Poulsen LM, Bendtsen A. Hydroxyethyl starch 130/0.42 versus Ringer's acetate in severe sepsis. N Engl J Med. 2012;367(2):124–34.
18. Myburgh JA, Finfer S, Bellomo R, Billot L, Cass A, Gattas D, Glass P, Lipman J, Liu B, McArthur C, McGuinness S. Hydroxyethyl starch or saline for fluid resuscitation in intensive care. N Engl J Med. 2012;367(20):1901–11.
19. Hartog CS, Kohl M, Reinhart K. A systematic review of third-generation hydroxyethyl starch (HES 130/0.4) in resuscitation: safety not adequately addressed. Anesth Analg. 2011;112(3): 635–45.
20. Lee MJ, Lee C, Kang H, Kim H. The impact of crystalloid versus colloid fluids on postoperative nausea and vomiting: a systematic review and meta-analysis of randomized controlled trials. J Clin Anesth. 2020;62: 109695.
21. Lewis SR, Pritchard MW, Evans DJ, Butler AR, Alderson P, Smith AF, Roberts I. Colloids versus crystalloids for fluid resuscitation in critically ill people. Cochrane Database Syst Rev. 2018;8(8):CD000567
22. Argalious M. Management of postanesthesia care unit emergencies. ASA Refresher Courses Anesthesiol. 2009;37(1):1–2.
23. Rivers E, Nguyen B, Havstad S, Ressler J, Muzzin A, Knoblich B, Peterson E, Tomlanovich M. Early goal-directed therapy in the treatment of severe sepsis and septic shock. N Engl J Med. 2001;345(19):1368–77.
24. Arise Investigators, ANZICS clinical trials group Goal-directed resuscitation for patients with early septic shock. N Engl J Med. 2014;2014(371):1496–506.
25. ProCESS Investigators A randomized trial of protocol-based care for early septic shock. N Engl J Med. 2014;2014(370):1683–93.
26. Mouncey PR, Osborn TM, Power GS, Harrison DA, Sadique MZ, Grieve RD, Jahan R, Harvey SE, Bell D, Bion JF, Coats TJ. Trial of early, goal-directed resuscitation for septic shock. N Engl J Med. 2015;372(14):1301–11.
27. Boulain T, Achard JM, Teboul JL, Richard C, Perrotin D, Ginies G. Changes in BP induced by passive leg raising predict response to fluid loading in critically ill patients. Chest J. 2002;121 (4):1245–52.

Part III
Physiology

Contents

Central and Peripheral Nervous Systems

16

Jia W. Romito, Ravi Bhoja, and David L. McDonagh

Abstract

The central nervous system (CNS) is composed of the brain and spinal cord. The peripheral nervous system (PNS) consists of the rest of the neuronal pathways outside the brain and spinal cord. Functionally, the brain is organized in two main sections: the cerebral cortex and the subcortical areas; the latter includes the basal ganglia, hippocampus, internal capsule, brainstem, and cerebellum. The spinal cord extends from the foramen magnum to the L1–L2 level in adults. It consists of neuronal tracts that carry signals between the brain and peripheral nervous system. Cerebral blood flow (CBF) fluctuates minimally with cerebral perfusion pressure (CPP) due to corresponding changes in cerebral vascular resistance (CVR) attributed to cerebral autoregulation. CPP and CVR are influenced by pH, $PaCO_2$, PaO_2, and cerebral metabolic rate for O_2 ($CMRO_2$). CPP below the lower limit of cerebral autoregulation can lead to cerebral ischemia. Anesthetic medications can affect CBF and $CMRO_2$ although no anesthetic drugs have definitively been shown to be neuroprotective in humans. During neurosurgical procedures, evoked potentials are the most commonly used neurophysiological monitors to detect ischemia or tissue injury in the central nervous system.

Keywords

Neurophysiology • Central nervous system • Peripheral nervous system • Brain anatomy • Anesthesiology

Key Points

1. Damage to Wernicke's area causes impaired language comprehension and a receptive aphasia. Damage to Broca's area causes an expressive aphasia with difficulty speaking and writing.
2. Cerebral blood flow equals cerebral perfusion pressure divided by cerebral vascular resistance (CBF = CPP/CVR). Cerebral perfusion pressure is equal to mean arterial pressure (MAP) minus the greater of intracranial pressure (ICP) or central venous pressure (CVP):

CPP = MAP−ICP (or CVP if greater than ICP)

Normal CPP in healthy adults is 80–100 mm Hg and is primarily dependent on MAP, given the generally low values of ICP and CVP in normal individuals.

3. The brain has the ability to autoregulate; however, this only occurs within a specific blood pressure (BP) range (~60–150 mm Hg). In order to maintain a constant CBF, the CVR will adjust accordingly: decreasing CVR at the lower BP range and increasing CVR when at the higher BP range. Once outside the autoregulation BP range, CBF becomes pressure-dependent. CPP below the lower limit of cerebral autoregulation can lead to cerebral ischemia, while CPP above the upper limit can cause bleeding and/or edema. In chronically hypertensive patients, the upper and lower limits of autoregulation are shifted to the right.
4. Any cause of inflammation/injury or ischemia, such as irradiation, sustained seizures, infection, stroke, tumor, or trauma, can disrupt the blood–brain barrier (BBB). Prolonged hypercapnia, hypoxia, or osmotic shock can also increase the permeability of the BBB and allow substances

J. W. Romito · R. Bhoja · D. L. McDonagh (✉)
Department of Anesthesiology and Pain Management, University of Texas Southwestern Medical Center, Dallas, TX, USA
e-mail: david.mcdonagh@utsouthwestern.edu

J. W. Romito
e-mail: jia.romito@utsouthwestern.edu

R. Bhoja
e-mail: ravi.bhoja@utsouthwestern.edu

M. Argalious et al. (eds.), *Basic Sciences in Anesthesia*,
https://doi.org/10.1007/978-3-031-60203-0_16

that are typically excluded to enter the brain and cerebrospinal fluid.

5. Therapeutic hypothermia, commonly called targeted temperature management (TTM), stands alone as the only direct neuroprotectant (acts directly on neural tissue) with human evidence for efficacy. Indirect neuroprotectants include agents, such as thrombolytics and thrombectomy for acute stroke. TTM is used in the setting of neonatal asphyxia and in adults following cardiac arrest (i.e., after global anoxic-ischemic injury).
6. No anesthetic or adjuvant medication has been proven to be neuroprotective in humans, either against global or focal ischemia. However, there have been demonstrated neuroprotective effects of certain anesthetic medications against ischemia in animal models.
7. CO_2 reactivity is preserved with both inhalational and intravenous anesthetics. The degree of cerebral vasodilation from inhalational anesthetics can be temporarily attenuated by hyperventilation along with maintaining the volatile agent at < 1.0 minimum alveolar concentration (MAC) (typically $\sim$ 0.5 MAC).
8. The spinal cord terminates at L1–L2 in adults. Lumbar punctures and spinal anesthetics must be performed below L2 in adults.
9. Evoked potentials have varying sensitivity to anesthetics, with the most affected to least affected as follows: visual evoked potentials (VEP) > motor evoked potentials (MEP) > somatosensory evoked potentials (SSEP) > brainstem auditory evoked potentials (BAEP).

16.1 Functional Organization of the Cerebral Cortex

The cerebral cortex is a convoluted, superficial layer of the cerebral hemispheres consisting of the gyri (ridges) and sulci (fissures) (◉ Fig. 16.1). This thin layer of gray matter covers the frontal, parietal, temporal, and occipital lobes of the cerebral hemispheres.

Multiple functional areas in the cortex interact to produce conscious behavior, which includes the abilities to process sensation, communicate, retain memory, and coordinate movements. The sensory cortices allow for awareness of the environment, while the motor cortices control voluntary movement. Each of the primary sensory and motor cortices have secondary and tertiary cortices nearby to connect to association areas. These association areas integrate complex information for purposeful action.

16.2 Sensory Cortices

The main sensory cortices include the somatosensory, visual, auditory, gustatory, vestibular, and olfactory cortices, along with Wernicke's (receptive speech) area (◉ Fig. 16.2). These primary cortices receive direct input from the peripheral sensory receptors. The sensory information is then transmitted from the primary cortices to the secondary cortices to perform higher order functions.

16.2.1 Somatosensory Cortex

Located in the postcentral gyrus of the parietal lobe, the somatosensory cortex and adjacent somatosensory

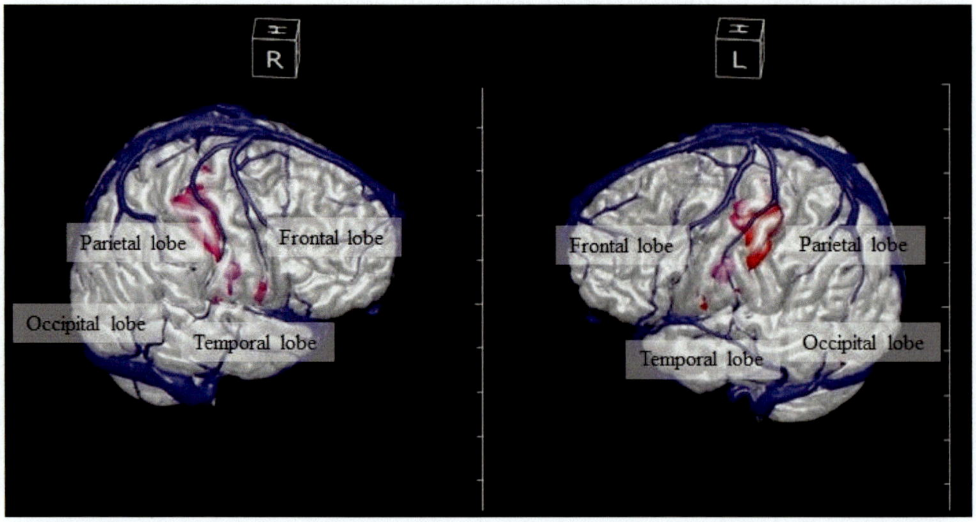

Fig. 16.1 Cerebral lobes depicted using a 3-dimensional (3D) reconstruction of functional brain MRI (fMRI)

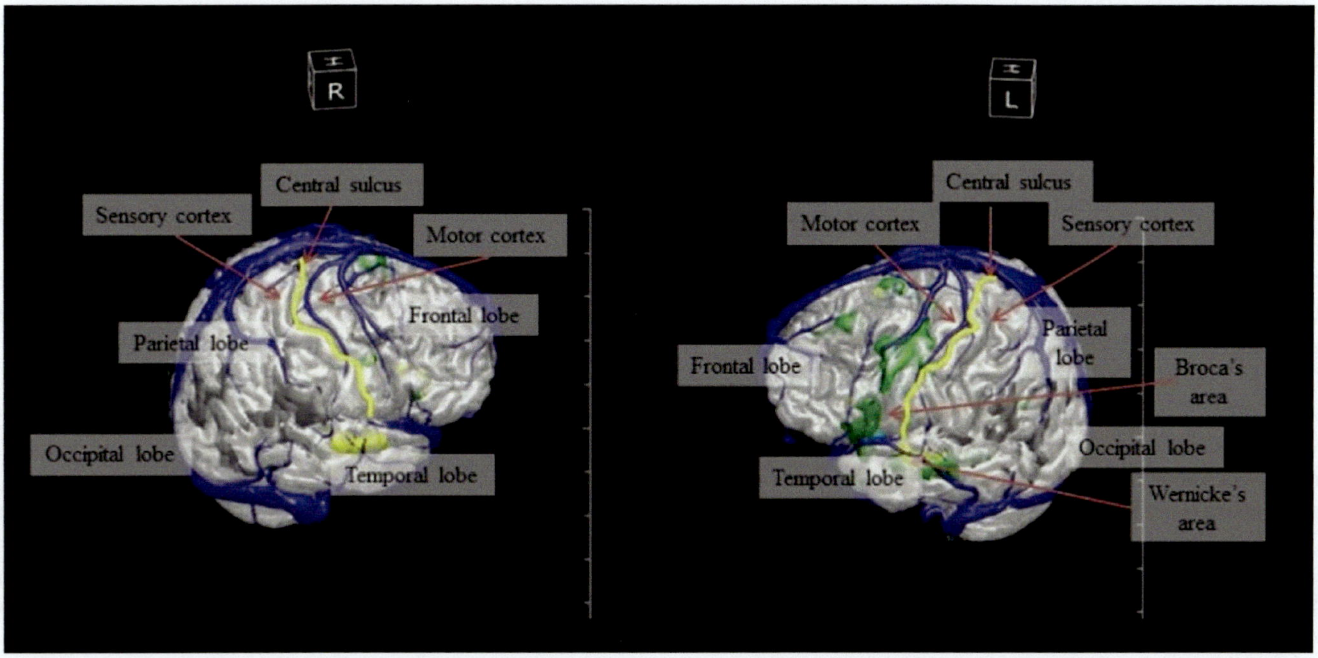

Fig. 16.2 Cerebral lobes and eloquent cortical areas depicted using a 3D reconstruction of functional brain MRI (fMRI)

association cortex are able to process information from cutaneous stimulation, proprioceptors, and tactile receptors.

16.2.2 Visual Cortex

The visual cortex is located in the occipital lobe. Damage to the occipital lobe (or to the subcortical optic radiations and/or the thalamic lateral geniculate nucleus) can cause cortical blindness, visual field deficits, and visual hallucinations.

16.2.3 Auditory Cortex

The auditory cortex is located bilaterally in the temporal lobes. Unilateral damage to the auditory cortex does not cause bilateral deafness due to bilateral sound representation from set neuronal pathways.

16.2.4 Gustatory, Vestibular, and Olfactory Cortices

The gustatory and vestibular cortices are located in the insular region of the parietal lobe and receive sensory input from the taste buds of the tongue and the ears, respectively. The olfactory cortex is located in the temporal lobes and receives sensory input from the nose.

16.2.5 Wernicke's Area

Wernicke's area, located in the language-dominant temporal-parietal lobe, is the receptive language area that is responsible for processing spoken and written language. Damage to this area results in impaired language comprehension and receptive aphasia. Preoperative testing before neurosurgical resection of a tumor in this area involves functional magnetic resonance imaging (fMRI) to identify this area in the individual patient (see the areas colored in green in ◉ Fig. 16.2 which are actual functional brain regions from a patient).

16.3 Motor Cortices

The motor cortices receive input from the sensory cortices and their respective association areas to allow for planning and execution of purposeful movement (◉ Fig. 16.2).

16.3.1 Primary Motor and Premotor Cortices

The primary motor and premotor cortices are located in the precentral gyrus and areas anteriorly adjacent in the frontal lobe. The corticospinal tracts originate in the primary motor cortex and travel caudally through the brainstem (decussate in the caudal medulla) and spinal cord to innervate skeletal muscle on the contralateral side. Stimulation of the primary motor cortex results in execution of a specific movement. Most of the synapses from the premotor cortex interface with the primary motor cortex to coordinate more complex movements. Stimulation of the premotor cortex results in a plan for a movement that can only be executed when the signal travels to the primary motor cortex. Damage to the motor cortex or corticospinal tracts causes a contralateral hemiparesis. It is important to be aware of the supplementary motor area (SMA) and the SMA syndrome. The SMA is in the dorsomedial prefrontal gyrus and involves a significant part of the frontal lobe [11]. This area is just in front of (anterior) to the primary motor cortex on the superior (dorsal) and medial aspects of the frontal lobe. Damage to this area, such as from a tumor resection, results in early postoperative motor (hemiparesis) and speech deficits. Importantly, these deficits are temporary and usually resolve over weeks.

16.3.2 Frontal Eye Fields

Projections travel from the visual association cortex in the occipital lobes to the frontal eye fields to produce eye movements. The frontal eye fields are on the lateral superior frontal lobes and drive the eyes (i.e., gaze) to the opposite side. Frontal lobe seizures classically cause gaze deviation to the opposite side along with clonic motor activity on the opposite side of the body. Acute frontal lobe strokes, most commonly from occlusion of the middle cerebral artery, with ischemic injury to the frontal eye fields cause the gaze deviation to the same side as the stroke.

16.3.3 Broca's Area

Broca's area is the expressive language area in the language-dominant frontal lobe (the left frontal lobe in *most* people). Damage to this area causes an expressive aphasia with difficulty speaking or writing.

The cortical areas serving motor or language function are termed eloquent cortex. Tumors or lesions in these areas often have to be removed during awake cranial surgery in order to continuously test the patient during resection of the lesion. Preoperative functional MRI is critical in identifying these areas and to allow for surgical planning.

16.4 Association Areas

There are multiple association areas that allow for higher level cognition, such as memory, judgment, emotion, and language, with coordination of sensorimotor data based on these interpretations. Perhaps, the most important association area is the prefrontal cortex. This cortex plays a critical role in executive control of goal-directed behavior, attention, and personality.

16.4.1 Subcortical Areas

The subcortical areas are the parts of the brain beneath and deep to the cortex. These areas include the basal ganglia, hippocampus, internal capsule (which includes the descending corticospinal tracts), cerebellum, brain stem, and the reticular activating system (◉ Fig. 16.3).

16.5 Basal Ganglia

The basal ganglia are a group of subcortical nuclei that regulate movement and posture by integrating motor processes associated with the cerebral cortex. The main components of the basal ganglia include the caudate nucleus, putamen, globus pallidus, subthalamic nucleus, and substantia nigra. The basal ganglia receive input from the cerebral cortex and send neuronal output to the thalamus. From the thalamus, the neurons travel to the frontal cortex, brainstem, and spinal cord to regulate movement. Damage to the basal ganglia results in dyskinesias and movement disorders, such as Parkinson's and Huntington's diseases.

Dopaminergic pathways are integral to the regulation of movement. Anti-dopaminergic therapies given in the perioperative period—such as metoclopramide, promethazine, and droperidol—can have dystonic side effects or exacerbate dopamine-deficient conditions, such as Parkinson's disease.

16.6 Hippocampus

Located in the temporal lobe, the hippocampus regulates short-term memory. A neuronal circuit connects the hippocampus and the rest of the limbic system, including the amygdala, to the hypothalamus and autonomic nervous system for cortical control of emotional behavior.

Lesions of the hippocampus and anterior temporal lobe (such as mesial temporal sclerosis) are particularly high risk for causing seizures.

16.7 Internal Capsule

The internal capsule contains the input and output pathways between the cerebral cortex and the rest of the central nervous system (CNS). These include the sensory pathways that run from the thalamus to the cortex and the motor pathways

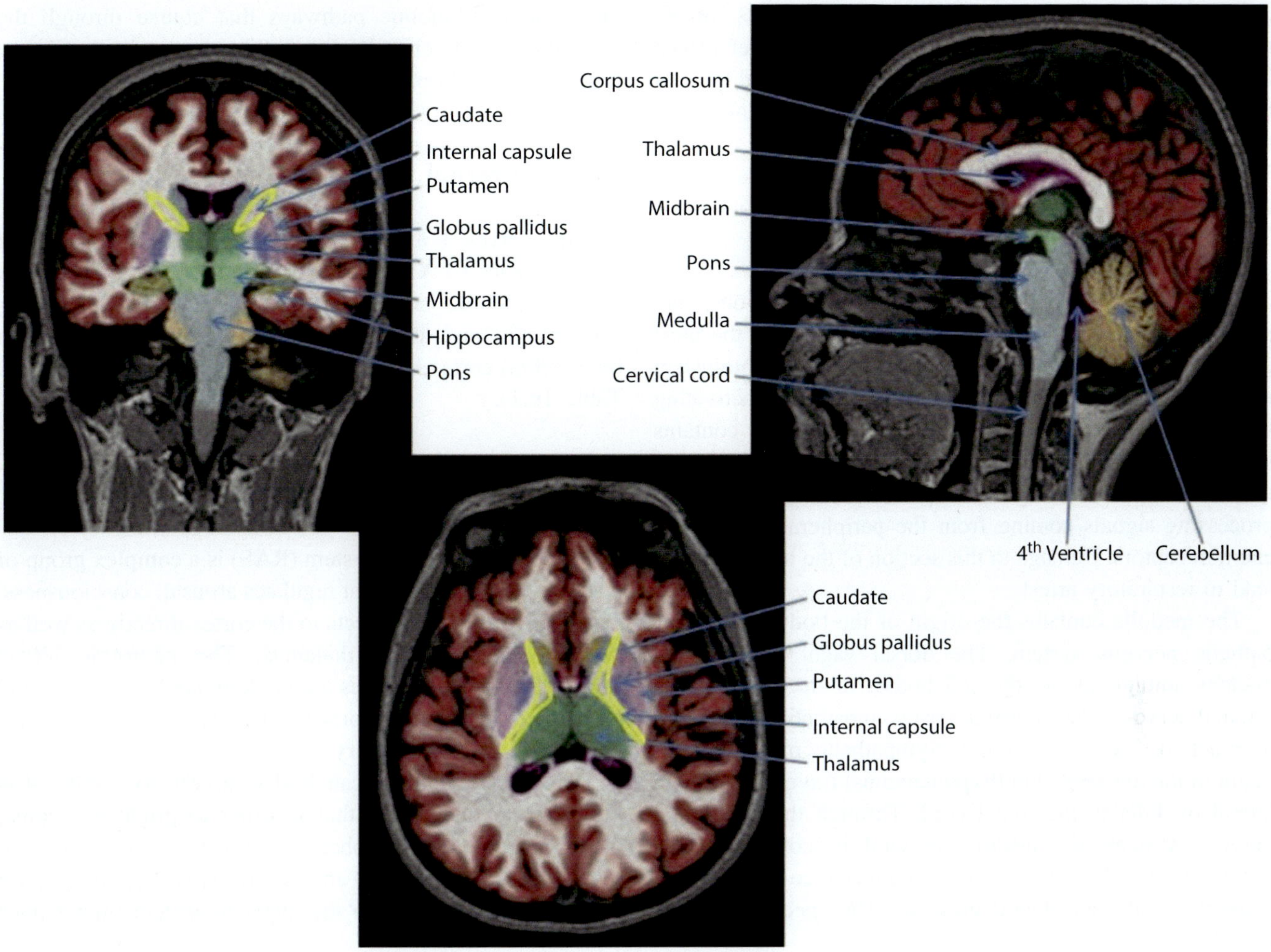

Fig. 16.3 Subcortical structures

that run from the primary motor cortex to the brainstem and spinal cord.

Patients with old strokes causing hemiparesis have damage to the corticospinal tracts. These patients are prone to hyperkalemia with depolarizing neuromuscular blockade (succinylcholine). When monitoring twitch count intraoperatively to titrate neuromuscular blockers, the monitor should be placed on the normal (non-paretic) limb as the paretic limb tends to be more resistant to non-depolarizing neuromuscular blockers (and leads you to give excessive doses).

16.8 Cerebellum

The cerebellum is located in the posterior cranial fossa (inferior to the occipital lobe of the cortex and dorsal to the brainstem). It is separated from the cortex by the tentorium cerebelli. It plays a vital role in motor coordination, posture, and balance. Functionally, the cerebellum can be divided into three components: cerebrocerebellum, vestibulocerebellum, and spinocerebellum.

The cerebrocerebellum includes the lateral aspects of the cerebellum that receive input from the cerebral cortex. It is involved in the planning of complex motor actions. The vestibulocerebellum includes the flocculonodular lobe of the cerebellum, and it receives input from the vestibular system. Its purpose is to control equilibrium. The spinocerebellum includes the vermis and intermediate hemispheres. The vermis receives somatosensory input from the head and proximal parts of the body to maintain posture, muscle tone, and control of the proximal muscles of the body and limbs. The intermediate parts of the hemispheres receive somatosensory input from the limbs to control the distal muscles of the limbs.

Note that damage to the cerebellum results in movement and balance problems ipsilateral to the site of the lesion. A cerebellar hematoma or edema can impose mass effect on the brainstem due to its close proximity to this structure. Moreover, cerebellar edema may compress the 4th ventricle, causing rapidly fatal obstructive hydrocephalus unless relieved with external ventricular drainage (catheter placed into the lateral ventricle through the skull and frontal lobe) or direct surgical decompression (suboccipital craniectomy removing bone from behind the cerebellum).

16.9 Brain Stem

The brain stem is divided into the midbrain, pons, and medulla and is responsible for controlling some of the most critical functions in the body (◉ Fig. 16.3). The brainstem maintains consciousness through the reticular activating system (discussed later). Moreover, the brainstem contains respiratory control centers (located in the medulla and pons) that are responsible for generating a respiratory rhythm and processing signals coming from the peripheral and central chemoreceptors. Damage to this section of the brainstem can lead to respiratory arrest.

The medulla contains the origin of the body's parasympathetic nervous system. The dorsal vagal nucleus and nucleus ambiguous are the cell bodies of the vagus nerve (cranial nerve X) that contribute parasympathetic innervation to much of the human body. Sympathetic pathways that begin in the diencephalon (hypothalamus) travel through the lateral medulla to the spinal cord. Through the autonomic nervous system, the medulla is vital in controlling the functions critical to life, including maintenance of heart rate, respiratory rate, and blood pressure. The specific sensory, motor, and autonomic pathways that course through the brainstem are described later in this chapter in the Spinal Cord Tracts section.

16.10 Cranial Nerves

Cranial nerves I and II arise from the cerebrum, while cranial nerves III-XII exit the brainstem. The cranial nerves control functions critical for survival and contain the sensory, motor, and autonomic pathways that travel between the cerebral cortex, cerebellum, and the rest of the body (◉ Table 16.1).

16.11 Reticular Activating System

The reticular activating system (RAS) is a complex group of nuclei in the brainstem that regulates arousal, consciousness, and sleep. The RAS projects to the cortex directly as well as indirectly through the thalamus. The neurotransmitters involved in these processes are predominantly serotonin and norepinephrine. Stimuli come from somatosensory, auditory, visual, and visceral sensory systems.

Damage to the RAS can lead to a comatose state. It is important to understand that in order to produce a coma, there must be bi-hemispheric dysfunction (such as from sedative agents, seizures, anoxic injury, or hypoglycemia); or damage to the RAS in the upper brainstem (upper pons

Table 16.1 Cranial nerves

Cranial nerve	Origin	Function
CN I (Olfactory)	Cerebrum	Smell
CN II (Optic)	Cerebrum	Vision
CN III (Oculomotor)	Midbrain	Motor to eye and eyelid; Pupil constriction
CN IV (Trochlear)	Midbrain	Motor to eye
CN V (Trigeminal)	Pons	Sensation of touch, taste; motor to lower jaw; cranial pain sensation
CN VI (Abducens)	Pons	Motor to eye
CN VII (Facial)	Pons/Pontomedullary junction	Sensation of taste; motor to muscles of facial expression; tearing; salivation
CN VIII (Vestibulocochlear)	Pontomedullary junction/Medulla	Hearing, balance, and equilibrium
CN IX (Glossopharyngeal)	Medulla	Sensation of taste, salivation; Motor to swallowing muscles
CN X (Vagus)	Medulla	Sensation of taste; sensory, motor, and autonomic functions of viscera (gastric secretion and movement, cardiac reflex, respiratory reflex)
CN XI (Accessory)	Medulla	Motor to trapezius and sternocleidomastoid
CN XII (Hypoglossal)	Medulla	Motor control of tongue

and midbrain) or diencephalon (hypothalamus or thalamus), such as from acute basilar artery occlusion. A unilateral lesion or tumor, in and of itself, will NOT produce coma.

16.11.1 Cerebral Blood Flow

Cerebral blood flow (CBF) varies in different parts of the brain depending on regional differences in metabolic activity because of a coupling mechanism between flow and metabolism. There is an intrinsic capability of the brain to deliver more blood flow to regions that have increased metabolic activity to match the heightened demand. Overall, the total CBF average is ~ 50 mL/100 g brain tissue/minute. CBF comprises approximately 15–20% of the cardiac output.

Decreased CBF rates are associated with cerebral impairment (20–25 mL/100 gbrain tissue/min), isoelectric electroencephalogram (EEG) (15–20 mL/100 g brain tissue/min), and irreversible brain damage (CBF < 10 mL/100 g brain tissue/min).

CBF is affected by the following parameters: cerebral metabolic rate, cerebral perfusion pressure, CO_2 reactivity ($PaCO_2$), O_2 reactivity (PaO_2), autoregulation, temperature, and anesthetic medications. Cerebral oximetry and EEG monitored over the frontal lobes (forehead; ◉ Fig. 16.4) are used as surrogates for CBF, which cannot be measured directly in the operating room with current technology. EEG can be used to derive depth of anesthesia data. Most commonly this involves signal processing to derive a numeric depth of anesthesia variable, but can be analyzed in its raw format or with density spectral arrays. The electroencephalogram (EEG) detects brain electrical activity recorded at the scalp, while electrocorticography (eCOG; used e.g., in epilepsy surgery) measures brain electrical activity recorded directly from the surface of the brain. ◉ Figures 16.5, 16.6, 16.7, 16.8, 16.9, and 16.10 show various examples of EEG and eCOG. Cerebral ischemia and anesthetics both cause slowing of the EEG and must be interpreted in the context of the clinical situation.

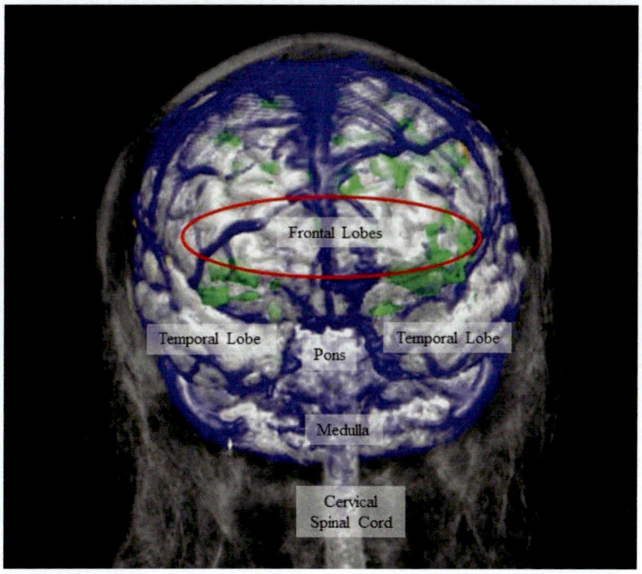

Fig. 16.4 Red ellipse notes area covered by processed electroencephalogram (EEG) and cerebral oximetry monitors. Major cerebral veins and sinuses appear *blue* in this fMRI image. *Green* areas represent areas of increased blood flow (i.e., increased metabolic activity causing coupled increases in blood flow) during functional MRI testing

16.12 Effects of Perfusion Pressure, pH, $PaCO_2$, PaO_2, & Cerebral Metabolic Rate for O_2

16.12.1 Perfusion Pressure

CBF is equal to the cerebral perfusion pressure (CPP) divided by the cerebral vascular resistance (CVR). CPP is the mean arterial pressure (MAP) minus the intracranial pressure (ICP), or central venous pressure (CVP), whichever is greater (◉ Fig. 16.11; ◘ Box 16.1). Normal CPP is 80–100 mm Hg and is primarily dependent on MAP given the generally low values of ICP and CVP. Normal adult ICP values range from 0 to 15 mm Hg; ICP is zero or negative in the normal patient in a sitting or standing position. Generally, 20 mm Hg is the threshold for treating pathologically elevated ICP.

CPP below the lower limit of cerebral autoregulation can lead to cerebral ischemia. This is generally thought to be < 60 mm Hg, whether due to decreased MAP or increased ICP. However, it is essential to remember that there is considerable inter-individual variability and that blood pressure goals intraoperatively should be chosen after consideration of the patient's baseline blood pressure. For patients with pathologically elevated ICP, CPP should generally be kept $\geq$ 60 mm Hg. Within normotensive blood pressure variations, CBF is maintained due to autoregulation of the CVR.

◘ **Box 16.1** CBF = CPP/CVR
CPP = MAP − ICP (or CVP)

CBF: cerebral blood flow
CPP: cerebral perfusion pressure
CVR: cerebral vascular resistance
MAP: mean arterial pressure
ICP: intracranial pressure
CVP: central venous pressure

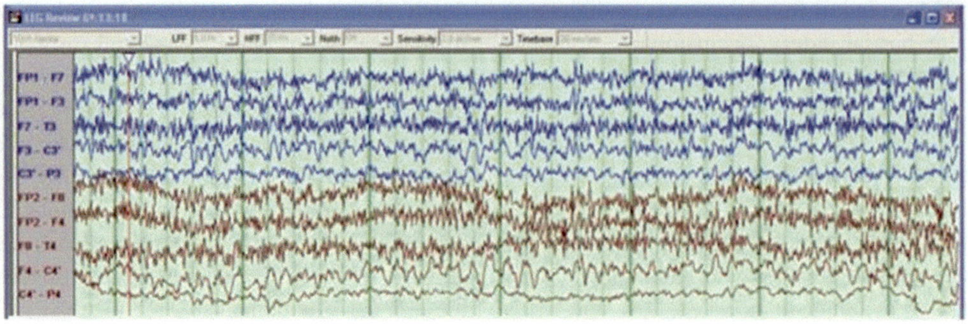

Fig. 16.5 Scalp electroencephalography (EEG) obscured by noise (usually due to muscle/EMG or electrocautery) (Courtesy of Biotronic Neuronetworks)

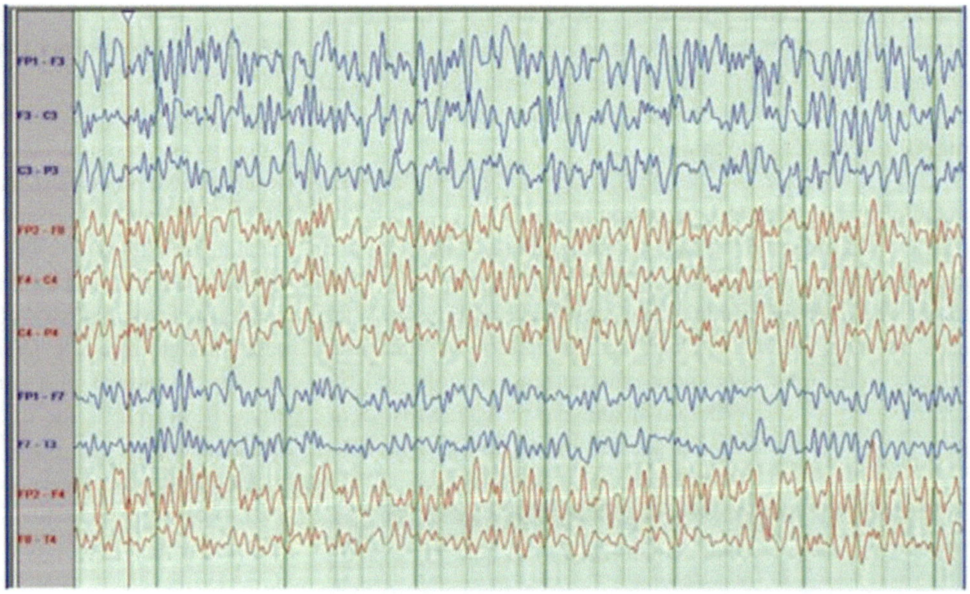

Fig. 16.6 Scalp electroencephalography (EEG)—normal (Courtesy of Biotronic Neuronetworks)

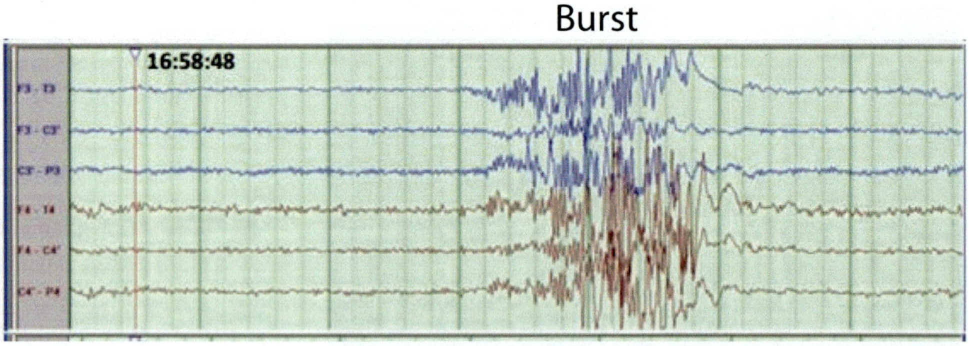

Fig. 16.7 Scalp electroencephalography (EEG) showing 6 channels (3 left and 3 right). Burst suppression pattern is seen (Courtesy of Biotronic Neuronetworks)

16.12.1.1 *$PaCO_2$ and pH*

$PaCO_2$ is the most significant extrinsic factor affecting CBF (◉ Fig. 16.11). Changes in pH and $PaCO_2$ can quickly alter CBF by changing CVR: Hypercapnia/acidosis increases CBF and hypocapnia/alkalosis decreases CBF. CBF changes 1–2 ml/100 g brain tissue/min per mm Hg $PaCO_2$ change between $PaCO_2$ 20–80 mm Hg. Hyperventilation is a very effective measure to help reduce cerebral blood

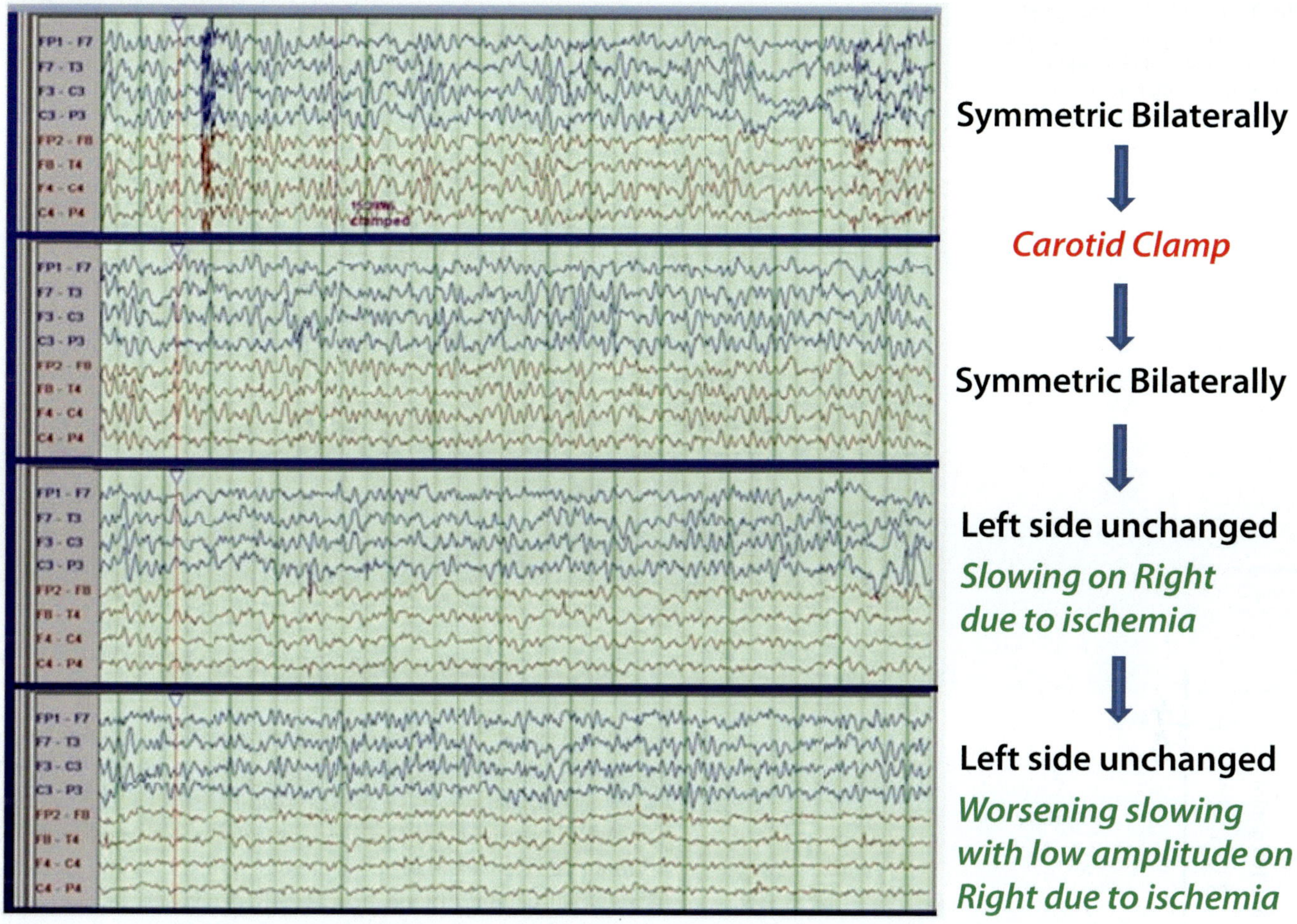

Fig16.8 Scalp electroencephalography (EEG) at 4 time periods following R carotid occlusion during endarterectomy. EEG from the left is in purple (1st 4 channels), and EEG from the right is in red (2nd 4 channels) (Courtesy of Biotronic Neuronetworks)

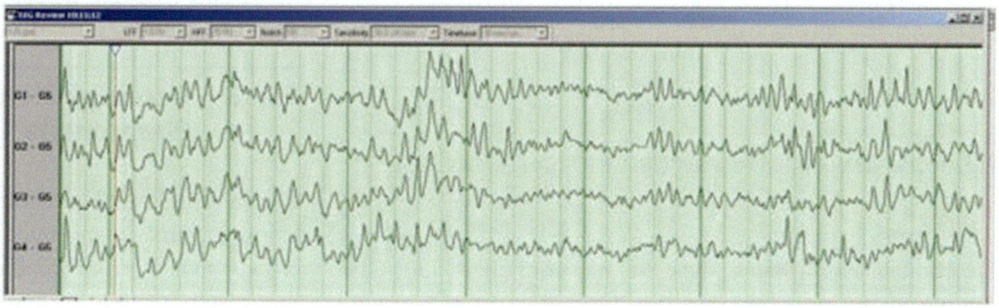

Fig. 16.9 Electrocorticography (ECoG) is EEG recorded directly from surface of brain. Here, you see 4 channels showing normal brain waves (Courtesy of Biotronic Neuronetworks)

volume in a patient with elevated ICP. However, excessive hyperventilation can lead to critically low CBF and cause cerebral ischemia. The effect of hyperventilation wanes with time so it is best used as an acute rescue modality for patients with elevated ICP. In operative neurosurgery, hyperventilation is used to control brain bulk (target $PaCO_2 \sim 30$ mm Hg) as needed and normocapnia is restored subsequently.

During acute metabolic acidosis, the increased hydrogen ions (H^+) cannot readily cross the blood–brain barrier (BBB), so it does not acutely affect CSF pH. However, with acute respiratory acidosis, an increase in $PaCO_2$ can quickly impact the CSF pH since the CO_2 can readily diffuse across the BBB. CSF bicarbonate takes up to 6 h to equilibrate across the blood–brain barrier to compensate for the pH change from the $PaCO_2$ changes. Once CSF

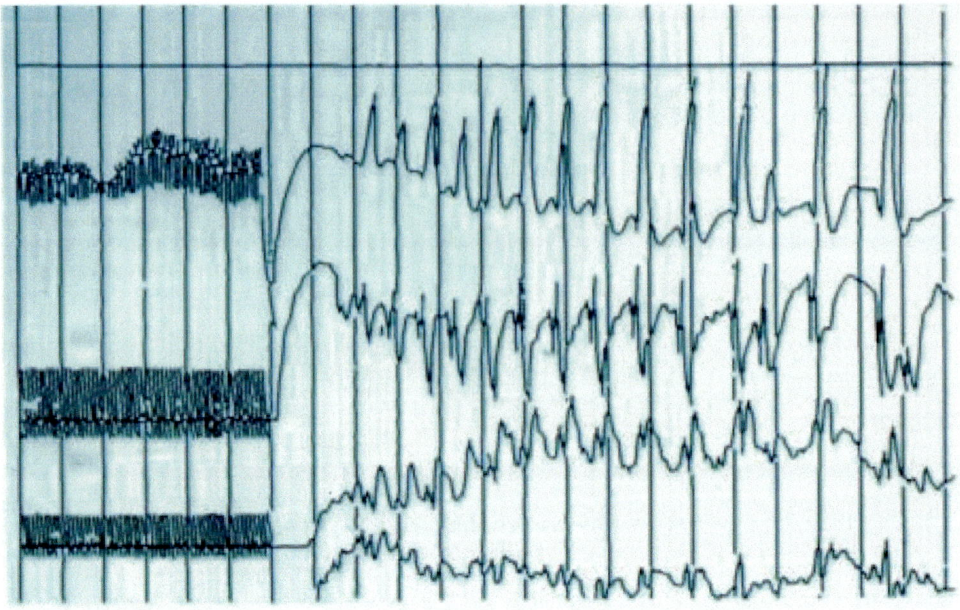

Fig. 16.10 Electrocorticography (ECoG). Here, you see 4 channels with initial stimulation artifact followed by "after discharges" (electrically induced seizures) (Courtesy of Biotronic Neuronetworks)

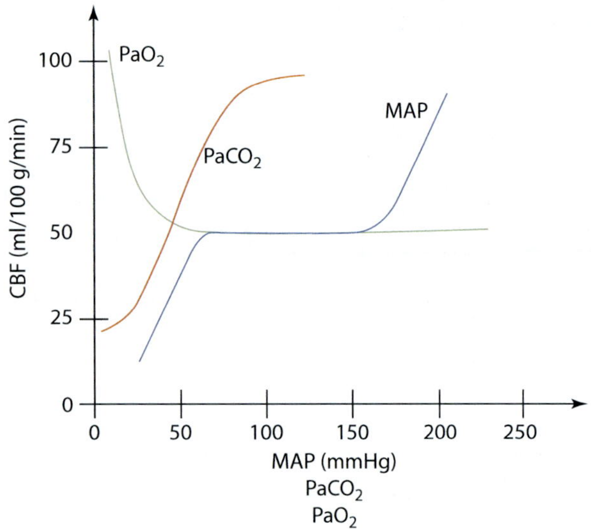

Fig. 16.11 Relationship between CBF, PaO_2, $PaCO_2$, and MAP

bicarbonate equilibrates, the CSF pH normalizes and CBF returns to the previous rate (i.e., the effect of hyperventilation wanes).

16.12.2 *PaO_2*

Extremes in PaO_2 can alter CBF (◉ Fig. 16.11). Hypoxemia ($PaO_2 < 50$ mm Hg) significantly increases CBF; however, hyperoxia ($PaO_2 > 300$ mm Hg) only slightly decreases CBF. The neurohumoral mechanisms for these effects are not well understood.

16.12.3 *Cerebral Metabolic Rate for O_2*

The concept of flow-metabolism coupling in the brain reflects the relationship between CBF and the cerebral metabolic rate for O_2 ($CMRO_2$) (◉ Fig. 16.11). The average $CMRO_2$ is 3–3.5 ml O_2/100 g brain/min. Elevated regional brain activity leads to local increases in CMR that increase regional cerebral blood flow. CMR decreases during sleep, comatose states, and hypothermia; CMR increases with seizure activity and hyperthermia. Hypothermia reduces CMR and decreases CBF by ~ 7% for every 1 °C reduction in body temperature. The effects of anesthetic agents on CMR and CBF are discussed later.

16.13 Cerebral Steal and Inverse Steal Phenomena

The cerebral steal phenomenon takes place when vasodilation occurs in normal regions of the brain, shunting blood away from pathologic regions with impaired vasoreactivity that are already vulnerable to ischemia (i.e., the 'reverse Robin Hood effect'). This can be relevant with hypercapnia and/or high concentrations (> 1 MAC) of volatile anesthetics. Inverse steal, also known as the Robin Hood effect, is the phenomenon where cerebral perfusion to pathologic regions increases. Hypocapnia can induce vasoconstriction in normal tissue, thereby increasing blood flow to the otherwise ischemic pathologic regions. The clinical relevance of both phenomena is unclear due to the inability to continuously measure regional cerebral blood flow.

16.14 Gray Versus White Matter

While the average CBF is ~ 50 ml/100 g brain tissue/min for the entire brain, gray matter has 4 times more CMR and CBF than white matter. Due to the inherent coupling mechanism between flow and metabolism, the CBF in the cortical gray matter is about 80 ml/100 g brain tissue/min while the CBF in the subcortical white matter is about 20 ml/100 g brain tissue/min (◘ Box 16.2).

> ◘ **Box 16.2** Average CBF = 50 ml/100 g Brain tissue/min
>
> - Gray matter CBF = 80 ml/100 g brain tissue/min
> - White matter CBF = 20 ml/100 g brain tissue/min

16.15 Autoregulation

16.15.1 Normal

Several organ systems in the body have autoregulatory capabilities, such as the brain, heart, kidneys, and spinal cord. This is an inherent, protective mechanism where an organ can adjust its vascular resistance to maintain a normal blood flow despite changing perfusion pressure. However, this only takes place when in a specific blood pressure range (◉ Fig. 16.12). For instance, in a normal brain, autoregulation takes place when within certain blood pressure (BP) parameters (e.g., MAP 60–150 mm Hg). While in this BP range, the CVR will automatically adjust, by vasodilating or vasoconstricting cerebral arterioles, in order to maintain a consistent CBF. The BP range for autoregulation has classically been designated as being between 50 and 150 mm Hg; however, this BP range in normal patients is now being challenged with consideration being given to raising the average lower limit of autoregulation to a higher value (60–80 mm Hg). Ultimately, what is clinically needed is a point-of-care continuous cerebral blood flow monitor.

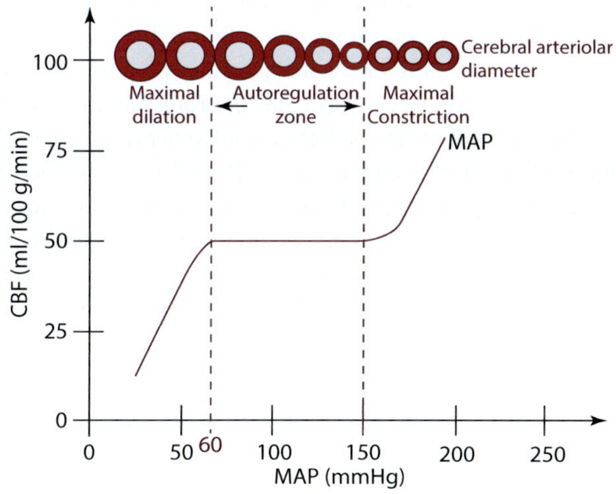

Fig. 16.12 Cerebral blood flow (CBF) autoregulation normally occurs between mean arterial pressure (MAP) ~ 60–150 mm Hg. Within these blood pressure limits, cerebral vascular resistance will automatically adjust by vasodilating or vasoconstricting cerebral arterioles in order to maintain a consistent CBF. Cerebral vascular tone (resistance) is maximally dilated below lower limit of CBF autoregulation and maximally constricted above upper limit of CBF autoregulation

CBF normalizes within seconds in patients with normal autoregulation, but those with impaired autoregulation can have a delayed response on the order of minutes or not at all. So, within the range of blood pressures at which autoregulation occurs, a rapid change in arterial pressure can lead to a brief period of hyperperfusion (with sudden hypertension) or hypoperfusion (with sudden hypotension) until the autoregulation takes place. Cerebral autoregulation is hypothesized to be due to a combination of myogenic and autonomic mechanisms. The myogenic mechanism involves the vascular smooth muscle of cerebral arterioles to respond to changes in MAP. The autonomic mechanism involves cerebral metabolic demands and neurogenic changes to determine cerebral arteriolar tone. With low or high MAPs (below 60 mm Hg or above 150 mm Hg), CVR (vessel tone) is either maximally dilated or constricted, respectively. Therefore, CBF becomes pressure-dependent and is directly/linearly related to CPP. At the low end, cerebral ischemia ensues; at the high end, cerebral hyperperfusion and subsequent BBB injury → edema → hemorrhage may occur.

16.15.2 Altered and Abolished

The most common cause of altered autoregulation occurs with chronic hypertension (◉ Fig. 16.13). With chronic hypertension, the limits of autoregulation are shifted to the right, which increases the lower limit and the upper limit of the autoregulatory zone. The changes with autoregulation allow for more cerebral protection on the high end, with stable cerebral blood flows at higher arterial pressures.

Other causes of altered or abolished autoregulation can be due to space occupying brain lesions (tumors, hematomas), stroke (ischemic, hemorrhagic, aneurysmal subarachnoid hemorrhage), traumatic brain injury, extreme hypertension (acute hypertensive encephalopathy, eclampsia, and posterior reversible encephalopathy syndrome [PRES]), long-term diabetes mellitus, and inhalational anesthetics (in concentrations greater than 1 MAC). When autoregulation is abolished, the CBF is entirely dependent on MAP (pressure-dependent).

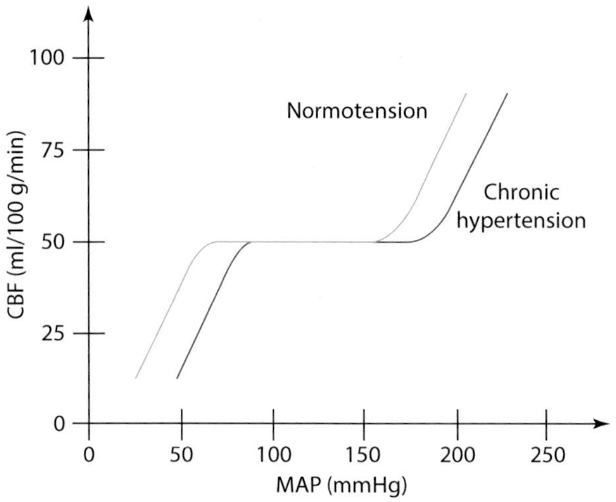

Fig. 16.13 Untreated chronic hypertension shifts cerebral blood flow autoregulation curve to right

16.16 Pathophysiology of Ischemia/Hypoxia

16.16.1 Global Versus Focal

The two types of ischemic brain injury are global and focal. Global ischemia takes place when both cerebral hypoxia and circulatory arrest occur. Focal ischemia occurs with arterial occlusion or edema/trauma/compression that causes regional areas of inadequate blood flow, such as stroke and traumatic brain injury. Both types of ischemic brain injury can result in cytotoxic edema with irreversible cell death and tissue infarction.

Reperfusion injury can occur after restoration of blood supply to ischemic tissue, following endovascular thrombectomy for stroke as an example. When CBF falls within 6–15 ml/100 g brain tissue/min in certain brain regions, these regions are referred to as ischemic penumbra. This term is used to describe 'stunned' brain tissue with reversible neuronal dysfunction if flow is restored in a timely matter.

16.16.2 Glucose Effects

Cerebral/neuronal function is dependent on a continuous supply of glucose for aerobic metabolism. Acute hypoglycemia can injure the brain. Hyperglycemia can exacerbate global and focal hypoxic brain injury, as well as the reperfusion phase after an ischemic insult, by accelerating cerebral acidosis and tissue damage. For this reason, it is optimal to maintain tight control of perioperative blood glucose levels while preventing iatrogenic hypoglycemia. Perioperative blood glucose levels are generally targeted in the 120–180 mg/dL range based on current evidence and guidelines.

16.16.3 Effects of Brain Trauma or Tumors

Both brain trauma and brain tumors can result in breakdown and increased permeability of the BBB, inflammatory damage to neurons, glia, and surrounding vasculature, cell death, and finally tissue infarction. Shear forces in brain trauma directly damage the brain, causing, among other injuries, cytotoxic edema. Brain tumors have considerable vasogenic edema causing inflammation by vascular space leakage of proteins, CSF flow obstruction, or venous obstruction. Vasogenic edema (i.e., from tumors) is responsive to corticosteroid therapy while cytotoxic edema is not.

16.16.4 Cerebrospinal Fluid

Cerebrospinal fluid is produced by the choroid plexus in the lateral, 3rd, and 4th ventricles, and is contained by the ependymal cells and blood–brain barrier. It bathes the CNS and provides a protective envelope for the brain and spinal cord.

16.17 Volume, Formation, Composition, Flow, and Pressure

In adults, the total volume of CSF at any given time is about 150 mL, with 500 ml of CSF being produced and reabsorbed every day at a rate of about 15–20 ml/h.

CSF is mainly formed in the ventricles by the ependymal cells of the choroid plexus. After formation, the active and passive transport of particles through the blood–brain barrier modifies the CSF composition to a solution that is isotonic to plasma, but with different concentrations of ions, proteins, and glucose. CSF flows from the choroid plexus into the lateral/3rd/4th ventricles, subarachnoid spaces, and then the cisterns of the subarachnoid space. The CSF is absorbed by the arachnoid granulations back into the venous bloodstream at the same rate as the fluid is produced. The brain was thought to have no lymphatic system, although current research is challenging this long-standing assertion. The glymphatic system consists of perivascular channels that are thought to be the "lymphatic system" of the brain.

Given the constraints of a rigid and closed calvarium, ICP and CSF pressures are in equilibrium. Normal mean ICP as well as correlating CSF pressure is 7–15 mm Hg in adults who are supine. Pressures of greater than 15 mm Hg are considered abnormal. ICP therapy is initiated at > 20 mm Hg. Elevation of the head is a method to reduce ICP; both by reducing hydrostatic pressure and venous blood volume.

CSF volume is most commonly increased by a blockage of CSF re-absorption, leading to increased ICP via communicating hydrocephalus. Blockage of CSF outflow from any of the ventricles is called obstructive hydrocephalus.

16.18 Blood–Brain Barrier

The blood–brain barrier (BBB) maintains the CSF composition to create a constant ambient environment for the CNS. The barrier consists of capillary endothelial cells that are connected by tight junctions, which generate resistance to the passage of ionized substances or large macromolecules, such as proteins. Non-ionized, lipid-soluble drugs penetrate the CSF and brain readily; ionized, non-lipid-soluble drugs enter the CSF and brain slowly unless facilitated by an active molecular transport system. Depending on their lipid solubility, drugs penetrate the blood–brain barrier in varying degrees.

16.18.1 Passive Molecular Transport

Passive molecular transport occurs by diffusion gradients from leaky epithelial tight junctions. Gradients between the blood, CSF, and intercellular spaces allow for water, non-ionized and lipid-soluble molecules, and gases, such as carbon dioxide, oxygen, and volatile anesthetics to pass through the blood–brain barrier freely.

16.18.2 Active Molecular Transport

The blood–brain barrier restricts movement of large-sized molecules (diameter > 20 angstroms), ionized and non-lipid-soluble compounds, proteins, glucose, and some electrolytes (such as sodium). These may only cross the blood–brain barrier with active molecular transport. Approximately 60% of the CSF is formed by active transport. Active molecular transport requires energy supplied by adenosine triphosphate (ATP) from the membrane Na^+-K^+ ATPase; thus, drugs that inhibit the ATPase pump will reduce CSF formation, such as digoxin. The term reflection coefficient is used to express the permeability of the BBB to a substance. For example, NaCl has a reflection coefficient of 1.0 (it does not get across an intact BBB), which makes it a good hyperosmotic agent for reducing brain water/bulk.

16.18.3 Causes of Disruption

Any cause of inflammation or ischemia, such as irradiation, sustained seizures, infection, strokes, tumors, or trauma, can disrupt the BBB. Prolonged hypercapnia, hypoxia, or osmotic shock can also increase permeability of the BBB and allow substances that are typically excluded to enter the brain and CSF.

16.19 Relation to Blood Chemistry and Acid–Base Balance

The osmolality is the same for CSF and blood: both ~ 289 mOsmol/kg H_2O. However, the concentrations of individual electrolytes and other molecules differ between the CSF and blood. The pH of CSF is primarily determined by the partial pressure of CO_2 and serum bicarbonate concentration. The BBB is freely permeable to gases, such as CO_2, while bicarbonate takes hours to reach a steady state and alter the pH of CSF. Due to the pCO_2 in CSF being ~ 6 mm Hg higher than arterial blood, the pH of CSF is ~ 7.3. Changes in pCO_2 can rapidly change the pH in the CSF as noted previously. Keep in mind that serum H^+ is not freely permeable through the blood–brain barrier and does not contribute significantly to the CSF pH.

16.19.1 Cerebral Protection

The goal of cerebral protection is to reduce neuronal injury from brain tissue ischemia. This is accomplished through manipulating oxygen supply and demand by increasing cerebral perfusion pressure and reducing cerebral metabolism. Avoidance of hypotension, hypoxia, and hypercapnia improves oxygen supply and demand balance. Hypothermia and anesthetic and adjuvant drugs are being studied regarding their ability to impart cerebral protection intraoperatively.

Direct cerebral/CNS protectants are therapies that act on the brain or spinal cord to guard tissue from injury (such as hypothermia). Indirect cerebral/CNS protectants are therapies that *do not* act on brain or spinal cord tissue to guard tissue from injury (such as tissue plasminogen activator to lyse intra-arterial clots in the setting of acute ischemic stroke).

16.20 Hypothermia

Hypothermia decreases both cerebral metabolic rate and CBF, with both $CMRO_2$ and CBF decreasing ~ 6–7% per 1 °C decrease in temperature. Therapeutic hypothermia stands alone as the only direct neuroprotectant successfully translated from bench to bedside. It has proven efficacy in survivors of neonatal asphyxia and adult survivors of cardiac arrest. Therapeutic hypothermia or controlled normothermia remains standard of care for comatose (unable to be aroused to the point of following commands) survivors of cardiac

Table 16.2 Anesthetic and adjuvant drugs' effects on $CMRO_2$ and CBF

Anesthetics	$CMRO_2$	CBF	Neuroprotective effect against focal ischemia[a]
Barbiturates	Decrease	Decrease	Yes
Propofol	Decrease	Decrease	Yes
Etomidate	Decrease	Decrease	Unclear
Benzodiazepines	Slight decrease	Slight decrease	Minimal
Opiates	Slight decrease	Slight decrease	Minimal
Ketamine	Slight Increase	Increase	Yes
Non-depolarizing Muscular Blockers	No effect	No effect	No effect
Volatile Agents (< 1 MAC + Hyperventilation)	Decrease	No effect or slight increase	Yes
Volatile Agents (> 1 MAC)	Decrease	Increase	Yes

[a] Neuroprotective effect found against focal ischemia in *animal* models. There is currently *no* high-level human evidence for pharmacologic neuroprotection

arrest. The term targeted temperature management (TTM) is used to encompass controlled body temperature; either therapeutic hypothermia or controlled normothermia. Hyperthermia exacerbates brain or spinal cord injury and should be avoided.

Hypothermia is routinely used in the operating room for patients undergoing cardiac surgery on cardiopulmonary bypass. Similarly, deep hypothermia ($\sim$ 18 °C) is utilized as a neuroprotectant for patients undergoing aortic surgery requiring circulatory arrest. TTM should be used in the setting of neonatal asphyxia following delivery, as well as in the adult patient who has a global hypoxic-ischemic brain injury in the operating room (such as prolonged cardiac arrest) and does not promptly regain consciousness (arousable and able to follow commands) after anesthetic effects should have dissipated. Therapeutic hypothermia has no proven role (in humans) in focal ischemia, such as during temporary vessel occlusion for cerebral aneurysm surgery. It is utilized in some neurovascular centers for cerebral vessel bypass surgery requiring prolonged vessel occlusion and cerebral ischemia. It is not indicated for routine cerebral aneurysm surgery.

16.21 Anesthetic and Adjuvant Drugs

No anesthetic or adjuvant medication has been proven to be neuroprotective, either against global or focal ischemia, in humans (◉ Table 16.2). Pre-clinical/non-human evidence is abundant. Most intravenous anesthetic agents reduce cerebral metabolic rate and CBF. Halogenated inhalational agents (sevoflurane, desflurane, isoflurane) reduce cerebral metabolic rate without a proportionate reduction in CBF, since they are vasodilators. However, in animal models these agents demonstrate neuroprotective effects, often both during the cerebral insult as well as in a pre- or post-conditioning scenario (delivered either before or after the insult). Human data is insufficient to make recommendations regarding clinical practice.

Barbiturates, specifically thiopental, have been shown to be protective against the effects of focal ischemia in animal models, producing burst suppression (inducing near electrical silence of the EEG), and decreasing $CMRO_2$. Hemodynamic support is typically needed after barbiturate administration to counteract hypotension. Like barbiturates, propofol can produce burst suppression, decrease $CMRO_2$, decrease ICP, and maintain cerebral autoregulation. It has been shown to offer neuroprotective effects against mild ischemic insults in animal models. Etomidate has similar characteristics, but its neuroprotective effect is uncertain.

Benzodiazepines and, to a lesser extent, opiates can lower the $CMRO_2$ and CBF. But both these drugs have minimal effects in this regard when compared to barbiturates, propofol, and etomidate. Ketamine is the only intravenous agent that increases $CMRO_2$ and CBF. Studies are evaluating ketamine and cerebral protection given its glutamate antagonist activity at the NMDA receptor.

Non-depolarizing neuromuscular blockers do not have a significant effect on $CMRO_2$ or CBF. Although succinylcholine can transiently increase CBF and ICP, these effects are not considered clinically significant and should not negate its use when deemed clinically appropriate.

Volatile agents, while able to decrease $CMRO_2$ and produce electrical silence in the brain, uncouple flow/metabolism and can increase CBF and ICP since they are potent cerebral vasodilators. Importantly, CO_2 reactivity is preserved with inhalational and intravenous anesthetics. Thus, the degree of cerebral vasodilation can be temporarily attenuated by hyperventilation along with maintaining the volatile agent at < 1.0 MAC (typically ~ 0.5 MAC).

16.22 Spinal Cord

16.22.1 General Organization

The spinal cord starts at the base of the skull (foramen magnum) and extends down to taper into the conus medullaris, and becomes the filum terminale, at the level of L1–L2 vertebrae in adults (lower in children). Note that lumbar punctures and spinal anesthetics must be performed below this level (below L2 in adults).

The vertebral column surrounds and protects the spinal cord. The vertebral column contains 5 sections: cervical, thoracic, lumbar, sacral, and coccygeal. There are 7 cervical vertebrae, 12 thoracic vertebrae, and 5 lumbar vertebrae, 5 fused sacral vertebrae, and the coccyx.

Each section contains a spinal cord segment that has 4 nerve roots (2 on each side), with a pair of ventral and dorsal roots on the left side and another pair on the right side. The first cervical segment does not typically have dorsal roots. For each spinal segment, the ventral and dorsal nerve roots join together to exit the intervertebral foramina. The first 7 cervical nerve roots arise in the space *above* their respective vertebrae while all the nerve roots below cervical nerve root 8 arise *below* their respective vertebrae, starting with cervical nerve root 8, which arises below cervical vertebrae 7.

There are two enlargements along the spinal cord: (1) The cervical enlargement contains the cervical nerve roots that become the brachial plexus and control the upper extremities; and (2) the lumbar enlargement, which contains the nerve roots that become the lumbosacral plexus and control the lower extremities. At the inferior end of the lumbar enlargement is the conus medullaris (ending at the L1–L2 vertebral level in adults). The filum terminale extends inferiorly from the end of the conus medullaris. The cauda equina extends inferiorly below the spinal cord and contains the nerve roots L2–L5, S1–S5, and coccygeal nerves.

The spinal cord is surrounded by 3 membranes, which are also continuous with the brain. The outermost is the dura mater (epidural catheters are placed just above this membrane), followed by the arachnoid membrane, and the pia mater, which is immediately adjacent to the spinal cord. The epidural space exists between the dura and the ligamentum flavum. Between the dura and arachnoid layers is the subdural space, a potential space. Deep to the arachnoid is the subarachnoid space, which contains CSF. The pia mater contributes to the filum terminale, which extends to the coccyx to stabilize the spinal cord.

16.22.2 Spinal Reflexes

A typical spinal cord reflex involves a stimulated receptor in the periphery (usually tendon, muscle, or skin), sensory afferent nerve, spinal cord interneurons, and a motor efferent nerve. These reflex arcs cause a stereotypical motor response to a certain stimulus. The spinal cord reflexes help the clinician localize lesions in the nervous system. Keep in mind that many autonomic responses and motor responses to pain reside at a spinal level and do not require conscious arousal (e.g., hypertension following skin incision).

16.22.3 Spinal Cord Tracts

16.22.3.1 Ascending Sensory Pathways

Sensory receptors use the ascending sensory pathways to transmit signals to the brain. The dorsal column system transmits proprioception, fine touch, and 2-point discrimination. The pathways ascend ipsilaterally and decussate in the medulla. Clinically, somatosensory evoked potentials (SSEPs) travel in the dorsal columns.

The spinothalamic tract ascends contralaterally (near the spinal level of origin) and transmits sharp pain and temperature, while the spinoreticular pathway transmits deep and chronic pain signals. The dorsal spinocerebellar tract and ventral spinocerebellar tract transmit movement and position data to the brain.

16.22.3.2 Descending Pathways

Descending pathways travel from the cerebral cortex and brain stem to modulate movement, reflexes, and autonomic functions. The motor pathways are divided between pyramidal tracts and extrapyramidal tracts.

The pyramidal tracts include the corticospinal tract and corticobulbar (i.e., travel to the pons—the bulb) tract (◉ Figs. 16.14 and 16.15). The axons of both tracts arise from the primary motor cortex and premotor area. The neurons of the corticobulbar tract decussate (cross) throughout the brainstem and travel to the different motor cranial nerves. The neurons of the corticospinal tract decussate in the caudal medulla and descend as the lateral corticospinal tract to the lower motor neurons of the spinal cord—for coordinated voluntary movements (which originate from the contralateral hemisphere). Some of the axons do not decussate and instead descend along the anterior corticospinal tract to reach the lower motor neurons.

Extrapyramidal tracts include vestibulospinal, rubrospinal, reticulospinal, and tectospinal tracts. These tracts control movement, posture, reflexes, and autonomic function. The vestibulospinal system modulates postural reflexes. The rubrospinal affects movement. The reticulospinal tract

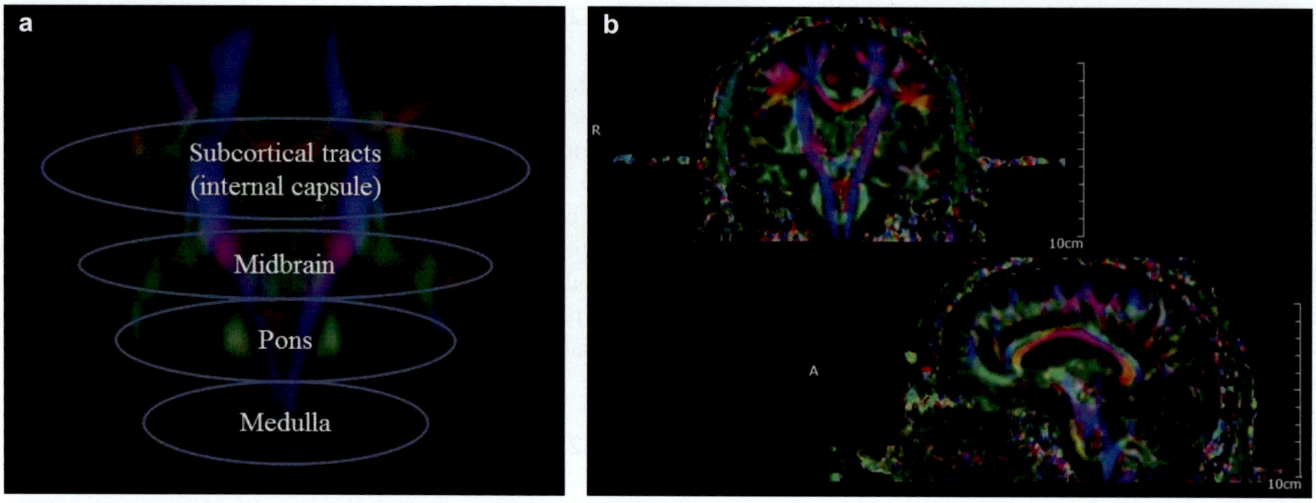

Fig. 16.14 Corticospinal tracts noted in *blue*, depicted by magnetic resonance diffusion tensor imaging. **a** Coronal view on left. **b** Coronal and sagittal views on right

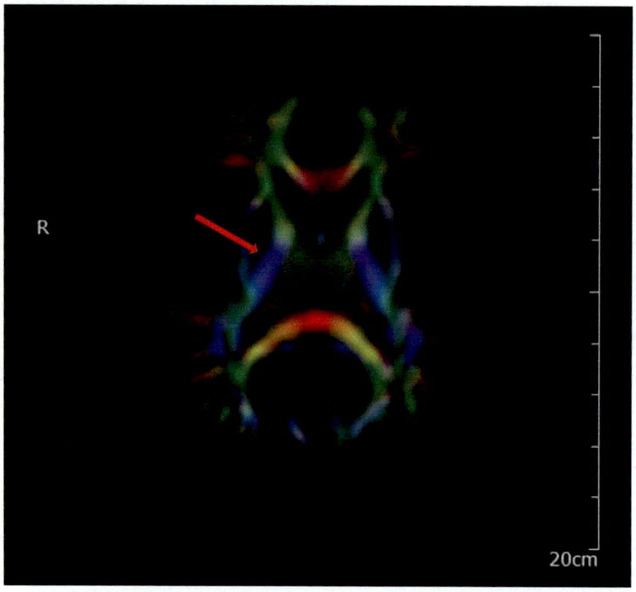

Fig. 16.15 Subcortical white matter tracts highlighted and depicted by diffusion tensor imaging. Axial mid-hemispheric view. Corticospinal tracts (*red arrow*) descend through posterior limb of internal capsule; seen in *blue/purple* just behind genu (*bend*) of internal capsule

modulates spinal reflexes. The tectospinal tracts cause reflex head movement in response to visual or auditory stimuli.

The medial longitudinal fasciculus (heavily myelinated tracts extending from the cervical spinal cord into the dorsal pons and midbrain) coordinates gaze and head movements with signals from the vestibular nuclei in the brainstem. The descending autonomic system arises from the hypothalamus and brain stem to control autonomic functions, including blood pressure and heart rate.

16.23 Evoked Potentials

Evoked potentials (EP) are the most commonly used neurophysiological monitors during neurosurgical procedures to detect ischemia/injury in the central nervous system. An evoked potential refers to the elicitation of a response following stimulation of the nervous system (central to peripheral or vice versa). The main types of evoked potentials are somatosensory, brainstem auditory, visual, and motor (◘ Box 16.3). These EPs monitor the integrity of the structures involved in a given sensory (visual, auditory, or somatic sensation) or motor pathway.

> ◘ **Box 16.3** Sensitivity to Anesthetics
> VEP > MEP > SSEP > BAEP.

The EP responses are measured in terms of *latency* (the time it takes for the stimulus to travel through the CNS and elicit a response; time to the start of the electrical wave) and *amplitude* (the magnitude of the response; the height of the electrical wave). The short-latency evoked potentials directly come from a stimulated nerve (such as brachial plexus response from median nerve stimulation) or from the brainstem. Intermediate- and long-latency evoked potentials come from the cerebral cortex. Neurologic injury typically results in prolonged latency and diminished amplitude. ◉ Table 16.3 outlines anesthetic effects on EPs.

Sensory EPs include somatosensory, brainstem auditory, and visual evoked potentials. A peripheral stimulus is applied and the EP is measured centrally to ensure that the signal transmits appropriately from the peripheral sensors,

Table 16.3 Anesthetic agent effects on motor evoked potentials, somatosensory evoked potentials, and brainstem auditory evoked potentials

Anesthetic agent	Motor evoked potentials (MEP)	Somatosensory evoked potentials (SSEP)	Brainstem auditory evoked potentials (BAEP)
Volatile anesthetics (Isoflurane, Sevoflurane, Desflurane)	↓↓ Amplitude	↓ Amplitude ↑ Latency	Negligible[a]
Nitrous oxide	↓↓ Amplitude	↓ Amplitude ↑ Latency	Negligible
Propofol	↓ Amplitude	↓ Amplitude ↑ Latency	Negligible
Etomidate	Negligible	↑ Amplitude ↑ Latency	Negligible
Ketamine	Negligible	↑ Amplitude	Negligible
Barbiturates	↓ Amplitude	Negligible	Negligible
Opioids	Negligible	Negligible	Negligible
Benzodiazepines	↓ Amplitude	Negligible ↑ Latency at higher doses	Negligible
Dexmedetomidine	Negligible or ↓ Amplitude	Negligible	Negligible
Neuromuscular blockers	↓ Amplitude	Negligible	Negligible

[a] Negligible at < 1 MAC concentrations

through the correspondent neurologic pathway, through the brainstem and to the sensory cortex (somatosensory–parietal lobe; auditory–temporal lobe; visual–occipital lobe).

Somatosensory evoked potentials (SSEPs) (◉ Figs. 16.16, 16.23, 16.24 and 16.25) monitor the functional integrity of the peripheral nerves (median nerve stimulation at the wrist; posterior tibial stimulation at the ankle), the spinal dorsal columns, subcortical structures, brainstem, thalamus, and primary sensory cortex (parietal lobe). After an electrical stimulus stimulates the peripheral nerve, evoked potentials are measured using electrodes on the scalp. SSEPs are used frequently during spinal surgery to ensure integrity of the spinal cord. SSEPs are somewhat sensitive to anesthetics. Volatile agents and nitrous oxide are suppressive, especially when administered at greater than 1.0 MAC. Intravenous anesthetics are less suppressive (ketamine actually improves SSEPs) and opiates have very minimal effects on SSEPs. Muscle relaxants do not impair SSEP signals. Rapid boluses or changes in anesthetic agents can cause disruption in EP signals.

Brainstem auditory evoked potentials (BAEPs) test the auditory pathways (◉ Figs. 16.17 and 16.18). The signals originate from the ear (external auditory canal) using a repetitive clicking sound. The response is assessed from scalp electrodes as the signal travels through cranial nerve VIII to the brainstem, lateral lemniscus, thalamus, and primary auditory cortex (temporal lobe). BAEPs are fairly resistant to most anesthetics, because only the subcortical signals are of clinical interest, and muscle relaxants do not impact signal transmission. These EPs are typically used in

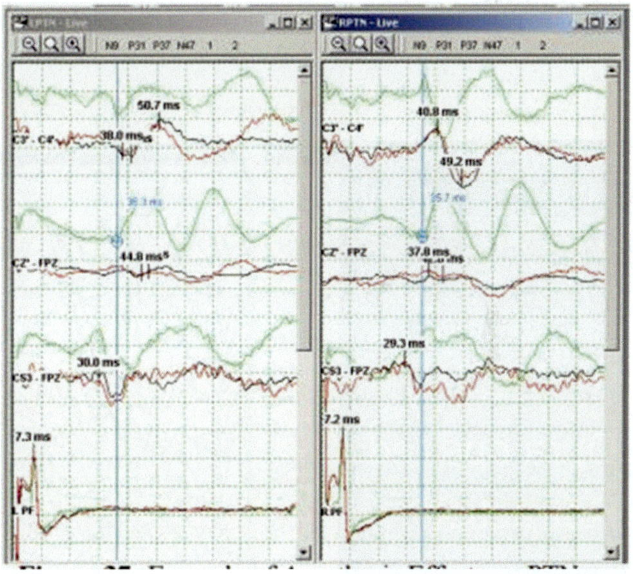

Fig. 16.16 Example of somatosensory evoked potentials (SSEPs) at posterior tibial nerve. Baseline tracing noted in *green*, and anesthetic effects noted in *red* and *black* (Courtesy of Biotronic Neuronetworks)

acoustic neuroma (cranial nerve VIII) resections and microvascular nerve decompressions of cranial nerves V or VII.

Visual evoked potentials (VEPs) test sensory input through the optic nerve (cranial nerve II) to the thalamus and subsequent transmission (via optic radiations) to the occipital cortex. The EPs can be useful in surgeries close to the optic nerve/chiasm or occipital cortex; however, they are

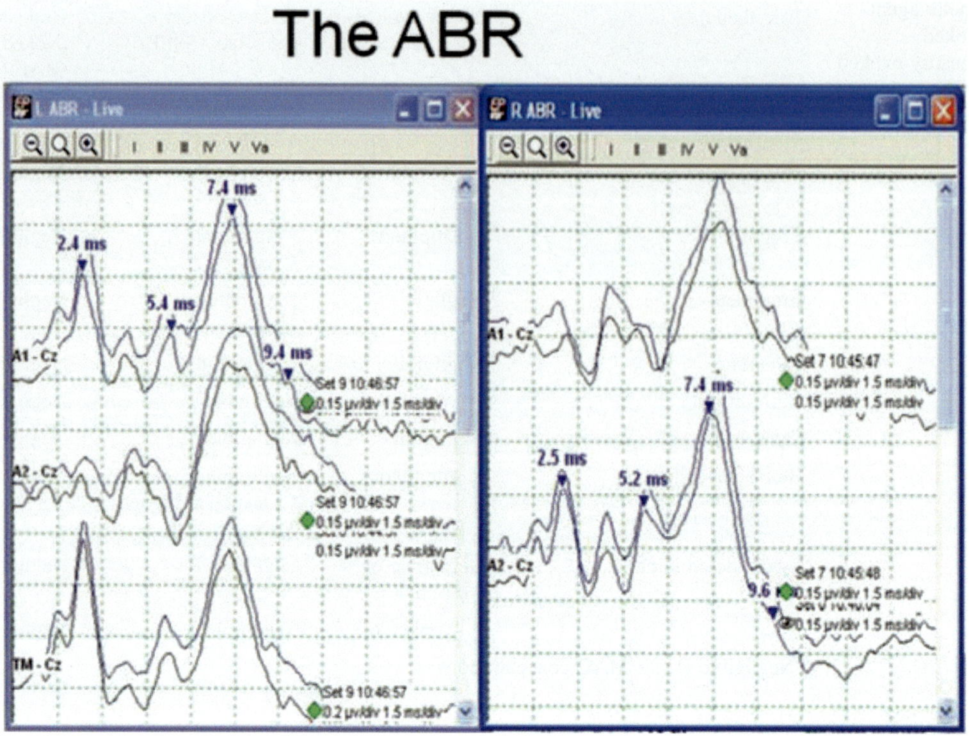

Fig. 16.17 Brainstem auditory evoked potentials or auditory brainstem responses (ABR) showing normal waveforms (designated I, II, III, IV, V) (Courtesy of Biotronic Neuronetworks)

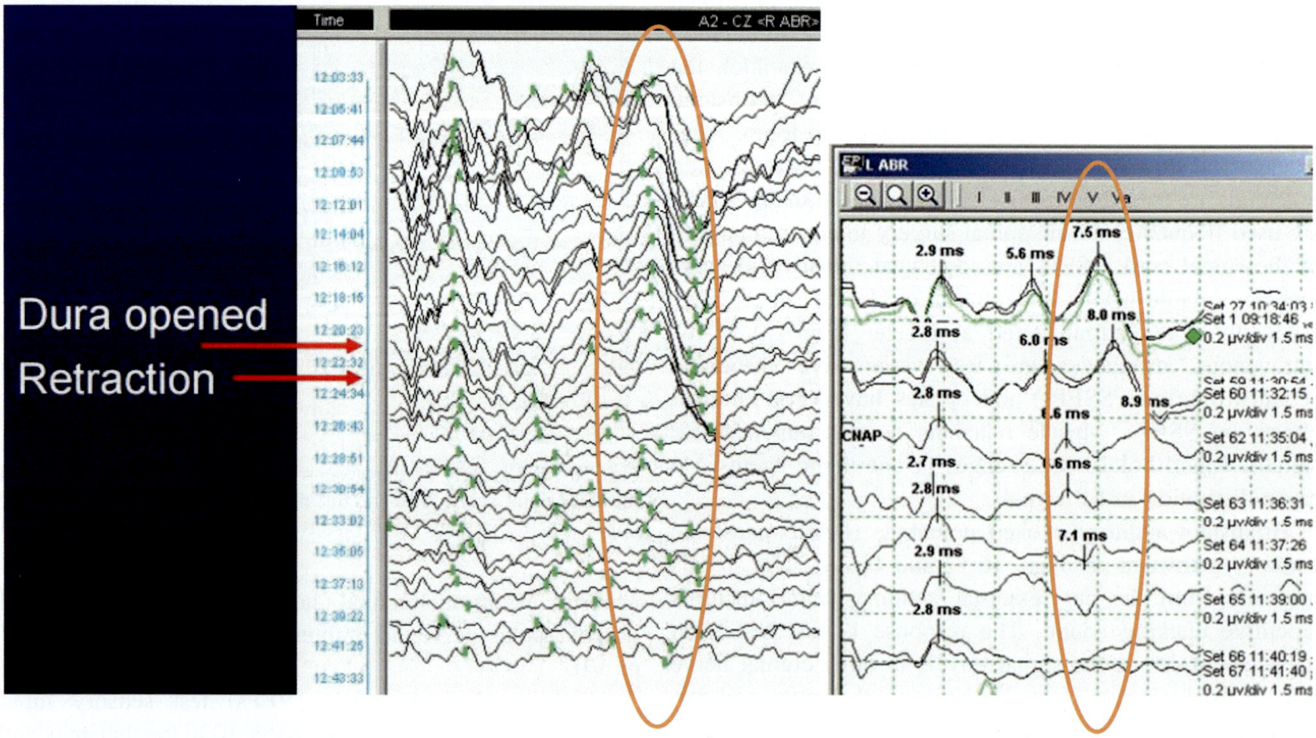

Fig. 16.18 Brainstem auditory evoked potentials showing loss of Wave V following brainstem retraction. Note that repetitive evoked potentials are stacked vertically with earliest recordings on top (Courtesy of Biotronic Neuronetworks)

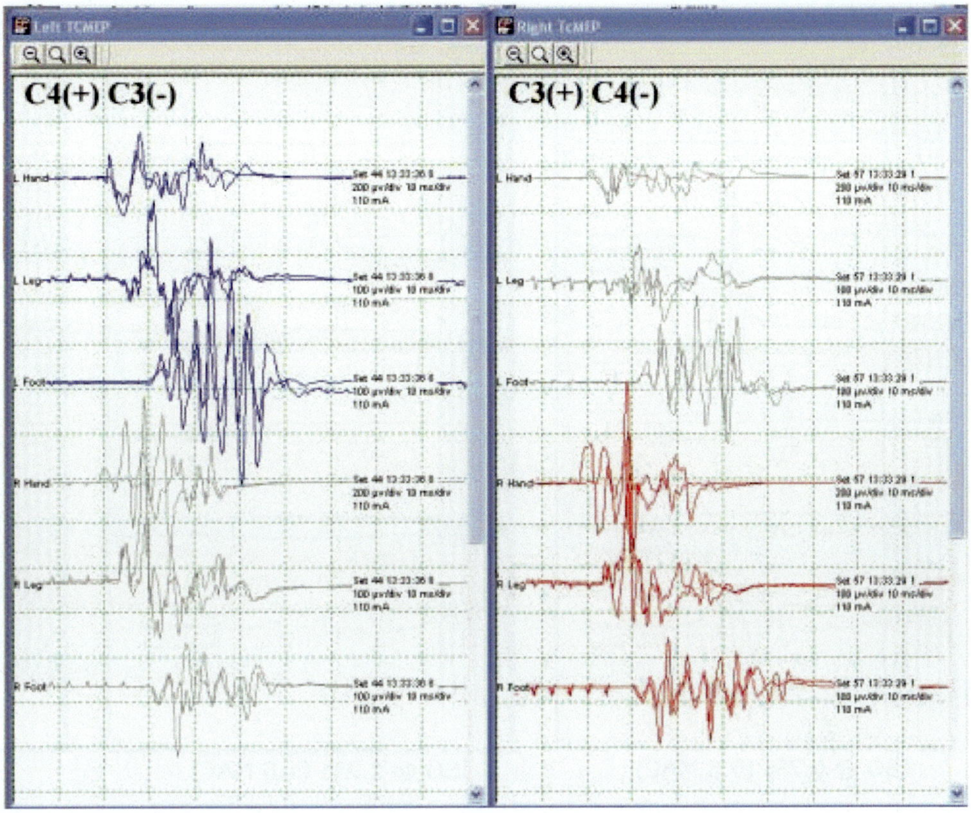

Fig. 16.19 Transcranial motor evoked potentials (TcMEPs): normal bilateral activation (Courtesy of Biotronic Neuronetworks)

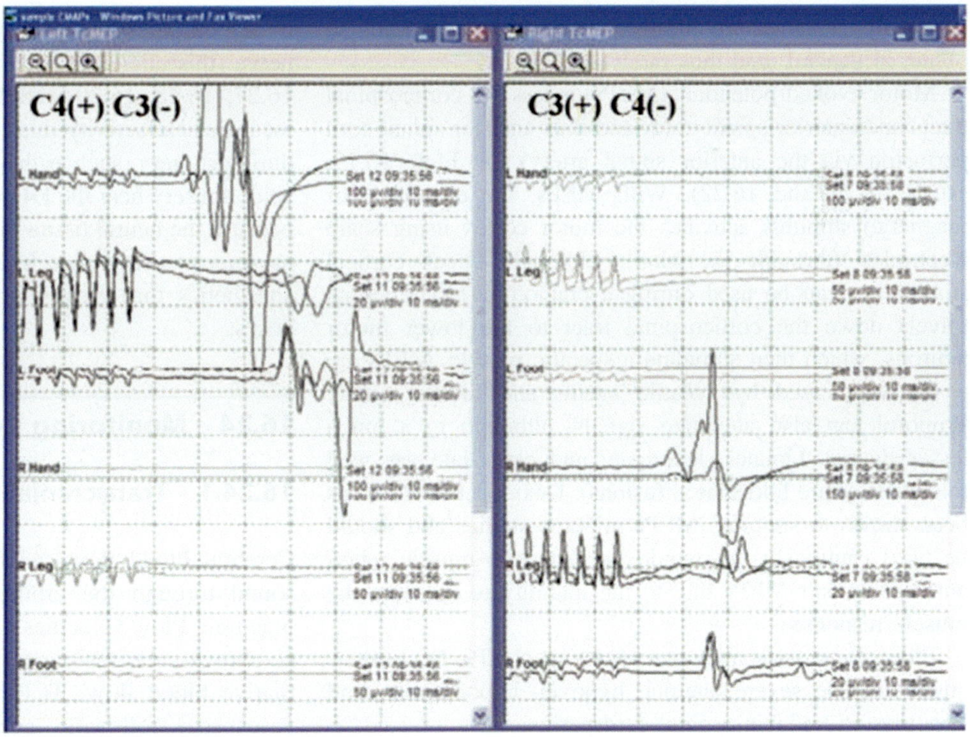

Fig. 16.20 Transcranial motor evoked potentials (TcMEPs): unilateral activation (Courtesy of Biotronic Neuronetworks)

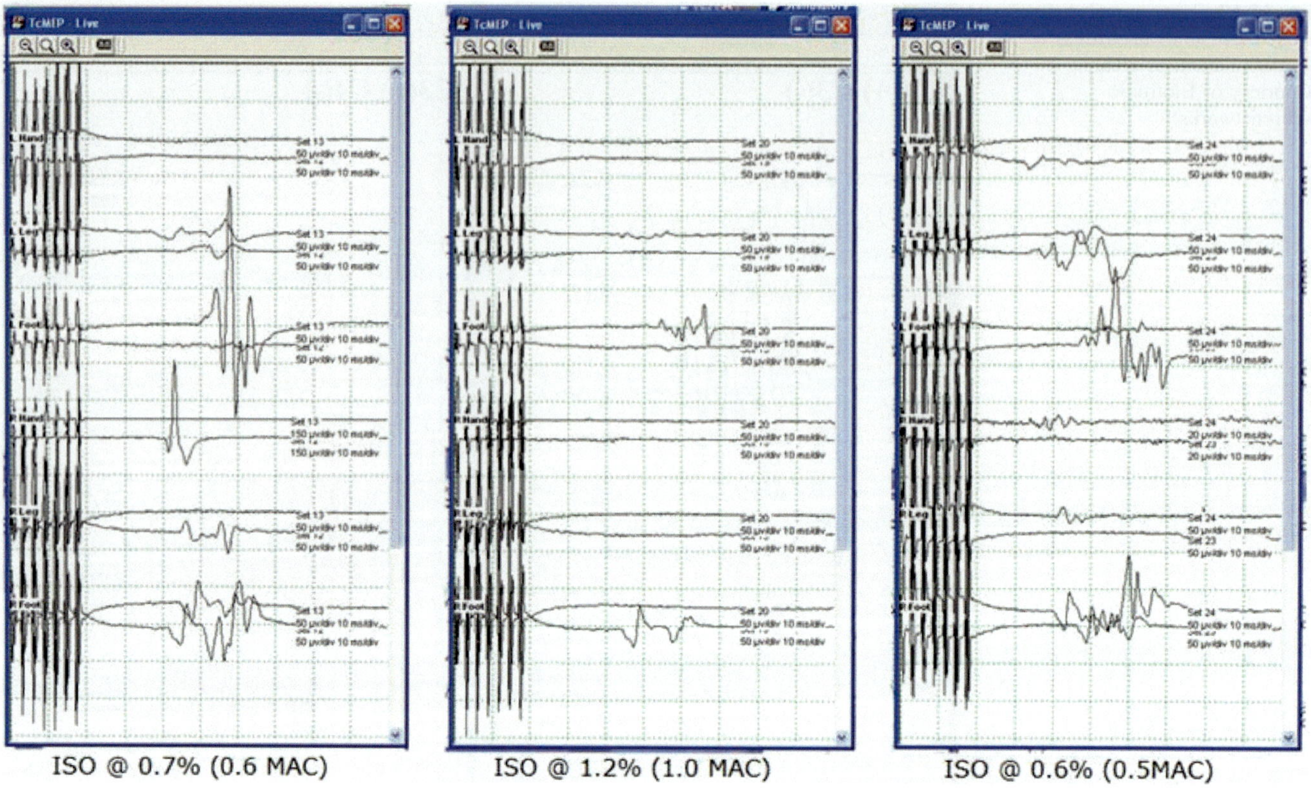

Fig. 16.21 Transcranial motor evoked potentials (TcMEPs): anesthetic effects (Courtesy of Biotronic Neuronetworks)

extremely sensitive to anesthetic agents and difficult to obtain in general (and thus rarely used).

Motor evoked potentials (MEPs) assess the corticospinal tracts and anterior spinal cord (and thus anterior spinal cord perfusion via the anterior spinal artery) (◉ Figs. 16.19, 16.20, 16.21 and 16.22). With MEPs, the electrical (or magnetic) stimulus activates the motor cortex using scalp electrodes (through the skull; although direct cortical stimulation can be used during a craniotomy). The signal travels down the corticospinal tract to the lower motor neurons, which then stimulate a specific muscle. MEPs are easily suppressed by volatile agents and nitrous oxide. Propofol can also attenuate signals, although to a much lesser degree. Opiates, ketamine, and etomidate are well tolerated (as are lidocaine infusions). Dexmedetomidine has been shown to suppress MEPs in some studies and should be used cautiously. As would be expected, muscle relaxants can impair MEPs due to the inability to measure the muscle response.

Physiologic anomalies can also impact EPs. Such alterations include severe anemia, hypoxia, hypothermia, and hypotension (reducing spinal cord perfusion).

Electromyography (EMG) involves placement of electrodes into specific muscles and monitoring the muscle response to stimulation of a nerve (such as the facial nerve during parotid surgery) or mechanical distortion/injury to the nerve (this elicits a distinct type of signal) (◉ Figs. 16.26, 16.27, 16.28, 16.29, and 16.30). EMGs continually assess local muscle activity due to irritation of a peripheral nerve during surgery (such as the quadriceps muscle during lumbar spine surgery near the L4 nerve root). EMGs differ from EPs because the neural tissue monitored is only in the *peripheral nervous system*. Aside from muscle relaxants, there are no anesthetics that greatly impair EMG responses at normal doses.

16.24 Monitoring Cerebral Blood Flow

16.24.1 Transcranial Doppler (TCD) Sonography

Cerebral blood flow can be assessed with Doppler ultrasound through the orbits, temporal bones, and foramen magnum. Flow velocities and pulsatility (a measure of distal cerebrovascular resistance) can be measured, but not quantitative blood flow. TCD is used to monitor for cerebral vasospasm following subarachnoid hemorrhage, among other indications. Here are waveforms from a normal patient and a patient with cerebral vasospasm, showing dramatically increased flow velocities (Figs. 16.31 and 16.32).

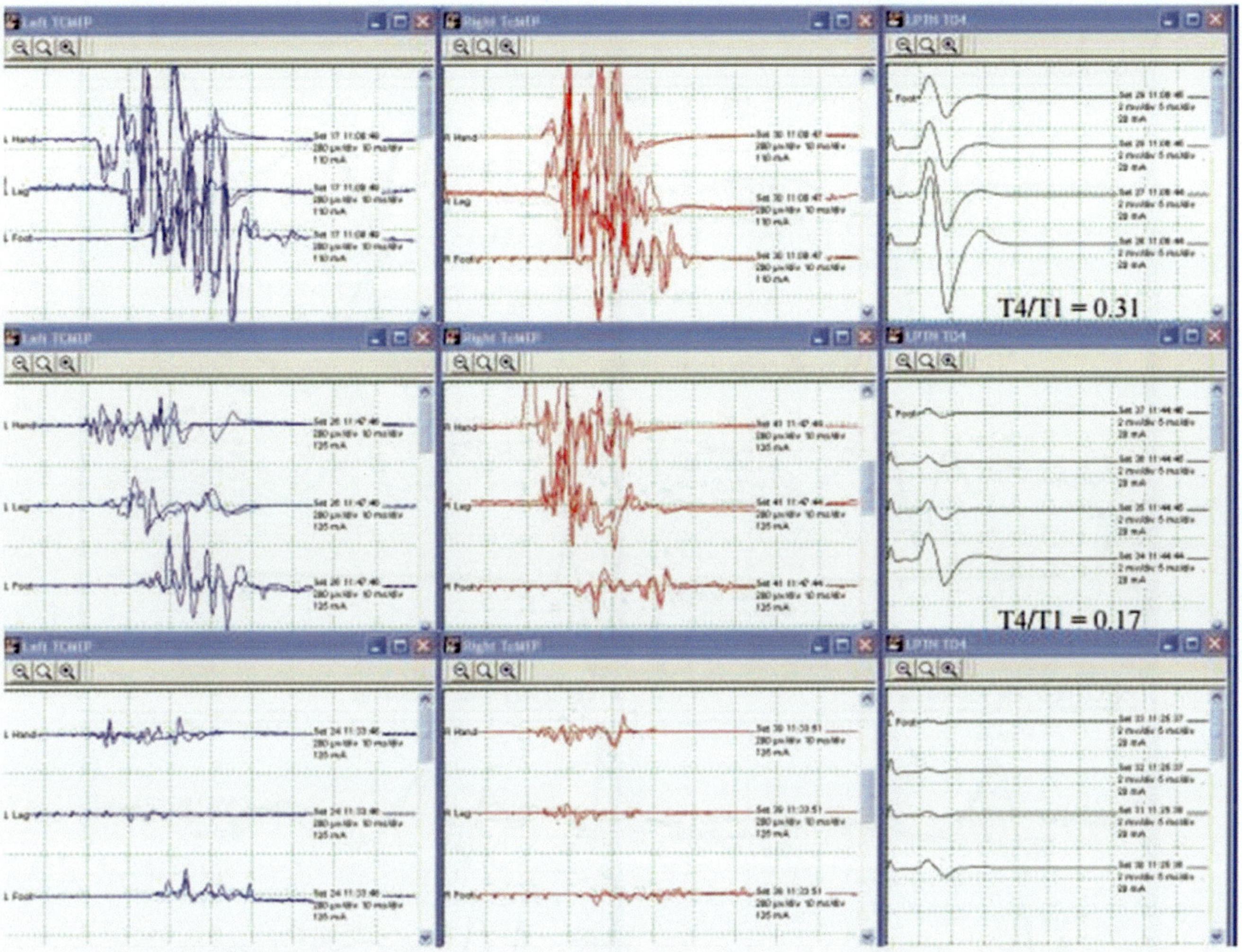

Fig. 16.22 Transcranial motor evoked potentials (TcMEPs): neuromuscular blocker effects (Courtesy of Biotronic Neuronetworks)

16.24.2 Perfusion Imaging

Quantitative cerebral blood flow measurements can be obtained with computed tomography (CT) or other imaging techniques (Fig. 16.32). In general, a contrast bolus is given during the head CT. Cerebral blood volume can be determined by the volume of contrast in a certain volume of brain tissue (i.e., the area under the signal intensity-time curve). Mean transit time is the time for contrast to traverse a given volume of brain tissue. Cerebral blood flow is the cerebral blood volume divided by mean transit time (CBF = CBV/MTT). This technology is currently used, for example, to triage patients for emergent stroke thrombectomy treatment. Good candidates are those with a small core infarct, identified as areas with CBF less than 30% of normal regions, and salvageable penumbral areas, identified by delayed time to peak perfusion greater than 6 s. In other words, when there is a large mismatch between core infarct and ischemic penumbra, the patient can benefit from clot removal and reperfusion.

16.25 Questions and Answers

Questions (Choose the Most Appropriate Answer)

1. Which one of the following is a goal of pharmacologic cerebral protective measures?
   A. Increase brain electrical activity to prevent a decline in long-term cortical functioning
   B. Minimize cerebral metabolic rate to decrease oxygen demand
   C. Therapeutic hyperthermia to prevent coagulopathy
   D. Decrease cerebral electrical activity with the use of glutaminergic or GABA-antagonist drugs
2. Which of the following is not true regarding evoked potentials?

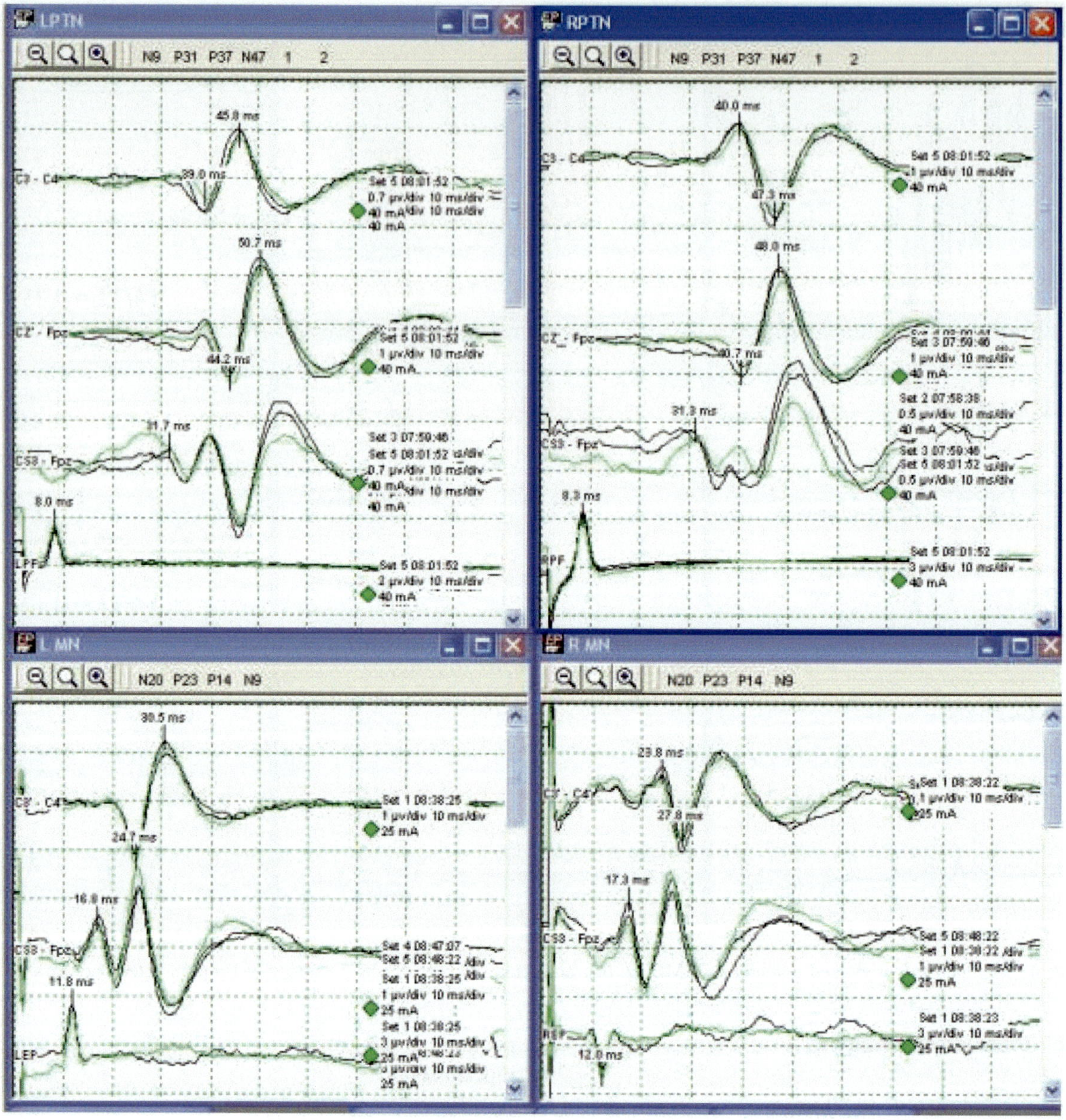

Fig. 16.23 Normal upper (median nerve) and lower (posterior tibial) somatosensory evoked potentials (Courtesy of Biotronic Neuronetworks)

A. Visual, auditory, somatosensory, and motor evoked potentials are examples of electrophysiological monitors used during surgery.
B. Short-latency evoked potentials directly originate from the stimulated nerve.
C. Intermediate-latency evoked potentials come from the brainstem.
D. Long-latency evoked potentials come from the cerebral cortex.

3. Mrs. Smith is a 79-year-old female who has progressively worsening anosmia. Where is the cranial nerve leading to her deficit located?
   A. Cerebrum
   B. Midbrain
   C. Pons
   D. Medulla
4. A patient has a blunt head trauma after a motor vehicle-pedestrian accident. His blood pressure is 90/60 mm Hg, HR 50 beats/min, respiratory rate 6 breaths/min, and ICP is 25. He is lethargic and responsive only to pain stimuli. What is his cerebral perfusion pressure?
   A. 65
   B. 55

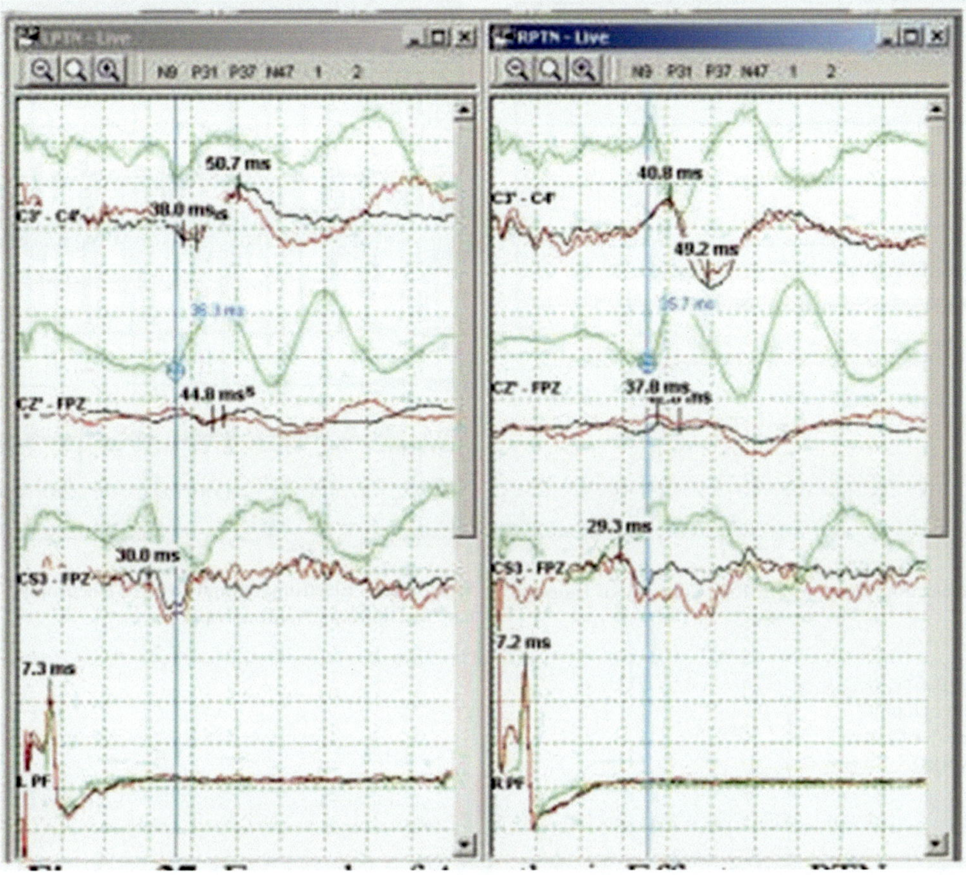

Fig. 16.24 Somatosensory evoked potentials (SSEP) from posterior tibial nerve (at ankle). Baseline tracings in green; anesthetic effects in *red/black* (Courtesy of Biotronic Neuronetworks)

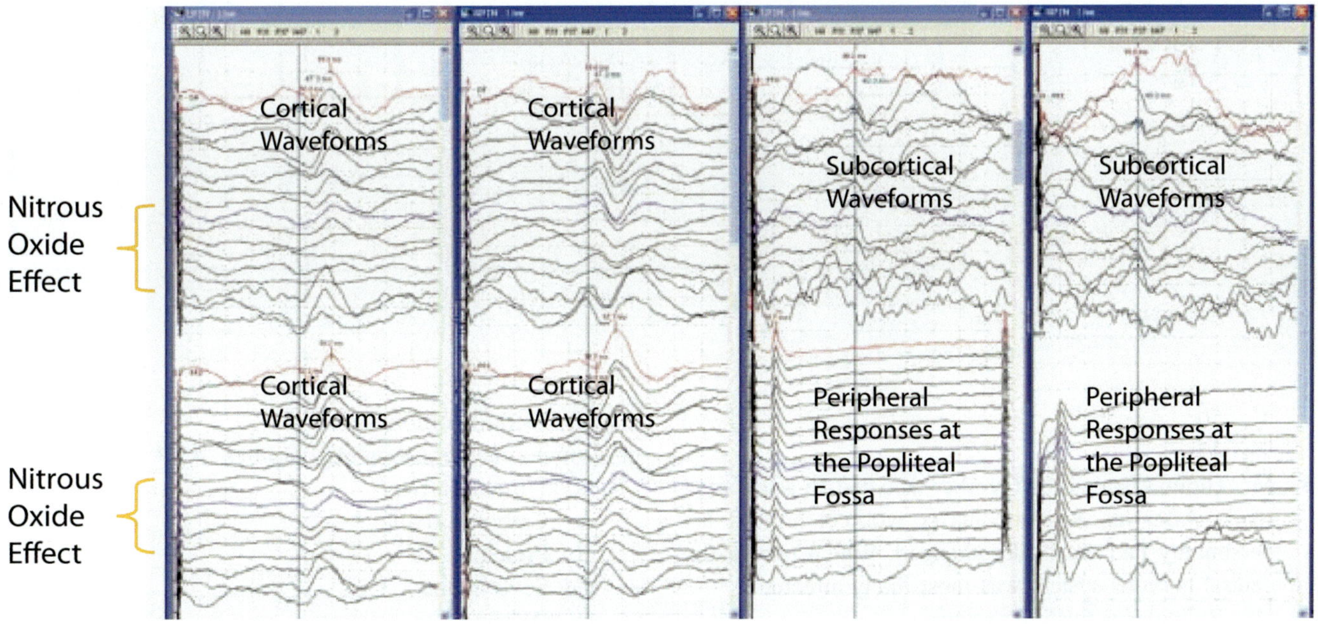

Fig. 16.25 Somatosensory evoked potentials (SSEP) from posterior tibial nerve (at ankle). Baseline tracings at bottom. Subcortical waveforms are unaffected by addition of nitrous oxide (N_2O) to desflurane. However, cortical waveforms disappear and then reappear with discontinuing N_2O (Courtesy of Biotronic Neuronetworks)

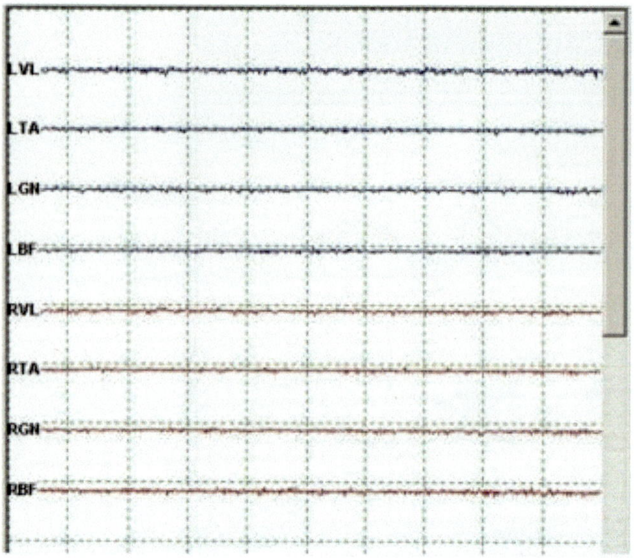

Fig. 16.26 Baseline electromyography (EMG) (Courtesy of Biotronic Neuronetworks)

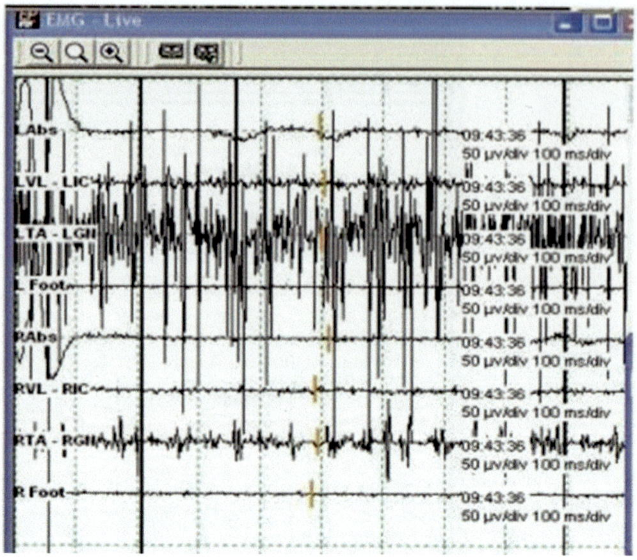

Fig. 16.28 Electromyography (EMG) neurotonic discharges (Courtesy of Biotronic Neuronetworks)

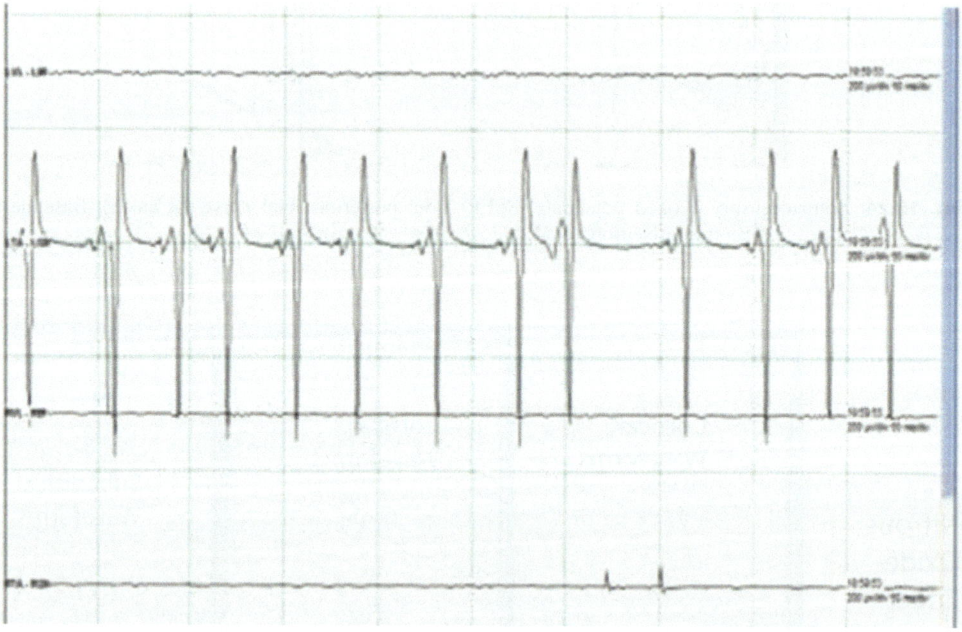

Fig. 16.27 Electromyography (EMG) spikes (Courtesy of Biotronic Neuronetworks)

C. 50
D. 45

5. Mr. Thomas is a railroad worker who had an accident at work. After his accident, his co-workers noticed his personality had drastically changed. Which part of the central nervous system was most likely affected?
   A. Reticular activating system
   B. Corticospinal tracts
   C. Prefrontal cortex
   D. Medulla oblongata
6. Which of the following requires ATP to cross the blood–brain barrier?
   A. Carbon dioxide
   B. Protein
   C. Sevoflurane
   D. Water
7. Which of the following is not accurate regarding cerebral blood flow?

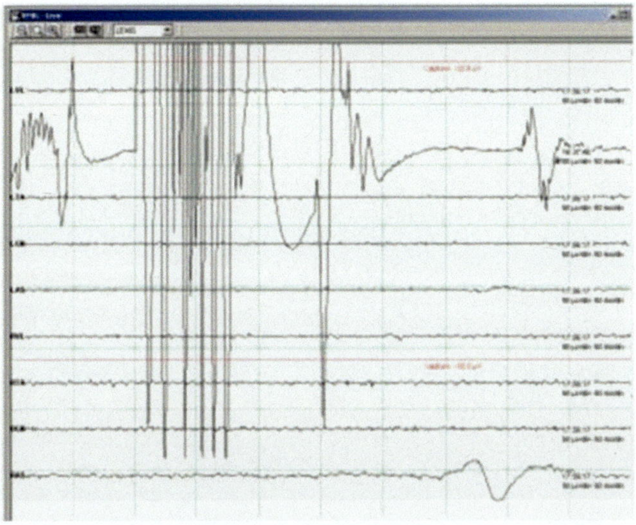

Fig. 16.29 Electromyography (EMG) burst (Courtesy of Biotronic Neuronetworks)

A. PaO_2 of 450 mm Hg increases CBF.
B. Gray matter has 4 times more CBF than the white matter.
C. $PaCO_2$ of 50 mm Hg increases CBF.
D. Cerebral blood flow equals the cerebral perfusion pressure divided by the cerebral vascular resistance.

8. A 61-year-old male with chronic uncontrolled hypertension, diabetes, and hyperlipidemia has a blood pressure of 200/100 in the preoperative holding area. Of the choices listed below, what would be the best goal for his blood pressure to maintain cerebral perfusion during surgery?
   A. MAP 60
   B. MAP 100
   C. MAP 200
9. Which of the following brain areas is not involved in a motor pathway?
   A. Hippocampus
   B. Basal ganglia
   C. Vermis
   D. Midbrain
10. Dr. Johnson is performing an intrathecal injection. Clear CSF leaks out and confirms he is in the correct location. Which 2 membranes surround the space he is in?
    A. Subcutaneous tissue and dura mater
    B. Pia mater and arachnoid membrane
    C. Dura mater and ligamentum flavum
    D. Arachnoid and dura mater

Answers

1. **B**. Pharmacologic cerebral protective measures in general suppress the cerebral metabolic rate with a concomitant decrease in oxygen and glucose utilization. This should make brain tissue more resilient to transient hypoxic-ischemic insults (such as temporarily clamping a cerebral blood vessel). Hyperthermia exacerbates acute brain or spinal cord injury and should be avoided. Therapeutic hypothermia is recommended as a neuroprotective therapy following anoxic brain insults (cardiac arrest or birth asphyxia). Cerebral electrical activity and metabolic rate are suppressed with anti-glutaminergic and/or GABA-agonist drugs.

2. **C**. Both intermediate-latency and long-latency evoked potentials come from the cerebral cortex. Short-latency evoked potentials can originate from a stimulated nerve or the brainstem. Visual, auditory, somatosensory, and motor evoked potentials are examples of neurophysiological monitors used during surgery; another neurophysiological monitor used is electroencephalography (EEG).

3. **A**. Anosmia is the loss of the sense of smell. The olfactory nerve (cranial nerve I) is located in the cerebrum. The optic nerve (cranial nerve II) is also located in the cerebrum. Cranial nerves III-IV are located in the brainstem midbrain, CN V-VII are located in the brainstem pons, and CN VIII-XII are located in the brainstem medulla.

4. **D**. After head trauma, autoregulation is often disrupted in a homogeneous or heterogeneous distribution. Cerebral perfusion becomes more directly related to mean arterial pressure. Cerebral perfusion pressure (CPP) is the mean arterial pressure (MAP) minus the intracranial pressure (ICP). In this patient, his MAP is 70, ICP is 25, and CPP is 45.

5. **C**. The prefrontal cortex is one of the most important association areas; it plays a critical role in personality, goal-directed behavior, and attention. The reticular activating system is a group of nuclei in the brainstem that regulates arousal, consciousness, and sleep. The corticospinal

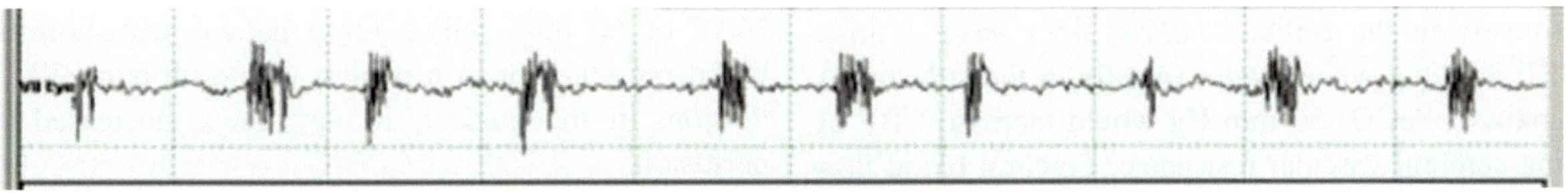

Fig. 16.30 Electromyography (EMG) myokymic discharges (Courtesy of Biotronic Neuronetworks)

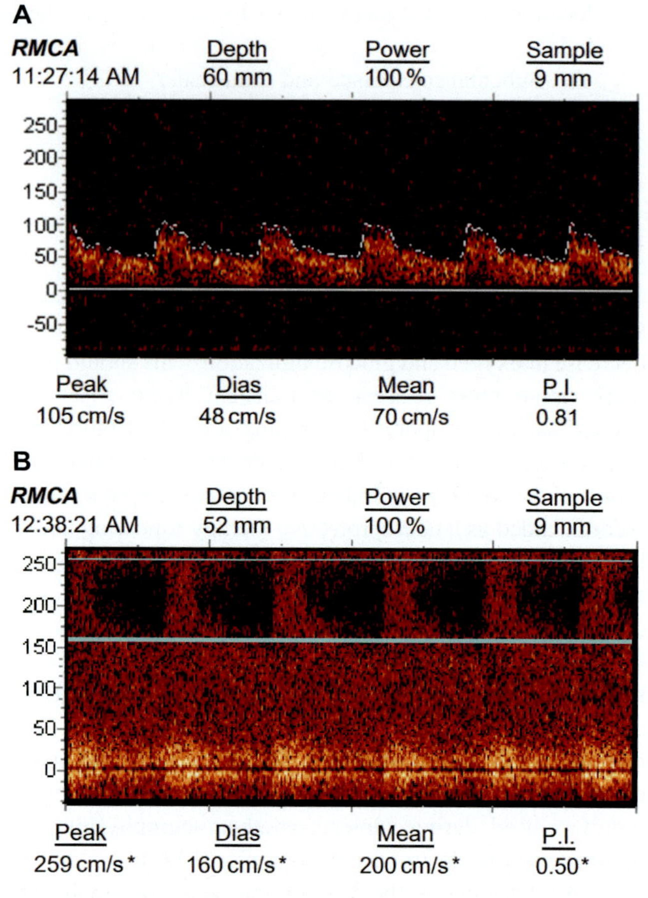

Fig. 16.31 A. Normal right middle cerebral artery waveform (2 MHz doppler ultrasound through the right temporal bone window). B. Right middle cerebral artery waveform showing severe vasospasm (vessel narrowing)

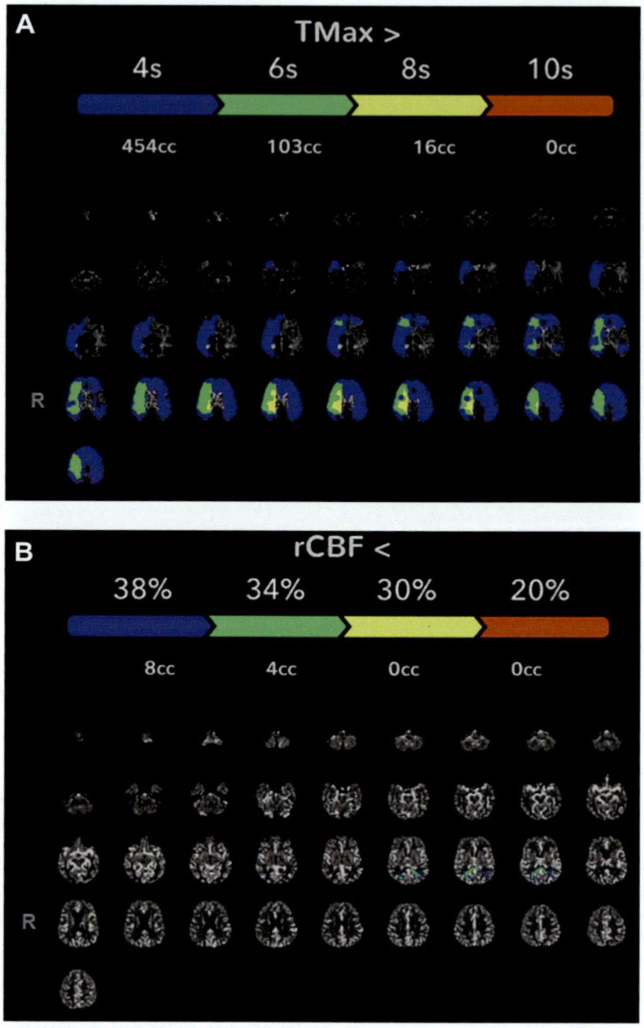

Fig. 16.32 A. Tmax in a patient with acute cerebral ischemia. The blue shading shows time to peak contrast intensity (Tmax) > 4 s; green > 6 s; yellow > 8 s. The green region is used to define the ischemic penumbra. B. Cerebral blood flow (CBF) in the same patient with acute cerebral ischemia. Yellow areas would indicate critically low CBF (absent here), or core infarct, that are not salvageable even with reperfusion. This large mismatch of ischemic penumbra to core infarct makes this patient an **excellent** emergent thrombectomy (clot removal) candidate

tract is a group of neurons that originate in the premotor and primary motor cortices in the brain that travels through the brainstem and spinal cord to connect to lower motor neurons to coordinate voluntary movement. The medulla oblongata contains the nuclei for both the parasympathetic and sympathetic nervous systems in the body, thus controlling the autonomic functions of the body to maintain its survival.

6. B. Out of the choices listed, only protein requires active transport with ATP to cross the blood–brain barrier. Water and all gases, including volatile anesthetics, cross the blood–brain barrier freely.

7. A. Hyperoxia (PaO_2 > 300 mm Hg) would only be likely to slightly decrease CBF while hypoxemia (PaO_2 < 50 mm Hg) significantly increases CBF. It is true that gray matter (mostly in the cerebral cortex) does have 4 times more CBF than the white matter (mostly in the subcortex). Hypercapnia of $PaCO_2$ 50 mm Hg would increase CBF by decreasing cerebral vascular resistance. Cerebral blood flow equals the cerebral perfusion pressure divided by the cerebral vascular resistance.

8. **B**. With a blood pressure of 200/100, his current MAP is 133. This patient has chronic uncontrolled hypertension. In patients with chronic hypertension, both the lower limit of cerebral autoregulation and the upper limit of the cerebral autoregulation are increased. These changes allow for stable cerebral blood flows at higher arterial pressures. While a MAP of 60 may suffice for a patient with normotensive blood pressures or in a patient with well-controlled hypertension; in this patient, it may cause decreased cerebral perfusion.

9. **A**. The hippocampus regulates short-term memory. The basal ganglia regulates movement and posture by

integrating motor processes associated with the cerebral cortex. The vermis is part of the spinocerebellum; it maintains posture, muscle tone, and modulates control of the proximal muscles of the body and limbs. The midbrain in the brainstem contains cranial nerves III and IV, which provide motor functions to the eye, as well as the cerebral peduncles, which contain the corticospinal tracts.

10. **D**. He is in the subarachnoid space in the lumbar cistern (below L2 to avoid injuring the spinal cord) that is surrounded by the arachnoid and dura mater. As he is placing the nerve block, his needle will pass through the layers of the back and spine in the following order: skin, subcutaneous tissue, ligamentum flavum, dura mater, and arachnoid membrane. The pia mater wraps around the spinal cord closely and a needle would not be able to inject between the pia mater and the spinal cord (or would injure the spinal cord). The space between the dura mater and ligamentum flavum is the epidural space. The space between the arachnoid membrane and the dura mater is the subdural space, a potential space.

References

1. Barrett KE, Barman SM, Boitano S, Brooks HL, editors. Ganong's review of medical physiology. 25th ed. New York: McGraw-Hill; 2015.
2. Benarroch EE. Basic neurosciences with clinical applications. Philadelphia: Butterworth-Heinemann; 2005.
3. Brain Trauma Foundation American Association of Neurological Surgeons Congress of Neurological Surgeons Joint Section on Neurotrauma and Critical Care, AANS/CNS, Bratton SL, Chestnut RM, Ghajar J, McConnell Hammond FF, Harris OA, Hartl R, et al. Guidelines for the management of severe traumatic brain injury. XIII. Antiseizure prophylaxis. J Neurotrauma. 2007;24 (Suppl 1):S83–6.
4. Butterworth JF IV, Mackey DC, Wasnick JD. Chapter 26 Neurophysiology & Anesthesia. In: Butterworth JF, Mackey DC, Wasnick JD, editors. Morgan & Mikhail's clinical anesthesiology. 5th ed. New York: McGraw-Hill; 2013. p. 575–92.
5. Costanzo LS, editor. Physiology. 5th ed. Philadelphia: Saunders; 2013.
6. Darby JM, Yonas H, Marion DW, Latchaw RE. Local "inverse steal" induced by hyperventilation in head injury. Neurosurgery. 1988;23(1):84–8.
7. Daroff RB, Fenichel GM, Jankovic J, Mazziotta JC, editors. Bradley's neurology in clinical practice. 6th ed. Philadelphia: Saunders Elsevier; 2012.
8. Hall JB, Schmidt GA, Kress JP, editors. Principles of critical care. 4th ed. New York: McGraw-Hill; 2015.
9. Hemphill J III, Smith WS, Gress DR. Neurologic critical care, including hypoxic-ischemic encephalopathy, and subarachnoid hemorrhage. In: Kasper D, Fauci A, Hauser S, Longo D, Jameson J, Loscalzo J, editors. Harrison's Principles of internal medicine. 19th ed. New York: McGraw-Hill; 2015. p. 1777–86.
10. Kleinman ME, Brennan EE, Goldberger ZD, Swor RA, Terry M, Bobrow BJ, et al. Part 5: adult basic life support and cardiopulmonary resuscitation quality: 2015 American Heart Association guidelines update for cardiopulmonary resuscitation and emergency cardiovascular care. Circulation. 2015;132(suppl 2):S414–35.
11. Palmisciano P, Haider AS, Balasubramanian K, Dadario NB, Robertson FC, Silverstein JW, D'Amico RS. Supplementary motor area syndrome after brain tumor surgery: a systematic review. World Neurosurg. 2022;165:160–171.e2. https://doi.org/10.1016/j.wneu.2022.06.080. Epub 2022 Jun 22. PMID: 35752423
12. Patel PM, Drummond J. Cerebral physiology and the effects of anesthetic drugs. In: Miller RD editors. Miller's anesthesia, vol. 2. 7th ed. Philadelphia: Elsevier; 2009. p. 2045–87.
13. Paulson OB, Strandgaard S, Edvinsson L. Cerebral autoregulation. Cerebrovasc Brain Metab Rev. 1990;2(2):161–92.
14. Purves D, Augustine GJ, Fitzpatrick D, Hall WC, LaMantia AS, White LE, editors. Neuroscience. 2nd ed. Sunderland: Sinauer Associates; 2001.
15. Ropper AH, Samuels MA, Klein JP. Chapter 30 Disturbances of cerebrospinal fluid, including hydrocephalus, Pseudotumor Cerebri, and low-pressure syndromes. In: Ropper AH, Samuels MA, Klein JP, editors. Adams & Victor's principles of neurology. 10th ed. New York: McGraw-Hill; 2014. p. 617–38.
16. The Hypothermia After Cardiac Arrest Study Group. Mild therapeutic hypothermia to improve neurologic outcome after cardiac arrest. N Engl J Med. 2002;346:549–56.
17. Waxman SG, editor. Clinical neuroanatomy. 27th ed. New York: McGraw-Hill; 2013.
18. Yao F-SF, Fontes ML, Malhotra V, Yao F editors Artusio's anesthesiology: problem-oriented patient management. 7th ed. Philadelphia: Lippincott Williams & Wilkins; 2011.

Cardiovascular Physiology

17

Sandeep Khanna, Roshni Sreedharan, and Carlos Trombetta

Abstract

Modern cardiovascular physiology is an evolving discipline. William Harvey published his classic treatise in 1628, describing the circulation of blood and the role of the heart. Since then, great strides have been made in the field of cardiovascular physiology. New insights in molecular and cellular biology are changing the way we think about the heart, the circulatory system, and their interaction. It is imperative for anesthesiologists to have a good knowledge of cardiovascular physiology as it plays a central role in patient care in the perioperative setting. The first part of this chapter focuses on describing the electrical activity of the heart and its interaction with the contractile apparatus to generate a cardiac cycle. The second part of the chapter deals with regulation of the heart and cardiac reflexes. The chapter concludes with a brief description of the circulatory system, the microcirculation, and important aspects of coronary blood flow.

Keywords

Cardiovascular physiology • Electrical activity • Contraction • Cardiac cycle • Excitation–contraction coupling • Circulatory system • Microcirculation • Coronary blood flow

Key Points

1. Excitation–contraction coupling of cardiomyocytes is a complex energy-dependent process that allows the heart to pump blood efficiently.
2. Mechanical coupling of adjacent cardiomyocytes occurs via intercalated disks, and electrical coupling occurs via gap junctions.
3. Sequential electrical and mechanical events occurring over the course of a heartbeat generate the cardiac cycle.
4. Action potentials in ventricular cardiomyocytes and sinoatrial node are different.
5. Spontaneous diastolic depolarization occurs during Phase 4 of the SA node's action potential.
6. The electrocardiogram is a representation of the electrical flow of ions in the heart during the cardiac cycle; electrical events precede mechanical events.
7. Various heart sounds, central venous pressure waves, and arterial pressure waves are generated as the result of the cardiac cycle.
8. Measurement of ejection fraction and ventricular strain on echocardiography help assess systolic function in clinical practice.
9. Diastolic function is defined by the ability of the heart to accommodate a normal preload at normal filling pressures.
10. End-diastolic volume, and not pressure, is a true measure of ventricular preload.
11. Wall tension and total peripheral resistance constitute left ventricular afterload.

S. Khanna (✉) · R. Sreedharan · C. Trombetta
Division of Multi-Specialty Anesthesiology, Cleveland Clinic Foundation, Cleveland, OH, USA
e-mail: khannas@ccf.org

R. Sreedharan
e-mail: sreedhr@ccf.org

S. Khanna · C. Trombetta
Division of Cardiothoracic Anesthesiology, Cleveland Clinic Foundation, Cleveland, OH, USA

S. Khanna
Outcomes Research Consortium®, Houston, TX, USA

R. Sreedharan
Division of Intensive Care & Resuscitation, Cleveland Clinic Foundation, Cleveland, OH, USA

M. Argalious et al. (eds.), *Basic Sciences in Anesthesia*,
https://doi.org/10.1007/978-3-031-60203-0_17

12. Generation of an adequate cardiac output depends upon five factors: heart rate, rhythm, preload, contractility, and afterload.
13. Cardiac reflexes, such as baroreceptor reflex, play an important role in immediate blood pressure control.
14. The venous circulation holds most of the blood volume while arterioles contribute the most to peripheral resistance.
15. Glycocalyx-generated endothelial surface layer plays an important role in the microcirculation.
16. Starling's forces may not be as important physiologically in the microcirculation as thought previously.
17. Mixed venous oxygen saturation can be used as a measure of oxygen extraction and global hypoperfusion.
18. Atrial natriuretic peptide and B-type natriuretic peptide are elevated in heart failure.
19. Coronary circulation is autoregulated between mean arterial pressures of 60–140-mm Hg.
20. Coronary perfusion can be compromised by fall in aortic diastolic blood pressure, rise in left ventricular end-diastolic pressure, tachycardia, or coronary artery blockages.

17.1 Introduction

Most cells in the human body utilize adenosine triphosphate (ATP) as a source of energy to maintain their integrity. The production of ATP in turn depends upon oxygen delivery. The heart is a unique volume-dependent stroke pump that is responsible for delivering oxygenated blood in a timely manner to cells. To lend perspective to the perseverance of the heart, let us consider the case of a 100-year-old person. This person's heart would have approximately beaten 3–4 billion times, delivering roughly 50 million liters (considering an average oxygen content of 20 ml/dl and stroke volume of 60 ml/beat) worth of oxygen to the body. Assuming 700 liters of oxygen weighs 1 kg; the heart would have moved a weight of about 70 tons in its lifetime. Given that the average weight of an adult human heart is 300 g, this is a superlative feat.

How does the heart do this? The focus of this chapter is twofold:

1. To present a synopsis of cardiovascular physiology.
2. To help the reader understand how these concepts are useful in the perioperative setting.

17.2 Anatomical Considerations

Anatomically, the heart is organized into four chambers: 2 atria (right and left, separated by the interatrial septum or IAS) and 2 ventricles (right and left, separated by the interventricular septum or IVS). The atria are separated from the ventricles by the atrioventricular (AV) groove or sulcus. The right atrium (RA) receives deoxygenated venous blood from the venae cava and empties into the right ventricle (RV). The RV in turn pumps the deoxygenated blood into the pulmonary artery (PA), divisions of which carry the blood to the alveoli. Oxygenated blood then flows into the left atrium (LA) via the pulmonary veins. The left ventricle (LV), which receives oxygenated blood from the LA, is responsible for ejection of oxygenated blood into the aorta (Ao) and rest of the body [1, 2].

Unidirectional flow is made possible by the presence of four valves in the heart:

1. The tricuspid valve (TV) between the RA and RV
2. The pulmonary valve (PV) between the RV and PA
3. The mitral valve (MV) between the LA and LV
4. The aortic valve (AoV) between the LV and the aorta.

Pictorially the heart is commonly represented in an upright position, with the atria being superior and the ventricles inferior. However, anatomically, the heart is obliquely placed in the thorax such that the RV forms the anterior surface, the RA forms the right lateral border, the LV forms the left lateral border, and the LA forms the posterior surface. The heart can be imagined as an inverted pyramid, with its base being formed by the AV groove and the apex being formed by its inferior angle. The heart, much like an onion, is a layered structure. From superficial to deep, these layers are (◉ Fig. 17.1):

1. The pericardium: This is a serous layer which invests the heart and typically has two components: an inner secretory visceral layer that is in contact with the myocardium and an outer parietal layer that separates the heart from other mediastinal structures. The layers are separated by the pericardial cavity.
2. The epicardium: This is formed by the visceral pericardium. The visceral layer's mesothelial cells secrete pericardial fluid into the pericardial cavity and this fluid, in turn, acts as a lubricant. The mesothelial cells adhere to the myocardium via fibroelastic and adipose tissue.
3. The myocardium: This is the muscle wall of the heart and consists of muscle fibers arranged in a circular and spiral manner.
4. The endocardium: This is the innermost layer of the heart and lines the chambers. It essentially consists of

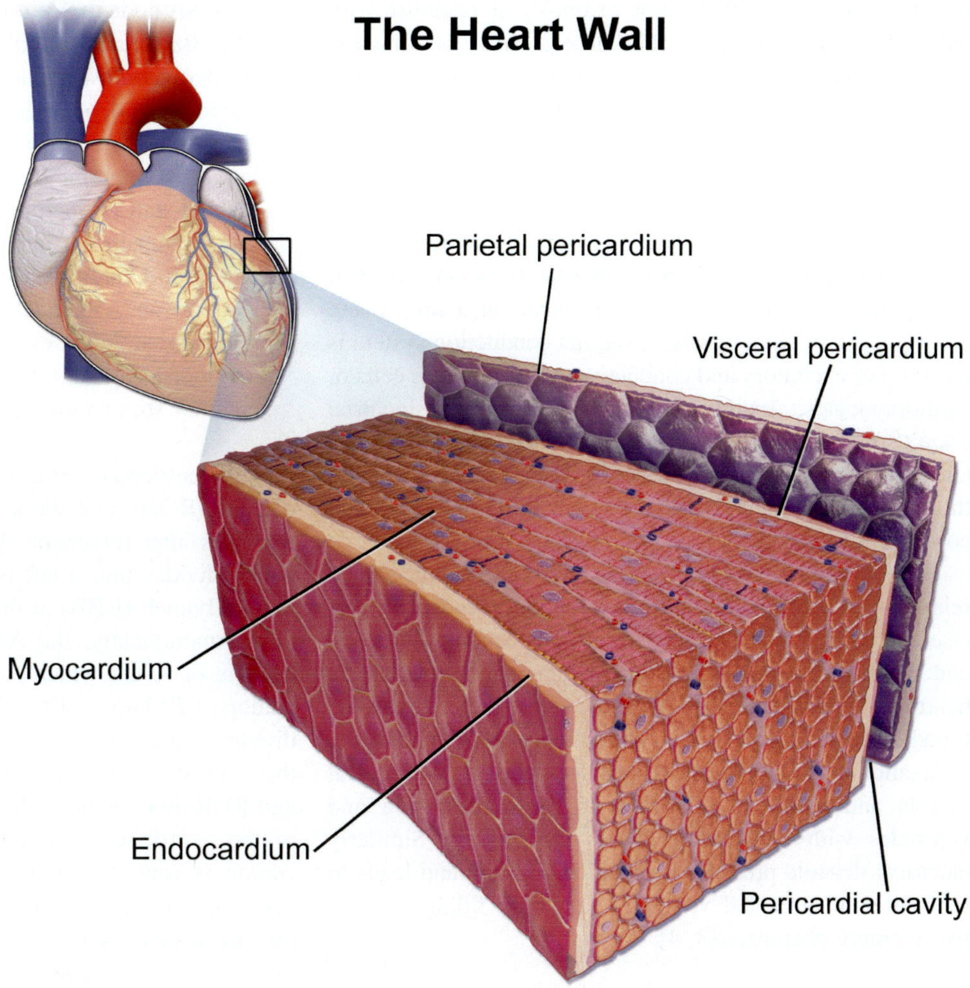

Fig. 17.1 Layers of heart (Reprinted under Creative Commons Attribution 3.0 Unported from Blausen.com staff (2014). "Medical gallery of Blausen Medical 2014". *WikiJournal of Medicine* **1** (2). https://doi.org/10.15347/wjm/2014.010. ISSN 2002-4436)

endothelial cells which are in continuity with the endothelium of the veins and the great arteries.

Similar to constructing a house, a backbone or scaffolding is required in the heart to attach components and provide a weight bearing infrastructure. This function is provided by the "skeleton" of the heart.

The "skeleton" is formed by flexible cartilaginous and dense connective tissue. This "backbone" typically consists of annuli of the cardiac valves, the trigones, the roots of the great vessels, and the central fibrous body. It forms an anchor for the valves and cardiac muscle bundles, allowing development of high intracavitary pressures without compromising the heart's structural integrity. Importantly, it electrically insulates the atria from the ventricles, allowing electrical impulses between both the structures to flow through the AV node only.

While the atria consist of two thin bands of myocardium, the ventricles contain deep and superficial spiral muscles. The organization of muscle bundles allow the ventricles to "twist and squeeze" as opposed to just squeezing, thereby enhancing their force. For example, if you take a wet piece of cloth, you can express more water out when you wring it as compared to just squeezing it. In heart failure with reduced ejection fraction, this ability to "wring" is diminished, leading to a decrease in contractility. During diastole, unwinding of the twisted ventricle contributes to pulling in blood from the atrial chambers and is known as diastolic suction.

Functionally, the heart has two parts connected in series: (1) a right heart, which receives and pumps out deoxygenated blood, and (2) a left heart, which receives and pumps oxygenated blood. Although both the LV and RV are efficient pumps, they differ in their organization, shape, and muscle content. The ellipsoid LV displays temporally uniform contraction and is thicker. The thinner RV is crescent shaped, has embryo logically distinct inflow and outflow tracts, and contracts in a peristaltic manner. The IVS couples RV and LV function and allows the RV to contract against it to generate force. The thinner RV, being compliant, adjusts easily to volume overload by dilating, but tends to fail when presented with an acute increase in afterload or pulmonary vascular resistance (PVR). For example, in response to a pulmonary embolus, the RV dilates and its function decreases. The thicker LV, on the other hand, can withstand acute and chronic afterload increases better compared to the RV.

The heart utilizes electrical input and converts it into a mechanical output. The electrical part of the heart is represented by a specialized conduction system that is responsible for generating the "spark" for a heartbeat. It also ensures that this spark travels to all parts of the heart in a timely and orderly fashion. On a cellular level, the conduction system is made up of excitatory and conductive cardiac muscle cells or cardiomyocytes. Anatomically, it is made up of sinoatrial node (SA), interatrial nodal pathways, atrioventricular node (AV), the bundle of His, and the Purkinje system. Broadly, the mechanical system consists of contractile myocytes and connective tissue.

Like skeletal muscle, cardiac muscle contracts and relaxes. This contraction and relaxation is preceded by precise electrical events. The interplay between the electrical and mechanical events, leading to generation of a single heartbeat, constitutes the cardiac cycle (CC). It can be broadly divided into systole (contraction phase) and diastole (relaxation phase). Electrical systole precedes mechanical systole and leads to sequential contraction of atria and ventricles with ejection of blood into vessels. Similarly electrical diastole precedes mechanical diastole and leads to relaxation of atria and ventricles, allowing filling of relatively empty chambers [3, 4].

17.2.1 Electrical Components and Activity of the Heart

Different parts of the conduction system are capable of spontaneously discharging and generating action potentials. The part that discharges most frequently, however, determines the rate at which the heart beats and is termed the cardiac pacemaker. The atrial conduction system consists of the:

1. **SA node:** Located at the junction of the superior vena cava (SVC) and RA. Normally, it acts as the cardiac pacemaker. It develops from the right side of the embryo and is predominantly innervated by the right vagus nerve. Sympathetic innervation comes from the stellate ganglion.
2. **Internodal atrial fibers:** These are arranged in three tracts: (1) anterior, which gives rise to the Bachmann bundle; (2) middle, or tract of Wenckebach; and (3) posterior, or tract of Thorel. These transmit impulses from SA node to AV node in about 30 milliseconds (ms). The Bachmann bundle is responsible for left atrial depolarization. Conduction via atrial fibers is fast, leading to atrial depolarization in about 100 milliseconds.
3. **AV node:** Located in the right posterior portion of the interatrial septum. It develops from the left side of the embryo and is predominantly innervated by the left vagus. Sympathetic innervation comes from the stellate ganglion. Conduction is slow in the AV node, and this leads to an AV nodal delay of about 100 milliseconds before ventricular excitation takes place. This delay is lengthened by stimulation of the vagus nerve and shortened by stimulation of sympathetic nerves.

The ventricular conduction system consists of the bundle of His (BOH) and Purkinje system (◉ Fig. 17.2). The impulses after traversing the AV node travel to the BOH, which divides into a left bundle branch (LBB) and a right bundle branch (RBB) at the top of the interventricular septum. Anatomically, the AV node and BOH reside in the triangle of Koch, which is bordered by the coronary sinus, tendon of Todaro, and the TV septal leaflet. The LBB further divides into anterior and posterior fascicles, which extend to the base of the left papillary muscles. Fibers from the LBB and RBB then merge with the Purkinje system supplying all of the ventricular myocardium, and this enables depolarization of ventricles in about 100 ms. Depolarization in the ventricles typically commences at the left side of the IVS, then moves across to the right side, followed by spread down the septum to the apex, and culminates by returning along the ventricular walls to the AV groove.

The discharging cells that act as dominant pacemakers determine two things: the heart rate and the heart rhythm.

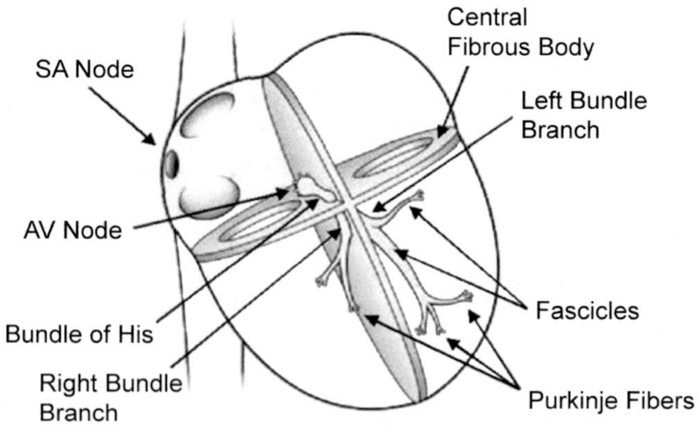

Fig. 17.2 Conduction system of heart. Normal excitation originates in sinoatrial node then propagates through both atria. Atrial depolarization spreads to atrioventricular node and passes through bundle of His to bundle branches/Purkinje fibers. *AV* atrioventricular, *SA* sinoatrial (Reprinted with permission from Iaizzo [5])

The rate is usually determined by the rate of discharge while the rhythm is determined by which group of cells is acting as the dominant pacemaker. The SA node discharges at about 60–100 times/min in adults. As this is higher than what other cells discharge at, the SA node acts as the dominant pacemaker. This phenomenon is called cardiac overdrive suppression, wherein other cells fail to discharge in the presence of a more rapidly discharging focus. Tonic vagal discharge influences the SA node leading to a resting heart rate of about 75 beats/min. Fluctuations in parasympathetic output during respiration, especially deep breathing, lead to acceleration of heart rate during inspiration and deceleration during exhalation. This sinus arrhythmia is a normal phenomenon. If for some reason the SA node stops discharging, other cells in the conduction system, such as AV nodal cells and cells of the His Purkinje system, can take over the pacemaker function. However, these cells discharge at lower rates of 30–50 beats/min. AV nodal rhythm is generated by AV nodal cells, and ventricular escape rhythms are generated by the His Purkinje system. Myocardial cells can also act as pacemakers, but they discharge sporadically and usually lead to ectopic or extra beats. This mechanism allows the heart to have multiple fallback options in case the SA node fails due to disease or degeneration [1, 2, 5].

17.2.2 The Cardiac Action Potential in Ventricular Muscle and Pacemaker Tissue

Ventricular myocardial cells and pacemaker cells have somewhat different electrical properties. Although both generate action potentials, the former group of cells produces a fast response action potential while the latter group demonstrates a slow response action potential. Myocardial cells have a resting membrane potential (RMP) of about − 90 millivolts (mV), which is determined mainly by ion fluxes across the plasma membrane. Although K^+ equilibrium potential predominantly determines the RMP, other ions, such as Na^+ , Ca^{2+}, and Cl^-, play an important role in generation of the action potential. Cells are mechanically connected via intercalated disks and electrically connected through gap junctions. This allows them to act as a syncytium and ensures rapid spread of electrical impulses. Fast response action potentials have 5 phases that are generated as follows:

1. **Phase 0:** Rapid depolarization due to Na^+ influx. Once the RMP is shifted to − 60 to − 70 mV (critical threshold), there is a rapid influx of Na^+ leading to a rapid upstroke.
2. **Phase 1:** This is followed by rapid repolarization due to a transient outward K^+ current, i_{to}.
3. **Phase 2:** The plateau phase occurs because of inward influx of Ca^{2+} through L type channels and efflux of K^+ via different channels: inward rectifier i_k, delayed rectifier i_{k1} and i_{to}.
4. **Phase 3:** Slow repolarization phase is characterized by predominance of K + efflux
5. **Phase 4:** Return to RMP or − 90 mV occurs in this phase. Ionic flow is minimal.

In contrast to the fast response action potential, the slow response action potential of pacemaker cells is characterized by a less steep Phase 0, absent Phase 1, shortening and merging of Phase 2 and 3 with repolarization occurring to firing levels (approximately − 40 mV), and a Phase 4 that is characterized by spontaneous diastolic depolarization (◉ Fig. 17.3). Phase 4 in the SA node occurs predominantly due to a mixed cation current (Na^+ and K^+). Because of its unusual activation following hyperpolarization, this channel has been termed the "funny" channel and the current I_f as the funny current. The membrane starts depolarizing because of the funny current, leading to activation of transient (T) and long (L) Ca^{2+} channels, which generates a Ca^{2+} influx leading to Phase 1. At the peak of the impulse, K^+ efflux ensues bringing about phase 3 or repolarization. When the membrane potential reaches firing levels, funny current kicks in and causes spontaneous diastolic depolarization during Phase 4, thereby ensuring automatic firing of pacemaker cells.

Action potentials generated at one region tend to depolarize neighboring regions and as myocytes are electrically continuous; this leads to rapid spread of depolarization as an electrical signal through the heart [3, 4].

Now that we know how the heart generates and spreads an "electric" spark, let us see how this spark is translated into a contraction.

17.2.3 Contractile Cardiomyocytes and Excitation–Contraction Coupling

Unlike the excitatory and conducting cardiomyocytes, which function as electric generators, the primary role of contractile cardiomyocytes is to function as force generators. Both these cells are supported by extracellular connective tissue, which predominantly contains collagen, elastin, proteoglycans, and metalloproteinases. A group of cardiomyocytes supported by this distinct extracellular matrix network constitutes a myofiber.

Cardiomyocytes typically have an outer plasma membrane, called sarcolemma, that becomes highly specialized at the junction of adjoining cells to form intercalated disks (◉ Fig. 17.4). These bind adjacent cells in series and parallel, thereby creating a syncytium of cells. This enables mechanical coupling between cells and effective

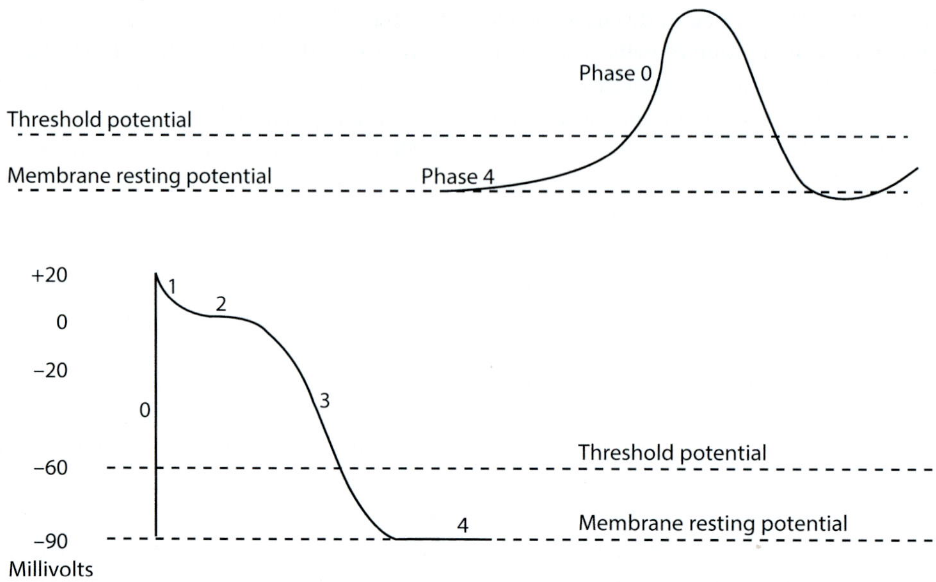

Fig. 17.3 Typical cardiac action potentials (slow on top and fast below). Resting membrane potential, threshold potential, and phases of depolarization (0–4) are shown (Reprinted with permission from Iaizzo [5])

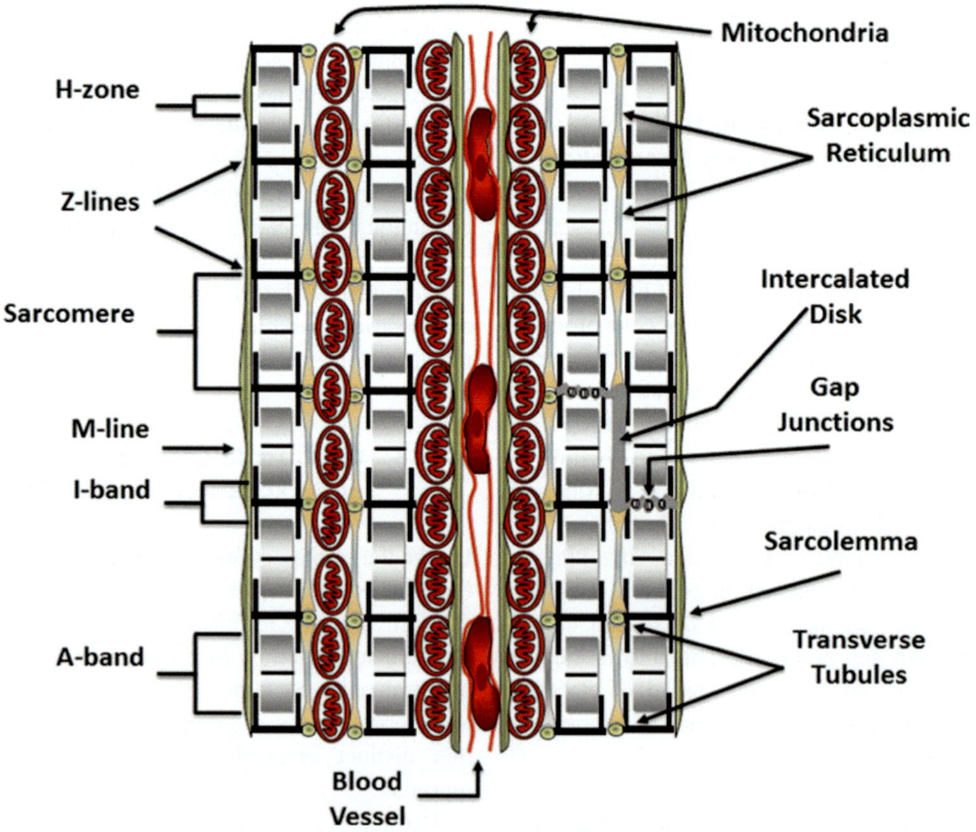

Fig. 17.4 A cross-section of cardiac tissue showing two cells separated by a blood vessel containing red blood cells. The repeating sarcomeric structure of the myofibrils and the names of the sarcomeric landmarks are highlighted on the left of the figure. On the right of the figure the legend points out the membrane specializations of the cell. These include the intercalated disks, gap junctions, the transverse tubules that punctuate the sarcolemma (plasma membrane), and the sarcoplasmic reticulum. Also shown are mitochondria compacted into a limited space because of the abundance of the myofibrils (Reprinted with permission from Iaizzo [5])

transmission of the force generated by the heart. Recall that electrical coupling between cells is provided by Gap junctions. The sarcolemma also invaginates into the cell to form an extensive tubular network called transverse tubules or T tubules.

Most of the contractile cardiomyocyte's cell volume is made of myofibrils. The rest is made up of cytosol, mitochondria, nucleus, and sarcoplasmic reticulum (SR). Unlike skeletal muscle cells, cardiomyocytes have a high density of mitochondria and strategic positioning of SR in the vicinity of T tubules.

Myofibrils consist mainly of two types of contractile proteins: thin filament actin and thick filament myosin. These are arranged in a specific pattern to generate the basic unit of contraction: the sarcomere. The arrangement of sarcomeres in turn gives cardiac muscle a distinct striated appearance when examined under the electron microscope. This is due to differences in refractive properties of the elements. These striations are identified by letters and represent either specific lines or bands of refraction. Z lines (from the German word *zuckung* or twitch line) are dark lines present at regular intervals along the myofibril. For the sake of understanding, let us imagine the sarcomere to be a square, with two lateral pillars, a roof, and a base (◉ Fig. 17.5).

The "pillars" then represent the Z lines. Now imagine a line running through the center of this square. This is the M line, which anchors the myosin filaments. Actin filaments

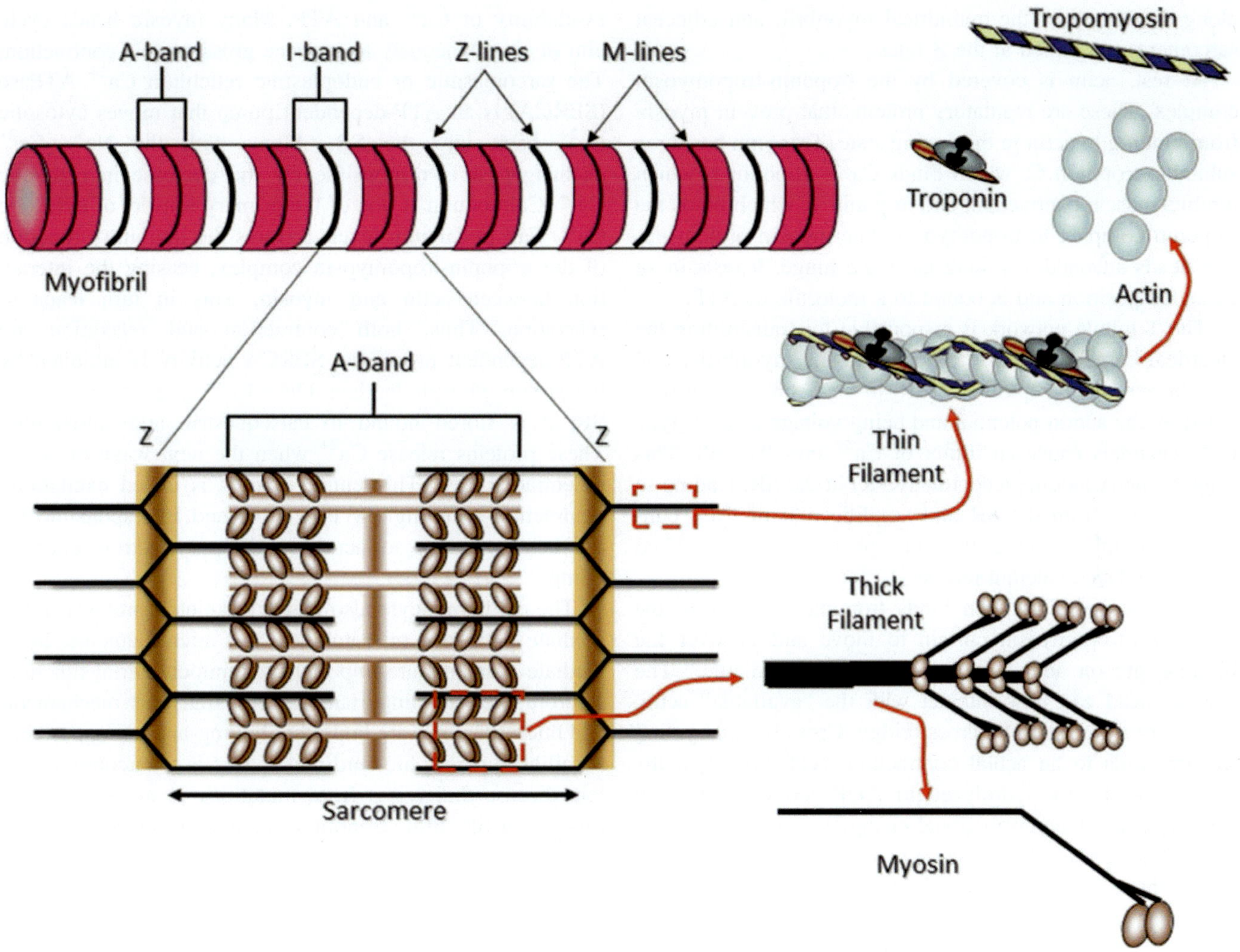

Fig. 17.5 Myofibrils are constructed of repeating sarcomeres within cardiac muscle cells. Each sarcomere is defined as the structures bounded on each end by Z-disks (Z lines). Thin filaments of the protein actin are attached to the Z line and reach toward the center of each sarcomere. Two regulatory proteins are found on the double-stranded actin thin filaments—tropomyosin and troponin. Tropomyosin is a double-stranded a-helical protein dimer that binds across 7 actin monomers on the thin filament obscuring a binding site for myosin. Troponin is a 3-subunit globular protein that binds 1 per tropomyosin. Thick filaments of the protein myosin are found in the center of the sarcomere. The area that contains the thick filaments is also known as the A band. The myosin molecules are asymmetrically shaped with a coiled-coil "tail" and two globular "head" domains. The head domains bind to actin to form crossbridges between the filaments and generate contractile force (Reprinted with permission from Iaizzo [5])

anchor onto Z lines via actinin and extend toward the M line, interdigitating with the myosin filaments. The region occupied by myosin filaments (with and without overlapping actin) is termed the A band (appears d**a**rk). The region occupied by actin filaments without any overlap with myosin is called the I band (appears l**i**ght). Z lines are connected to the sarcolemma via desmin. Scaffolding for the sarcomere is provided by the largest known protein, titin. Thus, each sarcomere consists of two half I bands and 1 A band between 2 Z lines. Sliding of the thin filaments over the thick filaments generates contraction. Actual lengths of the filaments do not change; shortening is brought about by increasing overlap between the thin and thick filaments. This is represented by lengthening of A band and shortening of I band during contraction. The sarcomeres are arranged in series along the length of the cylindrical myofibril, and adjacent sarcomeres are joined at the Z lines.

At rest, actin is covered by the troponin-tropomyosin complex. These are regulatory proteins that prevent myosin from binding to actin in the resting state. Troponin has three subunits: troponin C, which binds Ca^{2+}; troponin I, which inhibits muscle contraction; and troponin T, which binds the troponin complex to tropomyosin. The myosin protein has two heads attached to a long tail via a hinge. It rests in an extended position and is bound to a molecule of ATP.

The T tubule network is responsible for transmitting the electrical current or action potential to the myofibrils. The dihydropyridine receptors (DHPR) in the T tubules are activated by the action potential and being voltage gated L-type Ca^{2+} channels cause an influx of Ca^{2+} into the cell. This triggers the ryanodine receptors (RyR) in the SR, leading to Ca^{2+} release from the SR and amplification of Ca^{2+} concentration in the cytosol. This phenomenon is called calcium-induced calcium release.

The released Ca^{2+} then binds troponin C, causing the troponin I-tropomyosin curtain to move and uncover the binding site on actin, thereby making it "available." The myosin head can now interact with the "available" actin, leading to formation of a cross bridge. Cross bridge cycling in turn leads to an actual contraction. ATP bound to the myosin head gets hydrolyzed to ADP and energizes the myosin head. A conformational change occurs with release of ADP that causes the thin actin filament to move in relation to the thick myosin filament increasing their overlap, and producing a "power stroke." The myosin head goes from a resting "extended" to an active "flexed" position, moving the actin molecule along. ATP binds to the free site on myosin, interrupting the myosin–actin interaction. Rapid hydrolysis of ATP to ADP via myosin ATPase enzyme leads to "re-extension" of the myosin head and return to the original state. This myosin head is then ready for interaction with the next "available" actin. This can be visualized as follows: Lay your left arm supine on a table with palm facing the ceiling such that your elbow and wrist are in a straight line. Now make a fist and bend your elbow, making a 120° angle between your arm and forearm. Place the palm of right hand on top of your left fist. Your left fist represents a myosin head, your left elbow is the hinge, and your right palm is an actin molecule. Flex your left elbow to bring your right hand/palm toward your left shoulder. That represents the myosin head moving the actin molecule. Now disengage your left fist from your right palm. Let your right palm stay at the level of the left shoulder and bring your left fist back to its extended 120° position. Your left fist is ready to "cross bridge" with another palm (ask a friend to lend one). This is how myosin moves actin. Two ATPs are required: one to energize the myosin head and other to disengage from actin.

This process is repetitive and depends only on the availability of Ca^{2+} and ATP. Many myosin heads cycle almost simultaneously to produce gross muscle contraction. The sarcoplasmic or endoplasmic reticulum Ca^{2+} ATPase (SERCA) is an ATP-dependent pump that moves cytosolic Ca^{2+} back into the SR. Along with the Na^{+} –Ca^{2+} exchanger, it is responsible for the decrease in cytosolic Ca^{2+}. Calmodulin is one of the primary sensors of cytosolic Ca^{2+}. Fall in calcium levels restores the inhibitory function of the troponin-tropomyosin complex, ceasing the interaction between actin and myosin. This in turn leads to relaxation. Thus, both contraction and relaxation are ATP-dependent processes. SERCA activity is inhibited by the protein phospholamban. Once Ca^{2+} enters back into the SR, it is stored bound to calsequestrin and calreticulin. These proteins release Ca^{2+} when the next wave of action potential arrives. This entire process is called excitation–contraction coupling (◉ Fig. 17.6) and is responsible for the heart's ability to act as a tireless electromechanical pump.

The cardiomyocyte also has cytoskeleton proteins: intermediate filaments, microtubules, and microfilaments. Intermediate filaments are important for mitochondrial function. Microtubules are important for cell transport mechanisms and microfilaments are important linking-anchoring proteins. Familial hypertrophic cardiomyopathy is a sarcomeric protein disease that arises from mutations in genes encoding myosin, actin, titin, tropomyosin, and troponins. Familial dilated cardiomyopathy, on the other hand, is a cytoskeleton protein disease arising from mutations in genes encoding actin, desmin, lamin, and sarcoglycan [1–5].

17.3 The Electrocardiogram

Efficiency of contraction in the heart is achieved by precise timing of events during the cardiac cycle. The atria depolarize and repolarize before the ventricles. Thus at any given point of time, different parts of the heart are in different

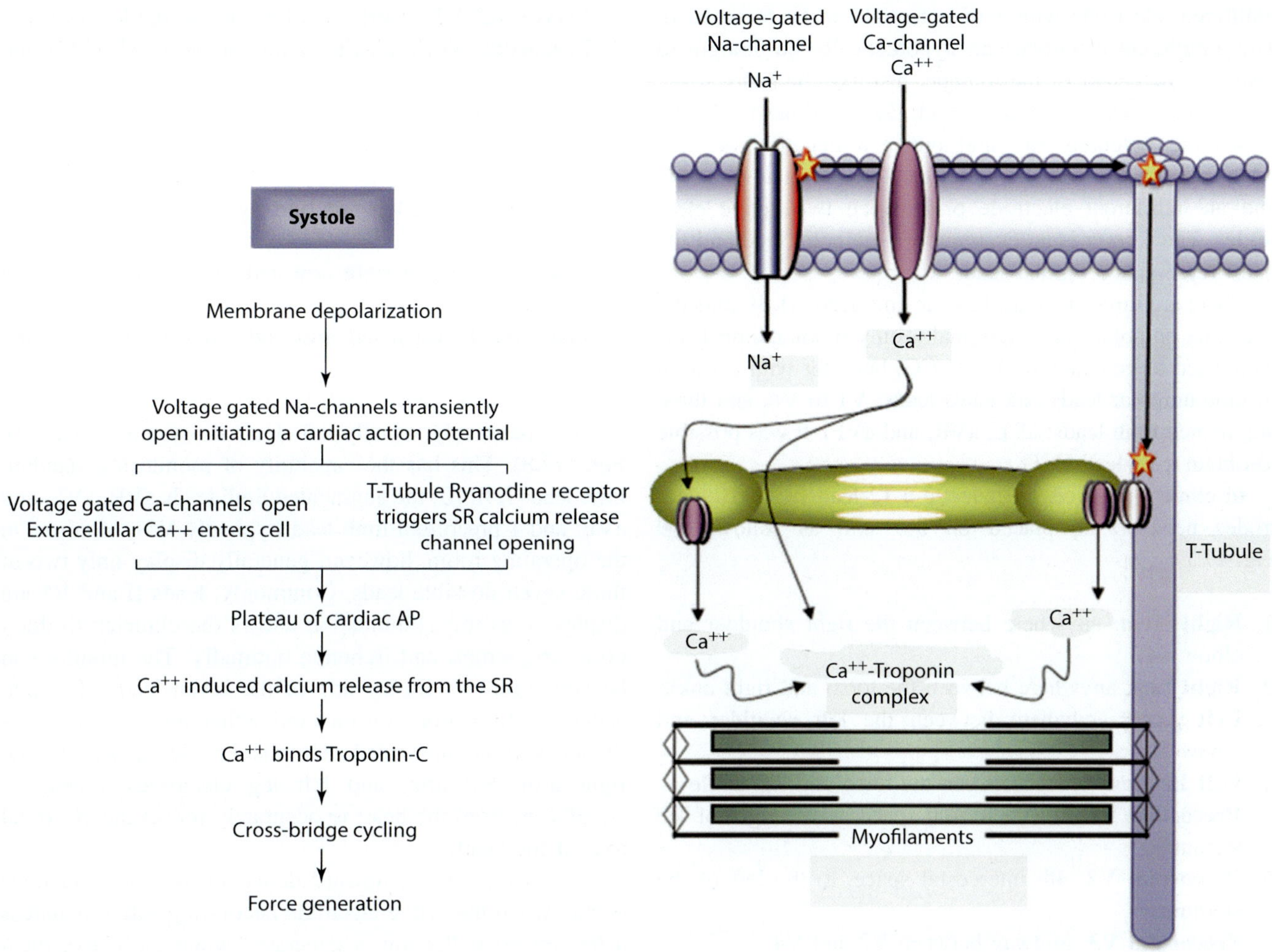

Fig. 17.6 Excitation–contraction coupling. In systole, an electrically depolarizing signal triggers the transient opening of voltage-gated Na-channels; the influx of positively charged Na ions further depolarizes the cell. This further depolarization causes the opening of L-type Ca-channels (long duration opening) and calcium enters the cell. This also causes ryanodine receptors in the T tubules to trigger the release of calcium from Ca-channels in the sarcoplasmic reticulum. This initiates the plateau of the cardiac action potential. The rise in intracellular calcium concentration triggers additional calcium release from the sarcoplasmic reticulum via Ca-channels. The calcium binds to troponin on the thin filaments, inducing the movement of tropomyosin. Crossbridge cycling begins generating tension in the cardiac myocytes (Reprinted with permission from Iaizzo [5])

phases of depolarization and repolarization. These discrepancies are responsible for generating a fluctuating potential difference. Given that the heart is enclosed by conducting fluid, much like a battery suspended in saltwater, it generates an electrical field around it. This can be measured and displayed by appropriately placed electrodes as an electrocardiogram (ECG). The ECG is not a display of individual action potentials occurring in the myocytes; it represents the cumulative change in electrical activity over time. When the ECG is measured by electrodes placed on skin, it is typically referred to as surface ECG. Electric potentials, other than that generated by the heart, can interfere or influence the net potential measured at the level of the skin. Patients are usually instructed to breathe quietly and lay still while an ECG is being recorded to minimize interference from skeletal muscle potentials. In the perioperative setting, it is difficult to get a good ECG trace from patients who are shivering or when electrocautery is being used.

William Einthoven did pioneering work in the field of electrocardiography and was awarded the Nobel Prize in 1924. His hypothesis: The Einthoven's triangle is used to obtain a surface ECG. According to the hypothesis, if a current source is placed in the center of an equilateral triangle, the sum of potential at the points of the triangle is zero at all times. Clinically this can be approximated by placing recording electrodes on both arms and the left leg. The heart then lies in the center of this imaginary triangle. If all these "active" electrodes are connected together, a fourth indifferent electrode with zero potential can be formulated. This indifferent electrode can hypothetically be thought to reside in the center of the triangle, just like the heart.

Two electrodes constitute a lead. Each lead has two ends: a positive potential end and either a negative or zero potential end. Current can therefore flow between an active and an indifferent electrode or between two active electrodes. The former is an example of a unipolar lead and the latter represents a bipolar lead.

There are three standard bipolar limb leads (I, II, and III) and nine unipolar leads. Originally only bipolar limb leads were used to generate a 3-lead ECG, but later with addition of nine unipolar leads (six chest leads: V1 to V6, and three augmented limb leads: aVL, aVR, and aVF), it was possible to obtain a 12-lead ECG.

In clinical practice, to generate a 12-lead ECG, 10 electrodes need to be placed on the skin as follows (◉ Fig. 17.7):

1. **Right Arm**: anywhere between the right shoulder and elbow
2. **Right Leg**: anywhere between the torso and right ankle
3. **Left Arm**: anywhere between the left shoulder and elbow
4. **Left Leg**: anywhere between the torso and left ankle
5. **Precordial V1**: 4th intercostal space, to the right of the sternum
6. **Precordial V2**: 4th intercostal space, to the left of the sternum
7. **Precordial V3**: midway between V2 and V4
8. **Precordial V4**: 5th intercostal space at the midclavicular line
9. **Precordial V5:** anterior axillary line at the level of V4
10. **Precordial V6:** midaxillary line at the level of V4 and V5.

Standard limb leads would then be:

1. **Lead I**: between left arm and right arm, left arm being positive
2. **Lead II**: between right arm and left leg, left leg being positive
3. **Lead III**: between left arm and left leg, left leg being positive.

Intraoperatively, usually a 5-electrode system is used (◉ Fig. 17.8). This has the capability of monitoring standard limb leads I, II, III; the augmented limb leads aVR, aVL, and aVF; and 1 precordial limb lead (typically V5). Monitors in the operating room, however, generally display only two of these seven possible leads. Commonly, leads II and V5 are displayed, as this combination allows the clinician to diagnose arrhythmias and ischemia optimally. The monitor can be configured to display any of the seven leads. To yield accurate information, it is imperative that the clinician places the leads in recommended anatomical positions. Ideally, the right arm, left arm, and left leg electrodes should be equidistant from the heart to accurately reflect the electrical axis of the heart.

By convention, an upward deflection on the ECG trace occurs when the active electrode becomes positive, whereas a downward deflection is generated when the active electrode becomes negative. The wave of depolarization moves from the SA node to the rest of the heart in multiple

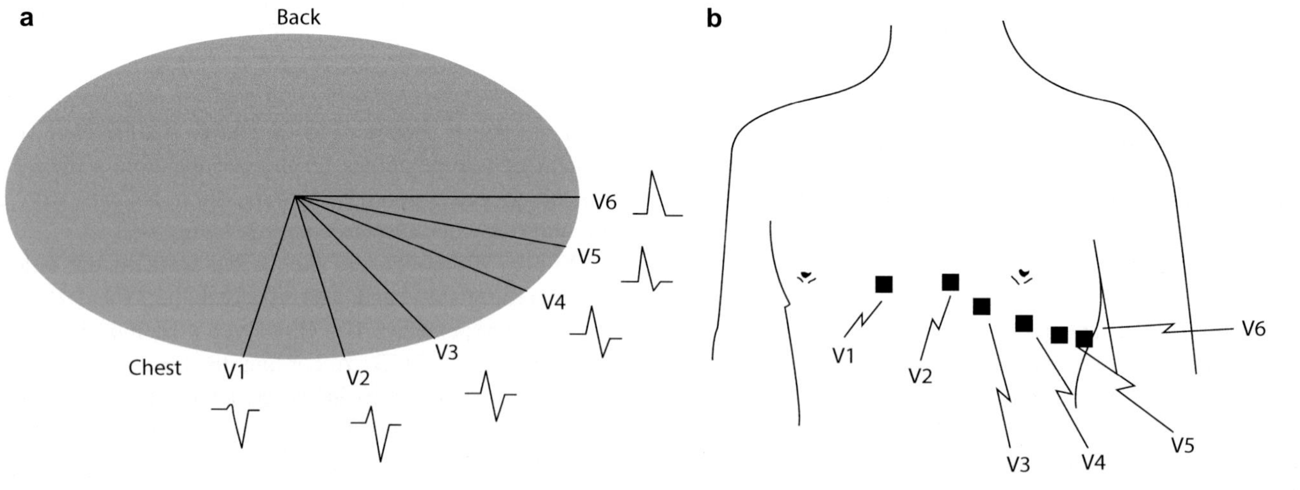

Fig. 17.7 **a** A cross-section of chest shows relative position of six precordial leads in traverse plane, along with a typical waveform detected for ventricular depolarization. **b** An anterior view of chest shows common placement of each precordial lead, V1 through V6 (Reprinted with permission from Iaizzo [5])

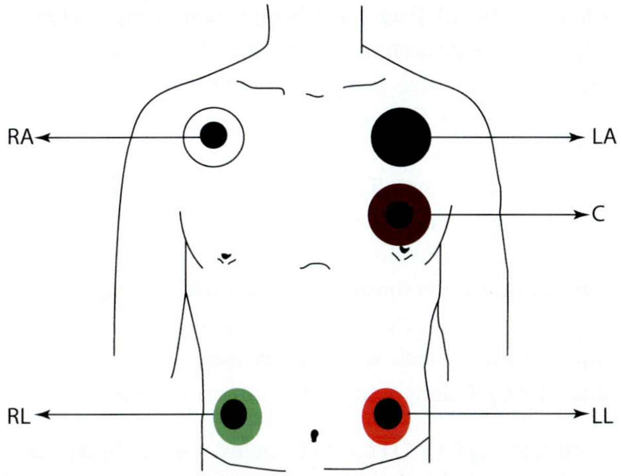

Fig. 17.8 Placement of common 5-wire ECG electrode system leads on shoulders, chest, and torso. Chest electrode is placed according to desired precordial lead position. *C* chest, *LA* left arm, *LL* left leg, *RA* right arm, *RL* right leg (Reprinted with permission from Iaizzo [5])

directions, but these can be summated to present a single electrical vector. The way the different leads are positioned to this vector determines if they record positive or negative deflections. These deflections give rise to the waves, segments, and intervals of the ECG. In a standard ECG strip, 1 mm square equates to 40 ms of duration on the horizontal axis and 0.1 mV of amplitude on the vertical axis. One mm square is often referred to as a "small" box. Five 1 mm squares form a 5 mm or large box (◉ Fig. 17.9).

The component waves are as follows:

1. **P wave**: Represents atrial depolarization. As it includes right and left depolarization, it may be biphasic or twin peaked. It is usually upright. Height in Lead II is less than 2.5 mm and duration is less than 0.11 s. Although the SA node is the first group of cells to fire, its electrical activity cannot be measured with surface electrodes. The cumulative activity of the atria can, however, be

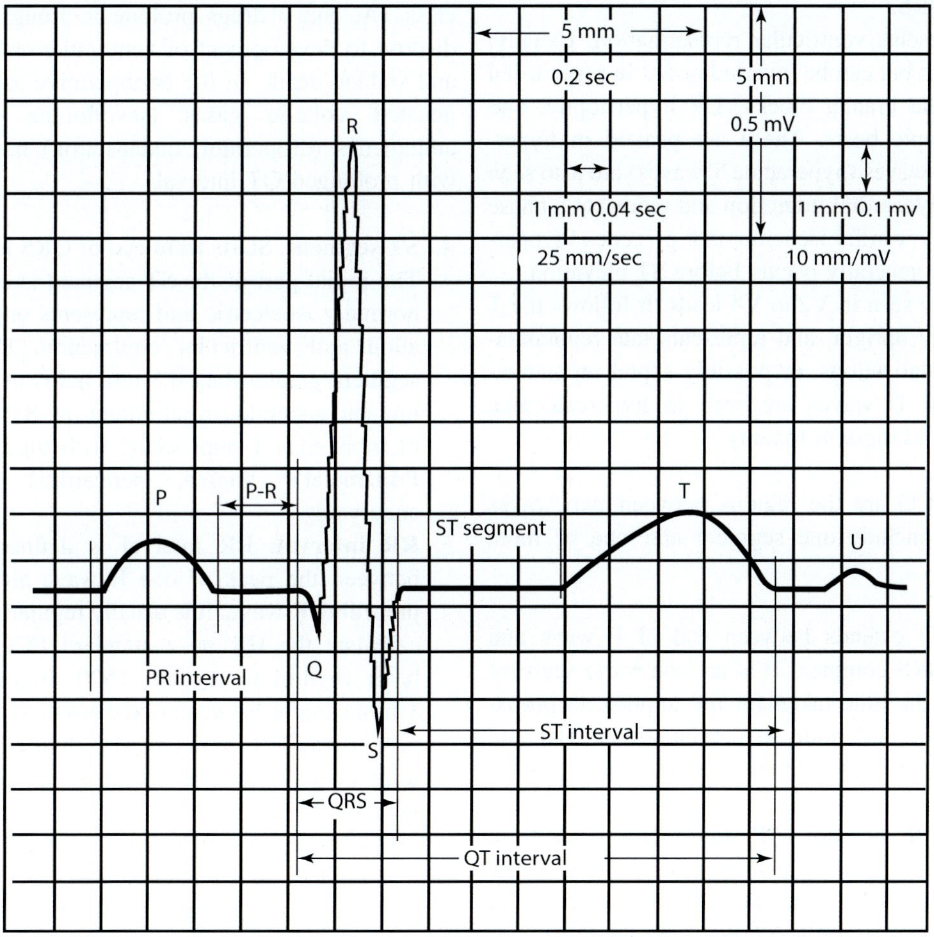

Fig. 17.9 Single components of an ECG and their temporal relations (Reprinted with permission from Romanò [6])

recorded. Taller P waves may be a sign of RA enlargement, and wider or M-shaped P waves may represent LA enlargement.

2. **Q wave**: It is a negative deflection that follows the P wave and represents septal depolarization. After myocardial infarction, pathologic Q waves develop (duration greater than 30 ms, depth greater than 0.1 mV) after a couple of days. These represent scar tissue; and as dead tissue does not conduct impulses, it produces a wide and deep negative deflection (pathological Q wave) representing flow of current away from the tissue.
3. **QRS complex**: Represents ventricular depolarization. As left ventricle has more muscle mass than right, it contributes more to the genesis of the QRS complex. Usually, duration is less than 0.12 s. R wave is upright and represents early ventricular repolarization whereas the S wave is negative and represents late ventricular depolarization. During the time when QRS is generated, the atria are repolarizing. This atrial repolarization wave or Ta is not usually seen due to the overwhelming signal generated by QRS.
4. **T wave**: Represents ventricular repolarization. Usually, these are upright but can be inverted or flat in myocardial ischemia, bundle branch blocks, LV hypertrophy, and ventricular ectopic beats. These are peaked in hyperkalemia. Tall T waves (hyperacute T waves) are also seen minutes after myocardial infarction and represent a phase of reversible myocardial ischemia that precedes myocardial necrosis. It generally occurs before ST elevation.
5. **U wave**: usually seen in V2 to V4 leads. It follows the T wave, is usually upright, and represents late repolarization, after depolarizations, or possibly septal repolarization. Prominent U waves are seen in hypercalcemia, hypokalemia, and digoxin toxicity.

Segments in ECG are the regions between two waves whereas intervals include one segment and one or more waves:

1. **PR segment**: It extends between end of P wave and beginning of QRS complex. It is an isoelectric segment and represents the time taken for the impulse to propagate through the AV node to the bundle of His and bundle braches. It is sometimes referred to as the P-Ta segment.
2. **PR interval (PR segment + P wave)**: It extends from beginning of the P wave to beginning of the QRS complex and represents the time taken for the impulse to reach the ventricles from the SA node. As the Q wave is frequently absent, it is called PR interval rather than PQ interval. Normal values lie between 120 and 200 milliseconds. It is shortened in pre-excitation syndromes, such as Wolff-Parkinson-White syndrome, where an accessory pathway between the atria and ventricles allows the impulse to bypass the AV node. It is greater than 200 ms in first-degree AV block.
3. **QT interval**: It begins at the onset of QRS and ends at the end of T wave. Thus, it includes the QRS complex, ST segment, and T wave. It represents the duration from depolarization to repolarization of the ventricles. Its duration depends upon heart rate (HR), gender, and age. It is usually corrected to the HR as it shortens with faster rates and lengthens with slower rates. This correction is done using Bazett's formula but is not error proof:

Corrected QT or QTc = QT/square root of heart rate

The normal value for the QTc in men is $\leq$ 0.44 s and in women is $\leq$ 0.45–0.46 s. Hypercalcemia, hyperthyroidism, hyperkalemia, digitalis toxicity, and class IB drugs shorten the interval. Myocarditis, hypokalemia, hypocalcemia, CHF, class 1A, and 3 drugs prolong it. Long QT intervals predispose to development of ventricular arrhythmias, torsade, and sudden death. In the perioperative setting, use of halogenated volatile gases (sevoflurane particularly) and antiemetics (droperidol, ondansetron) has been associated with prolonged QT interval.

4. **ST segment**: Starts from end of QRS to onset of T wave. The initial part of the ST segment is called J point. It is normally isoelectric and represents ongoing atrial relaxation and ventricular contraction. Depression of ST segment greater than 0.5 mm helps in diagnosing ischemia and subendocardial infarction. ST segment elevation of more than 1 mm occurs with transmural infarctions, Prinzmetal's angina, pericarditis, and ventricular aneurysms.
5. **RR interval**: RR interval is defined as the distance between the peak of one R wave and the peak of the preceding R wave. It is usually regular and can be used to calculate the HR on a standard ECG strip. Assuming heart rhythm is regular, 1500 divided by number of 1 mm squares between two consecutive RR intervals will give us the HR. You can also divide 300 by number of large boxes to get the HR. If the rhythm is irregular, do the following:
   A. Obtain a 6 s ECG strip. The ECG strip is usually marked at 3 s intervals. Recall, each small box is 40 ms, each large box is 200 ms or 0.2 s, and thus, 15 large boxes will constitute 3 s ($15 \times 0.2 = 3$ s).
   B. A 6 s strip will have 30 large boxes. Count the number of R waves in 30 large boxes (or 6 s) and multiply by 10 to get the HR per minute.

17.4 The Cardiac Cycle

The sequence of electromechanical events that take place during the course of a heartbeat constitutes the cardiac cycle (CC). As outlined before, CC can be broadly divided into systole (phase of contraction) and diastole (phase of relaxation). The atria as well as the ventricles undergo contraction and relaxation. However, we shall use the terms systole and diastole to denote ventricular contraction and relaxation, unless otherwise specified. Keeping this in mind, CC then comprises broadly of six events that occur sequentially: isovolumic (ventricular) contraction, ventricular ejection (rapid and slow phases), isovolumic (ventricular) relaxation, ventricular filling (early filling), diastasis, and atrial systole.

The QRS complex of the ECG represents ventricular depolarization. This triggers ventricular contraction and an increase in ventricular intracavitary pressures. This leads to closure of the tricuspid and mitral valves, which in turn generates the first heart sound or S1. This heralds the beginning of the isovolumic contraction phase wherein ventricular pressure increases without change in volume, and in this phase, all the valves are closed (beginning of R to end of S wave). The continuing increase in ventricular pressures eventually leads to opening of the pulmonary and aortic valves with rapid ejection of blood into the great arteries (rapid ventricular ejection phase). This leads to increasing pressures in the great arteries, and the rate of ventricular ejection slows down (end of S wave to approximately distal portion to end of T wave represents ventricular contraction). As action potentials are time-dependent, the LV and RV start repolarizing (T wave) and eventually stop ejecting. When the ventricles stop ejecting, the PA and aortic pressures briefly exceed ventricular pressures, leading to closure of PV and AoV. This generates the second heart sound (S2) and represents end systole (approximately at around peak of T wave). The RV being crescent shaped demonstrates peristaltic contraction and typically does not exhibit the isovolumic contraction phase like the LV.

The diastolic period has four phases: isovolumic relaxation, ventricular filling, diastasis, and atrial systole. The ventricular diastolic period (distal portion to end of T wave to beginning of QRS) starts after PV and AoV closure. The pressure in the ventricles decreases rapidly without an initial change in volume. This is called isovolumic relaxation, and all the valves are closed in this phase. Atrial diastole starts and continues during ventricular depolarization (QRS) and contraction (ST). Electrically, it is overshadowed by the QRS and is thus the atrial T wave or Ta (atrial repolarization wave) is not represented on the ECG. The ventricles continue to untwist and relax with continuing fall in their intracavitary pressures. On the other hand, the atrial pressures rise, given that they have been filling during atrial diastole. This pressure difference leads to opening of TV and MV, leading to rapid ventricular filling. Early filling is due to diastolic suction and contributes to about 70% of ventricular filling. It generates the third heart sound (S3). This phase is followed by diastasis, wherein rapid ventricular filling and subsequent ventricular pressure rise, impeding further filling from the atria to such an extent that the atria simply act as passive conduits for blood flow from the pulmonary veins into the left ventricle. This phase contributes about 5% to total ventricular filling and may disappear with tachycardia.

Atrial systole follows diastasis and is constituted by atrial depolarization (P wave) and contraction (PR segment) or "atrial kick." This "kick" contributes to about 20%–30% of ventricular filling and generates the fourth heart sound (S4). When the heart is hypertrophied or has low compliance, the atrial kick may be responsible for up to 40% of ventricular filling.

Atrial contraction is followed by atrial relaxation or diastole. Following atrial contraction, the propagating impulse leads to ventricular depolarization (QRS). This marks the beginning of ventricular systole. As the ventricles fill up during diastole, the intracavitary pressures rise, leading to closure of TV and MV and beginning of isovolumic contraction completing the cardiac cycle.

Thus, atrial systole occurs during ventricular diastole and ventricular systole occurs during atrial diastole. This mechanism of sequential activation is important to ensure forward flow of blood through the pulmonary and systemic circulation. Additionally, the kinetic energy of ventricular ejection is stored as potential energy in the great arteries and released to the distal vasculature during diastole ensuring forward flow through the entire CC [3, 4].

17.4.1 Timing of Events

Although the right and left hearts undergo similar events during the CC, the timing of events is asynchronous. RA depolarization precedes LA depolarization, but they contract almost simultaneously. As the LV depolarizes first, its contraction precedes RV contraction. However, as the PA pressures are lower compared to systemic pressures, the PV opens first allowing the RV to eject before the LV. The pulmonary vascular impedance is lesser than that of the aorta, and this allows the RV to eject for a longer time than the LV, leading to a later closure of the PV as compared to the aortic valve. This difference in timing of closures of aortic (early) and pulmonary valves (later) leads to splitting of the second heart sound (S2).

Table 17.1 Heart Sounds and their characteristics

Heart Sound	Characteristics	Notes
S1	• Frequency ≈ 30 Hz • Commonly heard as "lub." • Two components: one generated by closure of MV or M1 (occurs first) and the other by closure of TV or T1 (occurs later). However, the two events occur too closely to usually differentiate by auscultation • Occurs coincident with the upstroke of the carotid pulse and is best heard at the cardiac apex as its intensity is primarily determined by M1	• Accentuated in MS, TS, atrial myxoma, tachycardia & pre-excitation syndromes (short PR intervals) • Diminished when the valves are immobile due to fibrosis (mitral regurgitation/MR) or calcification and with long PR intervals • Splitting: split in pathological conditions such as complete RBBB, LV pacing, ASD, and Ebsteins anomaly. In ASD, the split is wide and fixed: it does not vary with the phase of respiration
S2	• Frequency: ≈ 50 Hz • Commonly heard as "dub." • Two components: A2 generated by Aortic Valve closure (occurs first) and P2 generated by PV closure (occurs later) • Coincides with the down stroke of the carotid pulse • A2 is best heard in the right second ICS and P2 in the left second ICS	• Ability to hear P2 at the apex signifies increased P2 intensity (PA hypertension or ASD) • Diminished P2 usually is present with PV stenosis or absent congenital PV • Accentuated A2 intensity can be appreciated in systemic HTN and coarctation of aorta • Diminished A2 intensity is present in AR as well as in calcific aortic stenosis AS • Splitting: Abnormal splitting present in conduction abnormalities (RBBB, WPW syndrome, pacing) and large ASD
S3	• Generated by rapid ventricular filling • Best heard at the apex with the patient positioned in the left lateral decubitus position	• Normally heard in young adults & high output states such as pregnancy • Presence in older individuals (> 40 years of age) is usually pathological • S3 gallop is usually present in chronic MR, chronic AR, and symptomatic heart failure
S4	• Generated by atrial systole • Best heard at the apex with the patient positioned in the left lateral decubitus position	• Presence in children and young adults, unlike S3, is usually pathological • Typically heard in HTN, AS, and hypertrophic cardiomyopathy

AR Aortic Regurgitation, *AS* Aortic Stenosis, *ASD* Atrial Septal Defects, *HTN* Hypertension, *MV* Mitral Valve, *MS* Mitral Stenosis, *PA* Pulmonary arterial, *PV* Pulmonary Valve, *RBBB* Right Bundle Branch Block, *TV* Tricuspid Valve, *TS* Tricuspid Stenosis, *WPW* Wolf Parkinson White

17.4.2 Heart Sounds and Waveforms Generated During the Cardiac Cycle

Heart sounds can be auscultated at the bedside using a stethoscope. A stethoscope usually has a bell and a diaphragm; the former is used to listen to low frequency sounds (S3 and S4) and the latter for high frequency sounds (S1 and S2). Characteristics of heart sounds are tabulated (Table 17.1).

The peak velocity of blood flowing through the aorta during systole ranges from 1 to 1.7 m/s. However, as noted before, the kinetic energy imparted by the LV also sets up a pressure wave that expands the arterial walls as it travels distally. This expansion is palpable as a pulse. The velocity of this waveform is far greater than that of the velocity of blood, and it increases as it moves distally. Typical velocities are 4 m/s in the aorta, 8 m/s in the large arteries, and 16 m/s in the small arteries in younger individuals. Thus, after LV systole occurs, a pulse can be felt at the wrist in about 0.1 s. As we age, the arteries lose elastin and become stiffer, and they conduct these pulses even faster. As the arterial tree branches, this pressure waveform keeps on reflecting in different directions and on itself, leading to amplification. This leads to increases in systolic blood pressure (SBP) and decreases in diastolic blood pressure (DBP) as we move distally from the heart. However, the mean arterial pressure (MAP) tends to remain similar if measured either centrally at the aorta or peripherally at the wrist or foot. Although, MAP can only be accurately measured by calculating the area under the pressure waveform, clinically it is often calculated as:

$$\mathrm{SBP} + \{(\mathrm{SBP} - \mathrm{DBP})/3\}$$

The CC typically generates a SBP of 100–120 mm Hg and DBP of 70–80 mm Hg. The pressure waveform exhibits a rapid upstroke during systole, a dicrotic notch that occurs due to AoV closure (reverberations from the valve interrupt the smooth descent of the arterial waveform), and a smooth diastolic downstroke. The pulse pressure (PP) is the

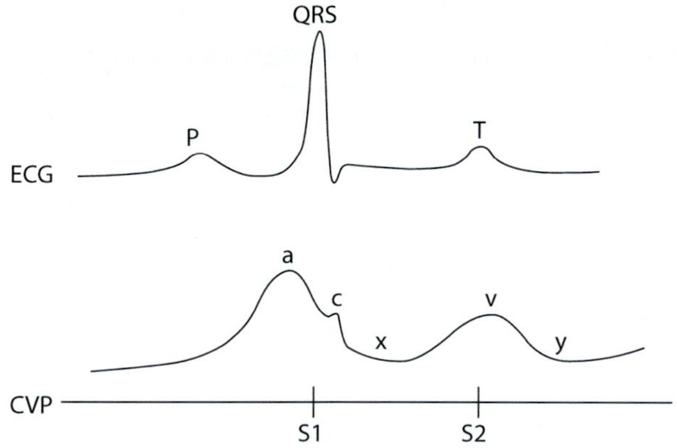

Fig. 17.10 A typical example of a central venous pressure wave form consisting of a, c, and v waves and x and y descents. The a wave is associated with atrial contraction. The c wave occurs as the tricuspid valve bulges up toward the *right atrium* during early ventricular systole. The v wave is associated with passive filling of the *right atrium* with closed valve. The x descent corresponds to the tricuspid valve being pulled down toward the *right ventricle* during late systole. The y descent corresponds with opening of the tricuspid valve as the *right atrium* begins to empty. *CVP* central venous pressure, *ECG* electrocardiogram (Reprinted with permission from Iaizzo [5])

difference between the SBP and the DBP and is normally 40–50 mm Hg. It determines the intensity or strength of the palpable pulse. The wider the pulse pressure, the stronger the palpable pulse. This is commonly seen in older people. In certain pathological conditions, such as severe AR, where the pulse pressure can be very wide (high SBP and near zero DBP), the intensity of the pulse can make the head nod. This is called Corrigan's sign.

Atrial systole and diastole also lead to characteristic changes in the central venous pressure (CVP) on the right side and LA pressure waveform on the left side (◉ Fig. 17.10). The "a" wave occurs due to atrial systole and backflow of blood into the SVC (or pulmonary veins on the left side). This is followed by the c wave, which occurs during early ventricular systole as the tricuspid valve is pushed into the RA. The "x" descent denotes the negative pressure generated in the RA by pulling down of the TV during late ventricular systole. The "v" wave occurs due to passive filling of the RA during atrial diastole or ventricular systole. This is followed by the "y" descent that represents opening of the TV and filling of the RV. Sometimes another wave representing diastasis, called "h" wave, is seen following the y wave, especially during slow heart rates. Thus, there are three waves that occur during ventricular diastole: y, h, and a (representing rapid filling, diastasis, and atrial systole) and there are three waves that occur during systole: c, x, and v (representing early systole, late systole, and atrial diastole).

The venous waveform can be examined by observing the internal jugular venous pulse (JVP) just adjacent to the trachea in the neck. Patients are semi-recumbent at 30–45° and turn their heads slightly to the opposite side to facilitate examination. The venous pulsation's predominant movement is inward (x or y descent), and this helps distinguishing it from the carotid pulse, which predominantly moves outward. The height of oscillation from the sternal border is measured and 5 cm is added to it to estimate RA pressures, as it is assumed that the RA lies 5 cm below the sternum.

Abnormalities of the CVP waves are presented below (Table 17.2) [3, 4].

17.4.3 The LV Pressure: Volume (P–V) Loop

The PV loop is generated by plotting LV pressure on the *y*-axis and LV volume on the *x*-axis and provides an assessment of LV function (systolic and diastolic) during a single cardiac cycle (◉ Fig. 17.11). The mechanical events during a single CC proceed in a counterclockwise manner over time. As denoted by the figure, the following events occur:

A: Mitral valve opens, begin ventricular filling
B: Mitral valve close, end diastole
C: Aortic valve opens, begin ejection
D: Aortic valve closes, end systole
A-B: Ventricular filling, diastasis, atrial systole
B-C: Isovolumic contraction
C-D: Ejection, rapid and slow
D-A: Isovolumic relaxation
E: Contractility

The area inside the loop is the myocardial energy or stroke work expended to generate a stroke volume/SV for a single beat. The width of the loop represents the SV and the slope of the end-systolic PV relationship (ESPVR) represents contractility (slope through point D). Slope AB represents the end-diastolic PV relationship (EDPVR). The PV loops are great diagnostic tools. A variety of conditions can be assessed with changes in their morphology, position of the loop, and position of ESPVR and EDPVR slopes. However, it is important to remember that these are generated over a single beat or CC, and although they help us understand different heart conditions, they are difficult to obtain clinically [1, 2]. The effect of common valvular lesions on the PV loop is demonstrated in **Fig.** 17.12.

17.5 Assessment of Cardiac Performance

Assessment of cardiac performance includes examining the systolic and diastolic function of the right and the left heart. Although this can be done invasively via right and left heart

Table 17.2 Central venous pressure waveforms

Waveform component and phase of cardiac cycle	Mechanism of generation	Conditions associated with accentuation	Conditions associated with diminution
A (Late Diastole)	Atrial systole and backflow of blood into the SVC	Tricuspid stenosis, RA myxoma, carcinoid heart disease, RA thrombus, tricuspid atresia, PV stenosis, and RV hypertrophy Very pronounced waves are called canon waves and are seen in complete AV block, junctional rhythms, and premature beats	Atrial fibrillation, severe Ebsteins anomaly (dilated RA cannot generate an effective systole)
C (Early Systole)	TV is pushed into the RA during early ventricular systole		
X descent (Mid to Late Systole)	Negative pressure generated in the RA by pulling down of the TV during late ventricular systole	Cardiac tamponade	
V (Late Systole)	Passive filling of the RA during atrial diastole or ventricular systole	TR (Lancisi sign), atrial septal defects without PA hypertension, arteriovenous fistulas	
Y descent (Early Diastole)	Opening of the TV and filling of the RV	Constrictive Pericarditis, restrictive cardiomyopathy, right heart failure. Rapid y descent without a prominent v wave suggests CP, but if accompanied by a prominent v wave it usually suggests TR	Cardiac tamponade
H (Mid Diastole)	Represents diastasis		

AV Atrioventricular, *CP* Constrictive Pericarditis, *PA* Pulmonary Arterial, *PV* Pulmonary Valve, *RA* Right Atrium, *RV* Right Ventricle, *SVC* Superior Vena Cava, *TR* Tricuspid Regurgitation, *TV* Tricuspid Valve

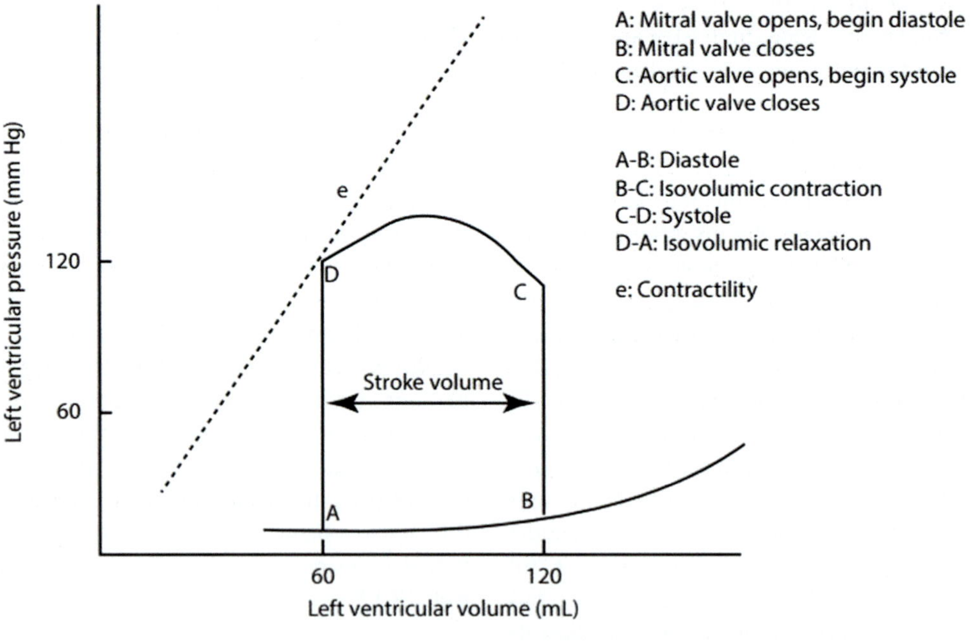

Fig. 17.11 Pressure–volume diagram of a single cardiac cycle (Reprinted with permission from Iaizzo [5])

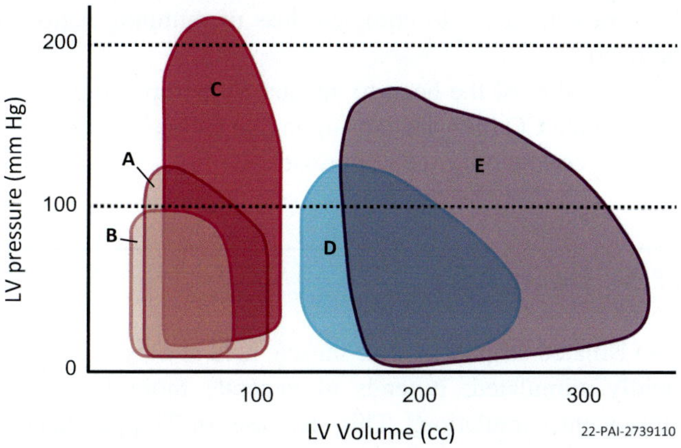

Fig. 17.12 LV Pressure–Volume loops in different valvular heart disease states with preserved systolic function. A: normal, B: mitral stenosis (under filled LV), C: Aortic stenosis (LV pressure overload), D: chronic mitral insufficiency (LV volume overload with reduced forward flow), E: chronic aortic insufficiency (LV volume overload). LV: Left Ventricle

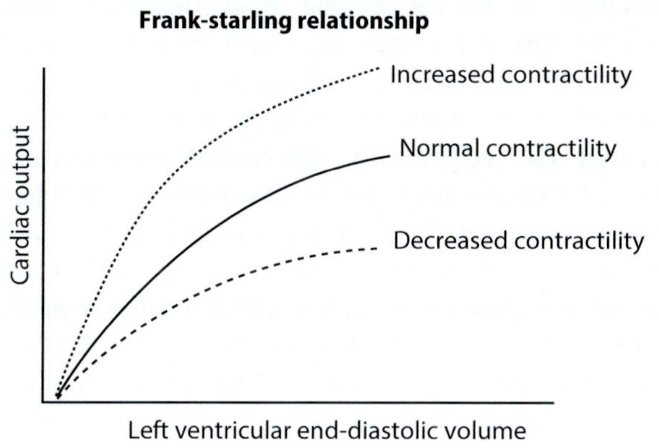

Fig. 17.13 "Frank–Starling relationship." As end-diastolic volume increases, cardiac output also increases. Excessive preload may eventually result in decreased cardiac output (Reprinted with permission from Iaizzo [5])

catheterization, it is commonly done non-invasively by echocardiography.

Usually, the right and left hearts pump the same amount of blood per unit time and this represents the cardiac output (CO). Mathematically then:

$$CO = \text{Stroke Volume (SV)} \times \text{Heart Rate (HR)}$$

where SV being the volume of blood pumped per beat or CC and the HR being the number of times the heart beats in a minute. When the CO is indexed to body surface area (BSA), it is referred to as cardiac index (CI). Normal CO in adults is about 5 L/min (range is 4–8 L/min) and CI is 2.5–4 L/min/m^2. *CO can be assessed by echocardiography, thermal dilution method via a pulmonary artery catheter, or via the Fick's principle.*

According to the Fick's principle, blood flow to an organ can be calculated using a marker substance if the following can be ascertained:

1. Amount of marker taken up by the organ per unit time
2. Concentration of marker in arterial blood supplying the organ
3. Concentration of marker in venous blood leaving the organ.

In Fick's original method, oxygen was the marker and the entire human body was the "organ." Mathematically, this can be represented as:

$$CO = \text{Oxygen consumption}/\text{concentration of oxygen in pulmonary venous blood} - \text{concentration of oxygen in pulmonary arterial blood.}$$

or

$$CO = VO_2/CpvO_2 - CpaO_2$$

Substituting $CpvO_2$ with CaO_2 (oxygen content of arterial blood) and $CpaO_2$ with CvO_2 (the oxygen content of mixed venous blood), the equation can be written as:

$$CO = VO_2/CaO_2 - CvO_2$$

or, oxygen consumption divided by the arteriovenous oxygen difference.

$$CaO_2 = 1.34 \times Hb \times SaO_2 + 0.003 \times PaO_2$$
$$CvO_2 = 1.34 \times Hb \times SvO_2 + 0.003 \times PvO_2$$

where Hb is hemoglobin concentration in g/dl, SaO_2 is the arterial oxygen saturation, and SvO_2 is the mixed venous oxygen saturation.

Assuming an Hb level of 15 g/dl, calculated CaO_2 is about 200 ml/Liter or 20 ml/dl, and CvO_2 is about 150 ml/dl or 15 ml/dl.

Oxygen consumption varies with stress, gender, and exercise capacity, but commonly is (erroneously) assumed to be 250 ml/min. It can be calculated as follows:

$$[\text{Concentration of inspired oxygen or } FiO_2 - \text{Concentration of expired oxygen or } EtO_2] \times \text{Minute Ventilation}$$

where minute ventilation is MV. For example, FiO_2 of room air is 0.21. Exhaled EtO_2 is 0.16 and MV is 5000 ml/min. Then, VO_2 is [0.21–0.16] × 5000 ml/min or 0.05 × 5000 ml/min or 250 ml/min. CO is then 250 ml/min divided by 200–150 ml/L or 250/50 or 5 L/min.

The left ventricle typically has about 120–130 ml of blood at the end of diastole (end-diastolic volume or EDV) and normally ejects about 70–90 ml (stroke volume or SV) in the aorta to yield an ejection fraction (EF) of about 65%. The 40–50 ml blood left after ejection is the end-systolic volume (ESV). Thus:

$$EF = EDV - ESV/EDV$$

EF is commonly used to assess systolic function of the heart and can be measured non-invasively with echocardiography. Other modalities to measure right or left ventricular systolic function include fractional area change, myocardial performance index, pulse wave tissue Doppler imaging (PW TDI), and strain.

Of note, heart failure (HF) can occur with or without decreases in EF as it is a symptom complex (dyspnea on exertion, fatigue, syncope) arising from the inability of the heart to contract (systolic) or relax (diastolic) appropriately. When the EF falls below 40%, HF is called HF with reduced EF (HFrEF). When symptoms of heart failure occur with an EF of more than 50%, it is called HF with preserved EF (HFpEF). The former usually occurs with systolic dysfunction and the latter with diastolic dysfunction. HF with an EF of 41–49% is referred to as HFpEF, borderline.

Systolic function typically depends upon preload, contractility, and afterload while diastolic function, among other factors, depends upon LV compliance. The HR influences both. In a single CC occurring with a normal HR, one-third of the time is taken up by systole and the rest by diastole. As tachycardia ensues, the diastolic time keeps on getting shorter. This leads to two things: less time for the ventricle to fill and impaired LV relaxation. The decrease in preload affects systolic performance while impaired LV relaxation adversely affects diastolic performance by decreasing LV compliance. Both processes, together or individually, can lead to HF. If the LV does not relax completely, it retains end-systolic volume in a smaller space and at a higher pressure. This makes it difficult to fill during diastole. For example, if you are manually inflating a basketball with an air pump, it is easier to pump initially when the ball is deflated but it takes more and more energy to pump as the ball starts filling up. Once the ball is all filled up, it takes a lot of force to over fill it. As it retains more volume, just like the LV, its compliance decreases and it becomes stiffer. *Transmitral pulse wave Doppler analysis in conjunction with PW TDI on echocardiography can be used to gauge diastolic function.*

Abnormal rhythms can dramatically affect heart function as the normal mechanical sequence of events depends completely upon presence of normal sequential electrical activation of the heart. An extreme example of this is ventricular fibrillation, wherein chaotic electrical activation of the ventricles leads to complete loss of pumping action of the heart.

The ability of the heart to adequately pump and generate an adequate CO then depends upon five factors: HR, rhythm, preload, contractility, and afterload.

17.6 Heart Rate

If an isolated strip of cardiac muscle held at a fixed length is rapidly stimulated, it tends to generate more force with subsequent stimulations. This staircase, or Treppe effect, is known as the Bowditch phenomenon. The basis of it is as follows: Each stimulus leads to transfer of calcium from the SR to the cytosol. This calcium initiates contraction, but before all of it can be pumped back into the SR or extruded from the cell via the Na+ /Ca^{2+} exchanger, the next stimulus arrives, leading to transfer of more calcium from the SR and thereby increasing cytosol calcium concentration. This mismatch in calcium influx and efflux leading to a stronger contraction is known as the force–frequency relationship. Clinically, it is commonly seen with post extrasystolic potentiation: Contraction following an extrasystole is stronger than a normal contraction. Does this mean that with increasing HR, contractility and cardiac performance will improve? Unfortunately, the muscle fibers in the heart are not always stimulated at a fixed length and often rapid heart rates lead to decreased diastolic filling and increased myocardial oxygen consumption. The activation of proteases and lipases by calcium leads to oxidative stress and injury. Eventually, cardiac performance falls due to diminishing preload, harmful effects of calcium on cellular structures, rapid depletion of ATP stores, and abnormalities of relaxation. Thus, in clinical practice, rapidly pacing the heart rate may initially improve inotropy or contractile force but the effect is limited. On the other hand, it is very common to see rapid HRs lead to hemodynamic collapse. Unstable rapid HRs should be synch ronized cardioverted to achieve a stable rate and rhythm. In contrast to rapid HRs, a slower HR can also adversely affect CO and lead to an unstable patient. Unstable slow HRs should be treated emergently with transcutaneous pacing, intravenous atropine, or epinephrine infusions to achieve an adequate perfusing rate.

17.6.1 Preload

Imagine a bodybuilder doing a bench press with a barbell. He or she lowers the barbell to the chest and then pushes it up. In this scenario, the barbell and gravity act as the afterload while the preload can be envisioned as the length of the pectoralis muscle fiber immediately before contraction. In the heart, the end-diastolic volume (EDV) acts as the preload. The relation between preload and SV is defined by the Frank–Starling law (◉ Fig. 17.13). As preload increases, the sarcomere gets stretched and can generate greater contraction force. However, if the sarcomere gets over stretched, its performance falls. Initially, it was thought that a greater stretch allowed for maximal myosin–actin cross-bridging, leading to an increased force of contraction. However, during overstretching, myosin–actin cross-bridging decreases, leading to fall in performance. This simplified force–length theory may hold true for skeletal muscle but is yet to be completely elucidated for the heart. Increased preload while maintaining normal contractility leads to an increase in SV. However, excessive increases lead to heart failure. Clinically, assuming normal biventricular function, pulmonary physiology, and biventricular compliance, preload or LV EDV is assumed to be related to the CVP by the following relationship:

$$\mathrm{CVP} = \mathrm{PADP} = \mathrm{PCWP} = \mathrm{LAP} = \mathrm{LVEDP} = \mathrm{LVEDV}$$

However, this is seldom the case and EDV is best measured non-invasively by echocardiography.

17.6.2 Contractility

It is the innate property of the heart to contract or eject when preload and afterload are kept constant. In an intact heart, it is nearly impossible to eliminate the effect of preload and afterload and consequently it is difficult to quantify contractility. PV loops generated after left heart catheterization are one of the best representations of contractility in an intact heart. Noninvasive methods, such as echocardiography, can measure EF as a surrogate measure of contractility. Contractility is affected by factors that influence intracellular calcium concentrations or utilization, such as exercise, sympathetic stimulation, drugs such as digoxin, temperature, and pH changes. Increases in preload and afterload also affect contractility. In systolic HF, initial increases in preload help maintain SV, but this eventually leads to fall in contractility and worsening of HF. This is reflected by a downward and rightward shift of the PV loop. If preload and afterload are kept constant, an increase in contractility leads to a leftward shift of the PV loop and an increase in SV.

17.6.3 Afterload

Afterload is represented by the systolic ventricular wall stress and impedance to ejection by the outflow valve and vessel. With regard to the LV, afterload is then represented by the LV wall stress and impedance offered by the aortic valve, aorta, and its branches. If there is no aortic valve stenosis, then the major contributor of afterload is the systemic vascular resistance (SVR).

Wall stress in a sphere is given by Young–Laplace's law:

$$T = p \times r/2h$$

where p is pressure generated in the ventricle, r is the radius of the ventricle, and h is the wall thickness. With acute increases in afterload, unchanged contractility, and preload, SV falls. Intact myocardium can respond by generating a higher intraventricular pressure, thereby restoring SV. This is represented by an upward and rightward shift of the PV loop.

In aortic stenosis or chronic hypertension, wall stress increases due to increased impedance to ventricular outflow necessitating an increase in intraventricular pressure. However, the wall thickness increases by concentric hypertrophy in presence of LV pressure overload and this decreases wall stress. In aortic or mitral regurgitation, the ventricular radius increases, thereby increasing wall stress. Eccentric hypertrophy occurs in these volume overload conditions, and the increased thickness tends to minimize wall tension.

SVR is determined by arteriolar tone and is calculated as:

$$\mathrm{SVR} = 80 \times (\mathrm{MAP} - \mathrm{CVP})/\mathrm{CO}$$

and is usually 900–1500 dyn s cm^{-5}.

Pulmonary vascular resistance or PVR is calculated as:

$$\mathrm{PVR} = 80 \times (\mathrm{PAP} - \mathrm{LAP})/\mathrm{CO}$$

and is usually 50–150 dyn s cm^{-5}.

PAP is the mean pulmonary artery pressure and LAP is the left atrial pressure (mm Hg). Pulmonary capillary wedge pressure (PCWP) is clinically used as a measure of LAP. CO is in L/min.

Clinically, a pulmonary artery catheter and arterial line are commonly employed to measure various hemodynamic data. These are shown in ◉ Tables 17.3 and 17.4.

17.6.4 Cardiac Work

Work occurs when a generated force moves an object in the direction of the force. The heart does external and internal work, with both processes contributing to myocardial oxygen consumption. External work is defined by stroke work, or the product of stroke volume and pressure developed during ejection of blood. Thus, more external work occurs if the stroke volume increases or resistance to ejection increases (AS, chronic HTN). Internal work is proportional to wall tension. Increases in wall tension occur when there is

Table 17.3 Relative intracardiac pressures in healthy heart

Pressures	Mean	Range
Left atrium	8	4–12
Left ventricle systolic	125	90–140
Left ventricle end-diastolic	8	4–12
Right atrium	5	2–12
Right ventricle systolic	25	15–30
Right ventricle end-diastolic	5	0–10
Pulmonary artery systolic	23	15–30
Pulmonary artery diastolic	10	5–15
Pulmonary capillary wedge	10	5–15
Mean pulmonary artery	15	10–20

Reprinted with permission from Iaizzo [5]

increased pressure inside the ventricle, increase in radius of ventricle, or wall thinning. Increase in left ventricular end-diastolic pressure (LVEDP) leads to greater pressure in the ventricle in diastole and increases internal work.

17.6.5 Cardiac Innervation and Control of Heart Rate

The heart is richly innervated by the autonomic system and exhibits predominance of parasympathetic influence at rest and of sympathetic system during exercise or stress. Autonomic regulation is provided by the medulla in the brainstem (central vasomotor center), which houses the cardio inhibitory and cardio acceleratory group of neurons. Afferents from the heart travel via the vagus nerve, while efferents travel via the cardiac nerves and the vagus nerves. Sympathetic efferents arise from the superior, middle, and inferior cervical ganglion and travel to the heart as superior, middle, and inferior cardiac nerves. These efferents supply the SA node, AV node, conducting tissue, atrial and ventricular myocytes. Sympathetic innervation of the ventricles is denser compared to the atria. Norepinephrine is the predominant neurotransmitter and acts on alpha (α) and beta (β) receptors. Although β(beta) 1, 2, and 3 receptors are present in the heart, β(beta)-1 receptors are the most numerous. However, β(beta)-2 receptors demonstrate more avid coupling to cAMP pathways. These receptors are coupled to G proteins, and their activation leads to stimulation of adenylyl cyclase, increased levels of cAMP, and protein kinase A activation. This in turn causes opening of more calcium channels in myocytes, increased influx of calcium, and longer duration of calcium channel opening. The increased influx of calcium in SA node increases spontaneous depolarization and hence the HR, while the increase in intracellular calcium tends to increase contractility. Noradrenergic α(alpha)-1 receptors are involved in signaling pathways that lead to cardiac hypertrophy; α(alpha)-2 receptors are prejunctional and modulate norepinephrine release. To summarize, sympathetic activation generally leads to increase in chronotropy (heart rate), inotropy (contractility), dromotropy (conduction velocity), and lusitropy (relaxation). Activation of the parasympathetic system demonstrates opposite effects. The vagus nerve is the main parasympathetic supply to the heart and innervates the atria, SA node, and AV node preferentially. Ventricular innervation is sparse. The right vagus nerve supplies the SA node and the left vagus nerve supplies the AV node but there may be significant overlap. Acetylcholine is the predominant neurotransmitter and acts on muscarinic receptors, mainly M2 [1, 2, 5].

Table 17.4 Cardiac hemodynamic parameters (with normal ranges)

Hemodynamic parameter	Derived formula	Range
CO	HR × SV	4–6 L/min
CI	CO/BSA	2.6–4.3 L/min/m^2
SV	CO × 1000/HR	50–120 mL/beat
SI	SV/BSA	30–65 mL/beat/m^2
SVR	(MAP−CVP) × 80/CO	800–1400 dyne s/cm^5
SVRI	(MAP−CVP) × 80/CI	1500–2300 dyne s/cm^5/m^2
PVR	(PAP−PCWP) × 80/CO	140–250 dyne s/cm^5
PVRI	(PAP−PCWP) × 80/CI	240–450 dyne s/cm^5/m^2
LVSWI	1.36 (MAP−PCWP) × SI/100	45–60 g m/m^2
RVSWI	1.36 (PAP−CVP) × SI/100	5–10 g m/m^2

Reprinted with permission from Iaizzo [5]

BSA body surface area, *CI* cardiac index, *CO* cardiac output, *CVP* central venous pressure, *HR* heart rate, *LVSWI* left ventricular stroke work index, *MAP* mean arterial pressure, *PAP* pulmonary artery pressure, *PCWP* pulmonary capillary wedge pressure, *PVR* pulmonary vascular resistance, *PVRI* pulmonary vascular resistance index, RVSWI—right ventricular stroke work index, *SI* stroke index, *SV* stroke volume, *SVR* systemic vascular resistance, *SVRI* systemic vascular resistance index

17.6.6 Cardiac Reflexes

Common cardiac reflexes include:

- **Baroreceptor Reflex**: This is primarily a negative feedback loop that plays a role in short-term regulation of arterial blood pressure. Baroreceptors are present in the carotid sinus and aortic arch in the adventitial layers. They respond to arterial distension by pulsatile pressure. Thus, hypertension increases baroreceptor discharge. This leads to inhibition of sympathetic outflow and increase in vagal influences to the heart. Consequently, there is slowing of HR, inotropy, and dromotropy, which results in normalization of blood pressure. The reverse is seen with hypotension.

Afferents from the carotid sinus form the carotid sinus nerve or Hering's nerve (branch of glossopharyngeal nerve), while those from the aortic arch form the aortic depressor nerve (branch of vagus nerve). These synapse in the medulla with the cardio inhibitory and acceleratory group of neurons. Efferents are via the cardiac nerves and vagus nerve.

The reflex gets activated once SBP increases to about 170 mm Hg and does not function if SBP is less than 50 mm Hg. It is inhibited by volatile anesthetics and anti-hypertensive drugs, such as calcium channel blockers. The reflex helps in normalizing blood pressure during postural changes, such as supine to sitting or standing. In the operative room, use of phenylephrine usually triggers a reflex bradycardia via this reflex.

- **Peripheral Chemoreceptor Reflex**: Stimulation of aortic and carotid bodies by hypoxemia (PaO_2 of less than 50 mm Hg) and fall in pH leads to activation of the chemo sensitive area of the medulla leading to increase in respiratory drive and ventilation. Usually, vagal efferents to the heart are also activated. However, if there is increased catecholamine secretion from the adrenal medulla due to hypoxia, it leads to tachycardia and increased contractility.
- **Cushing Reflex**: Increased intracranial pressure leads to medullary ischemia. This elicits an intense sympathetic response that initially causes a rise in blood pressure and tachycardia to restore blood flow to the medulla. The hypertension activates baroreceptors leading to bradycardia. Medullary compression also depresses respiration. The classic Cushing's triad consists of hypertension, bradycardia, and respiratory depression.
- **Oculocardiac Reflex**: Increased traction or pressure on the eye or surrounding structures (especially medial rectus muscle) leads to bradycardia (at least an HR decrease of 10%) via this reflex. Afferents flow via the ciliary nerves to the ophthalmic division of trigeminal nerve to the Gasserian ganglion and then to the visceral motor nucleus of the vagus nerve. Efferents travel to the heart via the vagus nerve leading to decrease in HR. In addition to sinus bradycardia, junctional rhythms, asystole, and ventricular tachycardia may also be seen. Hypoxia, hypercarbia, acidosis, and light anesthesia exacerbate the reflex, and it is elicited more frequently in the younger population. Interestingly, this reflex can occur in the absence of an eyeball.
- **Bainbridge Reflex**: This is elicited by stretch of cardiopulmonary receptors located in right atrial wall and atriocaval junction. Increase in right-sided filling leads to activation of vagal afferents and decrease in vagal discharge, eliciting increases in HR.
- **Bezold–Jarisch Reflex**: Following intravenous injection of veratrum alkaloids, a triad of apnea, hypotension, and bradycardia was reported by von Bezold in 1867 and later confirmed by Jarisch. Cardiac sensory receptors found in the left ventricle (especially the inferoposterior wall) mediate this reflex. Afferents are via nonmyelinated vagal C fibers, and the receptors are activated by stretch, drugs, or noxious stimuli leading to reflex bradycardia, vasodilatation, and hypotension. This is mediated via both inhibition of sympathetic discharge and increase in vagal discharge.
- **Valsalva Maneuver**: After a normal inspiratory effort, the subject is instructed to exhale against a closed glottis for about 15 s (strain period) and then breathe normally. Traditionally, this maneuver has been described as having 4 phases, beginning from initiation of strain to after release of strain:
  - Phase 1: brief increase in blood pressure (BP) and decrease in HR. This is due to increase in intrathoracic pressure.
  - Phase 2: BP falls slowly to normal with increase in HR. Possibly due to decreased venous return.
  - Phase 3: Strain is released, and it leads to fall in BP and rise in HR. This is due to decrease in intrathoracic pressure.
  - Phase 4: BP overshoots above the resting value and bradycardia. This is due to baroreceptor reflex.
- **The Transplanted Heart**: A transplanted heart is essentially completely denervated. The loss of parasympathetic tone leads to a higher resting HR of 90–100 beats/min. Drugs that act indirectly fail to elicit desired hemodynamic responses. Atropine does not lead to tachycardia and phenylephrine will not cause bradycardia. Response to direct acting agents, such as isoprenaline and epinephrine, is intact. Although HR increases after exercise, this response is delayed as it is mediated by catecholamines released by the adrenal medulla and not

by increased sympathetic stimulation that usually occurs with exercise. Transplant recipients do not experience angina due to loss of afferent fibers that carry sensation of pain. A donor heart is an example of post ganglionic denervation. The most common cause of such denervation in the non-transplant population is diabetes mellitus. Shy-Drager syndrome leads to preganglionic denervation [3, 4].

17.7 Systemic Circulation

The circulatory system consists of the pulmonary and systemic circulation. Systemic circulation broadly consists of:

- **Macrocirculation**: This consists of arteries and veins. The function of the macrocirculation is to transport oxygenated blood to organs via strong-walled arteries and deoxygenated blood back to the heart via thin-walled compliant veins.
- **Microcirculation**: This consists of arterioles, capillaries, and venules. Arteries divide into smaller arterioles, which regulate tissue perfusion and capillary flow. Arterioles being muscular contribute considerably to peripheral resistance or SVR. Capillaries participate in nutrient exchange with cells and venules collect blood from capillaries. Venules join to form veins that then empty into the heart via the venae cava.

17.7.1 Anatomical and Biophysical Considerations

Normal blood volume in adults is 70–75 ml/kg. Of this, about 60 ml/kg (80%–85%) is present in the systemic circulation, 6 ml/kg in the pulmonary (7%–9%) circulation, and 5 ml/kg (5%–7%) in the heart. Veins being capacitance vessels hold the majority of the systemic blood volume, up to 45 ml/kg; arteries hold up to 11 ml/kg; and capillaries hold up to 4 ml/kg. Although capillaries hold only about 5% of the total blood volume at any time, their cross-sectional area is staggering at about 2500 cm^2. This allows the red blood cells to form a "single line" as they traverse through the microcirculation.

Pressure (P) across a cylinder through which a fluid is flowing can simplistically be represented as product of flow (F) and resistance (R). Thus:

$$P = F \times R$$

Resistance is given by Poiseuille–Hagen formula:

$$R = 8\mu(\text{mu})L/\pi(\text{pi})r^4$$

where μ(mu) is viscosity, L is the length of the cylinder or tube, and r is the radius of cylinder.

Thus, resistance is determined not only by the radius but also by viscosity. In vivo, the primary determinant of viscosity of blood is the hematocrit, protein content of plasma, and rigidity of red blood cells. Viscosity is commonly increased in polycythemia vera, macroglobulinemias, and sickle cell disease (red blood cells are less deformable). Conversely, anemia often causes decreases in viscosity.

Flow is constituted by movement of a certain volume of fluid per unit time. It can be laminar or turbulent. Consider a slow stream of water flowing from an open faucet into a sink. When this stream hits the sink, it moves in different directions. The former is an example of laminar flow and the latter of turbulent flow. Imagine a bunch of red blood cells (RBCs) flowing slowly through a vessel. Laminar flow is characterized by a parabolic profile. RBCs in the center of the lumen have higher velocities than those that are in contact with the vessel wall. Such a flow pattern is layered and orderly; each layer moves at its own speed without disturbing the adjacent layer. Laminar flow patterns are associated with less energy losses and are commonly thought to be present in the aorta and larger arteries. Importantly, this flow creates high shear stress, which upregulates endothelial cell genes that produce proteins protective against atherosclerosis. When flowing fluids encounter an obstruction or branching, smooth flow gets disrupted and tends to become turbulent. This flow pattern is characterized by eddy currents. RBCs move in different directions and with different velocities. Turbulent flow is associated with more energy losses, and the low shear stress exerted on endothelial cells leads to production of proteins that promote atherogenesis. Thus, plaques are more commonly seen in branching points in the aorta, such as iliofemoral arteries. Type of flow can be predicted by the Reynolds number:

$$\text{Re} = d\text{Dv}/\mu(\text{mu})$$

D is the diameter of the tube, d is density of the fluid, v is the velocity of the fluid, and μ(mu) is the viscosity of the fluid. The Reynolds number is dimensionless. Laminar flow occurs with values less than 2000, transitional flow with values between 2000 and 4000, and turbulent flow with values above 4000.

As mentioned earlier, typical SBP and DBP in young adults measured at the brachial artery is usually 100–120- and 70–80-mm Hg. As BP is the product of CO and SVR, conditions that change CO and SVR affect BP. Conditions in which CO is increased, such as AR and MR, typically have high SBP. SVR is higher in stressed patients usually exhibiting "white coat hypertension." Also, BP is typically higher in the elderly population as explained earlier. BP readings should be taken with the arm at the level of the heart as gravity influences the measurement. The effect of gravity tends to increase pressures in vessels below the heart and decrease pressures in vessels above the heart. Changes are typically of the order of 0.7–0.77 mm Hg per cm change in height [1, 2].

17.7.2 Regulation of Blood Pressure

As perfusion pressures of most tissue beds depend upon generation of an adequate BP, various physiological mechanisms have developed to ensure its adequacy. Immediate and short-term (activated in seconds, lasting for few minutes) control of blood pressure is provided by the autonomic system and the baroreceptor reflex. Intermediate control (activated within minutes, lasting for a few hours) is exerted by activation of the renin–angiotensin–aldosterone system (RAAS) and release of arginine vasopressin (AVP). Both systems protect the body against hypotension and hypovolemia primarily. AVP is synthesized as a precursor protein in the hypothalamus and stored in the posterior pituitary. It causes vasoconstriction through V1a receptors, release of adrenocorticotrophic hormone (ACTH) via V1b receptors and exerts its antidiuretic effect via insertion of aquaporin-2 channels through its action on V2 receptors in collecting ducts of the kidney. AVP release is triggered by a fall in plasma volume; decrease in BP; rise in plasma osmolality; or increased stress, such as trauma, surgery, or pain. RAAS gets activated by an increase in sympathetic stimulation, fall in BP, and decrease in sodium chloride delivery to the macula densa in the distal tubules of the kidney. Renin is stored in specialized cells called juxtaglomerular cells (JG) of the afferent arteriole supplying the glomerulus. B-1 stimulation causes release of renin. Renin being an enzyme cleaves angiotensinogen to the decapeptide angiotensin (AT) I, which gets further cleaved to the octapeptide angiotensin II by the angiotensin converting enzyme (ACE). ACE is found mainly in the lung, kidney, and endothelial tissue. Angiotensin II is a potent vasoconstrictor, acts via AT 2 receptors, and stimulates aldosterone release from the adrenal glands leading to sodium and water retention. These actions tend to increase the BP. Long-term control (over days) of BP is provided by the kidneys, which alter sodium and water homeostasis to maintain normal BP. Increases in BP from excessive water or salt intake are prevented by the phenomenon of pressure diuresis and pressure natriuresis. Conversely, increased salt and water retention is seen in absolute or relative hypovolemic and hypotensive states (cirrhosis and HF).

17.7.3 Physiology of the Microcirculation

As fluids move along a high pressure to low pressure gradient, arterial and capillary pressures are usually higher than venous pressures. Resistance to blood flow in the large and medium arteries is low. Thus, pressure marginally changes as blood flows across them. At the arteriolar level, due to decreases in radius, there is greater resistance, leading to a drop in pressures to about 30–35 mm Hg. Capillaries have a functional pressure of approximately 17 mm Hg; pressures at the venular end are about 10 mm Hg and venous pressure varies from 2 to 7 mm Hg (◉ Fig. 17.14).

At the level of the microcirculation, arterioles communicate with capillaries. Their junction is encircled with a smooth muscle fiber that acts as a precapillary sphincter. Traditionally, it was thought as blood pressure increases, due to myogenic reflex, these sphincters contract maintaining normal capillary perfusion. When cells need more oxygen, the sphincters relax to increase blood flow and perfusion. This may be mediated by accumulation of local factors, such as adenosine and H^+ ions. As blood flows through the capillary, it exchanges nutrients with the interstitial fluid. This exchange occurs via diffusion, bulk flow, filtration, and vesicular transport. Fluid filtration across capillaries was described by Starling in 1896 using the Starling equation:

$$\text{Net fluid movement across the capillary} = k\left[(P_c - P_i) - (\pi[\text{pi}]_c - \pi[\text{pi}]_i)\right]$$

K capillary filtration coefficient

P_c capillary hydrostatic pressure (approximately 30–35 mm Hg on the arteriolar side and 15–18 mm Hg on the venular side of the capillary bed)

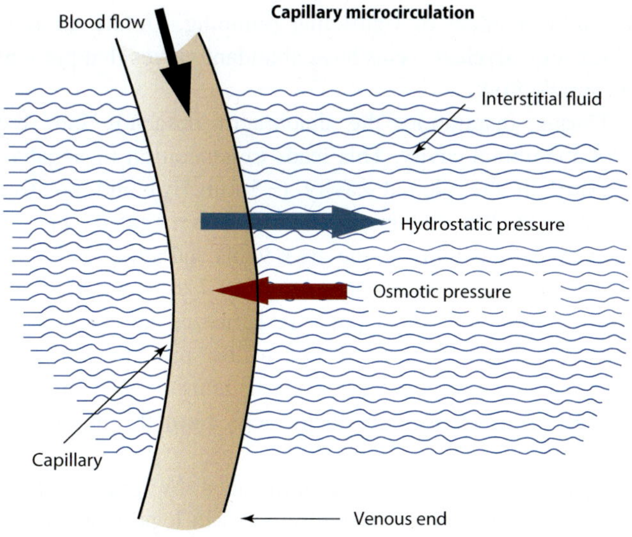

Fig. 17.14 Capillary microcirculation

P_i interstitial hydrostatic pressure (variable but usually considered to be −2 mm Hg to +2 mm Hg)

$\pi(\text{pi})_c$ capillary colloid osmotic pressure (approximately 25–28 mm Hg)

$\pi(\text{pi})_I$ interstitial colloid osmotic pressure (variable but usually considered to be 8 mm Hg)

A positive value denotes net outward movement of fluid from the capillaries, and a negative value represents inward movement of the fluid.

In the classic model, fluid egresses outward to the interstitium on the arteriolar side and moves back into capillaries on the venular side. Usually, more fluid moves out to the interstitium than returns to the venular side. This excess fluid is removed by the lymphatic system.

Research over the last two decades has questioned this rationale. The prevailing concept is that all vessels are lined by a glycocalyx layer along the endothelium. Glycocalyx is made up of syndecan and glypican (among other glycoproteins) and is associated with negatively charged compounds, such as sulfates (heparan and dermatan), hyaluronic acid, and albumin. Together, they make up an endothelial surface layer (ESL), which prevents egress of plasma proteins and fluid out of the vessel. Small amounts leak out to the interstitium via fenestrations. There is minimal or no reabsorption of fluid on the venular side. In addition to acting as a vascular permeability barrier, it has been postulated that the ESL protects the endothelium by inhibiting adhesion of leucocytes and coagulation.

17.7.3.1 Venous Circulation and Venous Return

After traversing the capillary bed, blood is collected by venules, which coalesce to form bigger veins that in turn empty into the vena cavae and the right heart. This heartward flow in the venous circulation is made possible by three mechanisms: thoracic pump, peripheral muscle pump, and the indirect effect of ventricular pumping. Unlike arteries, which are valveless, veins have abundant valves that prevent retrograde flow.

During inspiration, the diaphragm descends into the intra-abdominal cavity. This leads to generation of negative pressure in the pleural cavity (−5 mm Hg) and positive pressure in the abdominal cavity. The negative pleural pressure is transmitted to the great veins and atria, leading to a drop in central venous pressure from 7 to 2 mm Hg. The positive intra-abdominal pressure squeezes the mesenteric veins. As fluids move from high to low pressure, this thoracic pump mechanism aids in venous return. Valves prevent venous blood from going to the legs from the abdominal cavity.

Blood, like all fluids, is influenced by gravity. In a standing person, blood normally pools in legs generating a venous pressure of about 80 mm Hg. However, leg muscle contractions force venous blood toward the heart, reducing venous pressures to about 30 mm Hg. Retrograde flow is prevented by valves. In patients with varicose veins, these valves are faulty and this often leads to venous congestion in the lower extremities. Similarly in upper extremities, skeletal muscle pump mechanism propels venous blood back to the heart.

During ventricular systole, the tricuspid valve is pulled toward the RV, generating a negative deflection in the CVP waveform (x descent). This negative atrial pressure aids in right atrial filling. When the RV relaxes and untwists, it produces a diastolic suction force that pulls in blood from the vena cavae into the RA and then into the RV. This ventricular contraction pump mechanism is also responsible for venous return [1–5].

17.7.4 Assessment of Adequacy of Circulation: Lactate and Mixed Venous Oxygen Saturation

One of the primary functions of the circulatory system is to deliver oxygen to tissues and remove metabolic waste. However, in certain situations there is failure to provide adequate oxygen for meeting metabolic demands. Among other mechanisms, this can arise from global tissue hypoperfusion. Cells then switch from an aerobic mode of metabolism to an anaerobic mode, generating lactate and a state of metabolic acidosis ensues. This syndrome of abnormal decreased oxygen delivery or utilization by the cell is commonly referred to as shock. It can arise from inadequate circulating volume (hypovolemic shock: blood loss), failure of the cardiac pump to generate an adequate CO (cardiogenic shock: MI, arrhythmias), obstruction of normal circulatory flow (obstructive shock: cardiac tamponade, PE), or profound decreases in SVR (distributive shock: anaphylaxis, sepsis). In such situations, cells try to extract as much oxygen as possible from the arterial side and the normal arteriovenous oxygen difference widens. Clinically, this widening is commonly assessed by measuring SaO_2 from an arterial blood gas and SvO_2 (mixed venous oxygen saturation) from venous sample aspirated from the tip of an appropriately placed pulmonary artery catheter. Normally, SvO_2 is 68%–77%. It represents venous saturation of blood received from both the IVC and SVC. As the use of pulmonary artery catheters is declining, sometimes physicians use central venous oxygen saturation ($ScvO_2$) as a representative measure of mixed venous oxygen saturation. $ScvO_2$ can be measured from a central venous catheter in the SVC and is usually 5% higher than SvO_2. As oxygen extraction increases, the mixed or central venous oxygen saturations progressively fall.

Using Fick's equation:

$$CO = VO_2/CaO_2 - CvO_2$$

and then rearranging it, we get:

$$CvO_2 = CaO2 - (VO_2/CO)$$

This can further be written as:

$$SvO_2 = SaO_2 - [VO_2/(CO \times 1.34 \times Hb)]$$

Thus, fall in SvO_2 can be related to fall in SaO_2, increased oxygen consumption (VO_2), and decrease in CO or Hb. SvO_2 measurements can be used to track the adequacy of global circulation. In late sepsis, at the microcirculatory level, tissue cells are unable to utilize delivered oxygen due to abnormal mitochondrial function and microcirculatory shunting. In this scenario, the SvO_2 can be normal or increased even though the cell is not getting adequate oxygen. However, cells keep on producing lactate and increases in lactate can be used to track deficient oxygen utilization by cells.

17.7.5 Regulation of Circulation

Circulatory system is regulated by neural, local, endothelial, and neurohumoral factors:

- **Neural Control**: Except for capillaries and venules, all other blood vessels contain smooth muscle. This smooth muscle is densely innervated in arteries with noradrenergic fibers. Sympathetic activation leads to vasoconstriction via α(alpha) receptors in arteries and venoconstriction in veins. Cholinergic innervation is sparse and only found in some blood vessels of erectile tissue of reproductive organs, uterus, and salivary glands. Vasodilatation is mediated either through $\beta(\text{beta})_2$ receptor stimulation via epinephrine released from adrenal medulla (as occurs during exercise) or loss of α(alpha) sympathetic stimulation (spinal anesthesia).
- **Local Autoregulation**: Autoregulation is the ability of tissues to regulate their own blood flow. This capacity is most developed in the kidney. However, the brain, skeletal muscle, liver, and myocardium also demonstrate autoregulation. In contrast, uterine blood flow is not autoregulated. In pregnancy, it is pressure dependent. Two theories have been proposed to explain autoregulation: myogenic and metabolic. The myogenic theory postulates that as blood pressure rises, per Laplace's law to maintain normal wall tension, the radius of the vessel has to decrease. Smooth muscles demonstrate intrinsic contractile response to stretch. As pressure rises, vessels get stretched and decrease their radius by contraction, thereby limiting flow. The metabolic theory suggests that tissues generate a variety of vasodilatory metabolites (K^+, adenosine, and lactate). When blood flow decreases, these accumulate causing local vasodilation and increasing flow. The increased flow then "sweeps" these metabolites away. While the myogenic theory explains vasoconstriction better, the metabolic theory explains vasodilation better. Other local factors that influence vasodilation include increase in temperature, fall in oxygen tension, acidosis, and increase in carbon dioxide tension. Vasoconstriction can be caused by hypothermia and serotonin release (seen during vessel injury).
- **Effect of Endothelial Substances**: Common vasodilators secreted by the endothelium include prostaglandins, such as prostacyclin and nitric oxide (NO). Endothelial vasoconstrictors include thromboxane A_2 or TxA_2 and endothelin.

NO activates guanylyl cyclase in smooth muscles leading to increased cGMP that mediates relaxation and vasodilatation. It is inactivated quickly by hemoglobin. Increased NO production in sepsis and cirrhosis may account for the low SVR observed in these conditions. Prostacyclin commonly counteracts the platelet aggregating and vasoconstrictive effects of TxA_2. Mismatch in their production during placental ischemia may play a role in development of pre-eclampsia in pregnancy. Endothelin is a potent vasoconstrictor and acts via phospholipase. There are three types of endothelin, and they act on either ET_A or ET_B receptors. ET_A receptors are specific for endothelin-1 (ET-1). ET-1 levels are consistently elevated in patients with PA hypertension (PAH). Endothelin antagonists, such as bosentan (nonselective) and ambrisentan (selective action on ET_A receptors), are commonly used in treatment of PAH.

- **Effect of Neurohumoral Factors**: Prominent vasoconstricting factors include angiotensin, vasopressin, and norepinephrine. Vasodilators include bradykinin and histamine. Estrogen leads to vasodilation via stimulation of NO synthase and exerts a protective effect on the heart in ischemia reperfusion models. Testosterone, on the other hand, worsens myocardial injury after reperfusion. Substances secreted by cardiomyocytes include angiotensin, aldosterone, atrial natriuretic peptide (ANP), B-type natriuretic peptide (BNP), and adrenomedullin. Angiotensin levels are increased in HF. Increased levels lead to cardiac hypertrophy and fibrosis via its action on AT-1 receptors. The heart has an abundance of AT-1 receptors, unlike the blood vessels, which have an abundance of AT two receptors. Aldosterone has also been implicated in this process. Therefore, ACE inhibitors are used in HF to effect remodeling. ANP and BNP levels increase in response to hypervolemia and promote diuresis, natriuresis, and vasodilatation. Although normally atria secrete ANP and ventricles secrete BNP, in HF, ventricular cells secrete both hormones.

17.8 Coronary Circulation

Just like other organs, the heart is supplied by arteries, capillaries, and veins, and has a macro as well as microcirculation (◉ Fig. 17.15). The arterial macrocirculation is constituted by the right coronary artery (RCA) and the left main coronary artery (LM) that arise from the ostia in the right and left sinuses of the aortic valve, respectively. These divide into various branches as follows:

- **RCA**: After emerging from the aorta, it gives off 2 branches: the atrial branch to the RA and conus branch that supplies the RVOT. The atrial branch gives rise to the SA nodal artery in 50%–75% of adults. As the RCA descends in the AV groove traveling toward the apex of the heart, it gives off the marginal branch (supplies the right margin of the heart), AV nodal branch (supplies the AV node in 50%–60% of adults), and the posterior descending artery (PDA) or posterior interventricular artery that supplies the posterior one-third of the IVS in 80%–90% of adult hearts. Dominance of circulation depends upon which artery gives rise to the PDA. When the PDA arises from the RCA, it is called a right dominant circulation.
- **LCA or Left Main**: After emerging from the aorta, it travels a short distance between the pulmonary trunk and left atrial appendage and gives rise to the left anterior descending artery (LAD) and the left circumflex artery (LCx). In about 30%–50% of the population, there may be a third branch called the ramus intermedius. The LCx supplies the LA, the SA node in 25%–50% of the population, the lateral free wall of the LV, posterior wall of the LV, and both anterior and posterior papillary muscles of the LV. It gives rise to the obtuse marginal (OM) arteries. In 10%–20% of people, the LCx can give rise to the PDA, and when this happens, the circulation is termed left dominant. The LAD artery supplies the bulk of the heart and unfortunately is the most often occluded artery in atherosclerotic coronary artery disease. Its branches include the septal perforators and the diagonal arteries. The first septal perforator supplies the AV conduction system. The second and third septal perforators supply the bulk of the IVS (anterior two-thirds), bundle branches,

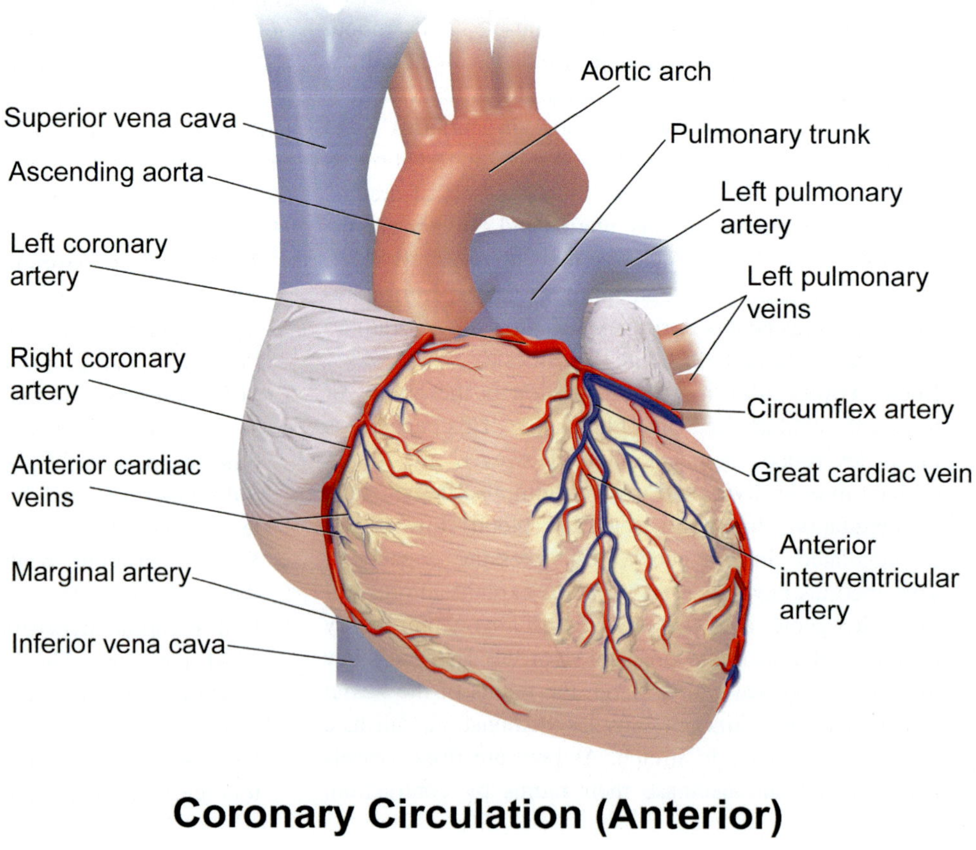

Fig. 17.15 Coronary vessels, anterior view (By Blausen Medical Communications, Inc. (Donated via OTRS, see ticket for details) [CC BY 3.0 (http://creativecommons.org/licenses/by/3.0)], via Wikimedia Commons)

and give rise to the moderator artery, which is responsible for supplying the moderator band of the RV. LAD also supplies anterior papillary muscles of the TV and MV. The diagonal arteries supply the anterior wall of the LV. LAD forms 4 important collateral anastomoses with the RCA: at the level of the conus artery (circle of Vieussens), at the level of IVS (septal perforators and PDA), at the level of the apex (LAD with PDA), and at the level of the crux of the heart (LCx with PDA).

As arteries supply specific regions of the heart, ECG changes can help to localize the region of the heart experiencing ischemia or myocardial infarction (MI). This is outlined below:

- Leads I, aVL, V5, and V6 represent the lateral wall of LV.
- Leads V1 and V2 represent the septal wall (LAD territory).
- Leads V3 and V4 represent the anterior wall of the LV (LAD territory).
- Leads II, III, and aVF represent the inferior wall of LV (RCA territory in right dominance, and LCx territory in left dominance).
- Anterior wall MI involves LAD territory and is manifested in Leads V1 to V6. Septal wall MI manifests with changes in V1 and V2. Lateral and anterolateral MIs manifest in Leads I, aVL, V5, and V6. Inferior wall MI manifests in Leads II, III, and aVF. Atrial MIs although uncommon can occur. RA infarction (RCA territory) occurs more frequently and presents with PR or P-Ta segment elevation in leads V1.

17.8.1 Venous Macrocirculation

Venous macrocirculation of the heart is made up the great, middle, and small cardiac veins that form the coronary sinus and the anterior cardiac veins. Both the coronary sinus and anterior cardiac veins empty into the RA.

17.8.2 Coronary Microcirculation

Arteries typically run beneath or within the epicardium but above the myocardium. These epicardial vessels branch into smaller arteries and arterioles that then supply the myocardium and endocardium. The arterioles deliver oxygenated blood (and other nutrients) to capillaries that are in close apposition to the cardiomyocytes and deoxygenated blood (and metabolic waste products) is carried by venules to veins that empty into the RA. The venules may also empty into the atrial and ventricular chambers directly via very small intramyocardial veins known as Thebesian veins.

17.8.3 Biophysics of Coronary Circulation

Recall that flow is pressure gradient divided by resistance. As the LV and RV are muscular pumps, when they contract, they compress intramyocardial vessels and impede flow by increasing resistance. In diastole when the ventricles relax, myocardial flow is restored. As blood moves from high to low pressure, it is necessary for aortic pressures to be higher than chamber pressures to allow blood to flow through the ostia and coronary arteries. However, LV systolic pressures are often higher than aortic systolic pressures. This impedes LV coronary flow. In contrast, the RV and atria usually have lower systolic pressures than the aorta and hence receive coronary flow during systole. In diastole, aortic diastolic pressures (AoDBP) is usually higher than diastolic pressures in all the heart chambers. This coupled with relaxation of myocardium, allows unimpeded coronary flow in diastole. Thus, the LV gets perfused mainly during diastole whereas all other heart chambers are perfused during the entire CC. The coronary perfusion of the LV can be represented as follows:

$$\text{Coronary perfusion pressure} = \text{Aortic diastolic blood pressure} - \text{LV end diastolic blood pressure}$$

or

$$\text{CPP} = \text{AoDBP} - \text{LVEDP}$$

Factors that will decrease aortic DBP (such as low SVR, presence of AR), increase LV EDP (such as HF or AS), and decrease the diastolic time (tachycardia) will lead to decreased coronary perfusion to the LV. As the subendocardial layer is exposed to high levels of LVEDP, it is most vulnerable to developing ischemia. The risk of ischemia is increased when the LV hypertrophies in conditions, such as aortic stenosis. The relative capillary density is reduced in hypertrophied myocardium, and due to diastolic dysfunction, LVEDP is very high. Thus drops in AoDBP, as seen commonly during induction of anesthesia due to vasodilatory effect of anesthetic drugs, predispose patients to coronary hypoperfusion and ischemia.

Resting coronary flow is about 250 ml/min. Cardiomyocytes normally extract 70%–80% of the delivered oxygen, leaving little room for more extraction. When the myocardial work load increases, the only way to match the increase in oxygen demand is to increase the supply. This supply–demand matching is essential for preventing ischemia.

The diastolic pressure time index (DPTI) is the product of the coronary perfusion pressure and diastolic time and represents oxygen delivery. Oxygen demand can be represented by the tension time index (TTI), the product of systolic pressure and systolic time.

The ratio DPTI/TTI is the endocardial viability ratio (EVR) and represents the myocardial oxygen supply–demand balance. A ratio < 0.7 is associated with subendocardial ischemia (normal EVR is 1).

In aortic stenosis and hypertrophic obstructive cardiomyopathy, the LV is commonly hypertrophied and generates enormous pressures during systole. Due to relatively decreased capillary density and increased LVEDP due to hypertrophy, these patients are at high risk for developing ischemia if their AoDBP falls.

Coronary circulation demonstrates autoregulation between MAPs of 60- and 140-mm Hg. Beyond this range, flow becomes pressure dependent. Metabolic autoregulation may be mediated by K^+, adenosine, fall in oxygen tension, and fall in pH. Neural control of coronary flow is complex. Epicardial arteries predominantly have α(alpha) receptors and intramyocardial vessels have β(beta) receptors. Predominant effect of sympathetic stimulation is to cause vasodilatation. Parasympathetic influences are weak and negligible.

17.9 Conclusion

Cardiovascular physiology is a complex discipline, but it is imperative for budding and practicing anesthesiologists to master its fundamentals.

17.10 Questions and Answers

Questions (Choose the Most Appropriate Answer)

1. A 70-year-old man with severe aortic stenosis is undergoing proctocolectomy under general anesthesia. After induction of anesthesia, his mean arterial pressure falls from 120 to 60 mm Hg. Heart rate is 70/min and other vitals are unchanged. There is no evidence of bronchospasm or skin rash. Intravenous administration of which of the following drugs is MOST appropriate?

A. Epinephrine
B. Phenylephrine
C. Dobutamine
D. Milrinone

2. Which of the following options BEST describes the most common pattern of sinoatrial (SA) node's innervation and blood supply?

Option	Innervation	Blood supply
A	Right Vagus Nerve	Right Coronary Artery
B	Left Vagus Nerve	Left Main Coronary Artery
C	Left Vagus Nerve	Ramus Intermedius Artery
D	Right Vagus Nerve	Left Anterior Descending Artery

3. Which of the following options BEST matches the SA node's phase of action potential with the ion channel responsible for facilitating electrical changes in that phase?

Option	Phase of action potential	Predominant channel or current
A	1	Sodium ion influx
B	0	Inward rectifier I_k current
C	3	Sodium ion efflux
D	4	Inward funny current

4. Which of the following proteins primarily functions as a cytosolic calcium sensor?

A. Calsequestrin
B. Calreticulin
C. Calmodulin
D. Phospholamban

5. With regards to the sarcomere, which of the following electron microscopy finding is MOST likely accurate?

A. The region occupied by Myosin filaments is termed the I band
B. Each sarcomere consists of two half I bands and an A band
C. Adjacent sarcomeres join at the M line
D. Actin filaments anchor to the M line

6. In the myocardial syncytium, which of the following structures MOST likely helps achieve electrical coupling between adjacent myocytes?

A. Intercalated discs
B. Ryanodine receptors
C. Gap junctions
D. Dihydropyridine receptors

7. Torsades de pointes is MOST likely to occur under which of the following circumstances?

Option	QT interval uncorrected (seconds)	RR interval (seconds)
A	0.4	0.49
B	0.3	0.64
C	0.4	0.81
D	0.3	1

8. Which of the following statements regarding Central Venous Pressure waveforms is MOST likely accurate?

A. A waves are accentuated in Atrial Fibrillation
B. Sinus tachycardia commonly leads to canon A waves.
C. Lancisi sign (tall V waves) is commonly seen in Tricuspid Stenosis
D. Cardiac tamponade is associated with a dominant X descent.

9. A 70-year-old male presents with New York Heart Association functional class IV dyspnea. He has a history of Heart Failure with reduced ejection fraction. His echocardiogram demonstrates an intact interatrial septum. His vitals are tabulated.

Vital parameter	Observed value or pattern
Heart rate (beats/min)	130
Heart rhythm	Atrial fibrillation
Mean arterial pressure (mm Hg)	55
Respiratory rate (breaths/min)	30

Which of the following parameters is MOST likely to be increased in this patient?

A. Left ventricular end diastolic pressure
B. Stroke volume
C. Diastolic filling time
D. Accentuated S1 Heart sound; wide and fixed split

10. 30-year-old female presents for emergent laparotomy after being involved in a motor vehicle accident. Pertinent laboratory and monitoring data are tabulated.

Parameter	Measured value
Arterial oxygen content (ml/dl)	20
Venous oxygen content (ml/dl)	12
Cardiac Output (L/min)	3
Respiratory rate (breaths/min)	30

Her calculated oxygen consumption VO_2 (ml/min) is MOST likely:

A. 250
B. 225
C. 240
D. 275

Answers

1. **B. Explanation:** In aortic stenosis, it is important to maintain coronary perfusion pressure (CPP) as the LV is prone to developing ischemia due to concentric hypertrophy, increased afterload, and increased LVEDP. These factors increase myocardial oxygen consumption. Myocardial capillary density is also relatively reduced. Additionally, the LV is perfused only in diastole. Compression of intramyocardial vessels during systole limits coronary blood flow during systole. Factors that will increase myocardial oxygen consumption while decreasing supply will lead to ischemia, worsening of both systolic and diastolic function, cardiogenic shock, and possibly cardiac arrest.CPP is the difference of aortic DBP and LVEDP. Factors that reduce aortic DBP (anesthesia induced hypotension), increase the LVEDP or reduce diastolic perfusion time (tachycardia) can lead to subendocardial ischemia. Anesthetic goals in AS include maintaining a normal preload, afterload, rhythm, and contractility. Decreases in afterload and tachycardia should be avoided. Phenylephrine increases SVR, restores vascular tone and coronary artery perfusion pressure. Increase in blood pressure activates the baroreceptor reflex leading to decrease in heart rate. Thus, it increases myocardial oxygen supply while reducing demand, minimizing risk of ischemia. Epinephrine can cause tachycardia and is not preferred. Milrinone and dobutamine decrease SVR and diastolic blood pressure and may precipitate LV ischemia in this patient. In the presence of fixed stenosis, milrinone and dobutamine are unlikely to increase CO.
2. **A. Explanation:** SA node is supplied by the right vagus nerve and the SA nodal artery, which in 50–75% of the population arises from the RCA. The AV node is supplied by the left vagus nerve and the AV nodal artery, which arises from the RCA in 50–60% of the population.
3. **D. Explanation:** SA node is a pacemaker and demonstrates slow response action potential as opposed to the fast response action potential of ventricular cardiomyocytes. This slow action potential is characterized by a less steep phase 0 (calcium influx),

absent phase 1, shortened phase 2 and 3 (K^+ efflux), and a phase 4 that is characterized by spontaneous diastolic depolarization (funny Corrected QT interval or QT_c is QT divided by the square root of the RR interval. The risk of torsades is highest when the QT_c is greater than 500 milliseconds or 0.5 s. Choice A when solved for yields a QT_c of 0.56 s.current: mixed ionic current mediated by Na^+ and K^+). In contrast, in the ventricular cell, phase 0 is mediated by Na^+ influx, phase 1 by K^+ efflux, phase 2 by calcium influx, phase 3 by K^+ efflux, and phase 4 was minimal ionic flow.

4. **C. Explanation:** The sarcoplasmic or endoplasmic reticulum Ca^{2+} ATPase or SERCA is an ATP-dependent pump that moves cytosolic Ca^{2+} back into the sarcoplasmic reticulum (SR). Along with the Na^+– Ca^{2+} exchanger; it is responsible for the decrease in cytosolic Ca^{2+}. Calmodulin is one of the primary sensors of cytosolic Ca^{2+}. Fall in calcium levels restores the inhibitory function of the troponin-tropomyosin complex, ceasing the interaction between actin and myosin. This in turn leads to relaxation. SERCA activity is inhibited by the protein phospholamban. Phospholamban performs this inhibitory function in the dephosphorylated state. Once Ca^{2+} enters back into the SR, it is stored bound to calsequestrin and calreticulin. These proteins release Ca^{2+} when the next wave of action potential arrives. Adrenergic β(beta) stimulation leads to phosphorylation of phospholamban and deactivation. This increases SERCA activity and improves relaxation or lusitropy.
5. **B. Explanation**: Myofibrils consist mainly of two types of contractile proteins: thin filament actin and thick filament myosin. These are arranged in a specific pattern to generate the basic unit of contraction: the sarcomere. The arrangement of sarcomeres in turn gives cardiac muscle a distinct striated appearance when examined under the electron microscope. This is due to differences in refractive properties of the elements. These striations are identified by letters and represent either specific lines or bands of refraction. Z lines (from the German word *zuckung* or twitch line), are dark lines present at regular intervals along the myofibril and connect adjacent sarcomeres. The M line anchors the myosin filaments. Actin filaments anchor onto Z lines via actinin and extend toward the M line, interdigitating with the myosin filaments. The region occupied by myosin filaments (with and without overlapping actin) is termed the A band (appears dark). The region occupied by actin filaments without any overlap with myosin, is called the I band (appears light). Thus, each sarcomere consists of two half I bands and 1 A band between 2 Z lines.
6. **C. Explanation**: Intercalated discs are mechanical couplers and ***gap junctions*** are electrical couplers in the myocardial syncytium. Ryanodine and dihydropyridine receptors are involved in calcium induced calcium release in the cell leading to actin-myosin interaction.
7. **A. Explanation:** Corrected QT interval or QT_c is QT divided by the square root of the RR interval. The risk of torsades is highest when the QT_c is greater than 500 milliseconds or 0.5 s. Choice A when solved for yields a QT_c of 0.56 s.
8. **D. Explanation**: Cardiac tamponade is characterized by a dominant x descent and attenuated y descent, while constrictive pericarditis (and diseases with restrictive behavior such as RV infarction) exhibits a steep x and y descent, producing an M or W configuration in the CVP waveform. Y descent represents rapid ventricular filling and is dependent upon the pressure differences between the RA and RV. In tamponade, because of external compression of all chambers (RA and RV), this filling is impaired from the get-go as the difference in pressures between the RA and RV is decreased. This leads to an attenuated y descent. In constrictive pericarditis, RA pressures are typically increased. This causes an increased pressure differential for filling. But as soon as the RV starts filling (steep y descent), the low RV compliance leads to attenuation of this pressure differential, quickly leading to a diastolic plateau or h wave. The combination of a steep y, followed by recovery to a diastolic plateau, typically inscribes a "square root sign" pattern on the CVP waveform.
9. **A. Explanation:** Decompensated heart failure can occur in both Heart Failure with reduced ejection fraction and Heart Failure with preserved ejection fraction. Increase is LV end-diastolic pressure either due to decreased forward LV ejection or compliance leads to increased left atrial pressure. This in turn gets transmitted across the valve less pulmonary circulation leading to increased egress of fluid into the pulmonary interstitium. This leads to sensation of dyspnea. As congestion worsens, the alveoli flood with transudate; this state is referred to as cardiogenic pulmonary edema. This patient is likely experiencing a fall in his SV and diastolic filling time due to atrial fibrillation with rapid ventricular response. Auscultation is likely to reveal a S3 gallop and bilateral lung rales. The S1 heart sound is split wide and fixed in patients with ASDs.
10. **C. Explanation**: Per Fick equation, Oxygen consumption VO_2 is the product of CO and Arteriovenous oxygen content difference {CO X (CaO_2–CvO_2)}. In this circumstance, it would be 3 l/min x (20−12) ml/dl or 30 dl/min × 8 ml/dl or 240 ml/min.

References

1. Hall JE, Hall ME, editors. Guyton and hall textbook of medical physiology. 14th ed. Philadelphia: Saunders Elsevier; 2021.
2. Barrett KE, Barman SM, Brooks HL, Yuan JJ. Ganong's review of medical physiology. 26th ed. New York: McGraw-Hill Education/Medical; 2019.
3. Sun LS, Davis NA. Ch 14. Cardiac physiology. In: Miller RD, editor. Miller's anesthesia. 9th ed. Philadelphia: Elsevier; 2020. p. 384–401
4. Pagel PS, Stowe DF. Ch 12. Cardiac anatomy and physiology. In: Barash PG, Cullen BF, Stoelting RK, Cahalan M, Stock MC, Ortega R, editors. Clinical anesthesia. 8th ed. Philadelphia: Lippincott Williams & Wilkins; 2017. p. 277–300.
5. Iaizzo PA, editor. Handbook of cardiac anatomy, physiology and devices. 3rd ed. Cham/Switzerland: Springer International Publishing; 2015.
6. Romanò M. Text atlas of practical electrocardiography. Milano: Springer-Verlag Italia; 2015.

Respiratory System Physiology

18

Siddharth Pawan Dugar, Mani Latifi, and Eduardo Mireles-Cabodevila

Abstract

This chapter will cover basic concepts of lung physiology in health and disease. The concepts we present are aimed toward the anesthesiologist, focusing on the topic to a degree of detail to encourage recall and practical knowledge. Understanding the respiratory system physiology is a key element in the work of the anesthesiologist. Not only does the anesthesiologist rely on the respiratory system to ensure appropriate gas exchange, but it is the means for drug delivery and allows us to obtain information about the body status with simple measurements.

Keywords

Perioperative pulmonary assessment • Gas exchange • Equation of motion • Control of ventilation • Diffusion • Compliance • Resistance

Key Points

1. Spirometry, lung volumes, diffusion capacity, and exercise testing can be performed preoperatively to better understand a patient's pulmonary mechanics and identify those at high risk for postoperative complications.
2. The equation of motion of the respiratory system helps understand the components that are involved in ventilation. It divides the components into elastic and resistive loads.
3. The pressure–volume curve can provide helpful information regarding the resistance and compliance of the respiratory system in an invasively ventilated patient.
4. Compliance of the respiratory system is a sum of lung compliance and chest wall compliance and is affected by lung, chest wall, or abdominal cavity pathology.
5. The surface tension is the force present at the air–liquid interface, which tends to minimize the surface area of a liquid. Surfactant reduces the surface tension, and this allows homogeneous ventilation and avoids atelectasis of the lung at low lung volumes.
6. The major determinant of airway resistance is the radius of the airway. A decrease in radius will increase the airway resistance to a power of 4.
7. The main determinants of gas exchange are ventilation and perfusion. Dead space occurs when ventilation is higher than perfusion. Shunt occurs when perfusion is higher than ventilation.
8. Diffusion of a gas through the alveolo-capillary membrane is dependent on the distance for diffusion, the pressure gradient, molecular weight, the thickness of the membrane, and the solubility coefficient of the gas.
9. The lung serves other functions besides gas exchange. It serves as a filter for both the circulation (emboli) and inhaled particles. It has the ability to metabolize endogenous compounds and secrete hormones.
10. Perioperative smoking has effects throughout the body. This will affect not only the physiologic characteristics of the patients, but their outcomes.

S. P. Dugar · M. Latifi · E. Mireles-Cabodevila (✉)
Respiratory Institute, Cleveland Clinic Foundation, Cleveland, OH, USA
e-mail: mirelee@ccf.org

S. P. Dugar
e-mail: dugars@ccf.org

M. Latifi
e-mail: latifim@ccf.org

M. Argalious et al. (eds.), *Basic Sciences in Anesthesia*,
https://doi.org/10.1007/978-3-031-60203-0_18

18.1 Introduction

The lungs are enclosed in the chest cavity, surrounded by chest wall, bones, and muscles. The lungs have a resting size (volume), which depends on the elastic characteristics of the lung and the chest wall. Figure 18.1 highlights the interaction between the chest wall and the lungs, the lungs recoil inward (always trying to collapse), while the chest wall is trying to expand outward. This relation reaches equilibrium when the distending pressure of the chest wall balances with the collapsing pressure of the lung, resulting in the resting volume or functional residual capacity. This is easily recognized after thoracotomy, the chest wall opens (outward) while the lungs collapse rapidly (no more negative pressure in the pleural cavity). The activity of the respiratory muscles, the habitus of the patient, and lung characteristics will affect this relationship. We use several physiological tests to evaluate this relationships.

We can assess the entire respiratory system physiology with three tests: (1) spirometry, (2) lung volumes, and (3) diffusion capacity. More complex tests, such as the cardiopulmonary exercise studies or ventilation perfusion studies, are also useful for some specific cases (e.g., lung resection). For most cases, the history and physical, spirometry, and a pulse oximetry will provide sufficient information on the status of the respiratory system to allow the anesthesiologist to understand the pulmonary mechanics and physiology of the patient.

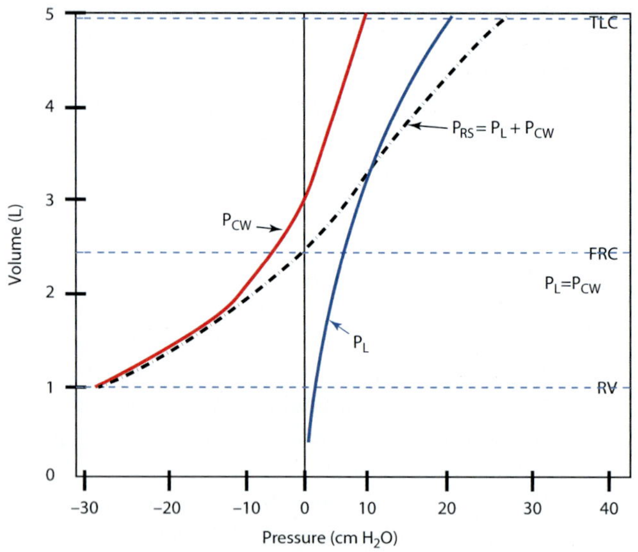

Fig. 18.1 This Fig depicts the pressure–volume curve of the lung (P_L), chest wall (P_{CW}), and total respiratory system (P_T). The diagram indicates the direction and magnitude of the elastic forces of the lung (*blue line*), chest wall (*red line*), and total respiratory system (*black dashed line*) at various lung volumes. At total lung capacity (*TLC*), the PCW is positive, trying to return to its resting state. The volume of lung and chest wall at zero pressure is different: lung has to be expanded and chest wall has to be compressed to reach resting volume. At resting volume (*FRC*), the inward elastic recoil of lung is equal to outward elastic recoil of chest wall. The residual volume is the lowest lung volume that the chest wall will allow to occur [1]

18.1.1 Spirometry

A spirometer is a device that measures the volume (flow) of inspired and expired air in terms of time. The values generated by the patient are compared to "normal" or predicted values, which are calculated using population-based equations using the patient's age, height, smoking status, gender, and race [2].

◉ Figure 2 depicts the different lung volumes measured with spirometry [3]. The *y*-axis represents the lung volumes, from being completely deflated (as if the thorax was open and the lung compressed to contain zero air) to completely inflated (total lung capacity; the lung cannot have any more air in it at maximal inspiratory pressure). ◉ Figure 18.2 initially displays a patient breathing at rest. This is called the tidal volume or tidal breathing. You can see that there is lung volume above and below the tidal volume; this is the "reserve" the patient can inhale or exhale. To measure it, the patient is instructed to take the deepest breath possible. The volume generated is the inspiratory capacity (if measured from end expiration) or the inspiratory reserve volume (if measured from the top of the tidal volume). To measure the expiratory reserve, the patient is asked to exhale as much as possible to the point where no further air comes out in spite of maximal effort (this is the expiratory reserve volume). Indeed, there is still air in the lungs; however, this air cannot come out due to the elastic recoil from the chest wall and negative pleural pressure. This "remnant air" is called the residual volume. The curve demonstrates the vital capacity, which entails the amount of air exhaled after a maximal inspiration (we add *forced*, as we ask the patient to "forcefully" exhale). The functional residual capacity is the expiratory reserve volume plus the residual volume, which is the amount of air that remains in the lungs at end of tidal breathing.

In summary, the lung has four basic lung volumes that constitute both inspiratory and expiratory phases and are as follows [1, 5, 6]:

1. Inspiratory reserve volume (IRV)
2. Tidal volume (Vt)
3. Expiratory reserve volume (ERV)
4. Residual volume (RV)

When two or more volumes are combined, they constitute four distinct lung capacities that are as follows [1, 5, 6]:

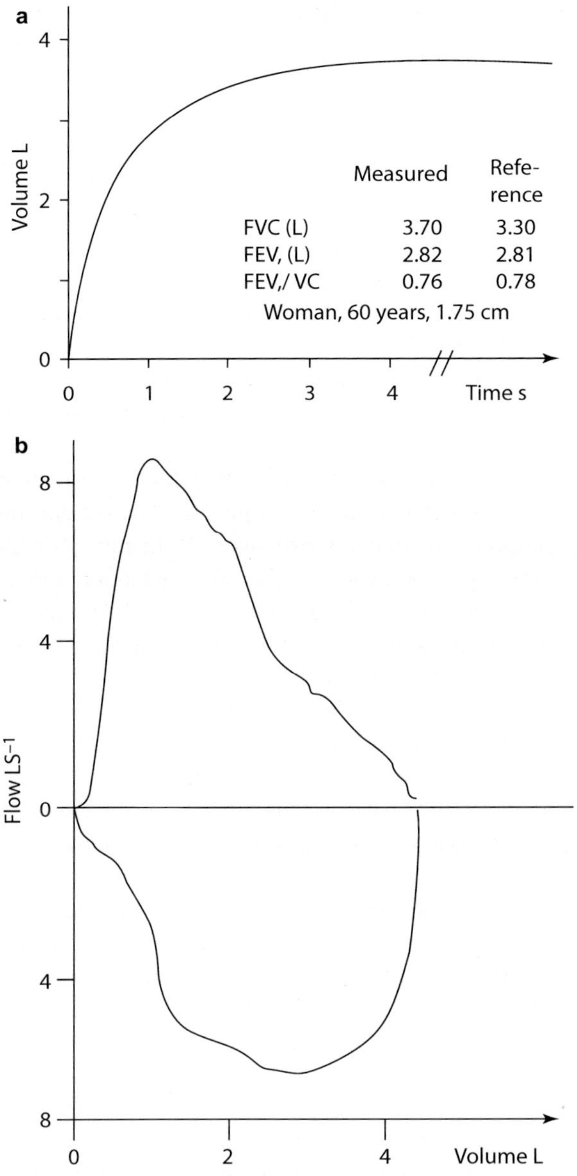

Fig. 18.2 **a** Depicts volume of air expired as a function of time in seconds with included examples of measured and expected values for FVC, FEV_1, and FEV1/FVC ratio. **b** Flow volume curve obtained with spirometry with expiration above the x-axis and inspiration below x-axis (Reprinted with permission from Madsen et al. [4])

1. VT + IRV = inspiratory capacity (IC)
2. RV + ERV = functional residual capacity (FRC)
3. VT + IRV + ERV = vital capacity (VC)
4. IRV + VT + ERV + RV = total lung capacity (TLC)

A typical spirometry tracing that displays the measured lung volumes is depicted in ◉ Fig. 18.2. Although the report will contain a large amount of data, the spirometry will only yield three values of interest for the anesthesiologist: The FVC (forced vital capacity), the FEV1 (forced expiratory volume in 1 s), and the ratio FEV1 to FVC. The absolute values are reported as percent of the predicted.

When interpreting spirometry, the first thing to check is that the patient values entered are correct as this will affect the predicted values. The next value to read is the FEV1/FVC ratio, which is a marker of obstruction. If the value is below the lower limit of normal for the patient, then the patient has obstructive airway disease (e.g., asthma, chronic obstructive pulmonary disease [COPD], tracheal stenosis) [7]. If there is obstruction, the next value to see is the FEV_1. This will help gauge the degree of obstruction present. The lower the value, the worse the obstructive physiology (in general, an $FEV_1 < 50\%$ predicted represents severe obstruction) [2]. The last value to see is the forced vital capacity (FVC). The FVC is subject to many influences (lung and chest wall elastance, pleura, airway resistance, patient effort, duration of effort). A reduction in FVC is interpreted as restriction (i.e., the lung cannot expand as much), which can be secondary to restrictive diseases of the lung itself (fibrosis, etc.) or due to factors outside the lung (decreased muscle strength, large abdomen displacing the diaphragm, obesity, pleural disease, spinal deformity, poorly compliant chest wall, or a poor patient effort). A decreased FVC requires clinical correlation, and if further clarification is needed to confirm restriction, then measuring lung volumes is the necessary next step. This can help differentiate restriction due to diseases affecting the lung parenchyma versus those outside the lung. It is worth noting that in the setting of severe airflow obstruction, the FVC may be reduced [2], a term called "pseudo-restriction."

18.1.2 Lung Volumes

We obtain all the lung volumes and capacities to better identify the type of physiological derangement the patient has. There are 3 methods available: (1) the plethysmography (body box), (2) the helium dilution technique, and (3) the nitrogen washout [1, 5, 6]. These techniques are used to measure the FRC and TLC (as these cannot be measured by spirometry alone). Each technique has its details and caveats, which can be read in pulmonary physiology books. In brief, plethysmography is based on Boyle's Law, which states that, under isothermal conditions, when a constant mass of gas is compressed or decompressed, the gas volume decreases or increases and gas pressure changes such that the product of volume and pressure at any given moment is constant [1, 6].

By placing the patient in a tightly enclosed box, we can measure the change in volume and pressure and calculate the FRC. The nitrogen washout and helium dilution rely on the volume of distribution of a known gas in order to determine FRC [7].

In the helium dilution technique, patients are attached to a spirometer that includes a known concentration of helium in a known volume. After several breaths, the concentration of the helium is distributed over an increased volume (that includes the patient's lung volume) and allowed to reach a new equilibrium. The final exhaled concentration can thus be measured and the FRC can be calculated based on the dilution of the gas [7].

Similarly, in the nitrogen washout technique, the patient is attached to a spirometer and allowed to breathe in 100% FiO_2 while measuring exhaled volumes and nitrogen concentration at timed intervals. With each breath, the exhaled concentration of nitrogen is decreased until after several minutes (approximately 7 min) the entire concentration of the nitrogen in the lung has been washed out [7]. Once this happens, FRC can be determined using a formula. A reduction of TLC below the lower limit of normal is consistent with restriction.

18.1.3 Diffusion Capacity

We measure the pulmonary diffusion capacity of carbon monoxide (DL, CO) to gain insight into gas exchange. CO is used due to its similarity to oxygen in both molecular weight and solubility coefficients. CO has an affinity for hemoglobin that is 210 greater than oxygen and thus able to maintain a very high pressure gradient across the alveolo-capillary interface as only the free unbound gas contributes to this gradient [8]. Therefore, in theory, the diffusion of CO would be a reflection of the alveolo-capillary interface itself (see later section in the chapter: Diffusion). The most common method for measuring DL, CO is by the single breath method. This test is done by having patients completely exhale to the level of RV followed by maximal inhalation of a gas mixture containing 0.3% CO to the level of the TLC [7]. The subject then holds their breath for 10 s followed by quick forceful exhalation. After the initial portion of gas is expired, which accounts for dead space, a sample of expired air is collected to calculate DL, CO [7]. It is measured in ml/min/mm Hg, using the volume of inhaled CO compared to exhaled volume of CO.

DL, CO is not only a manifestation of the alveolo-capillary interface, it depends upon several physiological factors (e.g., age, sex, height, hemoglobin, lung volumes, carboxyhemoglobin, and exercise and body position). To account for these changes, it is often reported with corrections to the absolute value using hemoglobin DL, hb and lung volumes $DL,_{VA}$.

18.1.4 Exercise Testing

In exercising healthy individuals, the supply of oxygen by the pulmonary system (minute ventilation) and the oxygen delivery by the cardiovascular system (cardiac output) are increased to provide oxygen to meet the demand of the skeletal muscle mitochondria. A cardiopulmonary exercise test is a physiological study that can identify defects in pulmonary ventilation, cardiovascular function, or skeletal muscle function. In complex patients, it can provide insight into the specific clinical limitations causing cardiopulmonary limitation. Exercise studies are also used to estimate preoperative morbidity and mortality in high-risk procedures [9].

Exercise testing is done with a metabolic cart connected via a non-rebreathing valve to a patient. The patient undergoes progressive exercise load over 10–15 min on either a stationary cycle or treadmill [7]. The metabolic cart measures the fractions of inspired and expired O_2 and CO_2, oxygen consumption (VO_2), CO_2 production (VCO_2), and minute ventilation (Ve) [9, 10].

The VO_2 is measured breath by breath during the exercise test. It reflects the amount of oxygen your body uses per kilogram per minute. In essence, it is the ability of a patient to deliver and use oxygen. Initially, during exercise, VO_2 increases linearly and is matched by linear increases in CO_2 production, which reflects the increased skeletal muscle function [10]. The linear increase in VO_2 continues until a maximum level is reached (VO_2 max) and represents the patient's aerobic capacity. If the patient continues to exercise after the VO_2 max, it results in the shifting of the skeletal muscle from aerobic to anaerobic metabolism. Anaerobic metabolism results in increased lactic acid, which is converted into lactate and CO_2. The point where the VCO_2 is higher compared to VO_2 is the anaerobic threshold (AT) [7].

VO_2 max is usually lower in women compared to men and increases with exercise training. Impairment in aerobic function is defined as abnormally low VO_2 max compared to predicted. A low VO_2 max can be due to decreased cardiac output, decreased oxygen level, decreased hemoglobin, or muscle condition/function/size. The patterns of cardiac, pulmonary, and muscle interaction help define the physiological defects. In addition to identifying exercise limitations, cardiopulmonary exercise testing can also be used to help gain insight in certain patient populations preoperatively. For example, a $VO_2max < 15$ ml/kg/min is associated with high-risk patients for thoracic surgery. An anaerobic threshold > 11 ml/kg/min is associated with decreased perioperative mortality after surgery [9, 10]. As a consequence, several protocols include cardiopulmonary testing to assess candidacy for surgery (lung volume reduction, heart transplantation, and high-risk lung resections).

18.2 Lung Mechanics

The best way to understand the mechanical characteristics of respiratory systems in our opinion is by using the equation of motion (the equation has been simplified for clarity). This equation illustrates the forces and their interaction during breathing:

$$P_{\text{mus}} + P_{\text{vent}} = (\text{volume} \times \text{elastance}) + (\text{flow} \times \text{resistance}) \quad (18.1)$$

where P_{mus} is the pressure generated by respiratory muscle activity and P_{vent} generated by a mechanical ventilator (if present). Pressure, volume, and flow are variables (i.e., change with time) while elastance and resistance are considered to be constant. The equation highlights the pressure needed from the respiratory muscles and/or the mechanical ventilator to overcome the loads from the elastic component (elastance × volume) and the resistive component (resistance × flow) [5, 6].

18.2.1 Elastance and Compliance

Elastance is the constant of proportionality between volume change and change in transrespiratory pressure (or the slope of the volume-pressure curve) [6, 7]. In practice, it may be calculated as the change in pressure difference across the system divided by the change in lung volume (i.e., tidal volume, V_{T}) between two points in time when flow throughout the respiratory system is zero and $P_{\text{mus}} = 0$ (i.e., the patient is paralyzed):

$$E_{\text{RS}} = \frac{\Delta P_{\text{vent}}}{\Delta V_{\text{T}}} \quad (18.2)$$

Compliance is the reciprocal of elastance (elastance = 1/compliance) [5, 7]:

$$C_{\text{RS}} = \frac{\Delta V_{\text{T}}}{\Delta P_{\text{vent}}} \quad (18.3)$$

With this understanding, now we know that compliance describes the ability of change in pressure to distend the respiratory system and is expressed in mL/cmH_2O. The respiratory system is not only comprised of lungs, it also includes the chest wall and abdomen. We need to recognize that a compliance obtained at the bedside includes this components [5, 11]. That is:

$$C_{\text{RS}} = \frac{C_{\text{L}} \times C_{\text{CW}}}{C_{\text{L}} + C_{\text{CW}}} \quad (18.4)$$

where C_{RS} is the respiratory system compliance, C_{L} is the total lung compliance, and C_{CW} is the chest wall compliance. The compliance calculated by the ventilator is C_{RS}, which is a global measure of the respiratory system. If we wanted to determine the C_{L} and C_{CW}, we need to know the transmural pressures (pressures across the lungs and the chest wall). This means that we need to measure the pressure in the pleural space (or its surrogate, esophageal pressure) [11]. Hence, the pressure across the lungs (transpulmonary pressure, P_{TP}) is the pressure at the airway opening minus esophageal pressure and trans-chest wall pressure, P_{TCW}, is esophageal pressure minus pressure on the body surface. Then, C_{L} and C_{CW} are calculated by substituting P_{TP} or P_{TCW} into Eq. 18.3.

18.2.1.1 Lung Compliance

The factors responsible for lung compliance are the elastin and collagen fibers present in lung parenchyma and the alveolar surface tension [5, 8]. To better understand the elastic components, we see a pressure/volume curve of the

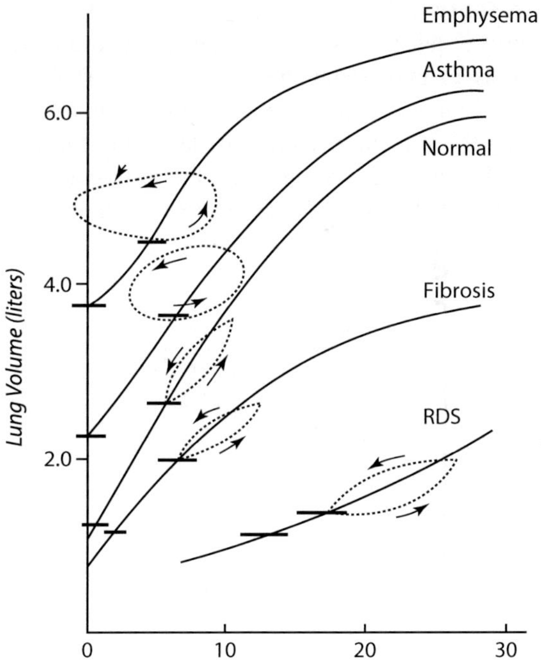

Fig. 18.3 This figure compares the compliance curve of the normal lung with various lung pathology. Note that in emphysema and asthma, the lungs are more compliant (i.e., a small change in pressure causes a large change in volume) while in fibrosis and RDS (respiratory distress syndrome), the lungs are less compliant (i.e., a large in pressure is needed for small change in volume) (Reprinted with permission from Hildebrandt [12])

lung under different conditions. ◉ Figure 18.3 compares the compliance curve of a normal lung with compliance curve of lung with different pathology.

The curves labeled fibrosis and RDS (respiratory distress syndrome) represent low lung compliance (i.e., a small change in volume for a large in change pressure). The curves labeled asthma and emphysema represent a lung with higher compliance (i.e., a large change in volume for a small change in pressure) from loss of elastic tissues. ◉Figures 18.3 and 18.4 highlight that the compliance of lung depends on the FRC from where the change in volume occurs. From ◉ Fig. 18.4, we can see that at the beginning or at the end of the inflation curve, minimal change in volume occurs with a large change in pressure. On the steeper part of the curve, a large change in volume occurs with less change in pressure. Clinically, this phenomenon is observed in patients with acute respiratory distress syndrome (ARDS) with too little positive end-expiratory pressure (PEEP) (under recruited) or very high PEEP (over distended). The other clinical condition is severe COPD, where the FRC is elevated due to air trapping and loss of elastic structures and is close to TLC, thus, small changes in volume require high amounts of changes in pressure.

Surface Tension

The surface tension is a little bit counterintuitive and requires us to understand the Laplace law (◉ Fig. 18.5). Surface tension is the force present at the air–liquid interface caused by the attraction of the particles in the surface layer of a liquid, which tends to minimize the surface area [8, 15]. In other words, liquids have an inherent elastic tendency to acquire the least surface area possible (i.e., a drop of water is circular in order to have the least surface area). The **Laplace equation** states that:

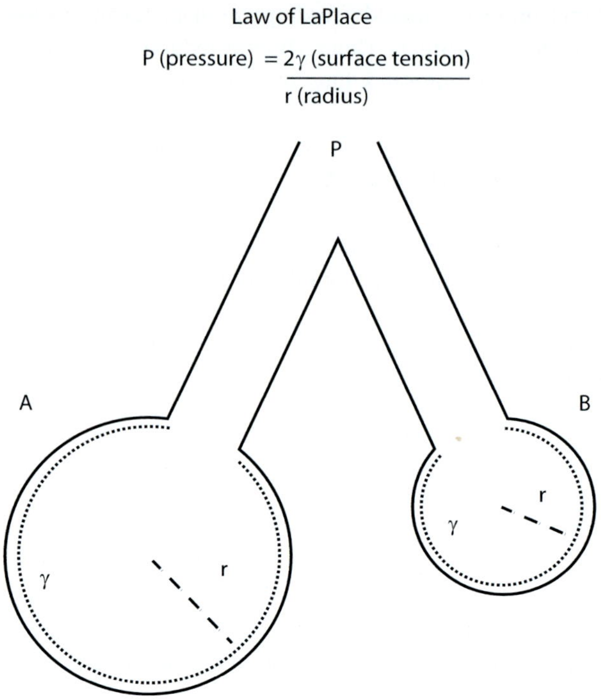

Fig. 18.5 Depicts 2 alveoli (*A* and *B*) with different radius. If the pressure inside both alveolus is same, the surface tension changes with change in alveolar radius to maintain stability. In this case, surfactant will lower the surface tension in alveoli *B*, reducing the pressure inside and preventing it from collapsing (Reprinted with permission from Haitsma [16])

$$P = \frac{2T}{r} \quad (18.5)$$

where, P is the pressure within the alveoli (dyn/cm^2), T is the surface tension inside the alveoli at air–liquid interface (dyn/cm), and r is the radius of the alveoli (cm).

Following this formula, for a constant surface tension, smaller alveoli will have higher pressure. The high pressure in smaller alveoli will force it to empty itself in large alveoli and collapse (atelectasis) while larger alveoli with less pressure would have preferential ventilation. This phenomenon is not observed under normal conditions due to the presence of pulmonary surfactant. The presence of pulmonary surfactant reduces the surface tension forces and results in lower pressure inside the alveoli [7, 8, 15]. Surfactant prevents atelectasis and allows even distribution of ventilation. The clinical correlate is ARDS in adults or RDS in premature neonates, where the absence of surfactant results in collapse of smaller alveoli and decreased total lung compliance.

The pulmonary surfactant is produced by type II pneumocytes and released by exocytosis in response to high-volume lung inflation, increased ventilation rate, or

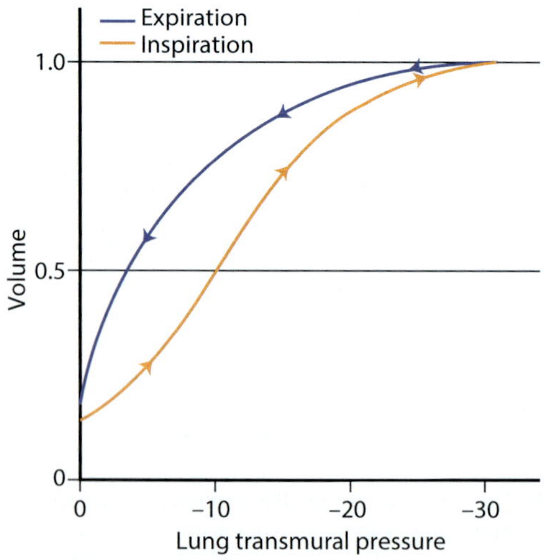

Fig. 18.4 Depicts the pressure volume curve during inspiration (inflation) and expiration (deflation) of a lung. Note the difference in lung volume at same pressure in inspiration and expiration limbs. This phenomenon is called hysteresis [5, 7, 13] see below. (Reprinted with permission from Nurok and Topulos [14])

endocrine stimulation [8, 15]. It is composed of 90% lipid in the form of phospholipids with the remainder of it being protein and carbohydrates. Dipalmitoyl phosphatidyl choline is the main constituent. The hydrophobic fatty acids project into the gas phase, while the hydrophilic end lies in the alveolar lining fluid. The surfactant gets packed densely together during exhalation when alveoli assume a smaller radius exerting a greater effect in reducing surface tension and preventing the alveoli from collapsing.

Hysteresis

The difference in shape between the inflation and deflation limbs of the pressure–volume curve is called hysteresis (◉ Fig. 18.4). That is, there is a higher lung volume, per unit of pressure, at any given point during deflation compared to inflation. Hysteresis is mostly due to the presence of pulmonary surfactant and its effect on surface tension forces at the air–liquid interface. The other factor responsible for hysteresis is opening of closed alveoli during inspiration [1, 7]. These alveoli remain open during exhalation, explaining why more than the expected pressure is required during inflation. The loop becomes progressively broader as the tidal volume increases or, in ARDS, due to loss of surfactant.

18.2.1.2 Chest Wall Compliance

The chest wall is composed of visceral pleura, rib cage, muscle (including the diaphragm), fat, and skin. The abdominal cavity also contributes to the chest wall compliance; this becomes evident in conditions such as ascites, abdominal compartment syndrome, or obesity.

To measure the chest wall compliance, one needs to measure pleural pressure by placing a pleural catheter (rarely done, if ever) or using surrogate of pleural pressure (classically using an esophageal catheter) [11]. The gradient between the pressure at the airway opening and the pleural pressure will provide the transpulmonary pressure, which is a reflection of the lung compliance. The chest wall compliance then will be the total respiratory system compliance minus the lung compliance. The contribution of the chest wall to the respiratory system compliance ranges from 20 to 50% in normal to severe ARDS patients. Normal chest wall compliance is 200 ml/cm H_2O.

18.2.1.3 Static and Dynamic Compliance

Static compliance is measured in absence of any air flow in the entire respiratory system with no muscle activity (muscle paralysis). Because, in some conditions, we can only hold it for a few seconds before we have to let the subject breathe, the system never reaches true static condition and thus is called quasi-static compliance. There are different methods to measure compliance [13]:

- **The Super Syringe**: In this method, a known amounts of gas (volume) is pushed into the lungs, and the pressure change is measured after flow has stopped. This is mainly used when trying to build a pressure volume curve. Another alternative is to use a very slow flow to increase the volume gradually while measuring the pressure change. Because the flow is low (<9 L/min), the resistive component is essentially eliminated.
- **Single Occlusion Test**: This is the most commonly used method at the bedside. An end inspiratory pause is performed in patients receiving mechanical ventilation. The pressure will decay to form a plateau, commonly known as plateau pressure (P_{plat}).
- **Multiple Occlusion Test:** Airway occlusions are performed several times at different points of expiration. This allows the building of a volume/pressure curve.

Dynamic compliance is measured during an active breath, but the changes in volume and pressure are measured between points in time when flow at the airway opening is zero. This can be done by hand, but a ventilator uses linear regression. Because there may still be flow among lung units even when flow at the airway is zero (i.e., pendelluft), the pressure difference may be larger than under true static conditions [5, 13]. Hence, dynamic compliance tends to be lower than static compliance to the degree that the mechanical properties in the lungs are heterogeneous.

18.2.2 Resistance

Resistance opposes the flow of gas in and out the respiratory system. Resistance is defined as the constant of proportionality between pressure (P) and flow ($\dot{V}$) in a flow conducting system and is usually expressed in units of cm H_2O/(L/s) [5, 7]:

$$R = \frac{\Delta P}{\Delta \dot{V}}$$

The total respiratory system resistance is the result of airway (natural and artificial) and tissue resistance [5, 17]. The lung parenchyma and chest wall viscoelastic resistance to motion gives rise to tissue resistance. The contribution is minuscule and in clinical practice, they are essentially ignored. Thus, this section focuses on airway resistance.

The airway caliber, nature of the gas flow, viscosity, and density of the gas determine airway resistance. Under normal conditions, the most decisive of them is airway caliber [5, 7]. Poiseuille's equation illustrates the relationship between airway caliber, laminar flow, and viscosity:

$$\dot{V} = \frac{\Delta P \pi r^4}{8 \mu L} \tag{18.6}$$

where, Δ(Delta) P is the pressure gradient across the flow path (airway), L is the length of the flow path, μ is dynamic viscosity, $\dot{V}$ is the flow, r is a radius, and π(pi) is a mathematical constant. This equation demonstrates that the pressure gradient is directly proportional to gas flow. Because of this, for any flow rate, the pressure gradient divided by the flow rate equals a constant, called resistance:

$$\text{Resistance} = \frac{\Delta P}{\dot{V}} \tag{18.7}$$

The equation can be rewritten to show the factors affecting resistance:

$$\text{Resistance} = \frac{8 \times \text{length} \times \text{viscosity}}{\pi \times (\text{radius})^4} \tag{18.8}$$

18.2.2.1 Airway Caliber

The Poiseuille's equation demonstrates that the major determinant of resistance is the airway radius. In normal subjects, the larger airway contributes to 80% of total airway resistance, while the rest stems from the smaller airways [1, 6, 8]. Although this seems counterintuitive (because the radius of the airway is the main contributor to resistance), the increase in cross-sectional area as the airways divide (bronchial subdivisions) compensates for the small diameter, such that because of the increased cross-sectional area of the distal airway, the resistance to flow is reduced [5]. In conditions such as airway edema, obstructive lung disease, or secretions where there is a decrease in airway radius, the airway resistance exponentially increases and so does the workload on respiratory muscles.

The airway caliber is also dependent on lung volume. Resistance is inversely proportional to lung volume. As lung volume decreases, there is a decrease in airway volume and thus in transmural pressure. This can result in the closure of smaller airway and increased airway resistance [1, 5]. During forced expiration, high intrathoracic pressures can exceed the transmural pressure, resulting in their collapse and increased resistance. The larger airway, due to presence of cartilage, has higher structural integrity and is less prone to collapse by changes in lung volume.

The airway caliber is mainly regulated by the autonomic system innervating the smooth muscle in the bronchus. The parasympathetic nervous system, via the vagal nerve, plays a critical role in maintaining the airway caliber. The afferent fibers in the bronchial epithelium are stimulated by noxious stimuli and cytokines [7, 8]. These stimuli cause the efferent fibers to release acetylcholine, which acts on muscarinic receptors (M3) leading to bronchoconstriction. As a counterbalancing measure, there are ß2 receptors in the bronchial epithelium that are responsive to circulating catecholamines. The activation of ß2 receptors causes bronchodilation as seen during stress, exercise, and with certain drugs.

18.2.2.2 Density, Viscosity, and Turbulent Flow

The other contributors to resistance, as demonstrated by Poiseuille's equation, are the characteristics of the gas (density and viscosity) and the nature of the flow (turbulent vs. laminar). From the equation, one can note that resistance, during laminar flow, is directly proportional to gas viscosity. Thus, helium (a low density, high viscosity gas) will not improve gas flow in conditions of laminar flow. However, in a condition where there is turbulent flow (i.e., upper airway obstruction), helium does improve flow [7, 18]. This is described by the Reynolds number (dimensionless unit):

$$\text{Reynolds number} = \frac{\rho d v}{\eta} \tag{18.9}$$

where ρ(rho) is the density of the gas, d is the diameter of the tube, v is the linear velocity of the gas, and η(eta) is the viscosity. It is known that turbulent flow occurs when the Reynolds number is greater than 2000. At that point, the pressure gradient to generate flow is proportional to the gas density but independent of viscosity. As a consequence, helium (low-density gas) may improve flow in airway stenosis.

In laminar flow, the gas flows in an orderly fashion as a series of concentric cylinders, which slide over each other forming the shape of a cone as they advance (◉ Fig. 18.6). The peripheral column of air in contact with the airway wall is stationary while the center column of air slides over them. This greatly reduces the frictional forces acting on the airflow and hence, the airway resistance is least with laminar flow. As can be seen from the diagram of laminar flow (◉ Fig. 18.6a), the center column of air will reach alveoli faster. During turbulent flow, the gas flows in a chaotic pattern with a square front (◉ Fig. 18.6b). This increases frictional forces acting on the flow and hence the resistance.

18.2.2.3 Measurement

In clinical practice, estimation of total respiratory system resistance (including the artificial airway) is often done during mechanical ventilation while delivering volume-controlled breath (at constant flow) with an end inspiratory pause (see ◉ Fig. 18.7). In light of Eq. 18.7, we can rearrange Eq. 18.1 to get:

$$R_{RS} = \frac{\Delta P_{\text{vent}}}{\Delta \dot{V}} \tag{18.10}$$

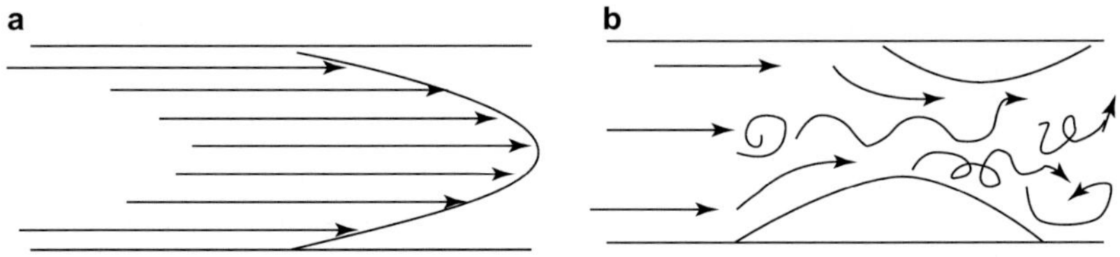

Fig. 18.6 **a** Shows a laminar flow with convex front. The arrows denote the direction and magnitude of air flow. **b** Turbulent flow with a square front (Reprinted with permission from Chatterjee and Fisher [19])

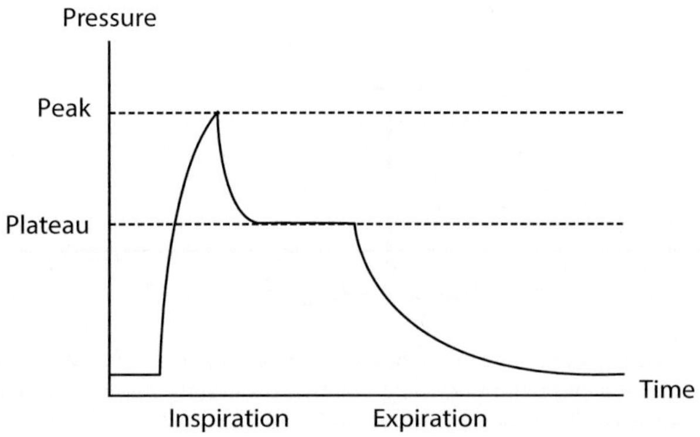

Fig. 18.7 The pressure time curve on constant flow with end inspiratory pause. The Δpressure between the peak and plateau pressure is the pressure required to overcome the resistive load, while the Δpressure between plateau and PEEP is pressure required to overcome the elastic load (Reprinted with permission from Rimensberger [20])

The pressure gradient, ΔP_{vent}, is the peak pressure minus the plateau pressure. The flow gradient, $\Delta \dot{V}$, is the set constant inspiratory flow relative to flow during the pause (i.e., zero). The peak airway pressure constitutes both the elastic and resistive component. After occlusion, there is a sharp drop in peak pressure followed by slow decline until it reaches plateau pressure. The plateau pressure constitutes the elastic component (as there is no flow). Thus, ΔP_{vent} is the pressure required to overcome the resistance at the set flow.

As with compliance, modern ventilators can use linear regression to calculate resistance under dynamic conditions [1, 7].

18.2.3 Work of Breathing

Work of breathing is the work (diaphragm or ventilator) required to move air in and out of the lungs by overcoming the elastic and resistive forces opposing it (◉ Fig. 18.8). Under normal conditions, the work of breathing is completely performed by the respiratory muscles. During respiratory failure, when respiratory muscles are unable to meet the demands, this work is partially or completely accomplished by the use of invasive or non-invasive mechanical ventilation.

Work occurs when force acting on an object causes displacement of the object in direction of force:

$$\text{Work} = \text{Force} \times \text{Distance} \tag{18.11}$$

Pressure is the force acting on a unit area of an object and volume is the product of area and distance. They can be expressed as:

$$\text{Pressure} = \frac{\text{Force}}{\text{Area}} \tag{18.12}$$

$$\text{Volume} = \text{Area} \times \text{Distance} \tag{18.13}$$

Rearranging the equation:

$$\text{Pressure} \times \text{Volume} = \text{Force} \times \text{Distance} = \text{Work} \tag{18.14}$$

Hence, work occurs when a change in pressure causes a change in volume and can be calculated from the pressure volume curve:

$$Work = \int P\mathrm{d}V \tag{18.15}$$

$\int P\mathrm{d}V$ Integral of applied pressure over a change in volume.

If you observe, at zero pressure, the resting volume of the lung and chest wall is different (◉ Fig. 18.8). The resting volume for lung is just above the residual volume. Hence, work is done to increase the lung volume to FRC. While the resting volume of the chest wall is above the FRC, the chest has to compress to FRC. This work done on the chest wall is stored as kinetic energy and utilized during normal tidal breathing [5, 22].

When the lung compliance is decreased (e.g., ARDS, pulmonary edema), the lung elastance curve is shifted to the left, requiring increased work of breathing. The increased work of breathing observed in obstructive lung disease is due to increased resistive component (i.e., diagonally hatched area) [5, 22].

The work of breathing can also be expressed as O_2 cost of breathing, which is the amount of oxygen consumed by the diaphragm and respiratory muscle during ventilation. The O_2

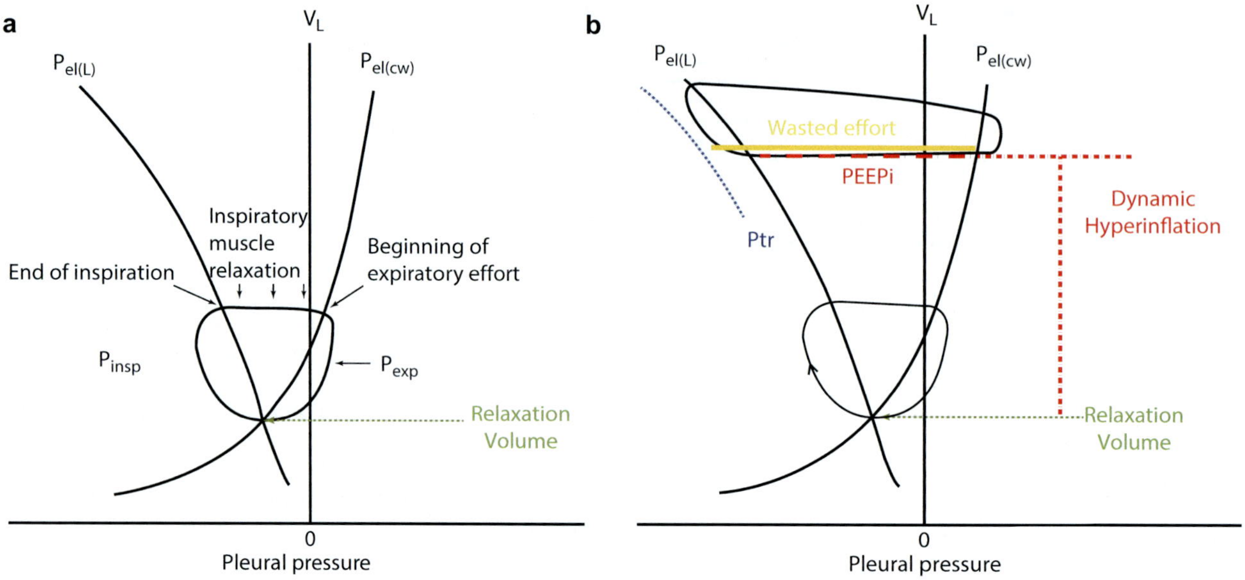

Fig. 18.8 **a** In normal subjects, inspiration starts from the relaxation volume of the respiratory system, where the passive pressure–volume curves of the lung [$P_{el(L)}$] and chest wall [$P_{el(cw)}$] intersect. Inspiratory muscle action results in pressure development (P_{insp}) on the left of the pressure–volume curve of the chest wall [$P_{el(cw)}$]. Inspiratory flow and thus increases in volume (V_L) take place on the left of the pressure–volume curve of lung and coincide with the beginning of inspiratory muscle action. Inspiration ends on the pressure–volume curve of the lung and the inspiratory muscles relax (so that pressure returns on the pressure–volume curve of the chest wall). In the case shown, expiration is active so that pressure develops on the right of the pressure–volume curve of the chest wall due to activity of expiratory muscles (P_{exp}). This returns volume back to the relaxation volume of the respiratory system. **b** In COPD patients with dynamic hyperinflation, inspiration starts from an increased end-expiratory lung volume. Inspiratory muscle action has to overcome the intrinsic positive end-expiratory pressure [PEEPi, red dashed line, horizontal distance between the $P_{el(L)}$ and $P_{el(cw)}$] before it results in inspiratory flow and thus increases in volume. In mechanically ventilated patients, inspiratory muscle action has to overcome PEEPi plus the trigger sensitivity (Ptr) before it results in inspiratory flow and thus increases in volume (V_L). When the magnitude of inspiratory muscle action is less than the sum of PEEPi + Ptr, this inspiratory effort (orange line) cannot trigger the ventilator and consequently does not result in inspiratory flow and thus increases in volume (VL). This inspiratory effort is called ineffective or wasted (Reprinted with permission from Vassilakopoulos [21])

cost of breathing in normal individuals is 0.5–1.0 mL of O_2 per liter of ventilation, which is less than 5% of the total body oxygen consumption. During increased respiratory demand, the oxygen consumption by respiratory muscles can exceed 30% of the total body oxygen consumption.

18.3 Ventilation Perfusion

The primary function of the respiratory system is exchange of oxygen and carbon dioxide. This depends on the gas inhaled and perfusion of the lungs. The ventilation and perfusion are not equally distributed throughout the lung normally, giving rise to a mismatch (V/Q = 0.8).

18.3.1 Ventilation

Ventilation involves convective movement of gas from the atmosphere into alveoli through the airways. Airways are divided into two zones (see ◉ Fig. 18.9):

1. **Conducting zone**, where there is no exchange of gas. It includes mouth, nose, trachea, and bronchi up to the terminal bronchioles.
2. **Respiratory zone**, where the airway participates in gas exchange. It includes the respiratory bronchioles, alveolar sacs, alveolar ducts, and alveoli.

18.3.1.1 Minute Ventilation

Minute ventilation is the amount of air entering the respiratory tree in a minute and is calculated as a product of respiratory rate (RR) and tidal volume (V_T). In literature and most mechanical ventilators, usually, the exhaled minute ventilation is reported:

$$\mathrm{MV} = \mathrm{RR} \times V_T \quad (18.16)$$

For a healthy adult breathing 10 breaths/min and having a V_T of 500 mL:

$$\mathrm{MV} = 10\ \mathrm{bpm} \times 500\ \mathrm{mL} = 5\ \mathrm{L/\,min} \quad (18.17)$$

A fraction of gas remains in the conducting airways and will not participate in gas exchange. The fraction of V_T that

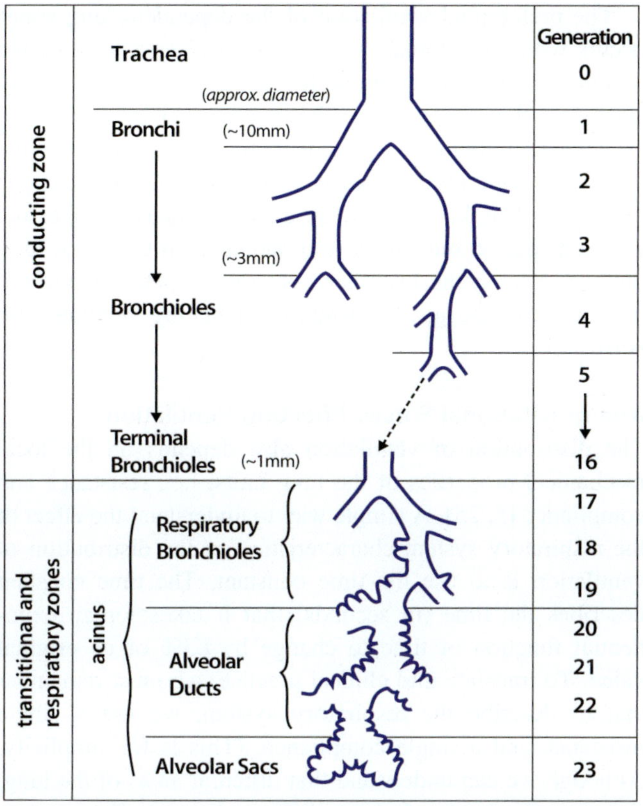

Fig. 18.9 Schematic representation of airway branching in adult human lung. Note that the airway branches a total of 21–25 times from trachea to alveoli. The exchange of gases occurs in respiratory bronchioles and alveoli (Reprinted with permission from Tu et al. [23])

participates in gas exchange is called "alveolar volume." The fraction of wasted breath in the conducting airway is called "dead space volume," and it is estimated as 2 mL/kg of ideal body weight. Thus:

$$V_T = V_D + V_A$$

V_D Dead space volume
V_A Alveolar volume

As a consequence, we can also calculate the alveolar minute ventilation as:

$$\text{Alveolar Minute Ventilation} = \text{RR} \times V_A$$

18.3.1.2 Dead Space

As stated above, dead space is the portion of the tidal volume that does not participate in gas exchange. Dead space occurs due to conducting airways (anatomical dead space) or from ventilation perfusion mismatch (alveolar dead space).

Anatomic Dead Space

The anatomic dead space—consisting of the nasopharynx, oropharynx, and the upper respiratory tract—does not participate in exchange of oxygen and carbon dioxide and is denoted by $V_{D\ anat.}$ It averages approximately 2 mL/kg of ideal body weight and is affected by age, posture, end-inspiratory lung volume, tidal volume, and respiratory rate [7].

The actual anatomic dead space can be calculated using the Fowler's method, also referred to as the single breath nitrogen washout test [5]. A patient is attached to a spirometer with 100% FiO_2 and instructed to take multiple deep breaths. The entire respiratory system along with dead space is filled with 100% FiO_2. The O_2 in respiratory zone engages in exchange of gases, while the O_2 in the conducting zone does not. Upon expiration, the amount of exhaled nitrogen concentration is measured. The initial part of exhaled air comes from upper airway. As no exchange of gases occurred, the exhaled air will not contain any nitrogen. As exhalation progresses, the gas from alveoli starts entering the airways and mixing with oxygen. The concentration of nitrogen rises sharply till a plateau is reached. This plateau represents the equilibrium of the exhaled nitrogen in the alveolar space when all the dead space volume has been washed out. Anatomic dead space can then be calculated as the area to the left of the curve after the plateau is reached (◉ Fig. 18.10).

Alveolar Dead Space

Absence or insufficient perfusion to ventilated alveoli results in them being unable to undergo gas exchange [6, 7]. This constitutes alveolar dead space and is denoted by $V_{D\ alv}$. It is seen in the normal healthy lung at the apices of lung with adequate ventilation but minimal perfusion in an upright position. Under normal circumstances, alveolar dead space is very small and not of any clinical significance. It assumes clinical importance during pulmonary hypoperfusion from low cardiac output states or pulmonary embolism.

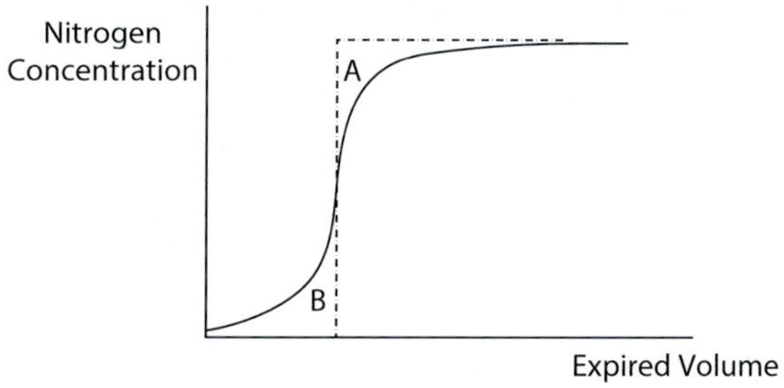

Fig. 18.10 Fowler's method to determine the anatomical dead space. The N_2 concentration is on y-axis and expired volume on x-axis. The deadspace volume is represented by the volume where the AB line intercepts the x-axis (Reprinted with permission from Sinha et al. [24])

Physiologic Dead Space
Physiological dead space is the sum of alveolar dead space and anatomic dead space. It is usually expressed as a fraction of tidal volume denoted as $V_{D\ phy}$:

$$V_{Dphy} = V_{Danat} + V_{Dalv}$$

Any factor that increases either the anatomical dead space or alveolar dead space will increase physiological dead space. Physiologic dead space is measured clinically by the modified Bohr's equation and assesses the functional ability of the lungs to eliminate carbon dioxide:

$$\frac{V_D}{V_T} = \frac{PACO_2 - PECO_2}{PACO_2} \tag{18.18}$$

V_T	tidal volume
V_D	dead space volume
P_ECO_2	Partial pressure of CO_2 in mixed expired air
P_ACO_2	Partial pressure of CO_2 in alveolus

In normal healthy lungs, alveolar and arterial PCO_2 are the same and hence, the equation can be modified as:

$$\frac{V_D}{V_T} = \frac{PaCO_2 - PECO_2}{PaCO_2} \tag{18.19}$$

$PaCO_2$ partial pressure of CO_2 in arterial blood

Any increase in physiological dead space will decrease the efficiency of lung to remove carbon dioxide from the body. Physiologic dead space increases in several conditions; classic examples are heart failure, pulmonary embolism, or increased anatomical dead space from insertion of artificial airway.

18.3.1.3 Distribution of Ventilation

The volume of air entering the lungs with each breath is not distributed equally in each lung units. This happens due to presence of multiple forces encountered by air as they move in the respiratory tree. These forces can be divided into gravitational and non-gravitational forces.

Gravitational Forces Affecting Ventilation
Gravitational forces play a key role in how the gas is distributed in the lungs. Due to the weight of the lung, the alveoli in the dependent region are smaller compared to the non-dependent region and are on the steeper part of pressure–volume curve. A small change in pressure causes a large change in volume at FRC and hence, the dependent areas receive higher ventilation. Thus, while standing, the ventilation per unit volume of lung is greatest in the bases and decreases as we move toward the apex. In supine, increased ventilation occurs in the dependent region; i.e., the posterior region compared to anterior lung regions [5, 7].

The preferential ventilation of the dependent lung zones occurs with concomitant increases in perfusion to the same region, so the ventilation/perfusion ratios are not greatly altered on changing posture. This is important to understand, as any local disease (e.g., pneumonia, atelectasis) of the dependent region will increase V/Q mismatch and affect gas exchange. This knowledge can also be utilized to alter the gas exchange in our favor. In a patient with unilateral lung disease, placing the healthier lung in a dependent position may improve the gas exchange by matching ventilation to perfusion.

Non-gravitational Forces Affecting Ventilation
The distribution of ventilation also depends on the local mechanical properties of the lung units; i.e., resistance and compliance [5, 25]. A simple way to understand the effect of the respiratory system characteristics on the distribution of ventilation is to use the time constant. The time constant describes the time (in seconds) that it takes for an exponential function of time to change by 63% of its original value. To translate into clinical practice, we must remember that to describe the respiratory system, we use a single resistance and a single compliance. (This is for simplicity. Although we can understand that different areas of the lung, and even single alveoli, have different values). These, when exposed to a change in pressure (step increase or decrease) in the airway opening, will lead to a change in alveolar pressure in an exponential function of time. That is, for a step change in airway pressure, the time constant is the time in seconds that it takes to inflate or deflate 63% of the alveoli (i.e., the lung). Alveolar pressure reaches its *near* steady state at 5 time constants.

The formula to calculate the time constant is:

$$\text{Time constant} = \text{Resistance}(cmH_2O/L/s) \times \text{Compliance}(L\ /cmH_2O)$$

(Be aware that compliance is usually presented in mL/cmH_2O, so you may need to multiply by 1000.)

If resistance or compliance increases, the time constant of that region increases and as a consequence, it takes longer to inflate/deflate, resulting in unequal ventilation [5, 13] (◉ Fig. 18.11). Another example is when respiratory frequency is increased in a patient with increased time constant. They might not be able to completely empty the lung before the next inspiration begins. This is observed in COPD as dynamic hyperinflation.

18.3.2 Perfusion

The pulmonary circulation is a low pressure and high capacitance system mainly determined at the level of the

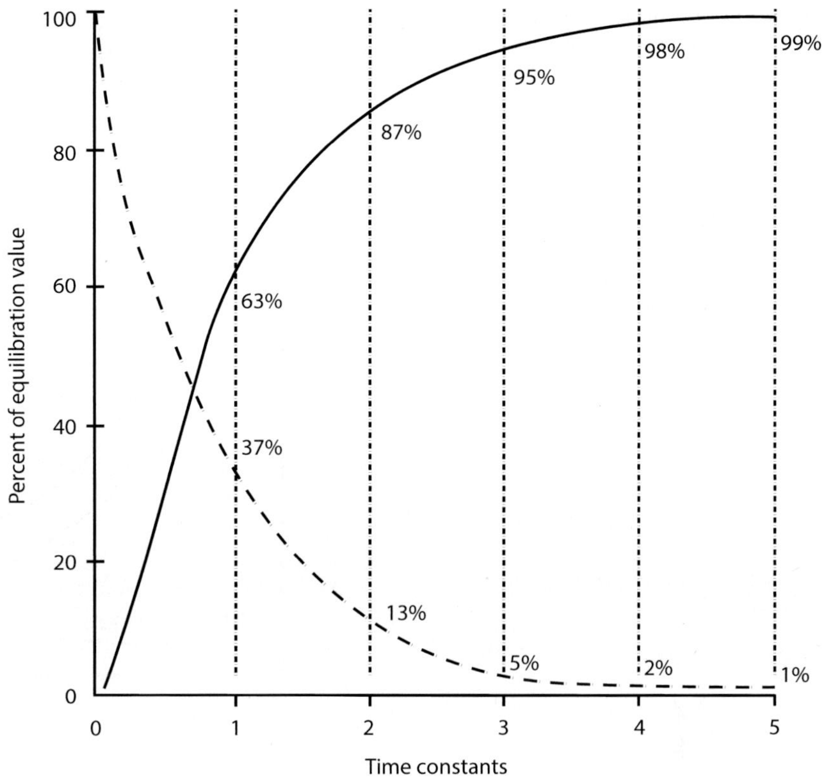

Fig. 18.11 This represents lung volume or pressure curve as a function of time constant during inspiration (*solid line*) and expiration (*dashed line*). Note that it takes 1 time constant to inflate or deflate 63% of the alveoli (i.e., the lung) and 5 time constant to inflate or deflate 99% of alveoli (Reprinted with permission from Martin [26])

pulmonary capillaries. The pulmonary capillaries are composed of alveolar and extra-alveolar vessels. The alveolar vessels are capillaries around the alveoli and are exposed to alveolar pressure, whereas the extra-alveolar vessels are more influenced by lung volume status [1, 7]. The caliber of these vessels is determined by the radial traction of the surrounding alveolar walls on the vessel. Extra-alveolar vessel resistance falls with lung inflation, whereas alveolar vessel (capillary) resistance rises with lung inflation. Similar to ventilation, gravitational and non-gravitational forces affect the distribution of blood flow.

18.3.2.1 Distribution of Perfusion

Gravitational Forces Affecting Perfusion

Gravity plays a very important role on distribution of blood flow. The average length of a healthy adult lung upright is 30 cm, providing a hydrostatic pressure difference of 30 cm of H_2O or 23 mm Hg the rom apex to the base. In upright position, the blood flow is highest in the dependent region and varies with posture as observed with ventilation.

Non-gravitational Forces Affecting Perfusion

The pulmonary vascular resistance is elevated at high and low lung volume and lowest at FRC (see ◉ Fig. 18.12). This is due to the effect of lung volume on alveolar pressure and traction on extra-alveolar vessels [5, 27]. At low lung volume, the extra-alveolar capillaries are collapsed due to lack of radial traction from the supporting lung tissue. As the lung volume increases, the vascular resistance falls with opening of extra-alveolar vessels. At high lung volume, the increased alveolar pressure causes collapse of alveolar capillaries along with stretching and distortion of extra-alveolar vessels, causing a rise in vascular resistance. In positive pressure ventilation, the increase in resistance is much more at high lung volume due to significant increase in alveolar pressure compared to arterial or venous pressure.

18.3.3 West Lung Zone

To better explain the blood flow based on the alveolar, pulmonary arterial, and venous pressure, John West et al. in 1964 divided the lung into three zones [27]:

- **Zone 1** is a lung region where alveolar pressure > arterial pressure > venous pressure. The high alveolar pressure causes the arterioles and alveolar capillaries to collapse, resulting in markedly decreased to no flow.
- **Zone 2** is a lung region where arterial pressure > alveolar pressure > venous pressure. The flow in this zone is described by arterial alveolar pressure difference. As we go down on zone 2, the hydrostatic effect causes the arterial pressure to increase but alveolar pressure remains

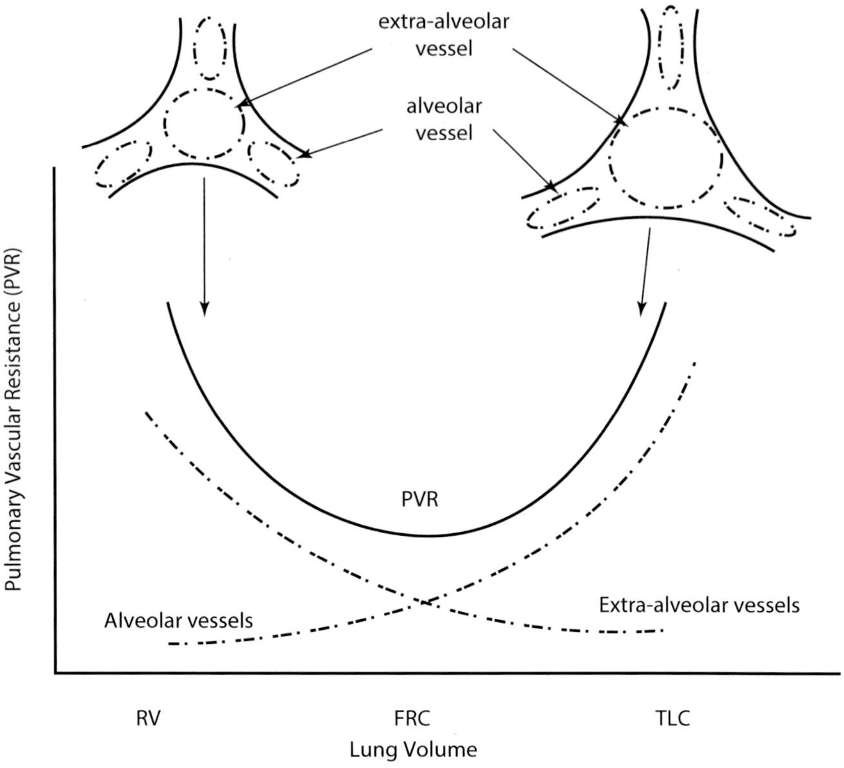

Fig. 18.12 This diagram shows the effect of lung volume on pulmonary vascular resistance. At low lung volume, the extra-alveolar vessels are compressed and at higher lung volumes, the alveolar vessels are compressed, increasing the pulmonary vascular resistance at both extremes of lung volume (Reprinted with permission from Jaeger and Blank [28])

constant, resulting in linear increase in flow. This effect is described as "waterfall" effect.

- **Zone 3** is a lung region where arterial pressure > venous pressure > alveolar pressure. The flow is dependent on arterial venous pressure difference. The blood flow increase in zone 3 is only partially because of increased hydrostatic pressure and more from increased transmural pressure, causing distension and recruitment of pulmonary capillaries.

18.3.4 Hypoxic Vasoconstriction

Another mechanism that affects perfusion distribution is hypoxic vasoconstriction. A drop in alveolar PaO_2 in a region of the lung is associated with contraction of the local pulmonary arterioles, leading to increased local vascular resistance and decreased blood flow to that region. This limits the ventilation perfusion mismatch and maintains arterial PO_2. The vasoconstriction is affected by alveolar PaO_2 and not arterial PaO_2.

The mechanism is not fully understood, but a multitude of local mediators are suspected to be the cause [29]. The vasoconstriction effect on hypoxia is non-linear, as no effect is observed when alveolar PO_2 is above 100 mm Hg. The vasoconstriction becomes prominent when alveolar PO_2 mm Hg falls below 70 and at lower levels, no blood flow is observed.

18.4 Diffusion

Simple diffusion is the process where there is gas exchange across the alveolo-capillary membrane in both directions. This process depends on the diffusion of molecules from either the gas to the fluid phase or vice versa based on pressure gradients. Several basic concepts, or laws, govern the process.

Dalton's law (partial pressures) states that the total pressure of a gas in a mixture is equal to the sum of all the individual partial pressures. That is, the partial pressure of each gas is the pressure it would exert if it occupied the entire volume alone [5]. This principle allows for the definition of the different partial pressures at various points along the respiratory tract:

$$\text{Partial Pressure of Gas} = \text{Barometric pressure} \times \text{fractional concentration of gas}$$

Henry's law (solubility) states that when a liquid and a gas are in equilibrium, the amount of gas in solution is directly proportional to the partial pressures of the gas if the temperature is constant. In the gaseous state, only the concentration of the gas determines the partial pressure; while the partial pressure of a gas in a liquid state is also influenced by the solubility coefficient of the gas. This is based on the principle that some molecules, based on their chemical properties, have different interactions with the fluids they are dissolved in. Recall that only unbound gas accounts for its partial pressure in a fluid (e.g., oxygen bound to hemoglobin does not exert a partial pressure) [5, 6]:

$$\text{Partial pressure ofgasdissolved in liquid} = \frac{\text{Concentration of dissolvedgas}}{\text{solubility coefficient}}$$

Graham's law (diffusion) states that the diffusion of a gas is inversely proportional to the square root of its molecular weight. An example is CO_2 (molecular weight is 44) versus O_2 (molecular weight is 32), thus, CO_2 has a greater molecular weight and diffuses slower than oxygen in the gaseous state.

18.4.1 Calculated Atmospheric, Tracheal Air, Alveolar Air

With the aforementioned formulas, the individual partial pressure of gases at atmospheric air can be determined by applying the known concentration of major gases (N_2 78.62%, O_2 20.84%, CO_2 0.04%, H_20 0.5%) multiplied by the total atmospheric pressure (760 mm Hg). Once air is inspired into the trachea, air is exposed to the moist mucosa of the airway and becomes humidified, which increases the partial pressure of H_2O (47 mm Hg at 37 °C) and thus dilutes the concentration of the other gases, since the sum of their combined total cannot exceed atmospheric pressure. Example:

$$(760 - 47) \times \text{Fractional concentration } O_2 = 149 \text{ mm Hg} O_2$$

Alveolar air concentration changes due to the fact that oxygen is constantly being absorbed by the pulmonary capillaries down the concentration gradient and with each breath, small amounts of atmospheric air is added with addition of O_2. The overall concentration of O_2 in the alveoli is thus dependent on the rate of absorption into the blood as well as the rate of addition of new O_2 that can vary extremely based on metabolic demands. In addition, the diffusion of CO_2 from the pulmonary capillaries into the alveolar air further changes their composition. The partial pressures of the gases in the atmosphere, tracheal air, alveolar air, arterial and venous blood and their relative percentages are outlined in Table 18.1.

18.4.1.1 Respiratory Membrane

In addition to the pressure gradients, molecular weight and solubility are determinants for diffusion. **Fick's law** summarizes the factors, and their impact, on the rate of diffusion [5, 8]:

$$D\alpha \frac{\Delta P \times A \times S}{d \times \sqrt{MW}} \quad (18.20)$$

where D is diffused gas flow, Δ(Delta)P is the pressure gradient across the gas–liquid interface, A is cross-sectional area, S is the solubility of the gas, d is the distance for diffusion, and MW is the molecular weight of the gas. Now, it becomes evident that the diffusion of a gas is proportional to the pressure gradient, solubility, and cross-sectional area, and inversely proportional to the distance for diffusion and the square root of the molecular gas. If we set the diffusion of O_2 as 1, the relative rates of diffusion of other gases follow. We can observe now that CO_2 diffuses faster than oxygen even though the molecule is larger because the solubility coefficient is much higher than oxygen.

18.4.2 Preoxygenation, Apneic Oxygenation, and Diffusion Hypoxia

Preoxygenation prior to endotracheal intubation has long been practiced in order to delay peri-intubation desaturation [30]. This is performed by administration of high concentrations of oxygen prior to intubation. The increase in the

Table 18.1 Partial pressures of respiratory gases at sea-level

	Atmospheric air	Tracheal air (Humidified)	Alveolar air	Arterial blood	Venous blood
Gas	Partial pressure (%)	Partial pressure (%)	Partial pressure (%)	Partial pressure (%)	Partial pressure (%)
N_2	596 (78.6)	573(75.4)	573(75.4)	573(75.4)	573(75.4)
O_2	159 (20.9)	158 (20.7)	104 (13.6)	95 (12.5)	40 (5.26)
CO_2	0.3 (0.04)	0.3 (0.04)	40 (5.3)	40 (5.3)	47 (6.2)
H_20	3.7 (0.5)	47 (6.2)	47 (6.2)	47 (6.2)	47 (6.2)
Total	760 (100)	760 (100)	760 (100)	760 (100)	760 00)

Reference: http://bjcvs.org/article/2044/en-us/Gaseous-microemboli-in-cardiac-surgery-with-cardiopulmonary-bypass–the-use-of-veno-arterial-shunt-as-a-preventive-method partial pressure of alveolar O_2 in relation to N_2 causes a "nitrogen washout" from the alveoli. This acts as a reservoir of oxygen and delays desaturation during intubation.

Apneic oxygenation refers to the administration of oxygen (via nasal cannula) during the period of apnea after induction and paralysis. During this period of apnea, air is entrained from the environment into the alveoli while oxygen reservoirs are depleted by extraction into the pulmonary circulation [31]. If time for successful intubation is greater than that of the oxygen reserves, desaturation will occur. The time to desaturation has been shown to delay even further with the administration of oxygen by nasal cannula in the peri-intubation phase [32].

Diffusion hypoxia (Fink or "third gas" effect) refers to the effect that a soluble gas has on the partial pressures of oxygen in the alveoli. Recall that the administration of any gas will affect the partial pressure of other gases and that highly soluble gases will diffuse rapidly. Thus, during administration of a soluble gas (the most commonly cited is nitrous oxide), the gas will diffuse faster than oxygen. As a consequence, the partial pressure of O_2 and CO_2 will increase. However, once the gas is no longer administered (postoperative period), it will be released from the tissues (due to pressure gradients) and will be eliminated through the lung. As the gas enters the alveoli, it will decrease the partial pressure of other gases (i.e., oxygen, CO_2, etc.) and thus, the patient may become hypoxemic [32].

The "second gas" effect was noted during the administration of inhaled anesthetics in conjunction with inhaled nitric oxide. Again, the rapid absorption of nitrous oxide leads to relatively higher partial pressures of other gases. However, this is relevant when the other gas is another anesthetic agent.

18.5 Transport of Gases

18.5.1 Transport of Oxygen

The transport of oxygen occurs mainly as a free dissolved oxygen and bound to hemoglobin.

18.5.1.1 Free Dissolved O_2

Similar to other fluids, blood is also subject to having gases dissolved into it upon exposure. Once equilibrated, the partial pressures of the gas in air will balance with the blood. Henry's law helps us define the amount of oxygen that the blood may carry:

$$\text{Concentration of dissolved} O_2 = \text{Solubility coefficient of oxygen} \times \text{Partial pressure of} O_2 \text{in blood}$$

Now, if the partial pressure of oxygen is 100 mm Hg, the solubility coefficient of O_2 in blood is 0.0031 ml O_2/mmHg O_2/dL blood (this is a constant, assuming 37 °C), then the total concentration of oxygen is 0.3 ml O_2/dl. If we consider a normal resting cardiac output of 5 L/min, the total delivery of oxygen from dissolved O_2 alone would be equal to 15 ml O_2/min (that is 6% of the normal adult O_2 consumption at rest, 250 ml O_2/min). Therefore, oxygen delivery is dependent on alternative transport methods to sustain even normal function at rest.

18.5.1.2 Oxyhemoglobin

Given the poor content of the dissolved oxygen in blood, the transport of oxygen is dependent on the reversible binding to hemoglobin (approximately 98% of the total oxygen delivery). In the oxygen-bound state, hemoglobin is referred to as oxyhemoglobin and conversely in the oxygen-free state is referred to as deoxyhemoglobin.

Hemoglobin consists of four subunits. Normal adult hemoglobin (Hemoglobin A, HbA) is comprised of two alpha and two beta subunits, each of which contains one heme molecule. Each heme molecule can reversibly bind to one molecule of O_2, totaling to four O_2 molecule for each molecule of hemoglobin [1]. At any given point, the total number of O_2 molecules that is bound is expressed as % saturation of hemoglobin. If on average all hemoglobin molecules in the blood are completely saturated with four molecules of O_2, then the % saturation would be 100%.

The total amount of O_2 content in the form of oxyhemoglobin can be determined by multiplying the hemoglobin level by the % saturation and the amount of O_2 carried by 1 g of hemoglobin (1.34 ml O_2/g Hg). The total O_2 content of blood is calculated by adding the amount of O_2 carried by oxyhemoglobin to the amount of O_2 carried dissolved in blood:

$$O_2\text{Content} = \begin{bmatrix} (\text{Hb}) \times (O_2\%\text{Saturation}) \\ \times 1.34\text{ml}O_2\text{mmHg} \end{bmatrix} + [\text{Partial Pressure of } O_2 \times 0.003 \quad (18.21)$$

18.5.1.3 Oxygen Hemoglobin Dissociation Curve

The oxygen hemoglobin dissociation curve is formed by the % saturation in the *y*-axis and the partial pressure of oxygen on the *x*-axis (◉ Fig. 18.13). The sigmoidal or S-shape of the Hb-O_2 dissociation curve is reflective of the avidity of hemoglobin for O_2. As 1 molecule of O_2 binds to a heme particle, it causes a conformational change that results in an increased affinity for adding additional molecules of O_2. With each additional O_2 molecule, affinity increases further until the hemoglobin molecule is maximally loaded to nearly 100%. The result is a steep portion of the curve where there is rapid rises in % saturation with minimal changes in partial pressures of oxygen. When approximately 90% of the hemoglobin is saturated, any further changes in partial pressure result only in minimal increases in O_2 saturation. The opposite effect also occurs during the unloading of oxygen, where the unloading of 1 molecule also causes conformational changes that quickly favor further oxygen unloading with minimal changes in partial pressures. The sigmoidal shape of the curve ultimately leads to efficient loading and unloading of oxygen in areas of high and low partial pressures, respectively.

The % saturation of hemoglobin is mainly dependent on partial pressures of O_2; however, these values are not fixed and can be affected by multiple variables. This is evident by evaluating the P50, which is the partial pressure for which hemoglobin is 50% saturated on the O2-Hb dissociation curve. There are some conditions (increased temperature, increased $PaCO_2$, and low pH) that decrease the affinity of hemoglobin for oxygen (favor unloading) (see ◉ Fig. 18.13). All of the conditions that result in a right shift occur in the peripheral tissues at times when metabolic activity, specifically of skeletal muscle, is increased requiring higher oxygen demands. The decreased affinity and further unloading of oxygen as a result of this right shift helps to provide this demand.

Another factor that causes right shift in the dissociation cure is the increase in 2,3–diphosphoglycerate (2,3 DPG), which is a byproduct of glycolysis inside red blood cells. Its concentration increases during times of hypoxia and binds to beta subunits on hemoglobin [5, 6]. This interaction causes a conformational change in hemoglobin resulting in decreased affinity of O_2 and thus results in increased unloading of O_2.

Once hemoglobin has left the peripheral tissues, it returns to the pulmonary capillaries where partial pressures of CO_2, temperature, and 2,3-DPG levels are lower relative to the peripheral tissues. The environment of the pulmonary capillaries is also associated with a higher pH. These relatively opposite values cause the opposite effect on hemoglobin, resulting in conformational changes that increase the affinity for hemoglobin. This results in a decrease in P50 and an overall left shift of the curve (favoring loading). The effect is to optimize the loading of oxygen back to hemoglobin.

18.5.2 Transport of CO_2

CO_2 is produced as a result of metabolic activity. It diffuses from the tissue to the venous blood, leading to a marginal increase from 40 to 47 mm Hg in arterial partial pressures of CO_2. The transport of CO_2 in the blood occurs in 3 methods: (1) dissolved in the blood, (2) bound to proteins, and (3) as carbonic acid.

18.5.2.1 Dissolved CO_2

Similar to oxygen, a small portion of this gas is transported back in the free dissolved state. The venous blood contains about 3 mL/dL of carbon dioxide. Now consider a normal resting cardiac output of 5 L/min. The total delivery of

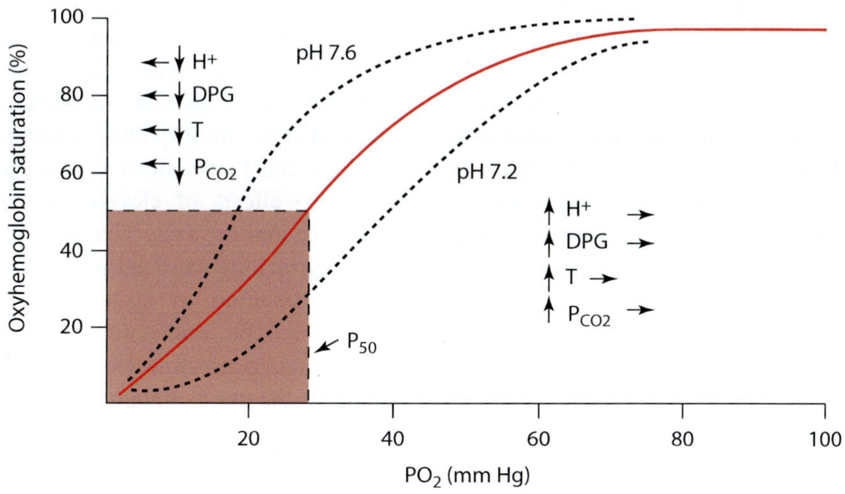

Fig. 18.13 The solid line depicts the characteristic Hemoglobin Oxygen Dissociation Curve, which is created by plotting oxygen saturation on the *y*-axis as a function of partial pressures of O_2 on the *x*-axis. The sigmoidal or S-shape curve of the hemoglobin oxygen dissociation curve represents the steep incline/decline in the oxygen saturation with relatively minimal changes in PO_2, which occurs in order to maximize loading/unloading of oxygen. Increases in H^+, DPG, Temp, and P_{CO2} (conditions favored in peripheral tissues) lead to a right shift in the curve which favors offloading of O2 in peripheral tissues. Conversely, decreases in H^+, DPB, Temp, and P_{CO2} (conditions found in lung) result in a left shift which favors loading of O_2 (Reprinted with permission from Sullivan and Nkromah [33])

carbon dioxide to the lung from dissolved CO_2 alone would be equal to 150 ml CO_2/min. However, because of carbon dioxide's high solubility and diffusing capacity, only about 25 mL will be exhaled. This amount contributes very little to the total amount of CO_2 content of the blood (approximately 5% of the total CO_2 transported) [1, 6].

18.5.2.2 CO_2Bound to Amine Groups

Another small portion of the CO_2 entering the venous system binds to amine groups of various plasma proteins and hemoglobin in a loose reversible bond producing carbaminohemoglobin. The amount of CO_2 transported in the form of carbaminohemoglobin also makes up a small portion of the total transported CO2—(roughly equal to 15–20%).

18.5.2.3 CO_2Transported as Carbonic Acid

The remainder of the 70–80% of transported CO_2 occurs in the form of bicarbonate (HCO_3-). Carbon dioxide and water diffuse into the red blood cell. There they form carbonic acid, in a reaction accelerated by the red cell carbonic anhydrase. Almost immediately, the carbonic acid dissociates into bicarbonate and hydrogen ions. Bicarbonate is transported across the membrane in exchange for chloride ions (AKA as the chloride shift). The H^+ molecule binds to deoxyhemoglobin, which acts as a significant acid–base buffer in venous blood. Once back into the oxygen-rich environment of the pulmonary circulation, this H^+ is released and replaced with oxygen. The free H^+ molecule combines with HCO_3- where the reverse reaction that takes place in the peripheral tissue occurs, resulting in free CO_2 that diffuses across the alveolar membrane and eventually expires.

The transport of CO_2 in all forms at various partial pressures can also be plotted in a CO_2 dissociation curve. The *x*-axis on this curve represents the total content of CO_2 in all forms plotted at partial pressures (*y*-axis). As the partial pressure of CO_2 increases from 40 mm Hg in the pulmonary capillaries to 45 mm Hg in the peripheral tissue, the total CO_2 content increases. Compared to the Hb-O_2 dissociation curve, the CO_2 curve results in a near linear appearance as the increase in CO_2 binds to hemoglobin and amino groups on proteins.

18.5.2.4 Bohr Effect

CO_2 is produced in the peripheral tissues as a result of ongoing metabolic activity. The increase in CO_2 when combined with H_2O, catalyzed by carbonic anhydrase results in a net increase in H^+ that is buffered by attaching to beta subunits on hemoglobin. The increase in CO_2, as well as H^+, causes a right shift of the Hb-O_2 association curve and an increase in P50 decreasing affinity for O_2. The changes to the curve from increased CO_2 and H^+ are referred to as the Bohr's effect [1, 6]. These changes ultimately help provide increases in O_2 supply in times of increased metabolic activity and thus increases in CO_2 and H^+.

18.5.2.5 Haldane Effect

When CO_2 that is transported bound to hemoglobin is returned to the pulmonary circulation where partial pressure of O_2 is 100 mm Hg, the binding of O_2 to hemoglobin is favored. The O_2 binding results in hemoglobin that is slightly more acidic. The more acidic hemoglobin has less affinity for CO_2 on the amine groups and also results in less affinity for buffered H^+ molecules. The displaced H^+ molecules, catalyzed by carbonic anhydrase, combine with HCO_3- and produce CO_2. Converse to the Bohr effect, where increases in CO_2 favor offloading of O_2 from hemoglobin, increases in partial pressures of O_2 result in the offloading of CO_2. This is referred to as the Haldane effect and similar to the Bohr effect is essential in transport of CO_2. The changes that occur in the setting of increased O_2 cause a downward shift in the CO_2 dissociation curve and a net increase in CO_2 offloading [5, 6].

18.5.3 Systemic Effects of Hypoxia and Hyperoxia

Hypoxemia has been shown to have deleterious effects, most notably cellular injury when the supply of oxygen is below the cellular demand. The threshold for cellular injury depends on the tissue. The most sensitive is the central nervous system. The mechanism of injury is a consequence of no longer being able to produce adenosine triphosphate (ATP) in order to provide the energy necessary for cellular function. This results in decreases in cellular pH that ultimately lead to cell death and tissue ischemia. In order to overcome these clinical situations, oxygen delivery is increased either by providing supplemental O_2 or by giving red blood cell transfusions if indicated. However, there are deleterious effects of elevated levels of O_2 with supplemental oxygen as well. The excess O_2 delivered by supplemental therapy can lead to the formation of oxygen-free radicals, resulting in systemic inflammation and tissue destruction. The threshold for hyperoxia-induced tissue injury is unknown. In order to prevent this from occurring, generally, the least amount of oxygen that is needed in order to maintain cellular function should be delivered. In addition to the possibility of oxygen toxicity, acute administration of oxygen increases displacement of CO_2 from hemoglobin, leading to changes in blood pH levels (Haldane effect). This effect is more marked in patients with hypercapnia and decreased pulmonary function (e.g., COPD).

18.5.4 Systemic Effects of Hypocarbia and Hypercarbia

There are systemic effects of both decreased and elevated levels of CO_2. As discussed previously, the partial pressure of CO_2 is maintained in a relatively narrow margin between the arterial and venous blood system. Increases in levels of CO_2 beyond the normal arterial range of 40 mm Hg may have several systemic effects. As levels of CO_2 increase, the CO_2 combines with H_2O, catalyzed by carbonic anhydrase, resulting in the HCO_3- as well as H^+. The net acid produced results in acidic blood pH (respiratory acidosis) that can cause significant impairment in skeletal and cardiac contractility, as well as metabolic changes. The CNS is also sensitive to increases in CO_2, which causes increases in cerebral blood flow and intracranial pressure as well as increased respiratory rate by triggering central receptors. These effects, if acute, can result in altered mental status, referred to as CO_2 narcosis. Conversely, low CO_2 levels have the opposite effects on the CNS, decreasing cerebral blood flow by vasoconstriction, which can also quickly result in CNS dysfunction. Similarly, with decreased levels of CO_2, the opposite reaction with HCO_3- occurs in order to maintain blood levels in normal ranges. This can result in depletion of H^+ molecules, leading to alkalotic blood pH (respiratory alkalosis). This can also cause dysfunction in cellular metabolic function of skeletal muscle.

18.6 Control of Ventilation

18.6.1 Respiratory Center

The respiratory center is a collection of neurons in the pons and medulla. This group of neurons generates uninterrupted rhythmic discharges similar to the pacemaker in the heart. The signal is transmitted via the phrenic nerve to the diaphragm and to the external and internal intercostal muscles via the by thoracic spinal cord. These groups of neurons are called: (1) dorsal respiratory group, (2) ventral respiratory group, and (3) pneumotaxic center.

Dorsal respiratory group neurons are located in the dorsal region of the medulla in the nucleus of tractus solitarius and mainly control inspiration. The sensory stimulus is carried from peripheral chemoreceptors, baroreceptors, and other receptors in the lung via the vagal and glossopharyngeal nerves to the tractus solitarius. These neurons discharge inspiratory neuronal action potentials mainly to the diaphragm in a "ramp" signal form. In a ramp signal, the action potential begins weakly and increases steadily until it reaches peak and then ceases abruptly, ending inspiration. Then, expiration occurs from elastic recoil followed again by an inspiratory ramp signal, and this cycle continues during normal quiet breathing. The pneumotaxic center transmits signal to inspiratory neurons and controls the rate and depth of breathing. The ventral respiratory group remains inactive during normal quiet breathing. It controls inspiration and active expiration by abdominal muscles.

18.6.2 Receptor

The main goal of the respiratory center is to maintain normal arterial PCO_2, PO_2, and H^+ concentration in arterial blood. There are numerous central and peripheral receptors that continuously monitor their concentration in arterial blood and regulate the respiratory center to maintain their concentration. Chemoreceptors are specialized nerve endings that are highly sensitive to changes in PCO_2, PO_2, and H^+ concentration.

1. **Central chemoreceptors** are a group of nerve endings present on the ventral surface of the medulla and collectively are called "chemosensitive area" or "medullary chemoreceptors." They monitor H^+ concentration of cerebrospinal fluid (CSF) and brain interstitial fluid. The blood brain barrier (BBB) and blood CSF barrier are not permeable to blood H^+, but CO_2 diffuses very easily through these barriers and enters the CSF. In CSF, CO_2 combines with water to form carbonic acid, which rapidly dissociates into H + and HCO-. This H^+ stimulates the chemoreceptors, which in turn activates the ventral respiratory neurons and controls inspiration and alveolar ventilation [34].
2. **Peripheral chemoreceptors** are a group of nerve endings present in the arterial wall bilaterally at the bifurcation of carotid arteries (carotid bodies) and on the aortic arch (aortic bodies). A few chemoreceptors are also found in thoracic and abdominal arterial wall. They are highly sensitive to changes in PO_2 and to a lesser extent to changes in PCO_2 and H^+ in arterial blood [35].
3. **Proprioceptive Receptors; Respiratory Muscles and Reflexes.** There are numerous receptors present in the respiratory tract, which are stimulated by the presence of chemicals or irritants and protect the lungs [5, 7]. There are also receptors that monitor the lung volume and regulate respiration accordingly. Here, we highlight some:
   - **Cough Reflex**: Cough reflex is mediated by C-fiber receptors with a primary aim of removing foreign bodies from the respiratory tree. It can be initiated from both the upper and lower respiratory tract.
   - **Hering-Breuer Reflex**: As the lung volume increases, it activates slowly adapting pulmonary stretch receptors present in lung interstitial tissue. These receptors inhibit phrenic nerve output and prevent overinflation

of the lungs. It increases respiratory frequency so minute alveolar ventilation is unaffected.

- **Sigh Reflex**: Sigh is a slow deep inspiration followed by a prolonged expiration and acts as a stimulus for surfactant release. Sighs open up closed alveoli and prevent atelectasis. Yawn is an exaggerated sigh and takes lung volume to total lung capacity for that breath.
- **Lung "J" Receptors** are sensory nerve endings found on the alveolar walls close to pulmonary capillaries. They are activated by the presence of pulmonary capillary engorgement or pulmonary edema and are considered to be the genesis of the sensation of dyspnea.

18.6.3 Voluntary Center

The voluntary control originates from the cerebral cortex and innervates the respiratory muscle via the corticospinal tract, bypassing the respiratory center in the medulla, and controls both inspiration and expiration (◉ Fig. 18.14). The voluntary control can alter the inspiratory or expiratory time,

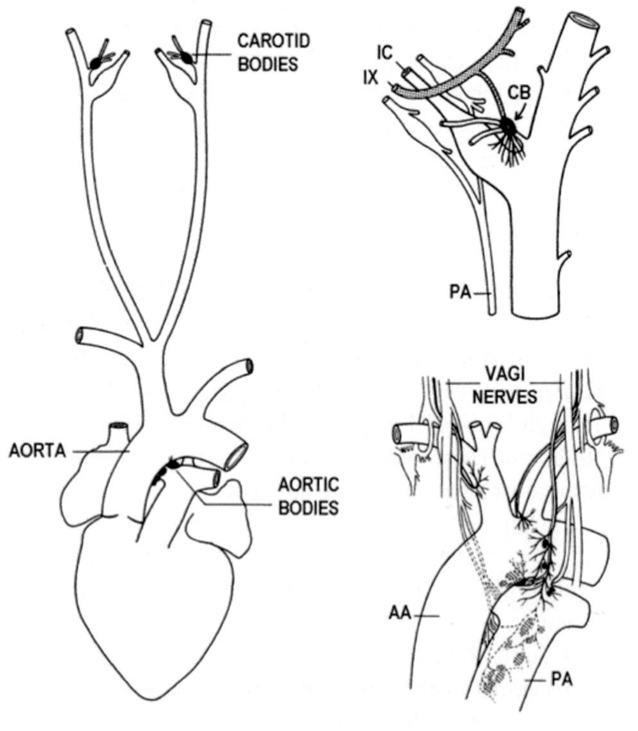

Fig. 18.14 The image shows the peripheral chemoreceptors, **a** aortic bodies and **b** carotid bodies (CB). They are a group of nerve endings present in the arterial wall, which detect changes in PO_2 and transmit the signal to central receptors. (IX) glossopharyngeal nerve, X vagus nerve, IC internal carotid, PA pulmonary artery, and AA ascending aorta (Reprinted with permission from Santos et al. [36])

intensity, or pattern. The limbic system and hypothalamus also exert some effect, as evidenced by hyperventilation in response to pain or emotional stimuli.

18.6.4 CO_2 and O_2 Response Curves

The goal of the respiratory system is to maintain an appropriate concentration of CO_2, O_2, and H^+ in arterial blood. The respiratory system is extremely sensitive to any changes in their concentration and alters breathing frequency or pattern to meet its goal.

18.6.4.1 Acute Carbon dioxide Response

A rise in $PaCO_2$ causes an equal rise in CSF and brain interstitial fluid CO_2 concentration, as blood brain barrier and blood CSF barrier are permeable to CO_2. This CO_2 dissociates and increases H^+ concentration and decreases pH in CSF. This activates the respiratory center and increases both the depth and rate of respiration and brings PCO_2 back to normal value [5, 34].

The peripheral chemoreceptors also respond to increase in arterial PCO_2. The response to rising PCO_2 is much stronger (7 times stronger) by the central chemoreceptors but quicker by peripheral chemoreceptors (5 times quicker). Their main function is to increase ventilation rapidly to increasing $PaCO_2$ followed by a stronger and sustained effect by central chemoreceptors.

18.6.4.2 Chronic Carbon dioxide Response

The stimulation of the respiratory center is greatest in the first few hours of $PaCO_2$ rise. The effectiveness in stimulation of the respiratory centers decreases to one-fifth in 1–2 days, as the blood and CSF pH is corrected by addition of bicarbonate by the kidneys [5, 8]. The bicarbonate neutralizes H^+ in CSF and brings pH closer to normal value with an elevated steady-state arterial PCO_2.

18.6.4.3 Acute Oxygen Response

Hemoglobin maintains adequate oxygen delivery to tissue for an arterial PaO_2 ranging between 60 and 100 mm Hg. The alveolar ventilation may decrease significantly without any change observed in PaO_2. Hence, the primary stimulus for respiration and alveolar ventilation is arterial $PaCO_2$. When PaO_2 falls below this critical level, it activates the respiratory center indirectly [37].

The carotid and aortic bodies have specialized glandular cells called glomus cells, which act as chemoreceptors [5, 35]. They have O_2-sensitive potassium channels, which are inactivated in absence of adequate oxygen causing depolarization of cells and opening of voltage-gated calcium channels. The increase in intracellular calcium concentration causes release of neurotransmitter and activation of afferent neurons. ATP or dopamine may be the key excitatory neurotransmitter released by glomus cells.

18.6.4.4 Chronic Oxygen Response

The response to chronically low oxygen state has been best studied in mountain climbers. The alveolar ventilation is initially increased due to hypoxia, but as $PaCO_2$ decreases from hyperventilation, it has an inhibitory effect on the respiratory center [38]. After 2–3 h, as central chemoreceptors lose their sensitivity to low $PaCO_2$, the alveolar ventilation often increases to 400–500% of normal. At normal or less than normal, alveolar ventilation does not increase until PaO_2 drops below 60 mm Hg. When $PaCO_2$ is held constant at a higher level, there is linear increase in ventilation with decreasing PaO_2 level.

18.7 Non-respiratory Functions of Lungs: Metabolic, Immune

The lung is primarily an organ involved in gas exchange. However, the importance of lung in the cardiorespiratory system accepting the entire right heart cardiac output and its constant exposure to environment necessitates it to perform additional functions to maintain a normal internal milieu.

18.7.1 Pulmonary Circulation as a Physical Filter

Thrombus, gas, and fat emboli formed in the body may enter the systemic circulation and cause devastating consequences in the coronary or cerebral circulation. The respiratory system acts as a physical barrier to various particle emboli and clears them. The effective clearance occurs due to the presence of a robust proteolytic system and endogenous anticoagulants. The pulmonary endothelium is rich in plasmin activator, which converts plasminogen into plasmin, which in turn converts fibrin into fibrin-degradation products. The pulmonary endothelium also contains thromboplastin, which converts prothrombin to thrombin and promotes coagulation.

18.7.2 Clearance of Inhaled Particles

The respiratory tree is in direct contact with atmosphere and constantly exposed to particles, pathogens, and chemicals present in inhaled air. The size of inhaled particle also affects their interaction with the respiratory system. Particles < 1 μm undergo diffusion by Brownian motion and are simply exhaled with minimum contact with airway. Particles 1–3 μm are either exhaled or deposited on alveolar walls by sedimentation and ingested by alveolar macrophages. Particles > 3 μm and particularly > 8 μm undergo inertial impaction and rarely reach beyond the pharynx [8].

The respiratory tree is lined by a pseudo-stratified ciliated columnar epithelium from the posterior two-thirds of the nose to the respiratory bronchioles. This is composed of two layers—the cilia arising from the columnar epithelium and the overlying mucous layer—and acts as the first line of defense. The mucous layer is formed by mucin, which is a highly viscous mucopolysaccharide secreted by goblet cells in the epithelium and mucous cells of the submucosal glands [39]. Mucin is secreted in response to direct chemical irritation, inflammatory cytokines, and vagal stimulation. The ciliated epithelial cells propel this mucous layer cephalad at an average rate of 4 mm/min [5]. The effective function of mucociliary escalator depends on the periciliary fluid volume; controlled by amiloride-sensitive Na^+Cl^- pump, also known as cystic fibrosis transmembrane regulator protein.

18.7.3 Clearance of Pathogens

The majority of inhaled pathogens are cleared by ciliated nasal epithelium, swallowed, or get trapped by the mucous layer, and removed by mucociliary escalator as discussed previously. If the particle enters deeper into the bronchioles or alveoli, then the defense mechanisms are surfactant, macrophages, and cytokines. Surfactant has a key role in innate defense against inhaled pathogens as the surfactant protein A and D are directly bactericidal [5, 7, 8]. Airway lining fluid contains defensins, which are antimicrobial peptides, and lysozyme with direct bactericidal activity. Immunoglobulins (Ig) are secreted by alveolar lining cells. The most predominant of them is secretory IgA in the larger airways and IgG in the alveoli. They act as an opsonin and induce complement activation and antigen recognition. They also activate the alveolar macrophages, resulting in recruitment of large numbers of phagocytic cells.

18.7.4 Metabolism of Endogenous Compounds

The lung may activate or inactivate certain endogenous compounds as they pass through the pulmonary circulation. Angiotensin is converted to vasoactive angiotensin II by angiotensin-converting enzyme (ACE), which is mostly present on the vascular surface of pulmonary endothelium. This is also responsible for removal of bradykinin, which, along with angiotensin II, provides a substantial role for the lungs in blood pressure control. The lung is also a major site of synthesis, metabolism, uptake, and release of arachidonic acid metabolites [40].

18.7.5 Drug Delivery and Elimination

The lung acts as an effective route for drug delivery for both topical action in the respiratory system and for systemic effect. The advantages are rapid onset of action, high concentration in the respiratory airway with minimal systemic side effect, and needle-free drug delivery for medications with poor oral bioavailability.

A particle size of 3 μm is optimal for alveolar delivery. Other factors influencing pulmonary uptake are lipophilicity, protein binding, ventilation, perfusion, oxygenation, ageing, lung pathology, and co-administration of other drugs. Nitrofurantoin, bleomycin, and amiodarone are taken up by alveolar cells and may result in lung toxicity.

The lung plays an important role in elimination of drug by metabolism or by retention in lung tissue acting as a reservoir and releasing the drug slowly. Certain inhaled drugs—such as theophylline, salmeterol, and budesonide—undergo significant metabolism in the lung due to high cytochrome P_{450}. This characteristic of medications has been used to minimize systemic side effects with improved airway selectivity.

18.7.6 Endocrine Lung

The airway mucosa contains pulmonary neuroendocrine cells and innervated cell clusters called neuroepithelial bodies constituting "pulmonary neuroendocrine system." They secrete peptide in response to hypoxia and cause central nervous system activation [41]. The lung is a rich source of nitric oxide, which regulates airway smooth muscle, pulmonary vascular resistance, and platelet function. It also secretes heparin, endothelin, and eicosanoids on exposure to allergens, resulting in immune and cardiovascular response.

18.8 Perioperative Smoking

18.8.1 Physiologic Effects

Smoking has long been associated with adverse postoperative outcomes for a multitude of reasons. In general, smoking causes a systemic pro-inflammatory state by increases in interleukin (IL)-1, IL-8, tumor necrosis factor-alpha, as well as others. The increase in systemic inflammation leads to a decrease in the ability to recruit local inflammation that is imperative in the wound reparative process. The increase in systemic inflammation also leads to vascular endothelial injury as well as platelet dysfunction [42]. In addition, the increase in pro-inflammatory cytokines has adverse effects on the ability of neutrophils and macrophages to produce bactericidal enzymes. Active smoking is also associated with tissue vasoconstriction and thus less delivery of peripheral oxygen. The decrease in oxygen delivery and increase in vasoconstriction also limits the ability to deliver necessary cells involved in tissue repair as well as promoting more ischemia to areas that have already sustained injury as a result of surgical trauma. The overall results are increases in rates of infection as well as delays in wound healing.

In addition to wound healing and infection, smoking is also associated with increased trends in pulmonary and cardiovascular complications. Smoking results in ciliary dysfunction, which acts as a primary defense mechanism for mucous and bacterial clearance. Increase in mucous production is also a result of ongoing inflammation in the bronchopulmonary tree that can also increase infection rates in the setting of decreased clearance. As a result, the postoperative pulmonary complications are increased compared to non-smokers, especially in those with underlying pulmonary disease. The increased rates in cardiovascular outcomes in the setting of long-term smokers are likely a consequence of vascular injuries that have been associated with increased postoperative cardiovascular events.

18.8.2 Cessation of Smoking

Many of the adverse effects that lead to increase in postoperative complications as a result of smoking can be minimized with the cessation of smoking. The most immediate of which is within hours of smoking cessation, the vasoconstrictive effects of smoking and thus peripheral O_2 delivery are returned to normal, in the absence of already present vascular disease [43]. Within 2–4 weeks of cessation, platelet dysfunction, neutrophil, and macrophage dysfunction are also improved as a result of decreases in oxidative stress. This leads to improvement in overall vascular endothelial function and bacterial fighting ability. However, the changes that result in an overall decrease in tissue proliferation and synthesis do not appear to reverse to the level of non-smokers. As evident in studies showing rates of complications in former smokers, although less than active smokers, they are still higher compared to never smokers [44]. While the timeframe for the ideal duration of cessation is unestablished, some studies have suggested that maximal outcomes in preventing complications as a result of smoking are at least 8 weeks. However, there is evidence that suggests some benefits compared to ongoing smoking with cessation as little as 1–2 weeks [44].

The overall effects of smoking cessation not only have improved clinical outcomes postoperatively but also proven financial/economic benefits to the healthcare system. This provides an excellent opportunity in the perioperative timeframe to discuss and advocate smoking cessation.

18.9 Questions and Answers

Questions (Choose the Most Appropriate Answer)

1. The Total Lung Capacity is the addition of the following:
   A. VT + IRV + ERV
   B. IRV + VT + ERV + RV
   C. VT + IRV
   D. RV + ERV
2. A reduced FEV1/FVC ratio is the manifestation of restriction
   A. True
   B. False
3. DL,CO is affected by the following, EXCEPT:
   A. Hemoglobin
   B. Lung volumes
   C. Age
   D. Body position
   E. PaO_2
4. The anaerobic threshold is the result of
   A. A boost of the aerobic metabolism
   B. A manifestation of mitochondrial dysfunction
   C. The moment where aerobic metabolism shifts to anaerobic metabolism
   D. The maximum level VO_2 can attain
5. Compliance of the lung will be decreased in the following conditions, EXCEPT
   A. Lung fibrosis
   B. Obesity
   C. Pleural thickening
   D. ARDS
6. The main determinant of airway resistance is
   A. Density of the gas
   B. Viscosity of the gas
   C. Length of the airway
   D. Caliber of the airway
7. Alveolar dead space increases in the following conditions:
   A. Increase in ventilation in relation to the local perfusion
   B. Decrease in ventilation in relation to the local perfusion
   C. Increase in perfusion in relation to local ventilation
   D. Increase in perfusion with proportional increase in local ventilation
8. To improve ventilation-perfusion matching in a patient with unilateral lung disease on mechanical ventilation
   A. You should sit the patient up
   B. Keep the patient supine
   C. Don't change the patient position, gravity has minimal effects on the V/Q matching
   D. Place the healthy lung down
9. Henry's law states that the total pressure of a gas in a mixture is equal to the sum of all the individual partial pressures
   A. True
   B. False
10. You should expect to see diffusion hypoxia at
    A. The beginning of the case when you are administering nitrous oxide
    B. At the end of the case when you are decreasing sevoflurane
    C. In the postoperative period
    D. 24 h after surgery
11. The Haldane effect can lead to hypercapnia in patients that are exposed to oxygen and already had chronic hypercapnia
    A. True
    B. False
12. The Hering-Breuer effect consists of:
    A. C-fiber receptors with a primary aim or removing foreign body from the respiratory tree
    B. Slow deep inspiration followed by a prolonged expiration and act as stimulus for surfactant release
    C. Pulmonary capillary engorgement leading to sensation of dyspnea
    D. Receptors inhibit phrenic nerve output and prevent over inflation of the lungs
13. The lung has effect on the following compounds passing through the lung, EXCEPT
    A. Angiotensin I
    B. Serotonin
    C. Bradykinin
    D. Dopamine
    E. Adenosine

Answers

1. **B**. The lung has four basic lung volumes that constitute both the inspiratory and expiratory phases and are as follows: Inspiratory reserve volume (IRV), Tidal volume (V_T), Expiratory reserve volume (ERV), and residual volume (RV). When two or more volumes are combined, they constitute four desiccant lung capacities that are as follows: V_T + IRV = Inspiratory capacity (IC), RV + ERV = Functional residual capacity (FRC), V_T + IRV + ERV = Vital capacity (VC), and V_T + IRV + ERV + RV = Total lung capacity (TLC).
   The TLC is the volume of air present in the lung at the end of maximal inspiratory effort (see ◉ Fig. 18.1) and can be calculated from the summation of all four basic lung volumes as above.

2. **B**. Vital capacity is the volume of air exhaled after maximal inspiration (from the point of TLC). If the expiration is performed with maximal effort, then it is referred to as forced vital capacity (FVC). The forced expiratory volume in 1 s (FEV_1) represents the total amount of the FVC that is expired in the first second; and in patients with healthy non-diseased lungs, the normal value is roughly 80%. In other words, 80% of the total FVC should be exhaled in 1 s. Reductions when compared to standard values of the FEV1/FVC ratio represent obstructive lung disease (asthma, COPD, tracheal stenosis). In restriction lung disease, both FEV_1 and FVC are decreased proportionally with near normal values the FEV_1/FVC ratio.
3. **E**. DL,CO (pulmonary diffusion capacity of carbon monoxide) is used clinically as a surrogate for gas exchange. CO is similar to oxygen in both molecular weight and solubility, hence, diffusion of CO would be a reflection of the alveolo-capillary interface itself. But certain physiological factors (e.g., age, sex, height, hemoglobin, lung volumes, carboxyhemoglobin, and exercise and body position) affect the diffusion of CO. This physiological factors are considered during calculation of DL,CO and reported.
4. **C**. Cardiopulmonary exercise testing can be performed to help identify defects in pulmonary ventilation, cardiovascular function, or skeletal muscle function in patients with undifferentiated shortness of breath or limitations in exertional capacity. It can also be performed in the preoperative setting to help identify high-risk patients for surgical interventions. It is performed by having patients exercise while connected to a metabolic cart that evaluates certain parameters that include heart rate, minute ventilation, O_2 consumption, and CO_2 production. Normally during exercise, O_2 consumption and CO_2 production are increased linearly and reflect increased metabolic demand and production of the tissues, respectively. However, there is a point in time at which CO_2 production is greater than O_2, which reflects the transition into anaerobic metabolism. The increase in CO_2 is a result of increased production of lactic acid that is converted to CO_2. This point is known as the anaerobic threshold.
5. **B**. Compliance is the change in volume per unit change in transmural pressure. The compliance measured at bedside is total compliance of respiratory system and is affected by compliance of lung, chest wall, and abdominal cavity. If you recall:

$$C_{RS} = C_{lung} + C_{CW}$$

Obesity decreases the total respiratory system compliance by decreasing the chest wall compliance with little to no effect on lung compliance.

6. **D**. Recall the equation for resistance is:

$$\text{Resistance} = \frac{8 \times \text{length} \times \text{viscosity}}{\pi \times (\text{radius})^4}$$

The airway resistance depends on the length of the airway, viscosity of the gas, and radius of the airway. If the other conditions remain constant, a decrease in radius of airway caliber by ½ will increase the resistance by 16-fold. Hence, caliber of the airway has the most significant effect on the resistance of system.

7. **A**. Alveolar dead space is the alveoli that are ventilated but do not contribute in gas exchange due to decreased or absent perfusion. A classic example is pulmonary embolism, where a blood clot partially or completely obstructs the pulmonary circulation. The alveoli downstream is ventilated but not perfused. These alveoli act like conducting airways and are called alveolar dead space.
8. **D**. The ventilation and perfusion are both affected by gravitational forces, as both flow to dependent regions of the lung. Hence, in a patient with unilateral lung disease, placing the healthy lung in a dependent position (i.e., down in lateral position) will increase the blood flow to the healthy lung, optimize V/Q matching, and improve oxygenation. The exception to this strategy is unilateral lung disease with excessive secretions or hemorrhage. In such a situation, the diseased lung should be placed in the dependent position to prevent overflowing of secretions or blood to the healthy lung.
9. **B**. Dalton's law (partial pressures) states that the total pressure of a gas in a mixture is equal to the sum of all the individual partial pressures. That is, the partial pressure of each gas is the pressure it would exert if it occupied the entire volume alone. This principle allows for the definition of the different partial pressures at various points along the respiratory tract. Henry's law refers to solubility and states that when a liquid and a gas are in equilibrium, the amount of gas in solution is directly proportional to the partial pressures of the gas if temperature is constant.
10. **B**. Diffusion hypoxia (Fink or "third gas" effect) refers to the effect that a soluble gas has on the partial pressures of oxygen in the alveoli. Recall that the adminis-

tration of any gas will affect the partial pressure of other gases and that highly soluble gases will diffuse rapidly. Thus, during administration of a soluble gas (most commonly cited is nitrous oxide), the gas will diffuse faster than oxygen. As a consequence, the partial pressure of O_2 and CO_2 will increase. However, once the gas is no longer administered (postoperative period), it will be released from the tissues (due to pressure gradients) and will be eliminated through the lung. As the gas enters the alveoli, it will decrease the partial pressure of other gases (i.e., oxygen, CO_2, etc.) and thus, the patient may become hypoxemic and hypoventilate once other gases are decreased at the end of a case.

11. **A**. The Haldane effect refers to the CO_2 carrying capacity of hemoglobin in the presence of oxygen (CO_2 hemoglobin dissociation curve). In the presence of oxygen, hemoglobin has a decreased affinity for CO_2, which results in offloading of CO_2, and thus an increase in unbound or dissolved CO_2. In patients with lung disease, specifically COPD with hypercarbia at rest, supplemental O_2 results in offloading of CO_2 by the hemoglobin. These patients, as a result of their underlying lung disease, are not able to increase minute ventilation in order to decrease this excess of dissolved CO_2, which ultimately can lead to increases in partial pressures of CO_2.
12. **D**. The Hering-Breuer reflex occurs due to presence of slow-adapting stretch receptors present in smooth muscle of smaller airways and lung interstitial tissues. They are activated during large inspiration, whereby they inhibit phrenic nerve output and prevent lung over inflation.
13. **D**. Angiotensin I is activated during its passage through pulmonary circulation, while serotonin, bradykinin, and adenosine are inactivated. Dopamine passes through the pulmonary circulation unchanged.

References

1. Ganong WF. Review of medical physiology. 6th ed. Los Altos, CA: Lange Medical Publications; 1973.
2. Miller MR, Hankinson J, Brusasco V, Burgos F, Casaburi R, Coates A, et al. ATS/ERS task force. Standardisation of spirometry Eur Respir J. 2005;26(2):319–38.
3. Al-Ashkar F, Mehra R, Mazzone PJ. Interpreting pulmonary function tests: recognize the pattern, and the diagnosis will follow. Cleve Clin J Med. 2003;70(10):866-81.
4. Madsen F, Mortensen J, Handel B, Pedersen OF. Ch 9. Lung function testing, spirometry, diffusion capacity and interpretation. In: Aliverti A, Pedotti A, editors. Mechanics of breathing. Italia: Springer; 2014.
5. Lumb AB, Nunn JF. Nunn's applied respiratory physiology. 7th ed. Edinburgh: Churchill Livingstone, Elsevier; 2010.
6. Milic-Emili J. Applied physiology in respiratory mechanics. Milano/New York: Springer; 1998.
7. Grippi MA, Elias JA, Fishman J, Kotloff RM, Pack AI, Senior RM, et al. Fishman's pulmonary diseases and disorders. 5th ed. New York, NY: McGraw-Hill Education; 2015.
8. Crystal RG. The lung: scientific foundations. 2nd ed. Philadelphia: Lippincott-Raven; 1997.
9. Beckles MA, Spiro SG, Colice GL, Rudd RM. American College of Chest Physicians. The physiologic evaluation of patients with lung cancer being considered for resectional surgery. Chest 2003;123(1 Suppl):105S–14S.
10. Datta D, Lahiri B. Preoperative evaluation of patients undergoing lung resection surgery. Chest. 2003;123(6):2096–103.
11. Gattinoni L, Chiumello D, Carlesso E, Valenza F. Bench-to-bedside review: chest wall elastance in acute lung injury/acute respiratory distress syndrome patients. Crit Care. 2004;8(5):350–5.
12. Hildebrandt J. Structural and mechanical aspects of respiration. In: Patton HD, Fuchs AF, Hille B, Scher AM, Steiner R, editors. Textbook of physiology. 21st ed. Philadelphia: Saunders, Elsevier; 1989., Chap. 52. p. 991–1011.
13. Lotti G.A, Braschi A. Measurement of Respiratory Mechanics during Mechanical Ventilation. Switzerland. Hamilton Medical AG. 1999
14. Nurok M, Topulos GP. Ch 2. Respiratory physiology. In: Hartigan PM, editor. Practical handbook of thoracic anesthesia. New York: Springer Science + Business Media; 2012.
15. Hamm H, Kroegel C, Hohlfeld J. Surfactant: a review of its functions and relevance in adult respiratory disorders. Respir Med. 1996;90(5):251–70.
16. Haitsma JJ. Physiology of mechanical ventilation. Crit Care Clin. 2007;23(117–134):vii.
17. Fry DL, Hyatt RE. Pulmonary mechanics. A unified analysis of the relationship between pressure, volume and gasflow in the lungs of normal and diseased human subjects. Am J Med 1960;29:672–89.
18. Rodrigo GJ, Rodrigo C, Pollack CV, Rowe B. Use of helium-oxygen mixtures in the treatment of acute asthma: a systematic review. Chest. 2003;123(3):891–6.
19. Chatterjee S, Fisher AB. Ch 54. Shear stress, cell signaling, and pulmonary vascular remodeling. In: Juan JX-J, et al. editors. Textbook of pulmonary vascular disease. New York: Springer Science+Business Media; 2011.
20. Rimensberger PC. Ch 13. Monitoring of the mechanical behaviour of the respiratory system during controlled mechanical ventilation. In: Pediatric and neonatal mechanical ventilation. Berlin/Heidelberg, Germany: Springer; 2015.
21. Vassilakopoulos T. Understanding wasted/ineffective efforts in mechanically ventilated COPD patients using the Campbell diagram. In: Pinsky MR, Brochard L, Hedensteierna G, Antonelli M, editors. Applied physiology in intensive care medicine 1. Berlin/Heidelberg, Germany: Springer; 2012.
22. Banner MJ, Jaeger MJ, Kirby RR. Components of the work of breathing and implications for monitoring ventilator-dependent patients. Crit Care Med. 1994;22(3):515–23.
23. Tu J, et al. Ch 2. The human respiratory system. In: Computational fluid and particle dynamics in the human respiratory system. Dordrecht: Springer Science+Business Media; 2013.
24. Sinha P, Flower O, Soni N. Deadspace ventilation: a waste of breath. In: Pinsky MR, et al. editors. Applied physiology in intensive care medicine 2: physiological reviews and editorials. Berlin/Heidelberg, Germany: Springer; 2012.
25. Otis AB, Mckerrow CB, Bartlett RA, Mead J, Mcilroy MB, Selver-Stone NJ, et al. Mechanical factors in distribution of pulmonary ventilation. J Appl Physiol. 1956;8(4):427–43.

26. Martin L. Ch 4. Mechanical ventilation, respiratory monitoring and the basics of pulmonary physiology. In: Tobias JD, editor. Pediatric critical care: the essentials. Armonk: Futura; 1999. p. 63.
27. West JB, Dollery CT, Naimark A. Distribution of blood flow in isolated lung; relation to vascular and alveolar pressures. J Appl Physiol. 1964;19:713–24.
28. Jaeger JM, Blank RS. Ch 4. Essential anatomy and physiology of the respiratory system and the pulmonary circulation. In: Slinger P, editor. Principles and practice of anesthesia for thoracic surgery. Verlag London: Springer; 2012.
29. Coppock EA, Martens JR, Tamkun MM. Molecular basis of hypoxia-induced pulmonary vasoconstriction: role of voltage-gated K+ channels. Am J Physiol Lung Cell Mol Physiol. 2001;281(1):L1-12.
30. Fink BR. Diffusion anoxia in clinical anesthesia. Acta Anaesthesiol. 1954;5(1):42–6.
31. Frumin MJ, Epstein RM, Cohen G. Apneic oxygenation in man. Anesthesiology. 1959;20:789–98.
32. Ramachandran SK, Cosnowski A, Shanks A, Turner CR. Apneic oxygenation during prolonged laryngoscopy in obese patients: a randomized, controlled trial of nasal oxygen administration. J Clin Anesth. 2010;22(3):164–8.
33. Sullivan JS, Nkromah TA. Ch 1. Fundamentals of gas exchange and the assessment of oxygenation and ventilation. In: Lucking SE, editor. Pediatric critical care study guide. Verlag, Italia: Springer; 2008.
34. Guyenet PG, Stornetta RL, Bayliss DA. Central respiratory chemoreception. J Comp Neurol. 2010;518(19):3883–906.
35. Nurse CA, Piskuric NA. Signal processing at mammalian carotid body chemoreceptors. Semin Cell Dev Biol. 2013;24(1):22–30.
36. Santos FB, Nagato LKS, Zin WA. Control of breathing. In: Lucangelo U, Pelosi P, Zin WA, Aliverti A, editors. Respiratory system and artificial ventilation. Milano: Springer; 2008.
37. Kiwull-Schöne H, Kiwull P. Hypoxia and the reaction theory of central respiratory chemosensitivity. Adv Exp Med Biol. 1992;316:347–57.
38. Easton PA, Slykerman LJ, Anthonisen NR. Ventilatory response to sustained hypoxia in normal adults. J Appl Physiol. 1986;61:906–11.
39. Houtmeyers E, Gosselink R, Gayan-Ramirez G, Decramer M. Regulation of mucociliary clearance in health and disease. Eur Respir J. 1999;13(5):1177–88.
40. Dahl AR, Gerde P. Uptake and metabolism of toxicants in the respiratory tract. Environ Health Perspect. 1994;102(Suppl 11):67–70.
41. Gosney JR. The endocrine lung and its response to hypoxia. Thorax. 1994;49(Suppl):S25-6.
42. Sansores RH, Pare P, Abboud RT. Effect of smoking cessation on pulmonary carbon monoxide diffusing capacity and capillary blood volume. Am Rev Respir Dis. 1992;146(4):959–64.
43. Sansores RH, Pare PD, Abboud RT. Acute effect of cigarette smoking on the carbon monoxide diffusing capacity of the lung. Am Rev Respir Dis. 1992;146(4):951–8.
44. Theadom A, Cropley M. Effects of preoperative smoking cessation on the incidence and risk of intraoperative and postoperative complications in adult smokers: a systematic review. Tobacco Control. 2006;15(5):352–8.

Physiology of the Autonomic Nervous System

19

Brian K. Johnson

Abstract

The autonomic nervous system is one of the most important systems in maintaining homeostasis of the human body. It is one of the two parts of the peripheral nervous system. The peripheral nervous system consists of the autonomic nervous system (ANS) and the somatic nervous system. The ANS controls automatic functions and responses such as heart rate and blood pressure. Understanding ANS physiology enables anesthesiologists to safely use medications while maintaining homeostasis. The ANS consists of two major subsets of systems: the sympathetic nervous system (SNS) and the parasympathetic nervous system (PSNS). This chapter will provide a comprehensive overview of the SNS followed by the PSNS. Each system overview will include a description of anatomy, ganglionic transmission, transmitter types, release, synthesis, storage, termination of effects, receptor types, effects, and, finally, reflexes and regulation. There will also be a brief discussion of the enteric nervous system at the end of the chapter.

Keywords

Autonomic nervous system (ANS) • Sympathetic nervous system (SNS) • Parasympathetic nervous system (PSNS) • Enteric nervous system • Neurotransmitters • Acetylcholine (ACh) • Norepinephrine • Adrenal medulla • Homeostasis • Ganglionic transmission

Key Points

- The practice of anesthesia requires a meticulous understanding of the autonomic nervous system physiology.
- The sympathetic nervous system (SNS) and the parasympathetic nervous system (PSNS) both use ganglionic transmission using acetylcholine (ACh) as the neurotransmitter.
- The SNS uses norepinephrine as its primary neurotransmitter at the nodal postganglionic location.
- The adrenal medulla is a specialized SNS organ that secrets epinephrine and norepinephrine into the blood.
- The PSNS predominantly uses acetylcholine (Ach) as its end neurotransmitter.
- The SNS predominately acts to increase energy expenditure for the fight-or-flight response. In contrast, the PSNS predominately acts to conserve energy.
- Both systems use feedback reflexes to help maintain homeostasis of the human body.
- The enteric nervous system is an additional component in the autonomic nervous system and constitutes a new and emerging area of study.

19.1 Introduction

The autonomic nervous system is one of the most important systems in maintaining homeostasis of the human body. It is one of the two parts of the peripheral nervous system. The peripheral nervous system consists of the autonomic nervous system (ANS) and the somatic nervous system. The ANS controls automatic functions and responses such as heart rate and blood pressure. The somatic nervous system sends sensory information to the central nervous system (CNS). The ANS can function rapidly to change the physiologic status of the body. The ANS can double the heart rate in 3–5 s, and in 10–15 s can elevate the arterial pressure to twice its normal level. On the opposite end of the spectrum, it can

B. K. Johnson (✉)
Department of Anesthesiology, Team Health, Akron City Hospital, Akron, OH, USA
e-mail: johnsob2@me.com

M. Argalious et al. (eds.), *Basic Sciences in Anesthesia*,
https://doi.org/10.1007/978-3-031-60203-0_19

decrease mean arterial pressure to a level that will induce fainting in 10–15 s.

One might ask why the ANS is important in the study of basic science in anesthesia. Anesthesia is the practice of autonomic medicine. Understanding ANS physiology enables anesthesiologists to safely use medications while maintaining homeostasis.

The ANS consists of two major subsets of systems [1–4]. These are the sympathetic nervous system (SNS) and the parasympathetic nervous system (PSNS). These two systems have vastly different effects on the respective end organs they innervate. The SNS, when activated, is responsible for the activation of the fight-or-flight response. This response redistributes blood flow from the viscera to the skeletal muscles, while increasing heart function, sweating, and dilating the pupils. The PSNS governs more of the body's maintenance needs such as digestive and genitourinary functions.

The anatomy of both systems varies in origin, pathway, and design. Both systems use several common neurotransmitters in some areas, and different transmitters and receptors in other areas, which is what allows anesthesiologists to pharmacologically manipulate each system. This chapter will provide a comprehensive overview of the SNS followed by the PSNS. Each system overview will include a description of anatomy, ganglionic transmission, transmitter types, release, synthesis, storage, termination of effects, receptor types, effects, and, finally, reflexes and regulation. There will also be a brief discussion of the enteric nervous system at the end of the chapter.

19.2 Anatomy

The anatomy of the ANS is complex and is comprised of multiple parts.

The outflow of both divisions (SNS and PSNS) consists of 2 neuron relays named after their anatomical locations relative to the autonomic ganglia, or relay centers.

The efferent (motor) ANS is a 2-neuron (bipolar) chain from the CNS to the effector organ. The first neuron of both the SNS and PSNS originates within the CNS but does not make direct contact with the effector organ. Instead, it relays the impulse to a second station known as an ANS ganglion, which contains the cell body of the second ANS (postganglionic) neuron. Its axon contacts the effector organ. Thus, the motor pathways of both divisions of the ANS are schematically a serial 2-neuron chain consisting of a preganglionic neuron and a postganglionic effector neuron. Pharmacologic manipulation, through the use of ganglion agonists and antagonists, produces many side effects. This is mainly related to their nonselective actions, since these drugs will affect the SNS and the PSNS ganglia equally. This limits the therapeutic usefulness of these drugs in clinical practice.

19.2.1 The Sympathetic Nervous System

The sympathetic nervous system originates from the spinal cord in the thoracolumbar region, from the first thoracic through the second or third lumbar segment, in 22 paired ganglia. The short myelinated preganglionic fibers project to the 22 paired ganglia for synaptic transmission. From here, they follow 1 of 3 different tracts:

1. Synapse with postganglionic fibers in ganglia at the level of exit.
2. Course upward or downward in the trunk of the SNS chain to synapse in ganglia at other levels.
3. Track for variable distances through the sympathetic chain and exit without synapsing to terminate in an outlying, unpaired, SNS collateral ganglion.

The adrenal gland is an exception to the rule as preganglionic fibers pass directly into the adrenal medulla without synapsing in a ganglion. The cells of the medulla are derived from neuronal tissue and are analogous to postganglionic neurons, by design. The majority of the preganglionic fibers lie closer to the spinal cord than the organs they innervate, whether in the paired sympathetic chain or in unpaired ganglia. The first 4 or 5 segments generate preganglionic fibers that ascend in the neck to form 3 special paired ganglia. These are the superior, middle, and cervicothoracic ganglia (stellate ganglion). The cervical ganglia provide sympathetic innervation of the head, neck, upper extremities, heart, and lungs. Pain fibers also trade with these preganglionic fibers, explaining why myocardial ischemic pain is often felt in referred locations in the head, neck, and arm. Postganglionic anatomy consists of longer nerve segments than the preganglionic segments. The sympathetic postganglionic neuronal cell bodies are located in ganglia of the paired lateral SNS chain or unpaired collateral ganglia in more peripheral plexuses, such as inferior mesenteric ganglia (plexus). Collateral ganglia are formed from the convergence of preganglionic fibers with many postganglionic neuronal bodies. Postganglionic sympathetic neurons are usually unmyelinated and send long fibers out to the peripheral organs that they supply. Postganglionic fibers pass back from the sympathetic chain into spinal nerves through gray rami at all levels of the spinal cord. These fibers control the blood vessels, sweat glands, and hair piloerector muscles. Almost 8% of the fibers in average skeletal muscle nerves are sympathetic fibers, indicative of their great importance in the flight-or-fight response.

19.2.2 The Parasympathetic Nervous System

The parasympathetic nervous system (PSNS) anatomy varies from that of the SNS in several important ways. It contains the same subsegments of preganglionic and postganglionic fibers, but similarities stop there. Preganglionic neurons of the PSNS are myelinated and extremely long. The origin of the fibers and their areas of innervation differ significantly as well. Preganglionic cell bodies originate and are found in cranial nerves III (oculomotor), VII (facial), IX (glossopharyngeal), and X (vagus). The fibers originate in three regions of the brain midbrain, medulla oblongata, and the sacral part of the spinal cord. About 75% of all parasympathetic nerve fibers are in the vagus nerve (cranial nerve X), passing down to the chest and abdomen. The ganglionic bodies also have differences from the SNS, typically passing directly to the organs of innervation. Except in the case of a few cranial parasympathetic nerves, the preganglionic fibers pass uninterrupted all the way to the end effect organ. This leads to a distinct lack of visual ganglia and short postganglionic nerves. Postganglionic parasympathetic neurons are generally unmyelinated and very short. One important similarity is that the unmyelinated postganglionic fibers in both the SNS and PSNS have slower action potential transmission times, precluding them from participation in the immediate phase of a somatic response.

19.3 Ganglionic Transmission

As discussed in the previous section, both SNS and PSNS use a system of preganglionic and postganglionic fibers, in most circumstances, to achieve end organ effects. One of the keys to this function is the transmission through the ganglia and into the postganglionic fibers. The nerve transmission at the ganglia is identical. In both sympathetic and parasympathetic ganglia, preganglionic stimulation leads to the release of acetylcholine (ACh), which activates postjunctional nicotinic acetylcholine receptors on postganglionic neurons to increase ion permeability, resulting in propagation of action potentials down the axon of the nerve to termination.

19.3.1 Transmitters Release, Synthesis, Storage, and Termination

The two systems do differ in the release of the final neurotransmitters at effector sites in the body. The vast majority of the postganglionic neurons of the parasympathetic system are cholinergic. In contrast, most of the sympathetic neurons are adrenergic, releasing norepinephrine. The only exception in the sympathetic system are some sweat glands and blood vessels. The body's use of differing transmitters for the two systems requires an understanding of the release, synthesis, storage, and termination of the three transmitters involved in the transmission of ANS impulses. First, the discussion will focus on the general release of the neurotransmitters at the site of action. Next, the discussion will discuss acetylcholine (ACh), the ganglionic transmitter, and transmitter of the PSNS. Finally, the focus will be on norepinephrine (NE), the primary transmitter of the SNS as well as on epinephrine (EPI), the primary output of the adrenal medulla.

The release of the neurotransmitters at the terminal effect zone is similar for both systems. The action potential arrives causing depolarization of nerve terminal, leading to the release of neurotransmitter into the extracellular fluid between presynaptic and postsynaptic cells (the synaptic cleft). The bulk of the ANS differs in its pathway of innervation of terminal organs when compared to the musculoskeletal system with its endplate design. The parasympathetic nerve fibers and almost all of the sympathetic fibers merely touch the cells of the organ they innervate as they pass by, or in some instances, they terminate in the connective tissues adjacent to the organ they innervate. These terminal filaments end in presynaptic enlargements called varicosities—the location of synthesis and eventual vesicular storage of the neurotransmitter. Varicosities contain large numbers of mitochondria that supply adenosine triphosphate, which is required to energize neurotransmitter synthesis. These varicosities contain small vesicles, $\sim$500 μ(mu)m in diameter, in which the neurotransmitters are stored, for release when an action potential depolarizes the cell. The varicosities also contain transmitter-specific reuptake mechanisms, which will be further discussed for each specific transmitter in the system.

The synthesis and storage of ACh is similar in all nerve cells that use ACh as the primary neurotransmitter. This includes the muscle terminals, PSNS, ganglionic cell bodies, and the few parts of the SNS that use ACh. Acetylcholine is synthesized and stored, in a highly concentrated form, in terminal nerve varicosities of cholinergic nerves. This process of the formation of ACh requires the mitochondria to produce acetyl coenzyme A as the acetyl donor. This is joined with choline provided by phospholipid hydrolysis within the cell or following uptake of cleaved choline from the extracellular fluid. Within the cell, these two components are acted upon by the enzyme choline acetyltransferase to form ACh, which is then stored in vesicles for release. The body continually releases small amounts of ACh, called quanta, during the resting state, yielding small changes to the endplate electrical potential without full depolarization. Upon release from the nerve terminal following the stimulation and depolarization described earlier, ACh is released into the synaptic cleft. Modulation of the function of an effector organ by a receptor is dependent upon rapid recovery of the receptor to its baseline state after stimulation. Therefore, the neurotransmitter must be quickly removed from the vicinity of the receptor. ACh removal occurs by rapid hydrolysis by acetyl cholinesterase, found in high quantities at the receptor junction. This rapid hydrolysis removes and deactivates the ability of the ACh to continue its effects at the nerve endplates and varicosities. The free choline released from the action of acetyl cholinesterase is rapidly taken up by the nerve varicosity for reuse in the synthesis of additional ACh. Acetylic acid diffuses from the synaptic cleft; the choline is taken back up into the nerve terminal by high-affinity choline transporter.

The primary neurotransmitters of the SNS are NE and EPI, which are produced and stored near nerve terminals and varicosities of the SNS, and the adrenal medulla. The synthesis process is more complex than the synthesis of ACh. A series of enzymatic processes take the precursor tyrosine created from phenylalanine and modify it as NE or EPI. The first step, which is the rate-limiting step of the process that takes place in the cytoplasm of the cell, involves the conversion of tyrosine into DOPA via the enzyme tyrosine hydroxylase (TH). The amount of stored NE stimulates or limits the functions of this enzyme, which increases activities with low levels of NE and decreases with high levels. There is also an effect on TH enzyme function that relates to oxygenation. TH depends on a pteridine cofactor and the presence of molecular oxygen. If the quantity of molecular oxygen is reduced, NE production may be decreased, which could account for changes in wakefulness. DOPA is then decarboxylated via the enzyme L-amino acid decarboxylase into dopamine (DA). The DA is readily taken into the storage vesicles. DA serves as a neurotransmitter in certain situations and has had use in the past as an intravenous infusion. In-vitro, most DA is β(beta)-hydroxylated within the vesicles to norepinephrine by the enzyme dopamine β(beta)-hydroxylase (Dβ[beta]H). Dβ(beta)H serves as the final enzyme in the synthesis of NE in the postganglionic sympathetic neurons, yielding the final neurotransmitter the SNS uses. The adrenal medulla, on the other hand, has to carry the reactions one step further to transform 80% of the NE into EPI. This step is achieved via methylation of NE by the enzyme phenylethanolamine N-methyltransferase. NE is stored in large, dense-core vesicles where the dense cores in these vesicles are filled not only with norepinephrine but also with binding proteins necessary for release. It is important to note that the primary release of NE occurs via exocytosis. Once released, the NE enters the synaptic cleft and begins to interact with the target cells and perform the excitation actions associated with the flight-or-fight phenomena for which the SNS is known.

The termination of NE at the receptor site is handled in three different ways, which explain the short duration of action of endogenous NE:

1. Reuptake into the adrenergic nerve endings by an active transport process, accounting for 50% to 80% of the secreted norepinephrine;
2. Diffusion away from the nerve endings into the surrounding body fluids and then into the blood account for the removal of most of the remaining norepinephrine; and
3. Destruction by local tissue enzymatic action (only a small amount).

The uptake mechanism is an important method to reduce the amount of NE that needs to be produced by the postganglionic nerve cells. This is important to conserve the overall energy needs to produce the NE. NE that is taken up by the extraneuronal tissue is metabolized by monoamine oxidase (MAO) and by catechol-O-methyltransferase (COMT) to form vanillylmandelic acid. Any remaining NE in the blood stream is metabolized by the liver using the COMT enzyme. Epinephrine is handled by the same enzymatic process as NE. The process of reuptake is the primary pathway for inactivation of the endogenous catecholamines, while metabolism by the liver and kidney is the predominant pathway for exogenous catecholamines. This allows us to use them as infusions with a longer duration of action of the exogenous catecholamines delivered at the synaptic cleft. The fact that reuptake does not occur with the use of exogenous administration of NE and EPI accounts for their usefulness as systemic medications in the support of homeostasis in the intensive care unit (ICU) or an operating room. In fact, they stay active in the blood for 10–30 s, with the effects lasting several minutes.

19.4 Receptors

The final part of the ANS is the receptor sites, where neurotransmitters trigger cells of a variety of organ systems into action. Receptors are protein macromolecules located in the plasma membrane and have a variety of actions when bound to the neurotransmitter or a synthetic agonist resulting in conformational changes. Alteration of the protein molecule excites or inhibits the cell by:

1. Changing the cell membrane permeability to one or more ions;
2. Activating or inactivating an enzyme attached to the other end of the receptor protein protruding into the interior of the cell.

The opening of ion channels can excite cells via calcium influx or inhibit cells via potassium outflow. The transmitters of the ANS, ACh, and NE use a multitude of different receptor enzymes to cause their effects. These receptors have undergone intense research, to define them for both understanding and pharmacological use. The receptors are divided into subtypes based on response to pharmacological studies and genetic testing.

The SNS has multiple different receptors that serve different features throughout the body, and in respect to what neurotransmitters they respond to. These receptors are traditionally known as adrenergic receptors and have been classified as alpha (α) or beta (β) or more specifically as α(alpha) 1, α(alpha)2, β(beta)1, or β(beta)2 based on responses to specific pharmacologic agents. NE excites alpha receptors more than beta, whereas EPI excites both equally. The α(alpha)1 receptor and its 3 subtypes use the Gq protein and phospholipid C-mediated diacylglycerol and inositol-1,4,5-triphospahte to produce its effects. The α(alpha)1 receptors are located on the postsynaptic organs that are affected by the SNS. They serve to either contract or relax various muscle systems related to these organs based on the need of the fight-or-flight response (see later section: End Organ Effects). The α(alpha)2-adrenergic receptors produce their effects predominately by inhibition of adenyl cyclase through inhibitory G proteins (G_i) via decreased intracellular cyclic adenosine monophosphate (cAMP). The α(alpha)2 receptor and its 3 subtypes are usually expressed presynaptically or even in non-neuronal tissue allowing them to serve as a feedback inhibitory function upon the release of NE. Stimulation of presynaptic α(alpha)2 receptors inhibits NE release into the synaptic cleft, serving as a negative feedback mechanism. The effects of the inhibition are primarily related to a reduction in sympathetic outflow with a concomitantly enhanced parasympathetic outflow (e.g., enhanced baroreceptor activity). This results in a decreased systemic vascular resistance, cardiac output (CO), inotropic state in the myocardium, and heart rate. Stimulation of each β(beta) adrenergic receptor subtype leads to activation of G_s increasing cAMP, which activates cAMP-dependent protein kinase, leading to the phosphorylating of various proteins in the effected cells. Beta-adrenergic receptors are not fixed; they change significantly in dynamic response to the amount of norepinephrine present in the synaptic cleft or in plasma, accounting for the changes in responsiveness to various adrenergic drugs. This variability allows for modulation of the effects of the levels of NE and EPI. Dopamine receptors (DA) represent a small, but vital, amount of adrenergic type receptors. DA1 receptors are postsynaptic in renal, mesenteric, splenic, and coronary vascular smooth muscle, mediating vasodilation via adenylate cyclase activation yielding cAMP. DA2 receptors are presynaptic, possibly inhibiting release of norepinephrine and acetylcholine. As will be demonstrated in the section on response to stimulus, some of the actions of the SNS excite some organs and some it relaxes.

The PSNS consists of three major systems of action: the ganglionic transmission, the muscle endplate, and the PSNS terminals. Cholinergic receptors are subdivided into muscarinic and nicotinic receptors based upon the response to either stimulation by muscarine or nicotine, respectively. Nicotinic receptors are ligand-gated ion channels allowing the influx of Na^+ and Ca + +, after activation by ACh. In contrast, muscarinic receptors are G-protein coupled receptors, which, when activated by ACh, activate G-proteins. ACh has affinity for both types of receptors equally despite physical differences with each subtype. Those physical characteristics allow for the design of drugs that affect each type of channel. Nicotinic receptors are found in the motor endplate, the ganglia of the ANS, and in the CNS. They are variably affected by pharmacologic agents, including the various types of non-depolarizing muscle relaxants. The muscarinic receptors are a family of five different subtypes: M1 through M5. M1, M3, and M5 stimulate diacylglycerol and inositol-1,4,5-triphosphate as do the α(alpha)1 receptors. M2 and M4 receptors act like α(alpha)2-adrenergic receptors, by inhibition of adenyl cyclase through G_i via decreased intracellular cyclic AMP. M1 receptors are located in autonomic ganglia (where they modulate the effects of nicotinic receptor activation), M2 receptors are located in the heart, and M3 receptors are located in many glands and smooth muscles. The location of the M4 and M5 receptors is poorly uncertain, though all five subtypes are known to exist within the CNS.

19.5 End Organ Effects

The majority of organ systems exhibit dual innervation, with input from the sympathetic and parasympathetic systems typically offering opposing effects. This dual innervation allows the two systems to provide different effects to different areas based on the needs of the body at the time. Organs innervated by both systems include the heart, eye, bronchial tree, gastrointestinal (GI) tract, urinary bladder, and reproductive organs (◉ Table 19.1). Some structures—including blood vessels, the spleen, and piloerector muscles—only receive sympathetic stimulation. There is no general scheme that describes the way each of these systems will stimulate a specific response to a stimulus. For this reason, each system must be discussed on its own.

19.5.1 Eyes

The eyes are innervated by both the SNS and PSNS, which yield opposing functional results. The systems control two functions related to the eye and sight. First, the pupillary constriction and dilation, which alters the gathering of light. Second, altering the shape of the lens allowing for focal plane adjustments. The pupillary opening is controlled by

Table 19.1 Effects of the sympathetic nervous system (SNS) and the parasympathetic nervous system (PSNS) on organs

Organ system	SNS response	SNS receptor	PSNS response	PSNS receptor
Eye				
Iris radial	Dilation	α(alpha)1		
Iris ciliary	Relaxation	β(beta)2	Miosis (contraction)	M3
Circular			Accommodation (contraction)	M3
Heart				
Rate of contraction	Increased	β(beta)1	Decrease	M2
Force of contraction	Increased	β(beta)1	Decreased	M2
Coronary artery	Constriction	α(alpha)1		
	Dilation	β(beta)1		
Blood vessels				
Arteries	Constriction	α(alpha)1 (α[alpha]2)		
Muscle	Vasodilation	β(beta)2		
Veins	Vasoconstriction	α(alpha)2 (α[alpha]1)		
Pulmonary				
Bronchial tree	Bronchodilation	β(beta)2	Bronchoconstriction	M3
Renal/GU				
Kidney	Renin secretion	β(beta)1		
Bladder detrusor	Relaxation	β(beta)2	Contraction	M3
Trigone	Contraction	α(alpha)1	Relaxation	M3
Ureter	Contraction	α(alpga)1		
Uterus	Contraction	α(alpha)1	Variable	
Vas deferens	Contraction	α(alpha)1		
Gastrointestinal system				
Intestines	Relaxation	α(alpha)2	Contraction	M3
Splenic capsule	Contraction	α(alpha)1		
Liver glycogenolysis	Increase	α(alpha)1 (β[beta]2) (β[beta]3)		
Glands and cells				
Fat cells	Lipolysis	β(beta)1 (β[beta]3)		
Hair follicles, Smooth muscle	Contraction (piloerection)	α(alpha)1		
Insulin release from pancreas	Decrease	α(alpha)2		
Nasal secretion	Decrease	α(alpha)1 (α[alpha]2)	Increase	
Salivary glands	Increase secretion	α(alpha)1	Increase secretion	
Sweat glands	Increase secretion	α(alpha)1	Increase secretion	

both the PSNS and SNS in different ways. The PSNS is responsible for putting into effect the constriction of the pupil in response to light hitting the retina. The SNS causes dilation of the pupil to let more light in during times of increased stimulation. Lens shape and focusing is almost exclusively a PSNS function. Stimulation of the PSNS causes excitation and constriction of the ciliary muscle, making the lens convex and suitable for near field vision. SNS stimulation, on the other hand, relaxes the ciliary muscle thinking the lens for distance vision. The aforementioned facts that both SNS and PSNS demonstrate both an excitation and relaxation effect in different areas prove that no generalized statement can be made regarding the final effects of either subsystem of the ANS.

19.5.2 Body Glands

Different glandular systems tend to respond in a different fashion, depending on location, intended function, and primary stimulation system. Nasal, lacrimal, salivary, and gastrointestinal glands are strongly stimulated by the PSNS, almost always resulting in copious quantities of watery secretion. This holds true for the upper part of the alimentary tract, but not the lower part, which is controlled predominantly by the enteric nervous system (to be discussed later). The SNS decreases blood flow to the alimentary glands, decreasing secretion rates, and causes secretion of concentrated, highly enzymatic secretions and mucus. Sweat glands are controlled by the SNS secreting sweat when stimulated by postganglionic *cholinergic fibers*. The process becomes even more contrary and confusing because the control of the stimulus originates in the hypothalamus, usually considered a PSNS controller. In summary, sweating is parasympathetic, in spite of its SNS distribution. The apocrine glands are purely sympathetic in nature.

19.5.3 Heart

The heart is innervated by both the SNS and PSNS, each acting in opposition to modulate function in three ways. The SNS and PSNS affect cardiac pump function in three ways. First, by changing the rate (chronotropism); SNS increasing the rate and PSNS decreasing it. Second, by changing the strength of contraction (inotropism); SNS increasing the strength and PSNS decreasing it. Finally, both systems modulate coronary blood flow. The PSNS, via the vagus nerve, predominantly innervates the sinoatrial and atrioventricular nodes, affecting choronotropy more than inotropy. Overall, the role of PSNS in cardiac contractility is poorly understood. Sympathetic stimulation increases overall activity of the heart, increasing rate and contractility. While the effects of the ANS on coronary artery blood flow are not well understood, it is known that the SNS, via α(alpha) receptors, can cause constriction of the large coronary vessels, which normally have no role in the coronary resistance. The SNS can also cause dilation via β(beta)2 receptor stimulation, providing balance to the effects of SNS stimulation.

19.5.4 Lung

The lungs receive innervation from both the PSNS and SNS. The effect of SNS stimulation leads to bronchial dilation and pulmonary vasoconstriction. The increased pulmonary vascular resistance may be important in maintaining the balance between right and left ventricular output during stress and exercise. PSNS stimulation leads to bronchial constriction with little to no vascular dilation.

19.5.5 Blood Vessels

SNS nerves are the most important regulators of the peripheral circulation and overall systemic vascular tone. Stimulation by the SNS generally causes vasoconstriction in all organs except the heart, brain, and muscle where there are less SNS fibers. PSNS has almost no effects on the blood vessels as far as direct stimulation of relaxation. SNS stimulation results in increased blood pressure via increased cardiac activity and increased flow resistance in the circulation. As stated before, the PSNS has little effect on the overall systemic resistance, but can render a rapid decrease in blood pressure via vagal stimulation of the nodal cardiac conduction for a brief period of time.

19.5.6 Other Organs

The rest of the body systems are affected in various ways by the SNS and PSNS. The kidneys decrease urine output and increase renin secretion following SNS stimulation, but have no change with PSNS stimulation. The urinary bladder has relaxed detrusor tone, increased trigone and sphincter tone, and ureter contraction with SNS stimulation. Increased detrusor tone with trigone and sphincter relaxation are PSNS effects. The SNS also has large effects on the liver, muscle, fat cells, and blood glucose levels. SNS stimulation causes glycogenolysis in the liver and skeletal muscle, increased lipolysis, decreased insulin release, and increased blood glucose levels. The brain responds to SNS stimulation by increases in mental activities.

19.5.7 Adrenal Medulla

The adrenal medulla is an organ that receives direct preganglionic fibers in the actual organ. Preganglionic fibers pass directly into the adrenal medulla without synapsing in a ganglion. Cells of the medulla, derived from neuronal tissue, are analogous to postganglionic neurons normally found in the paired SNS thoracic chain. It is also the site for the creation, storage, and release of EPI into the circulation, as opposed to the nerve terminal actions associated with the rest of the ANS. The organ releases a combination of EPI and NE in a ratio that averages 80% to 20%, respectively. This larger release of EPI has three very different effects than the direct, or circulatory, effects of NE. First, EPI acts on beta receptors with higher degree of affinity than does NE, thus EPI yields increased cardiac stimulatory effects when compared to NE. Second, EPI causes less constriction of muscle bed blood vessels, leading to a less robust vasoconstriction of NE alone. Third, EPI has 5–10 times more effect in metabolism than NE, yielding up to a 100% increase above normal rates. The effects of the circulatory release also last longer in the body than the nerve terminal actions. Stimulation of the adrenal medulla causes release of the hormones epinephrine and norepinephrine, whose effects can last 2–4 min beyond the initial stimulation. The adrenal medulla also provides a backup to the SNS, allowing either to fill most duties. Finally, the adrenal medulla allows for stimulation of structures with no direct SNS nerve endings.

19.6 Reflex and Regulation

The ANS is a regulated and reflexive pathway that maintains homeostasis via the aforementioned effects on end organs. This control system has sensors, afferent pathways, CNS integration, and efferent pathways from the receptors back to the efferent organs. Fine adjustments are made at the local level through positive and negative feedback mechanisms, such as with α(alpha)2 receptors. A prime example of these mechanisms is the baroreceptor reflex system that controls blood pressure. Blood pressure is sensed (carotid sinus), integrated (medullary vasomotor center), and adjusted through specific effector–receptor sites, throughout the body. The ANS is incorporated into several endocrine systems that ultimately control blood pressure and regulate homeostasis. These include the renin–angiotensin system, antidiuretic hormone (ADH), glucocorticoids, and insulin. The renin–angiotensin system acts to regulate water-electrolyte homeostasis as well as blood pressure. Glucocorticoids alter the production of EPI in the adrenal medulla. The pancreas has been found to have both α(alpha) and β(beta) receptors, which decrease and increase insulin release, respectively.

There also exists in the system the concept of adrenergic "sympathetic and parasympathetic tone," or the base rate of physical activity. Autonomic tone requires only low levels of nerve impulses to maintain normal function—only 1 every couple of seconds, and full stimulation requires only 10–20 impulses per second. Compare that to the full activation in the skeletal nervous system at 50–500 or more impulses per second. The SNS can regulate blood vessel constriction solo via its ability to either increase stimulation or decrease levels, constricting or dilating blood vessels as needed. The PSNS in the same way controls the GI tract. Without its normal tone, gastric atony and stasis occur.

The last concept of regulation is the return of baseline intrinsic organ function over time, albeit after many months in case of PSNS denervation. This denervation may also increase the responsiveness to exogenously administered agents. A classic example of deprivation is the denervated heart. NE infusion in the normal heart produces a slowing of the recipient's atrial rate through vagal feedback as the blood pressure rises. In the unmodulated donor heart, atrial rate increases, showing the abolishment of the baroreceptor reflex in the transplanted heart. Similar effects exist with beta agonists and blockers.

19.7 Enteric Nervous System

Also known as the intramural plexus, the enteric nervous system is the network of neurons and their supporting cells found within the walls of the gastrointestinal tract, including neurons within the pancreas and gallbladder. The SNS and PSNS interact with this system primarily by altering actions within the intramural plexus. The plexus has a large degree of independence in relation to the rest of the ANS. The SNS typically has only small effects on the GI tract, typically influencing the sphincters to close. Strong sympathetic stimulation inhibits peristalsis and increases the tone of the sphincters, resulting in a greatly slowed propulsion of food through the tract. SNS stimulation can lead to decreased secretion as well as causing constipation. The PSNS is responsible for easing the passage of food and increasing secretions as described earlier. Multiple neuroactive compounds participate in the autonomic control of intestinal function, not just NE and ACh. These include nitric oxide, substance P, opiate peptides, vasoactive intestinal polypeptide (VIP), and peptide hormones. Considering the importance of clinical phenomena such as nausea, vomiting, and alterations in bowel function associated with anesthesia, the enteric nervous system remains poorly understood.

19.8 Questions and Answers

Questions (Choose the Most Appropriate Answer)

1. Which of the following is a function of the sympathetic nervous system (SNS)?
   A. Vasoconstriction of arteries via α(alpha)1
   B. Vasoconstriction of arteries via β(beta)1
   C. Vasodilation of arteries via β(beta)1
   D. Vasodilatation of arteries via α(alpha)1
2. The adrenal medulla release EPI and NE into the circulation resulting in SNS stimulation. Following stimulation how long does this circulatory release of SNS neurotransmitters last in the circulation?
   A. 1–2 min
   B. 2–4 min
   C. 4–6 min
   D. 6–8 min
3. The bulk of SNS anatomy is made up of which of the following combinations?

A. Long myelinated preganglionic fibers with short non-myelinated postganglionic fibers
B. Short non-myelinated preganglionic fibers with long myelinated postganglionic fibers
C. Short myelinated preganglionic fibers with long non-myelinated postganglionic fibers
D. Long non-myelinated preganglionic fibers with short myelinated postganglionic fibers

4. Which of the following SSN sites is not innervated by adrenergic receptors?
   A. Pupil
   B. GI sphincters
   C. Sweat glands
   D. Piloerector muscles
5. The vagal nerve contains what percentage of PSNS fibers?
   A. 15%
   B. 50%
   C. 75%
   D. 90%
6. The cause of the majority of termination of effect of endogenous NE at the nerve terminal of SNS postganglionic nerve terminal is?
   A. Redistribution
   B. Enzymatic destruction
   C. Reuptake
   D. Protein binding
7. The α(alpha)2 receptor is located on the presynaptic side of the SNS ganglia and serves which of the following functions?
   A. Feedback loop increasing nerve terminal NE release
   B. Feedback loop decreasing nerve terminal NE release
   C. Feedback loop increasing nerve terminal NE reuptake
   D. Feedback loop decreasing nerve terminal NE reuptake
8. Which of the following nerves is **not** a carrier of the PSNS system?
   A. CN III
   B. CN V
   C. CN IX
   D. CN X
9. What percentage of skeletal muscle nerve fibers contain SNS fibers?
   A. 2%
   B. 4%
   C. 6%
   D. 8%
10. The stimulation of the SNS has which of the following effects on the enteric nervous system?
    A. Stimulation of peristalsis
    B. Stimulation of secretions
    C. Closing of sphincters
    D. No effect

Answers

1. **A**. Vasoconstriction of the arteries is a primary function of the SNS. It is predominately carried out via α(alpha)1 receptor, via G protein modulation. The SNS is the predominate moderator of the peripheral arterial tone. The SNS has the ability to self-regulate its degree of stimulation of arterial contraction via feedback mechanisms discussed in the chapter. The PSNS had minimal effects of arterial tone, although severe stimulation of the PSNS via vagal nerve can cause rapid drops in blood pressure leading to fainting.
2. **B**. 2–4 min following direct stimulation. This serves several purposes for the body. The first is to prolong the SNS stimulation longer than nerve terminal only excitation, allowing for prolonged fight-or-flight response. Second, it provides direct blood stimulation to areas of the body that do not have direct SNS nerve stimulation. Finally, the blood release of the adrenal medulla provides a back use system for the SNS in the event of central or peripheral nerve damage.
3. **C**. In the SNS, the fibers arise primarily from the thoracic and lumbar spines forming a 22-paired set of ganglia, known as the paravertebral chain. The bulk of anatomy consists of short myelinated preganglionic fibers and long unmyelinated postganglionic fibers that travel along with other nerves. The PSNS by contrast contains predominantly what is described in answer A: long myelinated fibers with the ganglia being located near the end organs.
4. **B**. The sweat glands and some artery muscle SNS activity are cholinergic in nature. In fact, the sweat glands are called a parasympathetic effect stimulated by the sympathetic system.
5. **C**. The vagal nerve is the main conduit of PSNS nerves carrying approximately 75% of the fibers related to the PSNS. The vagal nerve distributes all of the PSNS to the thoracic and abdominal organs. It contains preganglionic fibers directly to the organs that need innervation. These preganglionic fibers synapse close to the level of action and do not usually form visible ganglion.
6. **C**. The majority (50–80%) of termination of action of NE is due to reuptake by the nerve terminal itself. This reuptake is an active process that requires energy. It does, however, decrease the amount of NE synthesis that needs to take place in the nerve terminal

preserving the transmitter intact. Diffusion and enzymatic destruction are the other two mechanisms that take place to terminate the action of NE. Exogenous catecholamines are terminated not by reuptake but by the various other mechanisms. It is the fact that exogenous catecholamines do not get uptake that makes them useful in the OR and ICU.

7. **B**. The existence of the α(alpha)2 receptors acts to decrease the SNS outflow. The decreased SNS outflow acts in concert with the PSNS to decrease heart rate, CO, and arterial tone. This is a classic example of how a feedback system works to maintain the proper level of homeostasis needed in the body.
8. **B**. The four nerves are CN III (oculomotor), CN VII (facial), CN IX (glossopharyngeal), and CN X (vagal). These four nerves provide passage for the PSNS from its origin in the brain. The locations more specifically include the midbrain and medulla oblongata. These provide PSNS stimulation to the upper body and abdomen. The PSNS also has a second center of origin that is located in the sacral region of the body, which supplies the pelvic organs.
9. **D**. The fact that 8% of skeletal muscle nerve fibers are actually postganglionic SNS fibers demonstrates the need of SNS control to maintain homeostasis. The SNS allows for constriction at the muscle level via both adrenergic and cholinergic effects. Alpha-1 effects yield predominantly vasoconstriction. Beta-2 stimulation at the muscle body provides vasodilation. The muscle is the second location for cholinergic action by SNS aside from the sweat glands as previously mentioned.
10. **C**. Although the enteric plexus has a great degree of autonomy, it is effected by the rest of the ANS. The SNS has little effect on the plexus, usually only causing sphincters to close. Strong SNS stimulus can shut down the entire enteric process yielding constipation due to closed sphincters and no peristalsis. The PSNS on the other hand increases secretion of enzymes and movement of food products through the GI system.

Bibliography

1. Wecker L, Crespo L, Dunway G, Faingold C, Watts S. Introduction to the autonomic nervous system. In: Wecker L, editor. Brody's human pharmacology. 5th ed. Philadelphia: Mosby; 2010. p. 93–106.
2. Hall JE. The autonomic nervous system and the adrenal medulla. In: Hall JE, editor. Guyton and Hall textbook of medical physiology. 13th ed. Philadelphia: Elsevier; 2016. p. 773–5.
3. Grecu L. Autonomic nervous system: physiology and pharmacology. In: Barash PG, editor. Clinical anesthesia. 7th ed. Philadelphia: Lippincott Williams & Wilkins; 2013. p. 361–407.
4. Glick DB. The autonomic nervous system. In: Miller RD, Cohen NH, Eriksson LI, Fleisher LA, Wiener-Kronish JP, Young WL, editors. Miller's anesthesia. 8th ed. Philadelphia: Elsevier Saunders; 2015. p. 346–86.

Basic Principles and Consequences of Perioperative Hypothermia

20

Kurt Ruetzler and Maria-Jose Corrales-Martinez

Abstract

Perioperative hypothermia is common with an incidence ranging between 20 and 70%, and is conventionally defined by a body core temperature below 37.0 °C. Even severe intraoperative hypothermia was common during the previous centuries, as intraoperative warming was rare, and the negative impact of hypothermia was not fully understood yet. In the 1980s and 1990s, intraoperative hypothermia was identified as a significant and independent contributor to perioperative morbidity. Perioperative hypothermia causes impaired pharmacokinetics, surgical site infections, blood loss and coagulopathy, transfusion requirements, thermal discomfort, prolonged recovery, and prolonged duration of hospitalization. For many years, an intraoperative target threshold of 36 °C was considered effective, although only based on limited evidence. Most recent findings by a large RCT highlight that maintaining the patient in a slight hypothermic state at $\geq$ 35.5 °C is safe and won't affect patient outcomes. Core temperature should be measured in all patients having general or regional anesthesia lasting more than 30 minutes. Anesthesiologist should aim to maintain a core temperature $\geq$ 35.5 °C by actively (re-)warming patients. Several warming devices are commercially available, including active skin warming by forced air as the most commonly used, efficient, inexpensive, and easy-to-use technique for the majority of patients and surgeries.

K. Ruetzler (✉)
Department of Outcomes Research and General Anesthesiology, Anesthesiology Institute, Cleveland Clinic Foundation, Cleveland, OH, USA
e-mail: kr@or.org

M.-J. Corrales-Martinez
Department of Outcomes Research, Cleveland Clinic, Cleveland, OH, USA

20.1 Basic Principles of Perioperative Thermoregulation

Body temperature is tightly regulated by the thermoregulatory system, which consists of three major components:

- Afferent sensing,
- Central regulation, and
- Autonomic and behavioral defenses.

Figure from: [1] *actual body temperature is sensed by various receptors in the skin surface, deep tissues, spinal cord, brain, and hypothalamus. These inputs get processed in the hypothalamus, the most important controller of human temperature control. Efferent autonomic responses include sweating, vasoconstriction, and shivering.*

The actual body temperature is sensed by various receptors and nerves throughout the body in the skin surface, deep tissues, spinal cord, brain, and hypothalamus, with transient receptor potential proteins (TRPP) being the most important (Fig. 20.1). TRPP was identified relatively recently, and basic physiologic principles are still under investigation. Among them, there are at least 4 subtypes (TRPR 1-4), which are sensitive to and get activated by heat, and at least 2 subtypes (TRPM 1 and TRPA 1) sensitive to and get activated by cold [2]. Signals by TRPP are primarily processed in the anterior spinal cord and ultimately in the brain, specifically in the hypothalamus, which is the single most important controller of human temperature regulation.

After afferent sensing of the actual body temperature, and central regulation in the hypothalamus, autonomic and behavioral thermoregulatory defenses are activated as necessary.

Behavioral defenses are by far the most effective defense mechanism but are limited to awake patients and therefore not available in anesthetized patients.

Conceptually, there are two major *autonomic thermoregulatory defenses*: actively precapillary vasodilation and sweating [3] as the primary thermoregulatory response

M. Argalious et al. (eds.), *Basic Sciences in Anesthesia*,
https://doi.org/10.1007/978-3-031-60203-0_20

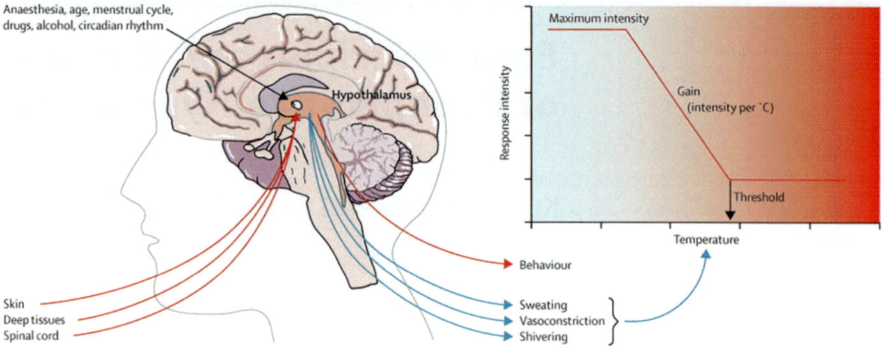

Fig. 20.1 Shivering, Vasoconstriction and Sweating physiological temperature thresholds in humans

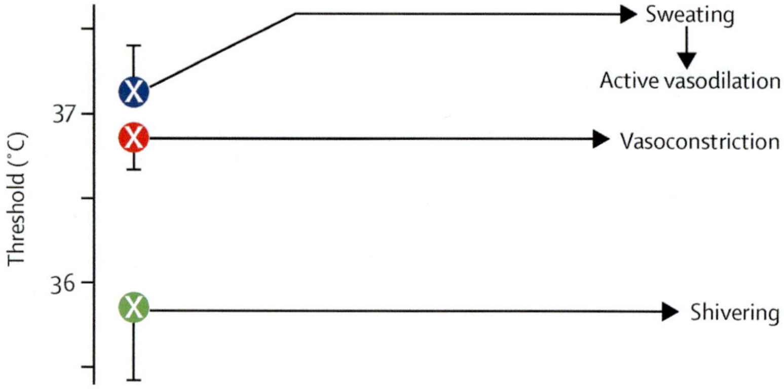

Fig. 20.2 From [1], based on [8]

to heat, and arteriovenous shunt vasoconstriction [4], and shivering [5] against cold. Thermoregulatory responses are well developed at birth, and infants have an addition primary defense against cold, the non-shivering thermogenesis (activation of brown fat by an uncoupling protein, thermogenin) [6], which is not important in thermoregulation of adults.

- *Sweating* as the primary response to heat is highly effective as adults can easily produce a liter of sweat per hour.
- *Arteriovenous shunts* in the limbs, and mostly in the fingers and toes, are the major target of thermoregulatory vasoconstrictions. These vessels are as small as about 100 μm and convey more than 10,000 times as much blood as 10 μm capillaries when dilated, but essentially no blood when vasoconstricted. Consequently, vasodilatation and vasoconstriction of the arteriovenous shunts does affect the blood flow of the entire extremities and is an effective response to heat (vasodilatation) and cold (vasoconstriction) [1].
- *Shivering* is the most important response to cold, can rapidly increase metabolic rate by a factor of five, and may endure a couple of hours until muscles exhaust [7]. The heat producing effect of shivering is constant, but limited, as shivering is mostly limited to the extremities and simultaneous vasodilation is necessary to compensate for the increased oxygen requirements in the muscles. This vasodilation counteracts the heat production effect and promotes heat loss to the periphery and ultimately into the environments. Shivering is extremely unsatisfying and unpleasant to patients, may cause post-shivering muscle cramps, and increases systemic oxygen requirements, which might be bothersome in cardiac and/or respiratory impaired patients.

Each autonomic thermoregulatory response is characterized by three individual properties:

- threshold (a triggering core temperature),
- gain (increase in response intensity with core temperature deviation beyond the triggering threshold), and
- a maximum response intensity.

Figure 20.2 displays the different threshold of the major thermoregulatory responses.

The thresholds for the primary responses to heat, precapillary vasodilation, and sweating have the same triggering core temperature and therefore occur synchronously.

The threshold of vasoconstriction, the primary response to cold, is usually a couple of tenths of a degree below the sweating threshold.

The threshold of shivering, the major response to cold, is usually about 1 °C below the vasoconstriction threshold.

The range of body temperature between the sweating and the vasoconstriction thresholds is usually about 1 degree C and is called the *inter-threshold range*. Although the

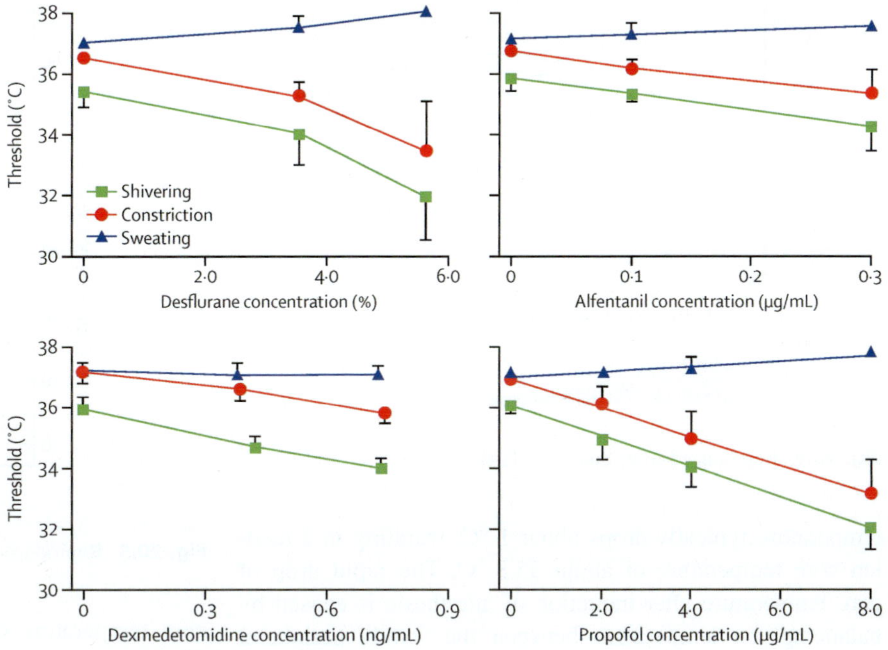

Fig. 20.3 Adapted from [1]: The major thermoregulatory responses to thresholds in volunteers given desflurane [11], alfentanil [12], dexmedetomidine [13], or propofol [14]

thermoregulatory system in principle is never switched on or off, thermoregulatory responses are minimal if the actual body temperature is within the inter-threshold range, usually a temperature roughly around 37° C.

The "normal" body temperature at any given time is therefore defined by the inter-threshold range, varies by at least 1 °C, and follows a circadian and menstrual/humoral cycle [9]. At the circadian nadir, usually at about 3 AM, core temperature is usually not below 36.5 °C, and at about 3 PM, core temperature is typically about 37.5 °C [9]. On average, then, normal core temperature in humans is about 37 °C, not the 36 °C widely accepted as suitable for perioperative patients [10].

General anesthesia affects thermoregulation by impairing thermoregulatory control. Most anesthetics used for general anesthesia including isoflurane, sevoflurane, nitrous oxide, opioids, and propofol do not have any significant effect on the sweating thresholds. But, all these medications greatly and synchronously lower the vasoconstriction and shivering thresholds. These reductions are mainly concentration dependent (the higher the concentration of the medication, the lower the threshold) and individual for each medication.

By decreasing these thresholds, the inter-thresholds range widens and thermoregulatory defenses against cold are not activated until the actual body temperature reaches the bottom of the inter-threshold range. In other words, in an awake patient, vasoconstriction is activated once the patient reaches a core temperature of roughly 36 °C, but might be delayed in anesthetized patient until the core temperature reaches 35 °C or even 34 °C. But once the actual core temperature reaches that certain threshold, the thermoregulatory response is activated.

Figure 20.3 *displays the concentration-dependent effect of lowering the vasoconstriction and shivering thresholds of four commonly used medications during anesthesia* [1].

20.2 Central Versus Peripheral Thermal Component

Importantly, there is no single body temperature as actual temperature varies from site to site. Traditionally, the human body is divided into two separate thermal components: The *core thermal component* including the trunk and head and is highly perfused and temperature is relatively homogeneous, and the *peripheral thermal component* including the arms and legs, which is less perfused, and temperature is usually 3–4 °C lower than the core thermal component. In patients having surgery, the anesthesia provider aims to maintain normothermia in the core thermal component, as many body functions critically depend on adequate normothermia in organs like the liver, heart, kidneys, or brain.

Perioperative hypothermia is common after induction of anesthesia, but not at the end of surgery.

Induction of anesthesia causes several physiological changes, affecting body core temperature. Within 60–90 minutes after induction of anesthesia, the body core temperature typically descends by about 1 °C. This phenomenon is mostly not based on heat loss, but on heat distribution instead.

Figure 20.4 displays the distribution of core temperature as a function of time after induction of anesthesia in a cohort of 58,814 patients having noncardiac surgery at the Cleveland Clinic [14]. During the first hour of anesthesia, the core

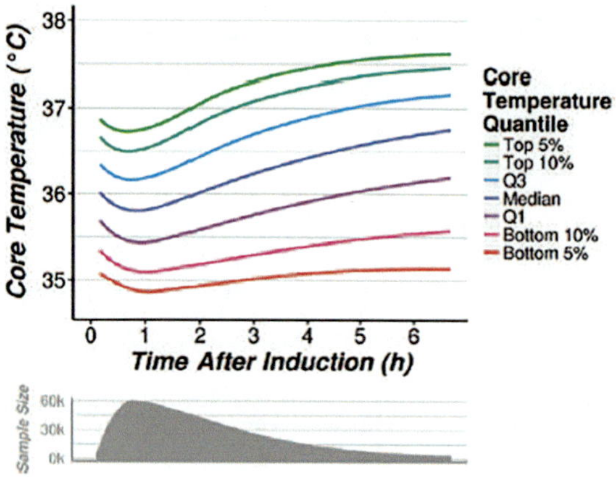

Fig. 20.4 Reproduced from Sun et al. [14]

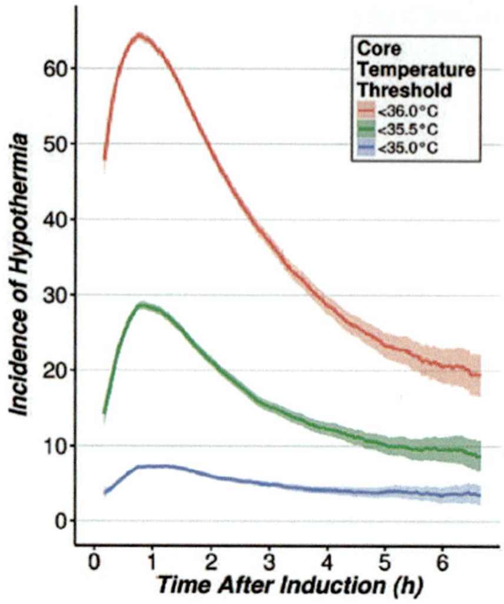

Fig. 20.5 Reproduced from Sun et al. [14]

temperature typically drops about 1 °C, resulting in a median core temperature of about 35.8 °C. The rapid drop of core temperature after induction of anesthesia is caused by balancing the temperature between the "cold" peripheral thermal compartment and the "warm" core thermal compartment. This period is therefore a shift of heat from the warm core to the cold peripheral thermal compartment and is accelerated by vasodilatation, caused by anesthetics. Thus, this period is called "re-distribution". This designation also makes clear, that the actual amount of heat is not decreased (or the least minimally) during this period, the overall amount of heat is just distributed.

Once the re-distribution effect is maxed out, core temperature of most anesthetized patients usually increases, which is a direct consequence of active warming. Depending on the surgical procedure and exposure to cold ambient temperature, surgical patients lose heat during surgery. This heat loss is counteracted by providing external heat to surgical patients. The extent of heat supply usually overcomes the constant heat loss, and the core temperature rises. As shown in Fig. 20.1, all patients under general anesthesia have a significant core temperature drop caused by heat re-distribution, but the overwhelming majority of most surgical patients are normothermic at the end of surgery.

Figure 20.5 displays the incidence of hypothermia under various core temperature thresholds. After 45 minutes of induction of general anesthesia, almost two-thirds of the patients reached the hypothermia threshold of 36 °C. In addition, more than one quarter reached the threshold of 35.5 °C within 51 minutes of induction. After 71 minutes, 7% of all patients reached 35 °C. Temporary hypothermia during general anesthesia is therefore common in surgical patients, but most patients are normothermic at the end of surgery. Still, after 6 hours of surgery, about 20% of patients are still hypothermic with a core temperature below 36.0 °C [14].

The duration of perioperative hypothermia varies between individuals (Fig. 20.6). Nearly half of all patients have a core temperature < 36 °C, and about 20% of all patients have a core temperature < 35.5 °C for more than 1 hour.

Most thermoregulation studies were performed in the 1990s, when patient warming was rare and scientific evidence about the consequences of perioperative hypothermia was weak. Consequently, moderate to severe hypothermia was common and identifying a threshold of core temperature of harm was challenging. For many years, maintaining a core temperature above 36 °C was considered the standard of care. However, a major randomized clinical trial, performed at the Cleveland Clinic and several Chinese hospitals, enrolled 5056 surgical patients and randomized them to a target core temperature of 37.0 °C or 35.5 °C [15]. The incidence of cardiovascular complications including Myocardial Injury after Noncardiac surgery (MINS) [16], cardiac arrest, or mortality was similar in both groups. Furthermore, intraoperative blood loss, need for transfusion, surgical site infections, and hospital readmission rate did not differ among the groups in this clinical trial [15]. These results therefore indicate that there is no evidence that mild hypothermia of about 35.5 °C throughout the surgery causes worse outcomes compared to patients who undergo an aggressive warming strategy (to maintain a core temperature of 37 °C). Consequently, targeting any core temperature above 35.5 °C appears to be sufficient.

Mild hypothermia (35–36 °C) seems to be of little clinical consequence, but moderate (< 35 °C) to severe hypothermia is undoubtedly worrisome. Most cellular functions and enzymatic activity are temperature dependent. Mild hypothermia prolongs actions of various drugs. By affecting drug metabolism, perioperative hypothermia is associated with delayed emergence from anesthesia and prolonged stay at the Post Anesthesia Care Unit (PACU). Hypothermia also provokes systemic responses, some of which are potentially

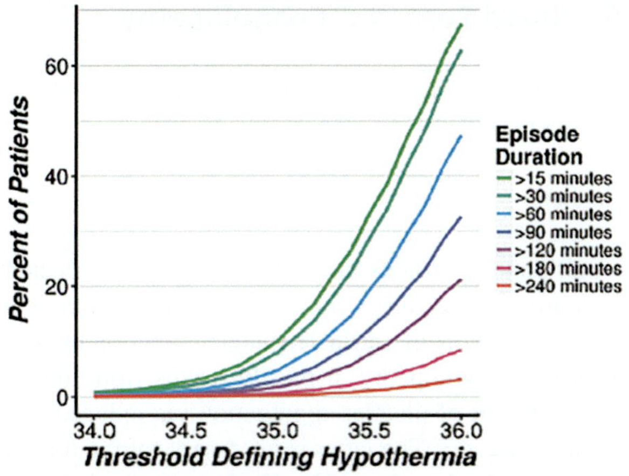

Fig. 20.6 Reproduced from Sun et al. [14]

harmful for the hypothermic patient. Hence, perioperative hypothermia significantly contributes to perioperative morbidity and mortality. Specifically, several randomized controlled trials have shown that moderate perioperative hypothermia (< 35 °C) causes impaired pharmacokinetics, surgical site infections, blood loss, coagulopathy, transfusion requirements, thermal discomfort, prolonged recovery, and prolonged duration of hospitalization.

20.3 Impaired Pharmacodynamics

a. Propofol and fentanyl

As plasma concentration of propofol and fentanyl is prolonged, clinicians should anticipate less requirements in hypothermic patients.

Propofol is one of the most commonly used intravenous anesthetics. A 3 °C decrease in core temperature results in an approximately 28% increase in plasmatic propofol concentration, largely because of the reduced hepatic blood flow [17]. However, mild hypothermia does not reduce propofol requirement during craniotomy surgery [18].

In a porcine model, the steady-state plasma concentration of fentanyl increased 5% per 1 °C drop of core temperature [19].

b. Muscle relaxants

Non-depolarizing muscle relaxants are markedly affected by perioperative hypothermia, resulting in a prolonged duration of action. Reasons include changes in volume of distribution, altered local diffusion receptor affinity, changes in pH at the neuromuscular junction, and the net effect of cooling on the various components of neuromuscular transmission.

The duration of action of vecuronium is approximately doubled in hypothermic surgical patients under nitrous oxide-isoflurane anesthesia [20]. Interestingly, hypothermia did not alter the clearance, maximum effect, or duration of action of neostigmine, when used as an antagonist of vecuronium [21].

Although atracurium appears to be not temperature sensitive, perioperative hypothermia prolongs the duration of action of atracurium by about 60% in patients that had a 3 °C core temperature decline [17].

Surprisingly, there is no difference in the recovery index (time for 25–75% twitch recovery) for both atracurium and vecuronium during normo- and hypothermia.

Rocuronium, another muscle relaxant, was reported to be affected in cardiac patients undergoing hypothermic cardiac bypass surgery [22]. Hypothermia led to a prolonged duration of action, reduced required maintenance doses, and altered plasma concentrations-response relationship of rocuronium. These effects were most likely a consequence of reduced plasma clearance during hypothermic cardiac bypass [11].

c. Volatile anesthetics

Anesthesia potency is driven by the steady-state plasma partial pressure opposed to the actual anesthetics concentration in the cells. Hypothermia increases the solubility of volatile anesthetics but does not appear to alter the potency [23]. However, the minimum alveolar concentration (MAC) is diminished, and thus, a lower amount of an inhalation agent is needed to prevent a reaction due to surgical stimulus. The MAC of halothane and isoflurane decreases by approximately 5% per 1°C drop of core temperature [24]. Simultaneously, in children, hypothermia decreases isoflurane requirements by 5.1% for every 1°C drop of core temperature [25].

20.4 Surgical Site Infections (SSI) and Complications (Wound Healing and Dehiscence)

Surgical site infections are the third leading cause of nosocomial infections overall, accounting for 14 to 16% of all hospital acquired infections, and the leading cause of nosocomial infections among surgical patients [26]. Considering all of the complications that may be triggered by anesthesia, surgical site infections are likely the most significant cause of morbidity. That's even greater than all other anesthetic complications combined. Perioperative hypothermia affects host defense against contamination via at least three mechanisms.

First, perioperative hypothermia triggers postoperative vasoconstriction to constrain metabolic heat to the core and speed rewarming. Vasoconstriction also reduces perfusion of wounded tissues. Hence, partial pressure of oxygen declines in tissues (even when blood is fully saturated). And, this is very important for the oxidative killing by neutrophils—the primary defense mechanism against bacterial, which mostly relays on the use of molecular oxygen [27].

Second, it reduces systemic immune activation, including T-cell-mediated antibody production and motility of key cells—including macrophages [28].

Third, vasoconstriction-induced tissue hypoxia impairs tissue healing and protein metabolism, which are important to prevent wound dehiscence and recontamination [29].

In a major landmark trial, 200 patients having colorectal surgery were randomized to routine (the standard of care in 1995) versus additional warming [30]. Surgical site infections were 3-fold (19% versus 6%) and duration of hospitalization was prolonged by 2.6 days in patients from the routine group (core temperature 34.7 °C ± 0.6 °C) compared to patients with additional warming (core temperature 36.6 °C ± 0.5 °C) (Fig. 20.7).

Surgical site infections increase postoperative hospitalization by an average of 4 days, resulting in an increased attributable cost of 8.000 USD to 25.000 USD for each patient, and are therefore a significant contributor to overall costs to the healthcare system [31].

As highlighted by the results of a review article, actively warming patients are highly beneficial to reduce the incidence of surgical site infections and associated complications (risk ratio RR 0.36, 95% confidence interval (CI) 0.2 to 0.66, $P = 0.0008$) [32].

20.5 Blood Loss and Coagulopathy

Perioperative hypothermia causes coagulopathy and consequently increases blood loss by several pathways:

a. Platelets

Although platelets counts are stable and are not affected by temperature, perioperative hypothermia affects function of platelets. Inhibition of intrinsic platelet function is not the cause of the coagulopathy; it mostly results from the reversible impairment of platelet aggregation via reduced release of thromboxane A3. The latter is necessary for the formation of an initial platelet plug [33]. Furthermore, perioperative hypothermia has been reported to induce morphological changes in platelets, and enhances their binding to fibrinogen, through the activation of GbIIb-IIa receptors.

b. Enzymes of the coagulation cascade

In addition, perioperative hypothermia impairs the function of several enzymes of the coagulation cascade and reduces clot formation. This is especially important, as this is frequently missed in the clinical setting, as coagulation laboratory studies including prothrombin time (PT) and partial thromboplastin time (PTT) are usually performed at a temperature of 37 °C, rather than the patient's actual *in-vivo* temperature [34]. These tests will be prolonged of up to 10%, if the testing is done at the actual patient's temperature (instead of 37 °C). However, it remains questionable if this prolongation is clinically relevant.

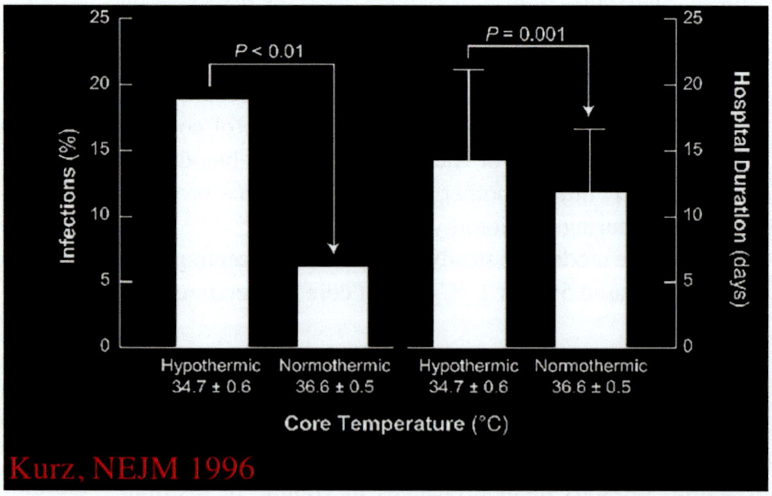

Fig. 20.7 Reproduced from Kurz et al. [30]

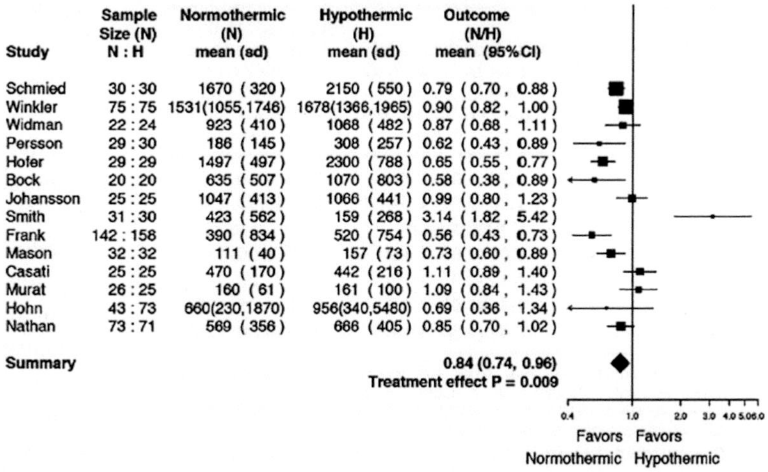

Fig. 20.8 From Rajagopalan et al. [36]

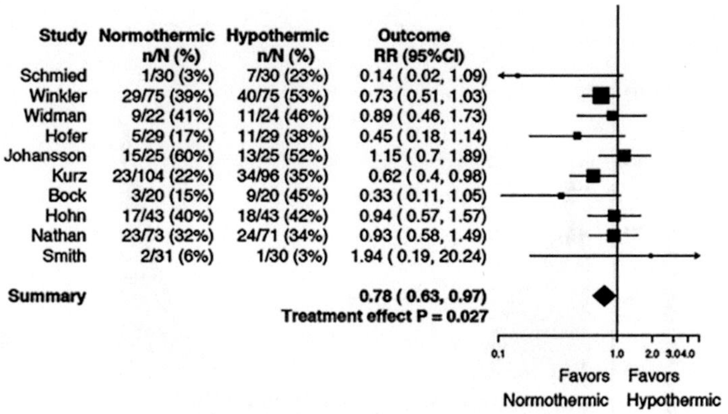

Fig. 20.9 From Rajagopalan et al. 36

c. Fibrinolysis

Generally, the fibrinolytic system regulates the balance between formation of hemostatic plugs and restoration of blood flow after clot formation [33]. Excessive fibrinolysis predisposes patients to hemorrhage, while inadequate fibrinolysis predisposes patients to thrombosis.

The most important structural element in formed clots is fibrin, but is subject to degradation by plasmin, which represents the activated form of plasminogen. Therefore, activation of plasminogen and conversion to plasmin represents the core step of the fibrinolytic system and is mostly mediated by tissue-type plasminogen. Findings of several studies suggest that fibrinolysis is not affected by mild perioperative hypothermia, while *hyper*thermia intensively affects fibrinolysis. As a conclusion, this might result in the assumption, that hypothermia-induced coagulopathy does not result from excessive clot lysis. Data from thromboelastogram (TEG) suggest that hypothermia impairs clot formation, rather than facilitating clot degeneration.

Although there are many divergent results from several retrospective studies, two randomized trials confirmed that a drop of only approximately 0.5 °C in core temperature increases the blood loss by 200–300 ml in patients undergoing hip arthroplasty [35].

A comprehensive meta-analysis included 14 studies to assess blood loss and 10 studies to assess transfusion requirements [36]. It showed that even mild hypothermia (<1) significantly increased operative blood loss by approximately estimated 16% (95% CI 4%, 26%) (Fig. 20.8), and increased the risk for transfusion by approximately 22% (95% CI 3, 37%) (Fig. 20.9).

20.6 Transfusion Requirement

There is no linear relationship between blood loss and transfusion requirements. Blood transfusion was thought to be safe for decades (besides the risk of HIV and hepatitis C), but now, we know that blood transfusion is more toxic than previously believed. Data of the before-mentioned meta-analysis by Rajagopalan et al. reported that mild hypothermia increased the relative risk for transfusion by approximately 22% (95% CI, 3–37%).

In a retrospective study performed at the Cleveland Clinic, about 4.6% of all patients were receiving a blood transfusion [14]. Based on a multivariable logistic regression

Area under 37°C (degree-hours)	Adjusted* Odds Ratio (Pointwise 95% CI) for Intraoperative Erythrocyte Transfusion (N = 45,866)	Adjusted* Ratio of Geometric Mean Duration of Hospitalization (Pointwise 95% CI) (N = 39,180)
0.25	1.34 (1.04, 1.73)	0.96 (0.90, 1.03)
0.50	1.10 (0.98, 1.24)	0.97 (0.93, 1.01)
1.00	(Reference)	(Reference)
2.00	1.00 (0.89, 1.13)	1.03 (1.00, 1.05)
4.00	1.12 (0.91, 1.39)	1.06 (1.03, 1.09)
8.00	1.41 (1.08, 1.84)	1.05 (1.01, 1.10)
16.00	2.02 (1.30, 3.14)	0.96 (0.86, 1.08)

*Estimates adjusted for year, type, and duration of surgery, body mass index, age, preoperative platelet count, preoperative hemoglobin, estimated blood loss, and individual anesthesiologist, as well as the Elixhauser comorbidities, which are listed in table 1.
CI = confidence interval.

Fig. 20.10 From Sun et al. [14]

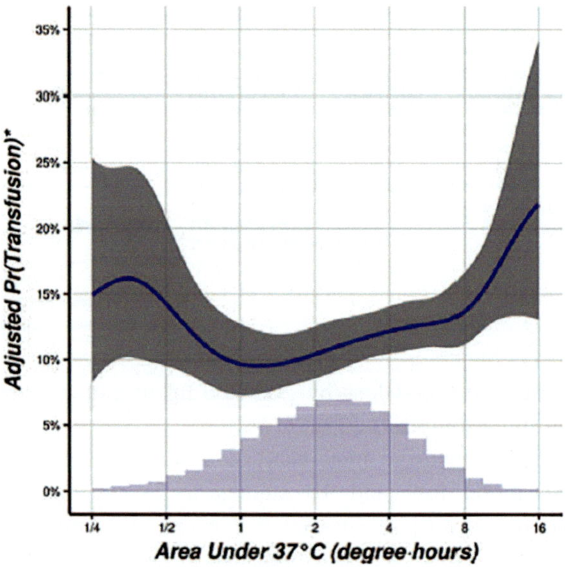

Fig. 20.11 From Sun et al. [3]

model, the authors found a significant association between core temperature < 37 °C and risk of having a transfusion (Fig. 20.10). The odds ratios relative to a reference value of 1 °C are presented in the Fig. 20.7.

Generally, the risk of transfusion significantly increases as a function of duration and dimension of perioperative hypothermia.

Figure 20.11 displays the adjusted probability of transfusion estimate versus the integrated area above the core temperature versus time curve and < 37 °C. The shaded regions represent pointwise 95% confidence intervals.

20.7 Shivering

Shivering is an autonomic thermoregulatory response, defined as rhythmic involuntary muscular activity. The ultimate goal of shivering is producing heat to restore normothermia.

Intraoperative shivering is rare, as most patients receive muscle relaxants and the shivering threshold is significantly reduced by anesthetic agents; only patients having serious hypothermia hit this threshold.

In contrast, postoperative shivering in hypothermic patients is common. Shivering intends to produce heat. However, thermoregulatory major muscular activity must be distinguished from low-intensity shivering-like muscular activity, which is common in patients in pain [37]. On average, postoperative shivering increases oxygen consumption by approximately 40% [38]. It seems to be evident that the increase of oxygen consumption might cause cardiac demand-ischemic complications—although not proven by any clinical study yet. Shivering is extremely uncomfortable for the patients and can be effectively treated by a variety of medication, including pethidine, clonidine, dexmedetomidine, and ketamine, by presumably lowering the shivering threshold as the assumed mechanism.

20.8 Thermal Discomfort and Anxiety

Thermal discomfort is a predictable and common consequence of postoperative hypothermia. Even mild hypothermia causes postoperative thermal discomfort and is therefore a significant source of patients' dissatisfaction [23]. Patients often identify that experiencing cold during the postoperative period was the worst part of their hospitalization, and sometimes even worse than surgical pain. Thermal discomfort is also stressful for the patients and it is reported to lead to higher blood pressure, heart rate, and plasma catecholamine concentrations [38]. Active warming improves thermal comfort in hypothermic patients, but prevention of postoperative hypothermia is clearly the preferable management strategy.

20.9 Cardiac Complications

Among the major complications of hypothermia, myocardial outcomes are least well established. An observational analysis suggested an association between Surgical Care Improvement Project-10 (SCIP-10) compliance and temperature and cardiovascular outcomes [10]. A single-center randomized trial of 300 patients evaluated cardiac outcomes, but unfortunately offers little insight of hypothermia-associated morbid cardiac complications [39]. This trial is limited by the inadequate small sample size, as only two hypothermic patients had a cardiac arrest and one had a myocardial infarction *versus* none in the normothermic group (36.7 °C). Ten hypothermic patients experienced cardiovascular events *versus* two normothermic patients. These fragile results, based on fewer than ten outcome events, are nearly as likely to be wrong as right, and a poor basis for health policy [40]. An additional limitation is that diagnosis was primarily based on Holter ECG findings rather than troponin concentrations, which are much more sensitive. Consequently, the overall myocardial infarction rate was < 1%, where the true rate of major cardiac events is about 13% in vascular surgery patients [41]. Another clinical trial included 100 surgical patients undergoing repair of infrarenal aortic aneurysms or aortoiliac occlusive disease [42]. Authors concluded that normothermia is protective for infrarenal aortic patients, but these findings are again only based on a few myocardial outcomes. Most recently, a large multicenter randomized controlled trial enrolled more than 5000 surgical patients, but reported no evidence that mild hypothermia (35.5 °C) causes any elevated risk of postoperative cardiac complications if compared to normothermic patients (37 °C) [15]. There, thus, remains considerable doubt as to the true effect of moderate to severe (< 35 °C) hypothermia on cardiovascular outcomes. However, mild hypothermia (> 35.5 °C) appears to be safe.

20.10 Delayed Discharge from the PACU

It may not be surprising that perioperative hypothermia is associated with delayed discharge from the Post Anesthesia Care Unit (PACU). In a randomized trial, Lenhardt et al. randomly assigned 150 patients undergoing elective major abdominal surgery to normothermia or hypothermia during anesthesia and assessed length of stay in the PACU, until reaching a sustained score of ≥ 13 [43]. The ability to discharge was based on modification of the Aldrete and Kroulik scoring system [44]. The score is based on activity,

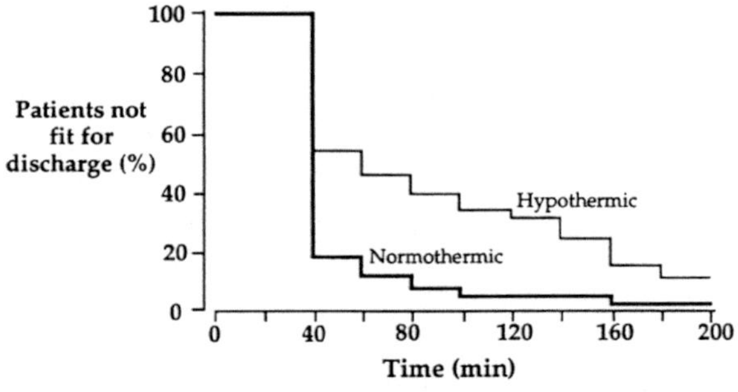

Fig. 20.12 From: Lenhardt et al. [43]

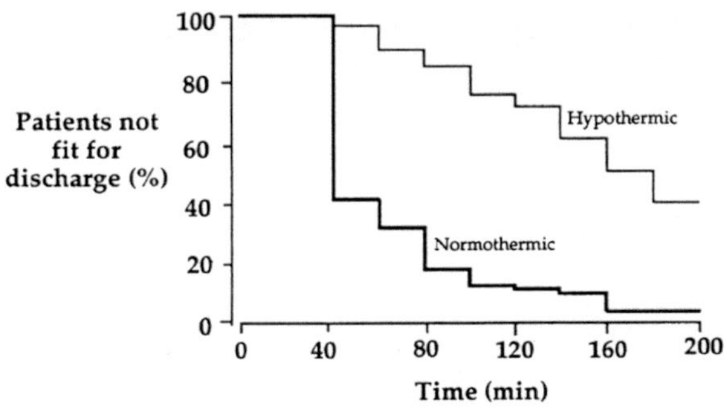

Fig. 20.13 From: Lenhardt et al. [43]

ventilation, consciousness, and hemodynamic responses; 0, 1, or 2 points were assigned for each of eight responses. In this study, hypothermic patients required about 40 min longer than normothermic patients to reach a sustained score ≥ 13, the defined criterion for discharge. Core temperature in the hypothermic patients required 134 ± 60 min to reach 36 °C (Figs. 20.12 and 20.13). Consequently, hypothermic patients required about 90 min longer than the normothermic ones to reach both a sustained score ≥ 13 and a core temperature > 36 °C ($P < 0.001$).

Kaplan–Meier "survival" analysis showing the percentage of patients not sustaining a recovery score ≥ 13. The probability value, using a Wilcoxon analysis, was < 0.0001.

Kaplan–Meier "survival" analysis showing the percentage of patients not sustaining a recovery score ≥ 13 and a core temperature ≥ 36 °C. The probability value, using a Wilcoxon analysis, was ≤ 0.0001 [43].

20.11 Prolonged Hospitalization

Moderate to severe hypothermia causes up to 3-fold higher incidence (6% versus 19% in patients having colorectal surgery) of surgical site infections [30]. It seems to be obvious that corresponding hospitalization in patient having a surgical site infection is prolonged. Interestingly, the important effect of prolongation of hospitalization is present in both all hypothermic (12.1 ± 4.4 versus 14.7 ± 6.5 days) and in infected hypothermic (11.8 ± 4.1 versus 13.5 ± 4.5 days) patients [30]. Therefore, perioperative hypothermia *per se* (beside the higher risk of having a surgical site infection) prolongs hospitalization (Fig. 20.14).

As is consistent with a delay in clinical healing, sutures were removed significantly later and the deposition of collagen (an index of scar formation and the strength of the healing wound) was significantly less in the hypothermia group than in the normothermia group (Fig. 20.11). Furthermore, that the patients assigned to hypothermia required significantly more time before they could tolerate solid food is also consistent with impaired healing.

Table 2. Postoperative Findings in the Two Study Groups.*

Variable	Normothermia (N= 104)	Hypothermia (N=96)	P Value
All patients			
Infection — no. of patients (%)	6 (6)	18 (19)	0.009
ASEPSIS score	7±10	13±16	0.002
Collagen deposition — μg/cm	328±135	254±114	0.04
Days to first solid food	5.6±2.5	6.5±2.0	0.006
Days to suture removal	9.8±2.9	10.9±1.9	0.002
Days of hospitalization	12.1±4.4	14.7±6.5	0.001
Uninfected patients			
No. of patients	98	78	
Days to first solid food	5.2±1.6	6.1±1.6	<0.001
Days to suture removal	9.6±2.6	10.6±1.6	0.003
Days of hospitalization	11.8±4.1	13.5±4.5	0.01

*Plus–minus values are means ± SD.

Fig. 20.14 From Kurz et al. [30]

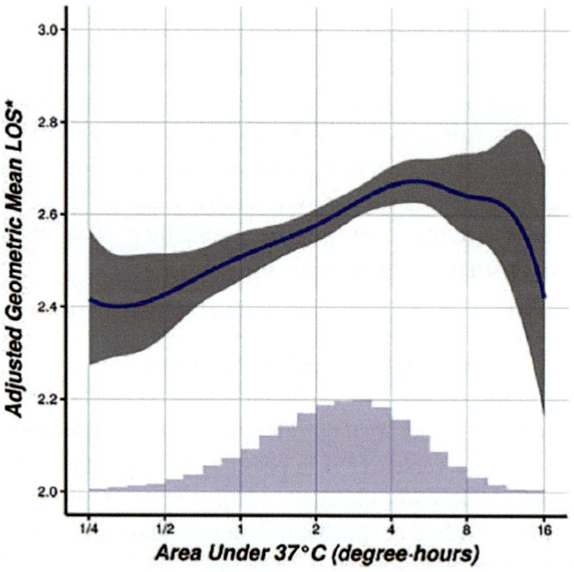

Fig. 20.15 From Sun et al. [14]

In another study consisting of 39,180 patients, Sun et al., reported a significant association between area < 37 °C core temperature threshold and geometric mean duration of hospitalization (Fig. 20.15).

Estimates of geometric mean duration of hospitalization in days versus integrated area above the core temperature versus time curve and < 37 °C core temperature. The shaded regions represent pointwise 95% confidence intervals.

Prolongation of hospitalization is an important concern, especially as healthcare-related costs tend to rise sharply. Even extremely cautious assessments of costs per in-hospital day of 1.000–2.000 USD represent increased overall costs of about 2.000 USD in every single patient experiencing perioperative hypothermia.

20.12 Strategies for Maintaining Normothermia During Anesthesia

a. Measurement of central core temperature

Measurement and continuous monitoring of central core temperature in all patients having noncardiac surgery under general anesthesia exceeding 30 minutes is essential. Core temperature can be reliably monitored on four different sites: [1]

- the pulmonary artery,
- nasopharynx with the probe inserted for 10–20 cm,
- distal esophagus,
- and tympanic membrane with a contact thermistor or thermocouple.

The temperatures measured at these four sites do not vary more than a couple of tenths of 1 °C and therefore, even a single measurement gives a reliable estimation of the actual core temperature [1]. Clinical decision-making should focus on central core temperatures only and shall not be based on peripheral including skin temperature.

b. Pre-warming

Core temperature drops during the initial hour of anesthesia, which is based on the principle of re-distribution (see above). The re-distribution effect might be partially attenuated by pre-warming the patients. It is important to understand that pre-warming does not increase patient's core temperature, but increases the temperature of the peripheral tissues and therefore decreases the amount of re-distribution hypothermia. Consequently, pre-warming alone does not prevent from perioperative hypothermia, but does reduce the drop of temperature during the initial period of anesthesia. Typically, the core temperature in pre-warmed patients stays about 0.42 °C (95% CI, 0.27–0.57) warmer compared to non-pre-warmed patients [45]. Giving the limited effect on core temperature, but high organizational effort, routine pre-warming should not be considered for all surgical patients and should be limited to patients at high risk for perioperative hypothermia.

c. Perioperative Warming Devices

Various perioperative warming devices are available and can be divided into 1. Passive insulation and 2. Active warming devices of the skin surface, fluids, inspired and peritoneal gases, and endovascular heat exchangers.

I. **Passive Insulation**: a single layer of passive insulation reduces cutaneous heat loss by 30%. However, it's essential to determine that the layer does not actively transfer heat into the body, even by adding several additional layers of insulation [46]. Consequently, passive insulation can decrease heat loss but will not add any benefit in maintenance of perioperative normothermia [1].

II. **Active Skin Warming**: Convective warming of the skin with forced air is by far the most frequently used and effective perioperative warming device. Forced-air warming is especially attractive, as it is easy to use, inexpensive, and for most patients and surgery, has a pretty good cost/benefit ratio. In order to achieve the highest effectiveness, the forced-air blankets should be directly placed on the patient's skin and should cover as much as possible. Alternate approach is conductive warming using resistive heating or circulating water [47, 48].

   a. **Fluid warming** is not efficient, as the temperature of the infusion can only slightly exceed core temperature (usually not warmer than 38–39 °C). Consequently, active rewarming of the patient is basically impossible unless very large amounts of fluids are given over a short period of time. The most important effect of fluid warming is decreasing the amount of heat loss. For example, one liter of crystalloid given at room temperature decreases core temperature by 0.25 °C. Equally, one unit of blood from the refrigerator decreases core temperature by 0.25 °C. In clinical practice, fluid warming should be considered if cold blood products are being transfused or large amounts of fluids are administered.
   b. **Warming inspired and peritoneal gases:** Warming patients by warming inhaled air is insufficient, as the heat capacity of air is low. Only a marginal amount of heat is lost via the respiratory system. Warming and humidification of insufflated carbon dioxide during laparoscopic procedures are comparably inefficient and unable to transfer considerable amount of heat into the human patient, although it was shown to be beneficial in a swine model [49, 50].
   c. **Vascular heat exchange catheters** transfer much more heat compared to skin warming devices. On the other hand, heat exchange catheters are quite expensive, and placement is invasive. Thus, their use is mostly restricted to patients requiring a rapid onset of hypothermia, for example, after distinct accidental hypothermia [1].

20.13 Summary

Perioperative hypothermia is common and significantly affects perioperative morbidity and mortality. Perioperative hypothermia causes impaired pharmacodynamics, surgical site infections, blood loss and coagulopathy, transfusion requirements, thermal discomfort, prolonged recovery, and prolonged duration of hospitalization.

Maintaining or restoration of normothermia/slight hypothermia ($\geq$ 35.5 ºC) is essential in all surgical patients and can be effectively achieved by consequent (re-) warming during surgery. Core temperature should be measured in all patients having general or regional anesthesia lasting more than 30 minutes.

Important points:

- Perioperative hypothermia is common in all surgical patients under general and regional anesthesia.
- Perioperative hypothermia is a significant contributor to morbidity and mortality.
- Maintaining a core temperature $\geq$ 35.5 ºC throughout appears to be sufficient.
- Core temperature should be measured in all surgical patients undergoing surgery exceeding 30 minutes.

20.14 Question and answers

1. Question: Perioperative hypothermia is broadly defined as a body core temperature
   a. Any temperature below 35.5 °C
   b. Any temperature below 36 °C
   c. Any temperature below 36.5 °C.

Comment: b. Hypothermia is usually defined as any body cire temperature below 36 °C.

2. Question: Regarding the "re-distribution" effect:
   a. Causes a redistribution of "warm" blood from the peripheral compartment to the "cold" central core compartment
   b. Causes a decrease of the body core temperature, usually within the first 60-90 minutes
   c. Can be avoided by adequate pre-warming.

Comment: **b**. The re-distribution effect causes a redistribution of cold blood from the peripheral compartment to the warm central core compartment. The effect is usually limited to the first 60-90 minutes, and cannot be avoided (but limited to some extent) by pre-warming.

3. Question: The "normal" body core temperature
   a. Follows a circadian rhythm
   b. Ranges between 35 °C and 37 °C
   c. Is usually 36 °C.

Comment: **a**. The normal body core temperature follows a circadian rhythm and usually ranges between 36 °C and 37 °C. A temperature of 36 °C is therefore never considered to be the optimal body core temperature,

4. Question: Intraoperative hypothermia
   a. Is associated with prolonged hospitalization
   b. Does not affect the incidence of surgical site infections
   c. Is associated with coagulopathy, but not with higher transfusion requirements.

Comment: **a**. Intraoperative hypothermia is associated with elevated morbidity, including higher incidence of surgical site infections, coagulopathy and increased transfusion requirements, and prolonged hospitalization.

5. Question: according to a recent major RCT
   a. Maintaining a body core temperature $\geq$ 35.0 °C is sufficient to avoid cardiac complications including MINS
   b. Maintaining a body core temperature $\geq$ 35.5 °C is sufficient to avoid cardiac complications including MINS
   c. Maintaining a body core temperature $\geq$ 36.0 °C is sufficient to avoid cardiac complications including MINS.

Comment: **b**. Results of the large RCT indicate, that maintaining a body core temperature $\geq$ 35.5 °C is sufficient to avoid cardiac complications including MINS. Traditionally, maintaining a temperature of $\geq$ 36 °C was considered to the optimal temperature goal.

6. Question: Effective strategies for (re)warming include
   a. Passive insulation
   b. Warming inspired and peritoneal gases
   c. Vascular heat exchange catheters.

Comment: **c**. Passive insulation does not help to rewarm a patient but does help to prevent heat loss. Warming inspired and peritoneal gases was reported to be insufficient. Vascular heat exchange catheters are highly efficient, but use is limited by the high costs and invasive nature.

7. Question: The body core temperature can be reliably measured in
   a. Pulmonary artery
   b. Urine bladder
   c. Axilla.

Comment: **a**. The body core temperature can be reliably measured in the pulmonary artery, distal esophagus, nasopharynx with the probe inserted 10 to 20 cm, and the tympanic membrane if measured with a contact thermistor or thermocouple. Measuring in the urine bladder is not reliable, as this technique critically depends of amount of urine. Measuring the temperature in the axilla is not reliable to measure the body core temperature.

8. Question: Intraoperative hypothermia is common and affects
   a. < 20 % of surgical patients.
   b. Between 20 and 70% of surgical patients.
   c. Only patients having surgery under general anesthesia.

Comment: **b**. Intraoperative hypothermia affects between 20 and 70 % of all surgical patients, no matter if under general and/or regional anesthesia.

9. Question: Non-depolarizing muscle relaxants are affected by intraoperative hypothermia
   a. Resulting in a shortened duration of action
   b. Resulting in a prolonged duration of action
   c. Resulting in inability toa adequately paralyze patients.

Comment: **b**. Hypothermia results in a un-predictable, prolonged duration of action of non-depolarizing muscle relaxants. Adequate dosing of neuromuscular agents is therefore more challenging.

10. Question:Shivering
    a. Primarily affects patients with postoperative hypothermia
    b. Is an autonomic response, caused by inhalative agents
    c. Is limited to the postoperative period only.

Comments: a. Postoperative shivering is an autonomic response with the intent to produce heat and ultimately increase body core temperature. Although shivering *in* *theory* is not limited to the postoperative period only, it is severely diminished/ non-existent during anesthesia by lowering the intertreshold range (ITR) and paralytic effects of anesthetics. Shivering primarily affects patients with postoperative hypothermia, independent of anesthetics used.

References

1. Sessler DI. Perioperative thermoregulation and heat balance. Lancet. 2016;387(10038):2655–64. https://doi.org/10.1016/S0140-6736(15)00981-2.
2. Feketa VV, Zhang Y, Cao Z, et al. Transient receptor potential melastatin 8 channel inhibition potentiates the hypothermic response to transient receptor potential vanilloid 1 activation in the conscious mouse. Crit Care Med. 2014;42(5):e355–63. https://doi.org/10.1097/CCM.0000000000000229.
3. Nadel ER, Stolwijk JA. Sweat gland response to the efferent thermoregulatory signal. Arch Sci Physiol (Paris). 1973;27(2):67–77.
4. Hales JR, Jessen C, Fawcett AA, King RB. Skin AVA and capillary dilatation and constriction induced by local skin heating. Pflugers Arch. 1985;404(3):203–7. https://doi.org/10.1007/BF00581240.
5. De Witte J, Sessler DI. Perioperative shivering: physiology and pharmacology. Anesthesiology. 2002;96(2):467–84. https://doi.org/10.1097/00000542-200202000-00036.
6. Affourtit C, Crichton PG, Parker N, Brand MD. Novel uncoupling proteins. Novartis Found Symp. 2007;287:70–80; discussion 80–91.
7. Eyolfson DA, Tikuisis P, Xu X, Weseen G, Giesbrecht GG. Measurement and prediction of peak shivering intensity in humans. Eur J Appl Physiol. 2001;84(1–2):100–6. https://doi.org/10.1007/s004210000329.
8. Lopez M, Sessler DI, Walter K, Emerick T, Ozaki M. Rate and gender dependence of the sweating, vasoconstriction, and shivering thresholds in humans. Anesthesiology. 1994;80(4):780–8. https://doi.org/10.1097/00000542-199404000-00009.
9. Sessler DI, Lee KA, McGuire J. Isoflurane anesthesia and circadian temperature cycles in humans. Anesthesiology. 1991;75(6):985–9. https://doi.org/10.1097/00000542-199112000-00010.
10. Scott AV, Stonemetz JL, Wasey JO, et al. Compliance with surgical care improvement project for body temperature management (scip inf-10) is associated with improved clinical outcomes. Anesthesiology. 2015;123(1):116–25. https://doi.org/10.1097/ALN.0000000000000681.
11. Annadata R, Sessler DI, Tayefeh F, Kurz A, Dechert M. Desflurane slightly increases the sweating threshold but produces marked, nonlinear decreases in the vasoconstriction and shivering thresholds. Anesthesiology. 1995;83(6):1205–11. https://doi.org/10.1097/00000542-199512000-00011.
12. Kurz A, Go JC, Sessler DI, Kaer K, Larson MD, Bjorksten AR. Alfentanil slightly increases the sweating threshold and markedly reduces the vasoconstriction and shivering thresholds. Anesthesiology. 1995;83(2):293–9. https://doi.org/10.1097/00000542-199508000-00009.
13. Talke P, Tayefeh F, Sessler DI, Jeffrey R, Noursalehi M, Richardson C. Dexmedetomidine does not alter the sweating threshold, but comparably and linearly decreases the vasoconstriction and shivering thresholds. Anesthesiology. 1997;87(4):835–41. https://doi.org/10.1097/00000542-199710000-00017.
14. Sun Z, Honar H, Sessler DI, et al. Intraoperative core temperature patterns, transfusion requirement, and hospital duration in patients warmed with forced air. Anesthesiology. 2015;122(2):276–85. https://doi.org/10.1097/ALN.0000000000000551.
15. Sessler DI, Pei L, Li K, et al. Aggressive intraoperative warming versus routine thermal management during non-cardiac surgery (PROTECT): a multicentre, parallel group, superiority trial. Lancet. 2022;399(10337):1799–808. https://doi.org/10.1016/S0140-6736(22)00560-8.
16. Ruetzler K, Smilowitz NR, Berger JS, et al. Diagnosis and management of patients with myocardial injury after noncardiac surgery: a scientific statement from the american heart association. Circulation. 2021;144(19):e287–305. https://doi.org/10.1161/CIR.0000000000001024.
17. Leslie K, Sessler DI, Bjorksten AR, Moayeri A. Mild hypothermia alters propofol pharmacokinetics and increases the duration of action of atracurium. Anesth Analg. 1995;80(5):1007–14. https://doi.org/10.1097/00000539-199505000-00027.
18. Leslie K, Bjorksten AR, Ugoni A, Mitchell P. Mild core hypothermia and anesthetic requirement for loss of responsiveness during propofol anesthesia for craniotomy. *Anesth Analg*. 2002;94(5):1298–303. https://doi.org/10.1097/00000539-200205000-00045
19. Fritz HG, Holzmayr M, Walter B, Moeritz KU, Lupp A, Bauer R. The effect of mild hypothermia on plasma fentanyl concentration and biotransformation in juvenile pigs. Anesth Analg. 2005;100(4):996–1002. https://doi.org/10.1213/01.ANE.0000146517.17910.54.
20. Heier T, Caldwell JE, Sessler DI, Miller RD. Mild intraoperative hypothermia increases duration of action and spontaneous recovery of vecuronium blockade during nitrous oxide-isoflurane anesthesia in humans. Anesthesiology. 1991;74(5):815–9. https://doi.org/10.1097/00000542-199105000-00003.
21. Heier T, Clough D, Wright PM, Sharma ML, Sessler DI, Caldwell JE. The influence of mild hypothermia on the pharmacokinetics and time course of action of neostigmine in anesthetized volunteers. Anesthesiology. 2002;97(1):90–5. https://doi.org/10.1097/00000542-200207000-00013.
22. Smeulers NJ, Wierda JM, van den Broek L, Gallandat Huet RC, Hennis PJ. Effects of hypothermic cardiopulmonary bypass on the pharmacodynamics and pharmacokinetics of rocuronium. J Cardiothorac Vasc Anesth. 1995;9(6):700–5. https://doi.org/10.1016/s1053-0770(05)80232-0
23. Reynolds L, Beckmann J, Kurz A. Perioperative complications of hypothermia. Best Pract Res Clin Anaesthesiol. 2008;22(4):645–57. https://doi.org/10.1016/j.bpa.2008.07.005.
24. Eger EI, Johnson BH. MAC of I-653 in rats, including a test of the effect of body temperature and anesthetic duration. Anesth Analg. 1987;66(10):974–6.
25. Liu M, Hu X, Liu J. The effect of hypothermia on isoflurane MAC in children. Anesthesiology. 2001;94(3):429–32. https://doi.org/10.1097/00000542-200103000-00011.
26. Esnaola NF, Cole DJ. Perioperative normothermia during major surgery: is it important? Adv Surg. 2011;45:249–63. https://doi.org/10.1016/j.yasu.2011.03.007.
27. Allen DB, Maguire JJ, Mahdavian M, et al. Wound hypoxia and acidosis limit neutrophil bacterial killing mechanisms. Arch Surg. 1997;132(9):991–6. https://doi.org/10.1001/archsurg.1997.01430330057009.
28. Jonsson K, Hunt TK, Mathes SJ. Oxygen as an isolated variable influences resistance to infection. Ann Surg. 1988;208(6):783–7. https://doi.org/10.1097/00000658-198812000-00018.
29. Carli F, Emery PW, Freemantle CA. Effect of peroperative normothermia on postoperative protein metabolism in elderly patients undergoing hip arthroplasty. Br J Anaesth. 1989;63(3):276–82. https://doi.org/10.1093/bja/63.3.276.

30. Kurz A, Sessler DI, Lenhardt R. Perioperative normothermia to reduce the incidence of surgical-wound infection and shorten hospitalization. Study of Wound Infection and Temperature Group. N Engl J Med. 9 1996;334(19):1209–15. https://doi.org/10.1056/NEJM199605093341901
31. Hart SR, Bordes B, Hart J, Corsino D, Harmon D. Unintended perioperative hypothermia. Ochsner J Fall. 2011;11(3):259–70.
32. Madrid E, Urrutia G, Roque i Figuls M, et al. Active body surface warming systems for preventing complications caused by inadvertent perioperative hypothermia in adults. Cochrane Database Syst Rev. Apr 21 2016;4(4):CD009016. https://doi.org/10.1002/14651858.CD009016.pub2
33. Valeri CR, Khabbaz K, Khuri SF, et al. Effect of skin temperature on platelet function in patients undergoing extracorporeal bypass. J Thorac Cardiovasc Surg. 1992;104(1):108–16.
34. Rohrer MJ, Natale AM. Effect of hypothermia on the coagulation cascade. Crit Care Med. 1992;20(10):1402–5. https://doi.org/10.1097/00003246-199210000-00007.
35. Winkler M, Akca O, Birkenberg B, et al. Aggressive warming reduces blood loss during hip arthroplasty. Anesth Analg. 2000;91(4):978–84. https://doi.org/10.1097/00000539-200010000-00039.
36. Rajagopalan S, Mascha E, Na J, Sessler DI. The effects of mild perioperative hypothermia on blood loss and transfusion requirement. Anesthesiology. 2008;108(1):71–7. https://doi.org/10.1097/01.anes.0000296719.73450.52.
37. Horn EP, Schroeder F, Wilhelm S, et al. Postoperative pain facilitates nonthermoregulatory tremor. Anesthesiology. 1999;91(4):979–84. https://doi.org/10.1097/00000542-199910000-00017.
38. Frank SM, Fleisher LA, Olson KF, et al. Multivariate determinants of early postoperative oxygen consumption in elderly patients. Effects of shivering, body temperature, and gender. Anesthesiology. 1995;83(2):241–9. https://doi.org/10.1097/00000542-199508000-00002
39. Frank SM, Fleisher LA, Breslow MJ, et al. Perioperative maintenance of normothermia reduces the incidence of morbid cardiac events a randomized clinical trial. JAMA. 1997;277(14):1127–34.
40. Ioannidis JP. Contradicted and initially stronger effects in highly cited clinical research. JAMA. 2005;294(2):218–28. https://doi.org/10.1001/jama.294.2.218.
41. Gualandro DM, Puelacher C, LuratiBuse G, et al. Prediction of major cardiac events after vascular surgery. J Vasc Surg. 2017;66(6):1826–35. https://doi.org/10.1016/j.jvs.2017.05.100
42. Elmore JR, Franklin DP, Youkey JR, Oren JW, Frey CM. Normothermia is protective during infrarenal aortic surgery. J Vasc Surg. 1998;28(6):984–92; discussion 992–4. https://doi.org/10.1016/s0741-5214(98)70024-2
43. Lenhardt R, Marker E, Goll V, et al. Mild intraoperative hypothermia prolongs postanesthetic recovery. Anesthesiology. 1997;87(6):1318–23. https://doi.org/10.1097/00000542-199712000-00009.
44. Aldrete JA, Kroulik D. A postanesthetic recovery score. Anesth Analg. 1970;49(6):924–34.
45. Akhtar Z, Hesler BD, Fiffick AN, et al. A randomized trial of prewarming on patient satisfaction and thermal comfort in outpatient surgery. J Clin Anesth. 2016;33:376–85. https://doi.org/10.1016/j.jclinane.2016.04.041.
46. Sessler DI, Schroeder M. Heat loss in humans covered with cotton hospital blankets. Anesth Analg. 1993;77(1):73–7. https://doi.org/10.1213/00000539-199307000-00014.
47. Ruetzler K, Kovaci B, Guloglu E, et al. Forced-air and a novel patient-warming system (vitalHEAT vH2) comparably maintain normothermia during open abdominal surgery. Anesth Analg. 2011;112(3):608–14. https://doi.org/10.1213/ANE.0b013e3181e7cc20.
48. Hasegawa K, Negishi C, Nakagawa F, Ozaki M. Core temperatures during major abdominal surgery in patients warmed with new circulating-water garment, forced-air warming, or carbon-fiber resistive-heating system. J Anesth. 2012;26(2):168–73. https://doi.org/10.1007/s00540-011-1306-1.
49. Sammour T, Kahokehr A, Hayes J, Hulme-Moir M, Hill AG. Warming and humidification of insufflation carbon dioxide in laparoscopic colonic surgery: a double-blinded randomized controlled trial. Ann Surg. 2010;251(6):1024–33. https://doi.org/10.1097/SLA.0b013e3181d77a25.
50. Noll E, Diemunsch S, Pottecher J, et al. Prevention of laparoscopic surgery induced hypothermia with warmed humidified insufflation: is the experimental combination of a warming blanket synergistic? PLoS ONE. 2018;13(7): e0199369. https://doi.org/10.1371/journal.pone.0199369.

Gastrointestinal/Hepatic Physiology

21

Allen Keebler

Abstract

Gastrointestinal (GI) physiology is a branch of human physiology addressing the physical function of the gastrointestinal system. The major processes occurring in the GI system are that of motility, secretion, regulation, digestion, and circulation. In anesthesiology, gastric emptying and the time from last oral intake (NPO status) become important. During the induction of anesthesia, the patient with a full stomach is at increased risk for gastric regurgitation and pulmonary aspiration, which can be lethal.

Keywords

Gastrointestinal physiology • Motility • Gastric emptying • Secretion • Ions • Digestive enzymes • Mucus • Bile • Hormones • Hepatic physiology • Liver • Blood supply • Bile flow • Coagulation • Protein synthesis • Lipid synthesis • Metabolic function • Immunologic function • Drug metabolism

Key Points

1. The liver produces both pro-coagulation and anticoagulation factors. Thus, the liver plays a major role in maintaining the balance within the coagulation system. With liver disease both are reduced, and homeostasis may often be seen even in the presence of abnormal laboratory tests.
2. The liver synthesizes thrombopoietin, which stimulates platelet production. A reduction in this hormone seen in liver disease is a major cause of thrombocytopenia.
3. The liver has a unique blood supply in that only 25% of the blood supply comes from the oxygen-rich hepatic artery. Roughly 75% of the blood supply comes from the relatively oxygen-poor portal venous system. This means that roughly 50% of the oxygen supply comes from arterial flow and 50% from venous flow.
4. The liver usually has four lobes. These are the left, right, caudate, and quadrate lobes. This anatomic distinction has little impact on surgical dissection. The liver can be divided into 8 segments each with its own blood supply and venous and biliary drainage. These are known as Couinaud segments and can facilitate relatively bloodless surgery.
5. Traditional liver function tests are a measure of hepatocyte injury not liver function. Liver function may remain normal in the setting of elevation of these lab values. To understand how well the liver is functioning, one should evaluate the synthetic function of the liver by checking lab values that are known to be affected in liver disease, such as serum albumin levels, platelet count, and coagulation parameters.

21.1 Gastrointestinal Physiology

Gastrointestinal (GI) physiology is a branch of human physiology addressing the physical function of the gastrointestinal system. The major processes occurring in the GI system are that of motility, secretion, regulation, digestion, and circulation. The function and coordination of each of these actions is vital in maintaining GI health, and thus the digestion of nutrients for the entire body [1].

A. Keebler (✉)
Department of General Anesthesiology, Cleveland Clinic, Cleveland, OH, USA
e-mail: KEEBLEA@ccf.org

M. Argalious et al. (eds.), *Basic Sciences in Anesthesia*,
https://doi.org/10.1007/978-3-031-60203-0_21

21.1.1 Motility

The gastrointestinal tract generates motility using smooth muscle subunits linked by small gap junctions. These subunits fire spontaneously in either a phasic or a tonic fashion. Tonic contractions are those contractions that are maintained from several minutes up to hours at a time. These occur in the sphincters of the tract, as well as in the anterior stomach. The other type of contractions, called phasic contractions, consists of brief periods of both relaxation and contraction, occurring in the posterior stomach and the small intestine, and is carried out by the muscularis externa. The patterns of GI contraction as a whole can be divided into 2 distinct patterns: peristalsis and segmentation. Occurring between meals, the migrating motor complex is a series of peristaltic wave cycles in distinct phases starting with relaxation, followed by an increasing level of activity to a peak level of peristaltic activity lasting for 5–15 min. This cycle repeats every 1.5–2 h but is interrupted by food ingestion. The role of this process is likely to clean excess bacteria and food from the digestive system. Peristalsis is one of the patterns that occurs during and shortly after a meal. The contractions occur in wave patterns traveling down short lengths of the GI tract from one section to the next. The contractions occur directly behind the bolus of food that is in the system, forcing it toward the anus into the next relaxed section of smooth muscle. This relaxed section then contracts, generating smooth forward movement of the bolus at a distance of 2–25 cm per second. This contraction pattern depends upon hormones, paracrine signals, and the autonomic nervous system for proper regulation. Segmentation also occurs during and shortly after a meal within short lengths in segmented or random patterns along the intestine. This process is carried out by the longitudinal muscles relaxing while circular muscles contract at alternating sections, thereby mixing the food. This mixing allows food and digestive enzymes to maintain a uniform composition, as well as to ensure contact with the epithelium for proper absorption [2].

21.1.1.1 Gastric Emptying and Anesthesia

In anesthesiology, gastric emptying and the time from last oral intake (NPO status) become important. During the induction of anesthesia, the patient with a full stomach is at increased risk for gastric regurgitation and pulmonary aspiration, which can be lethal. In general, the patient should be NPO for 8 h after a full meal before induction of anesthesia. Six hours after a light meal is considered adequate. Four hours after non-clear liquids and 2 h after clear liquids are also generally considered adequate. These are guidelines for normal healthy patients. Patients with delayed gastric emptying from any cause should be considered to have a full stomach.

Many patients have been found to have food in their stomachs on endoscopic examination even days after stopping oral intake. Patients who are considered to have full stomachs should be delayed as long as possible and should be considered candidates for antacid medications and pro-kinetic drugs.

Pulmonary morbidity from perioperative aspiration varies with the type and volume of the aspirate. Large volume, particulate, or acidic aspirates tend to carry the highest risk. If surgery is deemed emergent, a rapid sequence induction of anesthesia or an awake intubation is indicated with the knowledge that the patient is at increased risk for aspiration.

21.1.2 Secretion

Every day, approximately 7 l of fluid are secreted by the digestive system. This fluid is composed of four primary components: ions, digestive enzymes, mucus, and bile. About half of these fluids are secreted by the salivary glands, pancreas, and liver, which compose the accessory organs and glands of the digestive system. The rest of the fluid is secreted by the GI epithelial cells.

21.1.3 Ions

The largest component of secreted fluids is ions and water, which are first secreted and then reabsorbed along the tract. The ions secreted primarily consist of H^+, K^+, Cl^-, HCO_3^-, and Na^+. Water follows the movement of these ions. The GI tract accomplishes this ion pumping using a system of proteins that are capable of active transport, facilitated diffusion, and open channel ion movement. The arrangement of these proteins on the apical and basolateral sides of the epithelium determines the net movement of ions and water in the tract. H^+ and Cl^- are secreted by the parietal cells into the lumen of the stomach creating acidic conditions with a low pH of 1. H^+ is pumped into the stomach by exchanging it with K^+. This process also requires ATP as a source of energy; however, Cl^- then follows the positive charge in the H^+ through an open apical channel protein.

HCO_3^- secretion occurs to neutralize the acid secretions that make their way into the duodenum of the small intestine. Most of the HCO_3^- comes from pancreatic acinar cells in the form of $NaHCO_3$ in an aqueous solution. This is the result of the high concentration of both HCO_3^- and Na^+ present in the duct, creating an osmotic gradient to which the water follows.

21.1.4 Digestive Enzymes

The second vital secretion of the GI tract is that of digestive enzymes that are secreted in the mouth, stomach, and intestines. Some of these enzymes are secreted by accessory digestive organs, while others are secreted by the epithelial cells of the stomach and intestine. While some of these enzymes remain embedded in the wall of the GI tract, others are secreted in an inactive proenzyme form. When these proenzymes reach the lumen of the tract, a factor specific to a particular proenzyme will activate it. A prime example of this is pepsin, which is secreted in the stomach by chief cells. Pepsin in its secreted form is inactive (pepsinogen). However, once it reaches the gastric lumen, it becomes activated into pepsin by the high H^+ concentration, becoming an enzyme vital to digestion. The release of the enzymes is regulated by neural, hormonal, or paracrine signals. However, in general, parasympathetic stimulation increases secretion of all digestive enzymes.

21.1.5 Mucus

Mucus is released in the stomach and intestine, and serves to lubricate and protect the inner mucosa of the tract. It is composed of a specific family of glycoproteins termed mucins and is generally very viscous. Mucus is made by two types of specialized cells termed mucus cells in the stomach and goblet cells in the intestines. Signals for increased mucus release include parasympathetic innervations, immune system response, and enteric nervous system messengers.

21.1.6 Bile

Bile is secreted into the duodenum of the small intestine via the common bile duct. It is produced in liver cells and stored in the gall bladder until release during a meal. Bile is formed of three elements: bile salts, bilirubin, and cholesterol. Bilirubin is a waste product of the breakdown of hemoglobin. The cholesterol present is secreted with the feces. The bile salt component is an active non-enzymatic substance that facilitates fat absorption by helping it to form an emulsion with water due to its amphoteric nature. These salts are formed in the hepatocytes from bile acids combined with an amino acid. Other compounds such as the waste products of drug degradation are also present in the bile.

21.1.7 Gastrointestinal Hormones

GI peptides are signal molecules that are released into the blood by the GI cells themselves. They act on a variety of tissues including the brain, digestive accessory organs, and the GI tract. The effects range from excitatory or inhibitory effects on motility and secretion to feelings of satiety or hunger when acting on the brain. These hormones fall into three major categories: the gastrin and secretin families, with the third composed of all the other hormones unlike those in the other two families.

Gastrin is secreted by the G cells in the stomach and stimulates acid secretion and stimulates gastric motility. Cholecystokinin is secreted by the endocrine cells of the small intestine. It stimulates gall bladder contraction and pancreatic bicarbonate and pancreatic enzyme secretion. Secretin is secreted by the endocrine S cells of the small intestine. In response to luminal acid, it stimulates pancreatic bicarbonate secretion and inhibits acid secretion. Gastric inhibitory peptide is secreted by the endocrine K cells of the small intestine in response to luminal glucose, fatty acids, and protein. It stimulates insulin production and inhibits acid secretion. Motilin is secreted by the endocrine M cells of the intestine and stimulates the migrating motor complex.

21.2 Hepatic Physiology

21.2.1 The Normal Liver

21.2.1.1 Basic Anatomy

The liver usually has four lobes. These are the left, right, caudate, and quadrate lobes. This anatomic distinction has little impact on surgical dissection. The liver can be divided into 8 segments, each with its own blood supply and venous and biliary drainage. These are known as Couinaud segments and can facilitate relatively bloodless surgery. The functional microanatomy of the liver is a 6-sided lobule with branches of the hepatic artery, portal vein, and bile duct at the 6 points and a central venous channel for drainage into the caval system. Sinusoids connect the outer blood supply to the inner channel. These are lined with hepatocytes and macrophages.

21.2.1.2 Blood Supply

The liver receives approximately 25% of the cardiac output. It has a unique blood supply in that only 25% of the blood supply comes from the oxygen-rich hepatic artery. Roughly 75% of the blood supply comes from the relatively oxygen-poor portal venous system. This means that roughly 50% of the oxygen supply comes from arterial flow and 50% from venous flow. Thus, the liver is equally oxygen-dependent on both arterial and venous inflow.

21.2.1.3 Bile Flow

The biliary tract is derived from the branches of the bile ducts. The biliary tract, also known as the biliary tree, is the path by which bile is secreted by the liver then transported to the first part of the small intestine: the duodenum. The bile produced in the liver is collected in bile canaliculi—small grooves between the faces of adjacent hepatocytes. The canaliculi radiate to the edge of the liver lobule, where they merge to form bile ducts. Within the liver, these ducts are termed intrahepatic bile ducts, and once they exit the liver, they are considered extrahepatic. The intrahepatic ducts eventually drain into the right and left hepatic ducts, which exit the liver at the transverse fissure, and merge to form the common hepatic duct. The cystic duct from the gallbladder joins with the common hepatic duct to form the common bile duct. Bile either drains directly into the duodenum via the common bile duct, or is temporarily stored in the gallbladder via the cystic duct. The common bile duct and the pancreatic duct enter the second part of the duodenum together at the hepatopancreatic ampulla, also known as the ampulla of Vater [3].

21.2.2 Basic Physiology

The liver is a gland and plays a major role in metabolism with numerous functions in the human body, including regulation of glycogen storage, decomposition of red blood cells, plasma protein synthesis, hormone production, and detoxification. It is also an intricate part of the immune system and intimately involved in blood coagulation. Conceptually, it is easy to think about hepatic physiology in two parts: one part being the synthetic function and the other being the metabolic function.

21.2.2.1 Synthetic Function

Coagulation

The liver synthesizes both pro-coagulant and anticoagulant factors including factors 1, 2, 5, 7, 8, 9, 10, and 11 as well as protein C, protein S, and antithrombin. The liver also synthesizes thrombopoietin, which is the hormone that stimulates the bone marrow to produce platelets. Thus, the liver is important in maintaining the coagulation balance that naturally exists within the vascular system.

Protein and Lipid Synthesis

The liver plays multiple roles in lipid metabolism: it performs cholesterol synthesis, lipogenesis, the production of triglycerides, and a bulk of the body's lipoproteins are synthesized in the liver. The liver also plays a role in digestion, as it produces and excretes bile required for emulsifying fats and helps the absorption of vitamin K from the diet. Some of the bile drains directly into the duodenum, and some is stored in the gallbladder. The liver also produces insulin-like growth factor 1 (IGF-1), a polypeptide protein hormone that plays an important role in childhood growth and continues to have anabolic effects in adults.

21.2.2.2 Metabolic Function

The liver performs several roles in carbohydrate metabolism: The liver synthesizes and stores approximately 100 g of glycogen via glycogenesis—the formation of glycogen from glucose. When needed, the liver releases glucose into the blood by performing glycogenolysis, the breakdown of glycogen into glucose. The liver is also responsible for gluconeogenesis, which is the synthesis of glucose from certain amino acids, lactate, or glycerol. Adipose and liver cells produce glycerol by breakdown of fat, which the liver uses for gluconeogenesis.

The liver is responsible for the breakdown of insulin and other hormones. The liver breaks down bilirubin via glucuronidation, facilitating its excretion into bile. The liver is responsible for the breakdown and excretion of many waste products. It plays a key role in breaking down or modifying toxic substances (e.g., methylation) and drug metabolism. A key concept in drug metabolism is phase 1 and phase 2 biotransformation. Phase 1 is the oxidation, reduction, or dealkylization of substances to make them more polar. Phase 2 is attaching polar substances to the polar areas of phase 1 to make drugs even more polar. The more polar substances can then be excreted.

21.2.2.3 Immunologic Function

The liver is the largest organ in the reticuloendothelial system. It is lined with macrophages, which play a role in the immune system by clearing the blood of debris that gets translocated into the bloodstream from the gut.

21.2.3 Physiology of the Diseased Liver

There are many causes of liver disease. Regardless of the etiology, end stage liver disease results in cirrhosis with common manifestation. As the liver becomes fibrotic, it begins to lose its capacity to synthesize and metabolize substances. Blood flow through the liver is slowed and portal hypertension develops. This leads to ascites as the hydrostatic pressure into the postal system increases. As the blood supply attempts to find alternate routes around the fibrotic liver, varices develop throughout the body.

21.2.3.1 Synthetic Function

As synthetic function is impaired, coagulopathy develops as there is a decrease in the synthesis of clotting factors. Thrombocytopenia results from a decrease in the synthesis of thrombopoietin. Since anticoagulant factors are also decreased, a balance may be seen in these patients. Common coagulation tests, such as the pro-thrombin time, may be

Table 21.1 Common anesthetic drugs and the effect of decreased metabolism on their duration of action

Anesthetic	Effect of decreased metabolism on duration of action
Propofol	No effect
Etomidate	No effect
Morphine	Prolonged
Hydromorphone	Prolonged
Succinylcholine	Prolonged
Fentanyl	No effect
Midazolam	Prolonged
Vecuronium	Prolonged
Rocuronium	Prolonged
Neostigmine	Unchanged
Sugammadex	Mildly Prolonged

increased, which is suggestive of coagulopathy, but the patient may be asymptomatic. Perhaps, clotting studies, such as thromboelastography, may be more predictive of coagulopathy and bleeding than traditional methods. Care must be taken with these patients to avoid both coagulopathy and a hypercoagulable state as they are iatrogenically easily tipped into either state [2].

21.2.3.2 Drug Metabolism

Obviously, drugs that are highly metabolized by the liver will have a prolongation of their duration of action. Drugs that are metabolized by pseudocholinesterase will have a prolonged duration of actions secondary to the decrease in pseudocholinesterase production by the diseased liver. Volatile anesthetic agents are minimally metabolized in the liver. ◉ Table 21.1 lists common anesthetic drugs and the effect of decreased metabolism on their duration of action.

Water-soluble drugs, such as rocuronium, will be distributed into a larger volume of distribution because of the volume-overloaded nature of many liver disease patients. This accounts for the need for a larger initial dose to obtain the desired clinical effect despite the prolonged duration of action.

Ester local anesthetics are metabolized by pseudocholinesterase and may have a prolonged duration of action. Amide local anesthetics are metabolized by the liver so they may also have a prolonged duration of action. With either class, care should be taken to avoid toxicity and large volume blocks probably should be approached with caution or avoided.

Interestingly, the newer neuromuscular blocking agent reversal drug sugammadex seems to be prolonged in liver disease but remains faster and more complete than neostigmine [4]

21.3 Questions and Answers

Questions (Choose the Most Appropriate Answer)

1. Bile helps emulsify what substance in the GI tract?
   A. Fat
   B. Protein
   C. Sugars
   D. Complex carbohydrates
2. Gastrin is secreted by which cells in the GI tract?
   A. K cells
   B. G cells
   C. S cells
   D. P cells
3. Thrombocytopenia occurs in liver disease as a result of which of the following?
   A. Overall anemia of chronic disease
   B. Decreased overall protein synthesis
   C. Decrease in thrombopoietin production
   D. Peripheral thrombosis
4. Which of the following is metabolized by the liver?
   A. Ester local anesthetics
   B. Amide local anesthetics
5. True or False. Succinylcholine has a prolonged duration of action in liver disease?
   A. True
   B. False
6. True or False. Patients with liver disease may need a larger induction dose of rocuronium?
   A. True
   B. False
7. Which of the following clotting factors is not synthesized by the liver?
   A. Factor 2
   B. Factor 7
   C. Factor 8
   D. Von Willebrand Factor
8. The liver receives roughly how much blood supply from the hepatic artery and portal vein respectively?
   A. 25% and 75%
   B. 50% and 50%
   C. 75% and 25%
9. The liver receives roughly how much oxygen supply from the hepatic artery and portal vein respectively?
   A. 25% and 75%
   B. 50% and 50%
   C. 75% and 25%
10. True or False. Morphine has a prolonged duration of action in a patient with liver disease?
    A. True
    B. False

Answers

1. **A**. Bile is secreted into the GI tract to emulsify fat.
2. **B**. Gastrin is secreted by the G cells in the stomach.
3. **C**. Thrombopoietin, which is produced by the liver, is decreased in liver disease.
4. **B**. Amide local anesthetics are metabolized by the liver. Ester local anesthetics are metabolized by pseudocholinesterase. Both are prolonged in liver disease.
5. **A**. True. Succinylcholine is metabolized by pseudocholinesterase which is produced by the liver.
6. **A**. True. Water-soluble drugs such as rocuronium will be diluted into a larger volume of distribution due the volume-overloaded nature of many of these patients. It is partially metabolized by the liver so subsequent dosing requirements may be less.
7. **D**. All of the above except Von Willebrand Factor are synthesized by the liver. Von Willebrand Factor in synthesized by the vascular endothelium.
8. **A**. The hepatic artery supplies 25% of the blood supply. The portal vein supplies 75% of the blood supply.
9. **B**. Because arterial blood is significantly more oxygenated even though arterial blood supply is smaller in quantity, oxygen supply is roughly 50% from the artery and 50% from the portal vein.
10. **A**. True. Morphine is metabolized by the liver and thus has a prolonged duration of action in liver disease.

References

1. Barash PG, Cullen BF, Stoelting RK, editors. Clinical anesthesia. 5th ed. Philadelphia: Lippincott Williams Wilkins; 2005. p. 1393–5.
2. Bowen RA. Pathophysiology of the digestive system. July 5, 2006. http://www.freetextbooklist.com/pathophysiology-of-the-digestive-system/. Accessed 15 Jan 2017.
3. Silverthorn DU. Human physiology: an integrated approach. 4th ed. Upper Saddle River: Benjamin Cummings; 2006.
4. Deana C, Barbariol F, et al. SUGAMMADEX versus neostigmine after ROCURONIUM continuous infusion in patients undergoing liver transplantation. BMC Anesthestesiology. 2020;20:70.

Renal Physiology

22

Reem Khatib

Abstract

The kidney has a wide array of responsibilities that range from regulation of fluid volume and osmolarity, management of electrolytes, elimination of endogenous and exogenous toxins, metabolic functions including the production of hormones, and acid-base balance. This chapter will review the basic physiologic mechanisms by which the kidney accomplishes these tasks. Having an appreciation for the cellular mechanisms through which these responsibilities are achieved helps in understanding the effects of physiologic derangements and the body's defense of homeostasis.

Keywords

Renal physiology • Glomerular filtration rate • GFR • Acid-base balance • Drug excretion • Water homeostasis • Renal anatomy

Key Points

1. The kidney has a wide array of responsibilities that range from regulation of fluid volume and osmolarity, management of electrolytes, elimination of endogenous and exogenous toxins, metabolic functions (for example, the production of hormones), and acid-base balance.
2. The nephron is the functional unit of the kidney that is responsible for filtration, reabsorption, and secretion of compounds that the body must manage in order to maintain homeostasis.
3. The kidney receives approximately 20–25% of cardiac output.
4. The nephron is the functional unit of the kidney.
5. The glomerulus is responsible for filtration. The specialized filter allows water to flow freely through but acts as a barrier for particles based on both size and charge. Within the glomerulus, the amount of filtered fluid will depend on the counterbalancing forces of hydrostatic pressure and oncotic pressure.
6. Once the fluid filtered by the glomerulus exits Bowman's capsule it enters the proximal tubule, which is the major site of reabsorption. Through this process of reabsorption, the proximal tubule regulates the extracellular fluid volume of the body, reclaims important electrolytes and nutrients, and regulates acid-base balance.
7. The region from the corticomedullary junction to the papilla is characterized by an increasing osmolarity gradient that plays a critical role in the ability of the body to produce concentrated urine.
8. Water makes up approximately 50–60% of total body weight. The allocation of water within the body is divided into two basic compartments: intracellular and extracellular. Two-thirds of total body water is located in the intracellular compartment with the remaining one-third located in the extracellular space. The extracellular space is further divided into the intravascular space containing 25% of extracellular fluid and the interstitial space comprises of the remaining 75% of fluid. Thus, regulation of the body's fluid status is largely accomplished through its ability to manipulate serum sodium.
9. The bicarbonate/carbon dioxide buffer system is the most important buffering system in the body. The contribution that the kidney makes in regulating acid-base balance is accomplished through its handling of bicarbonate. The kidney has a variety of tools that it can employ in order

R. Khatib (✉)
Department of General Anesthesiology, Cleveland Clinic, Cleveland, OH, USA
e-mail: khatibr@ccf.org

M. Argalious et al. (eds.), *Basic Sciences in Anesthesia*,
https://doi.org/10.1007/978-3-031-60203-0_22

to compensate for different acid-base disturbances. As with any compensatory response, the effects are not able to completely correct for the original acid-base disturbance and take some time to fully develop.

10. The glomerular filtration rate (GFR) represents the cumulative functioning of all of the nephrons in the kidney and serves as an indicator of global renal function. This value represents the amount of plasma that is filtered through all the glomeruli per unit of time. A normal value for GFR ranges from 120 to 130 mL/min/1.73m^2. This value will vary from person to person depending on factors such as age, and sex. GFR cannot be measured directly. Instead, we must rely on surrogates that act as representative markers of filtration. These markers can either be produced endogenously by the body or be introduced exogenously. Although we use GFR as a measure of renal function, the degree of injury to nephrons does not translate to a proportional decrement in the GFR.
11. Inulin clearance remains the gold standard for determination of GFR. The convenience associated with the use of serum creatinine has led to its widespread use as an indicator of renal function. Creatinine is a product of skeletal muscle breakdown and is freely filtered by the kidney without being reabsorbed. Its serum levels correlate inversely with GFR. However, creatinine undergoes secretion by the proximal tubule in varying amounts depending on body conditions. It is not an ideal renal biomarker to assess glomerular filtration rates.
12. Creatinine clearance is not usually calculated based on plasma and urinary creatinine levels in clinical practice. Instead, an estimated GFR (eGFR) is calculated with equations that incorporate laboratory results with demographic data.
13. Cystatin C is a compound that is generated by nucleated cells and released into the blood. Because serum levels vary inversely with GFR like creatinine, it can be used to estimate GFR. While cystatin C levels are not impacted by factors such as diet and muscle mass in the manner serum creatinine levels are, they can be affected by conditions affecting cell turnover rate such as high doses of steroids and thyroid dysfunction.
14. The difficulties inherent in determining global renal function make it challenging to identify when the kidney has sustained an injury or is under stress. The current consensus definition for acute kidney injury has been described by the Kidney Disease Improving Global Outcomes (KDIGO) group. The classification system according to the KDIGO criteria describes three stages of acute renal injury. These stages are generally differentiated from one another based on two variables: increases in serum creatinine and changes in urine output.
15. Excretion of drugs is managed by both the glomerulus and the proximal tubule. The glomerulus filters cations and smaller molecules. The proximal tubule manages those compounds that are either too large or protein bound to be effectively filtered by the glomerulus. Multi-specific drug transporters then import the compounds into the peritubular cell. Once the compounds have been imported into the cell they are shuttled across into the tubular lumen. Variability in the clinical effects of drugs in different individuals may be partially explained by different variations or polymorphisms of these transporter proteins. Changes in the makeup of these proteins may lead to differences in rates of transport, which may affect drug efficacy and or toxicity.

22.1 Anatomy, Blood Flow, Glomerular Filtration, Tubular Reabsorption and Secretion

22.1.1 Renal Anatomy and Blood Flow

Before we drill down into events occurring at the cellular level, a quick review of the basic makeup and architecture of the kidney is needed [1]. The kidneys live in the retroperitoneal space at the level between the T12-L2 vertebrae and are surrounded by Gerota's fascia. Because of its proximity to the liver, the position of the right kidney is more caudal than that of the left kidney. Below Gerota's fascial plane lies a peritoneal fat pad. The organ itself is surrounded by the renal capsule, which is composed of fibrous connective tissue. Three main areas comprise the kidney: the outer renal cortex, renal medulla, and renal pelvis. The nephron is the functional unit of the kidney that is responsible for filtration, reabsorption, and secretion of compounds that the body must manage in order to maintain homeostasis. Each kidney contains roughly 1 million nephrons. The component parts of the nephron include the glomerulus, the proximal tubule, loop of Henle (comprised of thin and thick limbs), the distal tubule, the connecting tubule, and finally the collecting ducts (◉ Fig. 22.1) [2]. We will discuss the specific functions and characteristics of these areas subsequently. The renal cortex is the region that contains the glomeruli. Most glomeruli are located along the outer renal cortex and are thus referred to as cortical nephrons. Juxtamedullary nephrons are located further inside the kidney in the area adjacent to the renal medulla. The differences between these two nephron types are not limited to their placement in the renal cortex but also include modifications in the structure of the loop of Henle. Cortical nephrons have a short descending limb and the thick ascending limb begins shortly after the hairpin turn. The entire nephron remains mainly located in the renal cortex. In contrast, juxtamedullary nephrons have long descending and ascending limbs and dive deeper into the renal medulla. The thick ascending limb of these longer loops begins at the border of the inner and outer medulla. The renal medulla looks like an area organized into little pyramids. These pyramids are composed of the tubules draining urine into the renal pelvis. The renal pelvis then empties into the ureter.

The kidney receives approximately 20–25% of cardiac output. Blood enters the kidney from the aorta via the renal arteries, which divide into interlobar arteries. Each of these interlobar arteries travels through areas in which the renal cortex invaginates into the medulla between the medullary pyramids. Each interlobar artery is further divided into arcuate arteries, which travel parallel to the base of the renal pyramids at the junction of the renal cortex and medulla. Again, further division occurs into interlobular arteries that keep dividing until they become an afferent arteriole supplying a single nephron, which begins with the specialized capillary bed of the glomerulus. Blood exits the glomerulus via an efferent arteriole, before entering the peritubular capillary system. Drainage of the peritubular capillary system occurs via a small venue with venous drainage flowing back along a parallel path to the arterial system before finally emptying into a single renal vein and the vena cava. Of note, the left renal vein is longer than the right renal vein. This anatomical difference does have clinical implications. For example, donor nephrectomies can be done laparoscopically if the left kidney is being harvested because of this difference, whereas an open procedure may be performed for right donor nephrectomy.

22.1.2 The Glomerulus

Filtration begins in the glomerular capillary bed. This specialized capillary bed resides in a space called Bowman's

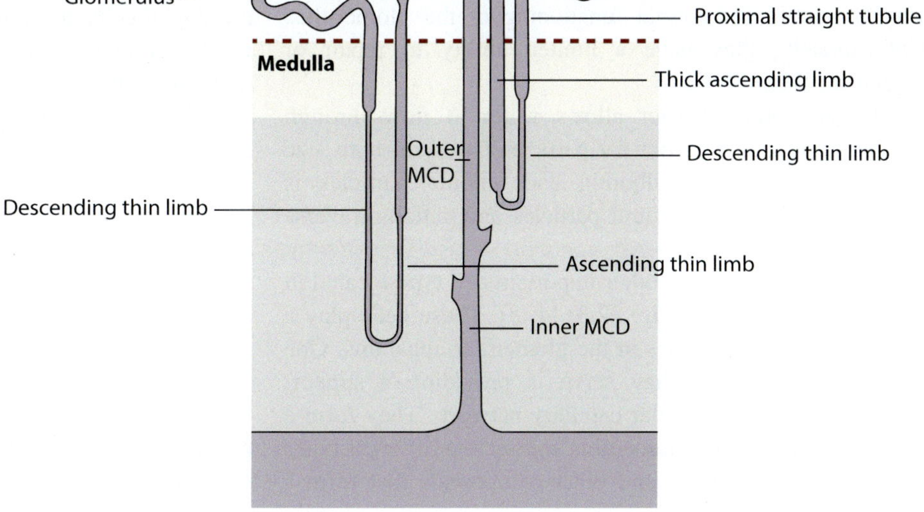

Fig. 22.1 Schematic of nephron. *CCD* cortical collecting duct, *MCD* medullary collecting duct (Adapted from [2])

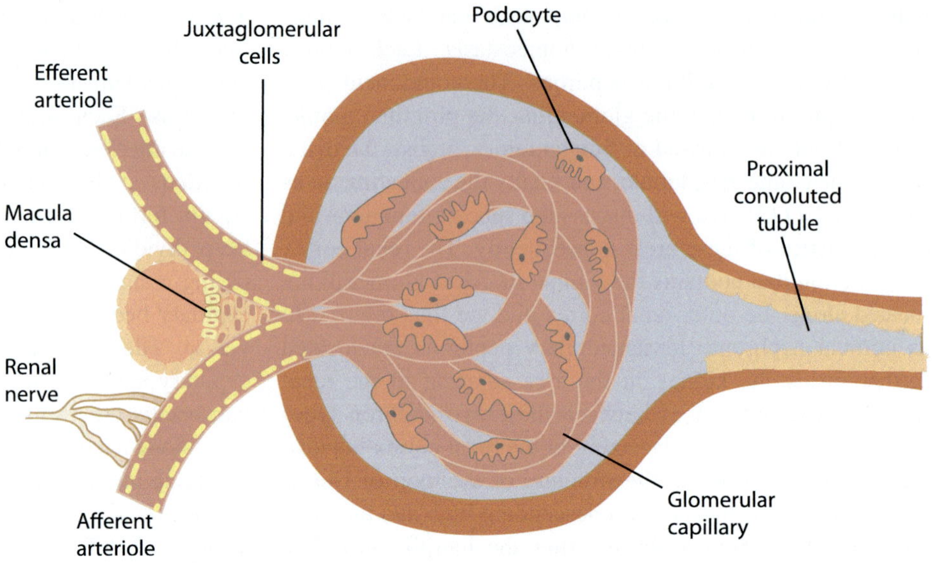

Fig. 22.2 Cross section of glomerulus (Adapted from [3])

capsule. The glomerular filter itself is made of three component parts: the endothelial cells of the glomerular capillary, the glomerular basement membrane, and specialized cells called podocytes or visceral epithelial cells (◉ Fig. 22.2) [3, 4]. The endothelial cells are different from those in other capillary beds in the body. They have fenestrations of roughly 70–100 nm in diameter that serve as a "size" filter. The glomerular basement membrane is an extracellular matrix of proteins created by fusion of the endothelial cell and podocyte basement membranes.

Podocytes provide support to the glomerular capillary complex and also form another slit type of filtration barrier by weaving together the little foot-like processes that extend from one cell to another. These foot-like processes support the glomerular capillary by wrapping around them and weaving together with the foot processes of adjacent podocytes. The areas between the adjacent "feet" form the slit filtration barrier that makes up the third component of the overall glomerular filtration barrier. Healthy podocytes are very important for normal functioning of the glomerulus. Unfortunately, they have a limited ability to repair or regenerate themselves.

The glomerular barrier allows water to flow through freely but acts as a barrier for particles based on both size and charge. Flow of albumin and anionic particles is restricted while small neutral particles and cations traverse the barrier freely.

Mesangial cells are another important cell type located in Bowman's capsule (◉ Fig. 22.3) [4, 5]. These cells play a number of important roles in the glomerular apparatus. One of the primary roles they serve is providing a support structure for the glomerular capillary network. They form a central tuft within the glomerulus and secrete different types of collagen, fibronectin, and other compounds that form a mesangial extracellular matrix. Mesangial cells help to support the structure of the glomerular loops and help to provide protection from high hydrostatic pressures. The mesangial cells have contractile properties that aid them in this task. Although the major regulation of blood flow to the glomerulus occurs as a result of changes in the efferent and afferent arterioles, the mesangial cells are thought to have the ability to fine-tune intraglomerular blood flow. The extracellular matrix produced by glomerular cells also has important immunologic and homeostatic functions. Production of free radicals, cytokines, and chemokines all occur when these cells become activated. Mesangial cells appear to "talk" with podocytes and endothelial cells through mechanisms that are still being investigated [6]. These interactions prove to be important during disease processes as dysfunction in one cell type can result in alterations in the others.

Two classic glomerular diseases that are associated with mesangial cell function are immunoglobulin A (IgA) nephropathy and diabetic nephropathy. In IgA nephropathy, mesangial cells are injured by the deposition of IgA, which results in mesangial cell proliferation and increased production of the mesangial matrix components through the work of cytokines and growth factors. In turn, this activation appears to result in changes in podocyte function leading to protienuria. Patients who develop diabetic nephropathy demonstrate pathologic changes in mesangial cells as well, as demonstrated by expansion of the mesangial matrix, mesangial cell hypertrophy and proliferation, and the development of inflammation. These changes contribute to the global renal dysfunction seen in this condition.

What determines the rate of flow through the glomerulus? Within the glomerulus, the amount of filtered fluid will depend on the counterbalancing forces of hydrostatic pressure and oncotic pressure. Thus at the beginning of the

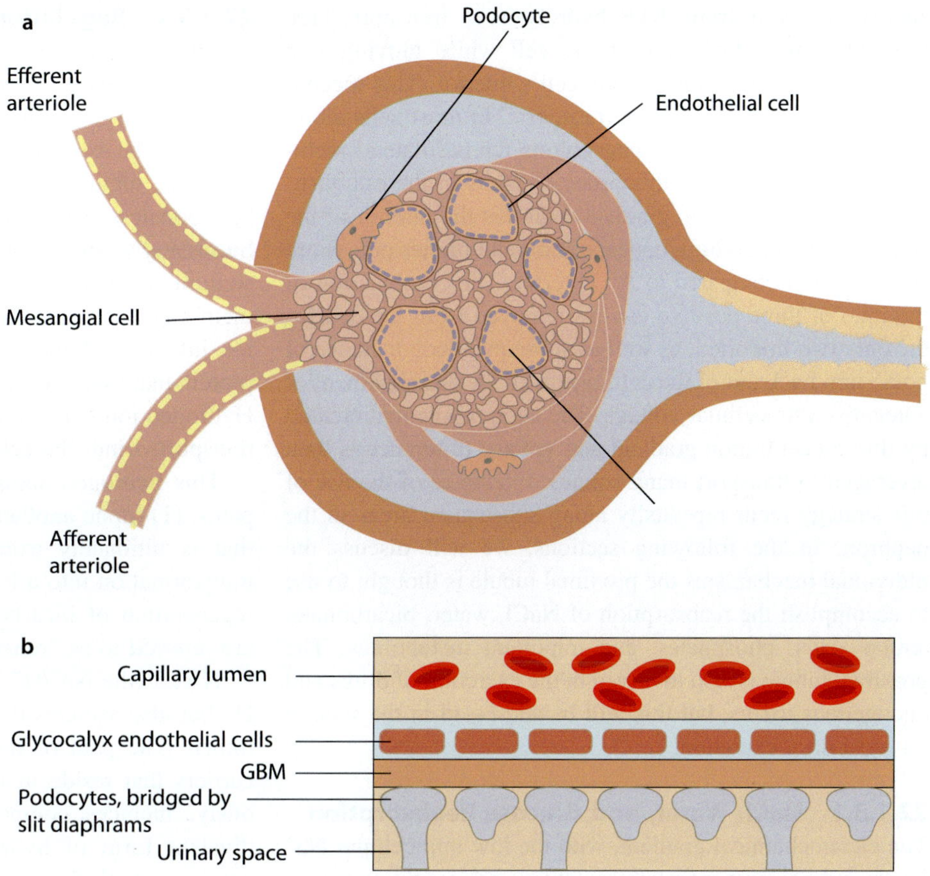

Fig. 22.3 **a** Cross section of glomerulus illustrating relationship between mesangial cells, podocytes, and endothelial cells. **b** Representation of the 3-part filtration barrier comprised of the podocytes, glomerular basement membrane (GBM), and endothelial cells (Adapted from [5])

glomerular capillary, the hydraulic force of fluid will overcome the oncotic pressures working to keep fluid within the capillary bed. As fluid exits the capillary, protein concentration and thus oncotic pressure will increase until the two forces balance and no further net filtration of fluid occurs. Another factor affecting flow is represented by ultrafiltration coefficient, K_f. This value represents factors such as the surface area available for filtration, and the "leakiness" of the capillary filter. One final component affecting the glomerular filtration rate (GFR) will depend on the rate of flow of fluid through the glomerular capillaries. When fluid is flowing slowly through the glomerulus, the point of equilibrium between the hydrostatic forces driving fluid out into Bowman's capsule and the oncotic pressure created by plasma proteins may occur earlier along the capillary path. Thus, for the remaining portion of the capillary bed left to traverse, no net filtration occurs. When fluid travels more quickly it takes more time for this point of equilibrium to occur. Thus, although there may be less net filtration at one single point, the longer path and thus greater time that filtration occurs leads to a net increase in the amount of filtered fluid. Differing resistances in the afferent and efferent arterioles modulate this rate of flow depending on hormonal factors, drugs, and other vasoactive substances.

22.1.3 Proximal Tubule

Once the fluid filtered by the glomerulus exits Bowman's capsule it enters the proximal tubule, which is the major site of reabsorption. Through this process of reabsorption, the proximal tubule regulates the extracellular fluid volume of the body, reclaims important electrolytes and nutrients, and regulates acid-base balance [7]. These proximal tubule cells can be thought of as bulk processing centers. They reabsorb the majority of the substances that were filtered, with the fine tuning of many processes accomplished further downstream of this component of the nephron.

To understand the manner in which proximal tubule cells accomplish all of the aforementioned tasks, we must first understand the general makeup of the tubular cells in the nephron. Each cell type, whether they be in the proximal tubule or the collecting duct, is oriented with two interfaces: one to the tubular fluid, and the other with blood from peritubular capillaries. The membrane lying at the interface with the tubular fluid is referred to as the apical membrane, while the basolateral membrane refers to the blood-cell interface. Many cellular processes in the nephron are powered by a protein transporter complex known as the Na^+-K^+-ATPase either directly or indirectly. The Na^+-K^+-ATPase uses the energy achieved from ATP hydrolysis to transport three molecules of sodium out of the cell while moving two molecules of potassium into the cell's interior. This mechanism is referred to as "active transport." In most cells along the nephron, this process occurs along the basolateral membrane. The net effect of this process results in the establishment of a concentration gradient such that the interior of the cell has a lower sodium concentration and higher potassium concentration compared to the exterior. The combination of the ratio of three positive cations removed from the cell for the only two imported, as well as subsequent conductance of potassium back out of the cell, results in the establishment of a negative intracellular voltage. The energy potential created by this concentration gradient and voltage difference is then leveraged to transport many solutes. Examples of the use of this strategy recur repeatedly along subsequent areas in the nephron. In the following sections, we will discuss the individual mechanisms the proximal tubule is thought to use to accomplish the reabsorption of NaCl, water, bicarbonate, amino acids, phosphates, and important metabolites. The proximal tubule is also involved in the excretion of drugs and endogenous toxins, but this will be addressed in the section on renal drug excretion.

22.1.3.1 NaCl, Water, and Glucose Reabsorption

The electrochemical gradient, with the low intracellular Na^+ levels and negative intracellular lumen, powers the transport of both sodium chloride and water into the cell at the apical membrane. This is accomplished by multiple different exchangers as there is no transporter protein that reabsorbs NaCl as a single unit. Instead, import of Na^+ is tied to organic compounds such as glucose, H^+, and sulfates. In a sense, Na^+ "catches a ride" with whatever transporter protein that can accommodate it. Chloride anion transport occurs through transporters tied to organic bases and other anions at the apical boarder and via a variety of transporters at the basolateral membrane. Also, a significant amount of chloride is reabsorbed via the paracellular pathway. In this route, chloride rides down the concentration gradient in passive transport between the proximal tubule cells. The net effect of all these processes results in the reabsorption of 60–70% of the filtered NaCl and water as well as reabsorption of > 99% of filtered glucose by the time the end of the proximal tubule is reached [7, 8]. Because water and solutes are reabsorbed together, the reabsorption occurring in the proximal tubule is generally isotonic in nature.

Another protein class that is integral to the process of water reabsorption is integral membrane proteins known as aquaporins. Many different types of aquaporin proteins exist. In the proximal tubules, the aquaporin AQP1 helps facilitate much of the water reabsorption in the proximal tubule. We will see another class of aquaporins, AQP2 which functions in the connecting tubules and collecting ducts [9].

22.1.3.2 Regulation of the HCO_3^- Buffer

Bicarbonate represents one of the most important buffers in the human body. Variations in the levels of bicarbonate contribute to the maintenance of the acid-base status, which needs to be regulated within a very precise range. The proximal tubule plays a major role in the regulation of bicarbonate, reclaiming 70–90% of filtered bicarbonate. Surprisingly, this is not accomplished by simply transporting sodium bicarbonate from the tubular lumen across the apical membrane. Instead, the proximal tubule secretes hydrogen ion into the tubular lumen through the work of NHE3, a protein that functions as an electroneutral Na^+/H^+ exchanger. Hydrogen ion is moved into the tubular lumen as the Na^+ is transported into the cell (◉ Fig. 22.4).

This hydrogen anion can then follow one of two basic paths: (1) titrate another substrate that acts as an acid carrier that is ultimately excreted in the urine, or (2) undergo transformation into a form that leads to the reclamation and regeneration of bicarbonate. Together these two processes are referred to as "renal acidification" [7].

NHE3 (the Na^+/H^+ exchanger protein) not only secretes H^+ but also secretes the acid NH_4^+ directly into the tubular lumen. The path of renal acidification through titration of carriers that reside in the tubular lumen, mentioned previously, includes compounds such as ammonium and the divalent form of hydrogen phosphate. When ammonium combines with the hydrogen ion, NH_4^+ is generated in the tubular lumen:

$$NH_3 + H^+ \rightarrow NH4^+$$

When hydrogen ion titrates phosphate to its monovalent form it functions as an acid that is secreted in the urine, much like the ammonium cation.

$$HPO_4^{2-} + H^+ \rightarrow H_2PO_4^-$$

The second path of bicarbonate reabsorption can be accomplished in a couple of different ways as well. The enzyme carbonic anhydrase catalyzes the combination of bicarbonate and hydrogen ion to form carbon dioxide, a substance that can easily diffuse across the apical cell membrane:

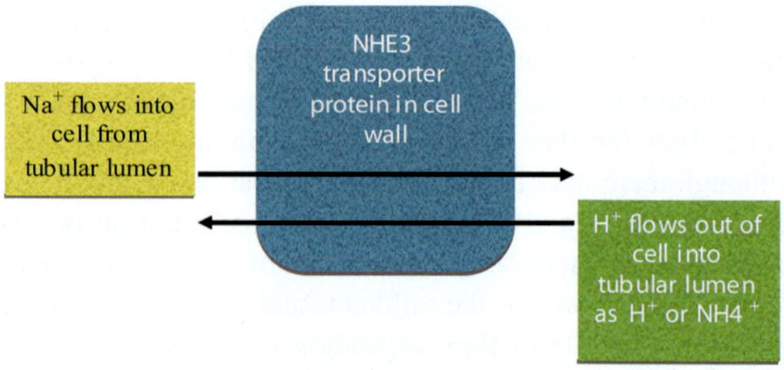

Fig. 22.4 Regulation of the HCO_3^- buffer

$$HCO_3^- + H^+ \xrightarrow{\text{CarbonicAnhydrase}} H_2O + CO_2$$

Once inside the cell, carbonic anhydrase regenerates both the hydrogen ion and bicarbonate. A transporter protein on the basolateral membrane called NBC1 then transports the bicarbonate into the peritubular capillary along with Na^+, thus reclaiming bicarbonate.

Alternatively, the secreted hydrogen ion can combine with citrate. The change in charge of citrate after its combination with hydrogen makes it compatible with a protein cotransporter called NaDC-1 (Na^+ decarboxylate cotransporter) that imports the citrate along with Na^+ ion into the cell. Citrate is then ultimately metabolized in the proximal tubule cell (in 1 of 2 manners) both resulting in the net generation of bicarbonate, which again can be transported across the basolateral membrane by NBC1. Thus, in summary, the hydrogen ion that was initially transported out of the proximal tubule cell combines with citrate allowing it to be transported from the tubular lumen into and across the proximal tubular cell where it is ultimately reabsorbed into the blood. ◉ Figure 22.5 portrays a nice summarization of these pathways and the transporter proteins involved [7].

22.1.3.3 Transport of Amino Acids

The majority of amino acids filtered by the glomerulus are neutrally charged and easily reabsorbed by a specific transporter protein at the apical membrane. Separate transporters exist for acidic and basic amino acids. One important amino

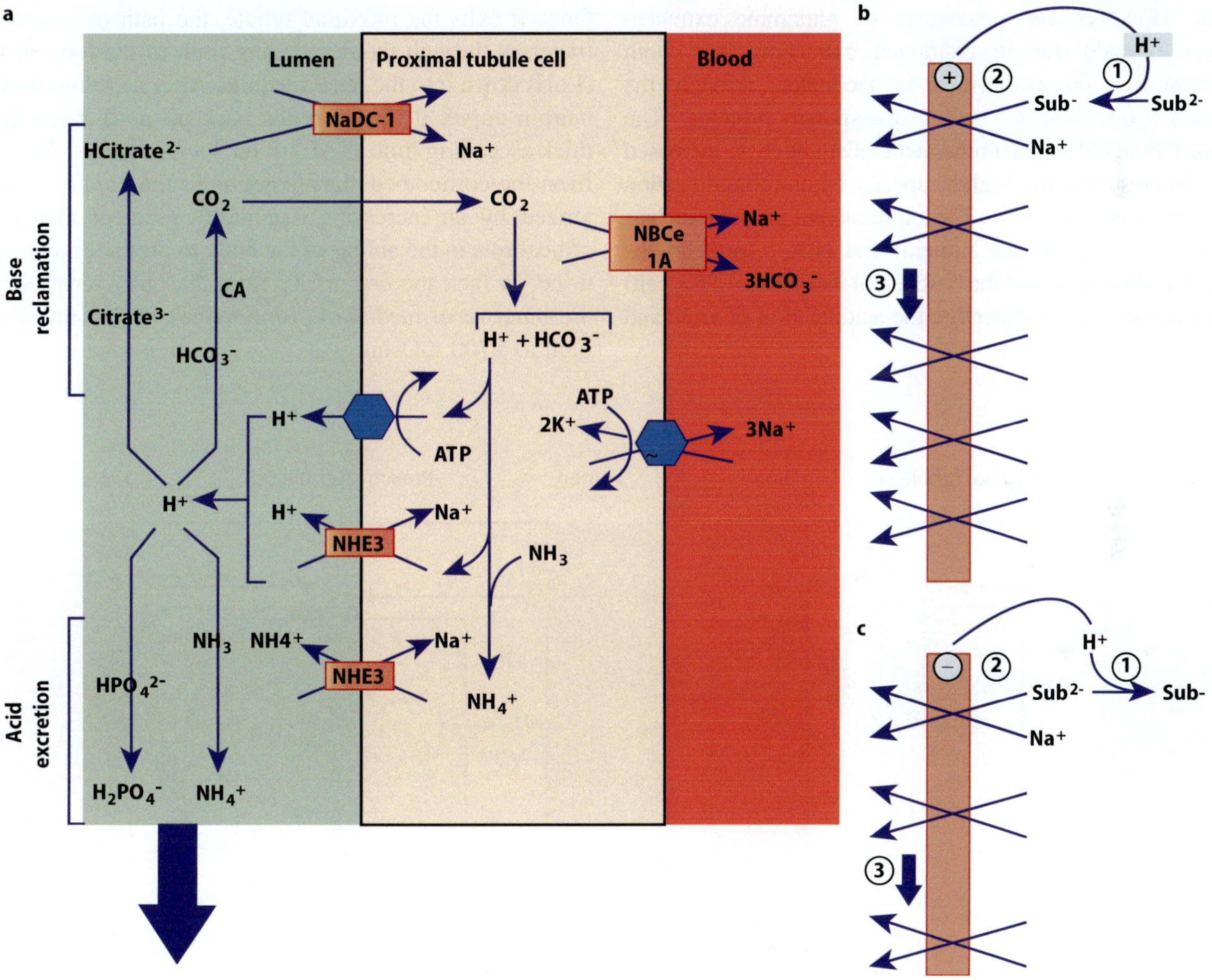

Fig. 22.5 Illustration of proximal tubule management of filtered bicarbonate. **a** Carbonic anhydrase catalyzes the luminal conversion of bicarbonate into CO_2 and water. The CO_2 diffuses through the cellular membrane where it again is converted by carbonic anhydrase into hydrogen ion and bicarbonate. Hydrogen ion can be secreted back into the tubular lumen by either the H^+-ATPase, or more commonly the Na^+/H^+ exchanger NHE3. NHE3 also has the ability to transport NH_4^+, which is generated intracellularly from NH_3 and H^+. Once hydrogen ion is secreted into the lumen it may be either recycled to participate again in the reabsorption of bicarbonate; may convert citrate to its bivalent form, which is transported into the cell; or may be used to titrate urinary acids, which are excreted. The degree to which the proximal tubule can reabsorb bicarbonate and acidify urine can be either unregulated or down regulated as illustrated in **b** and **c**, respectively. Sub-substrate (Adapted from [7])

acid to be familiar with is glutamine due to the role it plays in the renal response to metabolic acidosis [7]. Under normal physiologic conditions, only a small amount of glutamine undergoes uptake (approximately 20%) and metabolism (<3%). However, this picture rapidly changes under the acute onset of metabolic acidosis. During the onset of acute metabolic acidosis, the amount of glutamine that the kidneys are exposed to increases as a result of release from muscle tissue. The proximal tubule cell reabsorbs a greater amount of glutamine (roughly 35%) from the tubular lumen and also takes up glutamine from the peritubular capillary blood. This glutamine is then metabolized to generate greater amounts of ammonium cations (which are excreted in the urine), glucose, and bicarbonate (which undergoes reabsorption) (◉ Fig. 22.6) [7]. When metabolic acidosis becomes more chronic, the circulating levels of glutamine drop back to a level that is 70% of normal. However, the percentage of glutamine extracted remains elevated due to continued extraction from both membranes, a process which is facilitated through the increased expression of certain transporter proteins. The enzymes involved in glutamine metabolism have an increased expression resulting in a higher capacity for ammonium cation and bicarbonate production. The expression of proteins such as NHE3 (Na^+/H^+ exchanger protein) and NBC1 (protein that moves bicarbonate across the basolateral membrane of the cell) is increased as well, augmenting the acidification of urine and reabsorption of bicarbonate.

22.1.3.4 Phosphate

The renal component of phosphate balance is managed almost exclusively by the proximal tubule [7, 10]. Again the electrochemical gradient established by the Na^+-K^+-ATPase serves as the driving force for the apical reabsorption of phosphate via three separate transporters. The mechanism by which phosphate exits the basolateral membrane and is reabsorbed into the blood is not well understood. The amount of phosphate reabsorbed versus lost in the urine will depend on dietary intake as well as the input of signaling factors from parathyroid hormone, dopamine, fibroblast growth factor 23, and a transmembrane protein called klotho.

22.1.4 Thin Limbs of the Loop of Henle

Once it exits the proximal tubule, the path of tubular fluid traverses through the descending limb of the loop of Henle (LoH) down into the renal medulla. After traveling through a hairpin curve, it then ascends back up until it reaches the thick ascending limb (TAL) of the loop of Henle. The region from the corticomedullary junction to the papilla is characterized by an increasing osmolarity gradient that plays a critical role in the ability of the body to produce concentrated urine. In fact, the osmolarity from the outer renal cortex to the inner renal medulla is from values of 300 mOsm to as high as 2700 mOsms.

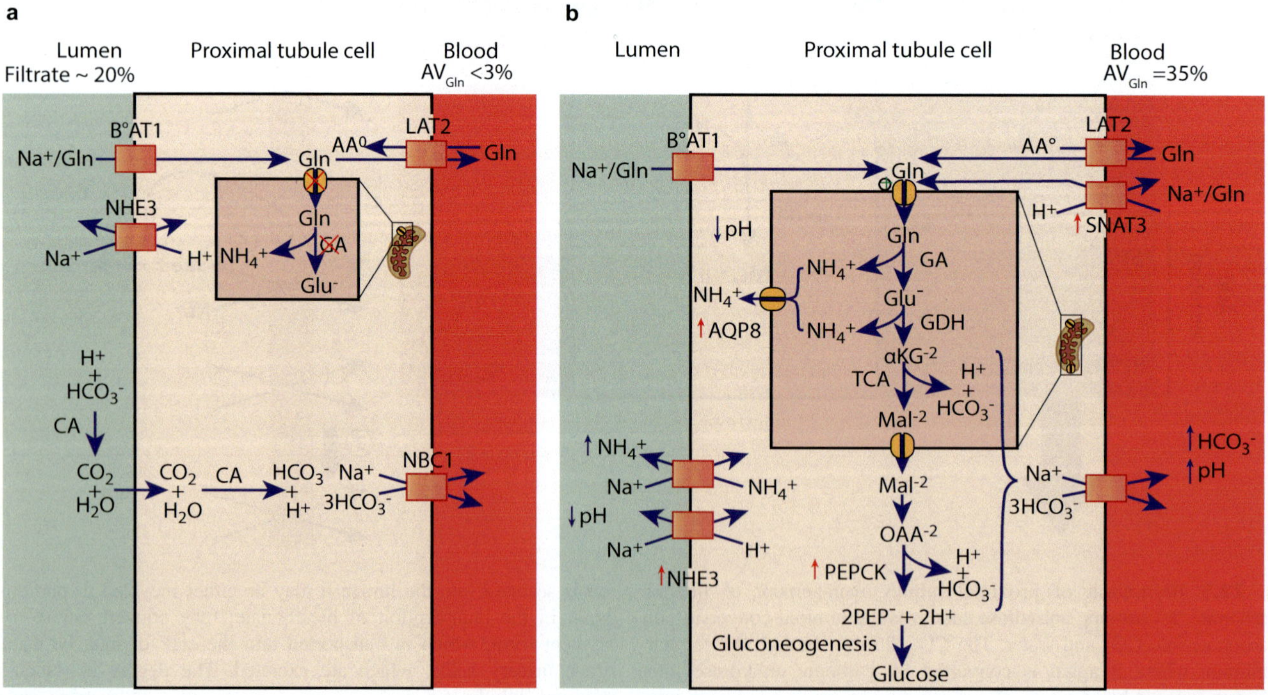

Fig. 22.6 Glutamine metabolism. **a** Represents handling of glutamine in a normal acid – base environment. **b** Illustrates the catabolism of glutamine during conditions of chronic acidosis demonstrating its catabolism to form bicarbonate, which is reabsorbed into the blood, NH4+ which acidifies the urine, and glucose (Adapted from [7])

The mechanism by which gradient is established and maintained is not entirely understood. Many structures participate in this process: both the thin and thick limbs of the loop of Henle, the collecting ducts, and the vasa recta. Traditionally the process has been referred to as "counter current multiplication", however, the traditional understanding of counter current multiplication has not accommodated data measured in experimental models. Also, the assumptions about the proximity of structures to one another and their physical relationship with the vasa recta appear to differ from the original assumptions [11]. Thus, the understanding of this process continues to evolve [12].

The best current understanding of how the kidney establishes the osmolar gradient begins with an acknowledgement of the special characteristic of the descending and ascending thin loops themselves (◉ Fig. 22.7) [12]. The first important characteristic relates to water permeability [2]. Contrary to prior models, it has been demonstrated that the descending thin limbs (DTLs) of short-looped nephrons fail to express the transmembrane protein aquaporin-1 (AQP1). AQP1, aquaporin, is a water channel that makes the tubule water permeable. For long-looped nephrons, the descending thin limbs only express AQP1 in the initial 40% of their length. Thus, most of the descending thin limbs are actually impermeable to water. Ascending thin limbs (ATLs) are water impermeable as well. While these segments have long stretches of impermeability to water, they do have a high degree of permeability to sodium chloride beginning from just before the hairpin bend and continuing on through the ascending thin limb. Finally, both the descending and ascending loops of Henle have a high permeability to urea along their entire lengths.

As tubular fluid flows down the descending thin limb, water exits the DTL lumen until it reaches the area in which AQP1 expression ceases, at which point water egress ceases. As the DTL dives into the renal medulla, the osmolarity of the tissue surrounding it increases due to increases in interstitial urea concentration. Thus, urea diffuses down its concentration gradient from its high concentration into the tubular fluid. As the bend of the LoH is approached, NaCl passively exits the cell, but due to the lack of water permeability, there is no concurrent egress of water. At the bend of the LoH, the tubular fluid is surrounded by the highest osmolar gradients it will see until it again descends back through the inner medulla via the collecting ducts. As the fluid exits the bend and rises back up toward the renal cortex, the concentration of urea begins to decrease the closer the fluid travels to the cortex. Urea will continue to travel down its concentration gradient. Thus, in the areas of the ascending limb that are deep, urea will diffuse into the tubule. However, at some point the fluid in the tubule will have a urea concentration that is greater than the surrounding intersitium, resulting in its diffusion back out into the interstitium. This process is referred to as "counter current multipication" [12].

22.1.5 Thick Ascending Limb of Loop of Henle

The mechanism described previously depends on a high osmolar gradient with a high concentration of urea and low concentration of NaCl in the inner medulla. How does this gradient become established and maintained? In order to understand this process, we must continue to understand the

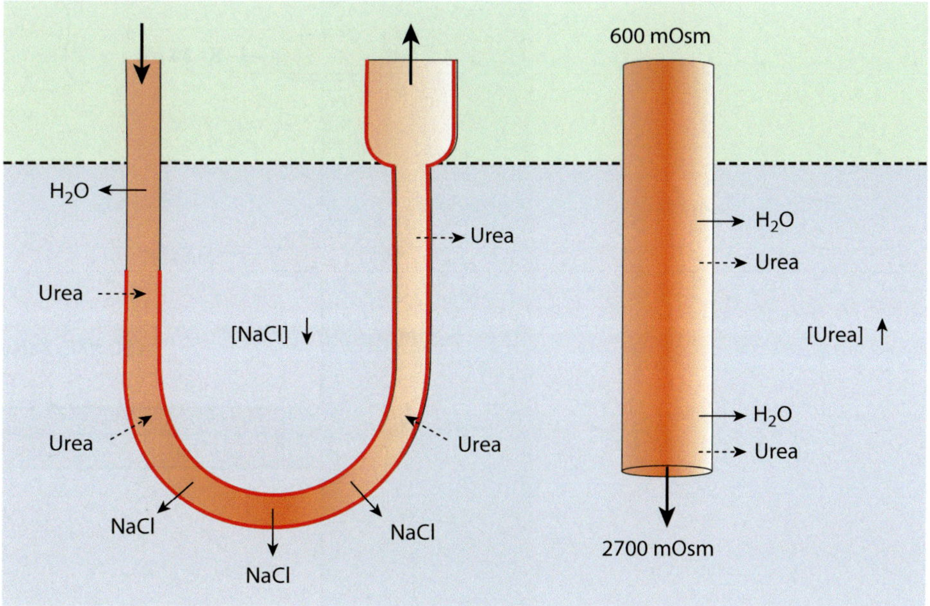

Fig. 22.7 Thin limb of loop of Henle. This figure demonstrates the current understanding of the role of water permeability and urea in creating the hypertonic environment that is responsible for the ability to concentrate urine. The *thick red line* demonstrates the portion of the thin limb that does not express aquaporin and is thus not permeable to water. In contrast, permeability of urea exists along the length of the tubule. Around the bend of the loop, NaCl is passively reabsorbed (Adapted from [12])

workings of the thick ascending limb (TAL) and collecting ducts (CD) (◉ Fig. 22.8) [2]. The TAL is impermeable to water and travels back up to the renal cortex where the cells of the macula densa abut the afferent and efferent arterioles of the glomerulus. The macula densa represents specialized cells in the TAL that play a role in tubuloglomerular feedback. While movement of NaCl occurs in a passive fashion in the thin limbs, it is actively transported out of the lumen in the TAL. The net result is an increasingly dilute luminal fluid that contributes to counter current multiplication.

Transport of NaCl is mediated by the protein complex NKCC2 at the apical membrane [2]. NKCC2 cotransports Na^+, K^+, and $2Cl^-$ to the intracellular space. This transport protein is of clinical importance because it is extremely sensitive to furosemide. Furosemide inhibits the transport of Cl^- across the cell and appears to have effects on the cells of the macula densa, which also contains NKCC2. In the macula densa, Lasix (furosemide) functions to inhibit tubuloglomerular feedback and suppress renin released by chloride in the tubular lumen.

Potassium plays a very important role in the TAL [2]. Its presence is necessary for the NKCC2 (furosemide-sensitive, electroneutral Na^+-K^+-$2Cl^-$ cotransporter) transporter to function. Since there is very little potassium in the tubular fluid at this point, in order for continued active transport of NaCl to occur, then the potassium must be recycled back across the apical lumen so that it may be reused. Renal outer medullary potassium channel (ROMK) and maxi-K (also

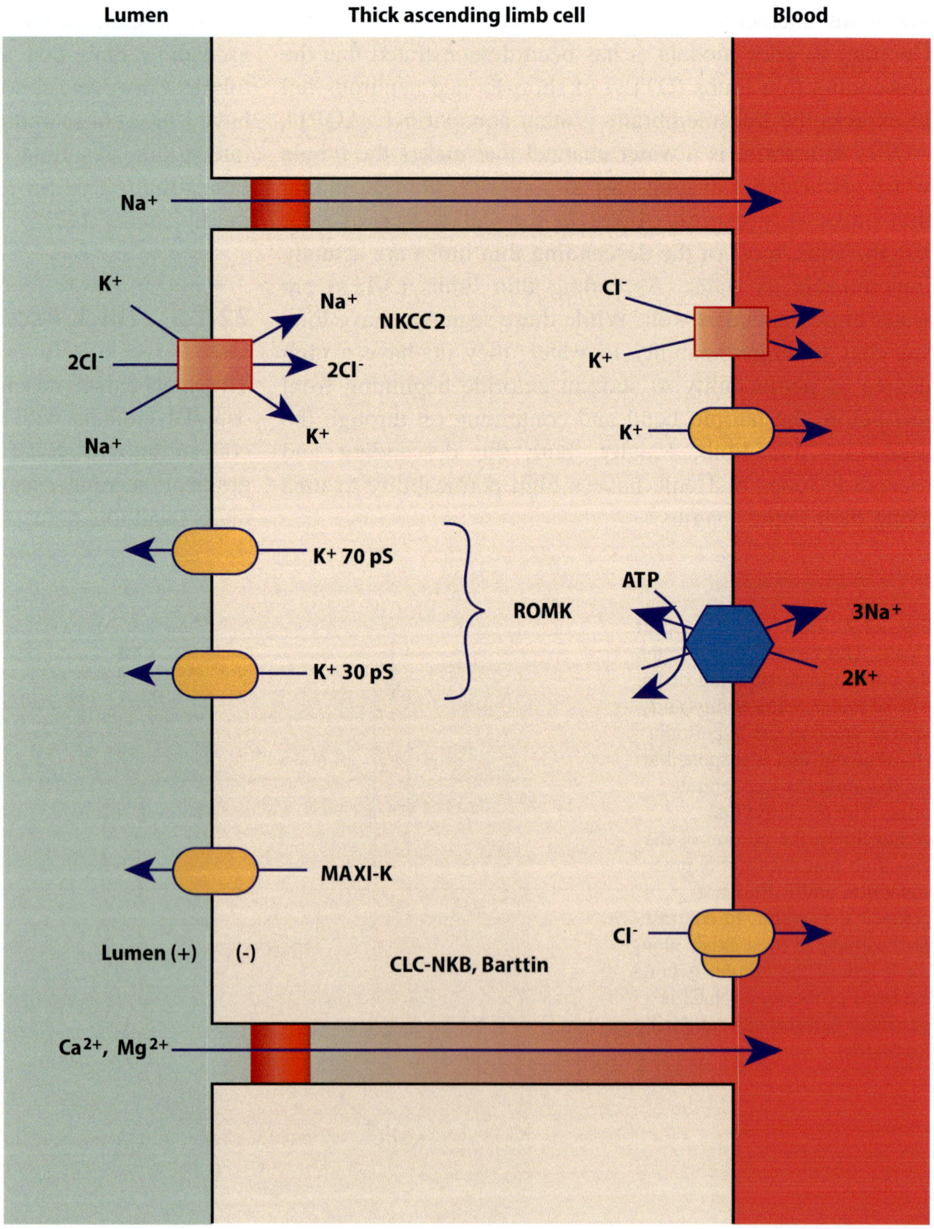

Fig. 22.8 Thick ascending limb of loop of Henle (Adapted from [2])

known as BK or "big" K) potassium channels at the membrane fulfill this task. The majority of the potassium transported across the apical membrane is recycled back into the tubular lumen, whereas the NaCl is transported across the basolateral cell membrane courtesy of the Na^+-K^+-ATPase and chloride channels. Thus, the active transport of NaCl in the TAL represents an example of secondary active transport. This process of NaCl reabsorption and K^+ recycling creates a positive potential difference in the tubular lumen.

Other functions of the TAL include reabsorption of more cations via the paracellular pathway [2]. This includes additional sodium, roughly 55% of filtered magnesium, and around 20% of filtered calcium. Part of the impetus for this movement is found in the positive-lumen potential difference established by furosemide-sensitive, electroneutral Na^+-K^+-$2Cl^-$ cotransporter (NKCC2), and is aided by channels in the tight junctions between cells that have an affinity for cations.

Additionally, the TAL contributes to maintenance of acid-base balance through the reabsorption of approximately 15% of filtered bicarbonate [2]. The mechanism by which this is accomplished involves electroneutral Na^+/H^+ exchanger (NHE3) as described earlier in the proximal tubule. The TAL also is important in the body's management of ammonia. When the ammonia produced by the proximal tubule reaches the TAL, a large percentage of it is reabsorbed back into the systemic circulation. This reabsorbed ammonium anion is transported to the liver where it undergoes metabolism to form urea. The reabsorption of ammonium anion is carried out mechanistically by apical transport of ammonium anion from furosemide-sensitive, electroneutral Na^+-K^+-$2Cl^-$ cotransporter NKCC2 (although NH_4^+ appears to be able to be transported by any transporter protein that handles K^+) and another protein transporter at the basolateral membrane called NHE4 (another electroneutral Na^+/H^+ exchanger). The capacity of the TAL to reabsorb ammonium anion increases under conditions of acidosis. Interestingly, NH_4^+ can be reabsorbed via the paracellular pathway as well. Ultimately, the transport of ammonium anion by the TAL establishes another gradient contributing to counter current multiplication, with the highest amounts of ammonia in the inner medulla and lowest levels located in the renal cortex.

The body's ability to adjust urine production and composition to meet metabolic needs depends on hormonal regulation [2]. Various hormones target the TAL to regulate ion transport. Substances such as vasopressin, parathyroid hormone, glucagon, calcitonin, and B adrenergic activation all increase ion transport through an increase in cyclic adenosine monophosphate (cAMP) levels. As an example, interaction of vasopressin with V2 receptors leads to an increased activity in electroneutral Na^+-K^+-$2Cl^-$ cotransporter (NKCC2) activity as well as an increase in the number of these proteins on the apical membrane. With prolonged exposure to vasopressin, the TAL cells hypertrophy and double their baseline activity of NaCl transport. In contrast, prostaglandin E2, extracellular calcium, and nitric oxide negatively influence ion transport.

22.1.6 Distal Convoluted Tubule

Once tubular fluid passes the macula densa it enters the distal convoluted tubule (DCT) [13]. Tubular fluid is now very dilute as a result of the active transport of NaCl and impermeability of the TAL. The measured transepithelial voltage, or the voltage difference between the DCT cells and the tubular lumen, remains very close to zero at the beginning of the DCT. The continued reabsorption of NaCl (described later) results in the formation of a negative charge in the tubular fluid. This negative voltage in turn helps to drive the secretion of K^+, along with the reabsorption of chloride, calcium, and magnesium.

The DCT is comprised of two distinct segments: the early or DCT1 segment, and the late, or DCT2 segment (◉ Fig. 22.9) [13]. These segments differ from one another in a number of ways. The first difference relates to the ability of the mineralocorticoid receptor (MR) to be stimulated by steroid hormones. In the DCT1 region, the MR responds to both glucocorticoids and mineralocorticoids. However, expression of an enzyme called 11-B hydroxysteroid dehydrogenase 2 in the DCT2 section prevents cortisol from exerting its effects at the mineralocorticoid receptor. Thus, the DCT2 segment is much more sensitive to the effects of aldosterone than the early DCT. A second difference relates to the manner in which NaCl reabsorption is executed. In the early DCT, sodium transport at the apical membrane occurs in an electroneutral manner. The transporter protein NCC (thiazide-sensitive NaCl cotransporter), transports both one Na^+ cation and one Cl^- anion together simultaneously. Activity of NCC also happens to be inhibited by thiazide diuretics. The coupled movement of sodium chloride maintains the zero voltage potential in the tubular lumen. In the late DCT, NCC continues to be expressed and function, but another transmembrane protein called the epithelial sodium channel (ENaC) also contributes to sodium reabsorption. The key difference lies in the electrogenic nature of this transport. Since there is no concomitant transfer of an anion to balance out the movement of the positively charged Na^+ in the epithelial sodium channel (ENaC), a voltage difference begins to occur and the tubular lumen develops a negative potential. The impetus for this influx of Na^+ at the apical membrane can again be traced back to our old friend the Na^+-K^+-ATPase functioning at the basolateral membrane. Remember, 3 Na^+ are transported out for every 2 K^+ carried into the cell creating a negative, low $[Na^+]$, high $[K^+]$ intracellular environment. The "leak" of potassium back

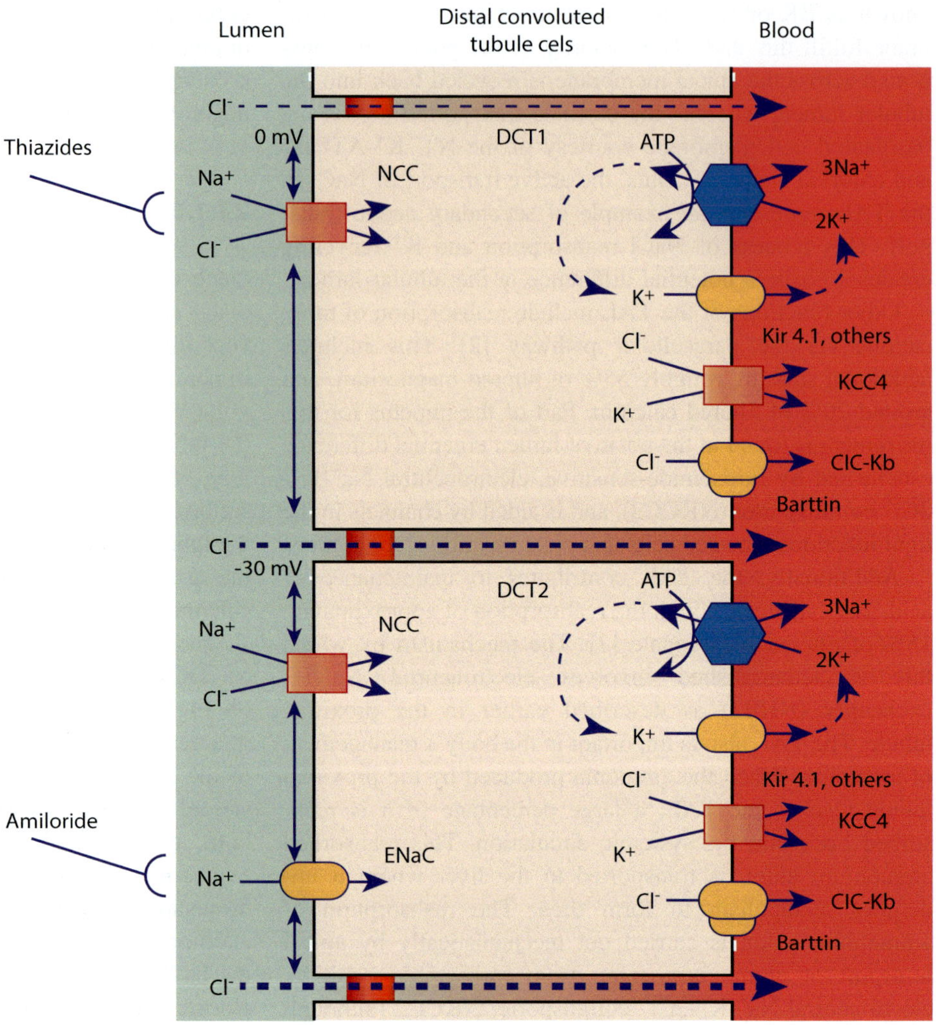

Fig. 22.9 Distal convoluted tubule. Illustration of NaCl reabsorption (Adapted from [13])

across the basolateral membrane by various potassium channels recycles the potassium and allows this electrochemical gradient to be regenerated and maintained. Basolateral chloride transport is mediated by a chloride-specific channel (ClC-Kb) as well as a KCl transporter protein (KCC4).

The voltage difference generated by the combined effects of an epithelial sodium channel (ENaC) and the Na^+-K^+-ATPase helps drive the movement of other solutes. Paracellular movement of chloride is one example. Other interesting examples are found in the active transport of calcium and magnesium, which will not be expanded upon here. Perhaps the most interesting example lies in the handling of potassium at the apical membrane. When tubular fluid exits the DCT2 it contains more potassium than was originally present due to secretion across the apical membrane [13]. The secretion of potassium increases the further down one travels in the DCT in proportion to the increasingly negative voltage potential. The faster the fluid travels down this path, the more potassium is secreted as well. These effects are mediated by two different potassium channels, which we have discussed previously: the renal outer medullary potassium channel (ROMK) and BK ("big" K or maxi-K). In the TAL, the function of these proteins at the apical membrane is to recycle potassium back into the tubular lumen to allow furosemide-sensitive, electroneutral Na^+-K^+-$2Cl^-$ cotransporters (NKCC2) to initiate the reabsorption of NaCl. In the DCT, however, their function at the apical membrane is to secrete potassium into the tubular lumen. Renal outer medullary potassium channel (ROMK) is voltage sensitive and it secretes more potassium as the voltage differential becomes more negative. When tubular fluid flows at an increased rate then the BK ("big" K) channel becomes activated due to the sheer stress. Intracellular calcium and nitric oxide are postulated to play a role in this. Thus, high flow rates and a high sodium load will activate both ROMK and BK channels leading to enhanced potassium secretion.

One final interesting fact about ROMK relates to the role that magnesium plays in the regulation of this transporter [13]. When magnesium binds to the renal outer medullary potassium channel (ROMK) on the intracellular side of the transport protein, it blocks the secretion of potassium. Thus, a lack of sufficient magnesium levels will lead to a more "open" ROMK channel and increased loss of potassium through the urine resulting in hypokalemia. This hypokalemia will not be corrected by simply administering exogenous potassium chloride. Instead, until the magnesium deficiency is corrected, the hypokalemic state will persist.

Knowledge of the receptors and mechanisms involved in sodium reabsorption in the nephron may seem overly detailed, but it does have implications on patient care and clinical practice. Diuretics play a very important role in the management of many patient populations, and medications such as furosemide are administered routinely. With continued administration of furosemide, its effectiveness wanes. The mechanism behind the phenomenon can be easily understood. NKCC2 (furosemide-sensitive, electroneutral Na^+-K^+-$2Cl^-$ cotransporter) sensitivity to furosemide leads to inhibition of NaCl reabsorption in the TAL, thereby increasing the sodium load delivered to NCC (thiazide-sensitive NaCl cotransporter) transporters in the DCT. Rates of flow in the tubular fluid will increase, as will the electrogenic reabsorption of sodium. As a result of the increasingly negative voltage and flow, ROMK and BK (both potassium transport channels) will increase potassium secretion. The hypokalemia that is observed with furosemide administration is thus explained [13].

If a patient is on Lasix (furosemide) chronically, the DCT1 segment adapts through cellular hypertrophy in order to increase the capacity to reabsorb sodium [13]. Remember, the distal convoluted tubule 1 segment's ability to reabsorb sodium occurs only as a result of the work of the thiazide-sensitive NaCl cotransporter. Hypertrophy of the cell leads to an increase in the number of thiazide-sensitive NaCl cotransporters (NCC). This leads to an ability to increase the amount of sodium reabsorbed. This process mitigates the effectiveness of the diuretic with furosemide thereby leading to diuretic resistance. However, since the action of NCC (the thiazide-sensitive NaCl cotransporter) may be inhibited by thiazide diuretics, then their administration may circumvent this adaptive response. In effect, the administration of the thiazide diuretic knocks out the ability of the kidney to reabsorb the increased sodium load that was delivered to the distal convoluted tubule from the administration of furosemide.

22.1.7 Collecting Ducts

Before tubular fluid exits the nephron it must finally pass through the collecting ducts (CD). The cells in the collecting ducts make the final set of fine-tuned adjustments in the areas of water balance, acid-base homeostasis, and inorganic solutes such as sodium, chloride, and potassium [14, 15]. Two cell types—principal cells and intercalated cells—carry out the responsibilities of this nephron segment and are interspersed with one another along the length of the epithelium.

The principal cell focuses its efforts on two main areas: sodium chloride and water reabsorption (◉ Fig. 22.10) [15]. The electrochemical gradient that acts as the driving force for sodium reabsorption is once again created by the Na^+-K^+-ATPase at the basolateral membrane. However, the ENaC protein channel acts as the vessel through which entrance occurs at the apical membrane [14]. Thus, in the CD, the sodium is not actively transported. The transport is electrogenic in nature, and contributes to the secretion of potassium through ROMK and hydrogen ion in a manner similar to what was described in the late DCT. The ENaC receptor is regulated by a number of hormones including aldosterone, atrial natriuretic peptide, and arginine vasopressin. After stimulating the mineralcorticoid receptor, aldosterone multiplies the number of receptors at the apical membrane, thereby magnifying its effects. Insulin also stimulates ENaC in the principle cell. Conversely, ANP inhibits the ENaC channel in addition to repressing secretion of renin and production of aldosterone.

Principal cells mediate water reabsorption through the aquaporin channels [14]. AQP2 is expressed at the apical membrane while AQP3 and AQP4 are located at the basolateral membrane. By this point in the nephron, approximately 90% of the water has already been reclaimed. The amount of fluid reabsorbed at this point is highly dependent on vasopressin levels. Vasopressin is able to modulate the water permeability of the collecting duct though its effects on AQP2. With vasopressin stimulation, AQP2 stores in the cell's interior are transferred to the apical membrane. Additionally, vasopressin can alter protein expression of AQP2 for a longer term effect. Dopamine and prostaglandin E2 antagonize these effects by initiating a mechanism that returns AQP2 from the apical membrane back to intracellular vesicles.

Intercalated cells (IC) make up the remaining population of the collecting duct [15]. One key difference between intercalated cells and almost every other cell described in this chapter lies in the power source driving transport events. Instead of the Na^+-K^+-ATPase, an H^+-ATPase serves as the generator of the electrochemical gradient in intercalated cells. Similar to cells within the distal convoluted tubule, intercalated cells are very rich in mitochondria and all IC contain the enzyme carbonic anhydrase. Three subtypes of intercalated cells exist: type A, type B, and non-A non-B. Type A intercalated cells help to acidify urine. Type B and non-A non-B cells secrete bicarbonate into the tubular lumen.

Type A intercalated cells position the H^+-ATPase at the apical lumen. In a combined effort with an H^+-K^+-ATPase

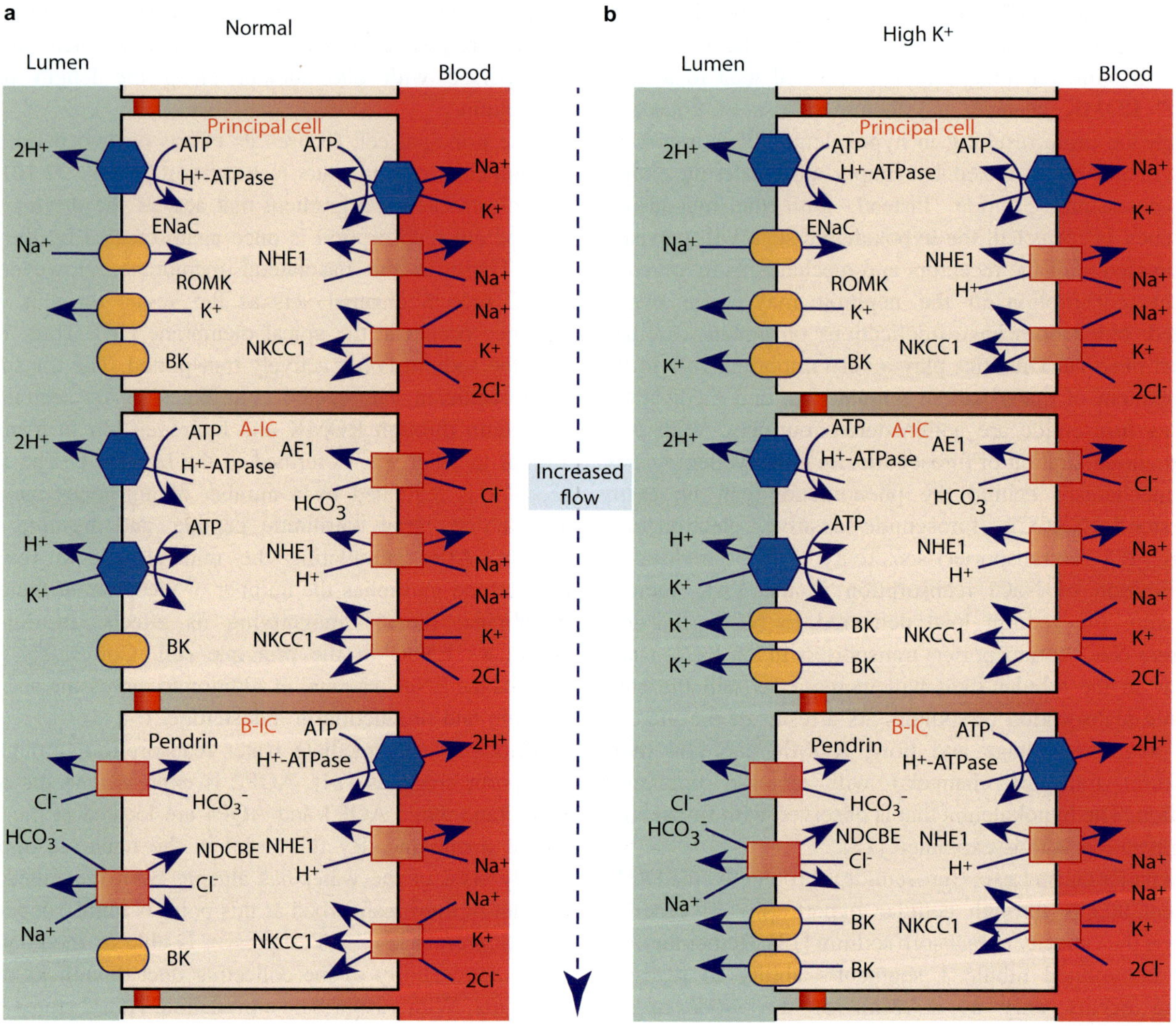

Fig. 22.10 Collecting duct principal cell, type A and type B intercalated cell. Illustration of receptors in each cell type as well as variability of potassium secretion depending on tubular flow. **a** Normal potassium secretion. **b** Potassium secretion as affected by high tubular flow (Adapted from [15])

pump, protons are secreted into the lumen [15]. The loss of the proton drives intracellular carbonic anhydrase to generate bicarbonate, which is reabsorbed by the transporter protein AE1 across the basolateral membrane in exchange for a chloride anion. A clinical example of the importance of this mechanism is found in the inherited forms of distal renal tubular acidosis. In these patient populations, the normal functioning of type A intercalated cells is upset, resulting in a lack of ability to acidify urine. This disruption leads to a state of acidemia, alkalization of urine, and often nephrolithiasis.

Potassium balance can be fine-tuned through the effects of type A IC. The cells can participate in both potassium reabsorption and potassium secretion depending on body conditions. The H^+-K^+-ATPase pump at the apical membrane creates a mechanism for the reabsorption of K^+ from the lumen [15]. However, in response to high luminal flow, a negative voltage gradient, or increased intracellular calcium potassium can be secreted through the BK (maxi-K) channel as has been previously discussed [16].

In type B intercalated cells the H^+-ATPase pump is positioned at the basolateral membrane [15]. The apical membrane contains a transporter protein named pendrin, which excretes a bicarbonate anion into the lumen in exchange for a chloride anion. The presence of an electroneutral $Na^+/HCO_3^-/Cl^-$ transporter allows these cells to play a role in NaCl reabsorption as well. Thus the two roles of the type B intercalated cells include volume expansion and bicarbonate secretion.

The final topic that needs to be addressed relates to the pivotal role that the collecting duct plays in the generation of the urea gradient necessary to drive counter current multiplication and the body's urine-concentrating ability. In the previous discussion of the LoH, we discussed the manner in which urea underwent a passive diffusion down its concentration gradient into the tubular lumen from the renal interstitium. What we neglected to mention, however, was genesis of the high concentration gradient in the renal interstitium. A number of urea transporters in the collecting duct establish and help to maintain the high concentration of urea in the inner medullary intersitium [17]. Located at the apical membrane, the urea transporter UT-A1 carries urea from the tubular lumen into the collecting duct cell. The urea is then transferred across the basolateral membrane by the urea transporter UT-A3. The activity and number of these transporters is regulated by vasopressin. In conditions of high osmolarity, or volume depletion, vasopressin increases the number and activity of the urea transporters thereby increasing the concentration of urea in the inner medullary intersitium. The increased osmolarity allows for increased reabsorption of water and further concentration of urine.

What prevents the concentration gradient established in the inner medulla from being diluted by the blood flowing down the vasa recta? Their permeability to all components (water, urea, and sodium) of the gradient and orientation to the tubular structures reinforce the counter current mechanism. Counter current exchange of urea plays a large role in this. The descending vasa recta and red blood cells contain the urea transporter protein UT-B1. This urea transporter allows the red blood cells to absorb urea as they descend into the inner renal medulla and effectively matches the osmolarity of the blood cells with that of the surrounding interstitium. Thus, no water flows out to dilute the surrounding tissue. As the red cells and vasa recta ascend back toward the renal cortex, UT-B1 helps the red cell to quickly eject urea back into the interstitium. This facilitated transport decreases the osmolarity of the red cells, prevents urea from being carried out of the inner medulla, and reinforces the medullary concentration gradient [11, 17, 18].

22.2 Integrated Processes in the Nephron

The aforementioned journey through all the sections of the nephron has demonstrated some of the cellular mechanisms and processing techniques that the kidney uses in order to adapt to the myriad of internal and external changes the body is confronted with (◉ Fig. 22.11) [8, 10, 16, 17, 19]. ◉ Tables 22.1 and ◉ 22.2 summarize key functions, characteristics, and receptors of each nephron segment. ◉ Table 22.3 delineates the handling of key electrolytes and solutes in the glomerular filtrate as they pass through the

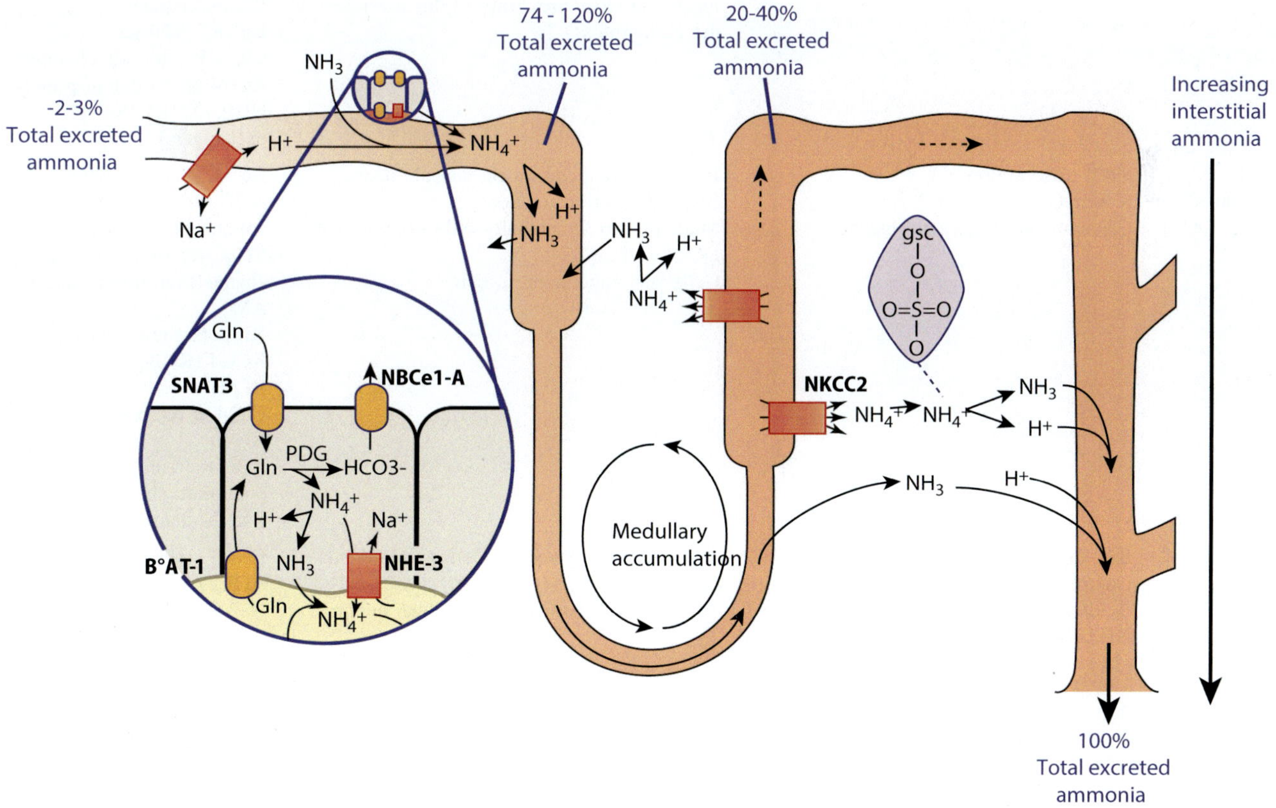

Fig. 22.11 Illustration of ammonia metabolism throughout nephron. See text for details (Adapted from [17])

Table 22.1 Key functions, characteristics, and receptors of each nephron component

Nephron component	Function	Characteristics	Important component receptors
Glomerulus	Filtering unit of kidney	Capillary bundle situated between efferent and afferent arteriole Structural components: fenestrated endothelium, glomerular basement membrane, podocytes, mesangial cells	
Proximal tubule	Reabsorption of large proportion of water, NaCl, $NaHCO_3$, Glucose, AA, phosphate, and citrate Hormone production Gluconeogenesis Synthesizes buffers (NH_3/NH_4^+) Excretion of drugs and endogenous toxins	Low-resistance Low transepithelial voltage High ion permeability High water permeability	Na^+-K^+-ATPase NHE3 receptor (Na^+/H^+ transporter) H^+-ATPase SGLT2/SGLT1 (Na^+-glucose transporter) NaDC-1 (Na^+-dependent dicarboxylic acid cotransporter) AQP1 (aquaporin, water channel)
Thin limb loop of Henle	Involved in counter current multiplication to exchange urea and create gradient to concentrate urine	Descending thin limbs (DTL) are permeable to water (upper 40%) Ascending Thin limbs (ATL) impermeable to water High permeability to urea Passive NaCl reabsorption from prebend segment to ATL	AQP1 (DTL)
Thick ascending limb loop of Henle	Extracellular fluid (ECF) volume Concentration of urine Calcium/Magnesium balance Bicarbonate reabsorption/Ammonium excretion	Water impermeable at apical membrane Actively reabsorbs NaCl leading to a dilute luminal fluid driving counter current multiplication Contains the specialized macula densa cells located in close proximity to the arterioles of the glomerulus	NKCC2 (furosemide-sensitive, electroneutral Na^+-K^+-$2Cl^-$ cotransporter) ROMK (renal outer medullary potassium channel) BK (K channel) Na^+-K^+-ATPase ClC-KB (chloride channel) KCC4 (K-Cl cotransporter) NHE3/NHE4 (Na^+-H^+ exchangers)
Distal Convoluted Tubule (DCT)	NaCl reabsorption K secretion Calcium and Magnesium balance	Begins downstream of the macula densa Shortest nephron segment Made of two functionally different segments: DCT1 and DCT2 Cells very mitochondria-rich	Na^+-K^+-ATPase (BLM) NCC (thiazide-sensitive NaCl cotransporter, AM) ENaC (epithelial sodium channel) (amiloride-sensitive, AM) Kir potassium channels (BLM) KCC4 (K-Cl- transporter, BLM) ClC-KB (chloride channel; BLM) ROMK (renal outer medullary potassium channel, AM) BK (K channel, AM)
Collecting duct	Salt and water transport Control of [K^+] Acid/Base regulation through excretion of NH3/NH_4^+, reabsorption/generation HCO_3	Two cell types: Principal Cells and Intercalated Cells Aldosterone sensitive part of distal nephron	ENaC (epithelial Na channel) AQP2 (water channel) Na^+-K^+-ATPase (principal cells) ROMK BK H^+-ATPase (Intercalated cells) Pendrin ($Cl^-$$HCO_3$ exchanger)

Table 22.2 Key functions of nephron segments and receptors

Hormone	Trigger	Receptor/nephron segment	Effect
Adenosine	Salt loading	Generated by interstitial fibroblasts, which metabolize ATP released by macula densa cells Activates A1 & A2 receptors Inhibition of ENaC in collecting ducts (CD)	Vasodilation of efferent arterioles and Vasoconstriction of afferent arterioles Overall reduction in glomerular filtration rate (GFR) Inhibits renin release
Aldosterone	Hyperkalemia Volume depletion	NCC in distal convoluted tubule (DCT) ROMK (renal outer medullary potassium channel) in DCT Increases # ENaC in DCT and CD Increase pendrin in CD Type B IC	Facilitates K^+ secretion directly Reabsorbs NaCl helping to increase extracellular fluid (ECF) volume Increases K^+ permeability
Angiotensin II	Volume depletion	NCC in DCT Activates ENaC in DCT and CD Increase pendrin and H^+-ATPase in CD Type B IC Inhibits ROMK	Reabsorbs NaCl helping to increase ECF volume Prevents K^+ wasting
Atrial natriuretic peptide	Atrial stretch receptors Angiotensin II Endothelin	Inhibits ENaC in CD Inhibits renin secretion Inhibits aldosterone production in adrenal gland	Inhibits reabsorption of Na^+
Erythropoietin	Decreased tissue oxygen tension	Produced by interstitial renal fibroblasts	Stimulates Erythropoiesis
Insulin	Hyperglycemia	Stimulates NHE3 dependent Na^+ in PT Activates NCC in DCT Stimulates ENaC in CD	Stimulates salt reabsorption
Parathyroid	Decreased in plasma concentration of ionized calcium	TRPV5 receptor in DCT Decreases the abundance of phosphate transporter proteins in proximal tubule	Increased renal reabsorption of calcium Stimulates bone resorption Enhanced intestinal calcium and phosphate absorption by promoting the formation of calcitriol in kidney Decreased renal reabsoption of phosphate
Renin	Atrial Natriuretic peptide Angiotensin II Sympathetic Activation (NaCl) in macula densa cells Nitric oxide Prostacyclin/Prostaglandin E2	Cleaves angiotensinogen to angiotensin I	Regulates the renin–angiotensin–aldosterone system (RAAS) Helps to maintain blood pressure and intravascular volume
Vasopressin	Increasing plasma osmolality Circulatory hemodynamics (i.e., CV collapse) Low sensed circulating volume NE/ Dopamine Pain Hypoxia Acidosis	NCC in DCT Stimulates ENaC in CD Induced an increase in AQP2 receptors in CD Increases permeability of inner medullary CD to urea by Increasing the number and ability of UT-A1/UT-A3 transporters	Stimulates salt reabsorption Increased water reabsorption Overall effect: lower Na^+ concentration

nephron. Now we will use this newfound understanding to broaden our perspective from the microscopic world of the single nephron in order to examine more global processes such as the defense of the body's fluid volume and acid-base status.

22.2.1 Water Homeostasis

Our body's composition consists mainly of water. In fact, water makes up approximately 50–60% of the total body weight [20]. The allocation of water within the body is

Table 22.3 Key electrolytes and solutes in the glomerular filtrate

Solute	Percent	Loop of Henle	Distal convoluted tubule (DCT)	Collecting ducts (CD)
Na^+	60–70% reabsorbed	25–30% reabsorbed: descending thin limb (DTL) and ascending thin limb (ATL) - passive reabsorption Thick ascending limb (TAL) - active reabsorption via NKCC2 and NH3	Reabsorbed via NCC and ENaC DCT and CD together only reabsorb 5–10% filtered Na^+	Reabsorbed via ENaC
Cl^-	60–70% reabsorbed	DTL and ATL – passive reabsorption TAL - active reabsorption	Reabsorbed by NCC and paracellular	Transport via: 1. paracellular transport
Bicarbonate	70–90% reabsorbed/generated	TAL- 15% reabsorbed via apical Na^+/H^+ exchanger		New generation in IC
K^+	Majority of filtered potassium is reabsorbed through paracellular pathway. Only ~ 10% reach distal nephron	TAL - Paracellular reclamation plus transcellular transport via NKCC2 transporter	Secreted into tubular lumen via ROMK (renal outer medullary potassium channel) and BK (K channel)	Secreted into tubular lumen via ROMK in PC May be secreted by BK receptor in Type A IC depending on conditions
Ca^{2+}	60–70% reabsorbed mainly by paracellular transport. Small amount actively transported	20% reabsorbed in TAL mainly via paracellular transport	7–10% actively reabsorbed	5% reabsorbed
Mg^{2+}	10–30% reabsorbed via paracellular pathway	40–70% reabsorbed in TAL via paracellular pathway	5–10% actively reabsorbed	
Phosphate	85% reabsorbed			
NH_4^+	Generates NH_4^+ from glutamine and secreted into lumen	Approximately 50% reabsorbed in TAL into peritubular space with formation of medullary gradient		Secretion of ammonium into lumen by intercalated cells
Urea	Concentration increases as salt and water are reabsorbed	Counter current multiplication, (urea) increases in thin limbs due to secretion but is reabsorbed as the thin limbs ascend; develops an equilibrium with medullary interstitium at TAL	Reabsorption of some of urea. Concentration changes from approximately 110% filtered load to roughly 70%	Excretion of urea into interstitium. Tubular fluid (urea) reduced to 50% filtered load
Water	60–70% reabsorbed	Some reabsorption in DTL ATL, TAL water impermeable	Impermeable	Reabsorbed via AQP proteins
Glucose	> 99% reabsorbed			

divided into two basic compartments: intracellular and extracellular. Two-thirds of total body water is located in the intracellular compartment with the remaining one-third located in the extracellular space. The extracellular space is further divided into the intravascular space containing 25% of extracellular fluid and the interstitial space comprised of the remaining 75% of fluid.

Water is able to flow freely across most cell membranes. Osmotic forces in the body will cause it to shift from one area into another (◉ Table 22.4). Generally, water flows from areas of low osmolality into areas of higher osmolality. The serum osmolarity of the body is tightly regulated and subjected to hormonal control [20]. Serum osmolarity can be calculated by the following equation:

$$\text{Serum Osmolality} = 2[\text{Na}^+] + ([\text{BUN}]/2.8) + ([\text{Glucose}]/18)$$

As illustrated by the equation, the serum sodium concentration exerts the largest effect on the serum osmolality. Thus, regulation of the body's fluid status is largely accomplished through its ability to manipulate serum sodium. Osmolarity is monitored through the presence of special receptors in portions of the brain such as the

Table 22.4 Mechanisms of action in homeostasis

Type of diuretic	Mechanism of action	Result	Example
Osmotic diuretic	Filtered at glomerulus with minimal reabsorption in proximal tubule. Offsets the passive reabsorption of water in the proximal tubule	Excretion of water	Mannitol
Loop diuretic	Inhibit Na and Cl reabsorption in the TAL by inhibiting the electroneutral Na^+-K^+-$2Cl^-$ cotransporter (NKCC2)	Increases excretion of filtered Na load. Increased Calcium and Magnesium excretion in urine Increases K^+ & H^+ excretion at DCT & CT	Furosemide Bumetanide Torsemide
Thiazides/Thiazide like diuretics	Inhibit sodium reabsorption through inhibition of the luminal NaCl cotransporter protein. (NCC) Augment Ca^+ reabsorption in distal tubule	Increase Na^+ excretion by a small amount Increased Na^+ excretion results in enhanced secretion of K^+ & H^+	Hydrochlorothiazide Metolazone Indaptamide
Potassium sparing diuretic	Collecting tubule: Inhibit Na^+ reabsorption and K^+ secretion by blocking epithelial sodium channel (ENaC). May inhibit Na^+ -K^+ -ATPase activity as well	May result in hyperkalemia and metabolic acidosis	Amiloride
Aldosterone Antagoinists	Antagonize aldosterone receptors in CT	Na^+ reabsorption and K^+ secretion are inhibited. This Can lead to hyperkalemia and metabolic acidosis	Spironolactone
Carbonic anhydrase inhibitors	Proximal tubule: inhibit carbonic anhydrase. Inhibits renal acidification (H^+ secretion and Na^+ / HCO_3^- reabsorption)	Weak diuretic due to ability of distal segments of nephron to compensate for the effects on Na^+ and HCO_3^-. End result is a mild hyperchloremic metabolic acidosis	Acetazolamide

organum vasculosum laminae terminalis (OVLT) and hypothalamus. When an increase in osmolality is detected, the osmoreceptors in these locales depolarize the membrane and lead to an activation of the thirst mechanism and release of vasopressin from the posterior hypothalamus. Binding of vasopressin to V2 receptors in the collecting duct actuates the insertion of the AQP2 channels into the apical membrane and the reabsorption of sodium.

22.2.2 Acid-Base Homeostasis

Normally, the serum pH is tightly regulated over a range of 7.36–7.44 to facilitate the optimal functioning of cellular metabolic processes. When physiologic derangements occur to drive the body's acid-base status outside of this range, compensatory responses are initiated in an effort to mitigate the perturbation from normal values [21]. Responses to alterations in pH are managed in a number of ways including the use of buffers, regulation of PCO_2, and manipulation of plasma HCO_3. Proteins and the bone act as important physiologic buffers. However, the bicarbonate/carbon dioxide buffer system is perhaps the most important buffering system in the body.

The Henderson-Hasselbach equation illustrates the relationship between pH, plasma bicarbonate, and PCO_2:

$$pH = 6.1 + \log HCO_3^- / (0.03 \times PCO_2).$$

In order to compensate for a specific change in pH, the body must manipulate values of either HCO_3 or PCO_2.

These values can be independently regulated by the kidneys and the lungs, respectively.

Through changes in ventilation, the lung is able to exert its effects on pH. The key to this effect lies in the interaction of carbon dioxide and water. When the two are combined, carbonic acid is formed, which then dissociates into hydrogen ion and bicarbonate. These forms of water and carbon dioxide exist in an equilibrium and are thus affected when the level of carbon dioxide changes:

$$CO_2 + H_2O \leftrightarrow H_2CO_3 \leftrightarrow H^+ + HCO_3^-$$

Hypoventilation results in an increase in PCO_2. This elevation in PCO_2 will drive the formation of carbonic acid, and thus hydrogen ion and bicarbonate. Changes in ventilation are triggered by specialized chemoreceptor cells within the medulla oblongata responding to alterations in pH and PCO_2. In the example of hypoventilation, the decrease in cerebral intrastitial pH causes the chemoreceptors to stimulate ventilation. As a result of this activation, PCO_2 decreases. Initially, ventilatory changes are most sensitive to changes in PCO_2. The maximal ventilatory response to changes in pH takes approximately 12–24 h. While PCO_2 is easily diffusible, the blood-brain barrier acts as hurdle slowing the response to nonvolatile acids and alterations in plasma bicarbonate. Generally speaking, there is a limit to the effect that ventilation can exert upon the pH via PCO_2, with decreases greater than 12 mm Hg unlikely.

The contribution that the kidney makes in regulating acid-base balance is accomplished through its handling of bicarbonate. Remember that bicarbonate is freely filtered by the glomerulus. The proximal tubule then reabsorbs about 80% of this filtered bicarbonate with the remaining amounts reclaimed in the thick ascending limb of the loop of Henle. The mechanism by which this reabsorption occurs was discussed in detail earlier [7], but essentially relies on the production of hydrogen ion and bicarbonate intracellularly through the work of carbonic anhydrase. The bicarbonate is then reabsorbed into the blood. Meanwhile, the hydrogen ion gets secreted into the luminal fluid. Here the hydrogen ion either gets bound as a titratable acid excreted in the urine or is recycled back into the proximal tubular cell as carbon dioxide (thanks to carbonic anhydrase again) or a form of citrate (remember that citrate can be converted into bicarbonate in the liver). The extent to which these processes occur in the proximal tubule will depend on the body's acid-base and volume status.

Final refinement of the body's acid-base balance is achieved in the distal tubule through the work of the Type A and Type B intercalated cells as previously mentioned. The ultimate effect on the urine, either acidification by type A intercalated cells, or bicarbonate secretion by type B intercalated cells will be influenced by a variety of factors [21]. For example, in type A intercalated cells, vesicles full of H^+-ATPase pump proteins lie beneath the cellular membrane awaiting the pH-induced signal to move to the apical membrane and insert themselves increasing the productivity of the cell. In a sense, these vesicles act as a type of SWAT team immediately responding to pH conditions sensed in the tubular fluid. While these vesicles act as a type of temporary workforce, if conditions persist more chronically, the cell begins to synthesize more transporter proteins, in a sense hiring a larger more permanent workforce. Factors such as potassium depletion, increased sodium reabsorption, and hormonal effects—such as those caused by mineralcorticoids, aldosterone, and angiotensin II—will all lead to increased tubular hydrogen ion secretion.

As illustrated, the kidney has a variety of tools that it can employ in order to compensate for different acid-base disturbances (◉ Table 22.4). As with any compensatory response, the effects are not able to completely correct for the original acid-base disturbance and take some time to fully develop. Chronic respiratory acidosis results in increased reabsorption of bicarbonate by the proximal tubule and its increased production in the distal tubule. Conversely, chronic hypocapnea decreases the reabsorption of bicarbonate by the proximal tubule and results in hydrogen ion secretion in the distal tubule. Large metabolic acid loads that overwhelm the kidney's ability to generate bicarbonate engenders a different set of responses. The plasma bicarbonate will fall despite increased reabsorption of bicarbonate by the proximal tubule. Concurrently, the distal tubule will increase both hydrogen ion secretion as well as secretion of NH_4^+. These responses will take approximately 3–5 days to become fully realized. In addition, a compensatory respiratory response to increase ventilation thereby decreasing PCO_2 will be stimulated. This respiratory response will fully manifest over a 12–24-h period, and again will not be able to fully correct for the metabolic derangement [7].

The response to metabolic alkalosis will depend on a variety of factors [7]. A pure alkali load, such as when a patient is given a bicarbonate infusion, is relatively easily dealt with by the kidney. Decreased proximal tubule reabsorption will lead to loss of bicarbonate in the urine and thus correct the derangement. From a respiratory standpoint, the compensatory response will be to decrease ventilation slightly leading to retention of PCO_2. However, when a metabolic alkalosis is caused by loss of acid such as with vomiting, the kidney's response may actually maintain the metabolic alkalosis until other factors such as hypokalemia, hypochloremia, and hypovolemia are corrected. Chronic hypokalemia results in secretion of hydrogen ion. In patients who are volume contracted, the effects of hormones (such as angiotensin II, aldosterone, and adrenergic agonists) will result in the increased reabsorption of sodium and bicarbonate. Until the volume depletion is corrected, the metabolic alkalosis may be maintained.

22.3 Renal Function Tests

To this point, we have focused on the function of a single nephron. This microscopic level is difficult for clinicians to measure, and considering that there are millions of glomeruli, knowledge of a single nephron's activity is not clinically relevant. As clinicians, we are more focused on the productivity of the kidneys as a whole unit. Unlike the cardiac myocytes, which leak troponin when injured and inflamed, we do not have any similar easily measurable, widely available, validated compounds that provide an early warning of injury to nephrons. This area is being actively researched, and it appears unlikely that a single biomarker will be able to encompass the heterogeneous nature of renal injury [22, 23]. Rather, the diagnosis of renal injury and monitoring of the progression of chronic renal disease may rely on a panel of many different biomarkers, each of which may provide information that helps determine the localization and underlying mechanism of disease [22–25].

At present, the glomerular filtration rate (GFR), which represents the cumulative functioning of all of the millions of nephrons in the kidney, is the parameter referred to as an indicator of global renal function. This value represents the amount of plasma that is filtered through all the glomeruli per unit of time, usually minutes. A normal value for GFR ranges from 120 to 130 ml/min/1.73m^2. This value will vary from person to person depending on factors such as age, and sex. Patients with Stage 5 kidney disease have end-stage renal disease requiring dialysis and have a GFR of less than 15 ml/min/1.73m^2.

A few challenges surround the use of the GFR by clinicians. First and foremost is the fact that the GFR cannot be measured directly. Instead, we must rely on surrogates that act as representative markers of filtration [26–32]. These markers can either be produced endogenously by the body or be introduced exogenously. In order to portray an accurate picture of renal function the concentration of these markers must not be altered by the kidney, i.e., they must not be metabolized, reabsorbed from, or secreted into the tubular lumen. Second, although we use GFR as a measure of renal function, the degree of injury to nephrons does not translate to a proportional decrement in the GFR. For example, a 10% loss of functioning nephrons does not result in a reduction of GFR by 10%. The kidney can be thought of as a stoic organ in the sense that early injuries to it are not easily visible. When nephrons are lost, the remaining units adapt by a "hyperfiltration" of the higher amounts of solutes and water. In this manner, nephron damage can occur without any perceptible change in GFR until this "functional reserve" has been exhausted.

Is it necessary to exactly measure GFR? Knowledge of this marker of kidney function allows us to accurately dose medications thereby reducing toxicity. While it may be imperfect, the GFR helps clinicians follow the progression of loss of renal function. Knowledge of the GFR may aid with issues in prognostication regarding need for renal replacement therapy or listing for renal transplant as well. Given this utility, how then do we reconcile the practical needs of this value with the fact that we cannot directly measure it? Fortunately, in many cases, an estimate of the GFR (eGFR) sufficiently answers many clinical queries [26–32]. For the instances in which a measured value is needed due to concerns of inaccuracies with estimated values, use of exogenous markers can be employed.

22.3.1 Exogenous Markers of Renal Function

Inulin clearance remains the gold standard for determination of GFR. Inulin is a polysaccharide, which is not protein bound. It is solely excreted by glomerular filtration and is neither secreted nor absorbed. The GFR is determined by the exogenous administration of inulin either by a bolus or an infusion. The specifics of how the calculation is determined depends on the method used, but does require multiple samples of blood, and may require a timed urine collection as well. Thus, the method is invasive, expensive, and time consuming [26–32].

The use of different radioisotope compounds largely replaced the use of inulin, but again were difficult to administer, not as accurate, expensive, and not safe in certain patient populations. The use of iohexol or iothalamate provides an alternative nonradioactive method. These compounds are radiocontrast agents. Iohexol is administered as an intravenous bolus injection and calculation of its plasma clearance provides a measurement of GFR. This spares the bedside clinician from having to perform a timed urine collection and deal with all of the special requirements of radioactive isotopes. Iohexol has been shown to underestimate GFR slightly compared to inulin. Renal clearance of iothalamate has also been demonstrated as an accurate method to measure GFR [26–32].

22.3.2 Endogenous Markers of Renal Function

The convenience associated with the use of serum creatinine has led to its widespread use as an indicator of renal function for many years. Creatinine is a product of skeletal muscle breakdown and is freely filtered by the kidney without being reabsorbed. Its serum levels correlate inversely with GFR. However, unlike inulin, creatinine undergoes secretion by the proximal tubule in varying amounts depending on body conditions. Thus it is not an ideal renal biomarker to assess glomerular filtration rates. While this secretion can be blunted by the administration of cimetidine, the use of plasma creatinine is problematic for other reasons as well. Evidence exists of external elimination of creatinine thus adding to inaccuracies. Also, the generation of serum creatinine will depend on factors such as muscle mass, obesity, and dietary intake. For example, a creatinine level of 1.2 may not have the same clinical implications in a body builder taking dietary supplements compared to a frail, wheelchair-bound 80-year-old woman. Patients who have a high volume of distribution from edema can have a "diluted" serum creatinine concentration which again may create a false impression of renal function. Nevertheless, use of creatinine is widely favored because of its ease of use, and cost effectiveness [26–32].

The creatinine clearance can be easily calculated by:

$$\mathrm{CrCl(mg/\,min)} = \frac{[\text{urine creatinine}(\mathrm{mg/mL})] \times 24\text{hour urine volume}(\mathrm{mL})}{\left[\text{plasma creatinine}\left(\frac{\mathrm{mg}}{\mathrm{mL}}\right)\right] \times 24 \times 60\,\mathrm{min}}$$

Performing a 24-h urine collection can be difficult, so in order to minimize inaccuracies, the equation can be modified for a shorter time period of urine collection. Unfortunately, the improvement in convenience and cost effectiveness comes at the price of decreased accuracy in the information obtained. Studies that have been performed comparing the accuracy of serum creatinine in relation to other renal markers have demonstrated that creatinine clearance consistently overestimates the GFR. Additionally, the amount of overestimation increases when the GFR is low.

In most instances, creatinine clearance is not calculated based on plasma and urinary creatinine levels but rather an estimated GFR, which is calculated with equations that incorporate laboratory results with demographic data. Various equations have been developed and evaluated for accuracy compared to measured GFR values. The familiar Cockcroft-Gault equation takes age, weight, and sex into account to calculate eGFR:

$$\begin{aligned}\mathrm{CrCl} &= (140 - \mathrm{YearsAge}) \times (\mathrm{Kgbodyweight}) \\ &\quad \times (0.85\mathrm{iffemale})/(72 \times \mathrm{sCrinmg/dL})\end{aligned}$$

Numerous other equations have been developed over time including the Modification of Diet in Renal Disease (MDRD) study equation, and the CKD-EPI (CKD epidemiology collaboration) equation. These equations have their strengths and weaknesses regarding their accuracy in predicting eGFR accurately and will vary depending on the patient population in question, cultural dietary factors, genetic factors, and level of kidney function.

The issues with serum creatinine described earlier have led to a search for other endogenous renal markers that do not suffer from the limitations described above. A lot of interest has surrounded cystatin C [27, 28]. This compound is generated by nucleated cells and released into the blood. Serum levels also vary inversely with GFR. In the kidney, it is freely filtered by the glomerulus and then reabsorbed and metabolized by the proximal tubules. As such it is not possible to calculate a cystatin C clearance in the way that we calculate one for creatinine. While cystatin C levels are not impacted by factors such as diet and muscle mass in the manner serum creatinine levels are, they can be affected by conditions affecting cell turnover rate such as high doses of steroids and thyroid dysfunction. There is also some evidence from animal studies of extrarenal elimination that may overestimate true GFR. As with serum creatinine, various equations have been developed to estimate GFR based on cystatin C levels. Additionally, equations have been developed that combine the use of both serum creatinine and cystatin C levels in an attempt to determine an equation that accurately reflects GFR and without needing modification due to race. In addition, cystatin C may help to better define and risk stratify patients with chronic kidney disease when compared to use of eGFR based on creatinine alone [27, 28].

Kidney Disease Improving Global Outcomes (KDIGO) has created guidelines for the evaluation of GFR [33]. These guidelines take into consideration the issues described above through a series of recommendations. While they advocate for the utilization of eGFR_{cr} expressed in units of milliliters per minute per $1.73\mathrm{m}^2$ as an initial test, they also recommend the use of confirmatory testing in situations where the presence of confounding factors may affect the accuracy of the initial test. This confirmatory testing can include clearance measurement, or the utilization of an alternate estimation method of GFR, (i.e., from serum cystatin or a combination of serum creatinine and cystatin C). There is still some debate about the role of race in GFR estimation, including which equation best accounts for any potential differences that may result [33].

22.4 Acute Kidney Injury and the Role of Emerging Biomarkers

The difficulties inherent in determining global renal function make it challenging to identify when the kidney has sustained an injury or is under stress. The clinical relevance of this reality is obvious. If one cannot identify that an injury has taken place, it is difficult to institute therapies or guide clinical decisions that reverse or arrest the pathologic process.

In the past, a lack of consensus regarding the definition of acute renal injury has further complicated the clinical picture. Prior research has utilized many different definitions and endpoints making it difficult to interpret research findings [34–40]. Fortunately, this issue is being addressed. A standardized criteria for the definition of acute kidney injury was proposed in 2004 by the Acute Dialysis Quality Initiative and is commonly referred to as the RIFLE criteria (Risk Injury Failure Loss End-stage renal disease) [34]. This definition has been refined over the years and the current consensus definition has been described by the Kidney Disease Improving Global Outcomes (KDIGO) group [35]. The classification system according to the KDIGO criteria describes three stages of acute renal injury. These stages are generally differentiated from one another based on two variables: increases in serum creatinine and changes in urine output. The KDIGO criteria is summarized in ◉ Table 22.5. The differentiation between the stages is relatively straightforward when one considers the urine output parameters. With a Foley catheter in place, it is not difficult to determine how much urine a patient has produced over the specified time period. On the other hand, the criteria for changes in serum creatinine are more difficult to interpret. Oftentimes, clinicians do not have the luxury of knowing what a patient's baseline creatinine is. This makes it difficult to interpret a given elevated creatinine level. A creatinine level that seems normal for the average individual may actually be pathologic in an older patient since they tend to produce less creatinine as a result of lower levels of muscle mass. Thus, an elevation in creatinine may either: (1) go completely unrecognized missing the acute renal injury completely, or (2) have a renal injury recognized but be underestimated in terms of its severity.

As mentioned previously, the desire to improve our clinical ability to both diagnose and improve prognostic prediction in acute kidney injury has led to a very active search to identify renal biomarkers. A number of different biomarkers have shown promise in helping to identify both acute kidney injury and kidney stress. Research into potential biomarkers has been very active. Multiple candidates have emerged and include proteins such as neutrophil gelatinase-associated lipocalin (NGAL), Kidney injury molecule-1 (KIM-1), Interleukin18 (IL-18), and liver-type fatty acid-binding protein (L-FABP). Molecules that act as mediators of cell-cycle arrest, such as tissue inhibitor metalloproteinases-s (TIMP-2) and insulin-like growth factor-binding protein 7 (IGFBP-7) may also serve as indicators of abnormal function. Finally, there has been a lot of work looking at the roles that microRNAs may play in the pathophysiology of the kidney and their potential utility in acting as biomarkers of function [22–25].

22.5 Renal Drug Excretion

Stop and think for a moment about the myriad of compounds that the kidney must handle over the course of a person's life. In addition to managing levels of electrolytes, amino acids, glucose, etc. that we addressed earlier, nephrons also manage the excretion of metabolic byproducts, both endogenous and exogenous toxins, as well as drugs and vitamins. The manner in which this impressive logistical feat is accomplished is not all that well understood and is being actively investigated. A discussion regarding the manner of disposal by the kidney of all the compounds of interest to the anesthesiologist is beyond the scope of this discussion. Instead, we will focus on developing an overall understanding of how drugs and endogenous toxins are manipulated by the kidney as well as the complexity of the interactions involved [41–43].

As discussed, the glomerulus is the site of initial filtration of most compounds with the exception of anions and large molecules. When the glomerulus is damaged, it may lose its ability to prevent these compounds from being filtered, leading to a loss of albumin and a subsequent alteration in binding and free fraction of protein-bound drugs.

The proximal tubule segment shares a significant portion of the responsibility for drug and endogenous toxin excretion as well, according to our current understanding of renal

Table 22.5 The Kidney Disease Improving Global Outcomes (KDIGO) criteria [35]

KDIGO stage of renal dysfunction	Serum creatinine	Urine output
1	Increase 1.5–1.9 × baseline *or* > 0.3 mg/dL increase within 48 h	< 0.5 mL/kg/h for 6–12 h
2	Increase 2.0 to 2.9 × baseline	< 0.5 mL/kg/h for > 12 h
3	Increase 3.0 × baseline *or* Rise serum creatinine to > or equal to 4.0 *or* Initiation of renal replacement therapy (RRT) *or* Decrease eGFR to < 35 mL/min per 1.73 m2 in patients < 18 years old	< 0.3 mL/kg/h for > or equal to 24 h *or* Anuria for > or equal to 12 h

eGFR estimated glomerular filtration rate

drug elimination. It manages those compounds that are either too large or too protein bound to be effectively filtered by the glomerulus. The sheer number of different compounds makes it impractical for a specific transporter protein to be created for every type of compound to which the body is exposed. Instead, the kidney appears to rely on specialized drug transporter proteins to process compounds depending on characteristics such as size and electrical charge. Compounds can be classified as positively charged organic cations, negatively charged organic anions, or containing both positive and negative charges.

Those drugs not undergoing glomerular filtration reach the proximal tubule through peritubular capillaries. Multi-specific drug transporters then import the compounds into the peritubular cell. Two general types of transporters exist and are differentiated from one another by the way that they fund the energy expenditure necessary for their actions. The first type, solute carriers or SLC carriers, either take advantage of a favorable concentration gradient or make use of secondary, or even tertiary active transport. (This again underscores the importance of the Na^+-K^+-ATPase.) The two most important members of this family of transporters are the organic anion transporters (OAT) and the organic cation transporters (OCT). The second general class is the ATP-binding cassette (ABC) transporters. These transporters make use of ATP hydrolysis to generate the energy needed for the transport process. Once the compounds have been imported across the basolateral (capillary-cell interface) membrane then they travel across the cell to the apical membrane where they are shuttled across into the tubular lumen.

Different transporters are involved in the handling of organic anions versus organic cations. For organic cations, OCT2 mediates transport on the basolateral membrane while proteins such as MATEs are involved in the apical transport. Transport of organic anions occurs via OAT1 and OAT3 on the basolateral membrane with OAT4 and ABC transporters such as MRP2 functioning at the apical interface.

The key here is not to get caught up in this veritable alphabet soup of transporters, but to have an awareness of the pathway drugs and toxins take in order to undergo secretion and elimination. This knowledge also helps us to understand the reasons for different drug-drug interactions and the variability of responses to medications in certain patients. With the many different substrates available to these transporter proteins it should not be surprising that they can become saturated. Fortunately, many of these compounds can be managed by more than one type of renal transporter. Still, the addition of a new substrate may alter the excretion of another one through its occupation of the renal transporter binding site. An example of this type of competitive inhibition was mentioned earlier when we discussed the ability of cimetidine to inhibit secretion of creatinine. Creatinine and cimetidine are both substrates of OCT2. Another example involves the interaction between methotrexate and nonsteroidal anti-inflammatory drugs (NSAIDs). The use of NSAIDs in preoperative care is very common. Many patients with Crohn's disease or other autoimmune diseases have been prescribed methotrexate. The elimination of methotrexate is mediated by OAT transporters, which can be inhibited by NSAIDs. Thus, the coadministration of these medications can result in methotrexate toxicity and bone marrow suppression.

Variability in the clinical effects of drugs in different individuals may be partially explained by different variations or polymorphisms of these transporter proteins. Changes in the makeup of these proteins may lead to differences in rates of transport, which may affect drug efficacy and or toxicity. Metformin is an example of a drug whose variable effectiveness may be explained by this mechanism.

Finally, the above discussion has mainly focused on drug elimination in healthy kidney. Chronic kidney disease results in many changes in drug elimination and excretion. These changes result from the accumulation of uremic toxins and have effects outside of the kidney itself. They can alter bioavailability of drugs, the expression and activity of cytochrome P450 3A enzymes in the liver, and drug transporter proteins in the liver. The transporter proteins in the kidney itself can also be affected leading to reduced excretion of drugs. Alterations in albumin levels affect free drug levels, and uremic toxins can affect the ability of the remaining albumin to bind to acidic drugs. Fortunately, it appears that the removal of uremic toxins by hemodialysis can reverse some of these effects.

22.6 Questions and Answers

Questions (Choose the Most Appropriate Answer)

1. Which of the following correctly pairs the highest degree of reabsorption of the indicated substance with the nephron segment?
   A. Proximal tubule: albumin
   B. Collecting duct: glucose
   C. Ascending thin limb loop of Henle: water
   D. Magnesium: loop of Henle
   E. Collecting duct: ammonium ion
2. The sodium potassium ATPase pump creates the electrochemical gradient responsible for cellular activities in all of the following cell types EXCEPT:
   A. Proximal tubule cell
   B. Descending thin limb loop of cell
   C. Thick ascending limb cell
   D. Principal cell in collecting duct
   E. Intercalated cell in collecting duct

3. Which of the following compounds/solutes is NOT reabsorbed in the proximal tubule?
   A. NH_4^+
   B. Amino acids
   C. Bicarbonate
   D. Water
   E. Sodium
4. Which of the following statements regarding renal anatomy is INCORRECT?
   A. The left kidney has a more cephalad position in the body compared to the right kidney.
   B. The body contains approximately 2 million nephrons.
   C. The kidney receives approximately 15% of total cardiac output.
   D. The majority of nephrons in the renal cortex are cortical rather than juxtamedullary.
   E. The left renal vein is longer than the right renal vein.
5. Which is the TRUE statement regarding the loop of Henle?
   A. The thin descending and ascending limbs are permeable to water.
   B. The thin descending and ascending limbs have limited permeability to urea.
   C. The area from the hairpin loop to the thick ascending limb of the loop of Henle is permeable to NaCl.
   D. Reabsorption of NaCl in the thick ascending limb occurs mainly via the paracellular pathway.
   E. More calcium than magnesium is reabsorbed in the thick ascending limb.
6. Which of the following statements about the distal convoluted tubule (DCT) is TRUE?
   A. Of the two segments of the DCT, the DCT2 segment is the most sensitive to the effects of aldosterone.
   B. Sodium reabsorption in the early DCT is electrogenic in nature, but electroneutral in the late DCT.
   C. The late DCT is an important mediator of potassium reabsorption in the nephron.
   D. Magnesium plays an important role in the mechanism through which potassium reabsorption is achieved in the DCT.
   E. None of the above
7. Which of the following patients would be expected to have a normal serum osmolality?
   A. An 18-year-old patient with type 1 diabetes was admitted with a blood sugar of 480.
   B. A 55-year-old patient who has been taking salt substitutes (KCl).
   C. An 81-year-old patient with end-stage renal disease (ESRD) prior to institution of dialysis.
   D. A 75-year-old patient with syndrome of inappropriate antidiuretic hormone secretion (SIADH).
   E. A 56-year-old patient treated with hypertonic saline in the neuro ICU secondary to elevated intracranial pressure (ICP).
8. Which of the following is a FALSE statement regarding inulin?
   A. Measurements of its clearance are considered to represent the "gold standard" for determination of renal function.
   B. Inulin is neither secreted, excreted, nor reabsorbed by the kidney.
   C. Measurement of GFR using inulin clearance is costly and effort intensive.
   D. Inulin clearance has been replaced by other methods in order to measure renal function.
   E. Inulin is an endogenous compound and is a polysaccharide.
9. Which of the following regarding endogenous markers of renal function is TRUE?
   A. Serum creatinine gives an accurate representation of renal function because it is not secreted or reabsorbed by the kidney.
   B. A serum creatinine level of 1.0 would be considered to be representative of normal renal function in all patients.
   C. Renal clearance of cystatin C acts as an alternative marker of renal function in a manner similar to creatinine clearance.
   D. Both cystatin C and creatinine levels vary inversely with GFR.
   E. Cystatin C levels are influenced by dietary factors in a manner similar to that of serum creatinine.
10. Regarding the handling of drugs and toxins by the kidney, which of the following represents an accurate pairing:
    A. Glomerulus: filtration of anions
    B. Proximal tubule: small, non-protein-bound drugs
    C. SLC carriers: make use of ATP hydrolysis to generate the energy needed for the transport process.
    D. Peritubular capillaries: Mechanism for transportation of large protein-bound compounds to the proximal tubule.
    E. ABC transporters: Depend on a favorable concentration gradient, secondary, or even tertiary active transport to drive the energy expenditure necessary for the transport of drugs.

Answers

1. **D**. The highest rate of reabsorption of magnesium occurs via the paracellular pathway in the loop of Henle. Under normal physiologic conditions, albumin is not filtered by the glomerulus and thus does not undergo reabsorption. Glucose is reabsorbed almost completely by the proximal tubule. The thin ascending limb of the loop of Henle is impermeable to water. The collecting duct secretes ammonium ion rather than reabsorbing it.
2. **E**. Instead of the Na^+-K^+-ATPase, an H^+-ATPase serves as the generator of the electrochemical gradient in intercalated cells.
3. **A**. All of the listed compounds/solutes undergo reabsorption by the proximal tubule with the exception of NH_4^+. Ammonium is actually *produced* by the proximal tubule not reabsorbed. Ammonium ion can be created in a variety of ways. Hydrogen ion secreted into the proximal tubule lumen can combine with NH_3 to form ammonium anion thus functioning as a titratable acid. Under conditions of acidosis, glutamine undergoes metabolism in the proximal tubular cell. The mitochondrial enzyme glutaminase interacts with glutamine to form glutamate and an ammonium ion. The glutamate then undergoes enzymatic conversion into alpha-ketoglutarate and another ammonium ion. The two ammonium ions can either be secreted into the lumen by the NH_3 transporter, or can undergo dissociation into a hydrogen ion and NH_3 with subsequent transport into the lumen. In summary, metabolism of glutamine under conditions of acidosis leads to the formation of two ammonium ions, and alpha-ketoglutarate. The ammonium is secreted into the tubular lumen and flows through subsequent nephron segments.
4. **C**. The kidney receives approximately 20–25% of cardiac output. The other statements are all correct.
5. **C**. The area from just prior to the hairpin loop to the thick ascending limb (TAL) is permeable to NaCl, which is passively reabsorbed. The ascending thin limb and the majority of the descending thin limb are impermeable to water due to a lack of expression of the aquaporin channel. The thin limbs of the loop of Henle are highly permeable to urea, which diffuses into the luminal fluid as the descending thin limb dives into the renal medulla. The urea then diffuses back out of the lumen as the tubule ascends back toward the renal cortex. In the TAL, the transport of NaCl occurs actively. While there may be a small amount reabsorbed from the tubular lumen via the paracellular pathway, the majority occurs as a result of secondary active transport. The paracellular pathway plays an important role in the reabsorption of both magnesium and calcium. However, 55% of filtered magnesium is reabsorbed by the TAL compared to only 20% of calcium.
6. **A**. It is true that of the two segments of the DCT, the DCT2 segment is the most sensitive to the effects of aldosterone.
7. **B**. Serum osmolarity can be calculated by the following equation:

$$\text{Serum Osmolality} = 2[\text{Na}^+] + ([\text{BUN}]/2.8) + ([\text{Glucose}]/18)$$

8. **E**. All of the answers are true with the exception of the fact that inulin is an exogenous compound administered to a patient in an effort to measure renal function.
9. **D**. Creatinine is not an ideal marker of renal function because it is secreted by the proximal tubule. Also, the generation of serum creatinine will depend on factors such as muscle mass, obesity, and dietary intake. For example, a creatinine level of 1.2 may not have the same clinical implications in a body builder taking dietary supplements compared to a frail, wheelchair-bound 80-year-old woman. Patients who have a high volume of distribution from edema can have a "diluted" serum creatinine concentration, which again may create a false impression of renal function. Cystatin C is generated by nucleated cells and released into the blood. In the kidney, it is freely filtered by the glomerulus and then reabsorbed and metabolized by the proximal tubules. As such it is not possible to calculate a cystatin C clearance in the way that we calculate one for creatinine. Cystatin C levels are not impacted by factors such as diet and muscle mass in the manner serum creatinine levels are affected. Both creatinine and cystitis C serum levels vary inversely with GFR.
10. **D**. The glomerulus is the site of initial filtration of most compounds with the exception of anions and large molecules. The proximal tubule manages those compounds that are either too large or protein bound to be effectively filtered by the glomerulus. Those drugs not undergoing glomerular filtration reach the proximal tubule through peritubular capillaries. Multi-specific drug transporters then import the compounds into the peritubular cell. Two general types of transporters exist and are differentiated by the way that they fund the energy expenditure necessary for their actions. The first type, solute carriers or SLC carriers, either take advantage of a favorable concentration gradient or make use of secondary, or even tertiary active transport. The second general class is the ATP-binding cassette (ABC) transporters. These transporters make use of ATP hydrolysis to generate the energy needed for the transport process.

References

1. Tanagho EA, Lue TF. Chapter 1. Anatomy of the genitourinary tract. In: MA JW, Lue TF, editors. Smith and Tanagho's general urology, 18e. New York, NY: McGraw-Hill; 2013. http://accesssurgery.mhmedical.com/content.aspx?bookid=508§ionid=41088078.
2. Mount DB. Thick ascending limb of the loop of Henle. Clin J Am Soc Nephrol. 2014;9(11):1974–86.
3. Pollak MR, Quaggin SE, Hoenig MP, Dworkin LD. The glomerulus: the sphere of influence. Clin J Am Soc Nephrol. 2014;9(8):1461–9.
4. Miner J. The glomerular basement membrane. Exp Cell Res. 2012;318(9):973–8.
5. Kitching AR, Hutton HL. The players: cells involved in glomerular disease. Clin J Am Soc Nephrol. 2016;11:1664–74.
6. Schlondorff D, Banas B. The mesangial cell revisited: no cell is an island. J Am Soc Nephrol. 2009;20:1179–87.
7. Curthoys NP, Moe OW. Proximal tubule function and response to acidosis. Clin J Am Soc Nephrol. 2014;9(9):1627–38.
8. Palmer LG, Schnermann J. Integrated control of Na transport along the nephron. Clin J Am Soc Nephrol. 2015;10:676–87.
9. Su W, Cao R, Zhang X, Guan Y. Aquaporins in the kidney: physiology and pathophysiology. Am J Physiol Renal Physiol. 2020; 318:F193–F203.
10. Blaine J, Chonchol M, Levi M. Renal control of calcium, phosphate, and magnesium homeostasis. Clin J Am Soc Nephrol. 2015;10:1257–72.
11. Zacchia M, Capolongo G, Rinaldi L, Capasso G. The importance of the thick ascending limb of Henle's loop in renal physiology and pathophysiology. Int J Nephrol Renovascular Disease. 2018; 81–92.
12. Dantzler WH, Layton AT, Layton HE, Pannabecker TL. Urine-concentrating mechanism in the inner medulla: function of the thin limbs of the loops of Henle. Clin J Am Soc Nephrol. 2014;9(10):1781–9.
13. Subramanya AR, Ellison DH. Distal convoluted tubule. Clin J Am Soc Nephrol. 2014;9:2147–63.
14. Pearce D, Soundararajan R, Trimpert C, Kashlan OB, Deen PMT, Kohan DE. Collecting duct principal cell transport processes and their regulation. Clin J Am Soc Nephrol. 2015;10:135–46.
15. Roy A, Al-bataineh MM, Pastor-Soler NM. Collecting duct intercalated cell function and regulation. Clin J Am Soc Nephrol. 2015;10(2):305–24.
16. Palmer BF. Regulation of potassium homeostasis. Clin J Am Soc Nephrol. 2015;10:1050–60.
17. Weiner ID, Mitch WE, Sands JM. Urea and ammonia metabolism and the control of renal nitrogen excretion. Clin J Am Soc Nephrol. 2015;10(8):1444–58.
18. Nawata CM, Pannabecker TL. Mammalian urine concentration: a review of renal medullary architecture and membrane transporters. J Comp Physiol B. 2018;188:899–918.
19. Zeisberg M, Kalluri R. Physiology of the renal interstitium. Clin J Am Soc Nephrol. 2015;10:1831–40.
20. Danziger J, Zeidel ML. Osmotic homeostasis. Clin J Am Soc Nephrol. 2015;10:852–62.
21. Hamm LL, Nakhoul N, Hering-Smith KS. Acid-base homeostasis. Clin J Am Soc Nephrol. 2015;10:2232.
22. Oh D. A long journey for acute kidney injury biomarkers. Renal Fail. 2020;42:154–65.
23. Perico L, Perico N, Benigni A. The incessant search for renal biomarkers: is it really justified? Curr Opin Nephrol Hypertens 2019;28:195–202.
24. Zhang WR, Parikh CR. Biomarkers of acute and chronic kidney disease. Annu Rev Physiol. 2019;10:309–33.
25. Bhatt K, Kato M, Natarajan R. Mini-review: emerging roles of microRNAs in the pathophysiology of renal diseases. Am J Physiol Renal Physiol. 2015;310:F109–18.
26. Lamba E, Stevens P. Estimating and measuring glomerular filtration rate: methods of measurement and markers for estimation. Curr Opin Nephrol Hypertens. 2014;23:258–66.
27. Shlipak MG, Mattes MD, Peralta CA. Update on cystatin C: incorporation into clinical practice. Am J Kidney Dis. 2013;62 (3):595–603.
28. Inker LA, Okparavero A. Cystatin C as a marker of glomerular filtration rate: prospects and limitations. Curr Opin Nephrol Hypertens. 2011;20(6):631–9.
29. Macedoa E, Mehta RL. Measuring renal function in critically ill patients: tools and strategies for assessing glomerular filtration rate. Curr Opin Crit Care. 2013;19:560–6.
30. Soveri I, Berg UB, Björk J, Elinder CG, Grubb A, Mejare I, et al. SBU GFR Review Group. Measuring GFR: a systematic review. Am J Kidney Dis. 2014;64(3):411–24.
31. Puzantian HV, Townsend RR. Understanding kidney function assessment: the basics and advances. J Am Assoc Nurse Pract. 2013;25(7):334–41.
32. Filler G, Yasin A, Medeiros M. Methods of assessing renal function. Pediatr Nephrol. 2014;29:183–92.
33. Levey AS, Titan SM, Powe NR, Coresh J, Inker LA. Kidney disease, race, and GFR estimation. CJASN. 2020;15:1203–12.
34. Bouman C, Kellum JA, Lamiere N, Levin N. Acute dialysis quality initiative. 2004. http://www.adqi.org/Upload/Reports/ADQI_2/ADQI2g1.pdf. Accessed 30 Nov 2016.
35. Kidney Disease Improving Global Outcomes (KDIGO). KDIGO clinical practice guideline for acute kidney injury. Kidney Int Suppl. 2012;2:8–12.
36. Goren O, Matot I. Perioperative acute kidney injury. Br J Anaesth. 2015;115(S2):ii3–14.
37. Vellum J. Diagnostic criteria for acute kidney injury. Crit Care Clin. 2015;31:621–32.
38. Golden D, Corbett J, Forni LG. Peri-operative renal dysfunction: prevention and management. Anaesthesia. 2016;71(Suppl. 1):S1-7.
39. Chen L, Koyner JL. Biomarkers in acute kidney injury. Brit Care Clin. 2015;31:633–48.
40. Washung ME, Lakhmir SC, Madero M. Biomarkers of renal function, which and when? Clin Chim Acta. 2015;438:350–7.
41. Naud J, Nolin T, Leflon FA, Pichette V. Current understanding of drug disposition in kidney disease. J Clin Pharmacol. 2012;52:10S-22S.
42. Joy MS. Impact of glomerular kidney diseases on the clearance of drugs. J Clin Pharmacol. 2012;52:23S-34S.
43. Nigam SK, Wu W, Bush KT, Hoenig MP, Blantz RC, Bhatnager V. Handling of drugs, metabolites, and uremic toxins by kidney proximal tubule drug transporters. Clin J Am Soc Nephrol. 2015;10(11):2039–49.

The Endocrine System and Metabolic Complications in Anesthesia

23

Ashley Miller, Trisha McGinnis, and Roshni Sreedharan

Abstract

This chapter outlines key aspects of endocrine physiology relevant to anesthesia practice. It discusses the functions of major endocrine organs, their hormonal regulation, and perioperative considerations. Highlighted disorders include acromegaly, diabetes insipidus, syndrome of inappropriate antidiuretic hormone secretion, hypothyroidism, hyperthyroidism, primary hyperparathyroidism, primary hyperaldosteronism (Conn syndrome), and primary hypercortisolism (Cushing's syndrome). The chapter underscores their implications for anesthesia management, stressing diagnosis, treatment, and perioperative strategies for optimal patient care.

Keywords

Hypothalamus • Pituitary • Acromegaly • Diabetes insipidus • SIADH • Thyroid gland • Parathyroid glands • Adrenal gland • Pancreas

Key Points

1. The neuroendocrine system within the brain consists of the hypothalamus and pituitary gland that regulates several physiologic processes including metabolism, volume status, stress response, growth, and reproduction.
2. Diabetes insipidus results in the inability of the kidney to concentrate urine due to deficiency in ADH. This can lead to profound hypovolemia and hypernatremia. Depending on the etiology, treatment involves fluid restriction versus desmopressin to restore fluid status.
3. Syndrome of inappropriate antidiuretic hormone is a disorder of excess ADH or vasopressin often resulting in euvolemic hyponatremia. Depending on the etiology, treatment involves electrolyte correction and fluid restriction.
4. Acromegaly is a condition resulting from excess growth hormone. Patients can be expected to have a difficult airway.
5. Hyperthyroidism and hypothyroidism have specific perioperative considerations. These pathologies carry significant morbidity and mortality including thyrotoxicosis and myxedema coma respectively.
6. The parathyroid glands control calcium homeostasis within the body. Hyperparathyroidism can result in altered mental status with EKG changes including QT shortening, ST segment elevation, and prominent U waves.
7. Primary hyperaldosteronism or Conn syndrome is a state of excess mineralocorticoids that results in hypertension and hypokalemia, with sodium and water retention. This pathology increases patients' morbidity and mortality from cardiovascular complications.
8. Primary hypercortisolism or Cushing's syndrome occurs due to an excess of glucocorticoids resulting in hypertension, impaired glucose metabolism, increased susceptibility to infections and poor wound healing. This pathology also increases morbidity and mortality due to cardiovascular complications.
9. Primary adrenal insufficiency or Addison's disease is a state of mineralocorticoid and glucocorticoid deficiency resulting in low blood pressure, hyponatremia, hyperkalemia, and metabolic acidosis. Patients are at an increased risk for a fatal

A. Miller (✉) · T. McGinnis · R. Sreedharan
Department of Intensive Care and Resuscitation, Anesthesiology Institute, Cleveland Clinic, Cleveland, OH, USA
e-mail: millere78@ccf.org

A. Miller · T. McGinnis · R. Sreedharan
Department of General Anesthesiology, Anesthesiology Institute, Cleveland Clinic, Cleveland, OH, USA

M. Argalious et al. (eds.), *Basic Sciences in Anesthesia*,
https://doi.org/10.1007/978-3-031-60203-0_23

Addisonian crisis during times of stress, presenting as catecholamine-resistant hypotension.

10. Iatrogenic adrenal insufficiency is due to chronic steroid therapy that results in suppression of the Hypothalamic-Pituitary-Adrenal (HPA) axis that can present as a life-threatening adrenal crisis during times of stress. Patients at greatest risk include those on an equivalent of 20 mg of prednisone a day for a duration greater than 3 weeks. Perioperative steroid supplementation should be provided in these patients.
11. Pheochromocytoma classically presents with hypertension, tachycardia and diaphoresis. Intraoperative management includes minimizing stressors that increase catecholamine release and use of alpha-adrenergic blockers prior to any beta 2 blockers to prevent a hypertensive emergency.
12. Diabetes mellitus, both type 1 and type 2, carries an increased risk of morbidity and mortality due to microvascular and macrovascular complications. Patients are at an increased risk for aspirationpositioning injuries, and cardiovascular complications such as myocardial injury.

23.1 Introduction

The endocrine system maintains homeostasis within the body by release of hormones that have modulatory effects on distant organs (Fig. 23.1). These pathways are regulated by feedback loops to maintain homeostasis and are involved in maintaining metabolism, intravascular volume status, stress response, growth, and reproduction to name a few. Endocrine glands are ductless secretory organs that release chemical messengers in the form of peptides, amines, steroids, and catecholamine's depending on the originating endocrine gland. This chapter focuses on the basic physiology and function of the major endocrine organs and perioperative considerations related to their dysfunction.

23.2 The Hypothalamus

The hypothalamus is located below the thalamus. Located inferiorly is the pituitary gland. The hypothalamus functions as the control center of the endocrine system via neurosecretory neurons which release hormones that act upon the pituitary gland (Fig. 23.2). These hormones are classified as releasing or inhibiting based on the response that is triggered by its action on the pituitary. The releasing hormones are

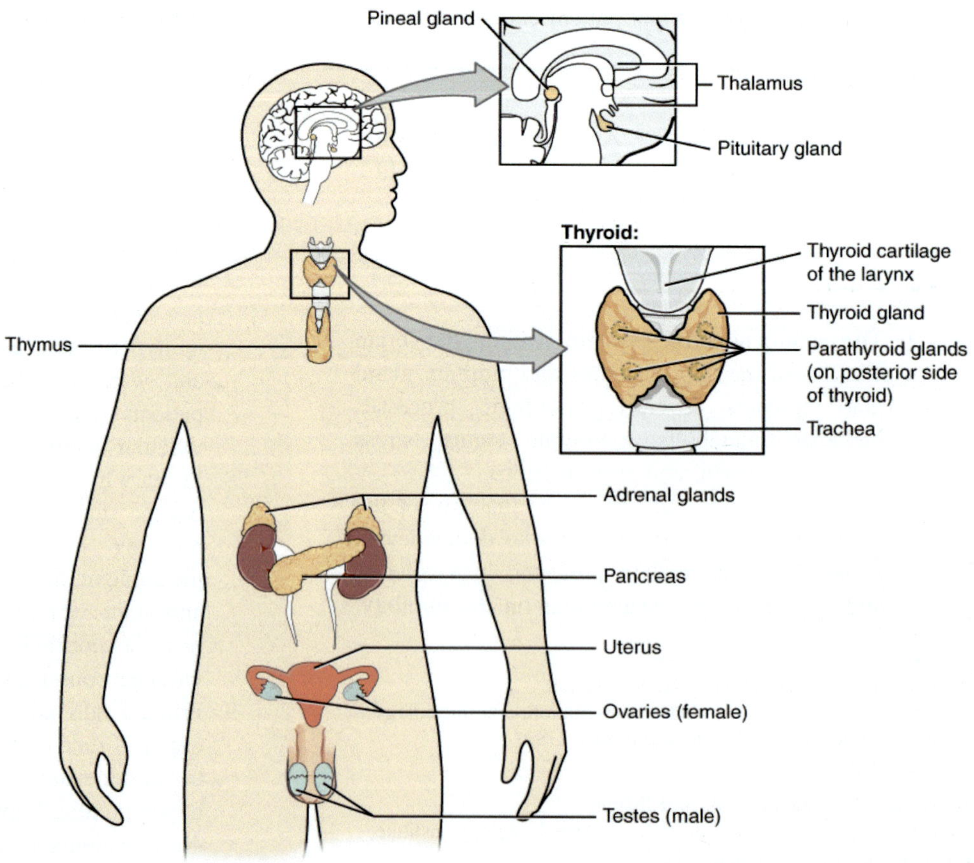

Fig. 23.1 The endocrine system (Reprinted from OpenStax, Anatomy & Physiology, OpenStax. 25 April 2013. Creative Commons Attribution 4.0 International License. Download for free at ► http://cnx.org/content/col11496/latest/

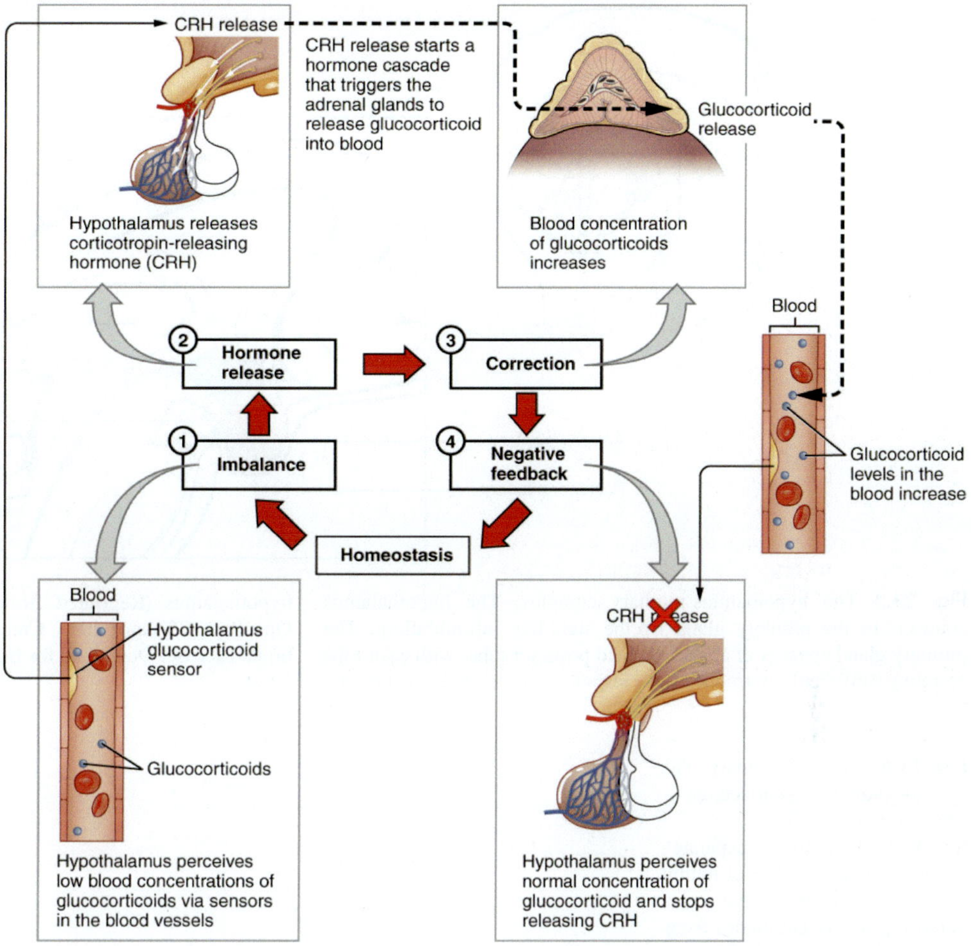

Fig. 23.2 The hypothalamus responds to different environmental stimuli and produces an endocrine response to maintain homeostasis (Reprinted from OpenStax, Anatomy & Physiology, OpenStax. 25 April 2013. Creative Commons Attribution 4.0 International License. Download for free at http://cnx.org/content/col11496/latest/

corticotropin-releasing hormone (CRH), gonadotropin-releasing hormone (GnRH), growth-hormone-releasing hormone (GHRH), and thyrotropin-releasing hormone (TRH) (Fig. 23.3). The inhibiting hormones are somatostatin and dopamine. Hormone release from the hypothalamus is regulated by negative feedback (Fig. 23.4). In addition to the function of secreting releasing and inhibiting hormones, the hypothalamus is responsible for producing antidiuretic hormone and oxytocin which are then stored in the posterior pituitary gland (Fig. 23.5) [1].

23.3 The Pituitary Gland

The pituitary gland is situated below the hypothalamus and is divided into the anterior pituitary and posterior pituitary. The anterior pituitary is connected to the hypothalamus by the hypophyseal portal system, whereas the posterior pituitary is comprised of hypothalamic neuronal axons.

The anterior pituitary is referred to as the adenohypophysis. It is made of five distinct cell types which produce and secrete hormones. Corticotrophs produce adrenocorticotropic hormone (ACTH) which acts on the zona fasciculata of the adrenal glands to stimulate glucocorticoid production. ACTH is regulated by the hypothalamic secretion of Corticotrophin Releasing Hormone (CRH). Gonadotrophs are responsible for the secretion of follicle-stimulating hormone (FSH) and luteinizing hormone (LH). These two hormones target reproductive function of the ovaries and testes. Gonadotrophin Releasing Hormone (GnRh) secreted by the hypothalamus regulates FSH and LH. Lactotrophs produce prolactin although secretion is tonically inhibited by dopamine. The purpose of prolactin is the development of the mammary glands and milk production. Somatotrophs secrete growth hormone (GH). GH plays an important role in the body guiding tissue growth and metabolism. Release of GH from somatotrophs is stimulated by Growth-Hormone-Releasing Hormone (GHRH) and inhibited by somatostatin, as well as other hormones. Thyrotrophs are the source of thyroid stimulating hormone (TSH) which acts on the thyroid gland to activate production and secretion of thyroxine and triiodothyronine. The release of TSH is controlled by TRH [2].

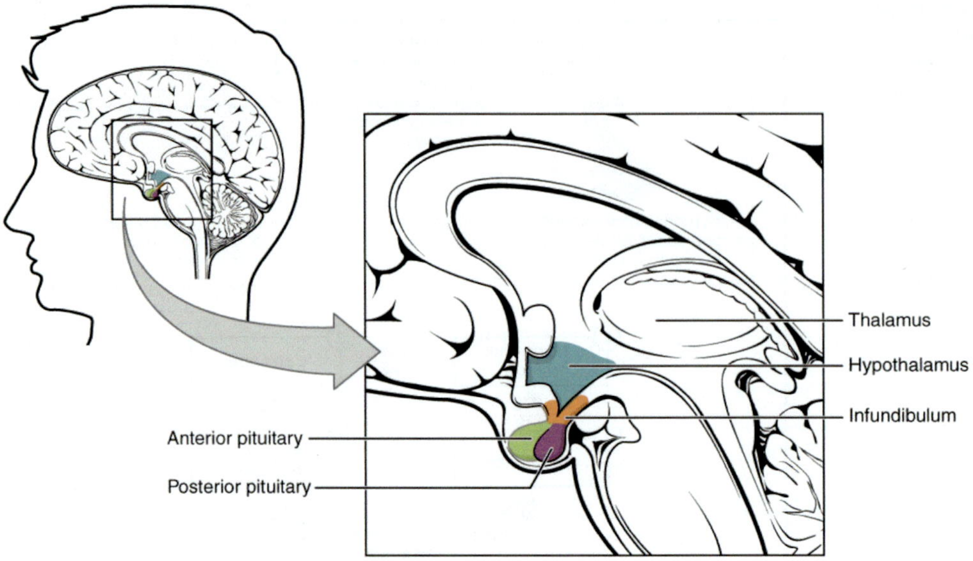

Fig. 23.3 The hypothalmus-pituitary complex. The hypothalamus connects to the pituitary gland by the stalk-like infundibulum. The pituitary gland consists of an anterior and posterior lobe, with each lobe secreting different hormones in response to signals from the hypothalamus (Reprinted from OpenStax, Anatomy & Physiology, OpenStax. 25 April 2013. Creative Commons Attribution 4.0 International License. Download for free at ► http://cnx.org/content/col11496/latest/

Fig. 23.4 Anterior pituitary. The anterior pituitary manufactures seven hormones. The hypothalamus produces separate hormones that stimulate or inhibit hormone production in the anterior pituitary.Hormones from the hypothalamus reach the anterior pituitary via the hypophyseal portal system (Reprinted from OpenStax, Anatomy &Physiology, OpenStax. 25 April 2013. Creative Commons Attribution 4.0 International License. Download for free at ► http://cnx.org/content/col11496/latest/

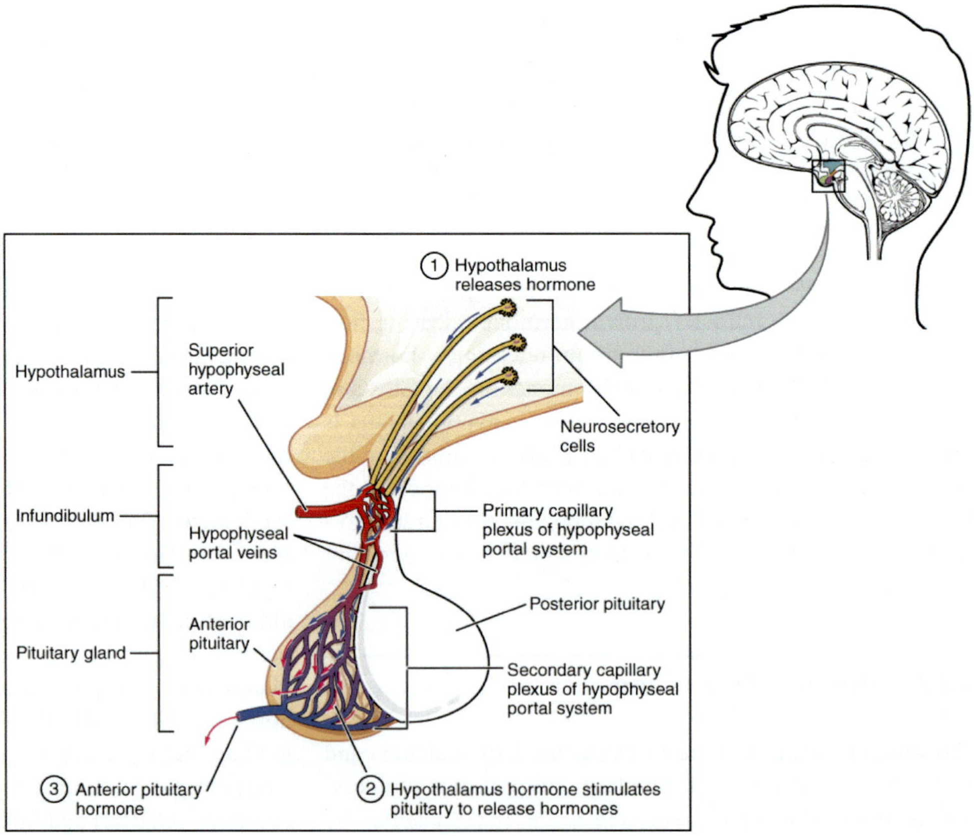

The posterior pituitary, also called the neurohypophysis, receives antidiuretic hormone (ADH) and oxytocin from the hypothalamus. Antidiuretic hormone, also known as vasopressin, is secreted in response to an increase in plasma osmolarity sensed by osmoreceptors or by a reduction in blood pressure sensed by baroreceptors. Antidiuretic

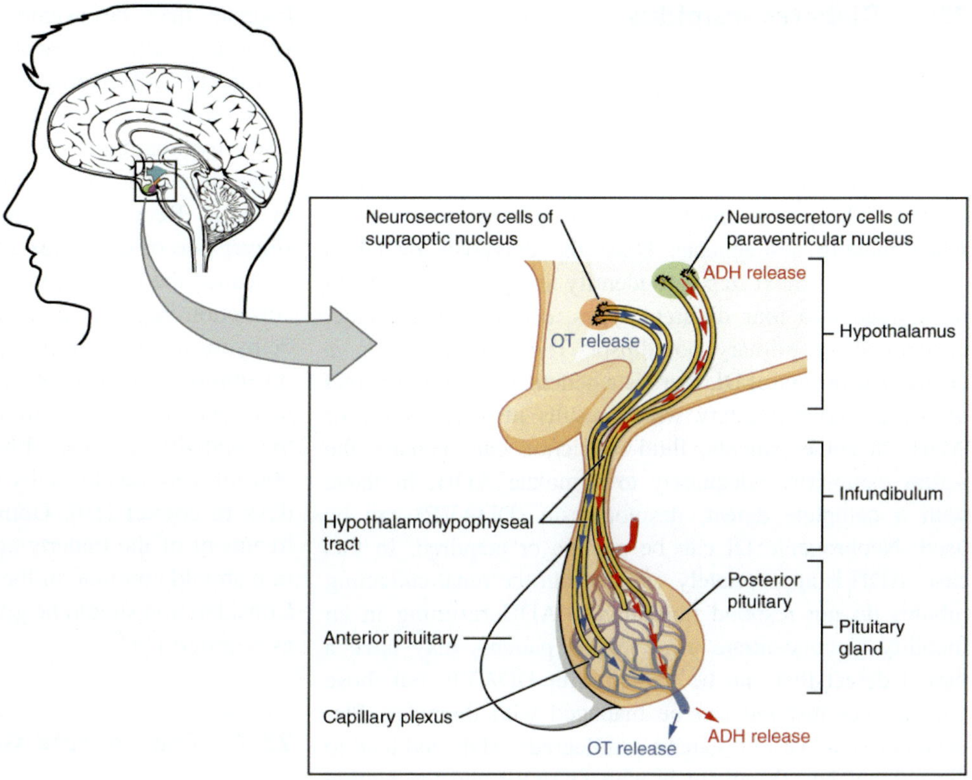

Fig. 23.5 Posterior pituitary. Neurosecretory cells in the hypothalamus release oxytocin (OT) or antidiuretic hormone (ADH) into the posterior lobe of the pituitary gland. These hormones are stored or released into the blood via the capillary plexus (Reprinted from OpenStax, Anatomy & Physiology, OpenStax. 25 April 2013. Creative Commons Attribution 4.0 International License. Download for free at ► http://cnx.org/content/col11496/latest/

hormone executes its action through the V1 and V2 receptors. Arteriolar vasoconstriction is mediated through ADH binding to V1. The antidiuretic effect comes from ADH binding to V2 leading to induction of aquaporins in the renal tubular cells. This allows for increased water reabsorption and plasma volume [3]. Oxytocin works to induce milk production in response to suckling and triggers uterine contraction during labor. The secretion of oxytocin is largely controlled by the presence of these stimulating events [2].

23.4 Acromegaly

Acromegaly is a rare disorder caused by excessive secretion of GH. Most often, this occurs from a somatotroph adenoma in the pituitary gland. This can lead to a variety of effects on the body. Growth of bone, soft tissue, and organs occurs to varying degrees and is often diagnosed about ten years after onset [4]. Changes in facial features resulting from acromegaly may include frontal bossing, prognathism, and macroglossia. These changes, in combination with hypertrophy of soft tissues in the airway, can result in a potentially difficult airway [5]. About half of patients with acromegaly develop obstructive sleep apnea, kyphoscoliosis, and hyperostosis. The cardiovascular system can be severely impacted by hypertension, biventricular hypertrophy, arrhythmias, and heart failure. Patients can develop concomitant renal failure and diabetes mellitus [4].

Diagnosis of acromegaly is done by performing a 75-g oral glucose load and testing for GH suppression two hours later. Inadequate suppression is considered diagnostic for acromegaly. Options for treatment include surgical resection, radiation therapy, somatostatin receptor ligands, and growth hormone receptor antagonists. The most common surgery to treat acromegaly is the endoscopic transsphenoidal resection of the pituitary tumor. Risks of surgery are bleeding, infection, CSF leak, diabetes insipidus, and incomplete resection. Postoperatively, non-invasive positive pressure therapy should be avoided due to risk for pneumocephalus. Treatment of acromegaly with radiation takes substantial time to normalize GH levels and about half of patients go on to develop some sort of pituitary deficiency. Somatostatin receptor ligands are octreotide and lantreotide. The goal of therapy is to control GH secretion and possibly reduce the size of the adenoma. The last therapeutic option is the growth hormone receptor antagonist, pegvisomant. This therapy can be added when adequate control is not achieved using maximum somatostatin receptor ligand dosing. Transaminitis is a potential side effect [4].

23.5 Diabetes Insipidus

Diabetes insipidus (DI) manifests with the excessive production of dilute urine. It is diagnosed when urine output is greater than 40 mL/kg in the setting of urine osmolarity less than 300 mOsm/L, normal oral intake, and negative urine glucose. The patient must not be on diuretic medications when making a diagnosis. Once the diagnosis of DI is established, the next step is to identify the type of DI. DI can be divided into four different types: central, nephrogenic, gestational, or primary polydipsia. The most common is central DI. In central DI, there is a genetic or acquired defect of the posterior pituitary which results in a deficiency of ADH. In some patients, fluid restriction can increase the serum osmolarity adequately to stimulate ADH. In those with a complete defect, desmopressin (DDAVP) can be used. Nephrogenic DI can be genetic or acquired. In this case, ADH is appropriately secreted but the renal collecting tubules do not respond normally to ADH resulting in an inability to concentrate urine. Some patients may have a partial defect that can be treated with DDAVP, but those who do not respond can be managed with thiazides. Placental enzyme vasopressinase can degrade ADH and lead to Gestational DI. Treatment is with DDAVP and the natural course is self-resolution 4–6 weeks postpartum. In primary polydipsia, an excessive amount of fluid intake leads to suppression of ADH. Treatment is on a case-by-case basis but ultimately requires fluid restriction [6]. DI affects electrolyte and fluid balance, impacting perioperative management. In patients with central DI who are treated with DDAVP, it is important to understand the baseline degree of polyuria. This will aid the anesthesiologist in gauging the patient's volume status, which is of utmost value because these patients are at risk of developing hyponatremia when administered intravenous fluids. If possible, fluid restriction should continue in the perioperative period to avoid this complication [7].

23.6 Syndrome of Inappropriate Antidiuretic Hormone

Hyponatremia is defined as a serum sodium level of less than 135 mEq/L and has been found to be a predictor of perioperative morbidity and mortality in healthy patients undergoing nonemergent surgeries [8]. One of the common causes of hyponatremia is the syndrome of inappropriate antidiuretic hormone (SIADH). Patients with SIADH present with euvolemic hyponatremia and urine sodium greater than 20 mEq/L with urine osmolality greater than 100 mOsm/kg. There are a variety of factors associated with SIADH including subarachnoid hemorrhage, traumatic brain injury, lung cancer, pneumonia, mechanical ventilation, and medications [9]. Hyponatremia may cause a range of symptoms. Patients may be asymptomatic or present with nausea, vomiting, altered mental status, seizures, or coma. Chronicity and severity of symptoms guide therapy. Altered consciousness or seizure is more often seen in those with acute hyponatremia and warrants consideration of hypertonic saline. The rate of correction of sodium is 8–12 mEq/L in 24 h. Recent guidelines have proposed that an even slower rate of correction of 4–6 mEq/L in 24 h is adequate to reduce the risk of cerebral edema and herniation. Rate of correction requires frequent monitoring to avoid osmotic demyelination syndrome, previously called central pontine myelinolysis. In patients with mild or no symptoms, treatment involves fluid restriction in combination with treating the underlying cause. Fluid restriction should start with 500 mL less than the daily urine output and may take several days to correct [10]. Optimization preoperatively involves treatment of the underlying cause of SIADH. Fluid restriction should continue in the perioperative period, if possible. Consideration should be given to the use of hypertonic saline as required [11].

23.7 The Thyroid Gland

The thyroid gland is located in the neck anterior to the trachea. It is in close proximity to the parathyroid glands, recurrent laryngeal nerves, vagus nerves, internal jugular veins, and carotid arteries (Figs. 23.6 and 23.7). The thyroid gland produces thyroxine (T_4) and to a lesser degree, triiodothyronine (T_3). This production occurs in response to the release of Thyroid Stimulating Hormone (TSH) from the anterior pituitary gland and is controlled by a negative feedback loop. Thyroid hormones play an important role in metabolism and growth [12].

23.8 Hypothyroidism

The most common causes of hypothyroidism are Hashimoto's thyroiditis, thyroidectomy, and radioiodine therapy. Loss of feedback to the hypothalamus from decreased circulating thyroid hormones results in an increased TSH. This increase in TSH leads to thyroid hyperplasia and the potential for developing a goiter [12]. Treatment is medical management with thyroid hormone replacement in the form of levothyroxine and, sometimes, liothyronine. Hypothyroidism can affect almost every system in the body. The clinical presentation could range from being asymptomatic to the occurrence of myxedema coma. Neurologically, patients may have lethargy or cognitive dysfunction. They are more sensitive to sedating medications and subsequently have decreased anesthetic requirements. The airway could be challenging due to unintentional weight gain as well as the

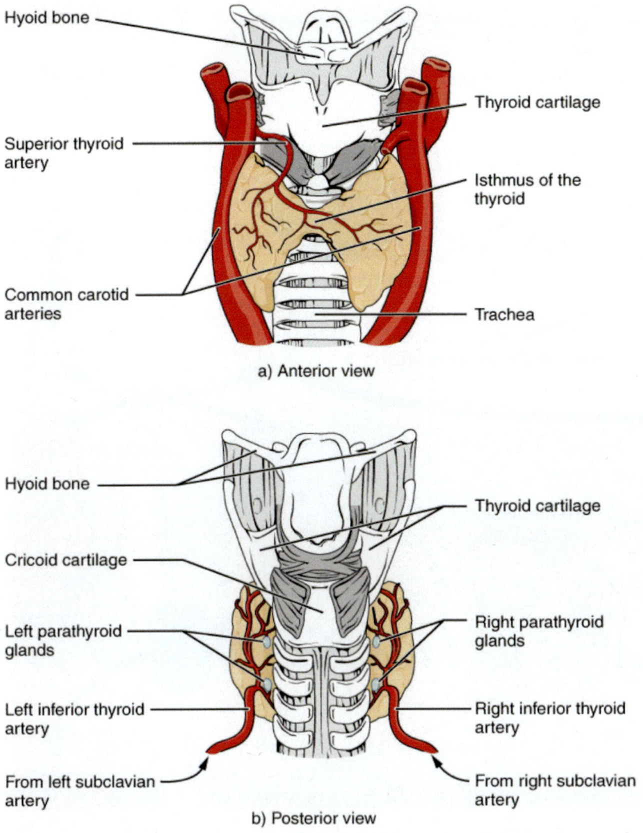

Fig. 23.6 Thyroid gland (Reprinted from OpenStax,Anatomy & Physiology, OpenStax.25 April 2013. Creative Commons Attribution 4.0 International License. Download for free at ► http://cnx.org/content/col11496/latest/

rare occurrence of laryngeal myxedema. They may also have delayed gastric emptying resulting in an increased risk of aspiration. The cardiovascular system can be seriously affected by hypothyroidism. Patients can have bradycardia, diastolic hypertension, prolonged QT, and systolic or diastolic dysfunction. Chronic hypothyroidism can result in increased circulating catecholamines and subsequent down-regulation of β-receptors. This can potentially lead to refractory hypotension. The respiratory system experiences a decreased response to hypoxia. Lastly, electrolyte abnormalities are common. Hyponatremia can be seen due to increased ADH [13].

23.9 Hyperthyroidism

Hyperthyroidism is most commonly caused by autoimmune disease. Graves' disease accounts for about 80% of hyperthyroidism and is followed by toxic multinodular goiter which is the cause in about 15% of cases. In Graves' disease, thyroid stimulating immunoglobin causes an increase in thyroid hormone production. It can be treated with anti-thyroid medication, β-antagonist, or thyroidectomy. Often a combination of these therapies is used. Thyrotoxicosis is a hypermetabolic state. Patients may present with anxiety or hyperactivity. They can also experience weight loss associated with an increased appetite and an intolerance to heat. Surgical stress can transform thyrotoxicosis into a thyroid storm. For this reason, it is recommended that patients achieve a euthyroid state prior to undergoing elective surgery [13]. Those with thyroid eye disease (TED) may have persistent corneal exposure and special precautions should be taken to protect the eyes. The anesthesiologist must pay special attention to the position of the mask during induction to avoid causing corneal abrasions. In addition to this, it is helpful to use an ophthalmic ointment or artificial tears for lubrication [14]. Like hypothyroidism, hyperthyroidism can have significant cardiovascular effects. A resting heart rate greater than 90 beats per minute is an indication to start therapy [13]. They may experience atrial fibrillation, left ventricular dysfunction, and pulmonary hypertension leading to right heart failure. Due to increased metabolism, anesthetic requirements can increase. The most dramatic presentation of hyperthyroidism is thyroid storm with a mortality rate of 10–20% [13]. Uncontrolled hyperthyroidism can be exaggerated by stress and hyperthermia [13]. Management of thyroid storm perioperatively requires supportive care and reducing production of thyroid hormone. This can be done using propylthiouracil (PTU), propranolol, and dexamethasone. Fever associated with thyroid storm may necessitate use of ice packs, cooling blankets, cooled intravenous fluids, and acetaminophen. With treatment, stabilization can be expected in 24–72 h [13] (Fig. 23.8).

23.10 The Parathyroid Gland

Parathyroid glands are found along the posterior borders of the thyroid. Most often, there is a superior and inferior pair, however up to 16% of the population may have an ectopic location in the neck or mediastinum [15]. Parathyroid hormone (PTH) acts on bones, small bowel, and kidneys in order to maintain calcium homeostasis. In bones, PTH mediates bone resorption via osteoclasts to mobilize calcium (Fig. 23.9). The role of PTH on the small intestine is indirect. First PTH acts on the kidneys to increase synthesis of 1,25-dihydroxycholecalciferol which then facilitates increased absorption of calcium in the small bowel. Additionally, PTH on the kidneys increases absorption of calcium in the ascending loop of Henle, distal convoluted tubule, and collecting tubules, as well as increasing phosphate excretion [16].

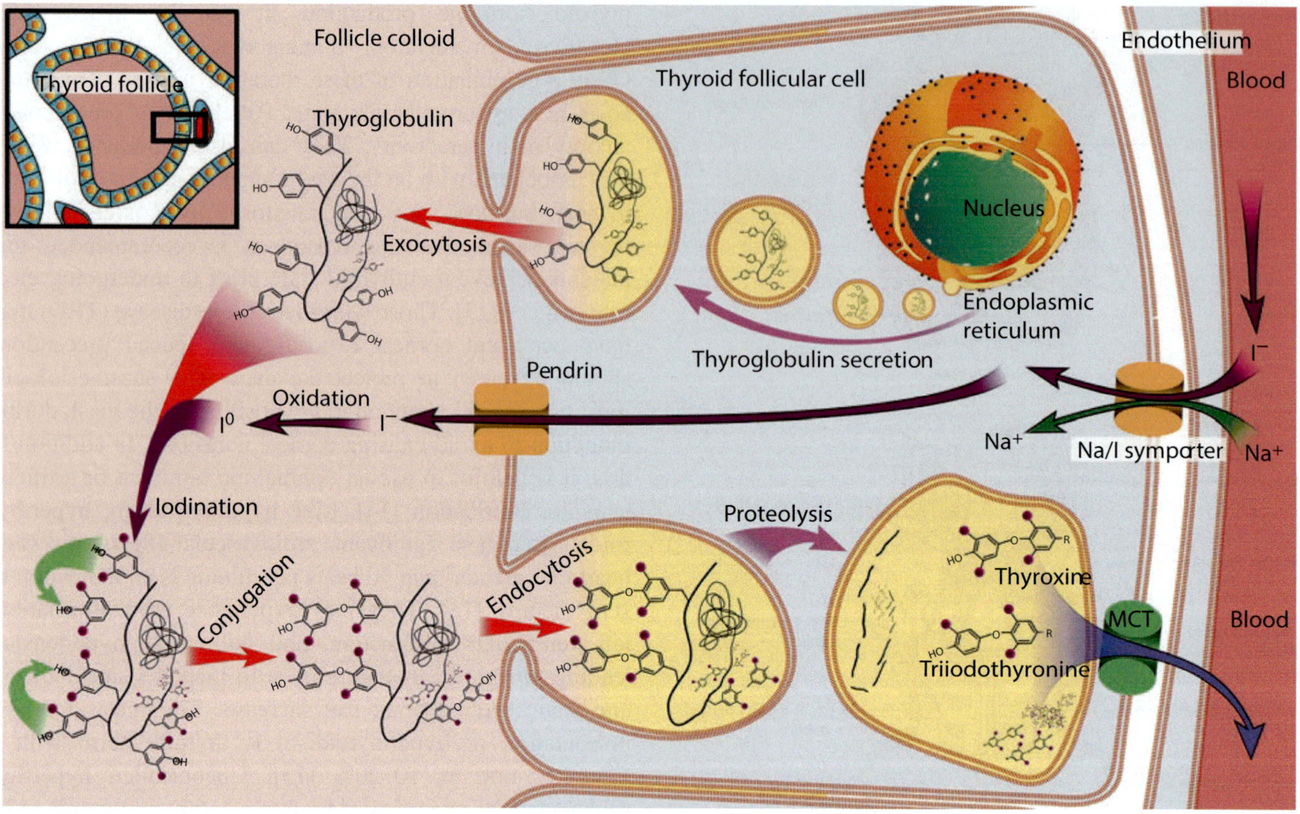

Fig. 23.7 Synthesis of the thyroid hormones, as seen on an individual thyroid follicular cell, monocarboxylate transporter (MCT) (Reprinted from Häggström)

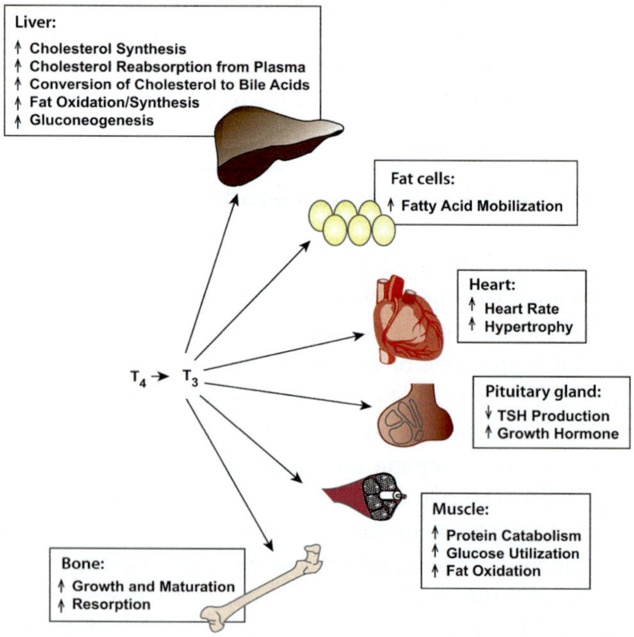

Fig. 23.8 The effects of thyroid hormone on different tissues of the body. T4 thyroxine,T3 triiodothyronine, TSH thyroid stimulating hormone (Adapted from Webb P, Phillips K, Baxter JD. Mechanisms of thyroid hormone action. ► Clinicalgate.com)

23.11 Hyperparathyroidism

Hyperparathyroidism leads to hypercalcemia and can be classified as primary, secondary, or tertiary. Primary hyperparathyroidism is most often caused by a parathyroid adenoma. It is rarely the result of a parathyroid carcinoma or as part of the multiple endocrine neoplasia type 1. Surgical parathyroidectomy is the treatment of choice. Secondary hyperparathyroidism occurs in response to sustained hypocalcemia and can lead to parathyroid hyperplasia. This may happen in chronic renal failure or those with vitamin D deficiency. With early diagnosis, the majority of these patients can be managed with calcium and vitamin D supplementation, although a small percentage may require parathyroidectomy. Tertiary hyperparathyroidism occurs as a result of progressive parathyroid hyperplasia despite medical management. In this case, parathyroidectomy is needed to control calcium levels.

Patients with undiagnosed or untreated hyperparathyroidism with hypercalcemia may have non-specific symptoms. They could be asymptomatic or present with memory loss, depression, fatigue, hypertension, decreased renal function, nausea, vomiting, peptic ulcer, or pseudogout [16].

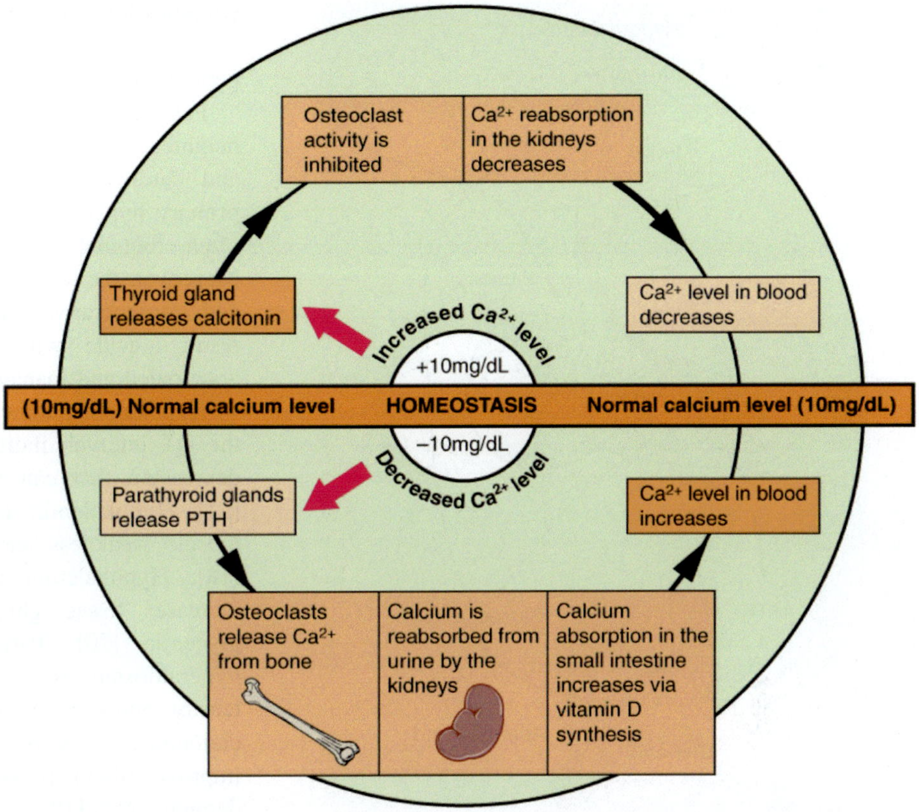

Fig. 23.9 The parathyroid glands regulate calcium homeostasis via 2 pathways: one turns on when blood calcium levels drop below normal and the other turns on when blood calcium levels are elevated.PTH —parathyroid hormone (Reprinted from OpenStax, Anatomy & Physiology, OpenStax. 25 April 2013. Creative Commons Attribution 4.0 International License. Download for free at ► http://cnx.org/content/col11496/latest/

Signs of hypercalcemia can potentially be seen on electrocardiogram as shortened QT interval, ST elevation, or prominent U waves [17]. In acute hypercalcemia, rehydration is of paramount importance. After the patient has been adequately volume resuscitated, loop diuretics may be given to increase calcium elimination in the urine.

When surgical parathyroidectomy is needed for management of hyperparathyroidism, the postoperative anesthetic concerns are similar to those patients having undergone thyroidectomy. There is potential for surgical site hematoma which can compromise airway and there is the possibility of recurrent laryngeal nerve injury [16].

23.12 The Adrenal Gland

The adrenal glands are located above the kidneys and play an integral role in (Figs. 23.10 and 23.11) modulating metabolism, regulating salt-water balance within the body, and mounting a stress response that affects the immune system. The adrenal glands are composed of an inner medulla and outer cortex, each with its own set of regulatory hormones. The medulla is embryologically derived from neural crest cells that develop into postganglionic autonomic nerve fibers called chromaffin cells [18]. Sympathetic stimulation or hormones, such as histamine, trigger release of catecholamines into the blood driving the fight or flight response.

The adrenal cortex is composed of three layers: the zona glomerulosa, zona fasciculata, and zona reticularis from outer to inner layers respectively. These layers secrete steroid hormones that affect transcription of protein synthesis within cells. The zona glomerulosa releases a mineralocorticoid called aldosterone in response to low blood pressure detected within the kidney via the renin angiotensin system. Circulating aldosterone targets the distal convoluted tubule and collecting duct to increase transcription of sodium potassium pumps. This results in avid reabsorption of sodium with loss of potassium and hydrogen ions to increase blood pressure [18]. ACTH stimulates the zona fasciculata to release glucocorticoids (cortisol) and the zona reticularis to release androgens such as testosterone. One of the main functions of cortisol is to stimulate the liver to release and create more glucose by gluconeogenesis, glycogenolysis, and proteolysis while also increasing tissue resistance to insulin.

23.13 Primary Hyperaldosteronism: Conn Syndrome

Primary hyperaldosteronism, also known as Conn's syndrome, is often an underrecognized cause for hypertension and patients can go undiagnosed for several years. Primary hyperaldosteronism is a disorder that arises from the adrenal cortex (zona glomerulosa) as a result of hyperplasia or

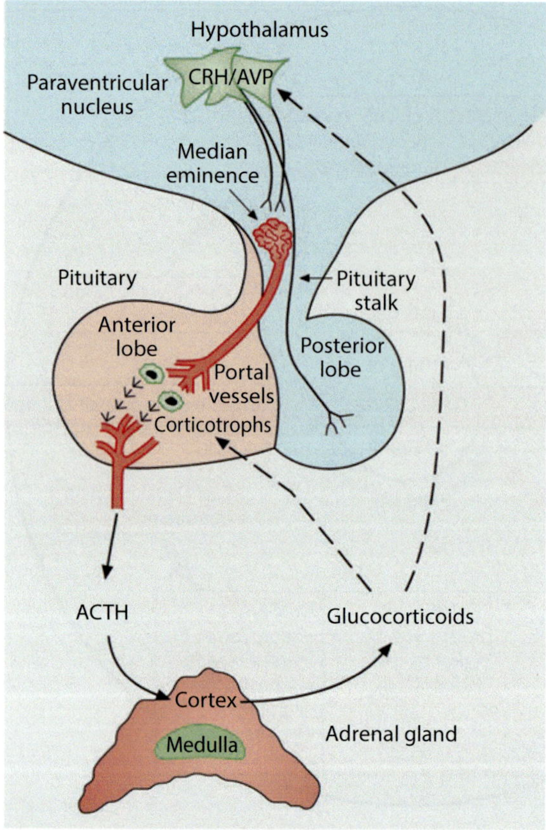

Fig. 23.10 A schematic representation of the components of the hypothalamic-pituitary-adrenal axis and their hormonal interactions. Stimulatory effects are represented by solid lines and inhibitory effects by dashed lines (CRH corticotropinreleasing hormone, AVP arginine vasopressin) (Reprinted with permission from Kyrou and Tsigos

adenomas. Patients classically present with hypertension and hypokalemia, although potassium could sometimes be normal [19]. It is diagnosed with imaging and hormonal assays. Low serum ACTH, high serum aldosterone, and low serum renin levels may indicate the presence of primary hyperaldosteronism.

Aldosterone increases sodium reabsorption in the renal cortical collecting tubules. With the retention of sodium, the gradient in the renal tubules then shifts to favor potassium excretion resulting in hypertension from sodium and water retention and hypokalemia from renal potassium loss. Metabolic alkalosis also accompanies these electrolyte derangements driven by urinary hydrogen ion excretion [19].

The deleterious effects of hyperaldosteronism are driven by the effect of hypertension on the cardiovascular system and kidneys. Persistent fluid retention and a direct effect mineralocorticoids on the vasculature results in increased systemic vascular resistance. Hypertension over a period of time can cause myocardial strain, left ventricular hypertrophy, and myocardial fibrosis. Overall, patients with primary hyperaldosteronism have a greater risk of cardiovascular complications including risk of atrial fibrillation, stroke, heart failure, and coronary artery disease compared to patients with primary hypertension [20].

Patients with primary hyperaldosteronism carry a heightened perioperative risk for electrolyte derangements and cardiovascular complications [20]. Hypertension in primary hyperaldosteronism can be difficult to control and often requires a multimodal antihypertensive regimen. Moreover, the use of antihypertensive drugs before surgery and intraoperative manipulation of the adrenal gland can result in wide swings of blood pressure which should be anticipated and managed perioperatively.

Hypokalemia affects cardiac conduction by prolonging the QT interval, flattening of the T wave, or causing ST depression that can potentiate lethal cardiac arrhythmias [21]. Hypokalemia and metabolic alkalosis can result in muscle weakness and potentiate neuromuscular blockade [18]. Hypokalemia also reduces insulin secretion and increases tissue glucose resistance resulting in hyperglycemia [20]. Perioperative management of primary hyperaldosteronism should include management of hypertension and correction of hypokalemia with use of a mineralocorticoid receptor antagonist such as spironolactone to improve blood pressure control and correct electrolyte derangements [18].

23.14 Primary Hypercortisolism: Cushing's Syndrome

Primary hypercortisolism or Cushing's syndrome is often caused by adrenocortical hyperplasia or adenomas resulting in excess glucocorticoid release from the zona fasciculata. Chronic hypercortisolism results in negative feedback to the HPA axis resulting in suppression of corticotropin-releasing hormone (CRH) and adrenocorticotropic hormone (ACTH).

Under normal physiologic conditions, the adrenal fasciculata releases cortisol following the circadian rhythm throughout the day, with a higher amount released in the morning and a lower amount released in the evening. While a majority of the lipid glucocorticoid molecules are protein bound, the free cortisol fraction is responsible for the physiologic effects. Cortisol increases endothelial alpha 1 receptors sensitivity to catecholamine and increases blood pressure [22]. Cortisol increases bone resorption, reduces calcium absorption in the gut, reduces reabsorption of calcium in the kidney, and reduces bone formation [23]. The metabolic effects of cortisol include proteolysis, lipolysis, gluconeogenesis, and increased insulin resistance within the tissues [24]. Furthermore, cortisol exerts its anti-inflammatory effect by suppressing the production and release of inflammatory mediators.

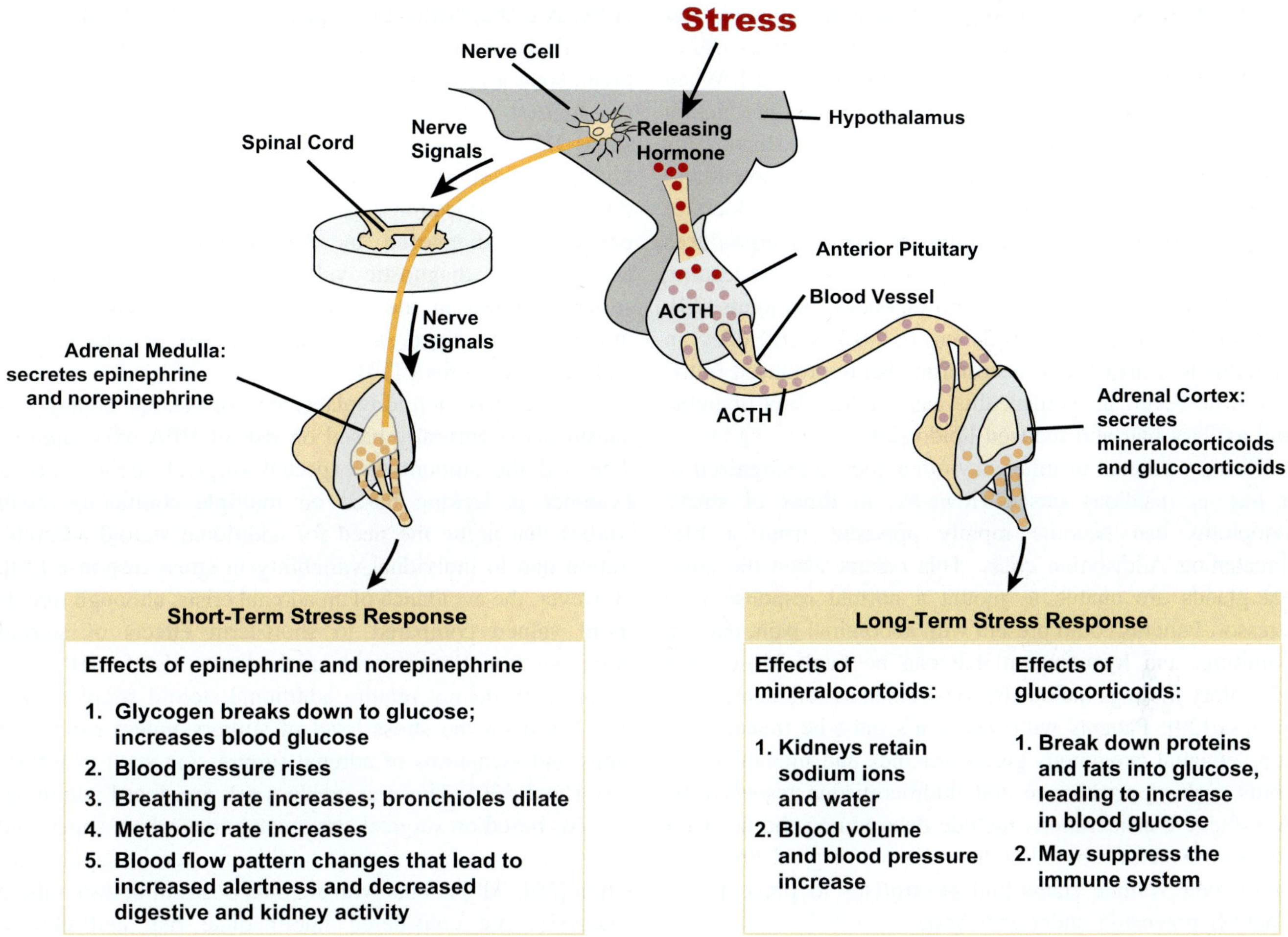

Fig. 23.11 Response of the adrenal glands to short-term and long-term stresses. ACTH adrenocorticotropic hormone (Adapted from ► http://www.proprofs.com/flashcards/story.php?title=bio-lecture-4-page-12411-lecture-pt-1

Chronic hypercortisolism increases the risk of developing hypertension including cardiovascular disease, diabetes, obesity, OSA, osteoporosis, vulnerability to infections, and poor wound healing [25]. Chronic metabolic derangements cause glucose intolerance, proximal muscle wasting, and increased fat deposition in the face, abdomen, and back resulting in the classic appearance of "moon face" and "buffalo hump" [26, 27]. Loss of subcutaneous fat from proteolysis and lipolysis leads to fragile atrophied skin that bruises easily and heals poorly [27]. In addition to increasing vascular sensitivity to catecholamines, due to structural similarity of the molecule, excess cortisol cross binds with mineralocorticoid receptors [28]. This results in retention of sodium and water and worsening hypertension.

Difficult airway consequent to obesity and long-standing diabetes is an important anesthetic consideration in these patients. Furthermore, these patients carry an increased risk of perioperative cardiovascular complications [25]. With increased skin fragility and osteoporosis in these patients, caution needs to be exercised with patient positioning.

Iatrogenic Cushing's syndrome due to exogenous glucocorticoid administration is a common cause of hypercortisolism. Feedback inhibition of ACTH in these patients results in adrenal atrophy. Consequently, under stress, the adrenal glands in these patients are not able to produce additional cortisol putting them at risk of life-threatening adrenal crisis.

23.15 Primary Adrenal Insufficiency: Addison's Disease

Primary adrenal insufficiency, also known as Addison's disease, occurs when the adrenal glands do not produce sufficient amounts of glucocorticoids and mineralocorticoids. The most common cause in developed countries is autoimmune destruction of the adrenal cortex [29]. Symptoms depend on which layer of the adrenal cortex has reduced function. When the zona glomerulosa is affected, there is a reduction in the production of aldosterone leading to hyponatremia, low blood pressure, hyperkalemia, and metabolic acidosis. This causes symptoms such as orthostatic hypotension, nausea, vomiting, and fatigue [29]. When the zona fasciculata is affected, there is reduced production of cortisol leading to an inadequate response to stress. This could present as weakness, fatigue, and potentially hypotension [29]. Without the negative feedback loop of adequate cortisol levels, the pituitary gland overproduces ACTH as well as melanocyte-stimulating hormone leading to darkening of the skin at the elbows, knees, and joints [29]. When the zona reticularis is damaged, this has little effect in men due to a majority of testosterone being produced in the testes, however, in women, this can produce loss of pubic and axillary hair and reduced libido [29].

Primary adrenal insufficiency often goes unrecognized as it has an insidious onset. However, in times of stress, symptoms can become rapidly apparent from a life-threatening Addisonian crisis. This occurs when the adrenal glands are unable to mount a normal response to a stressor. Patients could present with abdominal pain, nausea, vomiting, and hypotension that can be fatal. Most often laboratory findings include hyponatremia, hyperkalemia, and anemia [29]. Patients with Addison's must be treated with supplemental exogenous glucocorticoids and mineralocorticoids such as prednisone and fludrocortisone respectively. Anesthetic considerations include determining the need for stress dose steroids based on the expected surgical stress and optimizing volume status and electrolytes to prevent profound hypotension under anesthesia.

Iatrogenic adrenal insufficiency, also referred to as tertiary adrenal insufficiency, is due to chronic steroid therapy that results in suppression of the HPA axis. Patients on a dose equivalent to 5 mg prednisone or less for a duration less than three weeks are likely to have a non-suppressed HPA axis suggesting these patients are less at risk for an adrenal crisis. Patients on a dose equivalent to 20 mg prednisone a day for a duration greater than 3 weeks carry the highest risk for developing an adrenal crisis under stress [30]. This applies to all routes of steroid administration including oral, intravenous, inhaled, intranasal, intraarticular injections, or even topical. HPA axis suppression is diagnosed by the ACTH stimulation test, however, the diagnostic value of a short-acting ACTH stimulation test in the perioperative period has not been proven clearly diagnostic as this is a test of total cortisol and not free cortisol [30].

Perioperative steroid replacement for patients undergoing anesthesia is currently based on risk of HPA axis suppression and the amount of expected surgical stress. Current evidence is lacking based on multiple conflicting small studies that argue the need for additional steroid administration due to individual variability in stress response [30]. However, the avoidance of an adrenal crisis, although rare, is more valued compared to short-term effects of steroid administration. Patients who are the lowest risk for HPA axis suppression do not require additional steroid supplementation based on the stress level of surgery unless exhibiting signs and symptoms of adrenal suppression such as refractory shock [30]. Those at greatest risk are dosed additional steroids based on surgical stress categories where superficial procedures may not warrant additional steroid supplementation [30]. All patients with steroids doses in between these categories are considered intermediate risk and clinical judgement is used to administer stress dose steroids appropriately. Table 23.1 summarizes recommendations for perioperative steroid supplementation according to surgery type. Table 23.2 provides a guide for steroid activity and equivalent dosing.

Table 23.1 Recommendations for perioperative steroid supplementation

Surgery type	Recommended dosing
Superficial or low-stress surgery	**Continue daily dose**
Minor surgery	**Continue daily dose** + **Hydrocortisone 50 mg IV prior to incision** Continue 25 mg every 8 h for 24 h
Moderate surgery	**Continue daily dose** + **Hydrocortisone 50 mg IV prior to incision** Continue 25 mg every 8 h for 24 h
Major surgery	**Continue daily dose** + **Hydrocortisone 100 mg IV prior to incision** Continue 50 mg IV every 8 h for 24 h Reduced dose by half each day until tapered down to home dose

** According to the American Society of Anesthesiologist "Perioperative Steroid Management" 2017 Recommendations [30]

Table 23.2 Steroid activity and equivalent dosing

Steroid	Glucocorticoid Anti-inflammatory activity	Mineralocorticoid Salt retaining activity	Equivalent Dose	Duration of Action (t ½) (h)
Short acting				
Hydrocortisone = Cortisol	1	1	20	8–12
Cortisone	0.8	0.8	25	8–12
Intermediate acting				
Prednisone	4	0.8	5	12–36
Prednisolone	4	0.8	5	12–36
Methylprednisolone	5	0.5	4	18–36
Long acting				
Dexamethasone	30	0	0.75	36–72
Mineralocorticoid				
Fludrocortisone[a]	10	125	Replacement dose is 0.1–0.2 mg per day	12–36

[a] Fludrocortisone has no appreciable glucocorticoid activity at standard daily dose of 0.1–0.2 mg per day, thus it is solely used for mineralocorticoid replacement [24, 30]

23.16 Pheochromocytoma

The inner layer of the adrenal gland is called the adrenal medulla. This is embryologically derived from neural crest cells that form modified postganglionic sympathetic neurons called chromaffin cells. Chromaffin cells function to secrete catecholamines including epinephrine, norepinephrine, and dopamine in response to sympathetic adrenergic stimulation or hormones such as histamine and corticosteroids [31]. A neoplasm that arises from the adrenal medulla is termed a pheochromocytoma. It is a rare cause of hypertension that often goes unrecognized. The classic triad of presentation includes paroxysmal episodes of headaches, tachycardia, and diaphoresis [32]. Diagnosis is made most reliably by imaging and measurements of 24-h urine plasma fractionated metanephrins and catecholamines [33].

Long-standing complications arise due to catecholamine excess. Patients present with resistant paroxysmal hypertension and hypovolemia due to high vasomotor tone. This can present as orthostatic hypotension or perioperative hypotension. Chronic strain on the heart leads to development of cardiomyopathy that is similar to stress-induced or takotsubo cardiomyopathy [34]. Catecholamines also increase insulin resistance in the tissues and cause hyperglycemia. Patients with pheochromocytoma have and higher risk of developing diabetes and the complications that go along with chronic hyperglycemia [33].

Paroxysmal hypertension or hypotension can be triggered by different, foods, drugs, and stress. It is imperative to avoid beta 2 antagonist activity prior to alpha blockage when choosing antihypertensive therapies. This can cause a life-threatening hypertensive crisis leading to altered mental status, organ dysfunction, and possibly death. Patients are typically treated with a nonselective alpha blocker, phenoxybenzamine. Continuation of perioperative long-acting phenoxybenzamine has been shown to have increased chance of postoperative hypotension compared to short-acting alpha-adrenergic blockers [35]. Beta blockers can be safely administered after adequate alpha blockade to help control tachycardia. Attention to intravascular fluid repletion and attenuation of the pain response is advised. With bilateral adrenalectomies, patients require glucocorticoid and mineralocorticoid supplementation in the immediate postoperative period.

23.17 The Pancreas

The pancreas is a retroperitoneal organ that functions to release digestive enzymes and hormones. The endocrine pancreas is organized into islet cells that are composed of groups of cells (alpha and beta) with various functions that help regulate blood sugar. Alpha cells release glucagon which breaks down glycogen, a branched storage unit of glucose, to release glucose into the blood. Beta cells release insulin in response to hyperglycemia which converts glucose into glycogen. Somatostatin released by Delta cells stops the effects of glucagon, insulin, and other hormones such as cholecystokinin [36] (Fig. 23.12).

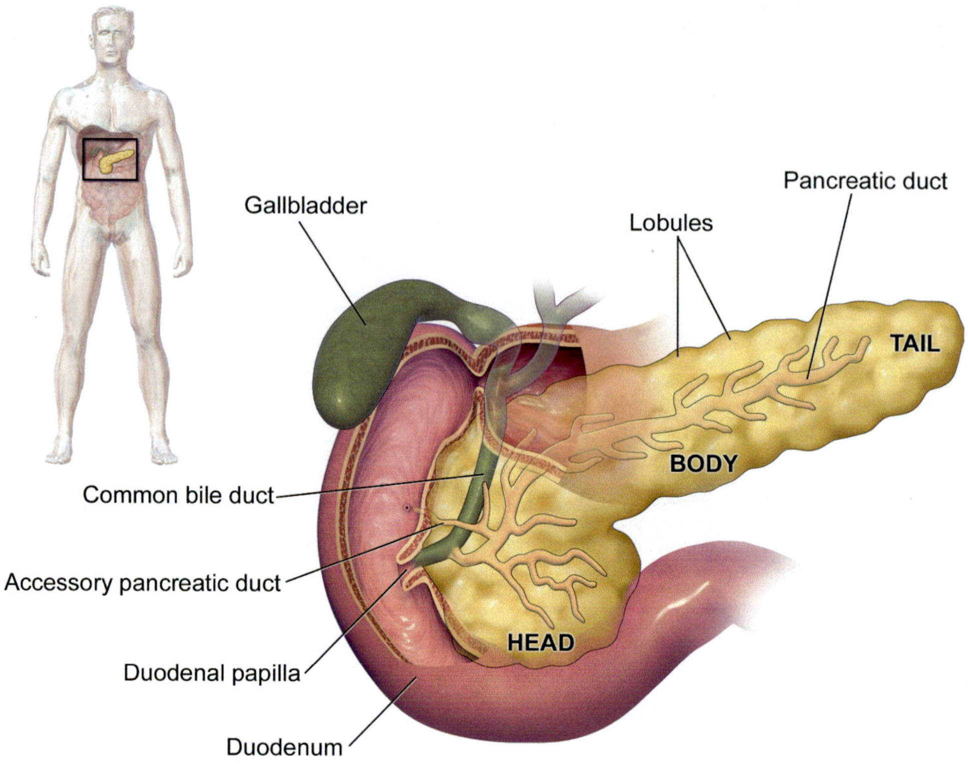

Fig. 23.12 The pancreas (Reprinted from Blausen.com staff)

23.18 Diabetes Mellitus

Diabetes mellitus is the most common of all endocrine disorders and continues to be the seventh leading cause of death in the United States [37]. Nearly 15% of the population over 18 years of age has a diagnosis of diabetes in the United States which has increased from 9% over the past decade [38]. Type 1 diabetes is a state of insulin deficiency due to beta islet cell destruction. Type 2 diabetes manifests with insulin resistance preventing uptake of glucose into the cells. Tissues most impacted by reduced insulin sensitivity include skeletal muscle, adipose tissue, and the liver. Endothelial cells have insulin receptors which are not glucose coupled but play a role in nitric-oxide synthase and other vasoactive substrates [39] (Fig. 23.13).

The pathogenesis of diabetes is driven by the deleterious effects of hyperglycemia on both micro and macrovascular endothelial cells resulting in multi-organ dysfunction over time. Persistent hyperglycemia causes cellular injury by altering cellular pathways, creating oxidative free radicals and advanced glycosylated end products [39]. The oxidative damage and deposition of glycosylated metabolites create an inflammatory state affecting connective tissue beds resulting in intimal thickening and fibrosis, vasoactive and immune dysfunction which greatly accelerates the development of cardiovascular disease, nephropathy, neuropathy, and obesity [39–41].

The most common cause of death in diabetic patients is cardiovascular disease. The risk is twice that of the non-diabetic population [40, 41]. Over time, lipid deposition and oxidative byproducts cause intimal thickening and fibrosis resulting in luminal narrowing and impaired blood flow [39, 41]. Non-compliant vasculature reduces blood flow and accelerates ischemic heart disease, peripheral vascular disease, and cerebrovascular disease. Diabetes remains an independent risk factor for stroke. The risk of ischemic stroke in diabetics is twice that of non-diabetic patients [42].

Chronic hyperglycemic damage to the microvasculature of the nervous system results in demyelination and axonal injury causing neuropathy [39]. Neuronal injury tends to be more pronounced in the sensory and autonomic fibers manifesting as autonomic dysfunction and the classic "stock and glove" peripheral neuropathy [39]. Persistent uncontrolled diabetes can affect motor neurons as well. The onset and progression of diabetic autonomic neuropathy is often insidious. It could manifest as resting tachycardia, reduced heart rate variability, orthostatic hypotension, gastroparesis, urinary retention, or erectile dysfunction [41].

Chronic persistent hyperglycemia causes renal dysfunction over time both from direct damage to the filtering organelles of the kidney and microvascular injury [43]. High concentrations of glucose filtered through the kidney are reabsorbed within the proximal convoluted tubule. This increases sodium-glucose coupled reuptake which subsequently affects how much sodium is delivered to the

Fig. 23.13 Ketogenesis pathway. The three ketone bodies (acetoacetate, acetone, and betahydroxy-butyrate) are marked within an orange box (By Sav vas [CC0], via Wikimedia Commons)

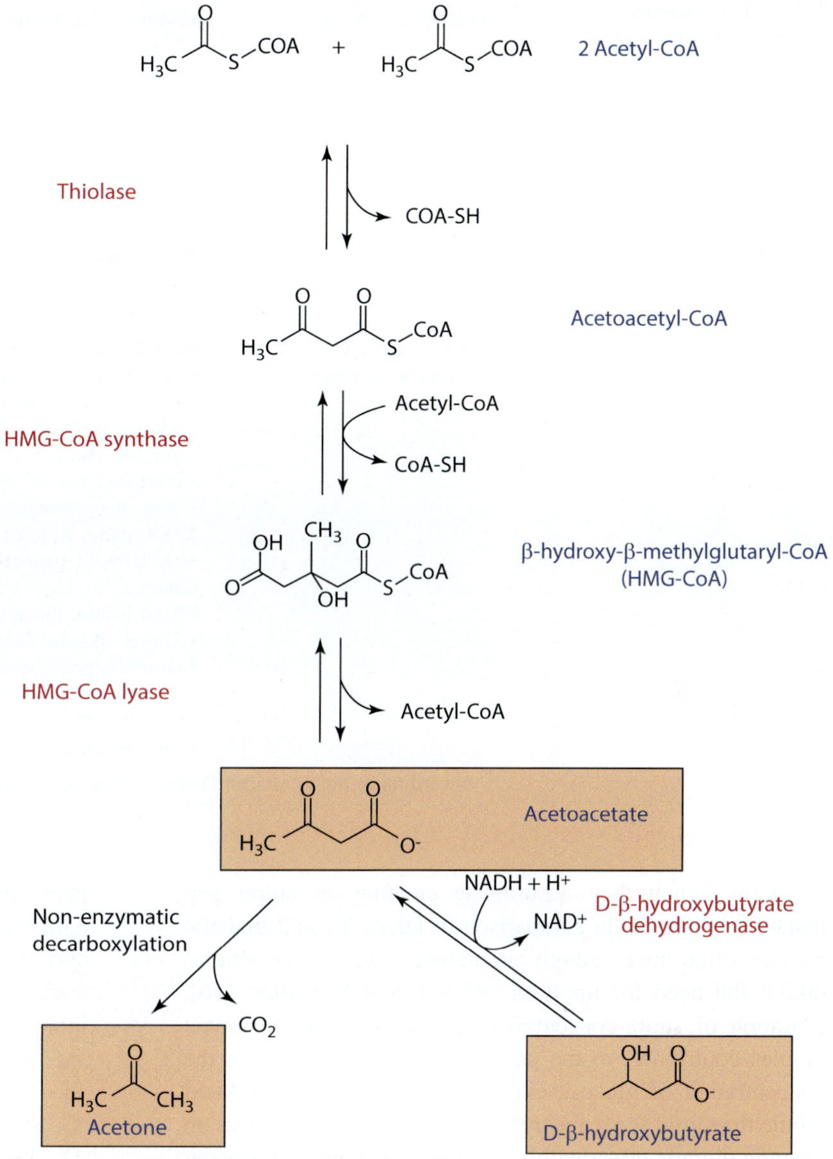

juxtaglomerular apparatus (JGA). Less sodium detected at the JGA results in activation of the renin angiotensin system (RASS) causing reduced vasoconstriction at the afferent arteriole, glomerular hypertension, and hyperfiltration [43]. Roughly 39% of adults 18 years or older with diabetes had chronic kidney disease based on data compiled by the CDC in 2021 [37].

Advanced glycosylated end products cross link with collagen proteins over time affecting the musculoskeletal system. Patients with long-standing or uncontrolled disease are at an increased risk for developing limited joint mobility leading to such complications as adhesive capsulitis, carpel tunnel, Charcot foot deformity, as well as ossification and calcification of spinal ligaments [44]. This is an important consideration during the preoperative evaluation of these patients and might indicate potential difficulty with airway manipulation. Perioperative glycemic control should include a baseline blood sugar perioperatively followed by routine intraoperative glucose monitoring with a target glucose of 140–180 mg/dl according to the American Diabetes Association [45].

Diabetic Ketoacidosis (DKA) (more common in Type 1 diabetes) and hyperosmolar hyperglycemic syndrome (HHS) (more common in Type 2 diabetes) are metabolic emergencies that can occur in patients with diabetes. Infections are the most common precipitating factor for the occurrence of DKA or HHS including pneumonia and urinary tract infections [46]. DKA is a state of absolute or relative deficiency of insulin in the setting of hyperglycemia. Peripheral tissues are unable to utilize glucose, forcing cells to shift to lipolysis to release free fatty acids for an energy source. Metabolism within the mitochondria releases

Table 23.3 Perioperative anesthetic considerations in diabetes mellitus

Preoperative phase	**History evaluation**: • Type of diabetes and long-term complications • Medication regiment (Oral vs Insulin requirements) • Glycemic control and average glucose levels • History of hypoglycemic episodes **Assessment**: • Physical exam • Baseline electrocardiogram • Appropriate additional cardiac testing based on risk and type of surgery **Blood glucose**: • A1C within 3 months • Renal function and electrolytes
Intraoperative and postoperative phase	**Risk factors to consider**: • Possible difficult airway from reduced cervical joint or jaw mobility • Increased aspiration risk from gastroparesis • Altered cardiac autonomic function can affect interpretation of pain and volume status • Increased risk of cardiovascular events • Risk of positioning injuries **Monitoring**: Routine blood glucose monitoring at least every 1–2 h, especially for patients on an insulin regiment **Goal**: • Start insulin therapy $\geq$ 180 mg/dl • Target Glucose 140–180 mg/dl[a] • Avoid hypoglycemia (most dangerous) • Avoid marked hyperglycemia • Targeted fluid and electrolyte replacement • Prevent metabolic derangements in patients at risk for DKA or HSS

* According to the American Diabetes Association in 2022 [45]

ketoacids which then accumulate creating an anion gap metabolic acidosis. In comparison to DKA, Type 2 diabetic patients often have enough circulating insulin to be able to inhibit the need for lipolysis and ketoacid formation [46]. Filtration of supra-concentrated glucose through the renal tubules contributes to the pathogenesis of HHS. When the concentration of glucose exceeds the proximal convoluted tubule threshold for reabsorption, the glucose load causes an osmotic diuretic effect within the nephron. This draws water and electrolytes into the urine creating severe dehydration which can progress to renal failure [46]. The metabolic derangements in HHS are not as severe as in DKA but it carries a mortality rate of about 20% which is higher than DKA [46]. Preoperatively if a patient is found to be in DKA or HHS, elective surgical procedures should be delayed to improve the state of volume depletion, electrolyte abnormalities, and metabolic acidosis to avoid potential hemodynamic instability and arrhythmias on induction of anesthesia. Table 23.3 outlines the perioperative anesthetic considerations in patients with diabetes mellitus.

Questions

1. A 26-year-old female who is G1P0 at 7 weeks gestation presents to the emergency department with the complaint of severe, progressive lower abdominal pain. She is diagnosed with a ruptured ectopic pregnancy and needs an emergency laparotomy. A week ago, she was diagnosed with hyperthyroidism and started on propylthiouracil (PTU). What should be included in this patient's perioperative plan?
   A. Start levothyroxine
   B. Continue beta antagonist and PTU
   C. Start radioactive iodine
   D. Discontinue PTU
2. A 57-year-old female with a history of multinodular goiter undergoes a total thyroidectomy. She was uneventfully extubated and transferred to the post-anesthetic care unit. Two hours later, she complains of difficulty breathing. What is most likely causing her symptoms?
   A. Post-thyroidectomy hematoma
   B. Hypocalcemia
   C. Recurrent laryngeal nerve injury
   D. Pneumothorax
3. What is the first step in management of a patient with symptomatic hypercalcemia?
   A. Thiazide diuretic
   B. Hemodialysis
   C. Normal saline bolus
   D. Loop diuretic

4. Where is antidiuretic hormone produced?
   A. Posterior pituitary
   B. Anterior pituitary
   C. Thalamus
   D. Hypothalamus
5. A 43-year-old male is postoperative day two from laparoscopic cholecystectomy and is noted to have hyponatremia (serum sodium 124 meq/L). He appears euvolemic. What is the most likely cause of his electrolyte abnormality?
   A. Syndrome of inappropriate antidiuretic hormone
   B. Diabetes insipidus
   C. Cerebral salt wasting
   D. Diuretic use

Question 1 of 2:

6. A 31-year-old male with acromegaly presents for planned transsphenoidal resection of a pituitary adenoma. He has been experiencing increased hoarseness and difficulty breathing over the past few weeks. What is the safest approach to securing his airway?
   A. Direct laryngoscopy
   B. Tracheostomy
   C. Awake fiberoptic intubation
   D. Video laryngoscopy

Question 2 of 2:

7. Two days later, the same patient is seen in the intensive care unit. He is confused. Upon further review, it is noted that his urine output was 3.5 L in the past 24 h and his sodium is now 154 mEq/L. What is the most likely diagnosis?
   A. Nephrogenic diabetes insipidus
   B. Neurogenic diabetes insipidus
   C. Syndrome of inappropriate antidiuretic hormone
   D. Cerebral salt wasting
8. Syndrome of inappropriate antidiuretic hormone (C) and cerebral salt wasting (D) lead to hyponatremia. Which of the following patients would most likely benefit from perioperative stress dose steroids?
   A. A 56-year-old male who routinely gets lumbar epidural steroid injections four times a year presenting for an open abdominal colectomy for a large bowel mass under general anesthesia.
   B. A 67-year-old female treated with a 14-day prednisone steroid taper for a COPD exacerbation one month ago is having a skin lesion removed under local anesthesia with MAC sedation.
   C. A 32-year-old male with severe asthma is on daily inhaled steroids and recently completed a high-dose prednisone taper two weeks ago is scheduled for a small bowel resection for colitis under general anesthesia.
   D. A 45-year-old female on 30 mg prednisone daily is scheduled for a dental extraction under MAC sedation.
9. Which medication is least likely to cause exacerbation of severe hypertension in pheochromocytoma?
   A. Glucagon
   B. Phenoxybenzamine
   C. Ketamine
   D. Metoclopramide

10. Which diabetic medication places a patient at risk for developing euglycemic diabetic ketoacidosis if continued perioperatively for a major surgery?
    A. Dapagliflozin
    B. Rosiglitazone
    C. Metoclopramide
    D. Sitagliptin

Answers

1. **ANSWER: B**—Treatment for hyperthyroidism should be continued in the perioperative period. Although euthyroid status will not be achieved until approximately 4–8 weeks of treatment with PTU, it may decrease the risk of developing thyroid storm. Starting radioactive iodine (C) may be an option for this patient in the future, but would not be safe until it is confirmed that she is no longer pregnant [47]. Starting levothyroxine (A) is inappropriate as this patient is hyperthyroid and not hypothyroid.
2. **ANSWER: A**—Although post-thyroidectomy hematoma is a rare complication, it can be life-threatening. It is important to consider symptoms and timing of onset when differentiating between nerve injury, hematoma, and hypocalcemia.
   Recurrent laryngeal nerve injury (C) is another rare, yet life-threatening potential complication after thyroidectomy. Unilateral nerve injury is unlikely to have serious effects, however, bilateral recurrent laryngeal nerve injury may present with immediate respiratory distress after extubation post-thyroidectomy [48].
   Hypocalcemia (B) is a common but often temporary complication post-thyroidectomy due to hypoparathyroidism. If severe, laryngospasm may occur [49].
   Pneumothorax (D) is a theoretical risk of thyroidectomy if dissection is carried down to the mediastinum. There is also the possibility of pneumothorax as consequence of positive pressure ventilation. This is unlikely to be the

culprit given an uneventful intraoperative course and rare incidence [50].

3. **ANSWER: C**—Hypercalcemia can lead to significant polyuria and dehydration. Restoring volume status is a priority in these patients and has a dilutional effect on calcium levels. Loop diuretics (D) can be used to increase urinary calcium excretion, although this practice is no longer recommended [51]. Hemodialysis (B) for hypercalcemia may be considered in patients who cannot safely receive intravenous fluids [52]. Thiazide diuretics (A) increase renal calcium reabsorption and would contribute to worsening hypercalcemia.
4. **ANSWER: D**—The hypothalamus is responsible for the production of antidiuretic hormone. It is then stored in the posterior pituitary and secreted in response to increased plasma osmolarity or decreased blood pressure. Posterior pituitary (A) is the site of antidiuretic hormone storage.
5. **ANSWER: A**—Surgical stress is known to increase secretion of antidiuretic hormone. This leads to retention of free water and dilutional hyponatremia. Cerebral salt wasting (C) results in hypovolemic hyponatremia. Diabetes insipidus (B) and diuretic use (D) both lead to hypernatremia.
6. **ANSWER: C**—Acromegaly is associated with prognathism, macroglossia, hypertrophy of airway tissues, and subglottic stenosis. These features can present a challenge in airway management. This patient's worsening hoarseness and shortness of breath are suggestive of potential upper airway obstruction and would be most safely managed using an awake fiberoptic technique with a smaller endotracheal tube.
7. **ANSWER: B**—Neurogenic diabetes insipidus is a common complication after pituitary surgery due to damage of the hypothalamus, pituitary stalk, or posterior pituitary. It typically presents within 1–2 days postoperatively and resolves within days. Nephrogenic diabetes insipidus (A) is a possibility, but less likely than neurogenic DI given the clinical scenario.
   Direct laryngoscopy (A) and video laryngoscopy (D) are options in acromegalic patients and have been described with successful use. However, this patient's airway symptoms raise concern for upper airway obstruction that would be managed most safely with (C) [53].
   Tracheostomy (B) equipment should be available in the event that the patient is unable to be orally intubated.
8. **ANSWER: C**—Perioperative steroid replacement aims to prevent catastrophic adrenal crisis. Patients at risk for adrenal insufficiency are most often caused by iatrogenic steroid administration followed by Addison's disease or primary adrenal insufficiency. Administration of stress dose steroids remains unclear based on conflicting studies but the avoidance of an adrenal crisis in appropriate patients is considered the primary goal over short-term side effects of steroid administration. Patients who are the lowest risk for HPA axis suppression include those on 5 mg or less of prednisone within the previous three weeks [30] This category does not require additional steroid supplementation based on the stress level of surgery unless exhibiting signs and symptoms of adrenal suppression such as refractory shock [30]. Those at greatest risk include patients on 20 mg or more of prednisone daily within the previous three weeks. These patients are dosed additional steroids based on surgical stress categories. Superficial procedures may not warrant additional steroid supplementation [30]. All patients with steroids doses in between these categories are considered intermediate risk and clinical judgement is used to administer stress dose steroids appropriately. These recommendations apply to all forms of steroids including oral, intravenous, inhaled, intranasal, intraarticular injections, or topical steroids.
9. **ANSWER: B**—Pheochromocytoma hypertensive crisis can be triggered by several mechanisms including anxiety, pain, and surgical stimulation. It is also important to recognize that several medications are to be used cautiously or avoided in this patient population. Glucagon receptors are unique to pheochromocytoma tumors that enhance epinephrine and norepinephrine release [54]. These receptors are not present in normal adrenal medulla cells.
   Metoclopramide acts to inhibit presynaptic dopamine receptors that function to reduce norepinephrine release. Because of the blockade, norepinephrine release is enhanced, and blockade of dopaminergic effects on the vasculature increases systemic vascular resistance causing hypertension. In addition, metoclopramide and similar drugs such as chlorpromazine directly stimulate the adrenal medulla to further release catecholamines [55].
   Historically, glucagon and metoclopramide have been previously used as a provocative test to assist diagnosis of pheochromocytoma [54, 55].
   Ketamine is considered a sympathomimetic drug and should be avoided in pheochromocytoma as it stimulates norepinephrine release. Other sympathomimetic drugs to avoid include cocaine and ephedrine. Histamine-releasing medications should also be used cautiously in patients with pheochromocytoma as histamine can directly stimulate the adrenal medulla.
   Phenoxybenzamine is a long-acting nonselective alpha blocker that can be safely used perioperatively. During adrenal resections, the alpha blockade effects will have

lasting effects into the postoperative period and can present with hypotension after the catecholamine-secreting tumors are resected.

10. **ANSWER: A**—Euglycemic DKA is a life-threatening metabolic emergency that can easily go unrecognized in the perioperative period due to the absence of hyperglycemia. Euglycemic DKA is precipitated by a class of medication called sodium-glucose cotransporter 2 (SGLT2) inhibitors such as dapagliflozin. This class of medication works to lower glucose independent of insulin by preventing renal tubular glucose reabsorption. In times of starvation or stress such as surgery, the body shifts its metabolic energy production to produce ketones much like in DKA, however with normoglycemia. This can present with profound metabolic acidosis, electrolyte derangements, and severe dehydration that can lead to death [56]. A heightened vigilance is needed for patients taking these medications into the perioperative and postoperative period to be able to recognize and promptly treat this condition.

References

1. Shahid Z, Asuka E, Singh G. Physiology, hypothalamus. In: StatPearls [Internet]. StatPearls; 2022. Available from: http://www.ncbi.nlm.nih.gov/pubmed/30571001.
2. El Sayed SA, Fahmy MW, Schwartz J. Physiology, Pituitary Gland [Internet]. StatPearls. StatPearls Publishing; 2022 [cited 2022 May 22]. Available from: https://pubmed.ncbi.nlm.nih.gov/29083639/.
3. Demiselle J, Fage N, Radermacher P, Asfar P. Vasopressin and its analogues in shock states: a review. Ann Intensive Care. 2020; 10(1).
4. Melmed S. Acromegaly pathogenesis and treatment. J Clin Investig. 2009;119(11):3189–202.
5. Menon R, Murphy PG, Lindley AM. Anaesthesia and pituitary disease. Continuing Educ Anaesthesia Critical Care Pain [Internet]. 2011;11(4):133–7. Available from: https://academic.oup.com/bjaed/article/11/4/133/266875.
6. Robertson GL. Diabetes insipidus: differential diagnosis and management. Best Pract Res Clin Endocrinol Metab. 2016;30 (2):205–18.
7. Achinger SG, Arieff AI, Kalantar-Zadeh K, Ayus JC. Desmopressin acetate (DDAVP)-associated hyponatremia and brain damage: a case series. Nephrol Dial Transplant [Internet]. 2014;29:2310–5. Available from: https://academic.oup.com/ndt/article/29/12/2310/1852258.
8. Leung AA, McAlister FA, Rogers SO, Pazo V, Wright A, Bates DW. Preoperative hyponatremia and perioperative complications. Archives Internal Med [Internet]. 2012;172(19):1474–81. Available from: https://jamanetwork.com/journals/jamainternalmedicine/fullarticle/1357514.
9. Braun MM, Barstow CH. Diagnosis and management of sodium disorders: hyponatremia and hypernatremia. Am Family Phys. 2015;91(5):299–310. Available from: www.aafp.org/afpAmericanFamilyPhysician299.
10. Cuesta M, Thompson CJ. The syndrome of inappropriate antidiuresis (SIAD). Best Pract Res Clin Endocrinol Metab. 2016;30 (2):175–87.
11. Summers J, Siadh SB. Diabetes insipidus, and transsphenoidal pituitary surgery. Essent Clinical Anesth. 2011;673–5. Available from: https://www.cambridge.org/core/books/essential-clinical-anesthesia/siadh-diabetes-insipidus-and-transsphenoidal-pituitary-surgery/64AD42F254B1703916EB44AA2382D836.
12. Nussey S, Whitehead S. The thyroid gland—endocrinology. In: Endocrinology: an integrated approach: chapter 3: the thyroid gland [Internet]. Oxford: BIOS Scientific Publishers; 2001. Available from: https://www.ncbi.nlm.nih.gov/books/NBK28/
13. Peramunage D, Nikravan S. Anesthesia for endocrine emergencies. Anesthesiol Clinics [Internet]. 2020;38(1):149–63. Available from: https://linkinghub.elsevier.com/retrieve/pii/S1932227519300886
14. Chua AWY, Kumar CM, Chua MJ, Harrisberg BP. Anaesthesia for ophthalmic procedures in patients with thyroid eye disease. Anaesthesia Intensive Care [Internet]. 2020;48(6):430–8. Available from: https://journals.sagepub.com/doi/full/https://doi.org/10.1177/0310057X20957018
15. Taterra D, Wong LM, Vikse J, Sanna B, Pękala P, Walocha J, et al. The prevalence and anatomy of parathyroid glands: a meta-analysis with implications for parathyroid surgery. Langenbeck's Archives Surg [Internet]. 2019;404(1):63. Available from: /pmc/articles/PMC6394670/
16. Mihai R, Farndon JR. Parathyroid disease and calcium metabolism. British J. Anaesthesia [Internet]. 2000;85(1):29–43. Available from: http://www.bjanaesthesia.org/article/S0007091217373348/fulltext
17. Chorin E, Rosso R, Viskin S. Electrocardiographic manifestations of calcium abnormalities. Ann Noninvasive Electrocardiol: The Official J Int Soc Holter Noninvasive Electrocardiol, Inc [Internet]. 2016;21(1):7. Available from: /pmc/articles/PMC6931435/
18. Davies M, Hardman J. Anaesthesia and adrenocortical disease. Contin Educ Anaesthesia, Critical Care Pain. 2005;5(4):122–6.
19. Mattsson C, Young WF. Primary aldosteronism: diagnostic and treatment strategies. Review [Internet]. Available from: www.nature.com/clinicalpractice/neph
20. Monticone S, Moretti C, Williams TA, Veglio F, Gaita F, Mulatero P. Cardiovascular events and target organ damage in primary aldosteronism compared with essential hypertension: a systematic review and meta-analysis. Diabetes-Endocrinol [Internet]. 2018;6. Available from: www.thelancet.com/
21. Diercks DB, Shumaik GM, Harrigan RA, Brady WJ, Chan TC. Electrocardiographic manifestations: electrolyte abnormalities. J Emerg Med. 2004;27(2):153–60.
22. Pirpiris M, Sudhir K, Yeung S, Jennings G, Whitworth JA. Pressor responsiveness in corticosteroid-induced hypertension in humans. Hypertension [Internet]. 1992;19(6):567–74. Available from: http://ahajournals.org
23. Lukert BP, Raisz LG. Glucocorticoid-induced osteoporosis: pathogenesis and management. Ann Intern Med. 1990;112:352–64.
24. Schimmer BP, Funder W. Adrenocorticotropic hormone, adrenal steroids, and the adrenal cortex. In: Goodman & Gilman's: the pharmacological basis of therapeutics [Internet]. 13th ed. McGraw Hill Medical; 2017 [cited 2022 Apr 9]. Available from: https://accesspharmacy-mhmedical-com.ccmain.ohionet.org/content.aspx?bookid=2189&sectionid=172482605#1162542130
25. Mancini T, Kola B, Mantero F, Boscaro M, Arnaldi G. 768 High cardiovascular risk in patients with Cushing's syndrome according to 1999 WHO/ ISH guidelines. Clin Endocrinol. 2004;61:768–77.
26. Wajchenberg L, Bosco A, Martins Marone M, Levin S, Rocha M, CARLOS LERkIO A, et al. Estimation of body fat and lean tissue distribution by dual energy X-ray absorptiometry and abdominal

body fat evaluation by computed tomography in Cushing's disease. J Clin Endocrinol Metabolism Copyright [Internet]. 1995(9). Available from: https://academic.oup.com/jcem/article/80/9/2791/2651125
27. Ferguson JK, Donald RA, Weston TS, Espiner EA. Skin thickness in patients with acromegaly and Cushing's syndrome and response to treatment. Clin Endocrinol [Internet]. 1983;18(4):347–53. Available from: https://onlinelibrary-wiley-com.ccmain.ohionet.org/doi/full/https://doi.org/10.1111/j.1365-2265.1983.tb00578.x
28. Stewart PM, Walker BR, Holder G, O'halloran D, Shackleton CHL. Lip-hydroxysteroid dehydrogenase activity in Cushing's syndrome: explaining the mineralocorticoid excess state of the ectopic adrenocorticotropin syndrome. [cited 2022 Mar 26]; Available from: https://academic.oup.com/jcem/article/80/12/3617/2649992
29. Charmandari E, Nicolaides NC, Chrousos GP. Adrenal insufficiency. www.thelancet.com [Internet]. 2014;383.
30. Liu MM, Reidy AB, Saatee S, Collard CD. Perioperative steroid management approaches based on current evidence. Anesthesiol [Internet]. 2017;127(1):166–72. Available from: https://pubs.asahq.org/anesthesiology/article/127/1/166/18755/Perioperative-Steroid-ManagementApproaches-Based
31. Carbone E, Borges R, Eiden LE, García AG, Hernández-Cruz A. Chromaffin cells of the adrenal medulla: physiology, pharmacology, and disease. Compr Physiol. 2019;9(4):1443–502.
32. Stein P, Black H. A simplified diagnostic approach to pheochromocytoma: a review of the literature and report of one institution's experience [Internet]. Endocrinol Cardiovascul Med. 1990 [cited 2022 Apr 11], 46–66. Available from: https://oce-ovid-com.ccmain.ohionet.org/article/00005792-199101000-00004/PDF
33. Krumeich LN, Cucchiara AJ, Nathanson KL, Kelz RR, Fishbein L, Fraker DL, et al. Correlation between plasma catecholamines, weight, and diabetes in pheochromocytoma and paraganglioma. J Clin Endocrinol Metab. 2021;106(10):4028–38.
34. Kassim TA, Clarke DD, Mai VQ, Clyde PW, Shakir KM. Catecholamine-induced cardiomyopathy. 2008
35. Prys-Roberts C, Farndon JR. Efficacy and safety of doxazosin for perioperative management of patients with pheochromocytoma. World J Surg. 2002;26:1037–42.
36. Chernobylsky DJ, Kaye AD, Hall SM. Clinical physiology in anesthetic practice: In: Clinical physiology in anesthetic practice: chapter 8: endocrine physiology. McGraw Hill; 2022.
37. Coexisting conditions and complications | diabetes | CDC [Internet]. [cited 2022 Feb 18]. Available from: https://www.cdc.gov/diabetes/data/statistics-report/coexisting-conditions-complications.html.
38. Prevalence of both diagnosed and undiagnosed diabetes | diabetes | CDC [Internet]. [cited 2022 Feb 18]. Available from: https://www.cdc.gov/diabetes/data/statistics-report/diagnosed-undiagnosed-diabetes.html.
39. Forbes JM, Cooper ME. Mechanisms of diabetic complications. Physiol Rev [Internet]. 2013;93:137–88. Available from: http://www.jdrf.org.au/about-jdrf-australia/media
40. Sarwar N, Gao P, Kondapally Seshasai SR, Gobin R, Kaptoge S, di Angelantonio E, et al. Diabetes mellitus, fasting blood glucose concentration, and risk of vascular disease: a collaborative meta-analysis of 102 prospective studies. The Lancet. 2010;375 (9733):2215–22.
41. Haas A, McDonnell ME. Pathogenesis of cardiovascular disease in diabetes. Vol. 47, Endocrinology and Metabolism Clinics of North America. W.B. Saunders; 2018. pp 51–63.
42. Arvanitakis Z, Schneider JA, Wilson RS, Li Y, Arnold SE, Wang Z, et al. Diabetes is related to cerebral infarction but not to AD pathology in older persons. 2006.
43. DeFronzo RA, Reeves WB, Awad AS. Pathophysiology of diabetic kidney disease: impact of SGLT2 inhibitors. Nat Rev Nephrol. 2021;17(5):319–34.
44. Le H, Wick JB, Van BW, Klineberg EO. Diffuse idiopathic skeletal hyperostosis of the spine: pathophysiology, diagnosis, and management. J Am Acad Orthopaedic Surg. NLM (Medline); 2021;29:1044–51.
45. Committee ADAPP. 16. Diabetes care in the hospital: standards of medical care in diabetes—2022. Diabetes Care [Internet]. 2022;45 (Supplement_1):S244–53. Available from: https://diabetesjournals.org/care/article/45/Supplement_1/S244/138924/16-Diabetes-Care-in-the-Hospital-Standards-of
46. Pasquel FJ, Umpierrez GE. Hyperosmolar hyperglycemic state: a historic review of the clinical presentation, diagnosis, and treatment. Diabetes Care. 2014;37(11):3124–31.
47. Ross DS, Burch HB, Cooper DS, Greenlee MC, Laurberg P, Maia AL, et al. American thyroid association guidelines for diagnosis and management of hyperthyroidism and other causes of thyrotoxicosis. Thyroid [Internet]. 2016 Oct 1 [cited 2022 May 31];26(10):1343–421. Available from: https://pubmed.ncbi.nlm.nih.gov/27521067/.
48. Bruch J, Kamani D. Hoarseness in adults [Internet]. UpToDate. 2021 [cited 2022 Jun 1]. Available from: https://www.uptodate.com/contents/hoarseness-in-adults?search=recurrent%20laryngeal%20nerve%20injury&source=search_result&selectedTitle=1~75&usage_type=default&display_rank=1#H24.
49. Lee YS, Nam KH, Chung WY, Chang HS, Park CS. Postoperative complications of thyroid cancer in a single center experience. J Korean Med Sci [Internet]. 2010;25(4):541. Available from: /pmc/articles/PMC2844597/
50. Lee SJ, Lee DJ, Kim MC, Im UJ. Pneumothorax in a post-anesthetic care unit after right thyroidectomy with left neck dissection—a case report. Korean J Anesthesiol [Internet]. 2010;59 (6):429. Available from: /pmc/articles/PMC3022139/
51. LeGrand SB, Leskuski D, Zama I. Narrative review: furosemide for hypercalcemia: an unproven yet common practice. Ann Intern Med [Internet]. 2008;149(4):259–63. Available from: https://pubmed.ncbi.nlm.nih.gov/18711156/
52. Koo WS, Jeon DS, Ahn SJ, Kim YS, Yoon YS, Bang BK. Calcium-free hemodialysis for the management of hypercalcemia. Nephron [Internet]. 1996;72(3):424–8. Available from: https://pubmed.ncbi.nlm.nih.gov/8852491/
53. Schmitt H, Buchfelder M, Radespiel-Tröger M, Fahlbusch R. Difficult intubation in acromegalic patients incidence and predictability. Anesthesiol [Internet]. 2000;93(1):110–4. Available from: https://pubs.asahq.org/anesthesiology/article/93/1/110/756/Difficult-Intubation-in-Acromegalic
54. Albertin G, Aragona F, Gottardo L, Malendowicz LK, Nussdorfer GG. Human pheochromocytomas, but not adrenal medulla, express glucagon-receptor gene and possess an in vitro secretory response to glucagon. 2001.
55. Guillemot J, Compagnon P, Cartier D, Thouennon E, Bastard C, Lihrmann I, et al. Metoclopramide stimulates catecholamine- and granin-derived peptide secretion from pheochromocytoma cells through activation of serotonin type 4 (5-HT4) receptors. Endocr Relat Cancer. 2009;16(1):281–90.
56. Modi A, Agrawal A, Morgan F. Euglycemic diabetic ketoacidosis: a review. Curr Diabetes Rev. 2016;13(3):315–21.

Part IV
Anesthetic Management Topics

Contents

24 Preoperative Evaluation of Patients Undergoing Non-cardiac Surgery

Elizabeth A. M. Frost and Daniel Katz

Abstract

Traditionally, routine tests have been considered important elements of preanesthetic evaluation to determine fitness for surgery. Over the past four decades, this practice has been scrutinized due to a low yield and high cost. In fact, routine tests such as complete blood count (CBC), chest X-ray, electrocardiogram (EKG), urinalysis, and electrolyte panel are of little value in detecting disease or changing management. Rather multiple investigations detect minor irrelevant abnormalities, increase patient risk, cause delay, and increase liability. Many reviews and studies have confirmed these findings that routine testing does little or nothing to aid in effective preanesthetic assessment. Rather, postoperative complications were linked to higher ASA classification, longer duration of anesthesia, more complex surgery, and poor nutritional status. More importantly recent studies indicate that risk assessment for cognitive dysfunction and prediction of other complications are important.

Keywords

Airway assessment • Preanesthetic evaluation • Choosing wisely • Herbal medications • Risk management

Key Points

1. Routine preoperative laboratory tests rarely change the course of anesthesia.
2. Approximately 1:500 tests reveal pertinent information.
3. Centers for Medicare and Medicaid Services (CMS) will not pay for solely age-based tests.
4. All medications should be documented, including over-the-counter drugs such as non-steroidal anti-inflammatory agents (NSAIDs) and herbal preparations.
5. An understanding of drug interactions, especially as they relate to herbals, is essential.
6. Multiple investigations detect minor irrelevant abnormalities, increase patient risk, cause delay, and increase liability.
7. Postoperative complications can be linked to higher American Society of Anesthesiologists (ASA) classification, longer duration of anesthesia, more complex surgery, and poor nutritional status.
8. Laboratory tests should be ordered only as indicated to discover a disease, verify a condition, or formulate a plan.
9. Current guidelines have no recommendations for starting calcium channel blockers in the perioperative period.
10. Mini-cog tests and risk assessment using the American College of Surgeons' National Surgical Quality Improvement Program should be applied preoperatively.
11. Frailty evaluation should be included.
12. Plans for pain management and postoperative nausea and vomiting prevention should be in place.

E. A. M. Frost (✉)
Department of Anesthesiology, Icahn Medical Center at Mount Sinai, New York, NY, USA
e-mail: elzfrost@aol.com

D. Katz
Icahn Medical Center at Mount Sinai, New York, NY, USA
e-mail: Daniel.katz@mountsinai.org

M. Argalious et al. (eds.), *Basic Sciences in Anesthesia*,
https://doi.org/10.1007/978-3-031-60203-0_24

24.1 Introduction

> On feeling the pulse of a gentleman about 21 years of age, in March 1855, who had just seated himself in the chair to take chloroform…I found it to be small weak, and intermitting and it became feeble as I was feeling it. I told the patient he would feel no pain and that he had nothing whatever to apprehend. His pulse immediately improved…Now if the inhalation had commenced without inquiry or explanation, the syncope which seemed approaching would probably have taken place, and it would have had the appearance of being caused by the chloroform, although not so in reality.
>
> —John Snow. *On Chloroform and other Anaesthetics*. London: John Churchill. 1858

Although the importance of examination of the patient, especially the pulse, had been emphasized since ancient times, Dr. Snow was one of the first to stress the need for physical contact and evaluation prior to anesthesia.

Traditionally, routine tests have been considered important elements of preanesthetic evaluation to determine fitness for surgery. Over the past four decades, this practice has been scrutinized due to a low yield and high cost. In fact, routine tests such as complete blood count (CBC), chest X-ray, electrocardiogram (EKG), urinalysis, and electrolyte panel are of little value in detecting disease or changing management. Rather multiple investigations detect minor irrelevant abnormalities, increase patient risk, cause delay, and increase liability [1].

Choosing Wisely was initiated in 2012 by the American Board of Internal Medicine to establish a national program to avoid unnecessary tests, treatments, and procedures through education of practitioners and patients [2, 3]. The initial 9 specialty boards and Consumer Reports were soon joined by some 70 other specialties, including anesthesiology in 2013. They were all charged with releasing 5 recommendations to facilitate decisions regarding appropriate care.

Recommendations from the American Society of Anesthesiologists (ASA) are as follows:

1. Do not obtain baseline laboratory studies ("routine tests") in patients without significant systemic disease (ASA I or II) undergoing low-risk surgery—specifically, complete blood count, basic or comprehensive metabolic panel, coagulation studies when blood loss (or fluid shifts) is/are expected to be minimal.
2. Do not obtain baseline diagnostic cardiac testing (trans-thoracic/esophageal echocardiography – TTE/TEE) or cardiac stress testing in asymptomatic stable patients with known cardiac disease (e.g., coronary artery disease [CAD], valvular disease) undergoing low or moderate risk non-cardiac surgery.
3. Do not use pulmonary artery catheters (PACs) routinely for cardiac surgery in patients with a low risk of hemodynamic complications (especially with the concomitant use of alternative diagnostic tools, e.g., TEE).
4. Do not administer packed red blood cells (PRBCs) in a young healthy patient without ongoing blood loss and hemoglobin of $\geq$ 6 g/dL unless symptomatic or hemodynamically unstable.
5. Do not routinely administer colloid (dextrans, hydroxyethyl starches, and albumin) for volume resuscitation without appropriate indications.

Nevertheless, many patients, surgeons, and internists as well as hospital protocols believe that the primary purpose of a preoperative evaluation is to give blood and urine samples, undergo an electrocardiogram, and have a chest X-ray. Routine testing, generally considered to include EKG, complete blood count, urinalysis, chest X-ray, electrolyte screen, blood urea nitrogen (BUN) and creatinine, blood glucose level, type and screen, and a coagulation profile (PT/PTT), is not only time consuming and but also extremely costly with little benefit. An early large study challenged the usefulness of routine preoperative laboratory screening in 1985. Over a four-month period, the authors assessed the value of screening 2000 patients of all ages, estimating that 60% of these routinely ordered tests would not have been performed if testing had only been done for specific indications. Abnormalities that might influence perioperative management were identified in 0.22% although they were not acted upon, and no changes were made to the planned procedure. No adverse anesthetic or surgical consequences were recorded. The authors concluded three decades ago that in the absence of specific indications, routine preoperative laboratory tests contribute little to patient care, and can be eliminated. Moreover, even when an abnormality was recorded, the results often were not read by the physician or nurse manager who had ordered the test—an oversight that could have serious malpractice consequences.

Some years later, one of the authors of the aforementioned study calculated that $40 billion a year was spent in the United States on preoperative testing and evaluation. Likening it to the statement that "if a little epinephrine is good, more is better," he remarked that additional testing caused iatrogenic disease by pursuit and treatment of borderline and false-positive results, thereby increasing medico-legal risks (especially if an abnormal result is obtained and not acted upon) and decreasing the efficiency of practice. Rather, he remarked, perioperative physicians could turn such inefficiency to advantage by successfully employing inexpensive technology to reduce costs substantially and improve the quality of care.

Over the past four decades, many reviews and studies have confirmed these findings that routine testing does little or nothing to aid in effective preanesthetic assessment [4, 5]. Rather, postoperative complications were linked to higher ASA classification, longer duration of anesthesia, more complex surgery, and poor nutritional status, especially low protein levels. In addition, increased age may also be a factor, although a weak one.

However, even now, hospitals and specialists are usually reimbursed for unnecessary testing, for example, stress testing, acknowledged by the American College of Cardiology (ACC) and the American Heart Association (AHA) to have restricted benefit in the majority of patients, amounts to around US$2300. A common test sequence that includes complete blood count, basic metabolic panel, chest X-ray, and EKG bills for about $1600, which does not include the cost of interpretation. In some instances, the Center for Medicare/Medicaid Services (CMS) and insurers will not reimburse for repeat testing and for tests based on age alone, placing the burden of payment on the patient. In other situations, CMS shoulders the enormous costs, almost arbitrarily. Change is slow to be realized and further studies, both larger and more diverse, must be undertaken.

24.2 Evaluation and Preoperative Preparation

Preanesthetic evaluation is the process of clinical assessment that precedes the delivery of anesthesia or ordering of tests for all procedures. It is the responsibility of the anesthesiologist or certified registered nurse anesthetist (CRNA) practicing alone. Consideration of information from multiple sources is essential, especially all medical records. Consultations should be sought as necessary. Further laboratory tests should be ordered only as indicated to discover a disease, verify a condition, or formulate a plan. Informed consent, as to risk–benefit of different types of anesthetic management, must be obtained. A plan for postoperative pain relief must also be in place [6].

The information sought must include at a minimum:

1. The procedure
2. Past medical and surgical history
3. Medications
4. Documentation of vital signs
5. Airway examination
6. Informed consent

24.2.1 ASA Physical Status Classification

The ASA Physical Status (PS) classification system was initially created in 1941 by the American Society of Anesthetists, an organization that later became the ASA. The grading system was intended simply to evaluate the degree of a patient's "sickness" or "physical state" before selecting the anesthetic and performing surgery. The preoperative physical status is used for recordkeeping, for communicating between colleagues, and to create a uniform system for statistical analysis. The grading system is not intended for use as a measure to predict operative risk. Standards, according to the ASA, that are required for all patients preoperatively include documentation of airway examination, vital signs, and ASA classifications.

The modern classification system consists of six categories, as follows:

- ASA PS 1—Healthy patients without systemic, physiologic, or psychiatric disease. No physical limitations. Good exercise tolerance.
- ASA PS 2—Patients with mild systemic disease that is well controlled. Controlled hypertension or diabetes with no physical effects. Mild obesity. Long-standing smoking without chronic obstructive pulmonary disease (COPD).
- ASA PS 3—Patients with severe systemic disease affecting > 1 body system. No immediate threat of death. Controlled congestive heart failure (CHF). Morbid obesity. Chronic renal failure. Bronchospastic disease.
- ASA PS 4—Patients with severe systemic disease that is a constant threat to life. Possible risk of death. Symptomatic CHF and COPD.
- ASA PS 5—Moribund patients who are not expected to survive > 24 h without surgery. Multiorgan failure. Sepsis with hemodynamic instability. Uncontrolled coagulopathy.
- ASA PS 6—Patients declared brain dead for organ donation.

24.2.2 Medical and Surgical History

Based on the medical and surgical history provided by the patient and the procedure to be performed, the American College of Surgeons, National Surgical Quality Improvement Program (ACS NSQUIP) has devised a Surgical Risk Calculator. Using standardized clinical data from almost 400 hospitals, a Web-based tool has been devised. By inputting 21 preoperative factors such as co-morbidities and demographics, surgeons can estimate the risks of surgery, chance of complications including death, and length of hospital stay. Not only does this mechanism afford better-informed consent for the patient, but it also allows decisions to be made regarding the type and even necessity for certain procedures. The Centers for Medicare and Medicaid Services are moving to incentivize surgeons through the Physician Quality Reporting System to discuss patient-specific risks and

Table 24.1 After entering a procedure, one or more CPT® codes are shown. The surgeon can then input information specific to the patient. A representative questionnaire for a patient undergoing colectomy is shown

Age	Diabetes
Sex	Hypertension treated
Emergency	Previous cardiac event
ASA class	Congestive cardiac failure within 30 days
Chronic steroid use	Dyspnea
Ascites within 30 days	Current smoker
Systemic sepsis within 48 h	Severe COPD
Ventilator dependent	Dialysis
Metastatic cancer	Acute renal failure
Height	Weight

ASA American Society of Anesthesiologists, *COPD* chronic obstructive pulmonary disease

Table 24.2 Based on the answers, the risk factors for a specific procedure, in this illustration, colectomy, are obtained. The predicted average length of hospital stay is then displayed

Outcomes	Average patient risk (on a sliding scale)	Chance of outcome (below, average, above)
Death		
Any complication (includes return to OR)		
Pneumonia		
Cardiac event		
Surgical site infection		
Urinary tract infection		
Blood clot		
Renal failure		

OR operating room
NSAIDs non-steroidal anti-inflammatory drugs, *MAO* monoamine oxidase

outcomes preoperatively. Using almost 3000 Current Procedural Terminology (CPT®) codes, several hundred operations over many subspecialties have been incorporated into the calculations. Thirty-day outcomes were ascertained from medical records or patient contact. Event rates were found to vary from 0.6% for renal failure to 9% for overall morbidity. Some of the patient and surgical information is shown in ◉ Table 24.1. Outcomes and risk factors are shown in ◉ Table 24.2.

While many surgical factors are taken into consideration, anesthetic factors are not addressed. History of previous difficult intubation or tracheostomy, or problems specific to anesthesia such as malignant hyperthermia or certain allergies might well impact outcome and hence risk. Nevertheless, this risk assessment can answer specific questions often asked of anesthetic care providers such as: "Am I at risk for a heart attack?".

24.2.3 Medications

All the medications that a patient is taking should be documented, including over-the-counter drugs such as non-steroidal anti-inflammatory agents (NSAIDs) and especially herbal preparations. The latter, while considered natural and thus safe, may have many interactions (◘ Box 24.1). Problems arise mainly in interference with the cytochrome p450 isoenzymes (CYP). Inhibition of this system decreases metabolism and increases drug levels and duration of action. Induction increases metabolism, while decreasing the effectiveness of the drug and its duration of action. Of most concern is the interference with CYP 3A4 in the liver as > 50% of current prescription drugs depend on this system. Some of the more commonly used herbal substances and their varied effects on the CYP system are shown in ◉ Table 24.3 * MERGEFORMAT.

Whether or not medications should be continued during the perioperative period should be made on a case-by-case basis for each individual patient by the patient care team. Of major concern are the cardiac medications. The ACC/AHA guidelines, however, can provide some guidance pertaining to cardiac medications that may directly affect perioperative morbidity and mortality [7].

Box 24.1 Several Interactions Have Been Identified with Herbal Medications and Anesthesia

- Echinacea offsets immunosuppression and inhibits hepatic microsomal enzymes (HME).
- Garlic augments heparin, NSAIDs, and increases perioperative bleeding.
- Ginger increases bleeding time.
- St. John's wort reacts with MAO inhibitors, tetracycline.
- Kava-kava reacts with ethanol, excessive sedation
- Feverfew inhibits platelet activity.
- Ephedra interacts with inhalation anesthetics.
- Ginseng causes hypertension, hypoglycemia, reacts with MAO inhibitors, increases bleeding.

24.2.3.1 Beta Blocker Therapy

Several studies have examined the risks and benefits of perioperative beta blocker therapy. Although each study was designed to answer the same question, most resulted in different answers. It does appear that beta blocker therapy in

Table 24.3 Many herbs affect the CYP system, some increasing the effectiveness of drugs, even to toxic levels while others prevent absorption and thus render the drug essentially useless

CYP3A4	Inhibition Induction	Chamomile, grapefruit, ginkgo, kava Garlic, ginkgo, St. John's wort
CYP1A2	Inhibition Induction	Chamomile, ginkgo, grapefruit St. John's wort
CYP2C19	Inhibition Induction	Feverfew, grapefruit, kava Ginkgo, St. John's wort
CYP2C9	Inhibition Induction	Feverfew, ginkgo, grapefruit, kava St. John's wort
CYP2E1	Inhibition Induction	Garlic, kava
CYP2D6	Inhibition Induction	Ginkgo, goldenseal, kava

the perioperative period decreases the number of cardiac events, such as myocardial infarction (MI). However, this benefit comes at the cost of increased hypotension, stroke, and, in some studies, composite death. The most recent systematic review examining the data came with the following recommendations [8]:

1. Beta blockers should be continued in patients undergoing surgery who have been on beta blockers chronically.
2. The management of beta blockers after surgery may be guided by clinical circumstances independent of when the agent was started.
3. In patients with intermediate or high cardiac risk, it may be reasonable to begin perioperative beta blocker therapy. If the decision is made to begin beta blocker therapy on a patient in the perioperative period, it is recommended that therapy be initiated at least 1 day prior to surgery, and preferably at least 2–7 days prior. Beginning beta blockers on the day of surgery is likely ineffective and may be harmful. Common sense would dictate that beginning a medication that could have significant changes in myocardial contractility and systemic blood pressure should occur days prior to surgery, such that the tolerability of the medication and its dose can be assessed by the patient and the physician. While there is no direct data to support this conclusion, it likely is best practice.

24.2.3.2 Statin Therapy

Statin therapy has been shown to be effective for primary and secondary prevention of cardiac events. Although most of the data related to statin therapy come from observational trials, the composite power suggests a protective effect on the preoperative use of these agents in either vascular surgery or high-risk patient populations [9]. The most recent guidelines therefore recommend that those on statins continue their therapy in the perioperative period. They also allow for the initiation of therapy in patients undergoing vascular surgery, as well as patients with clinical indications undergoing medium- or high-risk procedures. The mechanism of benefits from perioperative statin therapy are unknown but are likely related to pleiotropic, lipid-lowering effects, as well as anti-inflammatory effects. Additionally, it is not known when the optimal time is to begin therapy, nor is it clear what the duration of therapy should be.

24.2.3.3 Alpha-2 Agonists

Early data on the role of alpha-2 agonists such as clonidine and mivazerol suggested that the perioperative use of these agents, especially in vascular surgery was protective. The POISE-2 (PeriOperative ISchemic Evaluation-2) trial—a large, multicenter, international, blinded study—was unable to demonstrate the benefit of clonidine. Additionally, it was found that clonidine use in the perioperative period was associated with an increase in the rate of nonfatal cardiac arrest and clinically significant hypotension. It is therefore not recommended to use alpha-2 agonists in the perioperative period for the prevention of cardiac events. Patients who are on alpha-2 agonists for other indications (such as hypertension) should continue their dose of medication; or ideally, be weaned off their medication and started on other therapies prior to surgery. The abrupt discontinuation of these medications can result in rebound hypertension, headache, agitation, and tremor.

24.2.3.4 Calcium Channel Blockers

The most current guidelines have no recommendations for starting calcium channel blockers in the perioperative period. A meta-analysis from 2003 examined the use of calcium channel blockers in patients with coronary disease and found trends toward reduced death and MI. It should be noted that these differences were mostly attributable to the use of diltiazem. Neither dihydropyridines nor verapamil had effects on mortality or MI; however, the use of either verapamil or diltiazem seemed to be protective for the development of perioperative supraventricular tachycardia (SVT). The authors note that the results are trends and that larger more robust studies are needed to confirm the results. As such, although it would be prudent to continue these medications in the perioperative period it is not recommended to begin therapy unless otherwise indicated.

24.2.3.5 Low Does Aspirin

Recent guidelines have warned against routine use of aspirin in older patients (> 70 years). While there appears to be little benefit regarding cardiovascular protection, the risk of bleeding is increased.

24.2.3.6 Angiotensin-Converting Enzyme Inhibitors and Angiotensin Receptor Blockers

Approved for multiple indications from hypertension to prevention of diabetic nephropathy, ACE and angiotensin receptor blockers (ARBs) are some of the most commonly prescribed medications. Perioperative data on the risk/benefit profile of continuation of these medications is limited mostly to observational data. The largest study examined almost 80,000 patients (of which 13% were on ACE-I) and found that patients on therapy had an increased frequency of intraoperative hypotension. This has been found in other studies as well, with one showing an incidence of hypotension of 50% in patients on therapy. Despite the increase in hypotension, there appears to be no increased incidence of death, MI, or renal failure. The evidence on discontinuation of these medications prior to surgery is poor. There is data, however, on the risks of not restarting these medications in the perioperative period, which seems to be the greatest risk of discontinuation. In fact, maintaining the continuity of these medications in the setting of treatment for heart failure or hypertension is supported by other guidelines. Additionally, a more recent cohort study including 30,000 patients found an increased risk of mortality in patients in whom restarting ARB therapy was delayed. Due to the lack of demonstration of real harm to patients who continue therapy in the perioperative period as well as the potential risks of discontinuation, continuing these medications in the perioperative period is reasonable. If ACE/ARB therapy must be withheld, it should be restarted as soon as possible.

24.2.3.7 Medication

Recommendations to discontinue oral diabetic medication remain controversial. While elevated blood sugar levels have been shown to retard wound healing, an ideal blood sugar level has not been determined. While many laboratory scales consider hyperglycemia to be values above 120 mg/dl, it is probably more important to consider the individual and the level at which he most usually functions. Thus, values of 150–170 mg/dl may be considered normal for many. Should testing indicate values exceeding 180 mg/dl, oral medications should be discontinued, and an infusion of regular insulin commenced perioperatively? Further evaluation by an endocrinologist is indicated with repeated blood glucose checks.

24.2.4 Cardiac Evaluation

While nonspecific abnormalities are found on EKG tracings in about 30% of patients, the finding rarely predicts postoperative complications and is usually insignificant.

As part of *Choosing Wisely* and recommendations from the ACC/AHA, the need for further cardiac testing prior to non-cardiac surgery is limited to determination of 1 of 4 criteria [10]:

- Unstable coronary syndrome (MI, unstable angina).
- Decompensated heart failure (New York Heart Association [NYHA] class IV or worsening disease or new onset).
- Significant dysrhythmias; high grade or Mobitz II atrioventricular (AV) block, 3rd degree AV block, symptomatic ventricular dysrhythmias.
- Severe valvular disease.

Stress testing and cardiac consultation should only be requested if any of the above findings can be made on physical examination.

24.2.5 Airway Assessment

Evaluation of the airway begins with a comprehensive history and physical examination. It is very important to ascertain if the patient has been told of any difficulty with intubation in the past and if he/she had a sore throat after a procedure. A short list of factors that may be indicative of a difficult airway is shown in ◉ Table 24.4.

As well as assessment for any of the conditions listed in ◉ Table 24.4, physical examination requires a systematic approach as follows:

1. On nasal examination are there any polyps or a deviated septum?
2. Does the mouth open to allow at least 2 fingerbreadths between upper and lower teeth?
3. Is there good alignment with the upper and lower teeth? Protruding upper incisors or canines should be noted as well as carious or loose teeth and gum hypertrophy due to medication (usually dilantin). Edentulous patients often offer an easier airway, although a large tongue can cause hypopharyngeal obstruction.
4. Is the palate free of any clefts, high arch, or a long, narrow anatomy?
5. Can the lower jaw be protruded over the upper jaw?
6. Is there any limitation of temporo-mandibular joint movement?
7. Is the hyomental/thyromental distance at least > 6 cm?
8. Is the neck size < 17 cm?

Table 24.4 Many factors may contribute to a difficult airway and can usually be elicited by careful history and physical examination

Congenital	Trauma	Tumors	Body habitus	Infection	Arthritis
Down syndrome	Burns	Thyroid tumor	Obesity	Croup	Rheumatoid arthritis
Hunter-hurler syndrome	Facial fractures	Cystic hygroma	Dental caries	Intraoral abscess/tonsillar enlargement	Ankylosing spondylitis
Pierre-Robin syndrome	Cervical cord injuries	Lipomas	Facial hair/beard	Ludwig's angina	Temporo-mandibular joint disease
Marfan syndrome	Laryngeal trauma	Adenomas/polyps	Mandibular hypoplasia	Thrush	
Treacher Collins syndrome	Airway hematomas	Oral cancer	Acromegaly	Diphtheria	

9. Can a sniffing position be assumed?
10. Does the patient have any stridor, previous tracheostomy, or hoarseness?
11. Is the patient pregnant?

Some other specific tests can be made to determine anatomical criteria:

1. Mallampati test. The test is performed with the patient sitting, and the head in a neutral position. The mouth is opened wide, and the tongue protruded (◉ Fig. 24.1). The degree to which tongue size correlates to pharyngeal size is assessed. A review of 42 studies, with 34,513 participants, found that the score predicts difficult direct laryngoscopy and intubation, but does not predict difficult bag mask ventilation. Therefore, while useful in combination with other tests to predict the difficulty of securing an airway, it is not sufficiently accurate alone. Other assessments are indicated.
2. Comack and Lehane. Four grades of view are defined during direct laryngoscopy. Entire view of the laryngeal aperture is listed as Grade 1. Visualization of only the posterior commissure of the laryngeal aperture is graded as 2. If only the epiglottis is seen that is grade 3. Grade 4 view is just the soft palate.
3. Mandibular space assessment involves measurement of the thyromental space, and the sterno-mental and the mandibulo-hyoid distances. The thyromental distance is measured from the mentum to the thyroid notch with the neck extended. Alignment of the laryngeal-pharyngeal axes is optimal when the distance is > 6.5 cm. With the head and neck extended and the mouth closed the distance from the suprasternal notch to the mentum should exceed 12 cm. The mandibular length from the chin to the hyoid bone should be at least 4 cm (about 4 fingerbreadths). Distance between the lower and upper teeth is normally 4.5 cm.

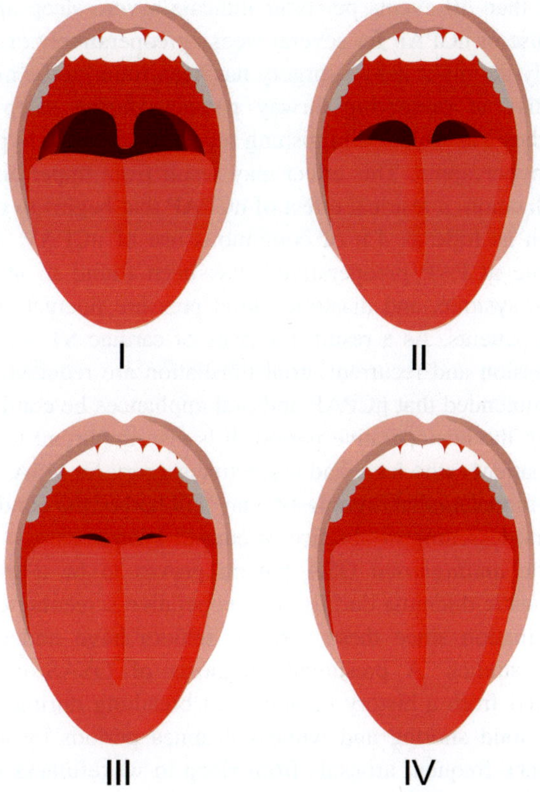

Fig. 24.1 Class I views allow visualization of the soft palate, fauces, uvula, and anterior and posterior pillars and indicate an easy intubation. Only the hard palate is visible in Class 4 (Illustration by Jmarchn—Own work, CC BY-SA 3.0, ► https://commons.wikimedia.org/w/index.php?curid=12842847. Reprinted under Creative Commons license. ► https://creativecommons.org/licenses/by-sa/3.0/)

24.2.6 Obstructive Sleep Apnea Syndrome

A complication often associated with obesity, but not exclusively, is obstructive sleep apnea syndrome (OSA or OSAS) [11]. The potential for airway difficulties in patients with OSA is more likely to be recognized by anesthesiologists even when the patient has not had a formal polysomnographic sleep study, which defines the patient's apnea/hypopnea index (AHI); categorizes the severity of OSA as mild, moderate, or severe; and makes recommendations for appropriate nasal continuous positive airway pressure (nCPAP). Apnea is defined as the cessation of airflow for at least 10 s. During hypopnea airflow decreases by 50% for 10 s or decreases by 30% if there is an associated decrease in the oxygen saturation or an arousal from sleep. To grade the severity of sleep apnea, the number of events per hour is reported as the AHI. An AHI of less than 5 is considered normal, 5–15 is mild, 15–30 is moderate, and more than 30 events per hour indicate severe sleep apnea. The use of nCPAP for several weeks preoperatively or even simply the night before surgery has been found to be highly effective at preserving airway patency during sleep and anesthesia as well as diminishing reflex responses to hypoxia and hypercapnia. This effect may result from upper airway stabilization, a residual effect of nCPAP that begins to occur within as little as 4 h of continuous use of nCPAP. Also, chronic nCPAP preoperatively has been found to abolish mean, systolic, and diastolic blood pressure fluctuations in OSA patients. As a result, the risks of cardiac ST segment depression and recurrent atrial fibrillation are reduced. It is recommended that nCPAP and oral appliances be continued during the postoperative period. It is also important to note that patients who have had corrective surgery for OSA, such as uvulopalatopharyngoplasty, may still harbor the condition despite lessening or absence of current symptoms.

The *undiagnosed* OSA patient proves to be a greater diagnostic dilemma during the preoperative screening clinic examination since these patients seldom have undergone sleep studies. A presumed diagnosis of OSAS can be inferred from a history of abnormal breathing during sleep (e.g., loud snoring and witnessed apnea periods by a bed partner), frequent arousals from sleep to wakefulness (e.g., periodic extremity twitching, vocalization, turning, and snorting), severe daytime sleepiness, a body mass index [BMI] of $\geq$ 35 kg/m^2, increased neck circumference ($\geq$ 17 inches for males, $\geq$ 16 inches for females), and the presence of coexisting morbidities (e.g., essential systemic hypertension, pulmonary hypertension, cardiomegaly). The STOP-Bang questionnaire has been shown reliable in correctly diagnosing the condition although age does not appear to be a significant factor (◉ Fig. 24.2).

The ASA task force on OSA recommended a risk scoring system as summarized (points are assigned for each of three categories [a, b, c] and then totaled [d]) [13]:

(a) *Severity of sleep apnea*: Based on a sleep study (i.e., AHI) or clinical indicators if a sleep study is not available (i.e., presumptive diagnosis). Points: 0 = None; 1 = Mild OSA; 2 = Moderate OSA; 3 = Severe OSA.
One point may be subtracted if a patient has been on CPAP or bi-level positive airway pressure (BiPAP) prior to surgery and will be using this consistently during the postoperative period. One point should be added if a patient with mild or moderate OSA has a resting $PaCO_2$ exceeding 50 mm Hg.
(b) *Invasiveness of the surgical procedure and anesthesia*: Based on type of surgery/anesthesia. Points: 0 = superficial surgery under local or peripheral nerve block, anesthesia without sedation; 1 = superficial surgery with moderate sedation or general anesthesia or peripheral surgery with spinal or epidural anesthesia (with no more than moderate sedation); 2 = peripheral surgery with general anesthesia or airway surgery with moderate sedation; 3 = major surgery under general anesthesia or airway surgery under general anesthesia.
(c) *Requirement for postoperative opioids*: Points: 0 = none; 1 = low-dose oral opioids; 3 = high-dose oral opioids or parenteral or neuraxial opioids.
(d) *Estimation of perioperative risk*: Based on the overall score (0–6) derived from the points assigned to (a) added to the greater of the points assigned to (b) or (c). Patients with overall score of $\geq$ 4 may be at increased perioperative risk from OSA. Patients with a score of $\geq$ 5 may be at significantly increased perioperative risk from OSA.

Clinical suspicion of OSAS may be the only preoperative tool available to the anesthesiologist as formal, widely used, preoperative-validated questionnaires have not been established.

In addition to the OSA risk factors presented above, the anesthesiologist should consider the patient's airway class and history of difficult intubation. To this end, a morphologic OSA prediction score has been developed that includes anatomical difficulties. Cardiovascular risk assessment may require an EKG (right ventricular hypertrophy secondary to cor pulmonale, left ventricular hypertrophy secondary to ischemic heart disease), echocardiography, cardiac stress testing, or preoperative cardiologist optimization. Pulmonary risk factors of morbid obesity and chronic obstructive pulmonary disease may prompt obtaining a radiograph or arterial blood gases to detect Pickwickian syndrome or hypercapnic chronic sleep apnea syndrome. These patients may have decreased sensitivity to CO_2 in the postoperative period and may need ventilatory support as their hypoxic drive to breathe may be abolished by O_2 as well as subanesthetic concentrations of inhaled anesthetics or sedatives.

STOP BANG Questionnaire
Height _______ inches/cm Weight _______ lb/kg Age _______ Male/Female BMI _______ Collar size of shirt: S, M, L, XL, or _______ inches/cm Neck circumference* _______ cm
1. *Snoring* Do you *snore* loudly (louder than talking or loud enough to be heard through closed doors)? Yes No
2. *Tired* Do you often feel *tired*, fatigued, or sleepy during daytime? Yes No
3. *Observed* Has anyone *observed* you stop breathing during your sleep? Yes No
4. Blood *pressure* Do you have or are you being treated for high blood *pressure*? Yes No
5. *BMI* *BMI* more than 35 kg/m2? Yes No
6. *Age* *Age* over 50 years old? Yes No
7. *Neck* circumference *Neck* circumference greater than 40 cm? Yes No
8. *Gender* *Gender* male? Yes No

* Neck circumference is measured by staff

High risk of OSA: answering yes to 3 or more items

Low risk of OSA: answering yes to less than 3 items Note that age is less important as OSA may occur in children.

Fig. 24.2 One of the simplest and easiest means to assess OSA and the one with most relevance to the anesthesiologist in a preanesthetic assessment clinic is application of the STOP-Bang questionnaire. The score is based on responding *yes* to three or more questions, which indicates a high probability of OSA: Snore, Tired, Observed (apnea), Pressure, Body mass index (BMI) (>35), Age (>50), Neck circumference > 40 cm or 17 in, and Gender male. This score is referenced but not illustrated in the guidelines. Age is probably a less important factor as many children are diagnosed with OSA (Adapted from [12])

OSA patients may be exquisitely sensitive to all preoperative central depressants. Respiratory arrest, coma, and death can occur. Avoidance of preoperative sedation with long-acting benzodiazepines and opioids may be wise. Premedication against aspiration may include histamine-2 receptor antagonists (such as famotidine) and pro-motility agents (such as metoclopramide). In addition, the anesthesiologist should ensure that the patient is monitored in a higher acuity setting postoperatively and should question whether same-day discharge is warranted.

24.2.7 Respiratory Evaluation

Postoperative pulmonary complications (PPCs) impact recovery after surgery. It is therefore important to identify risk factors and establish whether preoperative respiratory therapy combined with adjustments to intraoperative ventilatory management, such as addition of alveolar recruitment techniques, can decrease the risk of PPCs. Risk factors include smoking, surgical site (thorax or abdomen), previous lung disease, obesity, older age, malnutrition, and long anesthesia. Pulmonary function tests are of very limited value and should be used as management tools only. A simple test such as measurement of oxygen saturation on room air, giving a value > 90, may be all that is required. Chest auscultation is indicated in all patients. Should rhonchi be heard, in most instances, they can be cleared by coughing.

24.2.8 Neurologic Evaluation

A cursory review of the neurologic system usually suffices, checking for equal and bilateral motor strength and intact sensory perception. Any abnormalities should be referred for more advanced neurologic consultation. Any family history of neuromuscular disease or delayed awakening from anesthesia should be documented. Patients should be asked to extend their necks and paresthesias or limb weakness noted. Although multiple sclerosis is probably not worsened by anesthetic agents, symptoms that might relate to this disease should be documented. The ability of the patient to understand the procedure and the alternative anesthetic techniques should be assessed to obtain appropriate consent.

24.2.9 PostOperative Nausea and Vomiting Screening and Prevention

Postoperative nausea and vomiting (PONV) continues to have a negative impact on patient experience as well as potentially delaying discharge from the PACU [14, 15]. It can also delay postoperative oral intake as well as discourage early ambulation [16]. Although PONV has yet to be eliminated as a complication, risk stratification and mitigation strategies can eliminate much of the risk. An integral part of the preoperative evaluation must therefore include a thorough history of prior PONV as well as identification of risk factors for PONV (see Table 24.5).

Although universal PONV prophylaxis is recommended with two agents of different classes, those at high risk may benefit from three or four agents [14]. The Apfel risk score [17] is often used, with a score of 0, 1, 2, 3, and 4 which corresponds to PONV risks of 10, 20, 40, 60, and 80%. This scoring system uses only female gender, non-smoking, history of PONV or motion sickness, and postoperative opioids as risk factors. Utilization of this scoring system and application of appropriate therapy has been shown to reduce PONV rates and inform or guide management [18]. A thorough guide to PONV prevention and planning can be found in the fourth consensus guidelines for the management of postoperative nausea and vomiting [14].

24.2.10 Penicillin Allergy

A thorough history of prior adverse and allergic reactions to medications should be included in the perioperative evaluation. Each reaction should be evaluated individually and may impact perioperative care. A common allergic reaction reported by patients that may directly impact perioperative management is the penicillin (PCN) allergy. Prior literature reported cross-reactivity rates from PCN to cephalosporins

Table 24.5 Several risk factors have been associated with PONV

Impact	Risk factor
Increases risk	Female sex, history of PONV or motion sickness, non-smoking status, young age, use of general anesthesia, use of volatile anesthesia, use of nitrous oxide over 1-h duration, postoperative opioids, duration of anesthesia, surgical type (cholecystectomy, laparoscopic, gynecologic)
Conflicting evidence	ASA status, menstrual cycle, Anesthesiologist experience, perioperative fasting
Disproven or little evidence	BMI, anxiety, use of nasogastric tube, migraine history, supplemental oxygen

to be around 10%, which caused many anesthesiologists to utilize alternative regimens such as gentamycin and clindamycin for antibiotic prophylaxis for surgery instead of first-generation cephalosporins such as cefazolin [19]. It should be noted, however, that less than 10% of patients who report a PCN allergy have documented skin testing to verify despite recommendations from their doctors to be tested [20]. Furthermore, the cross-reactivity rate of 10% is not supported by the literature and is likely secondary to cross-contamination of early formulations of cephalosporins with PCN [21]. Finally, the allergic epitope that can cause cross-reactivity is related biochemically to the R1 sidechain of the amino acid which is different for several cephalosporins [22]. Cefazolin shares no similarity on the R1 chain to PCN and as such the risk of any cross-reactivity between cefazolin and PCN is minimal [22]. Given data that alternative regimens do not provide coverage that is effective and has more unfavorable side effect profiles, the benefits of using cefazolin in PCN allergic patients outweigh the risks. In fact, one retrospective cohort study demonstrated a 50% increased odds of surgical site infection in those who received alternative regimens due to PCN allergy [23].

24.2.11 Frailty

The purpose of the preoperative evaluation is to provide the anesthesiologist with information to risk stratify and mitigate risk in the perioperative period such as early ambulation, choice of regional or nerve block techniques if possible, enhanced and early nutrition and prompt removal or avoidance of catheters and intravenous lines among other measures. Recent literature has demonstrated that frailty is an important risk factor for postoperative complications and mortality [24]. These risks have been demonstrated in several surgical specialties as well as for both complex and simple surgery [25, 26]. In fact, a recent study of over 2 million surgeries from the National Surgical Quality Improvement Program (NSQIP) database demonstrated increase in both 30 and 180-day mortality rates across all surgeries and specialties in patients with identified frailty [27]. It should be noted that frailty is often assessed independently of patient age. Several frailty scales have been developed, one of the most popular being the Risk Analysis Index (RAI) which can be calculated prospectively from a questionnaire (RAI-C) or retrospectively from variables present in many healthcare databases (RAI-A) [28]. Shorter versions of these tools have been developed. A recent systematic review and meta-analysis of frailty scores found 35 different instruments. Of those only five were meta-analyzed. The Clinical Frailty Scale was most strongly associated with mortality and unfavorable discharge (odds ratio, 4.89; 95% CI, 1.83 to 13.05 and odds ratio, 6.31; 95% CI, 4.00 to 9.94, respectively). Perioperative complications were associated with the Edmonton Frail Scale (odds ratio, 2.93; 95% CI, 1.52 to 5.65). Delirium was mostly associated with the Frailty Phenotype (odds ratio, 3.79; 95% CI, 1.75 to 8.22). Of the tools that were measured, the Clinical Frailty Scale had the highest reported measures of feasibility [28–30] (See Table 24.6).

Table 24.6 Identification of frailty may help decrease risk of complications in the postoperative period

Frailty score	Description
1 Very fit	People who are robust, active, energetic, and motivated. These people commonly exercise regularly. They are among the fittest for their age
2 Well	People who have no active disease symptoms but are less fit than category 1. Often, they exercise or are very active occasionally, e.g., seasonally
3 Managing well	People whose medical problems are well controlled, but are not regularly active beyond routine walking
4 Vulnerable	While not dependent on others for daily help, often symptoms limit activities. A common complaint is being "slowed up", and/or being tired during the day
5 Mildly frail	These people often have more evident slowing and need help in high-order IADLs (finances, transportation, heavy housework, medications). Typically, mild frailty progressively impairs shopping and walking outside alone, meal preparation, and housework
6 Moderately frail	People need help with all outside activities and with keeping house. Inside, they often have problems with stairs and need help with bathing, and might need minimal assistance (cuing, standby) with dressing
7 Severely frail	Completely dependent on personal care, from whatever cause (physical or cognitive). Even so, they seem stable and not at high risk of dying (within ~ 6 months)
8 Very severely frail	Completely dependent, approaching the end of life. Typically, they could not recover even from a minor illness
9 Terminally Ill	Approaching the end of life. This category applies to people with a life expectancy < 6 months who are not otherwise evidently frail

24.2.12 Pain Management Strategy

Less than half of patients who undergo surgery report adequate pain management [31, 32]. The most recent guidelines put forth by the American Pain Society recommend that each patient receive a patient-centered tailored education about their treatment options for postoperative pain [31]. Although the quality of evidence is low, preoperative educational interventions may reduce postoperative opioid requirements, allay preoperative anxiety, and reduce length of stay [33, 34]. A complete preoperative assessment must therefore include a pain history including utilizing of chronic pain or anti-inflammatory medications as well as history of any substance use/abuse. Additionally, an assessment of the potential for multimodal analgesia should be completed, noting which modalities are likely to be efficacious or contraindicated. This information should be discussed with the patient in the preoperative period [31]. Whenever possible, shared decision-making with patient about their pain management plan should be undertaken. The plan should also be shared with the surgical team to avoid potential double dosing postoperatively. A table of potential interventions is seen below. Each of these may be discussed during the preoperative evaluation (Table 24.7).

24.2.13 Cognitive Dysfunction

As the need, importance and usefulness of laboratory testing has receded, emphasis has focused on the anesthesiologist as the perioperative physician, extending our care and involvement to the postoperative period. To this end, studies have centered on what might be done preoperatively to decrease the chance of postoperative complications [35, 36]. Recently, much work has been involved as to why some patients develop postoperative delirium or cognitive dysfunction and what, if anything, anesthetic care might be modified to decrease the incidence of these troubling complications. Assessment of multiple developments in the postoperative arena has also been studied in an attempt to uncover preoperative situations that can be modified to decrease the incidence of untoward events occurring. The role that frailty might play in postoperative complications and how it can be assessed has also come under scrutiny in recent years.

About 12–20% of apparently previously cognitively well patients undergoing anesthesia and non-cardiac surgery develop symptoms of cognitive dysfunction postoperatively that are usually self-limiting but may persist in the longer term. In addition, long-term sequelae of COVID-19 have been shown to include cognitive impairment that may be severe and long-lasting. Postoperative cognitive dysfunction (POCD) appear to affect, elderly patients specifically. Severe cases delay patient discharge and affect the patient's quality of life after surgery. Studies on POCD are ongoing, but the underlying pathogenesis is still unclear due to conflicting results and lack of evidence although the type of anesthesia employed (general, neuraxial, and regional) has not shown any specific linkage. The occurrence and development of POCD appears to be related to multiple factors. Among them, the pathogenesis of neuroinflammation in POCD has become a focus of research in recent years. Clinical and preclinical studies have confirmed the correlation between neuroinflammation and POCD. Central nervous system inflammation occurs and, may lead to POCD with changes in peripheral circulation and the pathological pathways between peripheral circulation and the central nervous system [37]. While there is not as yet a clear means to prevent POCD, assessment can be made as to the likelihood of

Table 24.7 Some schemes are presented for postoperative pain management

Intervention	Utilization
Oral opioids	Use as a component of multimodal analgesia
Patient controlled IV analgesia with opioids	Utilized only when parental route is needed
Acetaminophen	Use as a component of multimodal analgesia
Non-steroidal anti-inflammatory agents	Use as a component of multimodal analgesia
Gabapentin and pregabalin	Use as a component of multimodal analgesia in major surgery
Ketamine, melatonin	Use as a component of multimodal analgesia in major surgery
Lidocaine, magnesium	Use as a component of multimodal analgesia in major surgery
Peripheral, regional, neuraxial analgesia	Use as a component of multimodal analgesia in major surgery with evidence of benefit
Transcutaneous electrical nerve stimulation	Consider as an adjunct only
Cognitive modalities such as guided imagery or hypnosis, virtual reality, music	Consider as an adjunct only

patients developing the disorder [38]. The ASA has recommended that a min cog test, a 3 min evaluation, be applied to all patients over the age of 65 (Table 24.8). Scores below 4 indicate a higher risk suggesting that use of lighter planes of anesthesia, as indicated by entropy numbers and use of dexmedetomidine may be preferable choices.

Mini-Cog©

Instructions for Administration & Scoring

ID: __________ Date: ______________

Step 1: Three Word Registration

Look directly at person and say, "Please listen carefully. I am going to say three words that I want you to repeat back to me now and try to remember. The words are [select a list of words from the versions below]. Please say them for me now." If the person is unable to repeat the words after three attempts, move on to Step 2 (clock drawing).

The following and other word lists have been used in one or more clinical studies.[1-3] For repeated administrations, use of an alternative word list is recommended.

Version 1	Version 2	Version 3	Version 4	Version 5	Version 6
Banana	Leader	Village	River	Captain	Daughter
Sunrise	Season	Kitchen	Nation	Garden	Heaven
Chair	Table	Baby	Finger	Picture	Mountain

Step 2: Clock Drawing

Say: "Next, I want you to draw a clock for me. First, put in all of the numbers where they go." When that is completed, say: "Now, set the hands to 10 past 11."

Use preprinted circle (see next page) for this exercise. Repeat instructions as needed as this is not a memory test. Move to Step 3 if the clock is not complete within three minutes.

Step 3: Three Word Recall

Ask the person to recall the three words you stated in Step 1. Say: "What were the three words I asked you to remember?" Record the word list version number and the person's answers below.

Word List Version: ________ Person's Answers: ________________ ________________ ________________

Scoring

Word Recall: ______ (0-3 points)	1 point for each word spontaneously recalled without cueing.
Clock Draw: ______ (0 or 2 points)	Normal clock = 2 points. A normal clock has all numbers placed in the correct sequence and approximately correct position (e.g., 12, 3, 6 and 9 are in anchor positions) with no missing or duplicate numbers. Hands are pointing to the 11 and 2 (11:10). Hand length is not scored. Inability or refusal to draw a clock (abnormal) = 0 points.
Total Score: ______ (0-5 points)	Total score = Word Recall score + Clock Draw score. A cut point of <3 on the Mini-Cog™ has been validated for dementia screening, but many individuals with clinically meaningful cognitive impairment will score higher. When greater sensitivity is desired, a cut point of <4 is recommended as it may indicate a need for further evaluation of cognitive status.

Table 24.8 Mini-Cog Test: this test can be applied in 3 min and indicates those likely to experience postoperative cognitive dysfunction

1. Three-word registration	Patient asked to repeat and remember three words. If unable to repeat, go to 2
2. Clock drawing	Patient asked to draw a clock, insert the numbers, and indicate a time suggested by the healthcare professional
3. Word recall	Repeat the words given originally
Score	Words: 0–3 for each word repeated and recalled Clock drawing 0–2
Total	0–5

24.2.14 Miscellaneous

Several groups deserve special attention. Patients who are hard of hearing or have visual problems, as well as those for whom English may not be the primary language, should be identified and notation made on the chart and ongoing communication to subsequent caregivers. Pediatric patients also have different requirements. Whether the parents should accompany the child to the operating room should be determined on a case-to-case basis. Video games are generally more effective in calming small patients. Certainly, parents should have a clear understanding of the anesthetic process, including postoperative pain management that their child will undergo, and have ample time for questions. There are many rare diseases and situations that require consideration such as progeria, malignant hyperthermia, Tay Sachs, xeroderma pigmentosa, hemophilia, and porphyria, to name a very few. The transgender patient may have undergone laryngeal surgery or osteotomies. The complexities of these conditions are beyond the scope of this chapter beyond to say that members of the LGBTQ society deserve special understanding and consideration of their needs.

24.3 Conclusion

Tests and evaluations should have potential benefits that are greater than potential adverse effects. Benefits would include change in time or content of anesthetic care or perioperative resource use that would improve safety. Adverse effects include interventions that cause injury, discomfort, delay, cost, and inconvenience, all of which are not commensurate with benefit.

Preoperative laboratory evaluations and EKG testing should be driven by history, physical findings, and surgical risk. Tests are indicated only if the results can correctly identify abnormalities, and change the diagnosis, management plan, or outcome. Needless tests are expensive. Improved standardization is required, and it is important to remember that one size does not fit all.

24.4 Questions and Answers

Questions (Choose the Most Appropriate Answer)

1. Which finding best provides an easy and reliable means to diagnose obstructive sleep apnea syndrome (OSAS)?
   A. An apnea-hypopnea index of 4
   B. Morbid obesity
   C. A STOP-BANG score of 5
   D. A history of loud snoring
2. Routine preoperative testing:
   A. Remains a major expense within the health system in the United States
   B. Is on the increase
   C. Has been shown to be very useful for developing countries
   D. Must be studied further before conclusions can be drawn as to its usefulness
3. Which of the following statements best describes routine preoperative testing practices?
   A. It is standardized in all hospitals in the United States
   B. About 0.2% reveal abnormalities
   C. It is a useful screening measure
   D. Problems are immediately recognized and acted upon
4. Choosing Wisely:
   A. Was initiated by the American Board of Internal Medicine
   B. Nine specialty boards and Consumer Reports quickly joined
   C. Later 70 other specialties including Anesthesiology contributed by 2013
   D. All of the above
5. Ordering tests preoperatively only as indicated will:
   A. Decrease the number of tests performed only by 10%
   B. Improve hospital efficiency and cost savings
   C. Have major impact on patient care
   D. Certainly, be rejected by patients

6. Abnormality of the EKG tracing:
   A. Is found in up to 30% of patients
   B. Always signifies postoperative complications
   C. Changes management in almost half of patients
   D. Is frequently insignificant
7. Stress testing:
   A. Reliably indicates cardiac disease
   B. Is a good predictor of postoperative complications
   C. Should be used as a general screening test
   D. Is not recommended as a risk assessor in older patients based on age.
8. Regarding management of the diabetic patient:
   A. Blood sugar is best controlled at < 120 mg/dl
   B. Controversy remains as to whether all medications should be discontinued
   C. Normoglycemia may be an individual number
   D. An infusion of regular insulin should be started when blood sugar levels exceed 130 mg/dl
9. Use of nCPAP preoperatively can:
   A. Abolish fluctuations in blood pressure in OSA patients
   B. Require at least 24 h to be effective
   C. Not help in improving airway patency
   D. Increase reflex responses to hypoxia
10. Indicators of a potentially difficult airway are least likely to include:
    A. Pierre Robin syndrome
    B. Neck circumference of 18 cm
    C. Comack-Lehane grade 2
    D. Thyromental distance of 4 cm

Answers

1. **C**. A STOP-BANG score of 5 provides an easy and reliable means to diagnose obstructive sleep apnea (OSA). The score is based on responding *yes* to 3 or more questions, which indicates a high probability of OSA: snore, tired, observed (apnea), pressure, BMI (>35), age (>50), neck circumference > 40 cm or 17 inches, and male gender. Age is probably a less important factor as many children are diagnosed with OSA.
2. **A**. Routine preoperative testing remains a major expense within the U.S. health system. Traditionally routine tests have been considered important elements of preanesthetic evaluation to determine fitness for surgery. Over the past three decades, this practice has been scrutinized due to a low yield and high cost. One study author calculated that $40 billion a year was spent in the United States on preoperative testing and evaluation.
3. **B**. About 0.2% of routine preoperative testing reveals abnormalities. In fact, routine tests such as complete blood count, chest X-ray, electrocardiogram, urinalysis, and electrolyte panel are of little value in detecting disease or changing management. Rather, multiple investigations detect minor irrelevant abnormalities, increase patient risk, cause delay, and increases liability.
4. **D**. *Choosing Wisely* was initiated in 2012 by the American Board of Internal Medicine to establish a national program to avoid unnecessary tests, treatments, and procedures through education of practitioners and patients. The initial 9 specialty boards and Consumer Reports were soon joined by some 70 other specialties including anesthesiology in 2013. They were all charged with releasing 5 recommendations to facilitate decisions regarding appropriate care.
5. **B**. Ordering tests preoperatively only as indicated will improve hospital efficiency and cost savings. Preoperative laboratory evaluations and EKG testing should be driven by history, physical findings, and surgical risk. Tests are indicated only if the results can correctly identify abnormalities, and change the diagnosis, management plan, or outcome. Needless tests are expensive and improved standardization is required.
6. **A**. While nonspecific abnormalities are found on EKG tracings in about 30% of patients, the finding rarely predicts postoperative complications and is usually insignificant.
7. **D**. Stress testing is not recommended as a risk assessor in older patients based on age. Stress testing, acknowledged by the American College of Cardiology and the American Heart Association to have restricted benefit in most patients, amounts to around $2300. A common test sequence that includes complete blood count, basic metabolic panel, chest X-ray, and EKG bills for about $1600, which does not include the cost of interpretation. In some instances, the Center for Medicare/Medicaid Services (CMS) and insurers will not reimburse for repeat testing and for tests based on age alone, placing the burden of payment on the patient.
8. **C**. Regarding management of the diabetic patient, normoglycemia may be an individual number. Recommendations to discontinue oral diabetic medication remain controversial. While elevated blood sugar levels have been shown to retard wound healing, an ideal blood sugar level has not been determined. While many laboratory scales consider hyperglycemia to be values above 120 mg/dl, it is probably more important to consider the individual and the level at which he most usually functions. Thus, values of 150–170 mg/dl may be considered normal for many. Should testing indicate values exceeding 180 mg/dl, oral medications should be discontinued, and an infusion of regular insulin

commenced perioperatively? Further evaluation by an endocrinologist is indicated with repeated blood glucose checks.

9. **A**. Use of chronic nasal continuous positive airway pressure (nCPAP) preoperatively has been found to abolish mean, systolic, and diastolic blood pressure fluctuations in OSA patients. Also, the use of nCPAP for several weeks preoperatively has been found to be highly effective at preserving airway patency during sleep and anesthesia as well as diminishing reflex responses to hypoxia and hypercapnia. This effect may result from upper airway stabilization, a residual effect of nCPAP that begins to occur within as little as 4 h of continuous use of nCPAP.
10. **C**. Indicators of a potentially difficult airway are least likely to include Comack-Lehane grade 2. Using Comack-Lehane, 4 grades of view are defined during direct laryngoscopy. The entire view of the laryngeal aperture is listed as grade 1. Visualization of only the posterior commissure of the laryngeal aperture is graded as 2. If only the epiglottis is seen that is grade 3. Grade 4 view is just the soft palate.

References

1. Frost EA. Preoperative assessment: integrating information from divergent sources. Mt Sinai J. 2012;79(1):3–12.
2. Rao VM, Levin D. The overuse of diagnostic imaging and the choosing wisely initiative. Ann Intern Med. 2012;157(8):574–6.
3. Cassel CK, Guest JA. Choosing wisely—helping physicians and patients make smart decisions about their care. JAMA. 2012;307(17):1801–2.
4. Chung F, Yuan H, Yin L, Vairavanathan S, Wong DT. Elimination of preoperative testing in ambulatory surgery. Anesth Analg. 2009;108(2):467–75.
5. Katz RI, Dexter F, Rosenfeld K, Wolfe L, Redmond V, Agarwal D, et al. Survey study of anesthesiologists' and surgeons' ordering of unnecessary preoperative laboratory tests. Anesth Analg. 2011;112(1):207–12.
6. Committee on Standards and Practice Parameters, Apfelbaum JL, Connis RT, Nickinovich DG, American Society of Anesthesiologists Task Force on Preanesthesia Evaluation, Pasternak LR, Arens JF, et al. Practice advisory for preanesthesia evaluation: an updated report by the American Society of Anesthesiologists Task Force on Preanesthesia evaluation. Anesthesiol. 2012;116(3):522–38.
7. Fleisher LA, Fleischmann KE, Auerbach AD, Barnason SA, Beckman JA, Bozkurt B, American College of Cardiology, American Heart Association, et al. ACC/AHA Guideline on perioperative cardiovascular evaluation and management of patients undergoing noncardiac surgery: a report of the American College of Cardiology/American Heart Association Task Force on practice guidelines. J Am Coll Cardiol. 2014;64(22):e77–137.
8. Wijeysundera DN, Duncan D, Nkonde-Price C, Virani SS, Washam JB, Fleischmann KE, et al. Perioperative beta blockade in noncardiac surgery: a systematic review for the 2014 ACC/AHA guideline on perioperative cardiovascular evaluation and management of patients undergoing noncardiac surgery: a report of the American College of Cardiology/American Heart Association Task Force on practice guidelines. J Am Coll Cardiol. 2014;64(22):2406–25.
9. Ridker PM, Wilson PWF. A trial-based approach to statin guidelines. JAMA. 2013;310(11):1123–4.
10. Stone NJ, Robinson JG, Lichtenstein AH, Bairey Merz CN, Blum CB, Eckel RH, American College of Cardiology/American Heart Association Task Force on Practice Guidelines, et al. ACC/AHA guideline on the treatment of blood cholesterol to reduce atherosclerotic cardiovascular risk in adults: a report of the American College of Cardiology/American Heart Association Task Force on Practice Guidelines. J Am Coll Cardiol. 2014;63(25 Pt B):2889–934.
11. Gross JB, Bachenberg KL, Benumof JL, Caplan RA, Connis RT, Coté CJ, American Society of Anesthesiologists Task Force on Perioperative Management, et al. Practice guidelines for the perioperative management of patients with obstructive sleep apnea: a report by the American Society of Anesthesiologists Task Force on perioperative management of patients with obstructive sleep apnea. Anesthesiol. 2006;104(5):1081–93.
12. Meta-analysis. PLoS One. 2015;10(12):e0143697.
13. ASA Practice Guidelines for the Perioperative Management of Patients with Obstructive Sleep Apnea: An Updated Report by the American Society of Anesthesiologists Task Force on Perioperative Management of Patients with Obstructive Sleep Apnea Anesthesiology;2014: 120(2): 268–86.
14. Gan TJ, Belani KG, Bergese S, Chung F, Diemunsch P, Habib AS, et al. Fourth consensus guidelines for the management of postoperative nausea and vomiting. Anesth Analg. 2020;131:411–48.
15. Mc Loughlin S, Terrasa SA, Ljungqvist O, Sanchez G, Garcia Fornari G, Alvarez AO. Nausea and vomiting in a colorectal ERAS program: Impact on nutritional recovery and the length of hospital stay. Clin Nutr ESPEN. 2019;34:73–80.
16. Joshi GP, Kehlet H. Enhanced recovery pathways. Anesth Analg. 2019;128:5–7.
17. Apfel CC, Läärä E, Koivuranta M, Greim C-A, Roewer N. A simplified risk score for predicting postoperative nausea and vomiting. Anesthesiology. 1999;91:693–693.
18. Pierre S, Corno G, Benais H, Apfel CC. A risk score-dependent antiemetic approach effectively reduces postoperative nausea and vomiting—a continuous quality improvement initiative. Can J Anesth Can d'anesthésie. 2004;51:320–5.
19. Pichichero ME, Zagursky R. Penicillin and cephalosporin allergy. Ann Allergy, Asthma Immunol. 2014;112:404–12.
20. Jain V, Joshi N, Sidhu M, Kalicinsky C, Pun T. Penicillin allergies: referral and management practices of anesthesiologists. Allergy, Asthma Clin Immunol. 2014;10:A20.
21. Annè S, Reisman RE. Risk of administering cephalosporin antibiotics to patients with histories of penicillin allergy. Ann Allergy Asthma Immunol. 1995;74:167–70.
22. Vorobeichik L, Weber EA, Tarshis J. Misconceptions surrounding penicillin allergy. Anesth Analg. 2018;127:642–9.
23. Blumenthal KG, Ryan EE, Li Y, Lee H, Kuhlen JL, Shenoy ES. The impact of a reported penicillin allergy on surgical site infection risk. Clin Infect Dis. 2018;66:329–36.
24. George EL, Chen R, Trickey AW, Brooke BS, Kraiss L, Mell MW, et al. Variation in center-level frailty burden and the impact of frailty on long-term survival in patients undergoing elective repair for abdominal aortic aneurysms. J Vasc Surg. 2020;71:46-55.e4.
25. McIsaac DI, Bryson GL, van Walraven C. Association of frailty and 1-year postoperative mortality following major elective noncardiac surgery. JAMA Surg. 2016;151:538.
26. Shinall MC, Arya S, Youk A, Varley P, Shah R, Massarweh NN, et al. Association of preoperative patient frailty and operative

stress with postoperative mortality. JAMA Surg. 2020;155: e194620.
27. George EL, Hall DE, Youk A, Chen R, Kashikar A, Trickey AW, et al. Association between patient frailty and postoperative mortality across multiple noncardiac surgical specialties. JAMA Surg 2020:e205152.
28. Hall DE, Arya S, Schmid KK, Blaser C, Carlson MA, Bailey TL, et al. Development and initial validation of the risk analysis index for measuring frailty in surgical populations. JAMA Surg. 2017;152:175.
29. Aucoin SD, Hao M, Sohi R, Shaw J, Bentov I, Walker D, et al. Accuracy and feasibility of clinically applied frailty instruments before surgery. Anesthesiol. 2020;133:78–95.
30. Rockwood K. A global clinical measure of fitness and frailty in elderly people. Can Med Assoc J. 2005;173:489–95.
31. Chou R, Gordon DB, de Leon-Casasola OA, Rosenberg JM, Bickler S, Brennan T, et al. Management of postoperative pain: a clinical practice guideline from the American Pain Society, the American Society of Regional Anesthesia and pain medicine, and the American Society of Anesthesiologists' Committee on Regional Anesthesia. Executive Commi J Pain. 2016;17:131–57.
32. Apfelbaum JL, Chen C, Mehta SS, Gan and TJ. Postoperative pain experience: results from a national survey suggest postoperative pain continues to be undermanaged. Anesth Analg. 2003;97:534–40.
33. Butler GS, Hurley CAM, Buchanan KL, Smith-VanHorne J. Pre-hospital education: effectiveness with total hip replacement surgery patients. Patient Educ Couns. 1996;29:189–97.
34. Wilson JF. Behavioral preparation for surgery: benefit or harm? J Behav Med. 1981;4:79–102.
35. Needham MJ, Webb CE, Bryden DC. Postoperative cognitive dysfunction and dementia: what we need to know and do. Br J Anaesth. 2017;1(119):i115–25.
36. Kotekar N, Shenkar A, Nagaraj R. Postoperative cognitive dysfunction-current preventative strategies. Clin Interv Aging. 2018;8:2267–73.
37. Li Z, Zhu Y, Kang Y, Qin S. Neuroinflammation as the underlying mechanism of postoperative cognitive dysfunction and therapeutic strategies. Front Cell Neurosci. 2022;28(16): 843069.
38. Borson S. The mini-cog: a cognitive vital signs measure for dementia screening in multilingual elderly. Int J Geriatr Psychiatry. 2000;15(11):1021.

Premedication

25

Kenneth C. Cummings

Abstract

Many medications are administered prior to surgery to alleviate pain or anxiety and reduce the risk of postoperative complications. This chapter discusses the classes of medications used, their indications and contraindications, and considerations for special clinical circumstances. Perioperative management of chronic drug therapy and strategies for risk reduction are also discussed.

Keywords

Premedication • Anesthesia • Preoperative care • Antibiotic prophylaxis • Respiratory aspiration • Adrenergic beta-antagonists • Aspirin • Antiemetics

Key Points

- Premedication is often used to reduce discomfort, allay anxiety, or in an attempt to reduce perioperative risk.
- A simple score predicts the risk of PONV. Female gender, use of perioperative opioids, non-smoking status, and a history of PONV or motion sickness each yield 20% additive risk.
- Multiple antiemetic options are available. Each treatment reduces the risk of PONV by 20–25%.
- Droperidol in larger doses causes QTc prolongation and is associated with torsades de pointes. The first-generation 5-HT_3 antagonists also cause QTc prolongation but do not carry the same warning label as droperidol.
- The American Society of Anesthesiologists preoperative fasting guidelines do not recommend any routine prophylaxis against pulmonary aspiration of gastric contents. Antacids, acid-suppression agents, and prokinetic drugs are useful in patients considered to be at risk for aspiration.
- Chronic corticosteroid therapy can cause suppression of the hypothalamic-pituitary-adrenal axis. In patients with this condition, surgical stress may produce an adrenal crisis. Supplemental hydrocortisone can prevent this complication.
- Surgical antibiotic prophylaxis is given to reduce the microbial burden of the surgical wound. In most cases, skin flora are the causative organisms in surgical site infections.
- Most medications are continued through the perioperative period. Caution must be exercised, however, due to the potential for serious drug interactions.

Evidence from large randomized trials does not support starting beta blockers, alpha-2 agonists, or aspirin to reduce the risk of perioperative cardiac events. Patients taking beta blockers or alpha-2 agonists, however, should continue them through the perioperative period.

25.1 Introduction

Premedication refers to the administration of drugs to a patient shortly prior to anesthesia and surgery. These drugs are part of the perioperative plan but are not part of the anesthetic regimen per se. Premedication is often used in an effort to decrease anxiety, reduce the probability of postoperative nausea and vomiting, and mitigate the risk of complications such as pulmonary aspiration, adrenal insufficiency, and myocardial ischemia. Surgical antibiotic prophylaxis may also be considered premedication.

K. C. Cummings (✉)
Integrated Hospital Care Institute, Cleveland Clinic Foundation, Cleveland, OH, USA
e-mail: cummink2@ccf.org

M. Argalious et al. (eds.), *Basic Sciences in Anesthesia*,
https://doi.org/10.1007/978-3-031-60203-0_25

25.2 Analgesics

Opioid analgesics are not typically administered prior to anesthetic induction unless the patient is experiencing pain or is on a chronic opioid regimen. Respiratory depression from opioid use is the primary risk in this setting and many preoperative units do not have close patient monitoring. Consequently, opioids should be used cautiously, especially in patients with obstructive sleep apnea. Patients with increased intracranial pressure may also not tolerate the respiratory depressant effect of opioids due to increased cerebral blood flow from the resulting hypercarbia.

Non-opioid analgesics such as acetaminophen, non-steroidal anti-inflammatory drugs (NSAIDs), and cyclooxygenase-2 (COX-2)-specific inhibitors are often used preoperatively for their analgesic and opioid-sparing effects. The preoperative use of NSAIDs is limited by concerns about surgical bleeding due to inhibition of platelet thromboxane A_2 synthesis, although COX-2 inhibitors do not share this property [1].

Originally developed as anticonvulsants, the gabapentinoid drugs (gabapentin and pregabalin) are often used in enhanced recovery pathways. These drugs have been viewed as a safe method to improve analgesia and reduce perioperative opioid requirements. As more research has been conducted, however, it has become apparent that the risk-benefit ratio of using these agents is not as favorable as initially thought and some argue that their use should be abandoned [2, 3].

25.3 Anxiolytics

Preoperative anxiety is common and can be severe. Non-pharmacologic methods of anxiolysis (e.g., preoperative visit with an anesthesiologist) can be very helpful, but judicious use of anxiolytic drugs can improve patient satisfaction, decrease the physiologic consequences of excess anxiety, and improve patient compliance with necessary preoperative procedures.

25.3.1 Benzodiazepines

Benzodiazepines are effective anxiolytic and sedative drugs, as evidenced by their widespread use in the general population. Benzodiazepines facilitate activation of the $GABA_A$ receptor, inhibiting neuronal depolarization by increasing chloride conductance. Preoperatively, these drugs are useful because of minimal respiratory depression and hemodynamic effects when used alone. Caution is still warranted, however, in patients with obstructive sleep apnea as they have increased sensitivity to benzodiazepines. A specific benzodiazepine antagonist (flumazenil) provides a means to rapidly rescue patients from oversedation, although not without the risk of provoking withdrawal and/or seizures in patients physically dependent on benzodiazepines or ethanol.

With a clinical effective duration of less than 2 h and an elimination half-life of 2–7 h, midazolam is the benzodiazepine of choice for perioperative use. In adults, intravenous midazolam 1–2 mg typically provides anxiolysis and a variable degree of anterograde amnesia. Intravenous lorazepam is another reasonable choice. Alternatively, oral midazolam liquid (0.5–0.75 mg/kg) is useful for pediatric patients and does not appear to prolong emergence in moderate-length procedures [4].

25.3.2 Melatonin

Although study quality varies, orally administered melatonin has been shown in meta-analysis to produce sedation and anxiolysis roughly equivalent to benzodiazepines [5].

25.3.3 Clonidine and Dexmedetomidine

These centrally-acting alpha-2 adrenergic agonists also have sedative and anxiolytic properties that can be useful in the perioperative period. Their use as premedication may be limited by hemodynamic effects (hypotension, bradycardia) and prolonged duration of action.

25.3.4 Ketamine

Ketamine is an anesthetic drug that is thought to act primarily via inhibition of NMDA-type glutamate receptors in the CNS, although it interacts with multiple other receptor pathways. It has profound analgesic and amnestic properties when used at anesthetic doses but is often associated with negative psychological effects (dysphoria and hallucinations). These effects may be reduced by the concurrent administration of benzodiazepines.

Ketamine may be used for premedication in pediatric patients when a deeper level of sedation and analgesia is needed, such as in children with developmental delay or when uncomfortable procedures must be performed [6]. Ketamine produces significant salivation and is often given in combination with an anticholinergic agent such as glycopyrrolate or atropine.

25.4 Antiemetics/Postoperative Nausea and Vomiting

Postoperative nausea and vomiting (PONV) is a significant challenge in perioperative care. Using a simple risk stratification tool [7], it is possible to easily predict the likelihood of PONV given four risk factors:

1. Female sex
2. Non-smoker
3. History of PONV or motion sickness
4. Planned postoperative use of opioids

When 0 factors are present, the risk of PONV is 10%. One, two, three, and four risk factors yield PONV risks of approximately 20%, 40%, 60%, and 80%, respectively. Conversely, it has been demonstrated that each prophylactic intervention reduces the risk by approximately 20–25% [8].

25.4.1 Classes of Antiemetic Drugs

See Table 25.1.

Anticholinergic Drugs

Scopolamine is a muscarinic anticholinergic drug that readily crosses the blood-brain barrier and is an effective antiemetic [9]. In the CNS, it suppresses the emetic response to vestibular stimulation, one of the mechanisms of PONV. Typically, it is administered transcutaneously via a patch applied several hours prior to surgery. The patch formulation reaches peak effectiveness in 4 h and delivers approximately 1 mg of scopolamine over 72 h.

Dose-limiting side effects include dry mouth, mydriasis (leading to blurred vision), decreased gastrointestinal motility, urinary retention, and sedation/amnesia. Blockade of muscarinic receptors in the stomach delays gastric emptying and may increase gastric volume. Scopolamine should be used cautiously in patients with open-angle glaucoma due to the possibility of creating acute angle-closure glaucoma, an ophthalmologic emergency. Caution should also be used in elderly patients, as they are at increased risk for delirium from centrally-acting anticholinergic drugs.

Histamine H_1 Antagonists

Diphenhydramine and promethazine both have antihistamine effects and are thought to act via blockade of H_1 histamine receptors in the chemoreceptor trigger zone (CTZ). They both also exert anticholinergic effects similar to scopolamine, producing sedative and antiemetic effects. Diphenhydramine has also been shown to decrease the nausea associated with opioid administration.

Dopaminergic D_2 Antagonists

Several classes of drugs exert common antagonist effects at D_2 receptors in the CTZ. These include the phenothiazines (promethazine and prochlorperazine), the butryophenones (haloperidol and droperidol), and the benzamides (metoclopramide and amisulpride). These agents reduce both the

Table 25.1 Summary of antiemetic drugs used for PONV

Class	Examples	Dosing	Prophylaxis/treatment
Anticholinergics	Scopolamine	3 mg patch q 72 h (3–4 h prior to induction)	Prophylaxis
Antihistamines	Diphenhydramine	25–50 mg IV q 6 h (at emergence)	Both
Dopamine Antagonists	Prochlorperazine	5–10 mg IV/IM q 6 h (at emergence)	Both
	Promethazine	12–25 mg IM q 4 h (at emergence)	Both
	Droperidol	0.625–2.5 mg IV/IM q 6 h (at induction)	Both
	Amisulpride	5 mg IV (at induction) 10 mg IV (rescue)	Both
	Metoclopramide	10–20 mg (at emergence) 10 mg q 6 h (rescue)	Both
5-HT_3 antagonists	Ondansetron	4 mg IV q 6 h (at emergence)	Both
	Palonosetron	0.075 mg IV (at induction)	Prophylaxis
Corticosteroids	Dexamethasone	4–8 mg IV (at induction)	Prophylaxis
NK_1 antagonists	Aprepitant	40 mg PO 3 h prior to induction 100 mg IV (at induction)	Prophylaxis

sensation of nausea and actual vomiting. Metoclopramide's effect may largely lie outside the CNS, however, as it exerts a prokinetic cholinergic effect on the gastrointestinal tract.

Caution should be used when selecting these drugs. Generally, they should not be used in patients with Parkinson's disease, restless legs syndrome, or other movement disorders as they can interfere with drug therapy and prompt exacerbations of these conditions. Extrapyramidal effects (such as dystonia and akathisia) can limit these drugs' usefulness and may be very troublesome to patients. Other effects include sedation and orthostatic hypotension. Prolonged use of high-dose metoclopramide has been associated with tardive dyskinesia, although the true risk may be much lower than previously thought [10]. Its short-term perioperative use does not appear to carry this risk.

Much attention has been devoted to the effect of droperidol (and, to a lesser extent, haloperidol) on the QT interval. Droperidol (along with many other drugs) inhibits the delayed inward rectifier (I_{Kr}) potassium current in cardiac myocytes, thus prolonging the QT interval and rendering the myocardium more vulnerable to arrhythmias. Due to reports of torsades de pointes (TdP) in patients receiving larger doses of droperidol (such as for neuroleptanalgesia), the U.S. Food and Drug Administration (FDA) requires a "black box" warning on droperidol, including the requirement for cardiac monitoring for 4 h after drug administration. There has been much debate about the validity of this warning in light of the low doses of droperidol used for PONV prophylaxis (commonly less than 1.25 mg), its proven efficacy, and clinical evidence that supports droperidol's safety in low doses [11].

Used as an antipsychotic drug in Europe for many years, the D_2/D_3 receptor antagonist amisulpride has emerged as a useful agent for PONV prophylaxis. Given intravenously at low doses (5 mg), amisulpride has efficacy comparable to other antiemetics and does not appear to have significant effects on the QTc interval. It also carries a low risk of extrapyramidal effects [12]. In 2020, it received FDA approval for PONV prophylaxis as well as rescue therapy.

Corticosteroids

Although their exact mechanism of action is unclear, corticosteroids (usually dexamethasone) are commonly used for PONV prophylaxis. Dexamethasone (typically 4–8 mg IV) has been demonstrated to reduce the risk of PONV as well as decrease postoperative pain. It is presumed that it exerts anti-inflammatory effects in the CNS and peripherally to reduce inflammatory cytokine production.

A single perioperative dose of dexamethasone is generally well tolerated. Reported adverse effects include hyperglycemia, mood effects, headache, and edema. Hyperglycemia is unlikely in patients with normal glucose metabolism, however [13]. Overall, the risk-benefit balance supports the perioperative use of dexamethasone, as it does not appear to increase the risk of surgical site infection [14].

5-HT_3-Receptor Antagonists

The most commonly used drugs in this category include dolasetron, granisetron, and ondansetron. They bind to and inhibit activation of serotonergic receptors in the gastrointestinal tract, the solitary tract nucleus, and the CTZ. They are significantly more effective in preventing vomiting than nausea. No differences in efficacy or toxicity among the three drugs have been demonstrated at clinically-used doses. Contrary to many other prophylactic drugs, these agents are usually administered at the end of surgery. The second-generation 5-HT_3 antagonist palonosetron, however, is administered at the start of surgery due to its much longer half-life (40 h). Palonosetron may be more effective in preventing PONV than the first-generation drugs [15].

The 5-HT_3 antagonists are generally well tolerated. The most common side effect is mild headache (15–20%) followed by dizziness (10%). QTc prolongation also occurs with the first-generation drugs but not palonosetron. There have been case reports of TdP in patients receiving first-generation 5-HT_3 antagonists [16]. These drugs do not carry the black box warning that droperidol has, but the U.S. Food and Drug Administration does recommend cardiac monitoring for patients with electrolyte abnormalities or patients who are receiving other QTc-prolonging medications. These medications should also be used very cautiously (if at all) in patients taking class III antiarrhythmics such as dofetilide due to the risk of TdP.

NK_1 Antagonists

Substance P is a neuropeptide with a wide distribution in the CNS. It is found in particularly high concentrations in neurons innervating the solitary tract nucleus and CTZ. Acting through neurokinin type 1 (NK_1) receptors, it affects many functions including regulation of nausea and vomiting. The NK_1 receptor antagonist aprepitant was originally demonstrated to reduce delayed chemotherapy-induced nausea and vomiting. It has also been demonstrated to be an effective and long-lasting prophylactic antiemetic and is also available in a parenteral formulation. There is a related parenteral prodrug available (fosaprepitant) but its use for PONV prophylaxis is off-label. Common side effects of aprepitant include fatigue, abdominal pain, and diarrhea.

Caution is warranted with aprepitant because it is a moderate inhibitor of CYP3A4. Dexamethasone is a substrate of this enzyme and many clinical trials used reduced doses of dexamethasone in combination with aprepitant. Other substrates of CYP3A4 include macrolide antibiotics, many chemotherapeutic agents, opioids (including fentanyl), benzodiazepines (including midazolam), calcium channel blockers, statins, warfarin, and oral contraceptives. This long list of drug interactions and its high cost have dampened enthusiasm for aprepitant's widespread perioperative use.

Midazolam

In addition to its effects on anxiety, prophylactic midazolam (50 mcg/kg IV with induction of anesthesia) has also been shown to reduce the incidence of PONV compared to placebo [17].

25.4.2 Consensus Guidelines

The Society for Ambulatory Anesthesia has published guidelines outlining a strategy for managing PONV [18]. Patients should be assessed for the presence of risk factors for PONV. Patients with 1–2 risk factors should receive 2 prophylactic agents. Patients with additional risk factors should receive 3–4 agents. In all cases, risk mitigation should be considered, including strategies such as regional anesthesia and avoidance of inhalational anesthetics.

25.5 Aspiration Prophylaxis/Fasting Status

Perioperative pulmonary aspiration of gastric contents can lead to severe morbidity or mortality. The overall rate of clinically-evident aspiration is approximately 1:4000 for elective surgery and 1:900 for emergency surgery [19].

The main non-pharmacologic approach to reduce the risk of aspiration is preoperative fasting. The American Society of Anesthesiologists (ASA) publishes guidelines for the appropriate duration of fasting for otherwise healthy patients [20]. In general, clear liquids (without particulate matter or fat) may be consumed up until 2 h prior to surgery. The type of liquid is more important than the volume of liquid consumed. A "light meal" of non-fatty foods may be consumed 6 h preoperatively while heavier foods should be avoided for 8 h or longer. Infants may consume human milk up until 4 h preoperatively. Non-human milk, however, empties from the stomach at a similar rate to solid food.

The ASA guidelines do not recommend routine pharmacologic aspiration prophylaxis for healthy patients. For patients considered to be at increased risk for aspiration (anatomic abnormalities, gastroparesis, esophageal motility disorders, long-standing diabetes mellitus, and others), prophylaxis may be considered. Pharmacologic approaches to aspiration prophylaxis include prokinetic agents, antacids, and acid-suppression agents. Anticholinergic drugs are also discussed here.

25.5.1 Prokinetic Agents

Metoclopramide is a benzamide derivative with antiemetic and prokinetic properties. It acts on dopamine D_2 receptors in the CTZ to reduce nausea and vomiting. Additionally, it acts as an antagonist at the 5-HT_4 and muscarinic cholinergic receptors in the gastrointestinal tract. This activity increases the strength of peristaltic contractions in the small intestine and stomach while also increasing lower esophageal sphincter tone. The combined effect of these actions is to reduce gastric volume by propelling stomach contents forward through the small bowel.

Metoclopramide is not recommended for routine aspiration prophylaxis but may be useful in patients at increased risk for aspiration. Again, caution is advised in patients with Parkinson's disease or movement disorders. Also, the prokinetic effect of metoclopramide may be detrimental in cases of bowel obstruction.

25.5.2 Antacids

Although not strongly supported by clinical evidence, it is commonly believed that the acidic pH of aspirated stomach contents is associated with the development of aspiration pneumonitis. Thus, raising the pH of the gastric contents may be helpful in patients at risk for aspiration. Antacid medications are salts of alkaline ions (commonly citrate, bicarbonate, or hydroxide) combined with counterions to maintain neutrality. The ASA guidelines do not recommend the routine use of antacids for aspiration prophylaxis. In high-risk patients, however, preoperative oral administration of non-particulate antacids such as sodium citrate with citric acid may be a useful tool. Compared to other antacids (such as calcium carbonate), non-particulate antacids will raise the gastric pH without the risk of particulate matter aspiration.

25.5.3 Acid-Suppression Agents: H_2 Antagonists and Proton Pump Inhibitors

The histamine H_2 receptor is found on gastric parietal (acid-secreting) cells. Along with gastrin and muscarinic acetylcholine receptors, activation of the H_2 receptor stimulates acid secretion. The commonly used H_2 antagonists such as famotidine are very safe drugs with adverse reaction rates similar to placebo. Dose reduction in renal failure is indicated due to renal elimination (both filtration and tubular secretion) of these drugs. The H_2 antagonists have been shown to reduce gastric volume and acidity but no evidence exists to demonstrate a reduction in pulmonary aspiration risk. The ASA guidelines do not recommend routine use of these drugs but they may be useful in patients at increased risk.

Proton pump inhibitors (PPIs) such as omeprazole, lansoprazole, and pantoprazole inhibit the H^+-K^+-ATPase on the luminal surface of gastric parietal cells, thus directly decreasing acid secretion. To exert its effect, the drug is secreted into the gastric lumen, is activated by the acidic environment, and then forms a disulfide bond with a cysteine residue on the parietal cell H^+-K^+-ATPase. These drugs are more effective acid-suppression agents than the H_2 antagonists but no evidence exists to demonstrate efficacy in reducing pulmonary aspiration. The ASA guidelines do not recommend their routine use but, again, they may be useful in patients at increased risk of aspiration.

25.5.4 Anticholinergic Drugs

Gastric parietal cells have muscarinic acetylcholine receptors that, when activated, stimulate acid secretion. In principle, blocking these receptors should decrease acid secretion. Clinical trials, however, do not demonstrate a reduction in gastric volume or acidity when atropine or glycopyrrolate are administered. This fact, combined with the multiple undesirable effects of anticholinergic drugs, leads to the recommendation from the ASA that anticholinergic drugs have no role (routine or otherwise) in reducing the risk of pulmonary aspiration.

25.6 Corticosteroid Supplementation

Many patients take corticosteroid drugs for their anti-inflammatory effects. Long-term use of these medications is associated with suppression of the hypothalamic-pituitary-adrenal (HPA) axis (with resulting adrenal atrophy), leading to an inability of the body to produce sufficient cortisol to maintain homeostasis. This is of particular concern in the perioperative period due to the "stress response" to surgery, in which cortisol, catecholamines, and other mediators are produced to deal with the physiologic insult. Inadequate adrenal response to stress can lead to an acute adrenal crisis, manifesting as refractory hypotension, hyponatremia, and hyperkalemia.

Controversy exists as to the threshold doses of exogenous corticosteroids that would predictably cause HPA axis suppression and when perioperative supplementation is necessary. In general, patients taking 20 mg or more per day of prednisone for more than three weeks (or the equivalent dose of another corticosteroid) should be presumed to have HPA axis suppression. Conversely, patients receiving up to 5 mg prednisone daily (or equivalent) for any length of time are unlikely to have significant HPA suppression. Formal testing (e.g. ACTH stimulation test) can determine the patient's HPA axis status, but this is often not available preoperatively. For patients whose HPA axis status is unclear undergoing a stressful procedure, perioperative supplementation is reasonable in light of the low risk associated with a short course of a supplemental corticosteroid.

A typical regimen for corticosteroid supplementation in major surgery (laparotomy, thoracotomy) is 100 mg hydrocortisone intravenously followed by 50 mg intravenously every 8 h. This dosing is in addition to the patient's usual steroid regimen. The hydrocortisone is tapered postoperatively to return to the baseline corticosteroid dosing over 2–3 days. Less stressful procedures may require lower doses (e.g. 50 mg hydrocortisone followed by 25 mg every 8 h). Minimal-stress procedures (e.g. diagnostic endoscopy, surgery under local anesthesia) often do not require steroid supplementation.

25.7 Prophylactic Antibiotics

Surgical site infections (SSIs) are defined as infections occurring near a surgical site within 30 days of surgery or 90 days if material was implanted. SSIs occur in between 2 and 5% of surgical procedures, with the highest rates occurring in wounds classified as "dirty." The most commonly isolated pathogens are skin flora (*Staphylococcus* and *Streptococcus* species). Over time, the prevalence of methicillin-resistant *Staphylococcus aureus* (MRSA) isolates has increased, prompting efforts to identify MRSA carriers and eliminate their colonization prior to the day of surgery via nasal mupirocin ointment.

Along with maintenance of perioperative normothermia, proper hair removal, and appropriate skin antisepsis, timely perioperative antibiotic prophylaxis is a cornerstone of SSI prevention. Prophylaxis is indicated for procedures where the risk of infection is high (classified as "clean-contaminated," "contaminated," or "dirty") or in sites where an infection would be dangerous. The rationale for antibiotic prophylaxis is to decrease the bacterial burden introduced into the surgical wound, thus allowing host defenses a better opportunity to prevent overt infection. For most antibiotics, intravenous administration between 30 and 60 min before skin incision allows for therapeutic blood and tissue concentrations at the time of incision. For drugs with a longer infusion time (vancomycin and fluoroquinolones), 90–120 min is acceptable. Rapid infusion of vancomycin is not recommended, as it can provoke significant histamine release.

The specific choice of antibiotic varies by anatomic site and local antimicrobial resistance patterns. In general, first-generation cephalosporins (e.g. cefazolin) are recommended as they are active against the majority of skin flora. For surgeries involving the gastrointestinal tract, second- or third-generation cephalosporins are often chosen for their increased activity against Gram-negative bacteria and are often combined with metronidazole for activity against anaerobic pathogens.

For patients with true allergic reactions to penicillins, recommended alternative antibiotics include clindamycin, fluoroquinolones, and/or vancomycin. However, it is important to note that most patients with a documented penicillin allergy are not truly allergic: approximately 90% of these patients will have negative skin testing [21]. Even patients with true penicillin allergies can often receive cefazolin if indicated, as immune reactions are usually directed at the side chain ("R group") portions of the molecules, not the beta-lactam ring, and cefazolin has R group moieties that differ greatly from the penicillin drugs (as well as most other cephalosporins) [22].

Repeated antibiotic dosing is advised when the surgery is longer than more than two half-lives of the chosen drug or for procedures in which there is a large blood loss. Continued postoperative dosing beyond 24 h, however, is not recommended because of a lack of improved outcomes and the potential risk of fostering antibiotic resistance.

25.8 Perioperative Management of Chronic Drug Therapy

Withholding chronic medications during the perioperative period is a controversial topic. The goal of perioperative medication management should be to minimize the likelihood of any perioperative drug-drug interactions while at the same time minimizing disruption to the patient's chronic medical therapy. In general, medications with significant discontinuation effects or medications that are thought to be protective should be continued through the perioperative period. Specific drug classes will be discussed below.

25.8.1 Angiotensin Converting Enzyme Inhibitors (ACEI) and Angiotensin II Receptor Blockers (ARB)

Many clinicians prefer to withhold these medications on the day of surgery out of concern for refractory hypotension. In principle, blockade of the renin-angiotensin axis eliminates a powerful method for maintaining blood pressure in the setting of treatment with hypotensive agents (such as most anesthetic drugs). The bulk of available evidence suggests that continuation of these agents on the day of surgery increases the likelihood of intraoperative hypotensive episodes, which are associated with myocardial injury and acute kidney injury [23, 24].

25.8.2 Beta Adrenergic Antagonists

Beta adrenergic antagonists ("beta blockers") competitively bind to the different subtypes of beta adrenergic receptor, leading to effects such as decreases in heart rate and blood pressure. Patients chronically receiving beta blockers are at high risk for rebound tachycardia and hypertension if these drugs are stopped abruptly. In patients taking these drugs for the treatment of angina, sudden discontinuation can precipitate myocardial ischemia. In general, patients taking beta blockers should continue them throughout the perioperative period. Initiating beta blocker therapy in an attempt to reduce cardiac risk, however, is controversial (see below).

In patients presenting for urgent or emergent surgery with uncontrolled hyperthyroidism, the preoperative administration of beta blockers can be very useful to decrease the incidence of tachyarrhythmias, especially atrial fibrillation. Combined with an antithyroid drug such as propylthiouracil, beta blockers may reduce the risk of perioperative thyroid storm.

25.8.3 Alpha-2 Adrenergic Agonists

Alpha-2 adrenergic agonists act centrally to decrease sympathetic outflow from the CNS. Like beta blockers, abrupt withdrawal of clonidine can precipitate rebound hypertension and tachycardia. Thus, these agents should be continued through the perioperative period (see below).

25.8.4 Aspirin

Aspirin (acetylsalicylic acid) irreversibly inhibits both forms of cyclooxygenase, leading to inhibition of prostaglandin synthesis. This is of perioperative concern mainly due to inhibition of thromboxane A_2 production by platelets, thus decreasing platelet aggregation and potentially worsening perioperative blood loss. This risk is balanced by the beneficial effects of aspirin on cardiovascular morbidity in patients with coronary artery or cerebrovascular disease. In particular, aspirin is a key part of the antiplatelet regimens used after placement of intracoronary stents to prevent in-stent thrombosis. If (or when) it is permissible to withhold these agents after stent placement is an area of much debate and patients with recent cardiac interventions should definitely be evaluated by a cardiologist prior to surgery.

Because of convincing evidence (see below), it is reasonable to withhold aspirin in stable patients who do not require antiplatelet therapy for prevention of stent thrombosis.

25.8.5 Lipid-Lowering Medications

HMG-CoA reductase inhibitors ("statins") inhibit the rate-limiting step in the biosynthesis of cholesterol. Apart from their effects on lipid metabolism, these drugs have been found to have anti-inflammatory and plaque stabilizing effects. Initial concerns about an increased risk of perioperative rhabdomyolysis have not been borne out and these drugs should be continued through the perioperative period.

25.8.6 Psychoactive Medications

In general, most antidepressants, antipsychotics, anxiolytics, and mood-stabilizing drugs should be continued during the perioperative period. Discontinuation of these medications can lead to withdrawal symptoms or exacerbation of the underlying disorder. Although discontinuation was previously recommended, current practice is to continue these medications and use an appropriate anesthetic technique.

Selective Serotonin Reuptake Inhibitors (SSRIs) have been associated with increased surgical blood loss, likely due to their effects on platelet function [25]. Whether this is of clinical significance is unclear and the benefits of continuing the medication are usually thought to outweigh the risks of bleeding. Particular care, however, is indicated in patients receiving monoamine oxidase inhibitors (MAOIs). The 2 forms of monoamine oxidase are responsible for degrading catecholamines and inhibition of MAO leads to accumulation of biogenic amines in the CNS. These drugs are effective antidepressants but are used as third-line agents due to the unique risks involved in their use. The MAO-A isoform in the gut metabolizes ingested sympathomimetics such as tyramine (found in aged cheese, smoked meat, soy products, and draft beer). Use of these drugs thus requires a tyramine-free diet to prevent hypertensive crises.

Previously, patients taking MAOIs were instructed to hold the medication for 10–14 days prior to surgery. Because these are typically drugs of last resort in severe disease, withholding them may lead to an exacerbation of the underlying psychiatric condition, particularly depression, with the attendant risk of suicidal ideation [26]. Consequently, current practice is to continue these medications perioperatively. Patients on MAOIs are at increased risk of hemodynamic instability and drug interactions. In particular, meperidine must be avoided due to the risk of serotonin syndrome. If a vasoactive agent must be used, direct-acting drugs such as phenylephrine or epinephrine should be chosen instead of ephedrine.

25.8.7 Maintenance Therapy for Substance Abuse or Chronic Pain

Patients receiving therapy for opioid abuse or chronic pain present a particular challenge. Patients receiving methadone maintenance often have significant opioid tolerance and may require large doses of additional opioids. The basal methadone dose should be continued, either orally or intravenously (at one half the oral dose). Methadone prolongs the QTc interval and vigilance is required due to the number of drugs used perioperatively that also affect the QTc interval.

Patients receiving buprenorphine present a particular challenge. Buprenorphine is a semi-synthetic opioid that is a partial mu-opioid agonist and kappa- and delta-opioid antagonist. This drug will reduce the effectiveness of other opioids and has an inherent "ceiling effect" beyond which it will not provide additional analgesia. For patients undergoing minor surgery, the buprenorphine should be continued. For procedures associated with moderate to severe pain, the buprenorphine should ideally be tapered preoperatively and replaced with a pure mu-opioid agonist such as oxycodone. Alternatively, a non-opioid multimodal analgesic strategy may be chosen with options including NSAIDs, acetaminophen, regional anesthetic techniques, and adjuvant analgesics such as ketamine.

25.9 Cardiac Risk Reduction

25.9.1 Beta Adrenergic Antagonists

Despite early enthusiasm for perioperative beta blocker therapy as a means to reduce cardiac morbidity and mortality, it now appears that initiation of therapy in the perioperative period may not be beneficial and may in fact be harmful. The POISE trial [27] saw a reduction in cardiac events at the cost of an increase in ischemic strokes. Whether this is due to the regimen used (large doses of metoprolol started immediately before surgery) or is a true class effect is unclear. In general, therefore, patients on beta blockers should continue them through the perioperative period, but initiation of beta blocker therapy should be done carefully and several days prior to surgery if possible.

25.9.2 Alpha-2 Adrenergic Agonists

Because of their sympatholytic effects, it is believed that alpha-2 adrenergic agonists may provide perioperative protection against myocardial ischemia. To evaluate whether adding clonidine perioperatively reduces cardiac complications, a large trial (POISE-2) randomized patients at increased cardiac risk to perioperative clonidine versus placebo [28]. No reduction in cardiac morbidity was found. On the contrary, the clonidine group had more hypotensive episodes and cardiac arrests. Thus, analogous to beta blockers, patients receiving alpha-2 agonists should remain on them perioperatively but they should not be initiated without good reason.

25.9.3 Aspirin

Because of retrospective evidence associating aspirin use with improved cardiovascular outcomes after surgery, the POISE-2 trial included an arm testing whether adding (or continuing) aspirin perioperatively reduces cardiac morbidity in patients at risk for coronary artery disease [29]. Surprisingly, there was no improvement in the composite outcome of death or non-fatal myocardial infarction. There was, however, a higher incidence of major bleeding in the aspirin group. These results support withholding aspirin perioperatively in patients not taking aspirin as part of antiplatelet therapy for stents.

Questions

1. Which of the following is not a risk factor for postoperative nausea and vomiting (PONV)?
   A. Female gender
   B. History of PONV
   C. Smoking status
   D. Body Mass Index (BMI)
   Answer: D
   The Apfel risk score consists of 4 factors: Female gender, history of PONV or motion sickness, use of perioperative opioids, and non-smoking status. Baseline risk is 10%, whereas one, two, three, and four risk factors convey a PONV risk of 20%, 40%, 60%, and 80%, respectively.
2. Which of the following statements is FALSE regarding droperidol?
   A. It is a butyrophenone drug.
   B. Doses used for PONV prophylaxis are strongly associated with arrhythmias.
   C. It is an antagonist at dopamine D_2 receptors.
   D. It should be used very cautiously in patients with Parkinson's disease.
   Answer: B
   Droperidol is a butyrophenone derivative that acts as an antagonist at D_2 receptors in the central nervous system, particularly in the chemoreceptor trigger zone. Because dopamine D_2 receptors are involved in movement disorders, administration of this drug to patients with Parkinson's disease can worsen the patients' symptoms. Droperidol carries a "black box" warning about the risk of prolonged QTc interval and torsades de pointes, but there is reasonable evidence that the low doses used for PONV prophylaxis are safe.
3. Which of the following is TRUE regarding scopolamine?
   A. It must be administered intravenously.
   B. It has minimal effects in the central nervous system.
   C. It can precipitate acute angle-closure glaucoma.
   D. It is safe to use in elderly patients with a history of delirium.
   Answer: C
   Scopolamine is an anticholinergic drug that readily penetrates the blood-brain barrier. It is often administered as a transdermal patch for PONV prophylaxis. Like other anticholinergic drugs, scopolamine can cause CNS symptoms such as confusion and delirium. It should be used cautiously in elderly patients as they are particularly prone to postoperative delirium. Also, scopolamine should be avoided in patients with open-angle glaucoma because it can precipitate acute angle-closure glaucoma.
4. Which of the following drugs DOES NOT prolong the QTc interval?
   A. Ondansetron
   B. Dolasetron
   C. Droperidol
   D. Palonosetron
   Answer: D
   Palonosetron is a second-generation 5-HT_3 antagonist. It has a much longer duration of action than the first-generation drugs (ondansetron, dolasetron) and may be more effective at preventing nausea. Unlike the first-generation 5-HT_3 antagonists and droperidol, palonosetron has not been shown to prolong the QTc interval.
5. Which of the following statements about preoperative fasting is TRUE?
   A. The American Society of Anesthesiologists (ASA) recommends patients abstain from food or drink for at least 8 h prior to surgery.
   B. The ASA does not recommend routine prophylactic medications to reduce the risk of aspiration of gastric contents.

C. Cow's milk and human milk are treated the same in regards to duration of fasting.
D. Orange juice with pulp is considered a clear liquid.

Answer: B

For patients not at increased risk for aspiration, the ASA recommends allowing clear liquids up to 2 h prior to surgery. Clear liquids include water, juice *without* pulp, black coffee, plain tea, soft drinks, and so on. Cow's milk is treated as a light meal (6 h), whereas human milk is allowed up to 4 h prior to surgery. The ASA does not recommend routine premedication to reduce the risk of aspiration.

6. For patients considered to be at risk for aspiration of gastric contents, which medication is NOT useful to decrease the risk?
   A. Glycopyrrolate
   B. Sodium citrate/citric acid
   C. Famotidine
   D. Metoclopramide

Answer: A

Aspiration prophylaxis can consist of antacids, acid suppressive agents, and prokinetic drugs. The sodium citrate/citric acid combination is a commonly used non-particulate antacid that quickly raises gastric pH when administered orally. Histamine H_2 antagonists like famotidine reduce acid secretion indirectly by blocking the stimulatory effect of histamine on gastric parietal cells. Metoclopramide has a prokinetic effect on the gastrointestinal tract and may be useful to decrease the volume of gastric content. Anticholinergic drugs like glycopyrrolate have no role in aspiration prophylaxis.

7. Which of the following statements about surgical antibiotic prophylaxis is FALSE?
   A. Extending prophylactic antibiotic therapy beyond 24 h is not recommended.
   B. Skin flora are the most commonly-isolated organisms from surgical site infections.
   C. First-generation cephalosporins are recommended for all procedures.
   D. For most antibiotics, the optimal time of administration is 30–60 min before skin incision.

Answer: C

Most surgical site infections (SSIs) occur from skin flora being introduced into the surgical wound. The rationale for antibiotic prophylaxis is to have effective tissue concentrations of antibiotic present at the time of incision to decrease the microbial burden in the wound. First-generation cephalosporins are active against most skin pathogens and are recommended for most procedures. For procedures involving the bowel, however, increased activity against Gram-negative and anaerobic organisms is needed. For these procedures, a second- or third-generation cephalosporin is often chosen, typically in combination with metronidazole. Most antibiotics should be administered 30–60 min before incision. Vancomycin and fluoroquinolones, however, may be administered 90–120 min before incision due to longer administration times.

8. For which patient(s) would perioperative corticosteroid supplementation not be absolutely necessary?
   A. A patient taking prednisone 20 mg per day for 1 year for rheumatoid arthritis
   B. A patient taking methylprednisolone 2.5 mg per day for 1 month for Crohn's disease
   C. A patient using inhaled fluticasone metered dose inhaler for years for asthma
   D. B and C

Answer: D

It can be challenging to determine which patients are at risk for perioperative adrenal insufficiency. Patients taking 20 mg or more per day of prednisone (or equivalent) for more than three weeks should be presumed to have HPA axis suppression. Patients taking less than 5 mg per day of prednisone (in this case, 4 mg methylprednisolone) or using inhaled corticosteroids are much less likely to have adrenal suppression. The risks of perioperative stress dose hydrocortisone are low; thus, many clinicians err on the side of caution if uncertain.

9. Which medications should be continued perioperatively?
   A. Beta blockers
   B. Alpha-2 adrenergic agonists
   C. Monoamine oxidase inhibitors
   D. All of the above

Answer: D

Beta adrenergic antagonists and alpha-2 agonists should be continued perioperatively due to the risks of tachycardia and hypertension with abrupt cessation. Although it was previously recommended to stop therapy preoperatively, monoamine oxidase inhibitors should be continued perioperatively. These drugs pose particular challenges to maintaining hemodynamic stability. Additionally, drug-drug interactions should be kept in mind, particularly the risk of serotonin syndrome with the concurrent administration of meperidine.

10. Which statement is FALSE regarding perioperative cardiac risk reduction?
    A. Initiating clonidine preoperatively is an effective means to protect against myocardial ischemia.
    B. In randomized clinical trials, aspirin has not been shown to decrease the risk of perioperative cardiac ischemia.
    C. Initiation of perioperative metoprolol has been shown to reduce cardiac ischemic events but may increase the risk of stroke.
    D. Patients on beta blockers should continue them perioperatively.

Answer: A

The POISE-2 trial found no benefit for adding or continuing aspirin in the perioperative period for patients at risk for coronary disease. There was also no benefit demonstrated for clonidine; rather, there were more episodes of hypotension and cardiac arrest in the clonidine group. The POISE trial evaluated the effect of 100 mg of extended-release metoprolol started on the day of surgery. There were fewer cardiac events but more strokes in the metoprolol group. At present, therefore, patients on alpha-2 agonists and beta blockers should continue them but initiating therapy perioperatively is controversial. Withholding aspirin does not appear to increase cardiac risk in this population.

References

1. Huang Y-M, Wang C-M, Wang C-T, Lin W-P, Horng L-C, Jiang C-C. Perioperative celecoxib administration for pain management after total knee arthroplasty—a randomized, controlled study. BMC Musculoskelet Disord. 2008;9:77.
2. Verret M, Lauzier F, Zarychanski R, Perron C, Savard X, Pinard A-M, et al. Perioperative use of gabapentinoids for the management of postoperative acute pain: a systematic review and meta-analysis. Anesthesiology. 2020;133(2):265–79.
3. Kharasch ED, Clark JD, Kheterpal S. Perioperative gabapentinoids: deflating the bubble. Anesthesiol. 2020;133(2):251–4.
4. Feld LH, Negus JB, White PF. Oral midazolam preanesthetic medication in pediatric outpatients. Anesthesiol. 1990;73(5):831–4.
5. Melissa VH, Natalie LH, Rosenberg J, Gögenur I, Ann MM. Melatonin for pre- and postoperative anxiety in adults. Cochrane Database System. Rev. [Internet]. 2015;4.
6. Barkan S, Breitbart R, Brenner-Zada G, Feldon M, Assa A, Toledano M, et al. A double-blind, randomised, placebo-controlled trial of oral midazolam plus oral ketamine for sedation of children during laceration repair. Emerg Med J. 2014;31(8):649–53.
7. Apfel CC, Laara E, Koivuranta M, Greim CA, Roewer N. A simplified risk score for predicting postoperative nausea and vomiting: conclusions from cross-validations between two centers. Anesthesiol. 1999;91(3):693–700.
8. Apfel CC, Korttila K, Abdalla M, Kerger H, Turan A, Vedder I, et al. A factorial trial of six interventions for the prevention of postoperative nausea and vomiting. N Engl J Med. 2004;350 (24):2441–51.
9. Apfel CC, Zhang K, George E, Shi S, Jalota L, Hornuss C, et al. Transdermal scopolamine for the prevention of postoperative nausea and vomiting: a systematic review and meta-analysis. Clin Ther. 2010;32(12):1987–2002.
10. Al-Saffar A, Lennernäs H, Hellström PM. Gastroparesis, metoclopramide, and tardive dyskinesia: risk revisited. Neurogastroenterol Motil. 2019;31(11): e13617.
11. Tracz K, Owczuk R. Small doses of droperidol do not present relevant torsadogenic actions: a double-blind, ondansetron-controlled study. Br J Clin Pharmacol. 2015;79(4):669–76.
12. Kranke P, Bergese SD, Minkowitz HS, Melson TI, Leiman DG, Candiotti KA, et al. Amisulpride prevents postoperative nausea and vomiting in patients at high risk: a randomized, double-blind. Placebo-controlled Trial Anesthesiology. 2018;128(6): 1099–106.
13. Murphy GS, Szokol JW, Avram MJ, Greenberg SB, Shear T, Vender JS, et al. The effect of single low-dose dexamethasone on blood glucose concentrations in the perioperative period: a randomized, placebo-controlled investigation in gynecologic surgical patients. Anesth Analg. 2014;118(6):1204–12.
14. Kurz A, Fleischmann E, Sessler DI, Buggy DJ, Apfel C, Akca O. Effects of supplemental oxygen and dexamethasone on surgical site infection: a factorial randomized trial. Br J Anaesth. 2015;115 (3):434–43.
15. Park SK, Cho EJ. A randomized, double-blind trial of palonosetron compared with ondansetron in preventing postoperative nausea and vomiting after gynaecological laparoscopic surgery. J Int Med Res. 2011;39(2):399–407.
16. Turner S, Mathews L, Pandharipande P, Thompson R. Dolasetron-induced torsades de pointes. J Clin Anesth. 2007;19 (8):622–5.
17. Fujii Y, Itakura M. A prospective, randomized, double-blind, placebo-controlled study to assess the antiemetic effects of midazolam on postoperative nausea and vomiting in women undergoing laparoscopic gynecologic surgery. Clin Ther. 2010;32 (9):1633–7.
18. Gan TJ, Belani KG, Bergese S, Chung F, Diemunsch P, Habib AS, et al. Fourth consensus guidelines for the management of postoperative nausea and vomiting. Anesth Analg. 2020;131(2): 411–48.
19. Warner MA, Warner ME, Weber JG. Clinical significance of pulmonary aspiration during the perioperative period. Anesthesiol. 1993;78(1):56–62.
20. Practice guidelines for preoperative fasting and the use of pharmacologic agents to reduce the risk of pulmonary aspiration: application to healthy patients undergoing elective procedures: an updated report by the American Society of Anesthesiologists Task Force on preoperative fasting and the use of pharmacologic agents

to reduce the risk of pulmonary aspiration*. Anesthesiol. 2017;126 (3):376–93.
21. del Real GA, Rose ME, Ramirez-Atamoros MT, Hammel J, Gordon SM, Arroliga AC, et al. Penicillin skin testing in patients with a history of beta-lactam allergy. Ann Allergy Asthma Immunol. 2007;98(4):355–9.
22. Savic LC, Khan DA, Kopac P, Clarke RC, Cooke PJ, Dewachter P, et al. Management of a surgical patient with a label of penicillin allergy: narrative review and consensus recommendations. Br J Anaesth. 2019;123(1):e82–94.
23. Maheshwari K, Turan A, Mao G, Yang D, Niazi AK, Agarwal D, et al. The association of hypotension during non-cardiac surgery, before and after skin incision, with postoperative acute kidney injury: a retrospective cohort analysis. Anaesthesia. 2018;73(10): 1223–8.
24. Salmasi V, Maheshwari K, Yang D, Mascha EJ, Singh A, Sessler DI, et al. Relationship between intraoperative hypotension, defined by either reduction from baseline or absolute thresholds, and acute kidney and myocardial injury after noncardiac surgery: a retrospective cohort analysis. Anesthesiol. 2017;126:47–65.
25. Roose SP, Rutherford BR. Selective serotonin reuptake inhibitors and operative bleeding risk: a review of the literature. J Clin Psychopharmacol. 2016;36(6):704–9.
26. Abdi S, Fishman SM, Messner E. Acute exacerbation of depression after discontinuation of monoamine oxidase inhibitor prior to cardiac surgery. Anesth Analg. 1996;83(3):656–7.
27. Devereaux PJ, Yang H, Yusuf S, Guyatt G, Leslie K, Villar JC, et al. Effects of extended-release metoprolol succinate in patients undergoing non-cardiac surgery (POISE trial): a randomised controlled trial. Lancet. 2008;371(9627):1839–47.
28. Devereaux PJ, Sessler DI, Leslie K, Kurz A, Mrkobrada M, Alonso-Coello P, et al. Clonidine in patients undergoing noncardiac surgery. N Engl J Med. 2014;370(16):1504–13.
29. Devereaux PJ, Mrkobrada M, Sessler DI, Leslie K, Alonso-Coello P, Kurz A, et al. Aspirin in patients undergoing noncardiac surgery. N Engl J Med. 2014;370(16):1494–503.

Monitored Anesthesia Care

26

Ihab Adly Riad and Basem Abdelmalak

Abstract

The term "monitored anesthesia care" (MAC) does not describe a distinct type of anesthesia or a certain level of sedation. Rather, it describes a specific service where an anesthesia care provider has been requested to participate in the care of a patient undergoing a diagnostic or a therapeutic procedure. In MAC, the anesthesia care provider provides a number of services specific to patient care. These services include, but are not limited to, pre-procedure evaluation, intra-procedure care, as well as post-procedure management.

Keywords

Operating room • Anesthesia • Monitored anesthesia care • MAC • Gastroenterology • Electrophysiology • Interventional pulmonology • MRI • Radiology • Non-cardiac surgery

Key Points

1. Monitored anesthesia care (MAC) does not describe depth of sedation but rather an anesthesia service with a wide spectrum of levels of sedation.
2. Most anesthetics are used for sedation and pain control during MAC each with distinct advantages and disadvantages.
3. Same standards of preoperative evaluation, and NPO guidelines, should be followed in MAC cases as in general or regional anesthesia ones.
4. Oxygenation, ventilation, circulation, and depth of sedation should be continuously monitored in all cases. Same monitoring standards applied to MAC cases as in general and regional anesthesia.
5. As per the American Society of Anesthesiologists (ASA) practice guidelines, same standards of postoperative care should be provided to MAC cases as in general and regional anesthesia cases.
6. MAC is not generally safer than general or regional anesthesia.
7. ASA established several statements, guidelines, and positions on granting privileges for the administration of moderate and deep sedation by non-anesthesiologists.

26.1 Introduction

The term "monitored anesthesia care" (MAC) does not describe a distinct type of anesthesia or a certain level of sedation. Rather, it describes a specific service where an anesthesia care provider has been requested to participate in the care of a patient undergoing a diagnostic or a therapeutic procedure [1].

Historically, the American Society of Anesthesiologists (ASA) House of Delegates approved MAC as a new term in 1986 to replace the term "standby anesthesia" in an effort to demonstrate that the anesthesiologist was actively involved in the patient care, thus eliminating the confusion about the "standby" issue with third-party payers.

I. A. Riad
Cleveland Clinic Lerner College of Medicine,
Cleveland, OH, USA
e-mail: riadi@ccf.org

I. A. Riad
Regional Anesthesia, Cleveland Clinic, Cleveland, OH, USA

I. A. Riad
Department of Regional Anesthesiology, Lutheran Hospital,
Cleveland, OH, USA

B. Abdelmalak (✉)
Anesthesia for Bronchoscopic Surgery, Center for Sedation,
Department of Multispecialty Anesthesiology, Cleveland Clinic,
Cleveland, OH, USA
e-mail: abdelmb@ccf.org

M. Argalious et al. (eds.), *Basic Sciences in Anesthesia*,
https://doi.org/10.1007/978-3-031-60203-0_26

In MAC, the anesthesia provider offers a number of services specific to patient care. These services include, but are not limited to, pre-procedure evaluation, intra-procedure care, as well as post-procedure management [2].

During MAC, the anesthesiologist provides or medically directs specific medical services to the patient including:

- Support of vital functions.
- Administration of sedatives, analgesics, and even anesthetics as and if needed.
- Providing physical comfort and psychological support.
- Diagnose and treat clinical problems occurring during the procedure.

In other words, the term MAC does not denote a specific level of sedation, instead it includes different levels of sedation, analgesia, and anxiolysis required for different patients under different circumstances undergoing different procedures.

As per the ASA, the provider of MAC should be qualified and prepared to convert to general anesthesia (GA) if necessary. Thus, MAC should not be offered except by an anesthesia care provider.

If under MAC a patient loses consciousness and the ability to respond purposefully to stimuli, the care is considered general anesthetic, regardless of whether airway instrumentation is required, utilized or not.

26.2 Techniques of Monitored Anesthesia Care

26.2.1 Medications Used During Monitored Anesthesia Care

Almost all anesthetic and analgesic agents have been used during MAC with success. An ideal sedative has yet to be found, but should have certain properties [3]:

- Rapid onset of action and short duration.
- Easy titration to effect.
- Potent amnestic, sedative, and analgesic properties.
- Rapid offset and no residual effects.
- High safety profile with predictable pharmacodynamic and pharmacokinetic properties.
- Painless intravenous injection.
- Minimal to no effects on hemodynamics or respiration.
- Cheap.

26.2.2 Propofol

Propofol is an intravenous anesthetic agent that is widely used for sedation, both for MAC cases as well as in intensive care units (ICUs). In 1989, propofol was introduced commercially and since that time it has gained popularity due to its fast onset and recovery even after repeated dosing or extended use.

26.2.2.1 American Society of Anesthesiologists Statement on the Use of Propofol

The ASA stated that it is not always possible to predict individual responses to rapid-acting medications, such as propofol, that might cause a patient to unintentionally slip into deeper levels of sedation or even in a state of general anesthesia [4]. Due to these reasons, the ASA stated that when propofol is used the patients should receive care consistent with that required for deep sedation (Please refer to the ► Sect. 26.8 to see qualifications of deep sedation providers.)

The ASA also stated that non-anesthesia personnel who administer propofol should be qualified to rescue patients whose level of sedation becomes deeper than initially intended and who enter, if briefly, a state of general anesthesia. (Please refer to the ► Sect. 26.8 to see definition of rescue from deep sedation and general anesthesia.)

26.2.2.2 Advantages of Propofol in Monitored Anesthesia Care

1. Rapid onset and recovery.
2. Antiemetic action.
3. Easy titration.
4. Short stay in post-anesthesia care unit (PACU) due to the reduced residual sedation after continuous infusion.

Although it is generally expected that the recovery time and the discharge time after propofol sedation will be shorter [5], several studies in the gastroenterology literature dispute this [6].

26.2.2.3 Disadvantages and Side Effects of Propofol

1. Respiratory depression—In the subanesthetic doses needed for sedation, propofol infusion inhibits hypoxic ventilatory drive and depresses the normal response to hypercarbia. At higher doses, propofol can cause apnea and can inhibit airway protective reflexes.
2. Cardiovascular effects—Propofol decreases arterial blood pressure by decreasing systemic vascular resistance as well as decreasing myocardial contractility and preload. These effects are more profound with larger doses, poor cardiac function, extremes of age, and dehydration.
3. Painful injection and rarely thrombophlebitis—The incidence of pain with injection reported with propofol is

about 58%. Several methods are used to prevent or decrease the intensity of the pain, such as mixing propofol with lidocaine before injection or injecting lidocaine intravenously prior to propofol injection as a pretreatment.

4. Propofol infusion syndrome—It is a rare but serious side effect of prolonged (more than 48 h) propofol infusion especially in the pediatric population where acidosis, hepatomegaly, hyperlipidemia, rhabdomyolysis, as well as cardiac arrest were reported. Theories behind the mechanism of this syndrome include mitochondrial toxicity or abnormalities, impaired tissue oxygenation, and carbohydrate deficiency. This syndrome is more of a concern in the intensive care unit settings more than in the procedural sedation setting.

26.2.3 Benzodiazepines

Benzodiazepines are generally widely used in sedation due to their anxiolytic as well as their amnestic effects. In a MAC case, the short-acting member of this family, midazolam, plays a major role. Although, like most other anesthetics, the intravenous (IV) route is the preferred route, benzodiazepines can be administered orally, intramuscularly, or intranasally as well. Midazolam has many advantages, causing less respiratory depression than other sedatives used at the same level of desired sedation, has a reliable amnestic action, and it also increases the safety margins of local anesthetics in regards to central nervous system (CNS) toxicity by raising the seizure threshold. Moreover, a few studies pointed out the effectiveness of midazolam in the prevention of nausea and vomiting.

The onset as well as the duration of action of midazolam is dependent on the patient's age, route of administration, dose given, as well as the concurrent use of other medications. After a single use of IV midazolam, a peak effect is reached in 2–3 min. In MAC cases, it is used in incremental doses of 0.5–1 mg every 2–3 min to reach the desired level of sedation; it can be used also as a continuous IV infusion of 1–2 mcg/kg/min. Oral dose is 5–15 mgs for adults and 0.5–0.75 mg/kg for children. Due to the lack of analgesic effect of benzodiazepines, midazolam is usually used in conjunction with opioids during MAC sedation.

Remimazolam

Remimazolam is a new short-acting benzodiazepines recently approved by the FDA for procedural sedation [7]. Remimazolam is ester based that is metabolized by liver esterases to an inactive metabolite. With its short halflife, remimazolam combines an early restoration of cognitive function with very promising safety profile. A study [8] comparing remimazolam to midazolam showed the former to have faster recovery of neuropsychiatric function, and patients were ready for discharge earlier than the midazolam group.

Another recent study [9] evaluating the safety and efficacy of remimazolam in high risk patients undergoing colonoscopy showed that the drug is a safe sedative in both high and low risk patients, it also shows that remimazolam has the advantage of rapid onset and recovery of sedation.

Remimazolam recommended dose is 2.5–5 mgs IV initially over 30 s then 1.25–2.5 mgs IV boluses that can be repeated at least 2 min apart supplemental doses.

26.2.4 Opioids

Opioid analgesics have always been the mainstay of pain control in the perioperative period. Due to their potent analgesic actions and the unreliable amnestic effects, opioid analgesics have been used in MAC cases in conjunction with other sedatives such as propofol or benzodiazepines. Opioids have a central analgesic action both at the brain and at the spinal cord levels; they also have peripheral analgesic action at the tissue level. Several opioid receptors have been identified and their activation causes different effects (◉ Table 26.1) [10–12].

Table 26.1 Opioid receptors

Opioid receptors		
Receptor	Site of analgesic action	Action
Mu1	Supraspinal	Analgesia, euphoria, confusion, and nausea
Mu2	Spinal analgesia and supraspinal (brain stem) actions	Respiratory depression, cardiovascular (bradycardia) and gastrointestinal effects (slow motility), miosis, and urinary retention
Delta	Supraspinal and spinal	Analgesia, cardiovascular depression, and decreased brain and myocardial oxygen demand
Kappa	Supraspinal and spinal	Analgesia, dysphoria, and psychomimetic effects

Adapted from [10–12]

Respiratory depression, nausea, vomiting, pruritis, as well as chest rigidity are among the reported complications of opioid use even in a non-dose related fashion.

Several opioid analgesics are frequently used in MAC sedation cases, including morphine, fentanyl, meperidine, and hydromorphone, as well as the rapid onset opioids such as remifentanil, alfentanil, and sufentanil.

The onset as well as the duration of action is among the important factors that dictate which opioid to use in MAC sedation cases. Morphine has a slow onset and prolonged effect making it a poor choice for a MAC sedation case due to the difficulty in titration of its dose to the desired effect. Its long duration of action might make morphine a reasonable choice when significant pain is expected postoperatively.

Fentanyl has a relatively rapid onset and short duration of action, making it a good choice for analgesia in MAC sedation cases. It is commonly used in repeated intravenous boluses or as a continuous IV infusion. The bolus doses are usually 0.5–1 mcg/kg, and the intravenous infusion is usually 0.7–10 mcg/kg/h (usually the dose is in the range of 2–3 mcg/kg/h). Fentanyl is potent and has a relatively predictable effect, making it a drug of choice in procedural sedation by endoscopists, radiologists, and also by anesthesiologists.

Hydromorphone can be used as an IV bolus in increments of 0.2–0.4 mg combined with other sedatives. It is also reported to be used for mechanically ventilated pediatric patients for ICU sedation and pain control as a continuous IV infusion. The usual starting dose for IV infusion is 1 mcg/kg/h and can be titrated up to a maximum dose of 8 mcg/kg/h.

Meperidine used to be one of the most widely used analgesics in moderate procedural sedation for endoscopy—commonly used as an IV bolus of 25–100 mg. Meperidine causes tachycardia due to its atropine-like action that can confuse the picture of inadequate sedation and/or analgesia. In small doses, meperidine has a desirable anti-shivering action. Gastroenterologists were familiar with the use of meperidine but with the current practice, where more anesthesiologists are involved in the sedation of this patient population, the older medications with the slow onset characteristics are becoming rarely used in MAC sedation cases, as they are being replaced by more potent analgesics with a rapid onset and short duration of action. Relatively newer opioids such as remifentanil, alfentanil, and sufentanil are gaining more popularity in MAC sedation cases, as they all share in common a rapid onset and short duration of action, making them suitable for different procedures—especially those with an unpredictable duration—as these medications are used as continuous IV infusion. Remifentanil has been used frequently as a sole sedative as well as in combination with other short-acting sedatives such as propofol. Remifentanil has a unique property among other opioids, which is its metabolism by nonspecific esterases causing a rapid and uniform clearance even with a prolonged administration, especially in the sedation of ICU patients. Remifentanil is commonly used as a continuous infusion in a dose 0.05–0.1 mcg/kg/min with or without an initial bolus of 0.5–1 mcg/kg.

Alfentanil is another synthetic opioid analgesic with a rapid onset and short duration of action. It also can be used as IV boluses of 5–10 mcg/kg or as a continuous infusion of 0.25–1 mcg/kg/min. Alfentanil is usually combined with propofol in MAC sedation cases to provide successful sedation and adequate analgesia.

Both alfentanil and remifentanil have the disadvantage of the rapid offset of analgesic effect. So although they provide fast, potent, and reliable analgesia in painful procedures, their analgesic effects do not last for a long time after the termination of the infusion at the end of the procedure, leaving the patient in significant pain. Thus, it is recommended to give a longer acting analgesic during the procedure in addition to these opioids to ensure the patient's comfort in the post-procedure period.

Sufentanil is the most potent synthetic opioid, with an estimated potency of 5–15 times more than fentanyl. It can be used as IV boluses of 0.1–0.5 mcg/kg, and a continuous infusion of 0.005–0.01 mcg/kg/min sufentanil has the advantage of longer lasting post-procedure analgesic effect that lasts longer that fentanyl with less respiratory depression effects. Sufentanil causes non-dose-dependent bradycardia and hypotension due to its cardiovascular depressive action.

All opioids (especially rapid onset synthetic ones) suppress the gag reflex, which is beneficial in upper endoscopic procedures.

26.2.5 Ketamine

Ketamine is an IV anesthetic with significant analgesic, amnestic, and sedative effects. Ketamine exerts its action by blocking the membrane effects of the excitatory neurotransmitter glutamic acid at the N-methyl-D-aspartate (NMDA) receptor subtype, causing a dissociative anesthesia. It has the advantage of the preservation of spontaneous breathing and airway reflexes, but hypoventilation as well as a short period of apnea has been reported with larger doses. Its onset of action after a single IV bolus is 30–60 s, and its peak effects is in 1 min and duration is 15 min. Ketamine causes emergence phenomenon in 10–20% of cases where postoperative disorientation, sensory and perceptual illusions, and vivid dreams happen. Emergence phenomenon can be attenuated by the co-administration of other sedatives such as propofol, barbiturates, or benzodiazepines with ketamine during MAC sedation cases.

The IV general anesthesia induction dose of ketamine is 2 mg/kg, but sedation and analgesia can be provided by an

IV dose of 0.2–0.8 mgs/kg. The analgesic effect of ketamine lasts in the postoperative period, decreasing the need for postoperative analgesics.

Ketamine increases myocardial oxygen consumption, increases intracranial and intraocular pressures, and increases salivation. All these effects together with the possibility of emergence phenomenon make the use of ketamine in the MAC sedation cases less favorable.

26.2.6 Dexmedetomidine

Dexmedetomidine is a relatively new sedative with some analgesic and amnestic properties that was first introduced in 1999. It works on the α(alpha)2 receptors as an agonist. Dexmedetomidine is used as a continuous infusion at a rate 0.2–1 mcg/kg/h with or without an initial loading dose of 0.5–1 mcg/kg over 10 min. After the initial bolus, its onset of action is 5–10 min, with peak effect in 15–30 min. Duration of action is dose dependent.

Dexmedetomidine has several advantages:

- It has a moderate analgesic action, even when used in a small dose.
- Patients sedated with dexmedetomidine tend to be easily arousable and cooperative though still comfortable. This property is advantageous in cases where patients' cooperation is helpful, such as during awake intubation using the fiberoptic scope [13].
- It has a potent antisialagogue action making it desirable in cases of airway instrumentation.
- It has limited amnestic properties.
- It allows respiratory stability, even in deep levels of sedation, where patients usually maintain adequate ventilation.

The main disadvantages of dexmedetomidine are bradycardia and hypotension due to its α(alpha)2 agonist action. These cardiovascular effects are more pronounced in old age, especially when bolus doses are used and in cases of higher infusion doses. It also has slower onset and delayed recovery than other commonly used sedatives such as propofol.

With the recent introduction of generic formulation for dexmedetomidine, the medication cost decreased, making its use more favorable.

26.2.7 Fospropofol Disodium

Fospropofol is a water-soluble prodrug of propofol that was recently introduced as a sedative. It interacts with the enzyme alkaline phosphatase to release propofol. Its delayed and non-acute peak effects add to its safety. Its recommended dose is 4.9–6.5 mgs/kg as a bolus dose followed by supplemental doses of one-fourth the initial doses no more frequent than every 4 min as needed. Patients are dosed according to their weight if their weight is 60–90 kg, and patients who weigh less than 60 kg are dosed as if they are 60 kg. The dose per kg caps at 90 kg and patients who weigh more than 90 kg are dosed as if they weigh 90 kg.

Initial trials of fospropofol use in sedation were promising [14], due to its relatively good safety margins, and less painful injections compared to propofol, as well as the absence of the propofol lipid load in cases of prolonged use. But due to its delayed onset and slow recovery, in 2018, fospropofol was discontinued in the USA.

Fospropofol causes high incidence of pruritus and paresthesia (mainly perineal or genital), and it can also cause hypotension, headache, and hypoxemia.

26.3 Monitored Anesthesia Care Techniques

There are different techniques used to provide monitored anesthesia care to the patients. The choice of the appropriate technique is usually dependent on several factors:

- The experience and preference of the anesthesia care provider.
- The age and physical status of the patient.
- The length and nature of the procedure and the expected pain associated with the procedure.
- The needed level of patients' cooperation and level of sedation.
- Nature of the procedure room, setting, access to the patient, and its proximity to the recovery room.
- Special equipments availability, such as anesthesia machines and infusion pumps such as target-controlled infusion pumps (TCI).

26.3.1 Intermittent Intravenous Bolus Technique

This is one of the easiest, simplest, and most widely used MAC sedation techniques. The main advantage of this technique is its simplicity that makes it an attractive choice in minor, short procedures on young healthy patients who can tolerate the administration of intermittent IV boluses of relatively longer acting sedatives and analgesics (e.g., benzodiazepines, opioids, and fospropofol) to reach the desired level of sedation.

This technique might not be suitable for older, debilitated, or chronically ill patients where the safety margins with medications are narrow. Also, it is not a favorable technique in morbidly obese patients or patients with significant obstructive sleep apnea who can be oversensitive to the load of a bolus medication. In these patients, slow IV infusions provide a better titration option.

Patient-controlled sedation (PCS) is one of the intermittent bolus techniques tried for sedation with the suggested advantage of avoiding over- or under-sedation. In two trials comparing propofol PCS with anesthesiologist-controlled sedation, both methods provided comparable satisfaction levels. However, PCS was associated with lower mean calculated plasma concentrations of propofol in one report [15] and the second study reported significantly lower total propofol dose [16].

26.3.2 Continuous Infusion Technique

Providing IV sedatives, anesthetics, and/or analgesics in a continuous infusion pattern has several advantages:

- Provides a more predictable plasma drug concentration.
- Provides more cardiopulmonary stability, especially for older or debilitated patients, thus reducing the need for vasoactive medications.
- Reduces the need for supplemental anesthetics.
- Lowers the total agent's doses used, resulting in shorter recovery time.

This technique is mainly suitable for newer fast-onset and short-acting sedatives and analgesics, where these agents can also be used in combinations (propofol/remifentanil, propofol/alfentanil, or ketamine/propofol).

26.3.3 Target-Controlled Infusion Technique

The main concept of target-controlled infusion (TCI) is controlling a specific drug concentration in a specific compartment or end organ; this concentration is referred to as the target concentration. This target infusion rate needed to achieve a targeted concentration is determined using a complex computer system that uses the different pharmacokinetic models of the sedatives studied in volunteers or actual patients whose physical statuses are mostly ASA classes 1 and 2. These drugs' information are stored in the software of the machine and using multi-compartment kinetic models, as well as the variances in age, weight, height, and sex of different patients, calculated doses are determined by the TCI pumps according to the selected target level. Using this technique allows the computer in the pump to automatically calculate and control the infusion pump medication delivery rate to reach and maintain the target plasma concentration selected. Target concentrations can be adjusted over time based on the clinical need and patient response.

The accuracy and success of a TCI system is dependent on the medication's information data stored in the software. This information is derived from the medical literature and is, to a big extent, dependent on studies done on actual patients and volunteers who are usually healthy.

The TCI system can also incorporate a specific patient's cardiac output and hepatic function into the dosing models, making it unique in adjusting the sedatives needed to the patient's expected handling of these medications.

Due to the considerable inter-patient variability in both pharmacodynamics and pharmacokinetics, especially in older and chronically debilitated patients, the TCI systems are still dependent on data stored in the software that might not reflect the actual patient parameters.

Propofol is still the most used medication in this system.

26.3.4 Closed Loop Technique

The closed loop technique works by automatically administering sedatives guided by the Bispectral Index™ (BIS™) monitoring reading. It is still under investigation as a modification to the TCI system, which is considered an open loop system. The system adjusts the dose of sedative given and its target concentration according to the effect measured by the BIS number. The system is being evaluated both in the ICU as well as in the procedure room with promising results. The system aims at delivering minimum amounts of sedatives allowing for sedation, thus decreasing the side effects. Again, this technique is still under trial and not yet widely used in practice [17].

26.4 Perioperative Management

26.4.1 Fasting Time Guidelines

Sedation and general anesthesia is a continuum; so the same fasting duration required for general and regional anesthesia is also required for MAC sedation cases. The limited ability to predict different patients' responses to sedatives and to surgical stimulation necessitate that the patients who are planned to have sedation and MAC follow the same fasting guidelines as general anesthesia cases. Special attention should be paid to the level of sedation planned for patients with a history suggestive of gastroesophageal reflux disease (GERD), delayed gastric emptying, and potentially full stomach to minimize the risk of pulmonary aspiration.

26.4.2 Preoperative Evaluation

A significant number of cases done outside of the main operating rooms suite are cared for under MAC sedation. This fact caused a major and a common misconception that these patients do not need a formal pre-anesthesia evaluation like general anesthesia cases.

Pre-anesthesia evaluation guidelines should always apply to MAC sedation cases. Moreover, the pre-procedure evaluation of the procedure room, location, equipment, and personnel, as well as the availability of recovery rooms and emergency equipment, should all be evaluated before starting patient care.

Pre-procedure patient evaluation should focus on medical conditions, medication allergies, NPO status, and previous anesthesia-related complications for the patient or his family. Airway, chest, and cardiac examination should also take place. Relevant investigations should be reviewed.

Planned level of sedation, and degree of anesthesia intervention should be discussed with the patient and the physician performing the planned procedure before starting the sedation and the procedure. Questions and concerns from the patient's point of view should be addressed by the anesthesiologist at that time.

The anesthesiologist should also pay special attention to the candidacy of the patient for MAC sedation, as appropriate patient cooperation and motivation are of crucial importance to the success of the procedure and the patient's satisfaction as well.

There are certain conditions that make MAC sedation challenging or inappropriate such as:

- Impaired patient cooperation due to extremes of age, altered mental status, severe pain or discomfort, intoxication, or systemic or psychiatric diseases affecting the cognitive function of the patient.
- Factors related to the patient's positioning during procedure, such as inability to lie still or flat, or procedure requiring uncomfortable positioning for a prolonged period of time.
- Nature of the procedure, like in procedures where minor movements will be detrimental to the patient's safety, examination accuracy, or procedure success. Also procedure where expected blood loss or cardiopulmonary instability are highly expected.
- Suspected or known difficult airway management, when more than minimal sedation is expected to be required for the procedure.

26.5 Intraoperative Management

In the effort to improve, guide, and standardize the anesthesia and patient care practices, the ASA came up with recommendations, statements, and guidelines. In 1986, the ASA approved the standards of basic anesthetic monitored, which was last amended in 2010 and affirmed on December 13, 2020 [18]. They identified two standards:

- **Standard 1**—It stressed the importance of continuous presence of a qualified anesthesia care provider throughout the conduct of all general anesthetics, regional anesthetics, and monitored anesthesia care.
- **Standard 2**—During all anesthetics (including MAC sedation) oxygenation, ventilation, and circulation should be continually evaluated for all patients. They also identified the recommendations for ideal ways of monitoring that might differ from one type of anesthetic to the other. For oxygenation, although the inspired oxygen concentration in the breathing circuit should be monitored for patients under GA, only a quantitative method of measuring tissue oxygenation by a pulse oximetry is feasible and suitable for MAC sedation cases. They stressed the importance of audible variable pitch pulse tones and adequate illumination to assess the patients' color.

During moderate or deep sedation in MAC cases, the adequacy of ventilation should be evaluated by continual observation of qualitative clinical signs and monitoring for the presence of exhaled carbon dioxide, unless precluded or invalidated by the nature of the patient, procedure, or equipment.

Continuous assessment of circulation by means of heart rate and blood pressure monitoring at least every 5 min is mandated during all anesthetics.

Temperature monitoring is mandated in cases where significant body temperature changes are expected or intended.

26.5.1 Monitoring Depth of Sedation

Continuous monitoring of the depth of sedation is very important for ensuring the safety and effectiveness of sedation during MAC, both in the operating room as well as in procedure rooms. The most basic way of monitoring the depth of sedation is the continuous clinical assessment of the patient. Clinical assessment of a patient's response to verbal and tactile stimulation is very important. Observing eyelash reflexes, papillary responses, tearing, and the pattern of respiration are all helpful in evaluating the level of sedation.

Clinical scoring systems, such as Evan's score [19], are widely used, simple, and inexpensive. Assessing the autonomic responses of patients to procedure stimulation is of utmost importance. Although not all increased autonomic responses are caused by patient discomfort, but still these autonomic changes (tachycardia, tachypnea, and hypertension) together with the other quantitative measures help determine the actual level of sedation, and help prevent the sliding from a level of light sedation to deeper sedation and ultimately to a state of unintended general anesthesia.

Measuring skin conductance can help determine depth of sedation, as it increases with increasing depth of anesthesia. It is an indirect way of evaluating sympathetic nerve activity. Measuring skin conductance was found to correlate with the Modified Observer's Assessment of Alertness/Sedation (MOAA/S) scale as well as propofol plasma concentration. This method is not widely used due to its complexity and also due to the presence of several factors that affect its accuracy, such as sweating.

Heart rate variability observation plays a role in monitoring depth of sedation. Normally, heart rate increases during inspiration and decreases during expiration. This takes place through a parasympathetic reflex called respiratory sinus arrhythmia (RSA). Under sedation and anesthesia this RSA decreases. Measuring the RSA can be helpful to determine the depth of sedation [20], though it depends on an intact autonomic nervous system and is affected by autonomic neuropathy, sepsis, cardiac conduction abnormalities, and several medications that affect heart rate.

The Ramsay and MOAA/S scales are two clinical scales that are most widely used to determine depth of sedation and measure the patient's comfort level with the provided sedation. These scales have the advantage of simplicity and the disadvantage of relative inaccuracy. The Ramsay scale is widely used for ICU ventilated patients, whereas the MOAA/S scale is more used with good correlation to level of sedation during procedure sedations.

The need for an objective way of measuring the depth of sedation led to the development of brain activity measuring tools, basing its main idea onto measuring the effects of sedation on the patient's electroencephalogram (EEG) or auditory evoked potential (AEP). Examples of these monitors are:

- BIS monitor (single-channel EEG signal).
- Narcotrend monitor (computerized analysis of the raw EEG with less interference with electromyogram [EMG] interface than BIS).
- AEP monitor/2-derived, composite auditory evoked potential index (an AEP/EEG- derived hybrid index).
- PSA 4000 monitor (patient state analyzer, calculates the index from 4 EEG channels).
- Cerebral state monitor (another EEG-based monitor).
- Entropy module (based on the idea that EEG irregularities decrease as anesthesia and sedation depth increases).

The most widely used quantitative method of measuring the depth of sedation and general anesthesia is the Bispectral Index scale. BIS was introduced into clinical practice in 1992 by Aspect Medical Systems, and it evaluates the phase relations from a single-channel EEG signal measure from the patient's forehead. It gives a 0–100 scale where 0 denotes no cortical activity, 40–60 unconsciousness, 60–80 sedation, and 80–100 light sedation or awake. A BIS reading in the range of 60–80 is targeted in MAC cases.

The reliability of the BIS is affected by the sedative/anesthetic used. The BIS index correlates well with the level of sedation when propofol, midazolam, and even sevoflurane is used. BIS correlates poorly when ketamine, opioids, and nitrous oxide were used [21]. The poor correlation between the level of sedation and the BIS values when these anesthetics were used is explained by the fact that the BIS monitor measures the cortical activities, whereas these agents' consciousness inhibition is mediated through a subcortical action. The BIS monitor has another disadvantage in that it loses its accuracy in the presence of EMG activities.

26.6 Post-anesthesia Care

The ASA developed practice guidelines addressing post-anesthesia care [22], and they clearly stated that any patient receiving general anesthetic, regional anesthesia, as well as MAC should receive the same standards of post-anesthesia care. As discussed before regarding the criteria of an ideal sedative, it is important that the sedative would have a rapid onset and short duration of action, with little residual effects. These characteristics afford MAC sedation cases a faster recovery. During the stay in the post-procedure recovery area, the patients receive analgesics, antinausea medications, vasoactive medications to control circulation and heart rate, as well as supplemental oxygen as needed.

Different facilities follow different criteria and scoring systems for discharge readiness assessment. Most outpatient and post-procedure recovery areas have only one phase recovery room in contrast to surgical PACUs in hospitals where there are two phase recovery areas. Sometimes it is possible to bypass stage 1 recovery and patients go directly to phase 2 recovery after MAC cases.

Table 26.2 Modified Aldrete score

Motoric activity	
• Spontaneous movement when addressed	2
• Weak spontaneous movements when addressed	1
• No movement	0
Breathing	
• Coughs on comment or cries	2
• Keeps the airway open	1
• Obstructed airways	0
Blood pressure compared to reference measurement[a]	
• Δ < 20 mm HG	2
• Δ = 20–50 mm HG	1
• Δ > 50 mm HG	0
Consciousness	
• Awake	2
• Response to stimulus, reflexes intact	1
• No answer, reflexes absent	0
Oxygen saturation	
• 100–98%	2
• 97–95%	1
• < 95%	0

Reprinted with permission from Boellaard et al. [23]
[a]Reference measurement was performed 1 ½ min after administration of the spasmolytic agent

The most used scoring system to assess patients' readiness for discharge from recovery area is the modified Aldrete (◉ Table 26.2) [23].

It is beyond the scope of this chapter to discuss in details the different requirements for discharge, such as pain control, the management of nausea and vomiting, requirements of voiding, and tolerance of PO intake before discharge, which will be covered in other parts of the book.

26.7 Safety of Monitored Anesthesia Care

Contrary to the general belief, especially among radiologists, endoscopists, and surgeons, MAC sedation is not generally safer than general or regional anesthesia.

In the ASA closed claims analysis published in 2006 [24], the authors investigated about 7000 claims over a period of 20 years. Of these claims, there were approximately 2000 claims related to surgical anesthesia; 6% of these claims were associated with MAC, 78% were associated with general anesthesia, and 16% were associated with regional anesthesia.

Of these claims, death and permanent brain damage were more prevalent in MAC and general anesthesia cases than in the regional anesthesia group (◉ Fig. 26.1) [24].

Respiratory events were the most common causes of claims in the GA and MAC groups, where inadequate

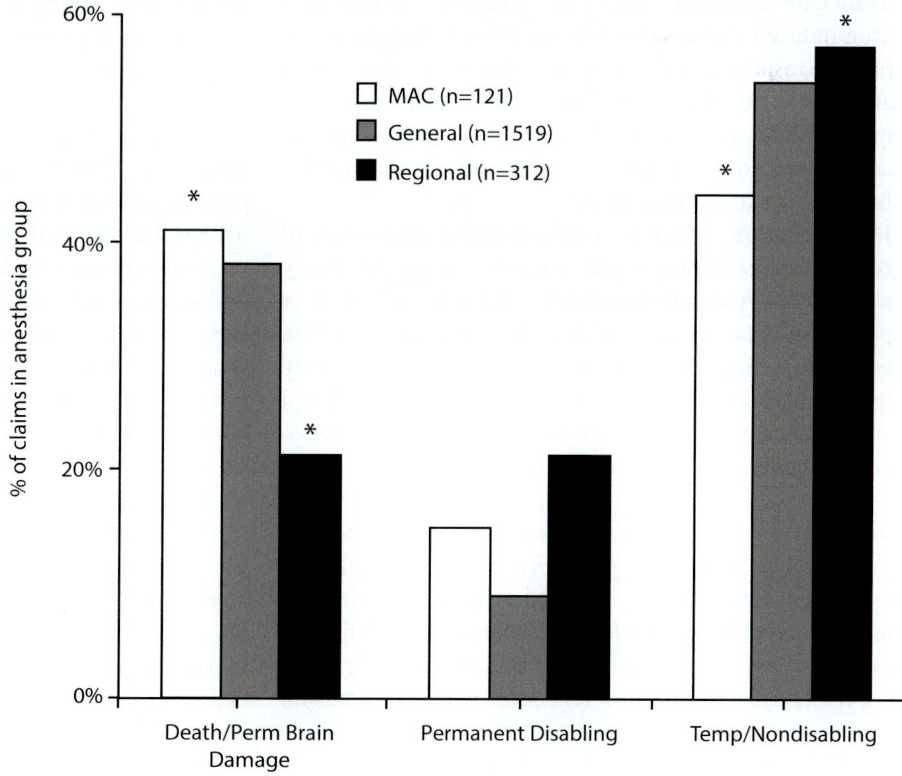

Fig. 26.1 Severity of injury in MAC, general, and regional anesthesia claims (Reprinted with permission from Bhananker et al. [24])

ventilation/oxygenation was the most common cause. The second most common events were cardiovascular adverse events.

In most of these events, patients were heavily sedated. Other contributing factors were:

- Procedure in the head and neck, with limited access to the airway by the anesthesia care provider.
- Poorly functioning monitors and alarms.
- Inattention from the anesthesia care provider.

Of note, many of the MAC sedation cases are performed in very sick patients who are deemed too sick to be surgical candidates or to receive general or regional anesthesia and as a result they receive a minimally invasive procedure under MAC sedation instead.

26.8 American Society of Anesthesiologists Guidelines for Sedation by Non-anesthesiologists

Over the years, the ASA developed and maintained several statements, guidelines, and positions on granting privileges for the administration of moderate [25] and deep sedation [26] by non-anesthesiologists, as well as qualifications for anesthesia care provider for office-based anesthesia care [27].

The ASA differentiated between:

- **Moderate sedation** "conscious sedation," which is a drug-induced depression of consciousness during which patients respond purposefully to verbal commands, either alone or accompanied by light tactile stimulation. No interventions are required to maintain a patent airway, and spontaneous ventilation is adequate. Cardiovascular function is usually maintained.
- **Deep sedation**, which is a drug-induced depression of consciousness during which patients cannot be easily aroused but respond purposefully following repeated or painful stimulation. The ability to independently maintain ventilatory function may be impaired. Patients may require assistance in maintaining a patent airway, and spontaneous ventilation may be inadequate. Cardiovascular function is usually maintained.

With regard to moderate sedation, the ASA stated that only physicians, dentists, or podiatrists who are qualified by education and training to administer moderate sedation should supervise the administration of moderate sedation by other supervised sedation professionals. Alternatively, they may personally perform these functions, with the provision that the individual monitoring the patient should be distinct from the individual performing the diagnostic or therapeutic procedure.

The ASA also stated that the non-anesthesiologist sedation practitioner who is to supervise or personally administer medications for moderate sedation should have satisfactorily completed a formal training program in: (1) the safe administration of sedative and analgesic drugs used to establish a level of moderate sedation, and (2) rescue of patients who exhibit adverse physiologic consequences of a deeper-than-intended level of sedation. This training may be a part of a recently completed residency or fellowship training, or may be a separate educational program.

They stressed several areas that should be covered in this training program such as:

- Ability to obtain informed consent.
- Skills to obtain personal history and physical examination (including airway examination).
- Assess and manage patients and medical situations that carry higher risks of aspiration of gastric contents.
- Pharmacology of sedatives and analgesics and their antagonists.
- Risks and benefits of supplemental oxygen.
- Airway management and ventilation.
- Monitoring of physiological variables.
- Use of audible alarms.
- Appropriate documentations of medications used and patients' physiological variances.
- Advanced cardiovascular life support (ACLS) or equivalent age-appropriate training to match the patient population served.

The ASA also identified guidelines to qualify non-physicians, dentists, or podiatrists to be supervised sedation professionals who can administer sedation under the supervision of a qualified moderate sedation provider [25].

As for the deep sedation, it is clearly stated that patients under deep sedation can easily and unintentionally slip into a state of general anesthesia, so privileges for deep sedation should only be granted to non-anesthesiologists (physicians, podiatrists, or dentists) who are qualified and trained to administer deep sedation, and can recognize and rescue from general anesthesia.

Rescue from general anesthesia means an intervention by a practitioner proficient in airway management and advanced life support. The qualified practitioner corrects adverse physiologic consequences of the deeper-than-intended level of sedation (such as hypoventilation, hypoxia, and hypotension) and returns the patient to the originally intended level of sedation.

These physicians should not supervise or delegate the administration of deep sedation or patient's monitoring to individuals who are not themselves qualified to recognize and rescue from general anesthesia.

26.9 Questions and Answers

Questions (Choose the Most Appropriate Answer)

1. Which of the following methods are not considered a quantitative way of monitoring depth of sedation and anesthesia?
   A. BIS
   B. AEP Monitor/2-Derived, Composite Auditory Evoked Potential Index
   C. Narcotrend Monitor
   D. Evans Score
2. When using which of the following anesthetics is the BIS monitor use accurate to monitor depth of anesthesia?
   A. Nitrous oxide
   B. Ketamine
   C. Remifentanyl
   D. Propofol
3. An ideal sedative should have all the following criteria except:
   A. Rapid onset
   B. Easy titration
   C. Prolonged effect
   D. Amnestic action
4. According to the ASA, which of the following scenarios are not appropriate in cases of providing deep sedation?
   A. An anesthesiologist supervising a nurse anesthetist or an anesthesiologist assistant.
   B. A non-anesthesiologist physician qualified and trained to recognize and rescue from general anesthesia
   C. A non-anesthesiologist physician qualified and trained to recognize and rescue from general anesthesia supervising an RN to monitor patient during a procedure deep sedation.
   D. A non-anesthesiologist physician qualified and trained to recognize and rescue from general anesthesia supervising a nurse anesthetist.
5. Safe use of propofol:
   A. Can be used by non-anesthesiologists who are qualified to provide deep sedation
   B. Can be administered by the endoscopist involved in the endoscopy procedure
   C. Can be administered by an RN under the supervision of the non-anesthesiologist who is qualified to provide deep sedation
   D. Can be used for patients in outpatient facility with no code cart but is linked to a hospital building.
6. All of the following are sedatives with a reliable amnestic action except:
   A. Propofol
   B. Midazolam
   C. Ketamine
   D. Remifentanil
7. The following medications used in MAC cases have an analgesic action except:
   A. Dexmedetomidine
   B. Ketamine
   C. Propofol
   D. Sufentanil
8. A sedation medication with the advantage of respiratory drive preservation:
   A. Dexmedetomidine
   B. Ketamine
   C. Fospropofol
   D. A & B
9. After an MRI done under MAC sedation, the 48-year-old ASA class 2 male should:
   A. Go directly to the regular nursing floor
   B. Wait outside the CT scan room under the supervision of the anesthesiologist till ready to be discharged home or to the RNF
   C. Follow the same guidelines of recovery and discharge criteria like general anesthesia cases in PACU
   D. Always be admitted to regular PACU phase 2 recovery bypassing phase 1
10. MAC sedation is not suitable in:
    A. A 3-year-old scheduled for BMT insertion
    B. MRI of C spine for a 37-year-old male after a MVA who was driving under alcohol influence and still combative.
    C. Pulmonary vein isolation scheduled for 8 h on a patient with mild orthopnea.
    D. Cerebral aneurysm coiling of the MCA scheduled for 2 h
    E. All of the above

Answers

1. **D**. BIS, AEP, and Narcotrend monitor are considered quantitative methods evaluating depth of anesthesia and sedation. BIS is a single lead EEG that measures the cortical activity over the forehead. It gives a number from 0 to 100, the lower the number, the lower

the cortical activity and the deeper the sedation/anesthesia. Narcotrend is another monitor that gives a pattern recognition of raw EEG and classifies it into different stages from A(awake) to F(electric silence). AEP monitor/2-derived, composite auditory evoked potential index is an auditory evoked potential and EEG-based index that is also a quantitative index. Evan's score is a score based on assessing the autonomic responses of patients to procedure stimulation. It is a qualitative method that is simple and inexpensive to evaluate depth of anesthesia and sedation.

2. **D**. The reliability of the BIS is affected by the sedative/anesthetic used. BIS monitor measures single lead cortical EEG from the forehead placed electrodes. Although the BIS number correlates well with the level of sedation when propofol, midazolam, and even sevoflorane are used, BIS correlates poorly when ketamine, opioids, and nitrous oxide were used. The poor correlation between the level of sedation and the BIS values when these anesthetics were used is explained by the fact that the BIS monitor measures the cortical activities whereas these agents consciousness inhibition is contributed to by a subcortical action.
3. **C**. An ideal sedative should meet the needs and expectations of both the patient and the physician performing the procedure. An ideal sedative should be easily titratable to meet the needs of the patients at different stages of the procedure performed, so if the patient's cooperation is needed the sedation is lightened and when the patient's cooperation is not needed the sedation is deepened. So an ideal sedative should have a rapid onset, short duration, and have an amnestic action to guarantee the patient's comfort. Discharge from recovery after procedures should be preferably fast, so the sedative should have a short duration of action and fewer hangovers.
4. **C**. The ASA identified specific guidelines for the qualifications of non-anesthesiologists to provide or supervise moderate and deep sedation. It is clearly stated that patients under deep sedation can easily and unintentionally slip into a state of general anesthesia, so privileges for deep sedation should only be granted to non-anesthesiologist (physicians, podiatrists, or dentists) who are qualified and trained to administer deep sedation, and recognize and rescue from general anesthesia and returns the patient to the originally intended level of sedation. These physicians should not supervise or delegate the administration of deep sedation or patient's monitoring by individuals who are not themselves qualified to recognize and rescue from general anesthesia. So no physician should supervise an RN, who is not qualified to recognize and rescue from general anesthesia.
5. **A**. The ASA stated that whenever propofol is used for sedation, the same guidelines as in deep sedation should be followed. Please refer to the answer of question 4 for the guidelines for deep sedation supervision.
6. **D**. Remifentanyl, as an opioid analgesic, has an unreliable amnestic action. Propofol, benzodiazepines such as midazolam, as well as ketamine have more reliable amnestic action by providing sedation, anxiolysis as well as antegrade amnesia.
7. **C**. Dexmedetomidine, an alpha2 selective agonist, has a moderate analgesic action, even when used in a small dose. Ketamine, an NMDA receptor blocker, has a significant analgesic action in the subanesthetic doses of 0.25 mgs/kg that even lasts in the post-procedure period. Sufentanyl, a synthetic analgesic that acts on the opioid receptors, producing strong analgesia in the intra-procedure as well as in the post-procedure period. Propofol is one of the most common IV anesthetics/sedatives with no analgesic action.
8. **D**. Although hypoventilation as well as short periods of apnea have been reported with the use of both dexmedetomidine and with the use of ketamine too, especially in larger doses or rapid injection or infusion, both dexmedetomidine and ketamine have the advantage of preserving the respiratory drive, thus maintaining spontaneous breathing and airway reflexes even in deep sedation in general. On the other hand, propofol infusion inhibits hypoxic ventilatory drive and depresses the normal response to hypercarbia, causing respiratory depression even in subanesthetic infusion rates. Due to these reasons, the ASA stated that when propofol is used the patients should receive care consistent with that required for deep sedation with the presence of a provider trained in rescuing from general anesthesia and trained in airway management.
9. **C**. The ASA developed practice guidelines addressing post-anesthesia care, and they clearly stated that patients receiving general anesthetic, regional anesthesia, as well as MAC should receive the same standards of post-anesthesia care. In MAC sedation cases, a patient needs to recover in a formal standardized recovery area that follows the standards and guidelines set by the ASA as well as the medical facility where the patient had his procedure done. In some cases, a patient might bypass phase one PACU and goes directly to phase two, but different facilities have different criteria qualifying a patient to bypass phase one.

10. **E**. There are certain conditions that make MAC challenging or inappropriate. A three years old would not be cooperative enough to have a bilateral myringotomy tubes inserted in his eardrums without moving. Combative patients under alcohol influence will unlikely lay still in an MRI machine to have C spine MRI done and in these imaging procedures even a minor movement will not allow an accurate diagnosis. Minor movements in cases like intracranial aneurysm coiling might be significantly detrimental for these patients; thus, it is generally recommended that these patients receive general anesthetic that would ensure that unintended patients movement be avoided. Pulmonary vein isolation procedures are generally long cases that require patients to stay for a long time in a relatively flat supine position. In cases of significant orthopnea, a patient might not be able to tolerate flat supine position for extended period of time making MAC sedation unsuitable in this case, necessitating general anesthetic. Changing to general anesthesia in the middle pf these procedures might not be an easy decision especially with poor access to the patient due to the continuous presence of the C arm over the patient for imaging.

References

1. American Society of Anesthesiologists. Continuum of depth of sedation: definition of general anesthesia and levels of sedation/analgesia. Approved by the ASA House of Delegates on October 13, 1999, and last amended on October 23, 2019.
2. American Society of Anesthesiologists. Position on monitored anesthesia care. Approved by the ASA House of Delegates on October 25, 2005, and last amended on October 17, 2018.
3. Riad I, Abdelmalak B. Ch 64 Monitored anesthesia care and non-operating room anesthesia. In: Longnecker D, Mackey S, Newman M, Zapol W, editors. Anesthesiology. 3rd ed. New York: McGraw-Hill Education; 2018. p. 1172–86.
4. American Society of Anesthesia. Statement on safe use of propofol. Approved by the ASA House of Delegates on October 27, 2004, and amended on October 23, 2019.
5. Koshy G, Nair S, Norkus EP, Hertan HI, Pitchumoni CS. Propofol versus midazolam and meperidine for conscious sedation in GI endoscopy. Am J Gastroenterol. 2000;95:1476–9.
6. McQuaid KR, Laine L. A systematic review and meta-analysis of randomized, controlled trials of moderate sedation for routine endoscopic procedures. Gastrointest Endosc. 2008;67:910–23.
7. Drug Trials Snapshots: Byfavo. FDA, 2020. Accessed 22 Sep, 2020, at https://www.fda.gov/drugs/drug-approvals-and-databases/drug-trials-snapshots-byfavo.
8. Rex DK, Bhandari R, Desta T, et al. A phase III study evaluating the efficacy and safety of remimazolam (Cns 7056) compared with placebo and midazolam in patients undergoing colonoscopy. Gastrointest Endosc. 2018. https://doi.org/10.1016/j.gie.2018.04.2351.
9. Rex DK, Bhandari R, Lorch DG, Myeres M, Schippers F. Safety and efficacy of remimazolam in high risk colonoscopy: a randomized trial. Dig Liver Dis. 2021;53:94–101.
10. Terrie YC. An overview of opioids. Pharmacy Times. June 13, 2011. http://www.pharmacytimes.com/publications/issue/2011/june2011/an-overview-of-opioids. Accessed 22 Apr 2016.
11. Schumacher MA, Basbaum AI, Way WL. Opioid analgesics & antagonists. In: Katzung BG, Masters SB, Trevor AJ, editors. Basic & clinical pharmacology. 12th ed. New York: McGraw-Hill Medical; 2012.
12. Yaksh TL, Wallace MS. Opioids, analgesia, and pain management. In: Brunton LL, Chabner BA, Knollman BC, editors. Goodman & Gilman's the pharmacological basis of therapeutics. 12th ed. New York: McGraw-Hill Medical; 2011.
13. Abdelmalak B, Makary L, Hoban J, Doyle DJ. Dexmedetomidine as sole sedative for awake intubation in management of the critical airway. J Clin Anesth. 2007;19:370–3.
14. Yen P, Prior S, Riley C, Johnston W, Smiley M, Thikkurissy S. A comparison of fospropofol to midazolam for moderate sedation during outpatient dental procedures. Anesth Prog. 2013;60(4):162–77.
15. Glass PSA. Intravenous infusion techniques: how to do it and why we should do it. Can J Anaesth. 1998;45:R117–37.
16. Newson C, Joshi GP, Victory R, White PF. Comparison of propofol administration techniques for sedation during monitored anesthesia care. Anesth Analg. 1995;81:486–91.
17. Le Guen M, Liu N, Bourgeois E, Chazot T, Sessler DI, Rouby JJ, Fischler M. Automated sedation outperforms manual administration of propofol and remifentanil in critically ill patients with deep sedation: a randomized phase II trial. Intensive Care Med. 2013;39(3):454–62.
18. American Society of Anesthesia. Standards for basic anesthetic monitoring committee of origin: standards and practice parameters. Approved by the ASA House of Delegates on October 21, 1986, last amended on October 20, 2010, and last affirmed on December 13, 2020.
19. Evans JM, Davies WL. Monitoring anesthesia. Clin Anesth. 1984;2:243–62.
20. Sinha PK, Koshy T. Monitoring devices for measuring the depth of anesthesia-an overview. Indian J Anesth. 2007;51:365–81.
21. Mi WD, Sakai T, Kudo T, Kudo M, Matsuki A. Performance of bispectral index and auditory evoked potential monitors in detecting loss of consciousness during anaesthetic induction with propofol with and without fentanyl. Eur J Anaesthesiol. 2004;21:807–11.
22. American Society of Anesthesiologists. Practice guidelines for postanesthetic care: a report by the American Society of Anesthesiologists Task Force on Postanesthetic Care. Adopted by the ASA in 2001 and published in 2002, last updated October 18, 2012.
23. Boellaard TN, van der Paardt MP, Hollmann MW, Eberl S, Peringa J, Schouten LJ, et al. A multi-centre randomised double-blind placebo-controlled trial to evaluate the value of a single bolus intravenous alfentanil in CT colonography. BMC Gastroenterol. 2013;13:94.
24. Bhananker SM, Posner KL, Cheney FW, Caplan RA, Lee LA, Domino KB. Injury and liability associated with monitored anesthesia care: a closed claims analysis. Anesthesiol. 2006;104(2):228–34.
25. American Society of Anesthesiologists. Statement on granting privileges for administration of moderate sedation to practitioners who are not anesthesia professionals. Approved by the ASA House of Delegates October 18, 2006, and amended on October 13, 2021.
26. American Society of Anesthesiologists. Statement on granting privileges to nonanesthesiologist physicians for personally administering or supervising deep sedation. Approved by the ASA

House of Delegates on October 18, 2006, and amended on October 25, 2017.
27. American Society of Anesthesiologists. Statement on qualifications of anesthesia providers in the office-based setting. Approved by the ASA House of Delegates on October 13, 1999; last amended on October 21, 2009; and reaffirmed on October 23, 2019.

27 Blood Products Transfusion

Jacek B. Cywinski

Abstract

Transfusion of blood products may be required during the perioperative period. Despite a well-established safety record, transfusion of blood and its components is not risk free. Indication for each of the blood components needs to be established based on the laboratory investigation and/or clinical picture. In general terms, when there is clinical evidence of a deficiency in oxygen-carrying capacity, red cell transfusion should be considered; and in the situations of clinically significant coagulopathy, hemostatic blood products (frozen plasma, platelets, cryoprecipitate, and factor concentrates) transfusion should be considered. Complications of blood administration range from rare but severe reactions (hemolytic transfusion reactions) to more common, and also associated with significant morbidity and mortality, such as transfusion-related acute lung injury (TRALI), transfusion-related circulatory overload (TACO), and changes in immune system (transfusion-related immunomodulation [TRIM]).

Keywords

Transfusion • Red blood cells • Frozen plasma • Platelets • Cryoprecipitate • Transfusion reaction • Crossmatch • Coagulopathy • Massive transfusion

Key Points

1. Transfusion of blood products can be lifesaving; however, it is not risk free. Therefore, it is the responsibility of the physician to use appropriate triggers for blood component therapy.
2. ABO and the Rh systems are the most important in the majority of blood transfusions, although human red cell membranes contain as many as 300 different antigenic determinants.
3. Indication for red blood cell (RBC) transfusion is the need to increase the oxygen-carrying capacity.
4. The US Food and Drug Administration (FDA) recommends avoiding HES in critically ill adult patients and septic patients requiring ICU care.
5. Transfusion-related acute lung injury (TRALI) is currently the leading cause of transfusion-related death. Clinical presentation of TRALI may be indistinguishable from acute respiratory distress syndrome (ARDS) and is characterized by acute onset, bilateral pulmonary infiltrates, and hypoxia without evidence of congestive heart failure (CHF).

27.1 Introduction

During the perioperative period, some patients may require transfusion of blood products. The most common cause and indication for administration of blood components is acute surgical blood loss. In such a situation, transfusion of blood products can be lifesaving, however, it is not risk free. Therefore, it is the responsibility of the physician to use appropriate triggers for blood component therapy. When there is clinical evidence of a deficiency in oxygen-carrying capacity, red cell transfusion should be considered; and if clinically significant coagulopathy is present, transfusion of hemostatic blood product should be considered. There are no mandatory thresholds for the transfusion; the clinician should take into consideration the patient's medical condition, the surgical procedure, symptoms, and the rate of blood loss when deciding if and when to start blood therapy.

J. B. Cywinski (✉)
Multi-Specialty Anesthesiology, Integrated Hospital-Care Institute, Cleveland Clinic, Cleveland, OH, USA
e-mail: cywinsj@ccf.org

M. Argalious et al. (eds.), *Basic Sciences in Anesthesia*,
https://doi.org/10.1007/978-3-031-60203-0_27

Although transfusion of whole blood is still used in certain clinical circumstances, blood components are transfused more often to correct specific deficiencies. The primary advantage of component therapy is that only the needed, specific fraction of the blood is administered, allowing several patients to benefit from 1 donation and administration of unnecessary or unneeded components is avoided. In addition, separation of the whole blood into components permits each to be stored under optimal conditions to enhance and preserve efficacy. The primary disadvantage of component therapy is encountered in treating patients with massive blood loss requiring massive transfusion, since these patients would benefit from whole blood to restore oxygen-carrying capacity as well as hemostatic function. Multiple components are more expensive and more difficult to transfuse in such situations as compared to whole blood, and exposure to various complications of transfusion can be increased as the number of donor exposures increases.

27.2 Donation of Blood

A blood donor may donate whole blood or donate a specific component of blood using apheresis technology. At the time of whole blood donation, blood is collected into a sterile plastic blood reservoir containing an anticoagulant and preservative. Integral tubing connected with satellite bags allows for the separation of whole blood into various components using differential speed centrifugation techniques. One whole blood unit may be separated into 1 unit of plasma, 1 unit of red cells, and 1 unit of whole blood-derived ("random donor") platelets. Each of these components is then stored under optimal conditions. Apheresis technology is used to collect needed components (red cells, platelets, or plasma) from a donor and then return the remaining constituents to the blood donor.

In order to provide adequate safety for the donors and recipients of blood, all blood donors are screened to determine suitability for donation. This process includes donor history and a physical examination, and then if the donor meets criteria, testing of the donor blood specimen. Donor blood is routinely tested for human immunodeficiency virus (HIV) 1/2, human T-cell lymphotropic virus (HTLV) I/II, hepatitis C virus (HCV), hepatitis B virus (HBV), West Nile virus, and *Treponema pallidum*. Since the use of the newest nucleic acid testing technology, the seroconversion window has decreased to 11 days for HIV and 8–10 days for hepatitis C. Hence, donation by seronegative individuals during the period of seroconversion can pose the risk of transmitting infection.

Some patients may request "designated donors": ABO compatible donors known to a patient and selected for donation with the stipulation that their blood be reserved for a specific patient's use. However, the concept that "designated donors" provide safer blood than units collected from the volunteer donors is not valid. Because of the potential increased risk for alloimmunization of an Rh-negative female who receives a blood transfusion from a Rh-positive male sexual partner and subsequent hemolytic disease of the newborn, blood transfusions from a male donor to a female sexual partner are not recommended. Cellular blood components from blood relatives carry an increased risk of causing transfusion associated graft-versus-host disease (TA-GVHD), even in an immunocompetent recipient, and should be irradiated to prevent TA-GVHD.

Limited donor exposure transfusion is based on the assumption that decreasing the number of donor exposures will result in a concurrent decrease in transfusion-related complications. This is most often used in the pediatric and neonatal patient populations. A donor, often a parent, may donate multiple units of blood over a period of time designated for a particular patient. Transfusion services may assign a particular RBC unit to a pediatric patient and take aliquots from the RBC unit for the shelf-life of the unit.

27.2.1 Compatibility Testing

Compatibility testing is done to prevent transfusion of incompatible blood that may result in a hemolytic transfusion reaction. ABO and the Rh systems are the most important in the majority of blood transfusions, although human red cell membranes contain many more different antigenic determinants. Individuals generate antibodies to the alleles they lack within each system or generate them in response to sensitization from a previous transfusion or pregnancy.

A type and screen (T&S) consists of typing the patient's red cells for ABO and Rh blood groups and screening the patient's plasma or serum for the presence of unexpected non-ABO antibodies. The ABO group is determined by typing the patient's red cells using anti-A and anti-B reagents (forward type) and by testing the patient's serum against A and B reagent cells (reverse type). The patient's RBCs are also tested with anti-D for the presence (Rh-positive) or absence (Rh-negative) of the D antigen. Also, the patient's plasma is screened for the presence of unexpected antibodies by incubating it with two selected screening cells that contain all of the critical non-ABO antigens using an antihuman globulin (AHG) technique (indirect antiglobulin test or Coombs test). If an antibody is detected in the patient's plasma, the screen is considered positive. ABO group, Rh type, and antibody detection screening take about 45 min to perform. If the antibody screen is negative and the patient has no history of detected antibodies, the patient may receive RBCs that are tested for

ABO compatibility by performing an immediate spin crossmatch or an electronic/computer crossmatch. ABO- and Rh-compatible blood is selected from the inventory and issued within 5–10 min. If the antibody screen is positive, the unexpected antibody or antibodies must first be identified before antigen negative-compatible RBC units can be found and then crossmatched—all of which usually takes several hours [1].

During a crossmatch, the patient's serum is incubated with red cells from a specific donor unit to verify in vitro compatibility. A crossmatch is performed with a short incubation time at room temperature (immediate spin) intended solely to verify ABO compatibility or as a long incubation time at 37 °C (AHG crossmatch) intended to verify compatibility for clinically significant non-ABO red cell antigens. The immediate spin crossmatch takes 5–10 min, while the AHG crossmatch takes at least 45 min. The electronic/computer crossmatch may be performed instead of an immediate spin crossmatch and uses a computer system to select an RBC unit based on a series of validated computer algorithms. Serologic testing of the donor RBC unit with patient specimen is not performed in this scenario. An AHG crossmatch is only required for patients with a current or past history of clinically significant unexpected antibodies in their plasma or when a patient develops unexplained, acute anemia after recent transfusion [1].

In an emergency situation when there is a need for transfusion, type-specific or type O Rh-negative red cells can be administered while awaiting a formal crossmatch to be performed. Type O Rh-positive red blood cells for males or postmenopausal females can be transfused in this setting as well. Administration of Group O uncrossmatched blood is safe as long as the patient has not been already alloimmunized to any non-ABO red cell antigens. Administration of a substantial number of Group O Rh-negative blood may potentially lead to hemolysis if multiple units of Group O whole blood (containing anti-A and anti-B antibodies) have been transfused to patients with Group A or B blood. The patient can be switched back to native type-specific blood after subsequent compatibility testing.

27.3 Whole Blood and Blood Components

27.3.1 Whole Blood

Indications

Restoration of oxygen-carrying capacity and restoration of hemostatic function in setting of massive blood loss.

Whole blood units contain approximately 450–500 mL donated blood plus approximately 70 mL of a citrate-based anticoagulant-preservative solution, which helps to maintain the viability of red blood cells. The whole blood collected and stored with citrate-phosphate-dextrose-adenine (CPDA-1) solution has a 35-day shelf-life and a hematocrit of approximately 35%. Whole blood is rarely transfused in a current clinical practice but it may be indicated for acute, massive blood loss. In cardiac surgery, transfusion of fresh whole blood was tested as an alternative to using red blood cells, platelets, and fresh frozen plasma (FFP) and it decreased need for component transfusion. Although one study showed less postoperative blood loss in infants, the majority of the studies concluded that the logistic problems of obtaining fresh blood from a prescreened donor (to be transfused within 12 h of collection) outweighed any advantages. Nonetheless, its indication for massive transfusion—particularly in combat and in disasters—is still under investigation. Because of the logistic, very few blood centers or hospitals maintain an inventory of CPDA-1 whole blood.

27.3.2 Red Blood Cells

Indications

Increasing the oxygen-carrying capacity.

One unit of whole blood is separated into red blood cells and platelet-rich plasma by centrifugation and collected in CPDA-1 anticoagulant-preservative solution with a hematocrit of approximately 70% and a shelf-life of 35 days. If 100 mL of Adsol® (AS-1), Nutricel® (AS-3), or Optisol® (AS-5) is added to red blood cells with CP2D or CPDA-1, shelf-life is prolonged to 42 days reducing the hematocrit to approximately 60%. Red blood cells are only indicated for raising the oxygen-carrying capacity, although they also provide volume when given to patients who are acutely hemorrhaging.

Glycerolized red blood cells are stored frozen at temperatures of − 65 °C or lower for up to 10 years. Glycerol is used to protect the red cells during freezing and thawing and is removed by washing before transfusion. An automated closed cell processing systems in conjunction with using nutrient-additive solutions, such as AS-3, have extended the post-wash storability of the blood to 14 days following thawing. This approach is indicated for prolonged storage of rare red cells for patients with antibodies to red cells with rare red cell antigen phenotypes and storage of Group O red blood cells to treat patients during times of shortage.

Leukocyte-reduced red blood cells were primarily indicated in the past for patients with a history of multiple febrile non-hemolytic transfusion reactions, for select patients who were frequent transfusion candidates and thus at risk for alloimmunization to leukocyte antigens, and for prevention of cytomegalovirus (CMV) infection in high-risk patients who were immunocompromised. For the same reasons, leukocyte-reduced red blood cells are increasingly being used in the USA general population of transfused patients, and universal leukocyte reduction is now mandated in Canada and many European countries as well. Certain patient populations at high risk (e.g., trauma, cardiac surgery), with systemic endothelial activation/dysfunction related to the systemic inflammatory response, may benefit from leukoreduced units to attenuate target organ injury. This is supported by randomized, controlled trials (RCTs) involving nearly 2500 patients, revealing a 50–70% reduction in mortality in patients who were randomly assigned to receive leukoreduced red blood cells (RBC) units [2]. Third-generation adsorption filters enable the removal of 99.9% of donor leukocytes and are more effective than the cell washing and centrifugation techniques used previously.

Washed red blood cells are prepared by centrifugation with saline to remove almost all plasma. They are indicated only for patients who have had severe allergic reactions associated with transfusion or immunoglobulin A (IgA) deficiency. Washed red blood cells must be given through a standard blood filter, and can be stored no longer than 24 h because of the risk of bacterial contamination following washing in an open system. Washing of red cells may be used to remove excess potassium from older units as well.

Irradiated whole blood or red blood cells are blood components that have been exposed to a standard dose of ionizing (gamma) radiation to render viable lymphocytes incapable of engraftment in premature newborns, highly immunocompromised patients (e.g., bone marrow or solid organ transplant), and blood relatives of directed donations to reduce the possibility of transfusion-related graft-versus-host disease. Increased membrane permeability has been noted after irradiation, with viability of the irradiated red cells leaking potassium at an accelerated rate. Mild functional impairment manifested by significant leakage of potassium and accumulation of plasma hemoglobin has been demonstrated subsequent to gamma irradiation. This issue can become especially problematic if blood is stored for extended periods of time following irradiation, resulting in rare but serious incidences of hyperkalemic cardiac arrhythmia or serious conduction abnormality. Washing the red cell component can be used to remove excess potassium. Irradiated red blood cells have a reduced storage period (not to exceed 28 days after irradiation) in order to limit the deleterious effects this treatment can have [3].

In general, red blood cells are indicated in symptomatic, anemic patients to restore oxygen-carrying capacity. Red cells may be used in the setting of severe bleeding (e.g., > 1–2 L/hour) in an attempt to manage ongoing hypovolemia/anemia. Transfusion volume required for individual patients can be estimated using the patient's hematocrit, blood volume, and state of hydration. In many cases, transfusion rates and/or amounts can be effectively reduced by employing blood conservation techniques. One unit of red blood cells will increase the hematocrit by approximately 3% and the hemoglobin by about 1 g/dL in the average adult. Ten mL/kg of red blood cells will raise hematocrit by 10%. The increase in the recipient's hematocrit will vary depending upon many factors, which include the donor's hematocrit, the recipient's fluid status and size, the anticoagulant-preservative solution utilized, the rate of active bleeding, and the duration of storage of the unit transfused.

Calcium-containing solutions must not be added to blood, particularly at slow infusion rates, because small clots may form due to the presence of calcium in excess of the chelating ability of the citrate anticoagulant. Hypotonic solutions such as 5% dextrose in water should not be used to dilute red cells since clumping of the cells or hemolysis may occur.

Even though an anticoagulant is added to blood at the time of the collection from the donor, small clots are occasionally present, which requires filtration at the time of infusion. Standard blood administration sets usually have a clot-screening filter with a pore size of 170–200 μ(mu)m. These filters permit rapid transfusion and should be used for administration of red cell components, platelet and granulocyte concentrates, FFP, and cryoprecipitate.

During storage of red cells, microaggregates consisting of platelets, leukocytes, and fibrin form. These microaggregates are able to pass through 170 μ(mu)m filters and lodge in the pulmonary circulation. For that reason, use of microaggregate (20–40 μ[mu]m) filters has become increasingly popular, although it has not been proven to reduce the incidence of respiratory distress syndrome in patients receiving multiple transfusions. The usefulness of microaggregate filters is still debated, and there is no firm indication for their use during routine transfusions, even when large volumes of blood are administered (massive transfusion).

27.3.3 Platelets

Indications

Correction of a deficiency in either platelet number or function in clinical situations of ongoing or anticipated bleeding.

Random-donor platelets can be prepared from whole blood stored at 22 °C within 8 h of collection. After the collection of approximately 500 mL of whole blood into citrate-based anticoagulant-preservative containing collection bags, the blood is centrifuged; the platelet-rich plasma (PRP) is separated into an attached empty satellite bag. This PRP is centrifuged again and separated into 1 unit of platelet concentrate and 1 unit of plasma. Each unit of platelets contains approximately 5×10^{10} platelets in 50–70 mL of plasma [4].

Platelets can be also isolated from the buffy coat layer, following centrifugation of whole blood in specific bags that remove RBC and plasma through tubing in the bottom and top of the bags. The platelet-enriched buffy coat is further processed (through centrifugation and/or leukoreduction filters) to eliminate white blood cells (WBCs) and remaining RBCs. This method is currently employed mostly in Europe and Canada, and it permits storage of whole blood at 22 °C for up to 24 h prior to platelet removal [4].

Another method to obtain platelet concentrate is apheresis. Platelets (single donor) are obtained by performing apheresis on volunteer donors. During this procedure, large volumes of donor blood are processed into an extracorporeal circuit and centrifuged to separate the components. The red blood cells and a certain percentage of the plasma are returned to the donor. A single donor donates the equivalent of $3–5 \times 10^{11}$, or 4–6 units, of platelets suspended in a volume of 200–400 mL of plasma. Pheresis-derived platelets minimize the number of donor exposures and increases the amount of collected platelets, and it has become the primary source of platelets in the US [4].

Platelets should be stored at room temperature (20–24 ° C) for up to 5 days with continuous gentle agitation to prevent platelet aggregation. All platelet products should be tested for bacterial contamination prior to transfusion. The administration of ABO-specific platelets is not strictly (i.e., usually limited to 300–500 mL of out-of-group plasma) required because platelet concentrates contain few red blood cells. However, administration of non-ABO-specific platelets may be of concern with transfusion of pediatric patients with a small blood volume because of anti-A and/or anti-B in the plasma. The administration of out-of-group pooled platelet components leads to transfusion of plasma-containing anti-A and/or anti-B, resulting in passive alloimmunization and may cause a weakly positive direct antiglobulin test due to anti-A and or anti-B from the plasma.

Platelets transfusion is indicated to correct a deficiency in either platelet number (thrombocytopenia) or platelet function (thrombocytopathy or qualitative platelet disorders). One unit of apheresis platelets or a pool of 4–6 whole blood-platelets (derived from 4 to 6 donors) increases the platelet count by approximately $3–5 \times 10^{10}$/L in the average adult. For pediatric patients, a dose of 10 ml/kg or 1 unit of platelets/10 kg will generally increase the platelet count to adequate levels. Factors to consider for the transfusion of platelets for counts between 5 and 10×10^{10}/L are the type of surgery, extent of actual blood loss or microvascular bleeding, presence of potent antiplatelet medications (e.g., clopidogrel, IIb/IIIa antagonists, etc.) and disorders, such as uremia, known to affect platelet function and coagulation. Operations at closed sites (e.g., neuro or ophthalmic surgery) usually require increasing the platelet count 100×10^9/L in order to ensure adequate hemostasis. Surgical procedures associated with insignificant blood loss may be undertaken in patients with platelet counts less than 50×10^9/L. The platelet count alone does not guarantee adequate platelet function and platelet transfusion may be indicated, even above 100×10^9/L count, if platelet dysfunction is suspected and/or there is a recent history of taking aspirin or other more potent or longer half-life platelet-inhibiting drugs (e.g., clopidogrel). Potent agents such as glycoprotein IIb/IIIb antagonists may require two or more apheresis platelet units to achieve normal hemostasis while effects of some other agents (e.g., clopidogrel) have not consistently been shown to be reversed with platelets. Whole blood coagulation tests such as thromboelastography or thromboelastometry testing can identify platelet dysfunction more precisely. The prophylactic administration of platelets is not recommended in patients with chronic thrombocytopenia caused by increased platelet destruction (e.g., idiopathic thrombocytopenic purpura) and, in fact, may be ineffective in a substantial percentage of these patients [3].

Platelets can be infused through a platelet or standard component administration set with a 170-micron filter; platelets should not be transfused through fluid warmers or rapid infusion systems. Microaggregate filters (20-micron to 40-micron) should not be used because they will remove most of the platelets.

27.3.4 Frozen Plasma

Indications

Correction of coagulopathy related to the deficiency of clotting factors.

After removal of red blood cells from the whole blood, the remaining platelet-rich plasma is further centrifuged to separate the platelets from the plasma. Separated plasma contains all the blood coagulation factors, fibrinogen, and other plasma proteins in a volume of 170–250 mL. The plasma is then frozen within 8 h of phlebotomy to prevent complete inactivation of temperature-sensitive ("labile") coagulation factors V and VIII and stored in temperatures colder than − 18 °C for up to 1 year with minimal loss of coagulant activity. Prior to the administration of FFP, the plasma must be thawed in a waterbath at 37 °C on, which takes approximately 30 min. After thawing, the units of FFP are stored at 1–6 °C and are generally transfused within

24 h. FFP that has been thawed but not used within 24 h can be relabeled as "thawed plasma" (TP) and stored at 1–6 °C for an additional 4 days. Thawed plasma maintains normal levels of all factors except factor V, which falls to 80% of normal, and factor VIII, which falls to 60% of normal. TP can be used as a substitute for FFP [5].

FFP is used for the treatment of microvascular bleeding due to congenital and acquired coagulopathies resulting in a prolongation of either the activated partial thromboplastin time (aPTT) or prothrombin time (PT) greater than 1.5 times normal, or a coagulation factor assay of less than 25%. Evidence-based data supporting administration of FFP in patients with international normalized ratio (INR) values < 2.0 are lacking. In emergent situations, FFP may be used to reverse the effect of warfarin prior to surgery or during active bleeding episodes. However, if time permits, oral or parenteral vitamin K will produce the same effect in 6–12 h without exposing patients to the risks associated with allogeneic blood components. In the patient who has been transfused with more than 1–2 blood volumes and PT and PTT cannot be obtained in a timely fashion, FFP may be administered after administration of platelets to correct microvascular bleeding believed to be due to coagulation deficiency. When FFP is indicated, it should be administered in a dose calculated to achieve a minimum of 30% of plasma factor concentration. Ten to 15 mL/kg of FFP will usually result in an increase of most coagulation factors by 25–30%. Transfusion of single unit of FFP in the adult patient should be avoided as it provides inadequate amount of clotting factors to correct coagulopathy. Whole blood coagulation tests such as thromboelastography or thromboelastometry testing can identify and quantify coagulation factors deficiency and provide guidance for replacement.

FFP should be administered through a blood administration set with a 170-micron filter [3].

27.3.5 Cryoprecipitate

Indications

Low fibrinogen levels or von Willebrand's disease (deficient or abnormal von Willebrand molecule).

Cryoprecipitate is prepared from a unit of FFP; it is the cold-insoluble white precipitate that forms when a bag of FFP is thawed at 1–6 °C. This cold-insoluble material is removed following centrifugation and immediately refrozen at − 18 °C to be stored at this temperature for up to 1 year. Each unit of cryoprecipitate contains 80–150 units of factor VIII, 150–250 mg of fibrinogen, von Willebrand factor, factor XIII, and fibronectin in a volume of 5–15 mL. Cryoprecipitate must be transfused within 4–6 h of thawing if given to increase factor VIII levels.

Cryoprecipitate is used primarily to augment fibrinogen levels depleted because of massive hemorrhage or disseminated intravascular coagulation (DIC). Rarely, it is used for the treatment of congenital or acquired factor XIII deficiency. For fibrinogen replacement therapy, 1 unit of cryoprecipitate per 10 kg body weight increases plasma fibrinogen by approximately 50–70 mg/dL in the absence of continued consumption or massive bleeding. The minimum hemostatic level of fibrinogen is more than or equal to 80–100 mg/dL, but many experts regard that minimal level as too low. The national guidelines in Germany and Austria recommend higher levels of 150–200 mg/dL [6]. Because cryoprecipitate does not contain factor V, it should not be the sole replacement therapy for DIC, which is almost always associated with a variety of factor deficiencies and thrombocytopenia. Hence, fresh frozen plasma also needs to be administered along with platelet concentrates in those settings where a coagulopathy secondary to DIC is likely occurring.

Cryoprecipitate should be infused through a 170- to 260-micron component filter.

27.4 Factor Concentrates

A number of plasma derivatives are available to treat coagulation deficiencies. The main advantage of their use is administration of specific deficient factor(s) and avoidance of transfusion of unnecessary blood components.

27.4.1 Factor VIII

Factor VIII concentrates are indicated to correct factor VIII deficiency (hemophilia A). Historically, administration of human concentrated factor VIII was associated with a relatively high incidence of infectious disease transmission; however, advances in purification techniques and screening tests have dramatically reduced that risk. Also the development of recombinant factor VIIIC in many instances has replaced human-based blood derivatives for the treatment of factor VIII deficiency. Recombinant factor VIIIC has the major advantage of not carrying the risk of transmitting viral diseases. Mild factor VIII deficiency and type 1 (80% of von Willebrand's disease) may be partially corrected with desmopressin (DDAVP). Administration of DDAVP is typically associated with a significant increase in both circulating factor VIII and von Willebrand's factor (vWf).

27.4.2 Factor IX

Factor IX concentrates were used to treat factor IX deficiency (hemophilia B, or Christmas disease). They contain negligible amounts of factors II, VII, and X and consequently are much less thrombogenic then factor IX complex (prothrombin complex). Recombinant factor IX is currently available and has the advantage of no infectious risk with transfusion.

27.4.3 Antithrombin III Concentrate

Antithrombin III (ATIII) deficiency is mostly a congenital defect but also can be acquired (i.e., in the setting of prolonged exposure to unfractionated heparin). Because ATIII is the major plasma inhibitor of thrombin, patients with ATIII deficiency are highly prone to thromboembolism. ATIII also has an important role as an inhibitor of the activated serum protease factors II, IX, X, XI, and XII. The anticoagulant effect of heparin is due to its ability to greatly increase the inhibitory activity of ATIII; patients with moderate to marked ATIII deficiency can display resistance to heparin. This is critically important for major cardiovascular procedures and surgeries involving cardiopulmonary bypass. Normal ATIII levels can be achieved by administering either human or recombinant preparation of ATIII concentrate. Prophylactic treatment with ATIII concentrate also is recommended for patients with a hereditary deficiency of ATIII (plasma level of 50% or less compared to normal) who have a history of thromboembolism or are undergoing surgical or obstetrical procedures associated with a high incidence of thromboembolism. ATryn is a recombinant antithrombin indicated for the prevention of perioperative and peripartum thromboembolic events in hereditary antithrombin deficient patients. It is not indicated for treatment of thromboembolic events in hereditary antithrombin deficient patients.

Coagulation factor concentrates such as purified human fibrinogen concentrate and prothrombin complex concentrates (PCCs) are thought to be valuable alternatives to plasma and cryoprecipitate, respectively.

27.4.4 Fibrinogen Concentrate

The administration of fibrinogen concentrate (FC) is approved only for the therapy of congenital hypofibrinogenemia in the United States. There is still ongoing debate regarding benefits of the perioperative administration of fibrinogen concentrate, and some studies suggest that substitution therapy with fibrinogen concentrate may reverse a dilutional coagulopathy by replacing the missing factor and restoring fibrin production and clot formation. Also fibrinogen concentrate significantly improves whole blood clot firmness and reduces the postoperative transfusion requirements in severely bleeding patients. Since adequate level of fibrinogen is crucial for optimal clot generation, administration of fibrinogen concentrate or cryoprecipitate might reduce postoperative bleeding and transfusion. However, the liberal fibrinogen substitution in the perioperative setting cannot be recommended. Plasma threshold levels for fibrinogen substitution of 80–100 mg/dL are still widely considered and recommended in guidelines, but many experts regard that minimal level as too low of a threshold for initiating exogenous fibrinogen replacement especially in a bleeding patient. The national guidelines in Germany and Austria recommend higher levels of 150–200 mg/dL in concordance with the Task Force of Advanced Bleeding Care in Trauma and the European recommendations in perioperative bleeding [6].

27.4.5 Prothrombin Complex Concentrate

Prothrombin complex concentrates (PCCs) are a human plasma-derived lyophilized product containing the vitamin-K-dependent coagulation factors: FII (prothrombin), FVII, FIX, and FX. PCCs are available as so-called three-factor PCCs with low levels of FVII or as four-factor PCCs with higher levels of FVII. PCCs may differ considerably in their contents of the anticoagulants protein C, protein S, and antithrombin as well as heparin. The most common indications for their use are the rapid reversal of oral anticoagulation (vitamin K antagonists) and the treatment of patients with a deficiency of vitamin-K-dependent coagulation factors, such as in liver failure. Recently, US and European guideline papers recommended the off-label use of PCCs in patients with trauma and massive bleeding after surgery.

Administration of PCCs might increase the risk of thromboembolic complications in the early recovery period due to prolonged elevation of thrombin generation potential together with the usual increases of fibrinogen level and platelet count and decreased levels of ATIII. Finally, standard coagulation tests including PT and aPTT do not adequately reflect the patient's thrombin generation potential and antithrombin levels; therefore, whole blood viscoelastic coagulation tests (such as ROTEM® or TEG®) may be more accurate to evaluate coagulation status. PCCs carry a prothrombotic risk and should only be administered in situations where the benefit of therapy outweighs this risk.

27.4.6 Recombinant Activated Factor VII

The FDA-approved indication for recombinant activated factor VII (rFVIIa) is the treatment of hemophilia in patients with antibody inhibitors to coagulation factors VIII or IX, congenital factor VII deficiency, and some rare inherited platelet dysfunctions. In the United States, rFVIIa has been used for off-label indications, such as prophylaxis or therapeutic agent to prevent or treat bleeding in patients without hemophilia. Thereby, rFVIIa was used prophylactically or as a treatment option in Jehovah's Witness patients undergoing cardiac surgery to prevent and control bleeding, or as a rescue medication in refractory bleeding in the postoperative period. Large reviews and meta analyses evaluating use of recombinant factor VIIa for the prevention and treatment of bleeding in patients without hemophilia did not show clinically significant benefits. The same was confirmed by RCT in patients undergoing liver transplantation. A more recent report on the off-label use of rFVIIa suggested an association with relevant increased morbidity and mortality. Meta-analysis of off-label use of rFVIIa in cardiac surgery suggested a higher rate of thromboembolic adverse events, especially in the arterial system. The current guidelines from the Society for Thoracic Surgery and the Society of Cardiovascular Anesthesiologists recommend the use of rFVIIa in patients with refractory microvascular bleeding after cardiac surgery. Further, in vitro data suggests a favorable effect of rFVIIa on thrombin generation in patients with recent intake of platelet inhibitors. Patients undergoing urgent or emergent cardiac surgery while treated with antiplatelet agents (e.g., clopidogrel, prasugrel, and ticagrelor) might potentially benefit from rFVIIa. Hemoglobin-Based Oxygen Carriers.

Hemoglobin-based oxygen carriers (HBOCs) solutions have been developed from animal, recombinant, and human sources. The main advantage of these agents involves potential use in hemorrhaging trauma patients or battlefield scenarios, and in patients who either refuse blood or who cannot get compatible blood (rare phenotypes or multiple antibodies). Some initial studies have demonstrated a substantial reduction in transfusion requirements when blood substitutes have been used with normovolemic hemodilution during cardiac surgery. While theoretically promising, there were many problems related to HBOCs use, mainly the toxicity of hemoglobin solutions, a short half-life, increased vasoactivity (i.e., vasospasm) and a relatively high colloid oncotic pressure and affinity for oxygen. Many research setbacks and disappointing results of the clinical trials caused cancellation of further development of a majority of HBOCs products. Natanson et al. examined clinical trials involving the following cell-free hemoglobin products: Hemassist, Hemopure (HBOC 201), Hemolink, Polyheme, and Hemospan. Since the results of this analysis were unfavorable, essentially all ongoing clinical trials involving HBOCs were stopped.

27.5 Albumin

Albumin, a protein solution of approximately 95% albumin and 5% other plasma proteins, is available as a 5% or 25% solution and has been widely used for its oncotic properties. The 25% solution has an oncotic equivalent to five times that of plasma. Serum albumin is prepared from pooled human plasma and is heat-treated to eliminate viral and bacterial contamination. Albumin (5%) can be used as a volume expander in patients with adequate oxygen-carrying capacity but should not be used to correct nutritional deficiencies. Recent meta-analysis of albumin vs. crystalloids in critically ill patients showed no difference in mortality or in other outcomes. The same was concluded in the Saline versus Albumin Fluid Evaluation (SAFE) trial as well. Considering that albumin is a blood product and as such a limited resource and its cost is much higher than that of crystalloids, it may be reasonable to suggest using crystalloids rather than albumin in general intensive care unit (ICU) patients. Pooling the data from the SAFE and the Albumin Italian Outcome Sepsis (ALBIOS) trials showed no benefit or harm from albumin compared with saline. Some Jehovah's Witnesses will not accept albumin administration.

27.5.1 Hydroxyethyl Starch

Hydroxyethyl starch (HES), a synthetic polymer derived from the starch amylopectin, is available in a 6% solution in normal saline. While it is a commonly used perioperative fluid, it should be used with caution in certain clinical situations. Evidence suggests that the use of HES in critically ill patients (including septic patients), increases the chance of renal injury and the requirement of renal replacement therapy (RRT) when compared to crystalloids. This effect has also been observed in patients with sepsis requiring critical care and has also been found to increase mortality irrespective of the need for RRT. Along the same lines, use of HES in cardiac surgery with cardiopulmonary bypass (CPB) was associated with acute kidney injury (AKI) and increased bleeding. Evidence suggests that HES, when used for large volume resuscitation, is associated with AKI, coagulation abnormalities, and increased transfusion rates. In a systematic review of studies that compared the effect of HES 130/0.4 on TEG as compared to saline or albumin, it was concluded that HES infusion resulted in a smaller and weaker clot. The FDA recommends avoiding HES in critically ill adult patients and septic patients requiring ICU care. The FDA also recommends avoiding these products in patients with preexisting renal dysfunction, bleeding disorders, and in those undergoing open heart surgeries with CPB [7].

Although systematic review did not demonstrate any harm associated with the use of 6% HES solutions in general surgical population, these findings should be interpreted with caution because some of the surgical patients receiving HES may be at high risk of both AKI and death and may require critical care support after surgery.

27.5.2 Dextrans

Dextrans, large glucose polymers, are available as dextran 40 (molecular weight 40KD) or dextran 70 (molecular weight 70KD). Dextrans can interfere with platelet function, red cell function, or blood crossmatching, and are associated with the potential for anaphylaxis. Therefore, dextrans are rarely used as volume expanders. Promit®, dextran 1 (molecular weight 1KD), should be administered prior to dextran 40 or dextran 70 to reduce the risk of anaphylaxis. Dextrans can improve microvascular circulation by decreasing blood viscosity and coating endothelial cells to minimize platelet and red blood cell aggregation.

27.6 Complications of Transfusion

27.6.1 Immune Reactions

Hemolytic transfusion reactions (HTRs) involve lysis of red blood cells, which can occur intravascularly (acute) or extravascularly (delayed) and can be caused by immunologic incompatibility between the donor and recipient. HTR causes destruction of the transfused red cells by the recipient's antibodies or, less commonly, hemolysis of a recipient's red cells as a result of transfusion of red cell antibodies.

Most serious HTRs are induced by transfusion of ABO-incompatible red blood cells. The incidence of fatal HTRs is 1 in 300,000 to 1 in 700,000 RBC transfusions; risk of acute HTR is estimated at 1 in 11,000 to as low as 1 in 1000,000 units. Signs and symptoms of HTRs present at the time of the transfusion and may occur after administration of as little as a few mL of incompatible blood. Clerical or system errors resulting in patients receiving the wrong red blood cells is the most common cause of acute HTRs. The severity of a reaction depends on the amount of incompatible blood transfused, the type of incompatibility, and the length of time before treatment is initiated. The patient usually develops with chills, fever, chest and flank pain, and nausea; however, in the anesthetized patient, the only signs may be hemoglobinuria, coagulopathy, and unexplained hypotension [8, 9].

In cases of suspected acute HTR, the transfusion must be stopped and the blood bank notified immediately to recheck all crossmatched. Treatment should be initiated without delay and is directed toward the most serious complications of HTR: acute renal failure and coagulopathy. Urine output should be maintained at a minimum of 1–2 mL/kg/h with intravenous (IV) fluids to prevent tubular system obstruction; alkalinization of the urine should be considered as well. Loop diuretics may be administered to promote urine flow only after adequate intravascular volume restoration, and vasopressors may need to be initiated to maintain optimal perfusion pressure. Laboratory investigation should include the direct antigen test, urine and plasma hemoglobin levels, other tests verifying hemolysis (elevations in lactate dehydrogenase [LDH], bilirubin, and/or undetectable haptoglobin) and baseline coagulation studies (platelet count, prothrombin time, activated partial thromboplastin time, and fibrinogen level).

Immune extravascular (delayed) reactions occur following transfusion of red blood cells containing an antigen other than ABO to a patient with an undetected alloantibody. Delayed hemolytic reaction is generally mild and is caused by antibodies to non-D antigens of the Rh system or to foreign alleles in other systems such as the Kell, Duffy, or Kidd antigens. Estimated risk of delayed HTR is much higher than acute HTR at about 1 in 1000 to 9000 units; the transfused red blood cells usually hemolyze within days to weeks. These reactions are caused by an antibody undetected during pretransfusion compatibility testing and may only become apparent because of a decreasing hemoglobin level, an unexplained poor therapeutic response from a red blood cell transfusion, or with detection of a new antibody (when an antibody screen is repeated). A positive direct antiglobulin (Coombs) test and an unexplained rise in bilirubin may be detected. The treatment of delayed hemolytic reactions is primarily supportive [10].

27.6.2 Febrile Reactions

Fever may be the first indication of either a hemolytic transfusion reaction (HTR) or administration of a bacterially contaminated blood component. Transfusion should be stopped and the cause investigated if a patient's body temperature increases by 1 °C or greater in association with blood transfusion (and is not explained by the patient's clinical condition). HTR always should be considered if red blood cells are being administered and the patient becomes suddenly febrile. If platelets are being transfused, bacterial contamination is more likely to be a cause of the fever.

27.6.3 Febrile Non-hemolytic Transfusion Reaction

The most common cause of fever in association with transfusion is febrile non-hemolytic transfusion reaction (FNHTR). About 0.1–1% of RBC transfusions are associated with FNHTRs, but the incidence is higher in chronically transfused patients. The reactions usually develop after most or the entire component has been transfused and are accompanied by chills and rigors. Other symptoms may include headache, nausea, and a feeling of discomfort. In some cases, symptoms might be limited to chills and rigors without any fever present.

FNHTRs are immunologically mediated, involving leukocyte antibodies in the patient's plasma (stimulated by previous transfusions or pregnancy) and antigens on donor leukocytes, causing release of endogenous pyrogens by the leukocytes. Cytokines released during component storage are also implicated in causing FNHTRs. Leukocyte reduction of RBC prevents most FNHTRs but has been less effective in preventing recurrent reactions associated with platelet transfusions. Prophylaxis and therapy of FNHTRs consists of pretransfusion administration of an antipyretic agent and treatment of chills (meperidine).

27.6.4 Allergic and Anaphylactic Reactions

Allergic, anaphylactoid, and anaphylactic reactions involve interaction between an allergen (usually a protein in the plasma of the transfused blood component to which the recipient was previously sensitized) and immunoglobulin E (IgE) antibody present on the surface of mast cells and basophils of the recipient. The antigen–antibody interaction takes place on the surface of the cells, activating them and causing release of various mediators of anaphylaxis (leukotrienes, histamine, bradykinin) that cause the signs and symptoms such as urticarial, bronchospasm, laryngeal edema, severe hypotension, and possibly death. The shorter the interval between initiation of transfusion and the onset of symptoms, the more severe the reaction. Minor allergic reactions occur in 1 per 20 to 2500 transfusions depending on the components used, definition of reaction, and the studied population. Similarly, major reactions range from 1 in 10,000 to 300,000 transfusions for components other than platelets, and much higher rates for plasma-containing components. Current estimates for the risk of minor allergic reactions after red cell transfusions and pooled platelet transfusions are 0.4% and 4.1% respectively. As for major allergic reactions (anaphylactoid and anaphylactic), risk estimates are 1 in 23,000 red cell transfusions and 1 in 1600 platelet pools–platelet transfusion.

When an anaphylactic reaction is suspected, transfusion must be discontinued immediately. Treatment is the same as for other anaphylactic reactions: epinephrine, diphenhydramine, and corticosteroids, in addition to appropriate fluid therapy and airway management.

Most anaphylactic and anaphylactoid reactions have no detectable cause. Although only a small percentage of allergic reactions are related to immunoglobulin A (IgA) deficiency in the recipient, laboratory evaluation should focus on the possibility that a patient is IgA deficient because of important implications for future transfusion management. Any patient who experiences an anaphylactic reaction should have a pretransfusion serum sample screened to quantify the IgA levels or to detect the presence of anti-IgA (i.e., observed in 30–50% of IgA-deficient patients). If anti-IgA is detected or IgA levels are undetectable, the diagnosis of IgA deficiency is confirmed. Until the diagnosis of IgA deficiency is confirmed, only washed or deglycerolized RBCs or washed platelets should be administered. Once the diagnosis is made; however, alloimmunized IgA-deficient recipients should only be transfused with components from IgA-deficient donors.

27.6.5 Bacterial Contamination

Bacteria present in stored blood can grow and may produce toxins. Contamination during collection, processing, or storage is possible but is most likely to occur at the time of phlebotomy or if the donor has bacteremia associated with unrecognized infection. Administration of a bacterially contaminated blood component may result in fever, tachycardia, hypotension, chills, vomiting, and diarrhea. In some patients, septic shock, oliguria, and DIC can develop. Since platelets are stored at room temperature, which facilitates bacterial growth, bacteremia is 40 times more frequent following platelet administration than transfusion of refrigerated components.

27.6.6 Post-transfusion Purpura

Post-transfusion purpura (PTP) is a rare disorder characterized by severe thrombocytopenia 5–10 days after transfusion in a patient sensitized by prior transfusion or pregnancy. In most cases, PTP follows administration of RBCs. The estimated risk is around 1 in 150,000 to 300,000 red cell units. Patients usually recover spontaneously, although plasmapheresis, corticosteroids, and intravenous immune globulin may need to be administered. The pathogenesis is unclear, but PTP is presumably related to the development of a platelet-specific antibody in patients who are deficient of a common platelet antigen (e.g., PLA-1) following transfusion.

27.6.7 Infections

27.6.7.1 Bacterial Infection

Current risk estimates of bacterial infection are 1 per 2000 to 8000 platelet units and 1 per 28,000 to 143,000 red cells units. Transfusion-associated sepsis is the most frequent cause of death from transfusion-transmitted infections and the second most common cause of transfusion-related death (20–30 deaths/million units transfused) as reported to the FDA, representing 17–22% of all reported fatalities (1 per 50,000–500,000 units platelets and 1 per 8000,000 red cell units.) The most common bacteria implicated in sepsis from red blood cells are *Yersinia enterocolitica* (46%), *Pseudomonas* spp. (25%), and *Serratia* spp. (11%). The common organisms identified in platelet units implicated in transfusion-associated sepsis include *Staphylococcus* spp. (42%), *Streptococcus* spp.

27.6.7.2 Hepatitis

Post-transfusion hepatitis may be evident clinically, but the majority of cases are subclinical. Introduction of testing for HCV in 1990 and subsequent implementation of an improved test have decreased the incidence of HCV. Current estimates are around 1 in 1,600,000 to 3,100,000 component units. It is estimated that up to 90% of infections become chronic, but clinical liver disease develops in only 10–20%. The incidence of transfusion-associated HBV, for which testing has been employed for many years, is estimated to be 1 in 31,000 to 220,000.

27.6.7.3 Human Immunodeficiency Virus, Types I and II

Testing for antibody to HIV-I and HIV-2 was implemented in 1985 and 1992, respectively. The most recent estimates of HIV infection are 1 in 1,478,000 to 4,700,000 units.

27.6.7.4 Human T-Lymphotropic Virus, Types I and II

The transmission of HTLV-I/II by transfusion is limited to cellular blood components, and data suggest that presence of viable lymphocytes is necessary for HTLV transmission. The estimated transfusion risk is 1 in 1,900,000 units. Two diseases are associated with HTLV-I infection albeit infrequently: (1) a chronic degenerative neurologic disease, HLTV-I-associated myelopathy (HAM) or tropical spastic paraparesis (TSP) characterized by progressive lower extremity weakness, spasticity, sensory deficits and urinary incontinence; and (2) adult T-cell leukemia/lymphoma. The lifetime risk of developing overt neurologic or neoplastic disease is thought to be less than 4%.

27.6.7.5 Cytomegalovirus

CMV can be transmitted by transfusion, but clinical disease in immunocompetent patients is rare. Infection can lead to life-threatening multisystem disease in immunocompromised patients such as low-birth-weight infants and bone marrow or solid organ transplant recipients. Use of leukocyte-reduced or CMV-seronegative cellular blood components is recommended to prevent infection in patients at risk for CMV disease.

27.6.7.6 West Nile Virus

Recently, cases of transfusion-transmitted West Nile virus have been confirmed in the US. Following these reports, nucleic acid testing for West Nile virus was widely implemented in the US in 2003, which resulted in identification and removal of around 1000 potentially infected donations in the same year. Transmission may still occur, however.

27.6.8 Massive Transfusion

There are some variations in definition of massive transfusion, however, the acute replacement of more than 1 blood volume or more than 10 units of PRBC within several hours are most widely used. Definitions accounting for the dynamics of clinical situations, such as the transfusion of 4 or more red cell concentrate within 1 h when ongoing need is foreseeable or the replacement of 50% of the total blood volume within 3 h, may be more appropriate. The most common clinical situation leading to massive transfusion is extensive trauma; but it also may occur in non-trauma settings during surgical procedures causing large blood loss. In trauma patients, the ideal solution to manage hypovolemia, anemia, and coagulopathy involves administration of fresh whole blood since this approach restores not only oxygen-carrying capacity but also hemostasis via maintenance of normal levels of coagulation factors and platelets. Fresh whole blood, however, is very difficult to maintain by the blood bank due to logistical and testing issues. Blood transfusion in resuscitation protocols for trauma victims is supported in the Advanced Trauma Life Support (ATLS) guidelines of the American College of Surgeons.

27.6.8.1 Coagulopathy During Massive Bleeding

Massive bleeding and fluid resuscitation are frequently complicated by coagulopathy; more often than not the etiology is multifactorial. Coagulation defects develop not only from dilution of platelets and coagulation factors when crystalloid, colloid, and red blood cells are used to replace lost volume, but also from hypothermia, tissue hypoperfusion with resultant lactic acidosis, and other trauma-related events (e.g., DIC triggered by release of tissue factor from apoptotic cells). Coagulopathy associated with massive transfusion is clinically characterized by the presence of microvascular bleeding or oozing from the mucosa, wound, and puncture sites. The development of acidosis, DIC, and hypothermia may parallel massive transfusion and complicate the ability to effectively manage the coagulopathy. Treatment of the coagulopathy should include restoration of systemic perfusion, maintenance of normal temperature, resolution of acid–base abnormalities, and blood component therapy when supported by abnormal laboratory tests in the setting of active bleeding. Viscoelastic analysis of whole blood clotting (thromboelastography, rotation thromboelastometry, and Sonoclot analysis) may be very useful in correction coagulation disturbances in trauma, liver transplantation, and cardiac surgical settings.

While thrombocytopenia may develop during massive transfusion, administration of platelets should be reserved for the patient exhibiting microvascular bleeding and a platelet count less than 50×10^9/L. Platelet transfusion may be necessary for patients with intermediate platelet counts ($50–100 \times 10^9$/L) if it is determined the risk for more bleeding is significant. FFP also should not be administered prophylactically; in the massively transfused patient, clinical bleeding associated with coagulation factor deficiencies is unlikely until factor levels fall below 20% of normal. In the clinical setting, this usually does not occur until greater than 1 blood volume has been replaced and the PT and PTT are greater than 1.5–1.8 times control values. Conversely, in a trauma patient with massive bleeding, a rise in the PT may be a late sign that the patient is developing a severe dilutional coagulopathy. In the event the PT and PTT cannot be obtained in a timely fashion, FFP may be administered for correction of microvascular bleeding in patients transfused with more than 1 blood volume.

For trauma patients presenting with exsanguinating hemorrhage, coagulopathy correction beginning with aggressive FFP administration early in pre-ICU phase may improve ICU resuscitation response and outcome. It may be appropriate to include the administration of PRBC, FFP, and plateletsat fixed ratio in early (pre-ICU) resuscitation protocols for bleeding trauma patients. It has to be emphasized that once bleeding is controlled and the patient is hemodynamically stable, the transfusion of the blood products should be guided by bedside and laboratory tests.

27.6.8.2 Hypothermia

Hypothermia (temperatures below 35 °C) is likely to occur during massive transfusion; therefore, all blood products and intravenous fluids should be warmed to normal body temperature. The potential effects of hypothermia include ventricular dysrhythmias, shivering, increased oxygen consumption, cardiac arrest, and citrate toxicity secondary to reduced metabolism of citrate and lactate; ventricular arrhythmias progressing to fibrillation often occur at temperatures close to 30 °C. Hypothermia also contributes to coagulopathy: it causes a reversible platelet dysfunction, activity of the coagulation factors and enhances fibrinolysis. Hypothermia also prevents the activation of platelets via traction on the glycoprotein Ib/IX/V complex by von Willebrand factor. In clinical practice, the contribution of hypothermia to coagulopathy may be overlooked because coagulation testing is usually performed at 37 °C. The use of blood and fluid warming devices during massive transfusion is essential to help prevent systemic hypothermia.

27.6.8.3 Citrate Toxicity

Transfusion of large volumes of blood or blood products results in hypocalcemia due to calcium binding by the citrate preservative. Clinically significant hypocalcemia, causing cardiac depression, usually occurs when the transfusion rate exceeds 1 unit every 5 min. In such situations, intravenous calcium preparations should be administered to restore normal calcium level. Also because citrate is metabolized in the liver, patients, with hepatic disease or dysfunction may demonstrate hypocalcemia and require calcium infusion during massive transfusion.

27.6.8.4 Acid–Base Balance

Although stored blood is acidic due to the citric acid anticoagulant and accumulation of red cell metabolites (carbon dioxide and lactic acid), metabolic acidosis due to transfusion is uncommon. However, acidosis interferes with the assembly of coagulation factor complexes involving calcium and negatively charged phospholipids. As a result, the activity of the factor Xa/Va prothrombinase complex is reduced by 50%, 70%, and 80% at pHs of 7.2, 7.0, and 6.8, respectively. The resulting delayed production and reduced concentrations of generated thrombin lead to delayed fibrin production, altered fibrin structure, and increased susceptibility to fibrinolysis. Citric acid and lactic acid are rapidly metabolized to bicarbonate by the liver in patients with liver dysfunction or undergoing liver transplantation accumulation of citric and lactic acid is possible due to decreased metabolism. In the situation of massive blood transfusion, acid–base status is largely dependent upon tissue perfusion, rate of blood transfusion, and citrate metabolism. Once normal tissue perfusion is restored, metabolic acidosis typically resolves, and metabolic alkalosis commonly occurs as citrate and lactate are converted to bicarbonate by the liver.

27.6.8.5 Hyperkalemia

As blood ages, the extracellular concentration of potassium steadily increases. The amount of extracellular potassium transfused with each unit is usually less than 4 mEq per unit transfused. However, hyperkalemia can develop regardless of the age of the blood when transfusion rates exceed 100 mL/min.

27.6.9 Transfusion-Related Acute Lung Injury

At a death rate of 30–40 deaths per million units transfused, transfusion-related acute lung injury (TRALI) is currently the leading cause of transfusion-related death. Clinical presentation of TRALI, in its severe form, is indistinguishable from adult respiratory distress syndrome (ARDS) and is characterized by acute onset (within minutes to 1–2 h after transfusion), bilateral pulmonary infiltrates, and hypoxia without evidence of congestive heart failure (CHF). However, some specific dissimilarities between the two entities exist: in comparison with ARDS, TRALI is characterized by a much shorter time interval between exposure to the precipitating risk factor (transfusion) and onset of clinical manifestations. TRALI resolves much faster and has a lower mortality rate when compared to ARDS. TRALI usually develops within 6 h (most often less than 2 h) of a transfusion, usually resolves within 24–48 h, and has a mortality rate of approximately 5–10%; however, ARDS does not usually develop until at least 24 h after exposure to 1 of the precipitating factors, has a duration often longer than 72 h, and a mortality approaching 30–60%. Because of increasing awareness and identification of TRALI and reductions in the incidence of infectious and hemolytic complications of transfusions, TRALI is now a primary cause of transfusion-associated mortality reported to the FDA. It can occur after the transfusion of a variety of blood components such as red blood cells, platelets, and FFP but is most often seen after transfusion of the plasma-containing blood components such as FFP and platelets [11].

Most cases of TRALI are due to passive transfer of donor-related anti-leukocyte antibodies directed at HLA or granulocyte-specific antigens on the patient's leukocytes. This promotes priming and activation of a patient's granulocytes leading to their pulmonary sequestration and release of proteases, oxidants, and leukotrienes, which cause alveolar epithelial and microvascular endothelial damage resulting in increased permeability and ultimate development of non-cardiogenic pulmonary edema. The 2-hit model of the specific causative agent in the blood component is unknown, although there is growing evidence implicating bioactive factors or white cell priming lipids: CD40 ligand released by platelets or several reactive lipid-like substances accumulating in red blood cells or platelets during storage. These compounds are referred to as biological response modifiers (BRM); the first insult or hit is generally systemic inflammatory condition secondary to major surgery, sepsis, trauma, or pulmonary aspiration that causes activation of the pulmonary endothelium and polymorphonuclear lymphocytes (PMN) priming leading to their sequestration in the pulmonary vasculature. The second hit occurs when the primed PMNs are activated by the BRM in the transfused component. Therapy for TRALI is generally supportive and includes administration of high FIO2, endotracheal intubation with mechanical ventilatory support in at least 70% of patients and either volume or vasopressor support of hemodynamics. The patient, however, is not at an increased risk of future TRALI reactions with future transfusion [11].

27.6.10 Transfusion-Related Circulatory Overload

Transfusion-related circulatory overload (TACO) has become a more frequently recognized clinical entity, and the most recent estimates suggest incidence rates as high as 11%. TACO has been implicated in 2–27% of the transfusion-related fatalities reported to the FDA, making it the second leading cause of transfusion-related death after TRALI. The actual incidence of perioperative TACO remains poorly defined and is likely much greater than that currently reported in other patient populations. Not only does this failure to appreciate TACO events contribute to our incomplete understanding of TACO epidemiology, but it may also result in suboptimal care delivery and unfavorable outcomes for patients.

According to the Biovigilance Component of the Centers for Disease Control (CDC) National Healthcare Safety Network, the following diagnostic criteria should be met to diagnose TACO—new onset or exacerbation of $\geq$ 3 of the following within 6 h of transfusion [12, 13]:

- Acute respiratory distress (dyspnea, orthopnea, and cough).
- Evidence of positive fluid balance.
- Increased brain natriuretic peptide (BNP).
- Radiographic evidence of pulmonary edema.
- Evidence of left heart failure.
- Increased central venous pressure (CVP).

27.6.11 Transfusion-Associated Graft-Versus-Host Disease

Transfusion-associated graft-versus-host disease (TA-GVHD) occurs when immunocompetent donor lymphocytes are transfused to an HLA-incompatible recipient or host (e.g., immunocompromised patients or patients receiving a blood donation from a relative) who is immunologically incapable of eliminating the donor cells. Among the immunocompromised patients at risk are individuals with congenital cell-mediated immunodeficiencies or Hodgkin's disease, recipients of bone marrow transplants, and patients receiving immunosuppressive therapy. Immunocompetent recipients of directed donations from biologic relatives may also develop TA-GVHD. Clinical manifestations are usually evident within 8–10 days after transfusion and include fever, skin rash, diarrhea, liver dysfunction, and pancytopenia, and death usually occurs within 3–4 weeks as related to bone marrow failure. Irradiation of blood components virtually eliminates the risk of TA-GVHD in susceptible patients.

27.6.12 Immunomodulation

The beneficial immunomodulatory effects of allogeneic transfusion in improving renal allograft survival have been known for many years, but considerable controversy exists regarding the question of adverse immunomodulatory effects related to transfusion. Numerous retrospective reports have suggested an increased incidence of postoperative infection and earlier recurrence of resected malignancies in transfused patients, but the same notion has not been confirmed by the available controlled trials. Critical evaluation of the reports has led some investigators to question whether transfusion causes these deleterious effects or whether the adverse effects are related to factors such as the need for transfusion of blood products. The donor leukocytes are the prime suspect in immunomodulation, and it has been indicated that leukoreduction may decrease postoperative infections in certain patient groups especially those undergoing cardiac surgery [14].

27.6.12.1 Transfusion-Related Immunomodulation

The concept of transfusion-related immunomodulation (TRIM) has been developed in an attempt to explain numerous clinical observations suggesting that RBC transfusion is associated with increased proinflammatory and/or immunosuppressive effects. These changes in immune system potentially may increase morbidity in some patient groups. It seems that the predominant mechanism of TRIM is likely related to an interplay of transfusion effects with the genetic predisposition and the current illnesses of the patient. TRIM has been associated with alterations in immune function in allogeneic transfusion recipients, including decreased helper to suppressor T-lymphocyte ratio, decreased NK cell function, defective antigen presentation, and reduction in cell-mediated immunity [14].

Platelets and vascular endothelial cells also potentially contribute to the "response" as both cell types are highly responsive to inflammatory signals and when activated release significant quantities of potent bioactive mediators.

The "2-insult" model of post-transfusion injury proposes that the first insult (i.e., the patient's underlying inflammatory condition) primes the patient's immune cells or endothelium, and frank inflammation is triggered by a second inflammatory insult—transfusion—resulting in full-scale activation.

27.7 Patient Blood Management

The concept of patient blood management (PBM) has been developed to improve patients' blood health and clinical outcomes. PBM can be defined as "a patient-centered, systematic, evidence-based approach to improve patient outcomes by managing and preserving a patient's own blood, while promoting patient safety and empowerment" [15].

PBM focuses on prevention of blood transfusion through a comprehensive approach to management of anemia and hemostatic derangements, setting evidence-based indications for blood components transfusion and establishing a team-based approach throughout the continuum of care. It can be divided into three periods: preoperative, intraoperative, and postoperative management. The preoperative period predominantly focuses on the diagnosis and management of anemia and its underlying causes. Anemia should especially be treated and corrected before procedures associated with moderate or severe anticipated blood loss (> 500 mL). Very often treatment involves iron supplementation, as iron deficiency is the most common cause of perioperative anemia. Several well-established protocols for perioperative management of anemia demonstrated both safety and efficacy and a reduced need for allogenic blood transfusions.

Intraoperatively, PBM efforts must focus on blood conservation strategies: cell salvage, in which shed blood is returned to the patient, is applicable for surgeries with moderate-to-high anticipated blood loss. Other intraoperative blood conservation strategies include the use of local hemostatic agents and meticulous surgical technique. Throughput the perioperative period, including postoperatively, blood loss, and exposure to allogeneic blood products can be reduced through treatment of coagulopathy, optimization of perioperative coagulation status, and preservation of normal physiology (maintenance of body normothermia, correction of acid–base status). Antifibrinolytic agents, such as tranexamic acid (TXA), have been shown to reduce blood loss during orthopedic, spine, and other types of surgical procedures [16, 17].

The Patient Blood Management International Consensus Conference, European Society of Intensive Care Medicine, American Society of Anesthesiologists, Eastern Association for the Surgery of Trauma, and the American Association of Blood Banks all recommend restrictive transfusion for non-bleeding anemia. For the vast majority of patients with non-bleeding anemia, a restrictive transfusion strategy targeting a hemoglobin concentration of 7–8 g/dL has been proven safe and effective (18).

27.8 Questions and Answers

Questions (Choose the most Appropriate Answer)

1. All are advantages of whole blood transfusion **except**:
   A. Provides of all blood components
   B. Increases exposure to multiple donors
   C. May be better for resuscitation of trauma victims
   D. It is less expensive compared to component therapy

2. A type and screen (T&S) consists of:
   A. Typing the patient's red cells for ABO and Rh blood groups
   B. Takes approximately 10 min to perform
   C. Crossmatch
   D. Screening patient's serum for ABO antibody only
3. Transfusion of red blood cells is indicated:
   A. In symptomatic patients to restore intravascular volume
   B. In symptomatic patients to restore oxygen-carrying capacity
   C. In patients with active bleeding
   D. When the hematocrit is below 26
4. Massive transfusion of Red Blood Cells can result in:
   A. Hyperkalemia
   B. Hypocalcemia
   C. Hypothermia
   D. All above
5. Platelets concentrate…
   A. Should be stored at room temperature
   B. Should be refrigerated
   C. Is indicated only when platelet count is below 50 k/dL
   D. Should be transfused through fluid warmer
6. Cryoprecipitate is indicated…
   A. For fibrinogen replacement therapy
   B. To restore adequate level of factor VIII
   C. To correct R time on TEG
   D. All above
7. The FDA recommends avoiding HES in…
   A. Patients undergoing organ transplant
   B. Patients undergoing elective surgery
   C. Non-critically ill adult patients
   D. Septic patients requiring ICU care
8. Complications of transfusion include:
   A. Febrile reactions
   B. Allergic and anaphylactic reactions
   C. Bacterial contamination
   D. All of the above
9. Transfusion-related acute lung injury (TRALI)…
   A. Is currently the leading cause of transfusion-related death
   B. Is a form of congestive heart failure
   C. Usually develops within days after transfusion
   D. It can only develop after transfusion of platelets
10. Diagnostic criteria for Transfusion-Related Circulatory Overload (TACO) include all except:
   A. Acute respiratory distress (dyspnea, orthopnea, cough)
   B. Evidence of positive fluid balance
   C. Evidence of left heart failure
   D. Anuria

Answers

1. **B**. Increased exposure to multiple donors is not an advantage of whole blood transfusion. Exposure to various complications of transfusion can be increased as the number of donor exposures increases.
2. **A**. A type and screen (T&S) consists of a group of tests performed on a patient's blood specimen. It includes typing the patient's red cells for ABO and Rh blood groups and screening the patient's plasma or serum for the presence of unexpected non-ABO antibodies. ABO group, Rh type and antibody detection screening take approximately 45 min to perform. If the antibody screen is negative and the patient has no past history of unexpected antibodies, the patient may receive red blood cells (RBCs) that are tested for ABO compatibility by performing an immediate spin crossmatch or an electronic/computer crossmatch. ABO- and Rh-compatible blood is selected from the inventory and issued within 5–10 min following immediate spin crossmatch or computer/electronic crossmatch. If the antibody screen is positive, the unexpected antibody or antibodies must first be identified before antigen negative-compatible RBC units can be found and then crossmatched—all of which usually takes several hours.
3. **B**. Transfusion of red blood cells is only indicated for raising the oxygen-carrying capacity, although RBCs also provide volume when given to patients acutely hemorrhaging.
4. **D**. Massive transfusion of red blood cells can result in hyperkalemia, hypocalcemia, and hypothermia:
   - Hyperkalemia—As blood ages, the extracellular concentration of potassium steadily increases. The amount of extracellular potassium transfused with each unit is usually less than 4 mEq per unit transfused. However, hyperkalemia can develop regardless of the age of the blood when transfusion rates exceed 100 mL/min.
   - Hypocalcemia—Transfusion of large volumes of blood or blood products results in hypocalcemia due to calcium binding by the citrate preservative. Clinically significant hypocalcemia, causing cardiac depression, usually occurs when the transfusion rate exceeds 1 unit every 5 min. In such situations intravenous calcium preparations should be administered to restore normal calcium level. Also because citrate is metabolized in the liver, patients with hepatic disease or dysfunction may demonstrate hypocalcemia and require calcium infusion during massive transfusion.
   - Hypothermia—Hypothermia (temperatures below 35 °C) is likely to occur during massive transfusion

therefore all blood products and intravenous fluids should be warmed to normal body temperature. The potential effects of hypothermia include ventricular dysrhythmias, shivering, increased oxygen consumption, cardiac arrest and citrate toxicity secondary to reduced metabolism of citrate and lactate; ventricular arrhythmias progressing to fibrillation often occur at temperatures close to 30 °C. Hypothermia also contributes to coagulopathy: it causes a reversible platelet dysfunction, activity of the coagulation factors and enhances fibrinolysis. Hypothermia also prevents the activation of platelets via traction on the glycoprotein Ib/IX/V complex by von Willebrand factor. In clinical practice, the contribution of hypothermia to coagulopathy may be overlooked because coagulation testing is usually performed at 37 °C. Warming of blood, as well as all other fluids during massive transfusion is essential to help prevent systemic hypothermia.

5. **A**. Platelets should be stored at room temperature (20–24 °C) for up to 5 days with continuous gentle agitation to prevent platelet aggregation. All platelet products should be tested for bacterial contamination prior to transfusion.
6. **A**. Cryoprecipitate is used primarily to augment fibrinogen levels depleted because of massive hemorrhage or disseminated intravascular coagulopathy (DIC). Rarely, it is used for the treatment of congenital or acquired factor XIII deficiency. For fibrinogen replacement therapy, one unit of cryoprecipitate per 10 kg body weight increases plasma fibrinogen by approximately 50–70 mg/dL in the absence of continued consumption or massive bleeding. The minimum hemostatic level of fibrinogen is less than or equal to 80–100 mg/dL, but many experts regard that minimal level as too low. The national guidelines in Germany and Austria recommend higher levels of 150–200 mg/dL in concordance with the Task Force of Advanced Bleeding Care in trauma and the European recommendations in perioperative bleeding. Because cryoprecipitate does not contain factor V, it should not be the sole replacement therapy for disseminated intravascular coagulopathy (DIC), which is almost always associated with a variety of factor deficiencies and thrombocytopenia. Hence, fresh frozen plasma also needs to be administered along with platelet concentrates in those settings where a coagulopathy secondary to DIC is likely occurring.
7. **D**. The US Food and Drug Administration recommends avoiding hydroxyethyl starch (HES) in septic patients requiring the intensive care unit. Evidence suggests that the use of HES in critically ill patients (including septic patients) increases the chance of renal injury and the requirement of renal replacement therapy (RRT) when compared to crystalloids. This effect has also been observed in patients with sepsis requiring critical care and has also been found to increase mortality irrespective of the need for RRT.
8. **D**. Complications of transfusion include febrile reactions, allergic and anaphylactic reactions, and bacterial contamination:
   - Fever is associated with several types of transfusion reactions and may be the first indication of either a hemolytic transfusion reaction (HTR) or administration of a bacterially contaminated blood component. In general transfusion should be stopped and the cause investigated when a rise in temperature of 1 °C or greater develops in association with blood transfusion and is not explained by the patient's clinical condition.
   - Allergic, anaphylactoid, and anaphylactic reactions involve interaction between an allergen (usually a protein in the plasma of the transfused blood component to which the recipient was previously sensitized) and immunoglobulin E (IgE) antibody present on the surface of mast cells and basophils in the tissues and circulation of the recipient. The antigen–antibody interaction takes place on the surface of the cells, activating them and causing release of various mediators of anaphylaxis (leukotriennes, histamine, bradykinin) that cause the signs and symptoms characteristic of the reactions. The severity ranges from mild urticaria to bronchospasm, laryngeal edema, severe hypotension, and possibly death.
   - Bacteria present in stored blood can grow and may produce toxins. Contamination during collection, processing or storage is possible but is most likely to occur at the time of phlebotomy or if the donor has bacteremia associated with unrecognized infection. Administration of a bacterially contaminated blood component may result in fever, tachycardia, hypotension, chills, vomiting, and diarrhea. In some patients, septic shock, oliguria and DIC can develop. Since platelets are stored at room temperature which facilitates bacterial growth, bacteremia is forty times more frequent following platelet administration than transfusion of refrigerated components.
9. **A**. At a death rate of 30–40 deaths per million units transfused, transfusion-related acute lung injury (TRALI) is currently the leading cause of transfusion-related death. It can occur after the transfusion of a variety of blood components such as red blood cells, platelets, and fresh frozen plasma (FFP) but is most often seen after transfusion of the plasma-containing blood components such as FFP and platelets. Clinical presentation of

TRALI, in its severe form is indistinguishable from adult respiratory distress syndrome (ARDS) and is characterized by acute onset (within minutes to 1–2 h after transfusion), bilateral pulmonary infiltrates, and hypoxia without evidence of congestive heart failure.

10. **D**. Anuria is not among the diagnostic criteria for transfusion-related circulatory overload (TACO). According to the Biovigilance Component of the Centers for Disease Control (CDC) National Healthcare Safety Network, the following diagnostic criteria should be met to diagnose TACO: new onset or exacerbation of $\geq$ 3 of the following within 6 h of transfusion:
    - Acute respiratory distress (dyspnea, orthopnea, and cough).
    - Evidence of positive fluid balance.
    - Increased brain natriuretic peptide (BNP).
    - Radiographic evidence of pulmonary edema.
    - Evidence of left heart failure.
    - Increased central venous pressure (CVP).

References

1. Shulman I, Downes K, Sazama K, Maffei L. Pretransfusion compatibility testing for red blood cell administration. Curr Opin Hematol. 2001;8:397–404.
2. Wallis JP, Chapman CE, Orr KE, Clark SC, Forty JR. Effect of WBC reduction of transfused RBCs on postoperative infection rates in cardiac surgery. Transfusion. 2002;42:1127–34.
3. Practice guidelines for perioperative blood management: an updated report by the American Society of Anesthesiologists Task Force on Perioperative Blood Management. Anesthesiol. 2015;122 (2):241–75.
4. Vassallo R, Murphy S. A critical comparison of platelet preparation methods. Curr Opin Hematol. 2006;13:323–30.
5. Downes K, Wilson E, Yomtovian R, Sarode R. Serial measurement of clotting factors in thawed plasma stored for 5 days. Transfusion. 2001;41:570.
6. Kozek-Langenecker SA, Afshari A, Albaladejo P, Santullano CA, De Robertis E, Filipescu DC, et al. Management of severe perioperative bleeding: guidelines from the European Society of Anaesthesiology. Eur J Anaesthesiol. 2013;30:270–382.
7. Myburgh JA, Finfer S, Bellomo R, Billot L, Cass A, Gattas D, et al.; CHEST Investigators, Australian and New Zealand Intensive Care Society Clinical Trials Group. Hydroxyethyl starch or saline for fluid resuscitation in intensive care. N Engl J Med. 2012;367 (20):1901–11.
8. American Association of Blood Banks. Blood transfusion therapy: a physician's handbook. 9th ed. Bethesda: American Association of Blood Banks; 2008. ISBN: 978-3-8055-9105-8.
9. Linden J, Tourault M, Scribner C. Decrease in frequency of transfusion fatalities. Transfusion. 1997;37:243–4.
10. Goodnough L. Risks of blood transfusion. Anesthesiol Clin North Am. 2005;23:241–52.
11. Clifford L, Jia Q, Subramanian A, Yadav H, Wilson GA, Murphy SP, et al. Characterizing the epidemiology of postoperative transfusion-related acute lung injury. Anesthesiology. 2015;122(1):12–20.
12. Centers for Disease Control. National healthcare safety network biovigilance component hemovigilance module surveillance protocol v2.4. 2017. http://www.cdc.gov/nhsn/pdfs/biovigilance/bv-hv-protocol-current.pdf. Accessed 17 Jan 2017.
13. Clifford L, Jia Q, Yadav H, Subramanian A, Wilson GA, Murphy SP, et al. Characterizing the epidemiology of perioperative transfusion-associated circulatory overload. Anesthesiology. 2015;122(1):21–8.
14. Committee on Transfusion Medicine of the American Society of Anesthesiologists, Brauer SD, Cywinski JB, Downes K, Johnson LN, Kindscher JD, Koehntop DE, et al. Questions and answers about blood management. 4th ed. Park Ridge: American Society of Anesthesiologists Committee on Transfusion Medicine; 2006–2007.
15. Shander A, Hardy JF, Ozawa S, et al. A global definition of patient blood management. Anesth Analg. 2022;135(3):476–88.
16. Levy JH, Koster A, Quinones QJ, et al. Antifibrinolytic therapy and perioperative considerations. Anesthesiology. 2018;128 (3):657–70.
17. Devereaux PJ, Marcucci M, Painter TW, et al. Tranexamic acid in patients undergoing noncardiac surgery. N Engl J Med. 2022;386 (21):1986–97.
18. Mueller MM, Van Remoortel H, Meybohm P, et al. Patient blood management: recommendations from the 2018 Frankfurt consensus conference. JAMA. 2019;321(10):983–97.

Complications in Anesthesia

28

Jonathan Korets and Fenghua Li

Abstract

Anesthesia-related complications still exist and account for significant morbidity. This chapter reviews common complications encountered throughout anesthesia practice, its etiology, and management. Trauma results from a variety of anesthesia procedures, such as airway manipulation, vascular access, positioning, and peripheral nerve blockade. Dental injury is the most common upper airway injury, but airway management can cause injury to all upper airway structures including the nostrils, tongue, pharynx, larynx, trachea, and esophagus. Esophageal perforation can lead to death. Vascular access is essential for anesthesia practice, but can lead to multiple complications including arterial and venous thrombosis, thrombophlebitis, sheared catheter, intra-arterial injections, air embolism, cardiac/vascular perforation, pulmonary artery rupture, etc. Anesthesiologists should be aware of preventing peripheral neuropathy resulting from excessive pressure applied to the mask, tourniquet use, positioning, and intraneural injection. Corneal abrasions are the most common eye injury during non-ophthalmologic surgeries, while postoperative vision loss is a rare, but devastating complication. Preventing an operating room (OR) fire is an important patient safety issue and anesthesiologists should use the lowest oxygen concentration in laser airway procedures to avoid airway burns, which is a disaster for the patient. Mild hypothermia is common during general anesthesia due to impaired thermoregulation and cold environmental exposure. However, it is important to keep the patient warm during surgery due to the many adverse effects that hypothermia has, including increased metabolic demand, shivering, increased surgical infection, and delayed wound healing. Both laryngospasms and bronchospasms are severe respiratory complications and require rapid treatment to avoid mortality. Post-obstruction pulmonary edema occurs most common after a laryngospasm and is treated with supportive measures and positive ventilation in severe cases. Anaphylaxis is defined as a serious, generalized or systemic allergic or hypersensitivity reaction that can be life threatening. The most common triggers of anaphylaxis during anesthesia are neuromuscular-blocking agents (NMBAs), antibiotics, latex, hypnotic agents, opioids, and colloids. Immediate recognition of anaphylaxis is a key to preventing mortality. Epinephrine is fthe first-line drug to restore circulation in the event of circulatory collapse. Perioperative pulmonary aspiration occurs after the induction of anesthesia, during a procedure, or in the immediate period after surgery. The American Society of Anesthesiologists (ASA) fasting guideline should be followed to prevent the aspiration of gastric contents.

Keywords

Anesthesia-related trauma • Laryngospasm • Peripheral nerve injury • Postoperative visual loss • Perioperative hypothermia • Operating room fire • Bronchospasm • Postobstructive pulmonary edema • Anaphylaxis • Aspiration

Key Points

1. Anterior nosebleeds are the most common complication; 90% of them occur within the vascular watershed area of the nasal septum, known as Kiesselbach's plexus.
2. The incidence of dental trauma in association with anesthesia is greater than 1:2073. Maxillary upper incisors are most likely to be injured, with

J. Korets · F. Li (✉)
Department of Anesthesiology, SUNY Upstate Medical University, Syracuse, NY, USA
e-mail: lif@upstate.edu

J. Korets
e-mail: koretsj@upstate.edu

M. Argalious et al. (eds.), *Basic Sciences in Anesthesia*,
https://doi.org/10.1007/978-3-031-60203-0_28

a majority of injuries occurring during the laryngoscopy.

3. Damage to pharynx, larynx, trachea, and esophagus is usually associated with the use of a laryngoscope, endotracheal tubeoropharyngeal/nasopharyngeal airway, laryngeal mask airway (LMA) or other supraglottic airway device, insertion of a nasogastric tube, and overzealous use of a suction catheter.
4. The most common etiology of corneal abrasion is simple drying of the corneal surface. It has been reported that dehydration of the cornea is demonstrable after 10 min of exposure without blinking. General anesthesia is associated with a significant reduction in tear production, which exacerbates the problem.
5. The main cause of postoperative visual loss (POVL) is ischemic optic neuropathy (ION) that happens in 83% of cases during spinal surgeries. Posterior ION (PION) occurs more often than anterior ION (AION).
6. The most common complication related to a central venous catheter during a closed claim study is a wire or catheter embolus followed by cardiac tamponade, carotid artery puncture/cannulation, hemothorax, and pneumothorax.
7. According to the American Society of Anesthesiologists (ASA) closed claims database, the most frequent sites of nerve injury are the ulnar nerve (28%), brachial plexus (20%), lumbosacral nerve roots (16%), and spinal cord (13%).
8. The National Institute for Occupational Safety and Health (NIOSH) recommended that waste anesthetic exposure should not exceed 2 ppm of halogenated agents when used alone, or 0.5 ppm of halogenated agents and 25 ppm of nitrous oxide.
9. Hypothermia is the most common perioperative temperature disturbance that results from a combination of exposure to a cold operating room environment and anesthetic-impaired thermoregulation.
10. Most perioperative bronchospasms occur during induction and maintenance of anesthesia, and it is less commonly encountered during emergence and recovery time.
11. The mechanisms of anaphylaxis involve either an immunologic or non-immunologic reaction.
12. Most perioperative aspirations happen immediately after induction of anesthesia; however, pulmonary aspiration can occur prior to induction due to trauma, active vomiting, or preoperative sedation; it also can occur after extubation in the post-anesthesia care unit (PACU), secondary to depressed consciousness from residual anesthetic effect. Silent aspiration can occur even while the patient is intubated with cuffed endotracheal tube

28.1 Introduction

Modern anesthesia has become safer for patients. However, anesthesia-related complications still exist and can expose patients to life-threatening situations. This chapter covers common complications encountered during anesthesia practice. Those complications include: anesthesia-related trauma, health concern due to anesthesia exposure, perioperative temperature disorder, respiratory-related adverse events (bronchospasm, laryngospasm, and obstructive pulmonary edema), anaphylaxis, and aspiration of gastric contents. Emphasis is put on etiology, prevention, and treatment of each complication associated.

28.2 Anesthesia-Related Trauma

Trauma to patients from anesthesia practice is not uncommon; airway and dental trauma as a result from a laryngoscopy and endotracheal tube or laryngeal mask airway (LMA) placement, peripheral neuropathy due to peripheral nerve blocks and inappropriate positioning during surgery, vascular access injuries, and burn injuries are described as follows.

28.2.1 Epistaxis

Epistaxis during anesthesia is a consequence of damage to the nasal mucosa, polyps, turbinates, or other tissues, due to instrumentation in the nasopharynx. Depending on the bleeding site, epistaxis can be classified as an anterior or posterior bleed.

Anterior nosebleeds are the most common. Ninety percent of them occur within the vascular watershed area of the nasal septum, known as Kiesselbach's plexus [1]. Anastomosis of three primary vessels occur in this area: (1) the septal branch of the anterior ethmoidal artery, (2) the lateral nasal branch of the sphenopalatine artery, and (3) the septal branch of the superior labial branch of the facial artery.

Posterior epistaxis arises from the posterolateral branches of the sphenopalatine artery, but may also arise from branches of the carotid artery.

28.2.1.1 Prevention

Vasoconstrictors, such as phenylephrine, should be used to shrink the mucosa of both nasal cavities before passage of the nasopharyngeal temperature probe/airway/endotracheal tube. A small-sized endotracheal tube with a diameter no larger than 7.5 mm for men and 7.0 mm for women should be chosen and be warmed before insertion. The tube should be passed directly back along the floor of the nose, as opposed to cephalad. Resistance may be overcome in the nasal passage by gentle rotation and use of a narrower tube. If not, insertion in the other nasal cavity should be tried. The risk of damage to nasal mucosa may be reduced if a flexible fiberoptic scope is used to view the nasal cavity [2, 3].

Treatment

Nasal bleeding usually responds to first-aid measures, such as compression. This can be achieved by grasping the alae distally and pinching them tightly against the septum, such that the mucosal surfaces are tightly apposed. Pressure should be maintained in this position continuously for 10–15 min without checking to see if the bleeding has stopped.

When epistaxis does not respond to simple measures, the source of the bleeding should be located and treated appropriately. Treatments to be considered include: topical vasoconstriction (oxymetazoline and phenylephrine), nasal packing (nasal tampon or gauze impregnated with petroleum jelly), posterior gauze packing, use of a balloon system (including a modified Foley catheter), electric cautery, and arterial ligation or embolization [4]. Consultation from an otolaryngologist is appropriate when bleeding is refractory, and complications (such as persistent bleeding) lead to hemodynamic instability, or specialized treatment (balloon placement, arterial ligation, and angiographic arterial embolization) is required.

28.2.2 Dental Trauma

The incidence of dental trauma in association with anesthesia is greater than 1:2073 [5]. Maxillary upper incisors are most likely to be injured, with most injuries occurring during the laryngoscopy. Dental injuries can also be caused by insertion, removal, and biting of the airway devices. These are common in patients who had difficult intubations in the past, have periodontal disease, have fixed dental work, and in small children with loose teeth.

28.2.2.1 Prevention

Preexisting dental conditions should be accurately documented, and the risk of dental injury should be discussed with the patient and family members during the perioperative period. Dental protection devices should be considered during the laryngoscopy, but keeping in mind that they may also hinder visualization. Use of alternative intubating equipment (trachlight/video laryngoscope) can help to minimize dental trauma.

28.2.2.2 Management

An immediate dental consultation should be sought when dental trauma is suspected. Serious injuries include subluxation, fracture, and avulsion of the teeth. If a fragment of tooth or restoration is displaced, it should be retrieved. Fluoroscopic pictures should be obtained to ensure no fragments are retained in the airway or in the lungs (antero-posterior [AP], lateral view). If replantation is planned within an hour, completely avulsed teeth should be saved in moist gauze or in normal saline.

28.2.3 Pharynx, Larynx, Trachea, and Esophagus Injuries

The most frequent sites of airway injury are the larynx (33%), pharynx (19%), esophagus (18%), trachea (15%), and temporomandibular joint (10%) according to an American Society of Anesthesiologists (ASA) closed claim study [6]. Damage is usually associated with the use of a laryngoscope, endotracheal tube, oropharyngeal/nasopharyngeal airway, LMA, or other supra-glottic airway device, insertion of a nasogastric tube, and overzealous use of a suction catheter.

Laryngeal Injuries

Laryngeal injuries include vocal cord paralysis, granuloma, arytenoid dislocation, and hematoma.

Pharyngeal Injuries

Pharyngeal perforation, contusions, localized infection, sore throat, and miscellaneous injuries (foreign body, burn, hematoma, and diminished taste sensation) are pharyngeal injuries. All claimed deaths due to a pharyngeal injury were related to the development of mediastinitis, which occurred from perforation.

Esophageal Injuries

Esophageal perforation usually occurs from esophageal intubation or placement of a nasogastric tube, use of an esophageal dilator or esophageal stethoscope, or a laryngoscope placed by the surgeon for conduct of surgery. Perforation of the esophagus is associated with poor outcomes, including delayed onset of subcutaneous emphysema, pneumothorax, fever, or sepsis which may be present.

Tracheobronchial Injuries

Perforation or rupture (as evidenced by a cough, sore throat, fever, dysphagia dyspnea when mediastinitis or pneumonia develop), granuloma, stenosis, and tracheomalacia.

Temporomandibular Joint Injuries

Pain and/or dislocation.

28.2.3.1 Prevention

Prevention results from gentleness and avoiding repeated use of techniques, particularly blind ones, when they prove to be ineffective. Unfamiliar techniques should not be used for the first time in an emergency situation.

28.2.3.2 Treatment

A high index of suspicion by the anesthesiologist and early signs of injury should be sought with vigilance. In esophageal/tracheal perforations, signs and symptoms may be delayed. Supportive management and appropriate consults with an ear-nose-throat (ENT), thoracic surgery, and other surgical specialties during the perioperative period must be done.

28.2.4 Eyes

Eye injuries range from simple corneal abrasion to blindness. They account for approximately 3% of cases reported in the closed claims database of the American Society of Anesthesiologists.

28.2.4.1 Corneal Abrasion

Corneal abrasion is the most common ocular complication following general anesthesia, accounting for approximately 35% of claims related to ocular injuries. In approximately 16% of the claims, corneal abrasions resulted in permanent injury [7, 8].

Potential causes of injury include chemical injury (skin antiseptic solutions); direct trauma during anesthesia; direct pressure from the surgeon, anesthetist, or instruments; injury from insertion of lubricant; and self-infliction (most associated with eye rubbing). Some studies have shown increased risk factors for corneal abrasions in the perioperative period include non-supine surgical position, Trendelenburg position, longer duration of anesthesia, and age [9, 10].

Pathophysiology

The most common etiology is simple drying of the corneal surface. It has been reported that dehydration of the cornea is demonstrable after 10 min of exposure without blinking. General anesthesia is associated with a significant reduction in tear production, which exacerbates the problem.

Clinical Presentation

It typically presents with acute ocular pain accompanied by the sensation of a foreign body in the eye. Other manifestations include photophobia, tearing, blurred vision, and blepharospasm.

Prevention

Unanimously accepted methods to prevent corneal abrasions during anesthesia are lacking:

1. The efficacy of eye ointment probably depends on the specifics of the ointment used. Petroleum-based ointments are associated with patient complaints regarding blurred vision and decreased visual acuity, which may stimulate rubbing of the eyes, subsequently causing a self-inflicted corneal abrasion. Methylcellulose drops are less likely to be associated with these complaints but have been reported to virtually “glue” the patient’s eyelids together.
2. Hypoallergenic paper tape can be used to secure the patient’s eyelids together, but even this approach has the potential to induce a corneal injury during removal.
3. Eyepads and goggles have been advocated, but there is no guarantee that the eyelids remain closed, and it has been suggested that the presence of the eyepad increases the risk of a corneal abrasion if the eyelids should open during the anesthetic period.

Treatment

This involves immediate consultation and confirmation of the diagnosis by ophthalmologic examination, which typically involves a slit lamp examination after instillation of fluorescein. Some hospitals have adopted protocols established by both the anesthesia and ophthalmology departments to work up patients with presumed corneal abrasions. Most algorithms begin with anesthesia staff using proparacaine ophthalmic drops to result in immediate relief of pain, confirming the presumptive diagnosis of corneal abrasion. Treatments with topical antibiotics and artificial tears may then be used for up to three days [9, 10].

28.2.4.2 Postoperative Visual Loss

Postoperative visual loss (POVL) is a rare but devastating complication. Patients may experience a range of vision changes, from transient blurring or loss of vision to permanent bilateral blindness. Transient visual changes are most commonly attributed to corneal abrasion; however, the most common causes of permanent POVL are central artery occlusion, ischemic optic neuropathy, and cerebral vision loss. Patients undergoing spine and cardiac surgery are at a higher risk of POVL. The incidence is about 3.09/10,000 to 9.4/10,000 in spinal surgical patients [11] while the cardiac surgical patient has an incidence of 6/10,000 to 8.64/10,000 [11]. POVL has recently been reported to have occurred in a patient who underwent robotic-assisted prostatectomy in the steep Trendelenburg position. Since the majority of reported POVL cases (67%) occurred in spine surgeries [12], our focus will be on POVL in spinal surgery in the prone position.

Types of POVL and Clinical Presentation

The main cause of permanent POVL is ischemic optic neuropathy (ION), which happens in 83% of cases during spinal surgeries [12]. Posterior ION (PION) occurs more often than anterior ION (AION). Other causes include central retinal artery occlusion (CRAO) and cortical blindness.

- **PION**: The most common form of POVL is PION that results from infarction of the optic nerve posterior to the lamina cribrosa. It manifests as a sudden onset of painless vision loss and can affect both eyes in two-third of cases. In patients with PION, physical exam shows poor pupil reaction to light, no light perception, central scotomas, and altitudinal vision defect. However, a fundoscopic exam is initially normal but optic nerve pallor and atrophy appear 4–6 weeks later.
- **AION**: It occurs at the optic nerve head anterior to the lamina cribrosa and happens primarily after cardiac and spine surgery. Patients with AION more often present with vision loss after a period of normal vision. Examination shows poor pupillary reaction to light, complete blindness, altitudinal field defect, and central scotomas. A funduscopic exam reveals a swollen optic disc with or without peripapillary hemorrhage at the optic disc margin.
- **CRAO**: It unilaterally occurs in the affected eye and is associated with periorbital trauma in surgeries done in the prone position. Patients complain of vision loss after waking from anesthesia, and a funduscopic exam reveals retinal whitening and pathognomonic cherry red spots in the macula.
- **Cortical Blindness**: It can occur in patients with a high risk of emboli to posterior cerebral arteries.

Risk Factors

The mechanisms that cause ION remain unclear. However, decreased optic nerve perfusion due to increased interstitial fluid accumulation and venous outflow reduction in the globe has been hypothesized to be the mechanism of ION [13]. A POVL study group in 2012 has identified risk factors that are contributory in spinal surgery patients [13]. The male sex, obesity, use of a Wilson frame, a long anesthesia time, greater estimated blood loss, and decreased percent colloid administration are risk factors. Anemia and hypotension were not confirmed to be risk factors of POVL in this study.

Prevention and Perioperative Management

To enhance the awareness, and to reduce frequency of POVL associated to spine surgery, the ASA published a practice advisory on POVL in 2012 and an updated version in 2019 [14]. Patients who undergo spine surgery in position prone and those who have long procedures and experience substantial blood losses are at high risk. High-risk patients should be identified preoperatively and POVL risk should be discussed with these patients. Intraoperatively, a patient's head should be positioned at or above the level of the heart whenever possible, and be maintained in neutral position. Direct compression of globes, hypotension, and severe anemia (hematocrit [HCT] < 28) should be avoided. Staging procedures may be considered in patients who have experienced significant blood loss. Colloid along with crystalloid is recommended for fluid resuscitation. Postoperatively, the anesthesiologists should check a high-risk patient's vision and be vigilant to its occurrence. An urgent ophthalmology consult should be obtained if any visual loss presents postoperatively. Patient hemodynamics and head position should be optimized until the patient is seen by an ophthalmologist. Consideration for magnetic resonance imaging (MRI) and computed tomography (CT) scan of the head to rule out intracranial causes should be taken.

28.2.5 Vascular Complications

28.2.5.1 Central Venous Access

Patient injuries from mechanical, infectious, and thrombotic complications are estimated to occur in more than 15% of patients in whom central venous catheters are used. Complications of central venous access and pulmonary artery catheter (PAC) are shown in ◘ Boxes 28.1 and 28.2, respectively.

The most common complication related to a central catheter during a closed claim study is a wire or catheter embolus followed by cardiac tamponade, carotid artery puncture/cannulation, hemothorax, and pneumothorax. The other complications involve hydrothorax/pleural effusion, fluid extravasation in the neck, air embolism, pulmonary artery rupture, a miscellaneous vessel injury (arteriovenous fistula, aorta injury, and subclavian artery injury resulting in arterial thrombosis, arterial aneurysm, and neck hematoma), or a non-vessel injury (phrenic nerve palsy and atrial fibrillation). The most common risk factors observed with vascular access complications include a body mass index (BMI) > 30 or < 20, prior surgery or prior radiotherapy of the vascular region, or prior catheterization of the region [15].

Prevention of complications related to central venous access [16]:

- **Choice of Insertion Site**—Internal jugular (IJ) and subclavian venous catheterization carry similar risks of mechanical complications. Subclavian catheterization is more likely than IJ catheterization to be complicated by pneumothorax and hemothorax, whereas IJ catheterization is more likely to be associated with an arterial puncture. Hematomas and arterial punctures are common during femoral venous catheterizations. Selection of the subclavian site appears to reduce the risk of infectious complications. Subclavian venous catheterization carries the lowest risk of catheter-related thrombosis.
- **Insertion Technique**
  1. Preparation: One should use maximal sterile-barrier precautions, including a mask, a cap, a sterile gown, sterile gloves, and a large sterile drape to reduce infection.
  2. Minimize the number of insertion attempts, since the incidence of mechanical complications after three or more insertion attempts is six times the rate after one attempt [15].
  3. Use of ultrasound guidance: The use of ultrasound guidance has been promoted as a method for reducing the risk of complications during central venous catheterization.
  4. Pressure transduction of introducer needle prior to the use of introducer to avoid arterial injury.
  5. Maintenance of the insertion site and catheter: Changing the end cap with each use is beneficial to reduce infection. Every catheter should be removed as soon as it is no longer needed, since the probability of catheter-related infections increases over time.
  6. Catheter hubs should be occluded at all times, and the patient should be placed in Trendelenburg's position during insertion to prevent air embolism.
  7. A chest X-ray is mandatory to confirm the catheter position and to rule out pneumothorax.

Management of acute complications:

1. Artery cannulation: vascular surgery should be consulted for management.
2. Air embolism: If an air embolism occurs, the patient should be placed in Trendelenburg's position with a left lateral decubitus tilt to prevent the movement of air into the right ventricular outflow tract; 100% oxygen should be administered to speed the resorption of the air. If a catheter is located in the heart, aspiration of the air should be attempted.
3. Tension pneumothorax: an immediate needle thoracotomy, followed by chest tube placement, should be done to relieve pressure. Thoracic surgery should be consulted immediately.
4. Pulmonary artery rupture: Management should focus on resuscitation and immediate control of the hemorrhage. The first priority is ensuring adequate oxygenation and ventilation, which may require endobronchial intubation with either a single- or double-lumen endotracheal tube to selectively ventilate and protect the unaffected lung. In addition, positive end-expiratory pressure (PEEP) applied to the affected lung may help control hemorrhage. Any anticoagulation should be reversed, unless the patient must remain on cardiopulmonary bypass. A bronchoscopy is performed to localize and control the site of bleeding. A bronchial blocker may be guided into the involved bronchus to tamponade the bleeding and prevent contamination of the uninvolved lung.

Box 28.1 Complications of Central Venous Access

- **Mechanical**:
  1. Vascular injuries: Arterial puncture, hemothorax, cardiac tamponade
  2. Respiratory compromise: Airway compression from a hematoma, tracheal and laryngeal injury, pneumothorax
  3. Nerve injury
  4. Arrhythmias
  5. Subcutaneous/mediastinal emphysema
- **Thromboembolic**:
  – Venous thrombosis, pulmonary embolism, arterial thrombosis and embolism (air, clot), catheter or guidewire embolism
- **Infectious**:
  – Insertion site infection, catheter infection, bloodstream infection, endocarditis
- **Misinterpretation of data**
- **Misuse of equipment**

Box 28.2 Complications of Pulmonary Artery Catheter Use

- **During catheterization**:
  - Arrhythmias, ventricular fibrillation, right bundle branch block, and complete heart block
- **Catheter residence**:
  - Catheter knots, thromboembolism, pulmonary infarction, infection, endocarditis, endocardial damage, cardiac valve injury, pulmonary artery rupture (0.02–0.2%), and pulmonary artery pseudoaneurysm
- **Misinterpretation of data**
- **Misuse of equipment**

28.2.5.2 Arterial Cannulation

Complications after arterial cannulations include distal ischemia, pseudoaneurysm, arteriovenous fistula, hemorrhage, hematoma, arterial embolization, local infection, sepsis, peripheral neuropathy, misinterpretation of data, and misuse of equipment [17].

Prevention and Treatment

Preventative measures to avoid complications include using ultrasound guidance for placement, post-placement imaging to confirm catheter tip placement, measuring intra-luminal pressure, and checking oxygen saturation. Early identification of accidental arterial placement [18, 19]. Vigilance should be maintained during and post-cannulation for complications and early management. Management algorithms have proposed that immediate treatment may include removal of the catheter and compression of the vessel [19, 20]. Vascular surgery consultation should be obtained to manage complications.

28.2.6 Neurologic Injuries

28.2.6.1 Injuries of Mask Use

A mask is an essential tool to ventilate and oxygenate the patient, but it is not devoid of any complications related to use. Excessive pressure and inappropriate application of the mask to a patient's face can result in soft tissue damage, injuries to the eyes and innervation of the face, and temporomandibular joints (TMJ) dislocation:

1. **Eye**: Corneal abrasion, retinal artery occlusion or blindness
2. **Nerves**: Mandibular branch of facial nerve leading to transient facial nerve paralysis. Mental nerves causing lower lip numbness.
3. **Temporomandibular Joint**: Lifting pressure on angle of mandible can sometimes subluxate the TMJ.

Prevention and Treatment

Appropriate use of masks during mask ventilation is the key to avoiding complications. It is important to ensure that the mask does not compress the eyes, and measures should be taken to avoid any unnecessary pressure against the face.

28.2.6.2 Nerve Injuries from Tourniquet Use During the Surgery

Tourniquets, including pneumatic Esmarch bandage tourniquets, are used by orthopedic surgeons to decrease blood loss and to provide favorable operating conditions during extremity surgery. However, its use can result in nerve injuries, ranging from paresthesia to total paralysis, if it is not used appropriately. Mechanic trauma due to tourniquet use and ischemia have attributed to nerve injuries. The upper limbs are more prone to nerve injury than the lower extremities. The radial nerve is the most vulnerable, followed by the ulnar and medial nerves in the upper limb, while nerve injury in the lower extremities most often involves the sciatic nerve [21].

Pathophysiology

Mechanical pressure under the cuff plays a more important role than ischemia in a nerve injury [21]. Nerve compression causes intraneural microvascular abnormalities and edema formation, and these subsequently compromise local tissue nutrition, resulting in axonal degeneration. Axial compression of the nerve causes damage at the nodes of Ranvier. Tissue trauma is most marked at the proximal and distal edges of a compression tourniquet, where shear stress forces are maximal [21].

Prevention

For prevention of nerve injury from tourniquet use:

- The lowest inflation pressure that causes arterial occlusion should be used. Pressure 50–100 mm of Hg above systolic is used for the arm; double systolic blood pressure is for the thigh; alternatively, standard pressures for the arm 200–250 mm Hg, leg 250–350 mm Hg (large cuffs are recommended for larger limbs instead of increasing pressure).
- Minimal duration of tourniquet should be used. The absolute maximum duration is 3 h (recovers in 5–7 days) but duration generally should not exceed 2 h.
- All tourniquets should undergo regular maintenance checks to ensure dependability and no faulty equipment. Calibration should be checked biweekly against a

mercury thermometer, and three-month maintenance is recommended.

- A tourniquet should be applied only to a healthy limb or with caution to an unhealthy limb.
- The size of tourniquet to be used on an arm is 10 cm, 15 cm for a leg, or wider in large arms and legs. Cuffs should exceed the circumference of the extremity by 7–15 cm, and should be positioned at the point of maximum circumference of the limb.
- Padding should be at least two layers of orthopedic wool. Prevent soaking of the wool after skin preparation.
- Keep the temperature cool, if feasible; keep tissues moist; and avoid heating (e.g., hot lights) on avascular limb.
- The duration, inflation pressure, and deflation duration need to be documented.

Management

Unresolved nerve injuries should be managed by consulting a neurologist within 48 h.

28.2.6.3 Perioperative Peripheral Neuropathies from Surgical Positioning

Nerve injury related to positioning while under anesthesia is a significant source of morbidity for patients. According to the ASA closed claims database, the most frequent sites of nerve injury are the ulnar nerve (28%), brachial plexus (20%), lumbosacral nerve roots (16%), and spinal cord (13%). Surgical positioning can result in peripheral neuropathies. The ulnar neuropathy is most common and is associated with general anesthesia. The most common nerve injury in a lower extremity associated with the lithotomy positioning is the superficial peroneal nerve that is vulnerable to compression from stirrups along the lateral aspects of the knee.

Mechanism of Nerve Injury

Nerve injury related to positioning during general anesthesia results from excessive pressure/compression, ischemia, stretching of nerves, toxins, metabolic/microvascular derangements due to coexisting diseases (preexisting neuropathy, diabetes, hypertension, smoking, and alcohol dependence), and direct trauma of the nerve and unknown factors. Other risk factors also included the male gender, a very thin or obese body habitus, and a hospital stay greater than 14 days.

During cardiac surgery, brachial plexus injury (C8-T1) can occur. It is postulated that excessive sternal retraction is a commonly accepted risk factor.

Prevention of perioperative peripheral neuropathy: The ASA published a practice advisory on how to prevent neuropathy in 2018 [22]. The recommendations are summarized in Box 28.3.

Management

Within 48 h, unresolved nerve injuries should be managed effectively by a consulting neurologist and followed up with nerve conduction studies to rule out preexisting neuropathy.

Box 28.3 ASA Recommendations for Prevention of Peripheral Neuropathy

1. A complete preoperative history and physical assessment will establish that patients can comfortably tolerate the anticipated operative position and identify preexisting illness
2. Positioning approaches for the upper extremities:
    1. Arm abduction in supine patients should be limited to 90°.
    2. Patients positioned prone may comfortably tolerate arm abductions greater than 90°.
    3. In supine position with arm on the arm board: The arm should be placed on a padded arm board. the upper extremity should be positioned to decrease pressure on the medial posterior condylar groove of the humerus.
    4. Either supination or the neutral forearm positions facilitates this action.
    5. For a supine patient with arms tucked at their side, the forearm should be in a neutral position and prolonged pressure on the radial nerve in the spiral groove of the humerus should be avoided. Hyperextension of the elbow beyond the range that is comfortable during the preoperative assessment may stretch the median nerve.
    6. Periodic perioperative assessments may ensure maintenance of the desired position.
3. Positioning strategies for the lower extremities:
    1. Positions that stretch the hamstring muscle group beyond the range that is comfortable during the preoperative assessment may stretch the sciatic nerve.
    2. As the sciatic nerve or its branches cross both the hip and the knee joints, limited extension and flexion of these joints should be considered. Neither extension nor flexion of the hip increases the risk of femoral neuropathy.
    3. Prolonged pressure on the peroneal nerve at the fibular head should be avoided.
4. Protective padding should be applied on arm boards. Chest rolls should be used in the laterally positioned patients, which might decrease

the risk of upper extremity neuropathy. Padding at the fibular head (peroneal nerve) may decrease the risk of peroneal neuropathy. Complications from inappropriate use of padding (e.g., too tightly padded) may increase the risk of perioperative neuropathy.

5. Equipment: The use of an adequately fit and properly functioning automated blood pressure cuff on the arm placed above the antecubital fossa does not change the risk of upper extremity neuropathy. Shoulder braces used during a steep, head-down position may increase the risk of perioperative neuropathies.
6. Postoperative assessment: A simple postoperative follow-up and assessment of extremity nerve function may lead to early recognition of peripheral neuropathies.
7. Documentation of specific perioperative positioning actions may be useful for continuous improvement processes and may result in improvements to patient care.
8. During open cardiac surgeries proper vigilance should be taken to minimize sternal retraction during internal mammary artery harvesting to reduce brachial plexus injury. If possible asymmetric retraction needs to be avoided. The head and neck should be maintained in a neutral position.

28.2.6.4 Nerve Injury Related to Peripheral Nerve Block

The incidence of a nerve injury from a peripheral nerve block is low, ranging from 2:1000 to 4:1000. As per the ASA closed claim analysis of 2008, nerve damage is the most common complication associated with peripheral nerve block.

The common nerves damaged in descending order are the brachial plexus, median, ulnar, and radial.

Mechanisms of nerve injury include mechanical and injection injury (traumatic), vascular (ischemic), chemical (neurotoxic), and inflammatory injuries.

Risk factors for peripheral nerve injury includes anesthetic risk factors, surgical factors, and patient factors:

- Anesthetic factors—Needle injury, intraneural injection, catheter trauma, hematoma, epinephrine use, and local anesthetic toxicity.
- Surgical factors—Mechanical stretch, direct trauma, malpositioning, hematoma, infection, and tourniquet use.
- Patient factors—Diabetes, multiple sclerosis, chemotherapy, polyneuropathies, obesity, and the male gender.

Prevention

Avoidance of deliberate trauma to nerves, including intraneural injection, is a key safety principle of regional anesthesia. Intraneural injections can cause direct needle and injection trauma, rupture of the perineurium, and loss of the protective environment within fascicle, with consequent myelin and axonal degeneration. Although ultrasound guidance has reduced the rate of local anesthetic systemic toxicity (LAST), it has not proven to reduce the incidence of peripheral nerve injuries associated with regional anesthesia [23]. However, there is evidence of ultrasound guidance reducing the incidence and intensity of hemidiaphragmatic paresis, but not eliminating it [24].

28.2.7 Burns

Burns during anesthesia can be secondary to surgical fire, explosions, and electrocautery use. Surgical fires can occur with or without warning; they generate tremendous heat, oftentimes leading to burns. The fire triangle includes that of an oxidizer, fuel, and an ignition source [25]. A common characteristic of a surgical fire is the use of supplemental oxygen via an open delivery system into an enclosed space (drapes), thus creating an oxygen-rich atmosphere close to an ignition source:

- Oxidizer: oxygen and nitrous oxide supports combustion.
- Fuel: cotton pledgets, endotracheal tube (ETT), gauze, OR drapes, and patient's hair act as fuel.
- Heat/ignition source: laser, electrosurgical unit (ESU), fiberoptic cables with light source, and defibrillators can provide the source of ignition.

28.2.7.1 Prevention

Education, training, and simulation drills are important in preventing OR surgical fires. The anesthesiologist should identify an oxygen-rich environment and assess the need by considering the risk benefit ratio to minimize the fraction of inspired oxygen (FiO2). During laser surgeries, the surgeon needs to minimize misdirection of the laser both inside and outside of the operative field. The patient's eyes should be covered with wet gauze pads only (no tape), plus laser-safe goggles, laser-safe ETT, and use of jet ventilation. The pooling of flammable solutions should be avoided; sufficient drying time should be allowed, and fire-resistant OR drapes must be used. With use of a bipolar ESU, move the cautery device away from patient/surgical drapes when not in use. Fire secondary to the use of carbon dioxide absorbents can be avoided by replacing desiccated absorbent.

28.2.7.2 Management of Operating Room Fire

- **Airway Fire Management** [25]: Eliminate all airway gases, extract ETT, extinguish the fire by flooding the area with normal saline, evaluate/remove debris, resume bag mask ventilation with room air if possible, examination with non-flexible laryngoscopy/bronchoscopy to look for tracheal tube/fragments, assess injury, and remove residual debris.
- **OR Drape Fire**: A fire extinguisher is to be used on OR drapes, as they are water resistant.
- **Carbon Dioxide Absorbent Fire**: Disconnect anesthesia circuit from patient, cease all fresh gas flow, maintain ventilation with ambu bag and replace CO2 absorbent canister.

28.3 Chronic Inhalational Anesthetic Exposure

Although the modern operating room is equipped with a scavenging system, OR personnel, including the anesthesiologist and nurses, may be at risk of exposure to trace anesthetic gases. Operating room contamination by waste inhalational anesthetics can be the result of a faulty flow-control valve, anesthesia circuit, hospital vacuum, scavenging system, unfitting masks, flushing breathing circuits, filling vaporizers, tracheal tubes without cuffs, and LMAs. However, no studies have proven that exposure to a trace concentration of currently used inhalational anesthetics including isoflurane, sevoflurane, desflurane, and nitrous oxide result in adverse health effects. Recent studies have suggested that exposure to high concentrations of anesthetic gases can result in DNA toxicity [26–31].

In 1977, the National Institute for Occupational Safety and Health (NIOSH) recommended [32] that waste anesthetic exposure should not exceed two parts per million (ppm) of halogenated agents when used alone, or 0.5 ppm of halogenated agents and 25 ppm of nitrous oxide. Gauger et al. found that female pediatric anesthesiologists were at an increased risk for spontaneous abortion due to the higher risk for exposure to anesthetic gases [33]. Rowland et al. [34, 35] reported there was reduced fertility and increased spontaneous abortions among female dental assistants exposed to nitrous oxide delivered to patients without the scavenge system. If nitrous oxide is used as a sole anesthetic agent, the U.S. Occupational Safety and Health Administration (OSHA) [36] recommends that no worker should be exposed to more than 8 h of concentrations greater than 25 ppm during anesthetic administration. For halogenated agents, no worker should be exposed to concentrations of those gases greater than 2 ppm for a period of more than 1 h. OSHA has no required standards but offers guidelines which recommend pre-placement medical exams with annual follow-up, a system for employees to report symptoms believed to be due to anesthetic gas exposure, documentation of an acute exposures, and educate employees on the possible reproductive effects.

28.3.1 Prevention

NIOSH recommends scavenging of waste anesthetic gases as work practices to reduce contamination and monitoring of trace anesthetic gases. However, OSHA recommends in its manual "Waste Anesthetic Gases: Work Place Exposure" that institutions should have a waste anesthetic gas management program including scavenging of waste gases, work practices to minimize exposure, and monitoring of trace gases. By maintaining the anesthesia machines and the OR ventilating system, the OR anesthesia gas exposure can be kept way below the recommended concentration.

28.4 Perioperative Temperature Disorders

28.4.1 Hypothermia

Normal body temperature is maintained between 36 and 38 °C. Core temperature monitoring sites include the pulmonary artery, tympanic membrane, distal end of esophagus, and the nasopharynx. Hypothermia is defined as the body core temperature (Tc) less than 36 °C. Hypothermia is classified into mild (32–35 °C or 32–36 °C), moderate (28–32 °C), and severe hypothermia (< 28 °C). In general, perioperative mild hypothermia is the Tc between 34 °C and 36 °C. It is the most common perioperative temperature disturbance that results from a combination of exposure to a cold operating room environment and anesthetic-impaired thermoregulation.

Mechanisms of hypothermia under general anesthesia:

- **Phase 1 (Internal Redistribution)**: Redistribution of heat from warm central core to cold periphery leading to 0.5–1 °C drop. The colder the skin temperature, the greater the central core temperature drops.
- **Phase 2 (Environmental Heat Loss)**: As normal physiologic response is depressed during anesthesia, phase 2 commences approximately after 1 h. As the core temperature decreases at a slower rate and proceeds in a linear manner as heat lost from the body through radiation, evaporation, conduction, and convection exceeds heat production. Compared to other mechanisms, radiation contributes the most heat loss at 60%.
- **Phase 3 (Core Temperature Plateau Phase)**: After 3–5 h, phase 3 commences as an equilibrium is reached

where heat loss is matched by heat production and thermo-regulated vasoconstriction commences to function.

Adverse effects of perioperative hypothermia [37] are as follows:

- Cardiovascular morbidity. Mild hypothermia can result in tachycardia, hypertension, increased peripheral vascular resistance, and myocardial ischemia. Moderate and severe hypothermia causes bradycardia and cardiac arrhythmias.
- Left shift of the hemoglobin-oxygen saturation curve that leads to the impairment of oxygen release to tissue.
- Hypothermia causes coagulation dysfunction and increases blood transfusion requirements.
- Delayed drug metabolism and prolonged recovery.
- Shivering.
- Surgical site infection and delayed wound healing.
- Thermal discomfort.

28.4.1.1 Prevention of Perioperative Hypothermia

Methods to warm patients include:

1. Increase ambient OR temperature.
2. Preoperative skin warming to minimize the heat redistribution.
3. Intraoperative temperature monitoring under general anesthesia > 30 min.
4. Use of patient warming systems, such as forced-air and resistive heating, fluid warmers, to warm fluids being given to patients.

28.4.2 Post-anesthetic Shivering and Its Management

Postoperative shivering is a common complication following general anesthesia. Its etiology is still not clear. Tremor from thermogenic shivering is usually tonic (continuous). The mechanism for thermogenic shivering is related to increased neuronal efferent outflow to skeletal muscle and subsequent feedback oscillations due to muscle spindle stretch reflexes. Non-thermogenic shivering is clonic and has been attributed to uninhibited spinal reflexes, decreased sympathetic activity, pyrogen release, adrenal suppression, and pain [38]. Clonic tremors are associated with recovery from volatile anesthetics. Shivering causes unpleasant discomfort that can be worse than pain for some patients. It increases oxygen consumption roughly 100% in proportion to intraoperative heat loss. However, myocardial ischemia is poorly correlated with shivering, suggesting that an increased metabolic rate is not the primary cause of this complication. Postoperative shivering possibly aggravates wound pain by stretching incisions. Treatment of postoperative shivering consists of warming patient with forced-air systems and medications including meperidine, clonidine, physostigmine, ketanserin, tramadol, and magnesium sulfate.

28.4.3 Non-malignant Hyperthermia

Perioperative hyperthermia is defined as core body temperature that is more than 38 °C. It occurs when the body produces or absorbs more heat than it can dissipate. It is more dangerous than a comparable degree of hypothermia. It results from a variety of causes outlined as follows:

- **Environmental**: very high ambient temperature, excessive warming by air warming blankets/ mattresses and warm IV fluids.
- **Drug-related**: neuroleptic malignant syndrome, serotonin syndrome, antibiotics, methylene dioxymethamphetamine agonists (ecstasy), cocaine, phencyclidine, LSD, and anticholinergic medications.
- **Patient-related**: sepsis, transfusion reactions, hyperthyroidism, pheochromocytoma, pulmonary embolus, and brainstem/hypothalamic injury

28.4.3.1 Consequences of Hyperthermia

Hyperthermia results in increased oxygen consumption/ carbon dioxide production and metabolic acidosis secondary to increased metabolic rate. It also causes tachycardia, hypertension, and arrhythmias secondary to increased sympathetic tone. Hyperthermia can produce generalized rigidity leading to rhabdomyolysis and hyperkalemia. Enzymatic deactivation due to hyperthermia leads to disseminated intravascular coagulation.

28.4.3.2 Management of Non-malignant Hyperthermia

Patient history should be reviewed and examined for possible causes. Measures for hemodynamic support need to be implemented and the underlying cause must be treated. Active cooling efforts such as lowering room temperature; cool air blower; cool IV fluids; ice in axilla, neck, or groin, should be initiated. Patient can be treated with antipyretic medication such as acetaminophen. Cardiac pulmonary bypass can be considered for rapid cooling for persistent hyperthermia.

28.5 Intraoperative Bronchospasm

A bronchospasm is a bronchoconstriction resulting from the contraction of the smooth muscle of bronchi and bronchioles. Bronchospasm results in the narrowing and shortening of the airway, and can cause hypoxia or even death. It can present alone, or as a component of a severe underlying pathology, such as anaphylaxis. A bronchospasm is the main feature of reactive airway disease including asthma and chronic obstructive pulmonary disease (COPD). Most perioperative bronchospasms occur during induction and maintenance of anesthesia, and it is less commonly encountered during emergence and recovery time. A bronchospasm during induction is most commonly caused by airway irritation, often related to intubation. Other triggers include recent upper airway infection, anesthetics, and drugs that cause histamine release, smoking, aspiration, and anaphylaxis.

28.5.1 Incidence

The overall incidence of bronchospasm during anesthesia is 1.7 per 1000 cases. Mamie et al. reported the incidence of perioperative bronchospasm of 1.6% [39] in pediatric patients. But a higher incidence was reported in both pediatric and adult patients with history of respiratory disease.

28.5.2 Pathophysiology

The parasympathetic nervous system is the dominant neural pathway that controls the airway smooth muscle tone. The predominant contractile innervation is parasympathetic and cholinergic in nature, while primary relaxant innervation of the airway is comprised of non-cholinergic (nitric oxide synthase- and vasoactive intestinal peptide-containing) parasympathetic nerves. Post-ganglionic parasympathetic fibers innervate the bronchi and bronchiole smooth muscles down to the level of terminal bronchioles. The normal human airway has a baseline mild contraction due to vagal activity. Airway smooth muscle is mediated by M3 muscarinic receptors on the airway smooth muscle. Stimulation of cholinergic nerves induces bronchoconstriction, mucus secretion, and bronchial vasodilation. Although there is no sympathetic innervation on airway smooth muscle, β(beta)-adrenergic receptors are abundant in airway smooth muscle; activation of these receptors causes bronchodilation.

Bronchospasm leads to increases in work of breathing (WOB), decreased airflow, increased air trapping, ventilation-perfusion mismatch, increased pulmonary vascular resistance (PVR), and right ventricular overload. If left untreated, bronchospasm causes severe hypoxia and heart failure.

28.5.3 Clinical Presentation Under General Anesthesia

Signs of acute bronchospasm include sudden increase in peak inspiratory pressure, wheezing on chest auscultation, decreased breath sound (or absent if severe), changes in end-tidal carbon dioxide ($EtCO_2$) (upsloping or shark-fin $EtCO_2$ waveform, decreased, or absent $EtCO_2$ waveform if severe), reduced tidal volume, and decreasing oxygen saturation.

28.5.3.1 Differential Diagnosis

Besides exacerbation of reactive airway disease (bronchial asthma and COPD), there are other non-bronchospastic causes that can mimic manifestations of bronchospasm. These clinical conditions are described as follows:

- **Endobronchial Intubation**: decreased breath sounds on one side of the chest and deep placement of the endotracheal tube.
- **Mechanical Obstruction**: A kinked, blocked, or misplaced endotracheal tube, or occlusion of breathing circuit can mimic a severe bronchospasm. It can be indicated by difficulty in passing the suction catheter, or removal of secretion upon suction.
- **Pneumothorax**: decreased breath sounds in one side, asymmetric chest rise, and trauma.
- **Pulmonary Edema**: frothy secretion in the endotracheal tube and cracks on auscultation.

28.5.4 Intraoperative Management

Once a bronchospasm is suspected, the initial management includes administering 100% oxygen, hand ventilation to test lung compliance, stopping any stimulation, and then considering anaphylaxis. An algorithm has been developed to manage a bronchospastic crisis [40].

Mild bronchospasms can be treated with deepening anesthesia, either by intravenous anesthetics (propofol or ketamine) or increasing the inhalation anesthetic concentration.

If the bronchospasm persists with difficulty of ventilation and desaturation, rapid, short-acting beta-agonists (such as albuterol) should be administered via a nebulizer connected to the breathing circuit, or by the metered dose inhaler (MDI) via endotracheal tube with an adapter. Help should be called.

If bronchospasm persist or worsens, other drug therapy is indicated. Those drugs are described here:

- **Anticholinergics**: Glycopyrrolate, atropine, and ipratropium have bronchodilatory properties. Since the onset of effects of anticholinergics takes 20–30 min, its use should be combined with more rapid acting medications, such as albuterol.
- **Epinephrine**: For refractory bronchospasms, epinephrine should be administered by an IV bolus of 10–50 mcg, or by continuous infusion 2–10 mcg/min.
- **Magnesium Sulfate**: Magnesium (up to 2 g IV over 20 min) may be helpful in a difficult bronchospasm; it can cause hypotension and muscle weakness.
- **Glucocorticoids**: High doses of glucocorticoids (hydrocortisone 100 mg or methyl prednisolone 60–80 mg IV) will not be effective for 4–6 h and should be combined with rapid acting drugs.

Extracorporeal Membrane Oxygenation

(ECMO) is reserved for the most severe bronchospasm that is refractory to maximal medical and mechanical ventilatory therapy.

28.5.5 Prevention

Patients with asthma and COPD should be optimized preoperatively by pulmonologists prior to elective surgery. Smoking cessation for 6–8 weeks before surgery reduces perioperative respiratory complications, including bronchospasms. Upper respiratory tract infections increase the risk of bronchospasm; elective surgery should be postponed until symptoms are completely resolved (approximately two weeks). Pretreatment with beta-agonist prior to surgery and adequate depth of anesthesia before airway manipulation reduces the risk of bronchospasm. In high-risk patients with active airway disease, use of laryngeal mask airway or regional anesthesia may be optional.

28.6 Anaphylaxis

Anaphylaxis is defined as a serious, generalized or systemic, allergic, or hypersensitivity reaction that can be life threatening or fatal. Anaphylaxis presents with acute onset of symptoms and signs in more than one body system within minutes to hours after trigger exposure. The most common affected systems are the skin, respiratory, gastrointestinal (GI), and cardiovascular (CV) systems. The symptoms and signs of affected systems are given in Table 28.1.

28.6.1 Epidemiology

Although most major studies on anaphylaxis during anesthesia are not conducted in the United States, most studies estimate the incidence to be from 1/10,000 to 1/20,000 [41]. The incidence in the pediatric population is estimated to be 1/37,000 [42]. Perioperative anaphylaxis occurs more often in women than in men, but occurs equally in both boys and girls [43]. More than half of perioperative anaphylaxis cases were identified as immunoglobulin E (IgE)-mediated [44]. Perioperative anaphylaxis is more likely to occur following anesthesia induction, but it can occur during the anesthesia maintenance and recovery period as well. The mortality from perioperative anaphylaxis is about 0–1.4% according to the most recent study [43]. The detection of anaphylaxis under anesthesia can be challenging due to masked symptoms under anesthesia and anesthesia-induced cardiovascular disturbances. Most anesthetics, such as propofol, can cause hypotension.

28.6.2 Pathophysiology of Anaphylaxis

The mechanisms of anaphylaxis involve either an immunologic or non-immunologic reaction. The immunologic reaction can be divided into IgE-dependent and non-IgE-dependent reactions. The previous exposure to a trigger is required for IgE-mediated immunologic reactions. When

Table 28.1 Symptoms and signs of anaphylaxis in affected systems

Affected systems	Symptoms and signs
Skin	Generalized hives, itching or flushing, swollen lips, tongue, and uvula, periorbital edema, and conjunctival swelling
Respiratory	Nasal discharge and congestion, change in voice quality, throat swelling, stridor, shortness of breath, wheeze, and cough. GI symptoms and throat swelling, stridor, shortness of breath, wheezing, and cough
Gastrointestinal (GI)	Nausea, vomiting, diarrhea, and crampy abdominal pain
Cardiovascular	Syncope, dizziness, tachycardia, and hypotension

antigens bind to IgE, the resulting IgE-mediated reaction activates mast cells and basophils to release inflammatory mediators such as histamine, leukotrienes, tryptase, and prostaglandin. In non-IgE-mediated mechanisms, the reaction is mediated through IgG or IgM antibody or antigen: antibody complexes and complement. Non-immunologic mechanisms cause direct release of histamine or other mediators from mast cells and basophils. The release of these mediators leads to generalized urticaria, angioedema, bronchospasm, and hypotension. Excessive activation of vasodilator mechanisms results in vasodilation that leads to severe hypotension and cardiovascular collapse.

28.6.3 Triggers

Many drugs can cause anaphylaxis during the anesthesia period, but the most common triggers of perioperative anaphylaxis are neuromuscular-blocking agents (NMBAs), sugammadex, antibiotics, chlorhexidine, latex, hypnotic agents, opioids, and colloids. Among them, NMBAs are the most identifiable causes of perioperative anaphylaxis. According to recent European studies, 50–70% of anaphylaxis cases related to anesthesia were due to NMBAs. Antibiotics appear to be the most common trigger of anaphylaxis during anesthesia in the United States [45].

28.6.3.1 Neuromuscular-Blocking Agents

NMBAs can cause anaphylaxis via both IgE-mediated and non-immunologic direct mast cell activation. The most implicated agents include atracurium, pancuronium, rocuronium, succinylcholine, and vecuronium. The ammonium ion of NMBAs is the main allergenic determinant. Anaphylaxis is more common with rocuronium and succinylcholine than with others. Suggamadex, a reversal agent for steroidal NMBAs (such as rocuronium) also causes anaphylaxis; cross activity exists among NMBAs.

28.6.3.2 Antibiotics

Antibiotics are often used to prevent wound infections during surgery, and were responsible for 12–15% of identifiable triggers in European studies. However, it accounts for 50% of IgE-mediated reactions and is the most common cause of perioperative anaphylaxis in the United States. β(beta)-lactam antibiotics (including penicillins and cepholosporins) as well as vancomycin are the most common triggers. Beta-lactam antibiotics cause IgE-mediated anaphylaxis while vancomycin causes a reaction secondary to direct histamine release from mast cells.

28.6.3.3 Latex Allergy

Latex anaphylaxis in the United States is less common since the introduction of latex-free products in surgical suites. However, occult exposure to natural rubber latex still accounts for a significant number of perioperative anaphylaxis. The latex allergy is an IgE-mediated process resulting from formation of a specific IgE against the protein in the natural rubber latex. The common latex resources are gloves, drains, and catheters. Latex allergy is likely to occur more often in patients with repeated exposure to latex gloves, or catheters from prior surgery or from occupational use, in patients with spina bifida, and in healthcare workers. Reactions to latex usually occur later in the surgical procedure, generally 30 min or more after the start of intervention.

28.6.3.4 Risk Factors

Risk factors for perioperative anaphylaxis include the female sex, past history of anaphylaxis, allergic drug reactions, allergic conditions such as eczema or hay fever, multiple past surgeries and procedures, and mast cell disorders. Patients with asthma are at a greater risk for perioperative anaphylaxis.

28.6.4 Diagnosis of Anaphylaxis

Anaphylaxis is a clinical diagnosis, and can likely be diagnosed if one of following criteria is met:

1. Acute onset of illness (minutes to hours) involved on the skin, mucosal or both; either respiratory compromise or reduced blood pressure; or associated symptoms of end organ dysfunction.
2. Two or more of following that will occur rapidly after likely antigen exposure (minute to hours): (a) involvement of skin-mucosal tissue, (b) respiratory compromise, (c) reduced blood pressure (BP) or associated symptoms, (d) persistent gastrointestinal (GI) symptoms.
3. Reduced BP after exposure to a known antigen for that patient.
4. Airway edema manifested by onset of stridor.

28.6.5 Severity Classification of Anaphylaxis

The severity of anaphylaxis is classified into three types based on the clinical manifestations:

1. **Mild**—involved in skin and subcutaneous tissue only.
2. **Moderate**—involved in respiratory, cardiovascular, or gastrointestinal system.
3. **Severe**—involved hypoxia, hypotension, or neurologic compromise.

The Ring and Messmer four-step grading scale classifies severity of anaphylaxis into four grades based on clinical presentations. Grade 1 involves cutaneous-mucosal signs, whereas grade 2 corresponds to mild cutaneous-mucous features that may be associated with cardiovascular and/or respiratory signs. Grade 3 involves cardiovascular collapse that may be associated with cutaneous-mucous signs and/or bronchospasms. Grade 4 is cardiac arrest. Grade 3 and 4 anaphylaxis are usually IgE mediated.

28.6.6 Perioperative Management of Anaphylaxis

Perioperative care depends upon the severity of anaphylaxis. Treatment during severe anaphylaxis should include cessation of anesthetic or drug, rapid volume resuscitation, and prompt epinephrine administration. Epinephrine is the first-line drug for anaphylaxis-induced cardiovascular collapse. The effects of epinephrine are mediated by both α(alpha)-adrenergic receptors and β(beta)-adrenergic receptors to produce vasoconstriction and an inotropic effect, and bronchodilation. Intravenous administration of 50–200 mcg epinephrine is recommended as an initial dose, followed by infusion as needed. Vasopressin is an alternative if epinephrine fails. Antihistamine receptor agents (such as diphenhydramine and cimetidine) and steroids (hydrocortisone) are second-line agents in the treatment of anaphylaxis.

28.6.7 Post-anaphylaxis Evaluation

Patients who had perioperative anaphylaxis should be referred to an immunologist for evaluation to determine the offender, and to prevent recurrent reactions in future surgery [46]. The safest perioperative care approach for patients with a history of anaphylaxis is the definitive identification, and complete avoidance of the trigger. If the evaluation did not reveal a specific agent causing anaphylaxis, then general precaution includes avoiding beta-blockers, angiotensin-converting enzyme (ACE) inhibitors, and drugs that release histamine, slowing the administration rate of antibiotics, and optimizing patients with asthma. Alternate anesthesia with local or regional anesthesia may be chosen if it is appropriate for the procedure.

28.7 Laryngospasm

Laryngospasm is a sustained glottis closure of the vocal cords resulting in a partial or complete airway obstruction during light anesthesia. It is the most frequent cause of post-extubation airway obstruction. If not treated quickly, it rapidly leads to hypoxia, hypercarbia, bradycardia, cardiac collapse, or even patient death.

28.7.1 Incidence

The overall incidence is under 1% in both adults and pediatric patients, but laryngospasm occurs twice as often in pediatric patients between birth and 9 years old, while three times as often during the newborn to three-month-old age. However, much higher incidence of laryngospasm (9%) is reported in pediatric patients with history of respiratory problems.

28.7.2 Pathophysiology

Glottic closure is a protective airway reflex that exists to prevent aspiration. A laryngospasm is an abnormal reflex that persists for a longer period. It is normally triggered by peri-glottic stimuli, mediated via the vagus nerve. Sensory fibers from the laryngeal mechanical, chemical, and thermal receptors ascend via the vagus nerve and via the internal branch of the superior laryngeal nerve (SLN). The motor response is mediated by the recurrent laryngeal nerve via the three intrinsic laryngeal muscles consisting of the lateral cricoarytenoids, thyroarytenoids, and cricoarytenoids. Glottis closure occurs by ether true vocal cord adduction alone or in combination with the false vocal cords. The supra-glottic soft tissues are thought to impact the glottis as they are pulled down by an increasing translaryngeal pressure gradient during obstructed inspiratory effort.

28.7.3 Risk Factors for Laryngospasm

- **Anesthetic Factors**: Light anesthesia at the time of stimulus, the use of potent irritant volatile agents such as desflurane during induction, the presence of blood or secretion in the airway, instrumentation of airway in the light plane of anesthesia, LMA malpositioning, and extubation during light anesthesia.
- **Patient Factors**: Young age, upper respiratory infection (URI), hypersensitive airway due to conditions such as asthma and smoking, preexisting airway abnormality,

ex-premature infants under 1 year of age, whooping cough, obstructive sleep apnea, and gastroesophageal reflux are risk factors for increased laryngospasm.
- **Surgical Risk Factors**: Upper airway surgeries, such as a tonsillectomy or an adenoidectomy, carry the greatest risk. Thyroid surgery and esophageal surgery also have higher risks.

28.7.4 Diagnosis of Laryngospasm

A laryngospasm must be considered if there is airway obstruction during anesthesia that was not relieved by basic airway maneuvers. Common signs of laryngospasm include inspiratory stridor, increased respiratory efforts, tracheal tug, desaturation with or without bradycardia, and airway obstruction that was not relieved by an upper airway device. Differential diagnoses include breath holding, bronchospasm, and pulmonary aspiration.

28.7.5 Management of Laryngospasm

Prevention of laryngospasm:

1. Patients with a higher risk for laryngospasm need to be identified preoperatively, and it must be ensured that adequate depth of anesthesia is achieved before triggering any stimulus.
2. Inhalational induction should be carried out by using non-irritating agents, such as sevoflurane; IV induction with propofol is less associated with laryngospasm.
3. Patients can undergo deep extubation while placed in lateral position, with the head down to keep the vocal cords clear of secretions during emergence.
4. Pharmacologic agents including magnesium, lidocaine, and atropine have been indicated to reduce the incidence of laryngospasm. Both topical and intravenous use of lidocaine is effective for preventing laryngospasm in children.

Once a laryngospasm is recognized, prompt therapy should be initiated and help may be called.

Treatment of laryngospasm:

1. Removing any triggering stimuli, relieving supra-glottic obstruction, removing obvious secretion and blood that is in the larynx, applying continuous positive airway pressure (CPAP) ventilation with 100% oxygen.
2. Jaw thrust and placement of a properly sized oral airway device will help to ensure the patency of the supra-glottic airway.
3. Larson's maneuver, a forcible jaw thrust with bilateral digital pressure on the body of the mandible just anterior to the mastoid process, may resolve laryngospasm by clearing the airway and stimuli.
4. If CPAP and the holding maneuver fail to stop the laryngospasm, deepening anesthesia with propofol or other drugs is required to diminish the exaggerated glottis closure reflex.
5. Despite all efforts mentioned above, if the patient continues to desaturate and the laryngospasm is ongoing, a small dose of succinylcholine (0.1–0.5 mg/kg) should be given to break the laryngospasm. If no IV is available, intramuscular succinylcholine 4 mg/kg can be administered.
6. In the case of refractory laryngospasm, a superior laryngeal nerve block and trans-tracheal block through cricothyroid membrane with lidocaine may break the laryngospasm [47].

28.8 Aspiration of Gastric Contents

Perioperative pulmonary aspiration is defined as aspiration of gastric contents that occur after induction of anesthesia, during a procedure, or in the immediate period after surgery [48]. Though it occurs infrequently, aspiration can lead to significantly increased morbidity and mortality rates. The incidence of aspiration during elective surgery is 1 per 2000–3000 anesthesia cases in adults and 1 per 1200–2600 anesthesia cases in children. However, a recent study demonstrated a much lower incidence of pulmonary aspiration with 1 per 4932 cases in pediatric populations. Most perioperative aspirations happen immediately after induction of anesthesia. However, pulmonary aspiration can occur prior to induction due to trauma, active vomiting, or preoperative sedation; it also can occur after extubation in the PACU, secondary to depressed consciousness from residual anesthetic effect. Silent aspiration can occur even while the patient is intubated with a cuffed endotracheal tube.

28.8.1 Pathophysiology

General anesthesia and anesthetics inhibit protective airway reflexes, including apnea with laryngospasm, coughing, expiration, and spasmodic panting that protects lungs from aspiration. Lower esophageal sphincter (LES) tone and barrier pressure are likely reduced under inhalational and propofol anesthesia. The upper esophageal sphincter (UES) of the cricopharyngeal muscle is reduced by most anesthetics, except ketamine. The depression of protective airway reflexes, in combination with reduction in LES and UES tone, makes anesthetized patients prone to aspiration.

Aspiration occurs once gastric contents (liquid or particulate matter, etc.) enter the tracheobronchial tree as a consequence of passive regurgitation or active vomiting. Depending on the composite of aspirates, patients can experience different clinical consequences: (1) acid-associated aspiration pneumonitis, (2) bacterial infection, and (3) particle-associated aspiration.

28.8.2 Acid-Associated Aspiration Pneumonitis

Aspiration results in parenchymal damage in two phases. The first phase is marked by direct toxic damage to respiratory epithelium by acid. The second phase is marked by an acute inflammatory response. Aspiration of gastric acid induces a chemical burn, triggering the release of various inflammatory mediators such as cytokines, chemokines, and adhesion molecules. These mediators cause inflammatory response and attract neutrophils and alveolar macrophages to activate leukocytes.

28.8.2.1 Aspiration Pneumonia

Aspiration pneumonia is an infection process secondary to aspiration of oropharyngeal and gastric contents contaminated with pathogenic bacteria. It has a slow onset and occurs more in elderly patients and in patients on ventilator support in the ICU. Aspiration pneumonia accounts for at least 10% of community-acquired pneumonia.

28.8.2.2 Particle-Associated Aspiration

Inhalation of gastric content particle matters can result in an acute obstruction of smaller (and possibly larger) airways with consequences of sudden arterial hypoxia and the development of atelectasis distal to the blockage site.

28.8.3 Risk Factors for Aspiration

Factors that increase the risk of perioperative pulmonary aspiration are as follows:

1. **Conditions that increase gastric contents**: full stomach (eating, non-fasting), emergency surgery, acute abdominal pathology, delayed gastric emptying (due to neuropathy or opioid use), diabetes, ileus, and pregnancy.
2. **Conditions that decrease the tone of the esophageal sphincter**: known uncontrolled gastroesophageal reflux disease (GERD), esophageal disorder (achalasia, stricture, Zenker's diverticulum), previous gastric banding, and gastric bypass surgery.
3. **Conditions that depress laryngeal reflexes**: brain injury, neuromuscular disorders (Parkinson's disease, multiple sclerosis, cerebral palsy, etc.).
4. A difficult airway and failed intubation strongly correlate with aspiration [49].

28.8.4 Diagnosis of Aspiration Pneumonitis

Visible gastric contents in the oropharynx always warrant suspicions of aspiration. Clinical manifestation of aspiration pneumonitis could be both asymptomatic and symptomatic. Aspiration of at least 0.4 ml/kg in volume and pH of contents of < 2.5 is required to produce symptoms. Classic symptoms associated with pulmonary aspiration include sudden onset of wheezing, shortness of breath (in awake patients), bronchospasm, desaturation, cyanosis, and tachycardia. The severity of bronchitis may relate to the pH and volume of the aspirated content; however, the presence of particles is most important. A chest X-ray (CXR) may be useful in diagnosing aspiration pneumonitis. However, CXR can be normal in patients with uncomplicated clinical cases. In one-third of aspiration cases, the initial CXR does not represent the full extent of lung involvement. Both the right and left lung can be affected; however, occurrence in the lower lobes is more common. CXR can show infiltrates as small, irregular opacities, confluent opacities, acinar opacities, or mixed patterns [49].

28.8.5 Prevention of Perioperative Pulmonary Aspiration

Prevention is the key to reduce morbidity and mortality of aspiration pneumonitis.

28.8.5.1 Preoperative Fasting

Patients undergoing elective surgery should be instructed to fast according to the ASA fasting guideline [48]. A minimum fasting period for clear liquids, breast milk, infant formula/nonhuman milk, and a light meal are 2 h, 4 h, and 6 h, respectively. Eight hours or more fasting time is required if a patient ingests meat, fried, or fatty foods. Both the amount and type of food must be considered when determining an appropriate fasting period.

28.8.5.2 Pharmacologic Prevention

Preoperative use of medications to prevent aspiration is not recommended for routine use. Common medications used for reducing gastric volume and acidity include gastrointestinal stimulants (metoclopramide), gastric acid secretion blockers (cimetidine, famotidine, ranitidine, etc.), antacids (sodium citrate, sodium bicarbonate, and magnesium trisilicate), antiemetics (droperidol and ondansetron), and anticholinergics (atropine, scopolamine, and glycopyrrolate).

These drugs have unwanted clinical side effects. However, treatment with antacids, H2-receptor antagonist, proton pump inhibitors, or pro-kinetics prior to elective cesarean delivery can rapidly reduce the acidity of stomach contents. A combination of antacids and H2-receptor antagonist is the most efficient technique.

28.8.5.3 Anesthesia Technique

A patient with a high risk of aspiration should be induced with a rapid sequence induction (RSI). Preparation of an RSI is important. The patient is usually positioned head up and IV access is established. Suction should be readily available. Preoxygenation is crucial to RSI to avoid hypoxia during later apnea. Application of cricoid pressure is still recommended to prevent regurgitation and aspiration. Cricoid pressure of 10 N ($\sim$1 kg) should be applied to awake patients and 30 N ($\sim$4 kg) after administration of induction agent, such as propofol. Succinylcholine is the main muscle relaxant to facilitate intubation because of its fast onset. If succinylcholine is contraindicated, a higher dose of a non-depolarizing muscle relaxant, such as rocuronium, can be substituted.

28.8.6 Management of Perioperative Pulmonary Aspiration Pneumonitis

Successful management of aspiration begins with immediate recognition of the occurrence of gastric contents in the oropharynx or the airway. Symptoms that indicate an aspiration of gastric contents are as follows:

1. Visible gastric contents in the oropharynx.
2. Hypoxia despite correct endotracheal intubation and ventilation.
3. Increased inspiratory pressure during mechanical ventilation.
4. Dyspnea, apnea, or hyperventilation during spontaneous breathing.
5. Bronchospasm, wheezing, crackles and laryngospasm.
6. Reduced compliance.
7. Desaturation/bradycardia/cardiac arrest.

Once the pulmonary aspiration is recognized during induction of anesthesia or laryngoscopy, the patient is positioned head down and the oropharynx is suctioned, followed by immediate endotracheal intubation. Once the patient is intubated, the endotracheal and bronchial tubes are suctioned. Controlled ventilation with 100% oxygen and positive end-expiratory pressure (PEEP) should follow suctioning. If the aspiration occurred after completion of intubation, the patient should be immediately positioned head-down and the trachea should be suctioned. Lavage via the endotracheal tube is usually not recommended after aspiration of liquids, since lavage may cause the aspirate to go deeper, perhaps into the peripheral lung sections. In the case of aspiration of particulate matter, a bronchoscopy should be performed to remove all particles to prevent airway obstruction. A sample of aspirate needs to be taken for pH determination and microbiological diagnosis.

Further treatment depends on the patient's symptoms. For bronchospasms, use of bronchodilators, such as albuterol, is recommended. If the patient is asymptomatic and oxygenation is adequate, the patient can be extubated and taken to the PACU. The patient can be discharged to the floor if they are stable after 2 h in the recovery room. If the patient is unstable, or saturation is not adequate, then intubation should be maintained and PEEP with protective ventilator strategy and the patient admitted to the ICU. Chest X-ray and a blood gas test should be performed. Continue PEEP and bronchodilators.

Steroids and antibiotics are not routinely recommended to treat pulmonary aspiration. Antibiotics may be indicated if aspiration pneumonia is suspected and cultures are positive for a bacterial infection.

28.9 Post-obstructive Pulmonary Edema (POPE)

Post-obstructive pulmonary edema (POPE) is noncardiogenic pulmonary edema that results from sudden relief of an upper airway obstruction. It was also referred to as negative pressure pulmonary edema (NPPE). The incidence of POPE is believed to be 0.05–0.1% during anesthesia, but higher incidences were reported in other clinical settings. Risk factors for POPE development during anesthesia include the male sex, young age, history of head and/or neck surgery, obesity with obstructive sleep apnea (OSA), and difficultly with intubation.

28.9.1 Type of POPE

POPE can be categorized to two types based on the respiratory phase against airway obstruction. Type 1 POPE is associated with forceful inspiratory effort against upper airway obstruction. The common causes for type 1 POPE during anesthesia include laryngospasm, endotracheal tube obstruction, LMA obstruction, and postoperative vocal cord paralysis. Type 2 POPE is associated with exhalation against chronic airway obstruction, and develops after relief of airway obstruction, such as post-adenoidectomy/tonsillectomy, post-laryngeal mass resection, and post-reduction of hypertrophic redundant uvula.

28.9.2 Pathophysiology

The pathology of Type 1 POPE involves negative pressure pulmonary edema (NPPE), hypoxia, and hyperadrenergic states resulting from acute airway obstruction and hypoxia. NPPE is triggered by inspiration against occluded airway. Inspiratory efforts to overcome obstructive airway can generates intra-thoracic negative pressure of up to − 140 cm H_2O. This large intra-thoracic negative pressure leads to sudden increase of venous return, resulting in increased preload and elevated pulmonary venous pressure, which in turn increases the capillary hydrostatic pressure. The negative intrapleural pressure is also transmitted to the interstitium and alveoli. The combination of elevated hydrostatic pulmonary capillary pressure and drop in interstitial and alveoli pressure causes an increase in the hydrostatic gradient, and finally, transduction of fluid from the pulmonary capillary to the interstitial space results in pulmonary edema. Hypoxia, as a result of airway obstruction, causes both hypoxic pulmonary vasoconstriction leading to an increase in pulmonary vascular resistance and disruption of capillary wall integrity that further facilitates the fluid transduction to interstitial space. A hyperadrenergic state is thought to redistribute blood flow to the pulmonary system, and thus increases pulmonary vascular resistance that contributes to increased hydrostatic capillary pressure.

Type 2 POPE's pathophysiology is related to exhalation against an obstructed airway. Expiration against an upper airway obstruction causes positive pleural and alveoli pressures, resulting in a decrease in venous return, cardiac preload, and pulmonary blood flow. Once the obstruction is relieved, such as post-adenotonsillectomy, the mechanism is similar to type 1. The sudden relief of chronic airway obstruction results in an abrupt fall in airway pressure, leading to an increase in venous return, cardiac preload, and pulmonary blood flow. This leads to an increase in hydrostatic capillary pressure and edema.

28.9.3 Clinical Manifestations

Common clinical presentation of POPE includes an immediate onset of respiratory distress occurring within minutes after relief of airway obstruction. But delayed presentation has been reported; clinical signs consist of tachypnea, dyspnea, paradoxical breathing, tachycardia, desaturation, wheezing, stridor, rales, ronchi, cyanosis, and pink frothy sputum in severe cases. Chest X-ray shows rapid bilateral changes, such as Kerley lines, peribronchial cuffing, and opacity that are consistent with pulmonary edema. A differential diagnosis in the setting of acute postoperative respiratory distress needs to include aspiration pneumonitis, pulmonary embolism, anaphylaxis, iatrogenic fluid overload, cardiogenic or neurogenic pulmonary edema.

28.9.4 Treatment of POPE

POPE treatment consists of supportive measures, respiratory therapy, and diuretic use depending on the severity of symptoms:

1. Supportive measures include ensuring adequate oxygenation with supplemental oxygen and maintaining patent airway.
2. Noninvasive respiratory therapy with PEEP or CPAP can be used to maintain the patient's oxygenation and leads to rapid resolution of pulmonary edema.
3. Mechanical ventilation with PEEP and 100% oxygen is required in severe cases.
4. Diuretics, such as furosemide, can be administered to decrease the intravascular volume and alter Starling equation intra-capillary filtration and resolution of edema. Caution should be paid, as diuretics may exacerbate hypovolemia and tissue hypoperfusion.

28.9.5 Prevention of POPE

POPE is a significant perioperative pulmonary complication associated with anesthesia. Prevention of POPE starts with avoidance of airway obstruction during anesthesia. Deep induction and awake extubation reduce the incidence of a laryngospasm. ETT biting by patients can be prevented by appropriate use of oral airways. In patients with difficult airways, awake intubation is the best way to ensure a secured airway without risk of an acute airway obstruction.

28.10 Questions and Answers

Questions (Choose the most Appropriate Answer)

1. After a long surgical procedure for carpal tunnel release with tourniquet use under general anesthesia, a patient developed radial nerve palsy. This persists > 5 weeks after the initial procedure. The most likely cause is:
   A. Direct surgical trauma
   B. Inappropriately high tourniquet pressure
   C. Prolonged application of tourniquet
   D. Post tourniquet syndrome secondary to edema

2. A 47-year-old male scheduled for laparoscopic cholecystectomy was intubated after induction with fentanyl and propofol. The patient was paralyzed with rocuroniun. At the beginning of the surgical incision, the surgeon noticed the nasopharyngeal temperature was 35 °C and asked to raise the patient's temperature. Which of the following mechanisms mainly contributes to the drop in the patient's temperature?
   A. Conduction
   B. Evaporation
   C. Radiation and Convection
   D. Redistribution
3. The most common complication of direct laryngoscopy and endotracheal intubation is:
   A. Dental trauma
   B. Esophageal intubation
   C. Pulmonary aspiration
   D. Laryngospasm
4. A 55-year-old female is admitted to the ICU for hypoxemic respiratory failure secondary to methicillin-resistant *Staphylococcus aureus* (MRSA) pneumonia. Past medical history is significant for coronary artery disease (CAD), hyptertension (HTN), fibromyalgia, and depression. Current medications include lisinopril, metoprolol, duloxetine, and oxycodone. After an infusion of the antibiotic she developed tachycardia, labile blood pressure, diarrhea, hyperreflexia, and hyperthermia. The causative agent for this syndrome is:
   A. Vancomycin
   B. Chloramphenicol
   C. Tigecycline
   D. Linezolid
5. A 52-year-old male underwent an elective lumbar spine fusion. Tracheal intubation was successful with direct laryngoscopy on the first attempt. On emergence, the patient accidently pulled the tube out before the ETT cuff was completely deflated. The patient was breathing spontaneously and with VSS upon transport to the PACU. In the recovery room with SpO2 of 97%, the patient was noted to have hoarseness, breathy voice, and decreased voice volume. His symptoms are mostly likely caused by:
   A. Airway edema
   B. Vocal cord paralysis
   C. Laryngospasm
   D. Arytenoid dislocation
6. Among the non-depolarizing neuromuscular-blocking drugs (NMBDs) listed below, which one has highest incidence of anaphylaxis?
   A. Atracurium
   B. Vecuronium
   C. Rocuronium
   D. Pancuronium
7. A 35-year-old female, otherwise healthy, with L4/5 disc herniation was scheduled for a lumbar discectomy. After an uneventful intravenous induction and intubation, the patient was positioned prone for surgery. Two grams of cefazolin were intravenously administered per the surgeon's request. The patient's blood pressure was 70/40 mm Hg prior to incision, and was not responsive to an intermittent IV bolus of phenylephrine treatment. In the meantime, the peak airway pressure increased from 15 cm H2O to 25 cm H_2O. The patient was turned supine, and facial edema and a rash were noticed. What medication should be administered first?
   A. Diphenhydramine
   B. Epinephrine
   C. Vasopressin
   D. Dexmethasone
8. A 3-year-old, 12.5 kg boy with a history of asthma underwent an uneventful tonsillectomy and adenoidectomy under general anesthesia with endotracheal tube intubation. The patient was found to have severe stridor immediately after extubation in the operating room. While he was being treated with positive pressure mask ventilation, the patient became cyanotic and his pulse oximeter saturation dropped to 75%. What is your next step for the management of this patient?
   A. Suction oropharyngeal area
   B. Administer 30 mg of propofol intravenously
   C. Larson's maneuver
   D. Administer succinylcholine 6 mg IV
9. A 45-year-old, 80 kg male with a history of hypertension is scheduled for an elective laparoscopic cholecystectomy. Which following method is best to prevent aspiration pneumonitis?
   A. Fasting for at least 8 h after the consumption of French fries.
   B. Preoperative oral ingestion of 40 ml of sodium citrate
   C. Cimetidine 150 mg IV 1 h prior to surgery
   D. Ondansetron 4 mg IV 30 min before the anesthesia induction
10. A 28-year-old, 75 kg, male healthy patient underwent endoscopic sinus surgery for his chronic sinusitis under general anesthesia. The patient developed a laryngospasm immediately after his extubation in the OR. His oropharynx was suctioned and a dose of propofol 50 mg was administered intravenously. Mask ventilation with positive airway pressure was able to break the laryngospasm. After the patent airway was assured, the patient was transferred to PACU with supplemental oxygen

through a facemask. While you were giving the report to the PACU nurse, the patient became tachypneic, had shortness of breath, and SpO2 dropped to 88%. Rales were heard on auscultation of both lungs. What is the most possible diagnosis?

A. Aspiration pneumonitis
B. Post-obstructive pulmonary edema
C. Congestive heart failure
D. Pulmonary embolism

Answers

1. **B**. High tourniquet pressure leads to tissue compression, which in turn effects nervous tissue. A pressure above systolic blood pressure leads to a physiologic conduction block 15–45 min after cuff inflation, which is reversible at the end of the procedure. Higher cuff pressures will lead to morphological changes, which include displacement of the nodes of Ranvier, stretching, and partial/complete rupture leading to demyelination of paranodal myelin in large myelinated nerves. This impaired nerve conduction can last up to 6 months. Surgical trauma at the distal forearm leads to no motor deficit. Poor patient positioning most commonly leads to ulnar nerve palsy at the elbow secondary to susceptibility to compression between the bone and a hard surface. During tourniquet use, muscle ischemia develops secondary to low PaO2 and an increase of PaCO2/lactate in muscles. After an hour, marked changes in mitochondrial morphology occurs. Once the tourniquet is released, interstitial and intracellular edema occurs as result of increased vascular permeability. This leads to post tourniquet syndrome, in which pale, swollen, stiff limbs with weakness (but no paralysis). This may persist for 1–6 weeks.
2. **D**. The administration of anesthesia is almost invariably associated with a drop in core temperature of 1 °C–3 °C, depending on the type and dose of anesthetics, the area of surgical exposure, and OR temperature. Intraoperative hypothermia has a characteristic pattern that consists of three distinct phases: redistribution, linear decrease, and Tc plateau. General anesthesia inhibits tonic thermoregulatory vasoconstriction by both a central and a peripheral vasodilating effect. Vasodilation promotes the redistribution of heat from the core compartment to peripheral tissue of the body, resulting in a relatively hypothermic core. Up to 80% of patients typically have a decrease of 1.5 °C in Tc during the first hour of anesthesia, which is attributed to heat redistribution.
3. **A**. Dental trauma is the most frequent complication of direct laryngoscopy and endotracheal intubation. Immediate dental consult should be sought for further advice. Though claims related to dental damage are statistically high, they contribute to a proportionally low total claim financially.
4. **D**. The development of life-threatening serotonin syndrome has been reported with serotonin and norepinephrine reuptake inhibitors (SNRIs) and selective serotonin reuptake inhibitors (SSRIs), such as duloxetine. Serotonin syndrome constitutes mental status changes (agitation, hallucinations, and coma), autonomic instability (tachycardia, labile blood pressure, and hyperthermia), neuromuscular aberrations (hyperreflexia, incoordination), and/or gastrointestinal symptoms (e.g., nausea, vomiting, and diarrhea). In its most severe form, serotonin syndrome can resemble neuroleptic malignant syndrome, with hyperthermia, muscle rigidity, autonomic instability and possible rapid fluctuation of vital signs, and mental status changes. Patients receiving SNRIs or SSRIs should be monitored for the emergence of serotonin syndrome or NMS-like signs and symptoms. Based on the mechanism of action, caution is advised when duloxetine is co-administered with other drugs that may affect the serotonergic neurotransmitter systems. Such drugs include triptans, linezolid (a reversible nonselective MAOI), lithium, tramadol, or St. John's Wort. Vancomycin, chloramphenicol and tigecycline are not MAO inhibitors.
5. **D**. Arytenoid dislocation is an uncommon, but underdiagnosed condition. Arytenoid dislocation easily can be misdiagnosed as vocal cord paralysis. Unlike vocal cord paralysis, arytenoid dislocation can be corrected with voice therapy and surgery. Early diagnosis and prompt treatment are more likely to reestablish normal joint mobility and restore voice quality. The cricoarytenoid joint is a diarthrodial joint with a synovium lined capsule composed of the pyramidal-shaped arytenoid positioned on top of the ellipsoid cricoid cartilage. The term *arytenoid subluxation* is used when the relationship of the cricoarytenoid articulation is abnormal but contact is maintained, whereas *arytenoid dislocation* refers to complete disruption of the joint. The arytenoid may be dislocated either anteriorly or posteriorly with respect to the cricoid. Anterior dislocation usually results in anteromedial displacement of the arytenoid cartilage, with an inferiorly located foreshortened and dysfunctional vocal cord. In contrast, with posterior dislocation, the vocal cord is often superiorly positioned, with

posterolateral displacement of the arytenoid cartilage. The most common symptoms of arytenoid dislocation are hoarseness, "wheezy" voice quality, decreased voice volume, and voice fatigue. Nearly 80% of reported cases are attributed to intubation trauma. Several authors suggest that the arytenoid cartilage is directly traumatized by the endotracheal tube or stylet during intubation or by an incompletely deflated cuff during extubation. Furthermore, it may be deduced that anterior arytenoid dislocation occurs from direct intubation trauma, while posterior dislocation can occur during extubation. Although the true incidence is unknown, arytenoid dislocation has been reported in less than 0.1% of endotracheal intubations. Airway edema may present with the aforementioned symptoms with decreased SpO2, responding to nebulized epinephrine. Vocal cord palsy is usually associated with trauma during difficult intubation.

6. **C**. Explanation: Neuromuscular-blocking drugs (NMBDs) are functional divalent, capable of crosslinking cell-surface IgE, and cause mediator release from mast cells and basophils without binding or haptenizing to larger molecules. NMBDs are responsible for most of the anaphylaxis related to anesthesia. The anaphylaxis rate for rocuronium is greater than other NMBDs. The most recent study confirmed that the anaphylaxis rate for rocuronium is 10 times higher than other non-depolarizing NMBDs, while the rate for succinylcholine is similar to rocuronium.
7. **B**. Explanation: Epinephrine is the initial drug to treat anaphylactic shock. Its α(alpha)-adrenergic effects constrict venous capacitance bed and arterial resistance vessels to reverse hypotension. Its β(beta)2-receptor stimulation produces bronchodilation and inhibits mediators release by increasing c-AMP in mast cells and basophils. Antihistamine, such as diphenhydramine, and corticosteroids, such as dexamethasone, are secondary treatment. If hypotension is refractory to epinephrine, vasopressin should be considered.
8. **D**. Explanation: Laryngospasm occurs more commonly in pediatric patients undergoing surgery under general anesthesia than in adults. It causes airway obstruction that could lead to hypoxia. Once a laryngospasm is suspected, initial treatment should include the removal of stimuli, positive mask ventilation, Larson's maneuver, and the deepening of anesthesia. In severe cases, neuromuscular-blocking drugs, such as succinylcholine, must be given to break the laryngospasm.
9. **A**. Following the ASA preanesthesia fasting guideline is the best prevention of perioperative aspiration. The minimum recommended hours of fasting after consumption of clear liquids, breast milk, formula and milk, nonfat light meal are 2 h, 4 h, and 6 h, respectively. Heavy meal and fatty food requires longer fasting times. Antacid, histamine blockers, proton pump inhibitors, serotonin antagonists are not indicated in healthy patients undergoing elective surgeries.
10. **B**. Post-obstructive pulmonary edema (POPE) results from sudden relief of airway obstruction that leads to a decrease in intra-thoracic pressure and an increase in venous return and pulmonary artery flow resulting in interstitial and alveolar edema. Common clinical presentations of POPE include an immediate onset of respiratory distress occurring within minutes after relief of airway obstruction; but, delayed presentation has been reported. Clinical signs consist of tachypnea, dyspnea, paradoxical breathing, tachycardia, desaturation, wheezing, stridor, rales, ronchi, cyanosis, and pink frothy sputum in severe cases. A chest X-ray shows rapid bilateral changes such as Kerley lines, peribronchial cuffing, and opacity that are consistent with pulmonary edema. Differential diagnosis in the setting of acute postoperative respiratory distress needs to include aspiration pneumonitis, pulmonary embolism, anaphylaxis, iatrogenic fluid overload, cardiogenic or neurogenic pulmonary edema.

References

1. Kucik CJ, Clenney T. Management of epistaxis. Am Fam Physician. 2005;71(2):305–11.
2. Kwon MA, Song J, Kim S, Ji S, Bae J. Inspection of the nasopharynx prior to fiberoptic-guided nasotracheal intubation reduces the risk epistaxis. J Clin Anesth. 2016;32:7–11. https://doi.org/10.1016/j.jclinane.2015.12.016.
3. Tong J, Tung A. A randomized trial comparing the effect of fiberoptic selection and guidance versus random selection, blind insertion, and direct laryngoscopy, on the incidence and severity of epistaxis after nasotracheal intubation. Anesth Analg. 2018;127(2):485–9. https://doi.org/10.1213/ANE.0000000000003396.
4. Newland MC, Ellis SJ, Peters KR, Simonson JA, Durham TM, Ullrich FA, et al. Dental injury associated with anesthesia: a report of 161,687 anesthetics given over 14 years. J Clin Anesth. 2007;19:339–45.
5. Rudmik L, Smith TL. Management of intractable spontaneous epistaxis. Am J Rhinol Allergy. 2012;26(1):55–60. https://doi.org/10.2500/ajra.2012.26.3696.
6. Domino KB, Posner KL, Caplan RA, Cheney FW. Airway injury during anesthesia: a closed claims analysis. Anesthesiology. 1999;91:1703–11.
7. Wilson SA, Last A. Management of corneal abrasions. Am Fam Physician. 2004;70:123–8.
8. Gild WM, Posner KL, Caplan RA, Cheney FW. Eye injuries associated with anesthesia. A closed claims analysis. Anesthesiol. 1992;76(2):204–8. https://doi.org/10.1097/00000542-199202000-00008. PMID: 1736697.

9. Segal KL, Fleischut PM, Kim C, Levine B, Faggiani SL, Banerjee S, Gadalla F, Lelli GJ Jr. Evaluation and treatment of perioperative corneal abrasions. J Ophthalmol. 2014;2014:901901. https://doi.org/10.1155/2014/901901. Epub 2014 Feb 4. PMID: 24672709; PMCID: PMC3941207.
10. Deljou A, Weingarten TN, Mahr MA, Sprung J, Martin DP. Postoperative corneal injuries: incidence and risk factors. Anesth Analg. 2019;129(3):737–42. https://doi.org/10.1213/ANE.0000000000003710. PMID: 31425215.
11. Shen Y, Drum M, Roth S. The prevalence of perioperative vision loss in the United states: a 10 year study from 1996 to 2005 of spinal, orthopedic, cardiac, and general surgery. Anesth Analg. 2009;109:1534–45.
12. Lee LA, Roth S, Posner KL, Cheney FW, Caplan RA, Newman NJ, et al. The American Society of Anesthesiologists postoperative visual loss registry: analysis of 93 spine surgery cases with postoperative visual loss. Anesthesiol. 2006;105:652–9.
13. [no authors listed], Postoperative Visual Loss Study Group. Risk factors associated with ischemic optic neuropathy after spinal fusion surgery. Anesthesiol. 2012;116(1):15–24.
14. Practice Advisory for Perioperative Visual Loss Associated with Spine Surgery 2019: An Updated Report by the American Society of Anesthesiologists Task Force on Perioperative Visual Loss, the North American Neuro-Ophthalmology Society, and the Society for Neuroscience in Anesthesiology and Critical Care. Anesthesiol. 2019;130(1):12–30. https://doi.org/10.1097/ALN.0000000000002503. PMID: 30531555
15. Mansfield PF, Hohn DC, Fornage B, Gregurich MA, Ota DM. Complications and failures of subclavianvein catheterization. N Engl J Med. 1994;331:1735–8.
16. McGee DC, Gould MK. Preventing complications of central venous catheterization. N Engl J Med. 2003;348:1123–33.
17. Bhananker SM, Liau DW, Kooner PK, Posner KL, Caplan RA, Domino KB. Liability related to peripheral venous and arterial catheterization: a closed claims analysis. Anesth Analg. 2009;109 (1):124–9.
18. Bowdle A. Vascular complications of central venous catheter placement: evidence-based methods for prevention and treatment. J. Cardiothoracic Vas. Anesthesia (1053-0770). 2014;28(2):358
19. Dixon OG, Smith GE, Carradice D, Chetter IC. A systematic review of management of inadvertent arterial injury during central venous catheterisation. J Vasc Access. 2017;18(2):97–102. https://doi.org/10.5301/jva.5000611.
20. Guilbert MC, Elkouri S, Bracco D, Corriveau MM, Beaudoin N, Dubois MJ, et al. Arterial trauma during central venous catheter insertion: Case series, review and proposed algorithm. J Vasc Surg. 2008;48(4):918–25; discussion 25.
21. Kam PC, Kavanaugh R, Yoong FF. The arterial tourniquet: pathophysiological consequences and anaesthetic implications. Anaesthesia. 2001;56:534–45.
22. Practice Advisory for the Prevention of Perioperative Peripheral Neuropathies 2018: an updated report by the American Society of Anesthesiologists task force on prevention of perioperative peripheral neuropathies. Anesthesiol (Philadelphia). 2018;128 (1):11–26. https://doi.org/10.1097/ALN.0000000000001937
23. Melnyk V, Ibinson JW, Kentor ML, Orebaugh SL. Updated retrospective single-center comparative analysis of peripheral nerve block complications using landmark peripheral nerve stimulation versus ultrasound guidance as a primary means of nerve localization. J Ultrasound Med. 2018;37(11):2477–88. https://doi.org/10.1002/jum.14603.
24. Neal JM. Ultrasound-guided regional anesthesia and patient safety: update of an evidence-based analysis. Reg Anesth Pain Med. 2016;41(2):195–204.
25. Apfelbaum JL, Caplan RA, Barker SJ, Connis RT, Cowles C, Ehrenwerth J, et al. American Society of Anesthesiologists Task Force on Operating Room Fires. Practice advisory for the prevention and management of operating room fires: an updated report by the American Society of Anesthesiologists Task Force on Operating Room Fires. American Society of Anesthesiologists Task Force on Operating Room Fires. Anesthesiol. 2013;118 (2):271–90.
26. Yilmaz S, Calbayram NC. Exposure to anesthetic gases among operating room personnel and risk of genotoxicity: a systematic review of the human biomonitoring studies. J Clin Anesth. 2016;35:326–31 (PubMed PMID:27871551. Epub 2016/11/23. eng).
27. Braz MG, Carvalho LIM, Chen CO, et al. High concentrations of waste anesthetic gases induce genetic damage and inflammation in physicians exposed for three years: a cross-sectional study. Indoor Air. 2020;30(3):512–20. https://doi.org/10.1111/ina.12643.
28. Costa Paes ER, Braz MG, Lima JT, Gomes da Silva MR, Bentes de Sousa L, Lima ES, Carvalho de Vasconcellos M, Cerqueira Braz JR. DNA damage and antioxidant status in medical residents occupationally exposed to waste anesthetic gases. Acta Cir Bras. 2014;29(4):280–6.
29. Turkan H, Aydin A, Sayal A. Efect of volatile anesthetics on oxidative stress due to occupational exposure. World J Surg. 2005;29(4):540–2.
30. El-Ebiary AA, Abuelfadl AA, Sarhan NI, Othman MM. Assessment of genotoxicity risk in operation room personnel by the alkaline comet assay. Hum Exp Toxicol. 2013;32(6):563–70.
31. Chandrasekhar M. Evaluation of genetic damage in operating room personnel exposed to anaesthetic gases. Mutagenesis. 2006;21(4):249–54.
32. National Institute for Occupational Safety and Health. Occupational Exposure to Waste Anesthetic Gases and Vapors: Criteria for a Recommended Standard. Cincinnati, Ohio: US Dept of Health, Education, and Welfare, Public Health Service, Center for Disease Control, National Institute for Occupational Safety and Health. 1977. Publication DHEW (NIOSH), 77–140.
33. Gauger VT, Voepel-Lewis T, Rubin P, Kostrzewa A, Tait AR. A survey of obstetric complications and pregnancy outcomes in paediatric and nonpaediatric anaesthesiologists. Pediatr Anesth. 2003;13(6):490–5. https://doi.org/10.1046/j.1460-9592.2003.01079.x.
34. Rowland AS, Baird DD, Weinberg CR, Shore DL, Shy CM, Wilcox AJ. Reduced fertility among women employed as dental assistants exposed to high levels of nitrous oxide. N Engl J Med. 1992;327:993–7.
35. Rowland AS, Baird DD, Shore DL, Weinberg CR, Savitz DA, Wilcox AJ. Nitrous oxide and spontaneous abortion in female dental assistants. Am J Epidemiol. 1995;141:531–8.
36. Safety O, Administration H. Waste anesthetic gases. Washington, DC: US Department of Labor; 1991. p. 91–138.
37. Sessler DI. Perioperative thermoregulation and heat loss. Lancet. 2016;387(10038):2655–64.
38. Diaz M, Becker DE. Thermoregulation: physiological and clinical consideration during sedation and general anesthesia. Anesth Prog. 2010;57:25–32.
39. Mamie C, Habre W, Delhumeau C, Argiroffo CB, Morabia A. Incidence and risk factors of perioperative respiratory adverse events in children undergoing elective surgery. Paediatr Anaesth. 2004;14(3):218–24.
40. Dobyns JB. Anesthesia for adult patients with asthma. UpToDate. 2022. http://www.uptodate.com/contents/anesthesia-for-adult-patients-with-asthma.
41. Mali S. Anaphylaxis during perioperative period. Anesth Essays Res. 2012;6(2):124–33.

42. Wakimoto M, Miller R, Kim SS, et al. Perioperative anaphylaxis in children: a report from the wake-up safe collaborative. Pediatr Anesth. 2021;31(2):205–12. https://doi.org/10.1111/pan.14063.
43. Gurrieri C, Weingarten TN, Martin DP, Babovic N, Narr BJ, Sprung J, et al. Allergic reactions during anesthesia at a large United States referral center. Anesth Analg. 2011;113(5):1202–12.
44. Dewachter P, Mouton-Faivre C, Hepner D. Perioperative anaphylaxis: what should be known? Curr Allergy Asthma Rep. 2015;15:21.
45. Kuhlen JL Jr, Camargo CA Jr, Balekian DS, Blumenthal KG, Guyer A, Morris T, Long A, Banerji A. Antibiotics are the most commonly identified cause of perioperative hypersensitivity reactions. J Allergy Clin Immunol Pract. 2016;4(4):697–704. https://doi.org/10.1016/j.jaip.2016.02.008. Epub 2016 Mar 30. PMID: 27039234; PMCID: PMC4939134.
46. Ledford DK. Perioperative anaphylaxis: evaluation and prevention of recurrent reactions. UpToDate. Waltham, MA. 2022. http://www.uptodate.com/contents/perioperative-anaphylaxis-evaluation-and-prevention-of-recurrent-reactions.
47. Al-alami AA, Zestos MM, Baraka AS. Pediatric laryngospasm: prevention and treatment. Curr Opin Anaesthesiol. 2009;22:388–95.
48. Practice Guidelines for Preoperative Fasting and the Use of Pharmacologic Agents to Reduce the Risk of Pulmonary Aspiration: Application to Healthy Patients Undergoing Elective Procedures: An Updated Report by the American Society of Anesthesiologists Task Force on Preoperative Fasting and the Use of Pharmacologic Agents to Reduce the Risk of Pulmonary Aspiration. Anesthesiology 2017; 126:376–393 Schultetus RR. Aspiration pneumonitis. In: Lobato EB, Gravenstein N, Kirby RR, editors. Complications in anesthesiology. Philadelphia, PA: Lippincott Williams & Wilkins; 2007.
49. Udeshi A, Cantie SM, Pierre E. Postobstructive pulmonary edema. J Critical Care. 2000;25(508):e1-5.

The Postoperative Period

29

Verghese T. Cherian and Robert J. Kerris

Abstract

Emergence from anesthesia is a transition from a controlled to an uncontrolled state and is rife with possibilities of complications. The patient may be distressed by inadequate pain control, nausea, or shivering. However, complications involving the respiratory, the cardiovascular, the renal, or the neurological systems can be associated with significant morbidity and even mortality. A brief summary of the potential complications to be anticipated in the post-anesthesia care unit is described here.

Keywords

Postoperative complications • Airway obstruction • Laryngospasm • Postoperative residual curarization • PONV • Delayed awakening • Serotonin syndrome • Postoperative visual loss • Oliguria • PACU discharge criteria

Key Points

- Airway complications at emergence and extubation have significantly increased over the years, with premature extubation, airway obstruction, and aspiration of gastric contents as the main causes.
- Laryngospasm occurs only under "light" anesthesia, when the patient is not deep enough to not respond to the stimulus, yet not awake enough to modify the response.
- A train-of-four ratio of <0.9 can be associated with upper airway obstruction, reduced airway tone, and an increased risk for aspiration.
- The incidence of postoperative nausea and vomiting can be up to 30% even with routine use of ondansetron.
- Postoperative delirium is associated with a nearly doubling of hazard ratio for mortality.
- The most common cause for postoperative visual loss is ischemic optic neuropathy.

29.1 Introduction

Emergence from anesthesia is a stage of re-establishing spontaneous respiration, airway reflexes, and consciousness. It is a transition from a controlled to an uncontrolled state and is rife with potential for complications (Box 29.1). Although hypoxia, pain, and nausea make up the majority of adverse events at emergence and extubation, the surge in sympathetic outflow could have significant cardiovascular effects, while the effect of residual anesthetics could lead to muscular weakness and confusion.

Box 29.1 Adverse Postoperative Events

Postoperative adverse respiratory events (PARE)

Airway obstruction
Laryngospasm, laryngeal stridor, airway injury
Hypoventilation
Postoperative residual curarization (PORC),
Residual anesthetics, sedatives
Ventilation-perfusion (V/Q) mismatch
Atelectasis and shunt
Gastric aspiration
Pulmonary embolism, pulmonary edema
Bronchospasm

V. T. Cherian (✉) · R. J. Kerris
Anesthesiology and Perioperative Medicine, Penn State Health, Milton S. Hershey Medical Center, Hershey, PA, USA
e-mail: vcherian@pennstatehealth.psu.edu

R. J. Kerris
e-mail: rkerris@pennstatehealth.psu.edu

M. Argalious et al. (eds.), *Basic Sciences in Anesthesia*,
https://doi.org/10.1007/978-3-031-60203-0_29

Postoperative adverse cardiovascular events (PACE)
Hypotension, hypertension,
Arrhythmia, Myocardial ischemia
Postoperative nausea and vomiting (PONV)
Postoperative inadequate analgesia
Postoperative adverse neurological events (PANE)
Delayed awakening, neuro-behavioral disturbances,
Serotonin syndrome
Postoperative visual loss (POVL)
Postoperative kidney complications (POKC)

29.2 Postoperative Adverse Respiratory Events (PARE)

According to the National Audit Project (NAP4), a UK-based self-reporting audit, 30% of the major complications in airway management occur at emergence [1]. The American Society of Anesthesiologists (ASA) Closed Claims Project has shown that, compared to before the 1990s, the incidence of difficult intubations, undetected esophageal intubations, and inadequate ventilation/ oxygenation has decreased—possibly as a result of wide use of pulse oximeters and end-tidal CO_2 monitoring and adherence to the ASA difficult airway algorithm [2]. However, airway complications at emergence and extubation have significantly increased over the years [3], with premature extubation, airway obstruction, and aspiration of gastric contents as the main causes [4].

The basic pathophysiology of postoperative adverse respiratory events (PARE) are airway obstruction, hypoventilation, and ventilation-perfusion mismatch.

29.2.1 Airway Obstruction

Laryngospasm

Laryngospasm is a "protective" reflex, mediated through the superior laryngeal nerve, causing closure of the glottis in response to a stimulus (blood, secretions, suctioning) to the larynx or the oro-pharyngeal mucosa. This results in dramatic desaturation. Signs of laryngospasm may include paradoxical chest movement, intercostal retractions, nasal flaring, inspiratory stridor, and diminished breath sounds resulting in hypoxemia and bradycardia. It occurs only under "light" anesthesia, when the patient is not deep enough to not respond to the stimulus, yet not awake enough to modify the response to the stimulus. Depending on the definition, ranging from complete airway obstruction to mild inspiratory stridor, the reported incidence varies from 0.1 to 5%. Patient-related factors for laryngospasm include young age, recent URI (usually within 2–4 weeks), and exposure to tobacco smoke. Secretions and bleeding or residual blood in the airway following surgery also increase a patient's risk of laryngospasm; therefore, gentle oropharyngeal suctioning is recommended prior to removal of the endotracheal tube.

The exaggerated inspiratory effort against the closed glottis can generate significant negative intrathoracic pressure that can result in extravasation of fluid into the alveoli (negative pressure pulmonary edema). This is associated with 2–40% mortality.

The management of laryngospasm:

1. Providing continuous positive airway pressure (CPAP) using a tight-fitting face mask and continuous oxygen flow.
2. Larson's maneuver is the application of firm, medially directed pressure, in the space between the mastoid process and the mandible, bilaterally. The possible mechanisms by which this maneuver helps could be: (1) anterior displacement of the mandible and opening of the airway, and (2) the intense stimulus of the pressure on the styloid process could awaken the lightly anesthetized patient.
3. Succinylcholine in a dose range of 0.1–1 mg/kg is sufficient to relax the laryngeal muscles and "break" the laryngospasm. It may be better to administer succinylcholine earlier than later, as it can lead to severe bradycardia and cardiac arrest in a severely hypoxic patient. Succinylcholine has been given intramuscularly (4 mg/kg) when intravenous (IV) is not available.
4. Small doses of propofol (20–30 mg) can be used to deepen the anesthetic and relieve the obstruction.

29.2.1.1 Prophylaxis

In adults, use of a laryngeal mask airway (LMA) is associated with a lower incidence of post-extubation coughing, desaturation, and laryngospasm. However, in children, LMA is associated with increased risk of laryngospasm. Administration of lidocaine (1.5 mg/kg) or magnesium (15 mg/kg) prior to extubation may reduce the incidence of laryngospasm. The application of a positive pressure breath at extubation may reduce the risk of laryngospasm. Positive intrathoracic pressure decreases the adductor response of the vocal cords.

Laryngeal Stridor

Laryngeal stridor is the vibration of the vocal cord apparatus caused by the passage of air through a narrowed glottis. Airway narrowing can be due to: (1) laryngeal edema due to airway injury following intubation or endoscopy or due to an anaphylactic reaction to a drug, (2) vocal cord palsy following injury to the recurrent laryngeal nerve (thyroid surgery, excessive endotracheal tube cuff pressure), or (3) collapse of the oro-pharyngeal soft tissue in obese patients and those with obstructive sleep apnea or due to the lingering effects of anesthetics or residual neuromuscular blocking agents. Airway narrowing could also happen due to paradoxical adduction of the vocal cords during inspiration, commonly seen in infants or in an anxious patient breathing rapidly.

Airway Injury

Airway injury could result from surgery (thyroid, endoscopy, anterior cervical spine), anesthesia (laryngoscopy, suctioning, prolonged intubation, high cuff pressure) or positioning (prone, Trendelenburg). Patients with C1 esterase inhibitor deficiency can develop severe angio-neurotic edema even after trivial airway injury or manipulation.

The majority of airway injuries are minor, resulting in sore throat and hoarseness and usually resolve within a few days. The management consists of conservative measures such as ice chips, lozenges or mild analgesics. In an acute and potentially life-threatening situation, management of oropharyngeal and laryngeal edema consists of nebulized racemic epinephrine and IV dexamethasone. However, if it progresses, emergent endotracheal intubation may be required and, in severe cases, cricothyroidotomy would be indicated. Airway injury resulting in tracheal perforation usually requires a surgical thoracotomy for repair and antibiotics to reduce the risk of mediastinitis.

29.2.2 Hypoventilation

29.2.2.1 Postoperative Residual Curarization (PORC)

PORC is a significant contributor to PARE in the post-anesthesia care unit (PACU). Residual paralysis of the pharyngeal muscles leads to collapse of the airway during inspiration, which manifests as retraction at the sternal notch and paradoxical movement of the abdominal muscles. At emergence, regular, spontaneous breathing through the endotracheal tube does not guarantee complete reversal of neuromuscular block, since the diaphragm recovers from effects of muscle relaxants earlier than the pharyngeal muscles. A train-of-four (ToF) ratio of <0.9 can be associated with upper airway obstruction, reduced airway tone, and an increased risk for aspiration. The variability of duration of action of neuromuscular blocking agents and the time for reversibility with acetylcholine esterase inhibitors are significant factors for PORC. Since, it is not possible to exclude clinically significant residual paralysis by subjective monitoring, the use of an accelero-myograph to monitor the neuromuscular blockade is recommended [5].

It is also recommended that neostigmine be given to all patients to reverse neuromuscular blockade, unless the accelero-myograph shows a T4/T1 ratio >0.9 measured at the adductor pollicis muscle [6]:

- No monitoring—routine reversal
- TOF count 1—delay reversal
- TOF count 2–3—routine reversal
- TOF count 4/fade—routine reversal
- TOF count 4/ No fade—neostigmine 20–30 μ(mu)g/kg

Sugammadex, a cyclodextrin molecule with a lipophilic core and a hydrophilic exterior, can effectively encapsulate rocuronium and vecuronium molecules, rendering them unavailable for neuromuscular blockade. It is effective even when a high dose of rocuronium is given, as for rapid sequence intubation. Since it does not have anti-cholinesterase activity, it does not have to be co-administered with anti-cholinergic agents. Sugammadex has been used to neutralize rocuronium in myasthenic patients.

- TOF count <1 with no post-tetanic twitch or following RSI dose—Sugammadex 16 mg/kg
- TOF count <1 with at least 1 post-tetanic twitch—Sugammadex 4 mg/kg
- TOF count <2 twitches—Sugammadex 4 mg/kg
- TOF count ≥ 2 twitches – Sugammadex 2 mg/kg

Appropriate counseling should take place when administering Sugammadex to women of child bearing age on hormonal oral contraceptives as Sugammadex may render the OCP ineffective for a period of 7 days. A rare but serious side effect of Sugammadex is bradycardia resulting in severe hypotension which may be treated with anticholinergic agents such as atropine or inotropic agents. It can also cause bronchospasm and anaphylaxis.

29.2.2.2 Residual Opioid, Benzodiazepine, Volatile, and IV Anesthetics

Residual sedatives (benzodiazepine), anesthetics (volatile and intravenous), and opioids decrease the sensitivity of the respiratory center to hypercapnia and depress the respiratory drive. Therefore, an intubated patient breathing spontaneously with raised end-tidal CO_2 indicates residual anesthetics. The diminished respiratory drive could be a decreased respiratory rate (opioids) or tidal volume (volatile anesthetics). Presence of renal or hepatic dysfunction increases the risk of persistent effects of sedatives, opioids, and neuromuscular blocking agents. Ketamine and dexmedetomidine have less suppressive effects. There are no pharmacological reversal agents for volatile anesthetics and propofol, but residual effects of benzodiazepine can be reversed with flumazenil (0.2 mg IV over 30 s and repeated to achieve the desired effect, up to a maximum of 1 mg) and of opioids with naloxone (40 mcg every 5 min IV). It is important to remember that the duration of effects of the antidotes may be shorter than that of the residual sedative and so may need to be repeated. Ventilator support and monitoring would be needed until effects of the anesthetic agents wear off. Adverse effects of naloxone include reversal of analgesic effects of opioids, sympathetic surge leading to myocardial ischemia in patients with cardiac disease, and pulmonary edema after large doses in young, muscular patients.

There is currently a rising trend in monitored anesthesia care (MAC), wherein a "conscious sedation" is provided for procedures such as gastrointestinal endoscopy, cardiac catheterization, radiation oncology, and diagnostic and therapeutic radiological studies. This has led to a rise in incidence of problems such as inadequate ventilation and oxygenation, in such non-operating room anesthesia (NORA) possibly due to over-sedation, inadequate monitoring of ventilation and oxygenation, and remote access to the airway [7].

29.2.3 Ventilation-Perfusion (V/Q) Mismatch

29.2.3.1 Atelectasis and Intrapulmonary Shunt

The functional residual capacity (FRC) reduces with induction of anesthesia and worsens with muscle relaxation and also in lithotomy and Trendelenburg positions. This raises the closing volume (lung volume at which the smaller alveoli start to close) above the FRC, leading to basal atelectasis and intrapulmonary shunt. The other causes for intraoperative atelectasis could be thoracic and upper abdominal surgery, morbid obesity, and unrecognized, inadvertent endobronchial intubation. This could persist into the postoperative period, especially with inadequate analgesia, limiting breathing excursion or in the morbidly obese who would have to be propped up to facilitate diaphragmatic excursion. Obesity is also associated with a higher incidence of postoperative myocardial infarction and infection [8]. Anesthesia-induced pulmonary atelectasis is more pronounced in morbidly obese patients and it remains atelectatic for a longer period of time. The STOP-BANG questionnaire (www.stopbang.ca) predicts the risk of obstructive sleep apnea. The early postoperative application of continuous positive airway pressure (CPAP) in the obese and patients with obstructive sleep apnea has been recommended [9, 10].

29.2.3.2 Gastric Aspiration

Analysis of the anesthesia Closed Claims Project [11] shows an increasing trend in the incidence of aspiration of gastric contents, contributing to 18% of adverse respiratory events. The analysis of these cases showed that aspiration occurred mainly with induction, but also intraoperatively (18%) and during emergence and extubation (17%). These patients were elderly, sicker, and having abdominal and emergency surgery. According to the 4th National Audit Project (NAP4) of the Royal College of Anaesthetists and the Difficult Airway Society, aspiration was the single most common cause of death due to airway complication and about 30% of aspirations occurred at extubation. In patients at risk for aspiration, a gastric tube should be sited and kept on continuous suction drainage prior to induction and through the intraoperative period. At emergence, it is crucial to ensure that the patient is conscious and has return of airway reflexes prior to extubation. In the author's personal opinion, upper airway obstruction at emergence could generate sufficient negative pressure to suck the gastric fluid into the oropharynx. In the event of aspiration, postoperative care is largely supportive. Standard extubation criteria apply for patients that have had an aspiration event. If the patient is extubated, an extended period of observation is recommended in the PACU to ensure the maintenance of adequate oxygenation and ventilation. A chest x-ray should be obtained which may demonstrate a consolidation which is usually on the right side due to the acute angulation of the left main bronchus. Antibiotics should only be used if pneumonia develops and the prophylactic use of corticosteroids to reduce inflammation has not been shown to be beneficial.

29.2.3.3 Pulmonary Embolism

During surgery, a dislodged venous clot, fat globules from a fractured long bone, or amniotic fluid in the parturient could embolize into the pulmonary circulation and present as pleuritic chest pain, tachycardia, tachypnea, and hypoxemia resistant to oxygen therapy in the immediate postoperative period. Diagnosis is based on clinical symptoms and a high index of suspicion, and confirmed with a computed tomography angiography (CTA). If the clinician is facile with bedside point of care ultrasound (POCUS), a bedside transthoracic echocardiogram (TTE) can help in rapid diagnosis. Signs of pulmonary embolism on TTE include right-sided heart failure such as right atrial dilation, right ventricular dilation, and bulging of the interventricular septum to the left during systole. Management of pulmonary embolism, depending on the severity of symptoms, could range from therapeutic anticoagulation to pulmonary angiogram with thrombolytic therapy to surgical pulmonary embolectomy.

29.2.3.4 Pulmonary Edema

Presence of pulmonary edema in the postoperative period could be due to exacerbation of congestive cardiac failure or iatrogenic fluid overloading. Patients who develop post-extubation airway obstruction or laryngospasm could develop a transudative edema due to the generation of excessive negative intrathoracic pressure. This is commonly seen in young, muscular patients who can generate sufficient negative pressure against a closed airway. The patient presents with tachypnea, hypoxemia, and respiratory rales on auscultation. The management consists of diuretics, oxygen, and a propped up positioning. Trans-thoracic echocardiography could be a handy tool to assess myocardial functioning and decide the need for inotropic medication.

29.2.3.5 Bronchospasm

Tachypnea and "wheezing" could be an exacerbation in a patient with reactive airway disease (asthma or chronic obstructive pulmonary disease [COPD]), a symptom of pneumothorax, or part of an anaphylactic reaction. It requires appropriate therapy.

Remember!

Although, oxygen should be provided to all patients recovering from anesthesia or sedation, it does not treat hypoxemia due to significant shunt and hypoventilation. All patients recovering from a general anesthetic should be administered oxygen, traditionally through a nasal cannula. As a general rule, each liter per minute of oxygen raises the inspired oxygen by 4%, making a FiO_2 of 0.44 with 6 L/m oxygen flow. If this oxygen supplementation fails to maintain reasonable oxygen saturation, escalation of ventilator care to continuous positive airway pressure (CPAP), non-invasive positive pressure ventilation (NIPPV), or intubation and mechanical ventilation should be considered. The important monitors to detect PARE are clinical vigilance, pulse oximetry, and end-tidal CO_2 monitoring.

29.3 Postoperative Adverse Cardiovascular Events (PACE)

Cardiovascular complications in the PACU are usually related to a pre-existing cardiovascular comorbidity such as coronary artery disease (CAD), hypertension, arrhythmia, and also a consequence of perioperative fluid balance and blood loss. The common cardiovascular complications seen in the PACU are hypotension, hypertension, and arrhythmia, any of which could progress to myocardial ischemia in a susceptible patient.

29.3.1 Hypotension

The most likely etiology of hypotension in the PACU is hypovolemia, but it could well be residual anesthetic effect, (over)effective epidural block, sepsis, myocardial ischemia, arrhythmia, ongoing bleeding, pulmonary embolism, or anaphylaxis. Therefore, a bolus of IV fluid is usually administered, while the other causes are being excluded. Although the treatment depends on the etiology, aliquots of vasoconstrictor agents such as phenylephrine, ephedrine, or norepinephrine would maintain the blood pressure in the meantime. Ongoing hemorrhage would need surgical control and transfusion.

29.3.2 Hypertension

A common cause of high blood pressure in the postoperative period is pre-existent hypertension, especially in patients who skipped their anti-hypertensive medications on the day of surgery. The other causes could be inadequate pain control, a distended urinary bladder, or anxiety. Hypoventilation is associated with increased sympathetic tone and hypertension. Narcotic abusers and alcohol-dependent patients could present with hypertension and tachycardia in the PACU as manifestations of withdrawal symptoms. If the treatment of any precipitating causes, such as pain or distended urinary bladder, does not help or the blood pressure is significantly high, antihypertensive medications (labetalol, hydralazine) should be administered.

29.3.3 Arrhythmia

Cardiac arrhythmia in the postoperative period could be a manifestation of sympathetic surge, hypertension, hypoxia, electrolyte imbalances or acute coronary insufficiency. The common postoperative arrhythmias are sinus tachycardia and premature ventricular contractions, which usually do not require specific treatment. Hypomagnesemia or certain medications that prolong QT interval (anti-arrhythmic, droperidol, ondansetron) could result in *torsade de pointes*, a polymorphic ventricular tachycardia, which could rapidly progress to ventricular fibrillation. New onset atrial fibrillation is common after cardiac or thoracic surgery. Management consists of treatment of the inciting factor and use of anti-arrhythmic agents to counteract cardiovascular instability. Severe cardiovascular instability would require electrical cardioversion.

29.3.4 4 Myocardial Ischemia

Although perioperative myocardial infarction (MI) is rare, it can be associated with significant morbidity and mortality, and a higher 30-day mortality. These patients may not present with classical chest pain, but may have tachypnea, hypotension, arrhythmias, or lethargy. A high index of suspicion is warranted in the elderly, and those with history of ischemic heart disease and recent MI. Analysis of leads II and V5 in a 12-lead electrocardiogram (ECG) can reflect 80% of the ischemic events and is recommended in patients with known or suspected coronary artery disease who have undergone a high-risk surgery. Measuring the serum troponin is indicated when myocardial ischemia or infarction is suspected. Routine monitoring of troponin levels in high-risk patients may become a norm in the future as >20% of high-risk patients will have postoperative troponin elevations. A number of cardiac risk indices exist, however, the most widely used index is Lee's Revised Cardiac Risk Index. This index risk stratifies patients into low risk (0 points), intermediate risk (1–2 points), or high risk (3 or more points) A point is awarded for high-risk surgery, history of cerebrovascular accident, history of known CAD, history of heart failure, use of insulin for diabetic control and chronic kidney disease with a creatinine greater than 2.0. High-risk patients have greater than an 11% risk of having a perioperative major adverse cardiovascular event such as MI or acute heart failure.

29.4 Postoperative Nausea and Vomiting (PONV)

The incidence of postoperative nausea and vomiting (PONV) can be up to 30% and is dreaded by the patients, even more than postoperative pain [12].

29.4.1 Pathophysiology of Nausea and Vomiting

The vomiting center (VC) lies in the medulla and receives impulses via cranial nerves from carotid baroreceptors (IX), middle ear (VIII), gastrointestinal receptors (X), aortic baroreceptors (X), and direct afferents from higher cortical areas involved in pain, olfaction, memory, and fear, as well as from the chemoreceptor trigger zone (CTZ), which is located in the floor of the fourth ventricle. The CTZ is stimulated by drugs and toxins present in the blood. The efferent fibers from the VC pass through the cranial nerves (V, VII, IX, X, and XI) to coordinate the actions of the smooth and striated muscles involved in vomiting and also through the spinal nerves to the diaphragm and abdominal muscles.

Numerous neurotransmitters are involved, both peripherally and centrally, in the modulation of nausea and vomiting. These include histamine (H_1 receptors at gastrointestinal tract), dopamine (D_2 receptors), serotonin (5-HT_3 at CTZ), acetylcholine (muscarinic receptors in vestibulocochlear apparatus), and the more recently discovered neurokinin-1 or Substance P (NK_1 receptor at the vomiting center).

The multifactorial etiology of nausea and vomiting and the involvement of numerous neurotransmitters are reflected in the range of medications that are available to prevent and treat nausea and vomiting. Anti-emetics can be classified according to their site of action:

- $5HT_3$ receptor antagonist; e.g., ondansetron
- Dopamine antagonist; e.g., droperidol, metoclopramide, domperidone
- NK_1 receptor antagonist; e.g., aprepitant
- Antihistamine; e.g., cyclizine, diphenhydramine, dimenhydrinate,
- Anticholinergic; e.g., hyoscine (scopolamine), phenothiazines (prochlorperazine)
- Steroids; e.g., dexamethasone
- Cannabinoids; e.g., dronabinol, nabilone, sativex

Some of these drugs act on more than 1 receptor, e.g., phenothiazine (anti-dopaminergic, anti-cholinergic, and anti-histaminic), and some are associated with significant side effects, e.g., extra-pyramidal symptoms, even 12–72 h after a single dose (metoclopramide, droperidol, phenothiazines), QT prolongation (droperidol, ondansetron), and tachycardia (cyclizine).

29.4.2 Risk Factors for PONV

Risk factors for PONV could be patient related (female, nonsmoker, history of motion-sickness, dehydration, anxiety, gastric distension), surgical (abdominal, ophthalmic, middle ear and gynecological), or anesthetic (inhalational anesthetics, opioids, neostigmine, hypotension).

The most commonly used risk stratification model for PONV is the Apfel score (female, nonsmoker, perioperative opioids, history of PONV or motion sickness—1 point for each factor present). The incidence of PONV increases with increasing score: 0 (10%), 1 (21%), 2 (39%), 3 (61%), 4 (79%) [13].

29.4.3 Management of PONV

In patients with moderate to severe risk of PONV, 2 drugs with different pharmacological actions are used. The common selection is dexamethasone 4 mg IV at induction and ondansetron 4 mg IV before emergence. In a patient with significant past history of PONV, a third antiemetic is added prior to induction of anesthesia—either aprepitant or transdermal scopolamine.

In the PACU, if the patient has PONV despite prophylaxis, a drug from a different class, such as promethazine, could be administered.

29.5 Postoperative Pain Management

Inadequately controlled pain during the immediate postoperative period is not only associated with patient distress and sympathetic overstimulation, but has also been shown to lead to long-term chronic pain problems. The mainstay of pain control in the PACU is usually intravenous administration of opioids. However, intravenous acetaminophen, regional and local anesthetic techniques, and physical therapy, such as ice packs or placing a pillow under the knees, to ease the abdominal muscle stretch could be useful. A large field of research is interested in the use of non-opioid adjuncts to help augment postoperative pain relief. Examples include the IV use of lidocaine or ketamine intra- and post-operatively as well as the use of IV dexmedetomidine, an alpha 2 agonist which has limited effects on respiratory drive.

Apart from a longer hospital stay, poorly controlled postoperative pain can result in increased morbidity and mortality. Patients may experience an increase in sympathetic output resulting in postoperative hypertension and tachycardia thus increase the possibility of postoperative MI in those at risk. The increased sympathetic surge may also result in ileus as well as nausea and vomiting. Poorly controlled pain within the abdominal area may result in "splinting" and inadequate respiration resulting in pulmonary complications.

29.6 Postoperative Adverse Neurological Events (PANE)

The two common neurological complications encountered, after general anesthesia, in the PACU are "delayed awakening" and "neuro-behavioral disturbances."

Delayed Awakening

The reason for prolonged unconsciousness after anesthesia is most likely to be the effect of residual anesthetics and sedatives. However, it could also be metabolic derangement or neurological causes, both of which could lead to serious outcomes. The pharmacological reasons for "delayed awakening" could be actual or relative overdose or synergic effect of anesthetic agents, opioids, and benzodiazepines. Opioids depress the sensitivity of brain stem chemoreceptors to CO_2, which leads to respiratory depression and hypercapnia. Benzodiazepines are effective anxiolytics and can cause prolonged unconsciousness in the extremes of age. Residual neuromuscular block can result from incomplete reversal or recurarization and it can lead to hypoventilation. Residual effects of opioids and benzodiazepine can be reversed with naloxone and flumezanil, respectively. The effect of a bolus induction dose of propofol is unlikely to linger to cause delayed awakening. However, with wider use of total intravenous anesthesia techniques, it is crucial to understand the concept of "context sensitive" half-life of drugs such as propofol and dexmedetomidine, which could be prolonged depending up on the duration of infusion [14]. The emergence from volatile anesthetic agent depends on pulmonary excretion and the minimum alveolar concentration (MAC) linked to eye opening to verbal command (MAC_{awake}), which is about 0.3 MAC. Elimination of volatile anesthetic depends on alveolar ventilation, partition coefficients (blood-gas and blood-fat) of the agent, and the duration of use. Desflurane is linked to rapid recovery, especially in an obese patient because of its low blood-fat solubility.

Non-pharmacological causes for delayed awakening could be hypoglycemia (40 mg/dL^{-1}), hypothermia (<33 °C), hyponatremia (<110 mmol/L^{-1}), or raised intracranial pressure.

Neuro-Behavioral Disturbances

Neuro-behavioral disturbances in the postoperative period manifest as delirium, a state of altered consciousness, and impaired cognition. Temporally, it can be immediately after emergence from anesthesia, lasting about 30 min (**emergence delirium**), or prolonged over a couple of hours (**postoperative delirium**). There may also be long-term subtle loss of cognition, attention, and memory (**postoperative cognitive decline**).

Emergence delirium (incidence of 5–21% among adults) is more common among younger males with history of preoperative anxiety and those who have been given a benzodiazepine premedication. Postoperative delirium is more common in the elderly following major orthopedic and vascular surgeries, with a reported incidence of 3–53%. Postoperative delirium is associated with a nearly doubling of hazard ratio for mortality (OR 1.95; CI 1.51–2.52) and also a higher risk of dementia. Deranged neurotransmission and neuro-inflammation with microglial activation are some of the theories suggested for the etiology of postoperative delirium. Although postoperative delirium may progress to long-term cognitive decline in some patients, present evidence does not suggest that it is the norm.

The diagnosis of delirium requires the presence of an acute onset of alteration in the mental status compared to the preoperative period and symptoms of inattention along with either disorganized speech or altered level of consciousness.

Postoperative cognitive decline is an adverse outcome that can impact a patient's quality of life. There is no set definition of postoperative cognitive decline in the Diagnostic and Statistical Manual for Cognitive Disorders (DSM) 5th edition; therefore, it is only diagnosed based on comparison between preoperative and postoperative neurocognitive testing. It is an area of great interest in research as patient populations are increasingly becoming more elderly.

Prevention and Treatment

Some of the steps that can be taken to reduce the incidence of postoperative delirium are avoiding benzodiazepine as premedication, good nursing care with regular orientation to time and place, and early access to spectacles and hearing aids if the patient is dependent on them. Dexmedetomidine, an α(alpha)2-agonist, has been shown to be associated with less postoperative delirium compared to midazolam or lorazepam. Addition of ketamine and dexmedetomidine in the anesthetic technique may reduce postoperative delirium, compared to benzodiazepine and propofol, which act through gamma-aminobutyric acid (GABA) receptors. Judicious use of opioids is indicated as both over-dosage of opioids and under-treatment of pain can contribute to delirium. Managing patients with delirium involves nursing care in a stable environment by familiar caregivers and constant reassurance; treatment of aggravating factors such as pain, hypoxia, electrolyte imbalance, or infection; and avoiding deliriogenic drugs. If general measures fail, haloperidol, a dopaminergic antagonist, in a dose of 0.5–5 mg may be used.

Regarding POCD, the single greatest risk factor for POCD is preoperative cognitive impairment. It is unclear if anesthesia, surgery or patient characteristics lead to POCD; however, the etiology is likely multifactorial. Unfortunately, no anesthetic regimen has been identified that reduces the risk of POCD thus no single anesthetic strategy can be recommended. The concept of preoperative cognitive optimization through a variety of cognitive training modalities is an active area of research.

Serotonin Syndrome

Serotonin syndrome is a potentially fatal condition that occurs due to excess serotonin in the central nervous system, secondary to an adverse drug reaction or a drug interaction. Numerous drugs that increase serotonin activity—such as monoamine oxidase inhibitors (MAOI), selective serotonin-reuptake inhibitors (SSRI), opioids, anti-emetics, etc.—have been associated with serotonin syndrome.

The classical clinical triad of altered mental status, autonomic hyperactivity, and neuromuscular abnormality is not universally present. The usual presentation is a spectrum ranging from mild symptoms such as shivering and drowsiness to tremor, altered sensorium, muscle rigidity, and hyperreflexia. In an extreme situation they could develop hyperthermia, rhabdomyolysis, metabolic acidosis, renal failure, and disseminated intravascular coagulopathy. In a postoperative patient, mild symptoms such as shivering, restlessness, or drowsiness are easily overlooked or treated with the drugs that can worsen the situation. The diagnosis requires a high index of suspicion in patients who have taken any of the precipitating drugs over the previous 5 weeks. The differential diagnosis includes anti-cholinergic overdose, malignant hyperthermia, and neuroleptic malignant syndrome.

The management of serotonin syndrome is mainly supportive with removal of the precipitating agent and administration of benzodiazepine for sedation [15]. Cyproheptadine, a $5HT_{2A}$ antagonist, in a dose of 12 mg followed by 2 mg every 2 h orally is recommended, but its efficacy is not conclusive. In patients who develop hyperthermia (>41 °C), in addition to the aforementioned therapy, sedation, neuromuscular paralysis, and endotracheal intubation with mechanical ventilation should be initiated.

Postoperative Visual Loss

Postoperative visual loss (POVL) is a rare but devastating complication, and is mainly associated with major spine and cardiac surgery. The most common cause for POVL is ischemic optic neuropathy (ION) [16]. This can occur with improper patient positioning, causing external compression of the eye, raising the intraocular pressure, and impairing flow in the retinal artery. This can occur in patients positioned prone for spine surgery. Prolonged surgery, excessive hemorrhage, and associated hypotension during the spine surgery could be contributing factors; although hypotension by itself seems to be a rare cause for retinal ischemia. Retinal artery occlusion can occur due to micro-embolus during an open-heart surgery. Other causes for POVL could be cortical blindness and acute glaucoma. Transient visual loss after transurethral resection of prostate can result due to excessive absorption of 1.5% glycine, used as the irrigation solution. Corneal abrasion could lead to irritation and redness of the eyes and cause impaired vision.

According to the practice advisory by the ASA, in a high-risk patient, vision should be assessed when the patient becomes alert, and an ophthalmology consultation obtained for any visual impairment.

29.7 Postoperative Kidney Complications (POKC)

Oliguria (<0.5 ml/kg/h) is the most common sign heralding renal dysfunction in the postoperative period. Although, the most common reason is depletion of intravascular fluid volume, it could be multifactorial. The causes could be "pre-renal" (hypovolemia, intra-abdominal hypertension, low cardiac output), "renal" (ischemia, contrast dye nephropathy, rhabdomyolysis), or "post-renal" (surgical injury to the ureters, blockade of urinary catheter). A judicial "fluid challenge" would be effective in restoring the urine output in most situations. Rhabdomyolysis is seen in patients who have suffered major crush injury, but may be seen in morbidly obese patients after prolonged surgery. Elevated serum creatine phosphokinase (CPK) levels would be diagnostic. Aggressive hydration and loop diuretics to flush the renal tubules are the mainstay of management.

29.8 Criteria for Discharge from the Post-anesthesia Care Unit

Perhaps the most important question to ask before discharging a patient from the PACU to the next lower level of care should be, "Is the patient safe to be left unmonitored for a period of time?" The patient should be oriented and be able to summon assistance, hemodynamically stable, adequately oxygenating, reasonably pain-free, and not nauseous.

The "Modified Aldrete Scoring System" is one of the commonly used objective discharge criteria (◘ ◉ Table 29.1). A score of ≥ 9 is required for discharge from the PACU [17].

Table 29.1 Modified Aldrete scoring system

	Score
Respiration	
Able to take deep breath and cough	2
Dyspnea/shallow breathing	1
Apnea	0
O_2 saturation	
Maintains $SpO_2 > 92\%$ on room air	2
Needs O_2 to maintain $SpO_2 > 90\%$	1
$SpO_2 < 90\%$ even with supplemental oxygen	0
Consciousness	
Fully awake	2
Arousable on calling	1
Not responding	0
Circulation	
Blood pressure ± 20 mm Hg preop	2
Blood pressure ± 20–50 mm Hg preop	1
Blood pressure ± 50 mm Hg preop	0
Activity	
Able to move all 4 extremities voluntarily	2
Able to move 2 extremities	1
Unable to move extremities	0

A score of ≥ 9 is required for discharge from the PACU

29.9 Questions and Answers

Questions (Choose the Most Appropriate Answer)

1. The most common early sign of myocardial ischemia in the PACU is
   A. ST-T wave changes on ECG monitor
   B. Diaphoresis
   C. Angina
   D. Dyspnea
   E. Tachycardia
2. All the following are recommended to treat the laryngospasm that occurs during emergence, EXCEPT
   A. Applying positive pressure by mask
   B. Larson's maneuver
   C. Succinylcholine 2 mg/kg dose
   D. Succinylcholine intramuscularly 4 mg/kg
   E. Small dose of propofol
3. According to the ASA and the Cardiac Anesthesia/Surgery Societies, patients who are not bleeding, are stable and euvolemic can tolerate a hemoglobin as low as:
   A. 6 g/dL
   B. 7 g/dL
   C. 8 g/dL
   D. 9 g/dL
   E. 10 g/dL
4. Which of the following tests reliably predicts recovery of airway protective reflexes?
   A. A negative inspiratory pressure of 25 cm H_2O or less
   B. Sustained head lift for 10 s
   C. Return of train-of-four response to preoperative levels
   D. A forced vital capacity of 10–12 ml/kg
   E. None of the above
5. Potential causes for prolonged unresponsiveness after anesthesia include all of the following, EXCEPT
   A. Pseudo-choline-esterase deficiency
   B. Hypoglycemia
   C. Hyperthermia
   D. Residual inhalational anesthetic
   E. Hypothermia
6. Regarding hypothermia and shivering in the PACU, which is FALSE
   A. Severe shivering may double the CO_2 production.
   B. Severe shivering can lead to myocardial infarction and ventilator failure.
   C. Inhalational anesthetic may accentuate shivering.
   D. Meperidine is an effective treatment for postoperative shivering.
   E. Non-shivering thermogenesis is effective in adults.

7. Management in patients with significant aspiration and hypoxemia, include
   A. Furosemide
   B. High-dose steroids
   C. Fluid restriction
   D. Mechanical ventilation with PEEP
   E. Prophylactic antibiotics
8. Pulmonary dead space decreases with which of the following
   A. Pulmonary embolism
   B. Endotracheal intubation
   C. Pulmonary hypotension
   D. Decreased cardiac output
   E. Transfusion related acute lung injury (TRALI)
9. Which of the following is true about serotonin syndrome?
   A. It is an idiosyncratic reaction.
   B. It presents as delirium and rigidity.
   C. Treatment include 5HT3 antagonists.
   D. Individuals have a genetic predisposition to develop this.
   E. It is seen in patients taking calcium channel blockers.
10. Which of the following should not be used to treat acute postoperative wheezing?
   A. IV steroids
   B. Aerosolized epinephrine
   C. Intramuscular terbutaline
   D. Ipratropium bromide
   E. IV epinephrine

Answers

1. **E**. In the PACU, the most common sign for acute MI is tachycardia and it is usually the reaction to, and not the cause of, MI. ST-T changes depends on lead placement and is usually a later sign on 12-lead ECG. Troponin levels could be used to confirm.
2. **C**. The usual recommended dose of succinylcholine is 0.1 mg/kg IV or 4 mg/kg IM if an IV access is not available. Propofol in doses of 20–30 mg can be used to deepen the level of anesthesia.
   Administration of lidocaine (1.5 mg/kg) or magnesium (15 mg/kg) prior to extubation may reduce the incidence of laryngospasm.
3. **A**. It is now well-accepted that patients who are not bleeding are stable, and euvolemic can tolerate a hemoglobin as low as 6 g/dL.
4. **E**. All these imply adequacy of muscle strength and not recovery of airway protective reflexes.
5. **C**. The common causes for delayed awakening after an anesthetic are residual anesthetic and residual curarization, hypothermia, and hypoglycemia. Pseudo-choline-esterase deficiency can lead to prolonged action of succinylcholine.
6. **E**. Non-shivering thermogenesis is ineffective in adults. Severe shivering may increase oxygen consumption and CO_2 production by 200%. This increases cardiac output and minute ventilation leading to myocardial ischemia and ventilator failure. Inhalational anesthetics cause tremors, which accentuate postop shivering. Meperidine is an effective treatment for shivering.
7. **D**. Significant aspiration can lead to hypoxemia, increased airway resistance, and pulmonary edema. Management includes endotracheal intubation and suctioning of trachea followed by mechanical ventilation with positive end expiratory pressure (PEEP). Pulmonary edema is usually secondary to increased capillary permeability and do not require diuretics or fluid restriction. Bacterial infection is rare and prophylactic antibiotics are not indicated nor are steroids.
8. **B**. Any decrease in pulmonary blood flow INCREASES pulmonary dead space and pulmonary embolism, hypotension, low cardiac output, and TRALI will all decrease pulmonary blood flow. Anatomical dead space can be reduced by 75% by endotracheal intubation and almost eliminated by tracheostomy.
9. **B**. Serotonin syndrome is a potentially lethal condition that occurs due to excess serotonin in the central nervous system, secondary to an adverse drug reaction or a drug interaction. Numerous drugs that increase serotonin activity, such as monoamine oxidase inhibitors (MAOI), selective serotonin-reuptake inhibitors (SSRI), opioids, and anti-emetics (5HT3 antagonists) have been associated with serotonin syndrome. The classical clinical triad of altered mental status, autonomic hyperactivity, and neuromuscular abnormality is not universally present. The usual presentation is a spectrum ranging from mild symptoms such as shivering and drowsiness to tremor, altered sensorium, muscle rigidity, and hyper-reflexia. The terminal events are hyperthermia, rhabdomyolysis, metabolic acidosis, renal failure, and disseminated intravascular coagulopathy.
   Cyproheptadine, a $5HT_{2A}$ antagonist, is a recommended treatment.
10. **A**. The treatment of acute bronchospasm include inhaled or IM terbutaline, anticholinergic medication such as ipratropium, and, finally, epinephrine (inhaled or IV) for severe bronchospasm. Steroids are not effective for acute improvement but may prevent later recurrence.

References

1. Cook TM, Woodall N, Frerk C, Fourth National Audit Project. Major complications of airway management in the UK: results of the fourth National Audit Project of the Royal College of anaesthetists and the difficult airway society. Part 1: anaesthesia. Br J Anaesth. 2011;106:617–31.
2. Metzner J, Posner KL, Lam MS, Domino KB. Closed claims' analysis. Best Pract Res Clin Anaesthesiol. 2011;25:263–76.
3. Cavallone LF, Vannucci A. Extubation of the difficult airway and extubation failure. Anesth Analg. 2013;116:368–83.
4. Peterson GN, Domino KB, Caplan RA, Posner KL, Lee LA, Cheney FW. Management of the difficult airway: a closed claims analysis. Anesthesiology. 2005;103:33–9.
5. Murphy GS. Neuromuscular management and patient outcomes. ASA Refresher Course. 2015;43:80–6.
6. Viby-Mogensen J, Claudius C. Evidence-based management of neuromuscular block. Anesth Analg. 2010;111:1–2.
7. Xará D, Santos A, Abelha F. Adverse respiratory events in a post-anesthesia care unit. Arch Bronconeumol. 2015;51:69–75.
8. Eichenberger AS, Proietti S, Wicky S, Frascarolo P, Suter M, Spahn DR, Magnusson L. Morbid obesity and postoperative pulmonary atelectasis: an underestimated problem. Anesth Analg. 2002;95:1788–92.
9. Mendonça J, Pereira H, Xará D, Santos A, Abelha FJ. Obese patients: respiratory complications in the post-anesthesia care unit. Rev Port Pneumol. 2014;20:12–9.
10. Bamgbade OA, Rutter TW, Nafiu OO, Dorje P. Postoperative complications in obese and nonobese patients. World J Surg. 2007;31:556–60.
11. Bailie R, Posner KL. New trends in adverse respiratory events from ASA closed claims project. ASA Newsl. 2011;75:28–9.
12. Gan TJ. Postoperative nausea and vomiting d can it be eliminated? JAMA. 2002;287:1233–6.
13. Blackburn J, Spencer R. Postoperative nausea and vomiting. Anaesth Intensive Care Med. 2015;16(9):452–6.
14. Sanders RD, Pandharipande PP, Davidson AJ, Ma D, Maze M. Anticipating and managing postoperative delirium and cognitive decline in adults. BMJ. 2011;343:d4331.
15. Boyer EW, Shannon M. The serotonin syndrome. N Engl J Med. 2005;352:1112–20.
16. American Society of Anesthesiologists Task Force on Perioperative Visual Loss. Practice advisory for perioperative visual loss associated with spine surgery: an updated report by the American society of anesthesiologists task force on perioperative visual loss. Anesthesiology. 2012;116(2):274–85.
17. Aldrete JA. The post-anesthesia recovery score revisited. J Clin Anesth. 1995;7:89–91.

Perioperative Pain Management

30

Andrzej P. Kwater and Juan P. Cata

Abstract

This chapter highlights the prevalence of inadequate pain control in surgical patients, emphasizing the need for a multimodal approach to address nociceptive, inflammatory, and neuropathic pain. This involves integrating regional anesthesia techniques with systemic analgesics throughout the perioperative period. Understanding pain mechanisms from nociceptor activation to central modulation informs effective interventions. Factors such as gender, age, psychological influences, and social experiences significantly impact pain perception and outcomes. Persistent postoperative pain (PPP) arises from complex sensitization processes, warranting a multifaceted preventive strategy. Pharmacologic interventions, including opioids, gabapentinoids, dexamethasone, ketamine, and NSAIDs, are key components, but their judicious use is crucial to mitigate adverse effects. Regional anesthesia techniques offer promise for opioid-sparing analgesia, though rebound pain post-block resolution remains a concern. Overall, optimizing perioperative pain management requires a comprehensive understanding of pain mechanisms and tailored interventions to improve patient outcome.

Keywords

Pain management • Perioperative • Multimodal analgesia • Transduction • Transmission • Perception • Nociceptors • Persistent postoperative pain • Pharmacology • Regional analgesia • Opioids • Cryotherapy • Acupuncture • Transcutaneous electrical nerve stimulation (TENS) • Hypnosis

Key Points

- Transduction, transmission, and perception are necessary steps in pain physiology. Peripheral and central sensitization are key elements of acute and persistent pain formation.
- The concept of multimodal analgesia involves the blockade of peripheral and central nociceptors involved in transduction, transmission, and perception of pain.
- A comprehensive preoperative evaluation and ongoing postoperative assessment of patients, comorbidities, and pain intensity are crucial to provide adequate postoperative pain management.
- Regional analgesia can be used for a wide variety of surgical procedures. A careful selection of the technique, local anesthetic concentration, and adjuvant analgesic is important to maximize the efficacy of each technique while minimizing adverse events.
- Continuous intravenous infusion of opioids is not recommended in patients not previously exposed to these medications or those with advance age, sleep apnea, and obesity due to the increased risk of respiratory depression.
- The transmucosal and transdermal routes of administration are not the optimal choice for treating postoperative acute pain. Iontophoresis delivery of opioids has recently been described and shown some efficacy in postoperative pain management. Acupuncture, TENS, and cryoanalgesia are considered non-pharmacological techniques that can be implemented in multimodal analgesic strategies.

It is estimated that 75% of patients undergoing any surgery in the United States experience inadequate pain control [1]. Surgical pain has the features of nociceptive,

A. P. Kwater · J. P. Cata (✉)
Department of Anesthesiology and Perioperative Medicine, The University of Texas – MD Anderson Cancer Center, Houston, TX, USA

J. P. Cata
Anesthesiology and Surgical Oncology Research Group, Houston, TX, USA

M. Argalious et al. (eds.), *Basic Sciences in Anesthesia*,
https://doi.org/10.1007/978-3-031-60203-0_30

inflammatory, and neuropathic pain [2]. Therefore, it has been recommended that more than one analgesic modality (multimodal analgesia) will be necessary to achieve adequate perioperative pain control, thus avoiding the unwanted effects of large doses of single analgesics, in particular opioids [3]. A multimodal analgesic technique entails the preoperative initiation, intraoperative continuation, and postoperative maintenance of a combination of regional anesthesia/analgesia techniques (when applicable) with two or more systemic analgesics [4]. In the postoperative period, the addition of systemic analgesics is important; in particular when regional anesthesia techniques are discontinued, as during this time, patients may experience severe distress and discomfort ("analgesic gap period") [5].

30.1 Pain Mechanisms and Pathways (Fig. 30.1)

(a) Nociceptors and Nociceptive Afferent Neurons

Transduction is the first necessary step to convert a noxious stimulus (mechanical, chemical, and thermal) into electrical neural activity. The sensors responsible for detecting noxious stimuli are called nociceptors. Although nociceptors are located in the terminals of sensory afferent fibers with different diameters and velocities of conduction (Aδ and C fibers), they can also be found in non-neuronal cells such as keratinocytes [6]. After surgical trauma, not one single substance, but a myriad of inflammatory mediators (glutamate, ATP, prostaglandins, cytokines, bradykinins, neurokinins, and growth factors) act on nociceptors to initiate the transduction process. Nociceptors are either ionotropic (ion channel) or metabotropic (second messenger-signaling cascade). The former rapidly transmit sensory information while the latter are slower responders. A particularly important group of inotropic receptors are the transient receptor potential vanilloid (TRPV) receptors and purinergic receptors [6–8]. Metabotropic receptors involved in transduction include tumor necrosis factor (TNF) receptor, prostaglandin receptors (EP1-4), leukotriene receptors (BLT1, BLT2, CysLT1, and CysLT2), neurokinin receptors (NK1 and NK2), and growth factor receptors (BDNF and NGF) [7, 9–12]. The action of the inflammatory mediators on peripheral nociceptors is responsible for the so-called peripheral sensitization. Once the transduction process and peripheral sensitization have been initiated, neurons remain in a hyperexcitable state even after cessation of noxious stimulation.

Once a nociceptor is activated, the second necessary step is the **transmission** of pain impulses from the periphery, in the form of electrical signals, to the dorsal horn of the spinal cord. Sodium voltage-gated channels located in Aδ fibers (small myelinated) and C fibers (unmyelinated) are key in

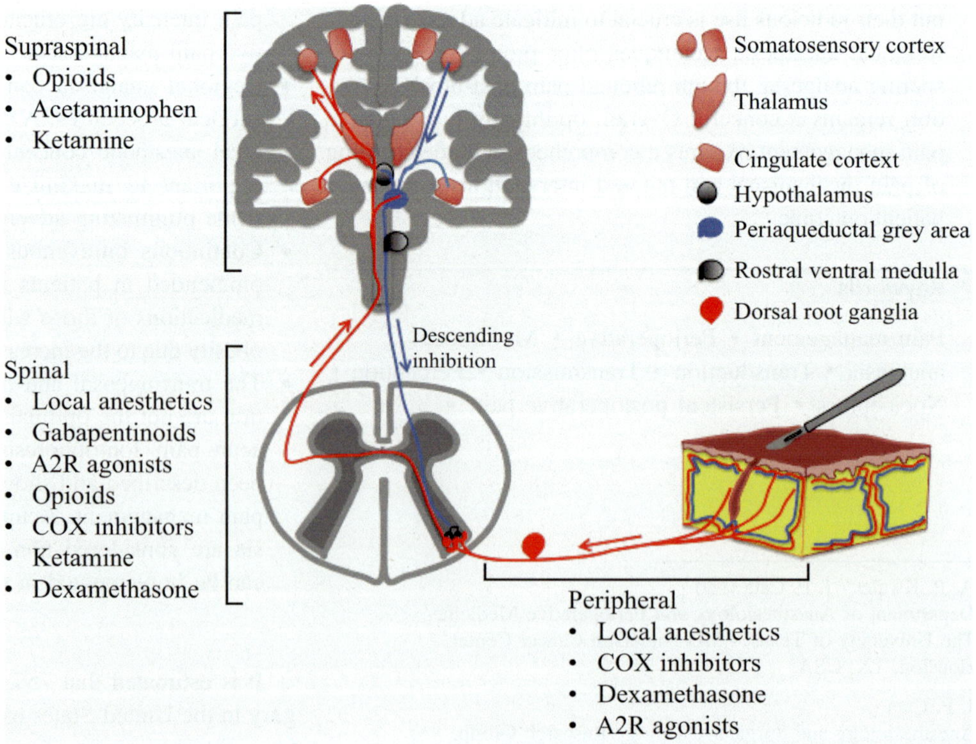

Fig. 30.1 The figure illustrates the nociceptive pathways and the site of action of routinely used analgesic and anesthetics

the transmission of electrical impulses [13]. These ion channels are of particular importance because they are the sites of action of local anesthetics [14]. Other ion channels involved in the transmission process include voltage-gated calcium (the site of action of gabapentinoids) and potassium channels [15].

(b) Dorsal Horn Transmission and Modulation; Wind-Up Phenomenon

Once peripheral sensitization (also known as ***primary hyperalgesia***) takes place, the spinal cord functions to receive a barrage of impulses and serves as a relay station. Sensory afferents, interneurons, and ascending and descending projection neurons located in the dorsal horn work in coordination to modulate the sensory information by muting, attenuating, limiting, amplifying, and transmitting pain signals back to the periphery or to supraspinal centers. Wide dynamic range neurons are of particular importance because they participate in the process of central sensitization (***secondary hyperalgesia***) and "wind-up," which refers to the frequency dependent facilitation of spinal neuron excitability induced by repetitive electrical stimulation of afferent C fibers [16]. Glutamate is one of the main neurotransmitters in the dorsal horn. There are two major types of glutamate receptors: ionotropic (AMPA and NDMA) and metabotropic. Although both types of receptors contribute to pain transmission, the NMDA receptor has particular clinical relevance because it is the site of action of drugs like ketamine, methadone, and magnesium sulfate [17–19]. Thrombospondin-4 (TSP4) is another excitatory neurotransmitter that is upregulated after nerve injury. TSP4 interacts with voltage-gated calcium channels, in specific the $\alpha 2\delta 1$ subunit that serves as the site of action of gabapentin [20].

(c) Spinal and Supraspinal Neurotransmission and Modulation; Opioid Receptors

From the dorsal horn to cortical structures, sensory pain information is transmitted by the spinothalamic tract and spinobulbar projections. From the thalamus, information regarding location, quality, and intensity of pain reaches cortical structures **(perception),** which are activated in a coordinated manner to differentiate between discriminative (somatosensory cortex) and emotional (anterior cingulate and insular cortex) aspects of pain [21]. Activation of the specific brainstem areas is responsible for the autonomic responses and descending modulation of pain. The periaqueductal grey and the rostral ventral media areas of the brainstem are of the utmost importance because they modulate afferent signaling by descending facilitation or inhibition and act as the site of action of drugs like opioids (descending inhibition) [21].

(d) Autonomic Contributions to Pain; Visceral Pain Perception and Transmission

A significant interaction exists between the autonomic nervous system and pain responses. Acute pain creates a response characterized by an increase in sympathetic activity proportional to the noxious stimulation and a relative decrease of parasympathetic activity [22]. The magnitude of autonomic response not only correlates with the degree of activity of cortical areas such as the medial prefrontal cortex, but also with surgical pain responses [23]. Clinical investigations have found that there is a negative correlation between preoperative baroreflex sensitivity and early postoperative persistent pain [24]. In fact, it has been suggested that activation of baroreceptors would induce antinociception [25]. Moreover, recent evidence indicates that the contribution of the sympathetic system on acute postoperative pain is significant. For example, the use of preoperative stellate ganglion blockade resulted in a significant reduction in pain scores and analgesic requirements following upper extremity surgery [26, 27].

Inflammation, ischemia, and distention (tension receptors) of the gut activate afferent sensory fibers located in the mucosa, muscle, and serosa [28]. The same chemical mediators that activate somatic nociceptors, including TRP receptors, stimulate visceral nociceptors [29]. For instance, ATP, bradykinins and prostaglandins are able to induce depolarization of visceral sensory afferents [30]. Vagal afferents have their cell bodies in the nodose and jugular ganglia, and innervate all thoracic and abdominal viscera including part of the colon. On the other hand, spinal afferents have their cell bodies in the dorsal root ganglia and uniformly innervate all the viscera [29]. Ultimately, both vagal and spinal nerve afferents are responsible for conveying information from the gastrointestinal tract to the central nervous system. It has been postulated that vagal fibers transmit physiological information while spinal nerves are responsible for conveying noxious stimulation. Once the afferent neurons reach the spinal cord, they make synaptic connections with second-order neurons that will project to the thalamus and nucleus tractus solitarius via the spinothalamic, spinoreticular, and dorsal column pathways. Significant interactions between somatic and visceral afferents are responsible for the clinical manifestation of referred pain [28]. Descending inhibition also plays a role in visceral pain. It has been demonstrated that low doses of opioids can activate descending pathways and cause antinociception [31].

(e) Social, Vocational, and Psychological Influences on Pain Perception

Preoperative social experiences, psychological factors (i.e., anxiety and depression), and patients' expectations have a significant impact on postoperative pain perception and development of persistent postoperative pain. For instance, alexithymia, the inability to identify and express emotions, predicts the development of persistent postoperative pain after mastectomy [32]. Along with this evidence, a preoperative diagnosis of severe/definite depression or preoperative self-perceived risk of addiction is also associated with a significant increase in the risk for persistent postoperative pain after surgery [33, 34]. Patients' coping strategies can also be useful to predict postoperative pain outcomes. For example, catastrophizing patients may misinterpret and exaggerate situations that are perceived as threatening and report worse quality of life and activity levels following surgery [35, 36].

Lastly, inadequate postoperative pain management can be associated with the development of psychiatric disorders after surgery. For instance, patients with high postoperative pain scores appear to be at risk for depression and post-traumatic stress disorder 1 year after surgery [37]. On the other hand, perioperative cognitive interventions targeted to improve depression postoperatively have been shown to decrease pain scores and improve quality of life after cardiac surgery [34].

(f) Gender and Age Differences in Pain Perception

Overall, women are more likely to report a variety of recurrent pain that is more severe and frequent when compared to men. In the context of surgery, women reported higher pain scores than men after a variety of surgical interventions [38, 39]. Furthermore, women exhibit slower recovery and have a higher risk of developing postoperative persistent pain when compared to men [40, 41]. This can be explained by (a) biological factors: signs of central sensitization are less pronounced in men than women while descending inhibition control is less efficient in women than men, (b) psychological factors: differences in coping strategies, (c) social factors (expectations), and d) past medical history [42, 43].

(g) Persistent Postoperative Pain (PPP)

Persistent Postoperative Pain (PPP) is defined as pain that persists after surgery longer than 3 months in duration, following exclusion of other identifiable causes [44]. The incidence of PPP ranges from 5–50% [44]. Persistent postoperative pain can occur after major and minor surgery, as well as open and laparoscopic procedures; however, its incidence appears to be lower after video-assisted surgery [45, 46]. Risk factors for PPP include female gender, preoperative pain, diabetes mellitus, poorly managed acute postoperative pain, prolonged operative time, tissue ischemia, anxiety, and depression (Table 30.1) [2, 47, 48].

PPP and chronic postsurgical pain typically present clinically with neuropathic components [49]. Direct nerve injury (transection, stretching, or crushing) in addition to a persistent inflammatory state has been indicated as the cause ("primary injury") for PPP [44]. This primary injury to the nerve is the initial step in a series of events resulting in both peripheral and central pain sensitization, which ultimately leads to the development of chronic postsurgical pain. Peripheral pain sensitization results from nociceptive inputs stimulating the release of mediators, including prostaglandins, nerve growth factor, and cytokines, in addition to an increase in glutamatergic activity in the spinal cord [50]. Central pain sensitization subsequently progresses as changes in pain signaling in the spinal cord lead to central neuroplasticity and a state of signal potentiation as well as increased pain sensitivity. These factors in addition to a variety of molecular and cellular changes in the setting of persistent inflammatory signaling, ultimately lead to the development of PPP.

Persistent postoperative pain (PPP) is common after thoracic surgery (post-thoracotomy pain syndrome), breast surgery (post-mastectomy pain syndrome), limb amputations (phantom limb syndrome), and total knee replacements [44, 47, 51]. PPP has features of neuropathic pain, thus patients usually report pain as burning, tingling, numbing, or characterized by electric-like shocks in one or two dermatomes surrounding the surgical incision. The effects of PPP extend into a patient's overall health and quality of life following surgery.

Despite the publication of various studies in recent years, at this time there are no pharmacological agents that have demonstrated consistent efficacy in preventing chronic postsurgical pain, otherwise known as PPP. While gabapentinoids (pregabalin), IV lidocaine, and NSAIDs have been identified in a subset of studies as providing some level of benefit in the prevention of PPP, there is significant uncertainty in these findings as it relates to overall clinical relevance [52]. On the other hand, regional anesthesia techniques (neuraxial and peripheral nerve blocks) have demonstrated promising results in reducing the incidence of chronic postoperative pain, especially in the context of breast surgery, thoracotomies, and cesarean section [53–55]. Preventive mechanisms of regional anesthesia involve pain signaling modulation, decreased central sensitization, and anti-inflammatory effects during the perioperative period [55].

(h) Rebound Pain

Regional anesthesia in the form of spinal anesthesia and peripheral nerve blockade provides notable benefits to perioperative pain management in the form of opioid-sparing analgesia, improved patient satisfaction and pain scores,

Table 30.1 Predictor factors and causes of persistent postoperative pain

Causes	Predictors
Nerve injury	Female gender
Prolonged tissue ischemia	Preoperative pain
	Anxiety–Depression–Catastrophizing
	Diabetes mellitus (TKA)
	Operative time
	Open > minimally invasive procedures
	Type of surgery (thoracotomy, mastectomy, TKA and limb amputations)
	Exaggerated acute postoperative pain

TKA Total knee replacement

reduced opioid-related side effects (nausea, vomiting, sedation), and shorter hospital length of stay. However, peripheral nerve blocks (PNBs), especially as single-shot injections, are limited by the duration of analgesia, even with the use of local anesthetic additives or adjuncts [56]. Upon resolution of regional anesthetic effects, patients are at risk of experiencing severe pain as underlying noxious stimuli from the surgical site exhibit unopposed pain signaling, a phenomenon referred to as rebound pain [57]. Overall incidence of rebound pain is unclear due to various underlying factors such as type of surgical intervention and associated postoperative pain trajectory, but it could be as high as 40% in patients following resolution of peripheral nerve blockade [57, 58]. This translates to potential unwanted hospital admissions following ambulatory surgery or prolonged hospital stays after surgery secondary to inadequate pain control. Of note, recent findings examining brachial plexus PNBs demonstrate that the use of perineural dexamethasone as an adjunct not only serves to prolong the duration of nerve blockade, but also appears to reduce the incidence and severity of rebound pain. The mechanism is likely attributed to a prolonged reduction in nociceptive input with PNBs following surgery [59, 60].

30.2 Pain Management

(1) ***Pharmacologic Interventions***

(a) **Drugs**

Opioids provide adequate postoperative analgesia, but their routine use is often limited by adverse effects. The mechanism of action of opioids occurs through binding mainly to mu-opioid receptors, which result in hyperpolarization of sensory neurons, thus decreasing the release of neurotransmitters involved in nociception. In the perioperative period, opioids are typically administered intravenous, neuraxial, oral, and less often sublingual and transdermal. Intravenous patient-controlled analgesia (IVPCA) is a commonly used technique in the postoperative period following major surgery. Fentanyl, morphine, and hydromorphone are the most commonly used opioids for IVPCA (Table 30.2). Intrathecal opioids also provide adequate analgesia during and after surgery. In particular, fentanyl, sufentanil, morphine, and hydromorphone are often used for neuraxial analgesia. Oral opioids are also available and are often used in the ambulatory setting. Oxycodone, hydrocodone, tramadol, and codeine are frequently used as oral formulations when patients are able to tolerate at least liquids by mouth. Opioids are associated with a multitude of side effects including respiratory depression, nausea and vomiting, ileus, drowsiness, urinary retention, confusion, and hyperalgesia [61–63]. Therefore, the judicious use of these drugs is recommended in the perioperative period. Tramadol is a weak mu-opioid agonist as well as norepinephrine and serotonin reuptake inhibitor with questionable efficacy as a single agent. On the other hand, it has proven to be effective when given in combination with other analgesics [64].

Opioids are associated with adverse effects including sedation, tolerance, addiction, tolerance, and respiratory depression. These side effects, particularly respiratory depression, are thought to be mediated by activation of beta-arrestin signaling. **Oliceridine** is a G protein selective (biased) agonist of the mu-opioid receptor indicated in opioid naïve adults to manage acute postoperative pain moderate-to-severe enough to require intravenous conventional opioid analgesics [65]. Oliceridine is structurally distinct from traditional opioids (e.g., morphine) or synthetic derivatives (e.g., fentanyl or hydromorphone). Thus, it has been theorized that mu-opioid receptor ligands such as oliceridine may constitute more effective analgesic therapy with reduced adverse effects [66]. Specifically, the G protein selectivity or biased activity of oliceridine results in potent analgesia with substantially reduced (about 14%) recruitment of β-arrestin, a signaling pathway associated with opioid-related adverse effects [66].

Methadone (intravenous or oral) is an opioid that provides analgesic benefit with the advantage of exhibiting a long and variable half-life. It functions as a mu-receptor agonist,

Table 30.2 Common solutions for intravenous patient (adult) controlled analgesia

Solution	Bolus	Interval	Basal rate*	Max. dose hour
Morphine	0.5–2 mg	5–10 min	1 mg/h	6 mg
Fentanyl	5–20 μ(mu)g	5–10 min	10 μ(mu)g/h	60 μ(mu)g
Hydromorphone	0.1–0.2 μ(mu)g	5–10 min	0.2 mg/h	1.2 mg

Solutions and type of opioid used for IVPCA should be administered considering patients' expectations, comorbidities and type of surgery

serotonin and norepinephrine reuptake inhibitor, and potent NMDA receptor antagonist. This pharmacological effect is of clinical significance as upregulation of NMDA receptors has been attributed to the subsequent development of opioid tolerance and chronic postsurgical pain. Thus, methadone is often used for the treatment of opioid abuse disorder but is also beneficial in the setting of perioperative pain management. Intraoperative administration of methadone (0.2–0.3 mg/kg as a single dose) has been shown to provide prolonged analgesic effect in patients undergoing major surgery (orthopedic, spine, gynecologic/obstetric, cardiac) over the course of the first 3 postoperative days [67–69]. In relation to its safety profile, methadone has not been shown to increase the incidence of common opioid-related side effects, such as sedation, postoperative nausea and vomiting, and decreased bowel function. However, the potential for prolonged respiratory depression remains a consideration when combined with other opioids, as well as the risk of serotonin syndrome (when used in conjunction with other serotonergic medications) and QT prolongation [67].

Gabapentinoids (pregabalin and gabapentin) are adjuvant drugs with analgesic benefit and opioid-sparing effects [70, 71]. Their mechanism of action is through the binding of α2δ and thrombospondin receptors in the central nervous system [72]. Pregabalin (75–150 mg) is commonly given orally before surgery and in the postoperative setting every 12 h. In comparison to gabapentin, pregabalin is associated with less sedation and cognitive disturbances. Gabapentin can be administered orally three times a day (100–1,200 mg); however, the side effects of sedation and cognitive impairment associated with larger doses are disadvantageous when being considered in the perioperative period, especially in elderly patients [3]. In recent developments, following a meta-analysis of randomized controlled trials, the perioperative use of gabapentinoids was demonstrated to offer no clinically significant analgesic effect in the management of acute pain and was associated with greater risk of adverse events, including dizziness and visual disturbances [73]. Therefore, current evidence does not support the routine use of gabapentinoids as part of a perioperative multimodal analgesic regimen, unless continued for patients already taking these medications for other medical indications [74].

Dexamethasone (intravenous) is a potent glucocorticoid that has anti-inflammatory and analgesic properties [75]. The exact mechanism of analgesia is still not clear but it appears to be related to the anti-inflammatory effects (down-regulation of cyclooxygenase-2 mRNA). Epidural dexamethasone may be acting at spinal sites by inducing the synthesis of the phospholipase-A2 inhibitory protein lipocortin, and modulating the activity of the glucocorticoid receptor at the level of the substantia gelatinosa [76, 77]. Doses of 4–10 mg commonly used for postoperative nausea and vomiting prophylaxis are effective in providing analgesia and have been demonstrated not to interfere with wound healing or to cause an increase in the rate of complications after major surgery [3, 78, 79]. Dexamethasone does not provide any preventive benefit in relation to the onset of persistent postoperative pain [80]. Dexamethasone has also been shown to prolong and enhance the quality of peripheral nerve blockade [81, 82]. The mechanism of action is likely related to stimulation of neuronal glucocorticoid receptors, and the subsequent increased expression of inhibitory potassium channels (thus decreasing neuronal excitability), in addition to systemic anti-inflammatory effects [83].

Ketamine (intravenous or epidural) is an NMDA receptor antagonist that has strong analgesic and opioid-sparring properties [84]. Other mechanisms for ketamine-induced analgesia include direct action on monoaminergic, cholinergic, and mu receptors. Subanesthetic (or analgesic) doses of 3–5 mg/kg/min given during surgery and/or postoperatively as a continuous intravenous infusion have been shown to provide effective analgesia for a wide range of procedures [84]. Nystagmus, diplopia, blurred vision, and hallucinations are potential side effects reported even with low doses of ketamine, although the incidence is low (<1%) [84]. The preventive effects of ketamine on postoperative persistent pain formation have been observed after intravenous but not epidural administration [85].

Non-steroidal anti-inflammatory drugs (NSAIDs) are adjuvant analgesics with proven efficacy in the context of multimodal analgesia for surgery (Table 30.3) [86–88]. Their mechanism of action is inhibition of COX-1/COX-2 enzymes. The concept of COX enzyme selectivity denotes the extent to which these drugs are able to inhibit one enzyme isoform relative to the other at half-maximal inhibitory concentrations [89]. Interestingly, the same drug might show COX-1/COX-2 ratios at distinct inhibitory concentration levels, therefore, demonstrating that each

Table 30.3 Recommended solutions for epidural and peripheral nerve catheter patient controlled analgesia

Route	Local anesthetic	Additives	Basal rate	Bolus	Interval
Epidural	Ropicavaine 0.05–0.2%	Fentanyl 5–10 μ(mu)g/mL	3–8 mL/h	3–5 mL	10–15 min/4–6 doses/hr
	Bupivacaine 0.0625–0.125%	Sufentanil 0.25–2 μ(mu) g/mL Hydromorphone 3–10 μg ml Clonidine 1.5 μ(mu)g/mL			
Peripheral nerve catheter	Lidocaine 1%	Fentanyl 1–2 μ(mu)g/mL	3–10 ml/h	10–12 mL	60 min/1 dose/hr
	Bupivacaine 0.125–0.25% Ropivacaine 0.1–0.2%	Sufentanil 0.1 μ(mu)g/mL Hydromorphone 3–10 μg/ml Clonidine 1–2 μ(mu)g/mL			

Solutions and doses of local anesthetics and additives should be administered considering patients' expectations, comorbidities, and location and type of surgery

COX inhibitor has its own selectivity (Table 30.3) [90]. In other words, one analgesic can be more or less selective depending on the dose used. NSAIDs have several routes of administration depending on the type of drug. Ketorolac is one of the most commonly used NSAIDs in the perioperative period because of its strong analgesic properties and the fact that it can be administered via oral, sublingual, and intravenous routes [91]. Other intravenous NSAIDs, although not all available in the United States, include diclofenac, ibuprofen, dexketoprofen, flurbiprofen axetil, and lornoxicam [92–95]. Overall, NSAIDs can be administered safely in the perioperative period. However, their use, in particular ketorolac, should be limited to short periods of time and avoided in patients with coagulopathy, renal failure, or a history of peptic ulcers [3].

Among the selective COX-2 inhibitors (parecoxib, eterocoxib, and lumiracoxib), celecoxib (oral formulation) has been the most commonly used in the perioperative period after rofecoxib and valdecoxib were withdrawn from the United States market. Although their main advantage over non-selective COX inhibitors is a lower incidence of gastrointestinal complications, recent concerns regarding an increase in major adverse cardiovascular events and anastomotic leaks after colorectal surgery have been raised with the use of non-selective and selective COX-2 inhibitors [3, 96–100].

Acetaminophen (intravenous, rectal, or oral) is widely used in the context of multimodal analgesia. The mechanism of analgesia of acetaminophen is still unclear; however, it can be related to a dose-dependent reduction of prostaglandin E levels and activation of $5HT_3$ receptors in the central nervous system [101–103]. Acetaminophen reduces morphine consumption by 20% in addition to reducing postoperative nausea and vomiting. This combined effect can be attributed (a) to its analgesic effect and (b) increase in anandamide levels [104]. Acetaminophen has a duration of action of 4–6 h and can be administered every 6–8 h for maximal benefit [105, 106]. A maximum dose of 4 g per day in adults is advised to avoid hepatoxicity. The lack of interference with platelet function and safe administration in patients with a history of gastrointestinal bleeding, peptic ulcers, or asthma makes acetaminophen preferable over NSAIDs [3, 106]. Although initially presumed to provide superior analgesic efficacy secondary to increased plasma and effect site concentration, intravenous acetaminophen has more recently been shown to have no clinically significant advantage over the oral formulation [97, 107–111]. For instance, in a large retrospective study of open colectomy patients, the use of intravenous acetaminophen demonstrated no clinical benefit when compared to oral acetaminophen as it relates to decreasing postoperative opioid consumption [109].

Intravenous infusions of ***lidocaine*** are commonly used in protocols of multimodal analgesia because it reduces intraoperative requirements of opioids and postoperative nausea and vomiting, improves gastrointestinal motility, and shortens length of stay although these beneficial effects appear to be surgery specific [112–114]. The mechanism of action of lidocaine is related to its properties as a local anesthetic in addition to anti-inflammatory effects. A continuous infusion (1.5–4 mg/kg/h) of this amide local anesthetic can be used intraoperatively and/or postoperatively although the maximum benefit appears to be when used during surgery as opposed to short-term postoperative infusions [112, 113]. Adverse events associated with the use lidocaine are very low and mostly related to its actions on the central nervous system (perioral numbness, confusion, and visual disturbances) [112]. In addition, the use of perioperative intravenous lidocaine can reduce the incidence of postoperative persistent pain [115].

Esmolol (a *selective ultra-short-acting beta-blocker) has* been used in intravenous infusions (loading dose of 0.5 mg/kg followed by 5 μg/kg/min) to provide analgesia in major surgery [116, 117]. The mechanism of analgesia of esmolol is not fully understood, although it appears to be related to the activation of G proteins at a central level which resembles the effect of clonidine [118]. Intraoperative infusions of esmolol have not only shown to provide adequate analgesia and hemodynamic stability but also have opioid- and anesthetic-sparing effects [116, 117]. Bradycardia and hypotension are observed during infusions of larger doses than recommended.

Intravenous or intrathecal ***magnesium sulfate*** has analgesic effects that appear to be exerted by at least two mechanisms: (a) regulation of calcium influx into neurons and (b) antagonism of the NMDA receptors at central levels [18]. It can also significantly potentiate the antinociception of drugs like ketamine and reduce the overall consumption of opioids [119]. It is commonly used intraoperatively and administered as a bolus (30–50 mg/kg) followed by a continuous infusion (8–15 mg/kg/h) [119]. Intrathecal administration of 50 mg of magnesium sulfate can delay the onset of sensory block and prolong the duration of motor block produced by local anesthetics[120–123]. Hemodynamic instability (bradycardia and hypotension) and muscle weakness are commonly reported adverse effects associated with the use of intravenous magnesium. Thus, caution should be advised in the dosage of muscle relaxants or in the use of other anesthetics that can trigger hemodynamic instability when used in conjunction with magnesium sulfate during surgery.

Dexmedetomidine and clonidine are $\alpha 2$-adrenoreceptor agonists with known analgesic effects. The mechanism of action is through activation of the $\alpha 2$-adrenoreceptor, which results in depression of the release of presynaptic C-fiber transmitters and hyperpolarization of postsynaptic dorsal horn neurons. Both agents have anesthetic and opioid-sparing properties and can be used systemically (intravenous) or as adjuncts with local anesthetic solutions in regional analgesia [124]. As adjuvants for peripheral nerve blocks or neuraxial analgesia (intrathecal or epidural) both drugs can a) accelerate onset and prolong the duration of the motor and sensory blockade, b) decrease the concentration of local anesthetics needed for surgical blockade, c) prolong the time to first rescue analgesic requirement, and d) improve patient satisfaction. However, it is worth noting that these effects are not consistent across clinical outcomes [125–128]. Although bradycardia, hypotension, and sedation are side effects associated with the use of both drugs, when compared to clonidine, dexmedetomidine may avoid the undesirable cardiovascular effects due to $\alpha 1$ adrenoreceptor activation [125, 127, 128].

Neostigmine is an acetylcholinesterase inhibitor that can be administered in the epidural (1–10 μg/kg) or intrathecal (1–100 μg) space [129, 130]. Neostigmine causes dose-dependent analgesia, potentiates opioid-induced analgesia, and reduces the requirements of other analgesics. It does not influence the dynamics of nerve blockade provided by local anesthetics [129–134]. The mechanism of action appears to be related to an increase in the concentration of the neurotransmitter acetylcholine that, in turn, acts on muscarinic M1, M3, and presynaptic nicotinic receptors located on interneurons at the laminae II and V of the dorsal horn [135]. Side effects are dose-dependent and include nausea and vomiting, headache, and hemodynamic disturbances [131–133].

Despite being used primarily as an anxiolytic, intrathecal ***midazolam*** (1–2 mg) has shown analgesic properties [136–138]. The mechanism of action is still unclear but is likely related to the activation of $GABA_A$, benzodiazepine receptors, and the release of endogenous opioids [139–142]. Midazolam causes dose-dependent acceleration of the onset of motor/sensory block, prolongation of the duration of analgesia, and a reduction in opioid consumption [136, 138, 143, 144]. Sedation has been reported as an adverse effect associated with the use of intrathecal midazolam [136, 137].

Antidepressants are commonly used for the treatment of chronic pain syndromes and several trials have been conducted to evaluate their efficacy in the context of surgical pain. Antidepressants can be grouped into three different classes: (1) tricyclic antidepressants, (2) selective serotonin reuptake inhibitors, and (3) serotonin and norepinephrine reuptake inhibitors. Their mechanism of analgesia can be explained by central and peripheral actions and include an increase in the synaptic concentrations of serotonin and norepinephrine, modulation of peripheral sodium channels, and NMDA receptors. The literature does not support the use of antidepressants for treatment of acute pain, or prevention of chronic postoperative pain [145]. Adverse effects appear to be drug specific and include somnolence, dizziness, nausea, diarrhea, constipation, shivering, and tingling of extremities [145].

(b) **Routes**

Intravenous, Subcutaneous, and Intramuscular Analgesia

Intravenous analgesia is the preferred analgesic modality in patients with a non-functional gastrointestinal tract, those in whom regional analgesia is not indicated, or to treat severe breakthrough pain. Based on these factors, intravenous patient-controlled analgesia (IVPCA) is still one of the most common used analgesic techniques to manage acute postoperative pain. It consists of the intravenous administration of analgesics, most commonly opioids, that is self-controlled by the patient. A particular concern is that IVPCA cannot be considered in all patients (i.e., infants or patients with dementia). Although IVPCA provides superior analgesia compared to "around the clock" techniques, it is still not better than regional anesthesia or multimodal analgesic techniques [146]. Furthermore, opioid consumption is higher in patients treated with IVPCA when compared to regional analgesia; thus patients are at constant risk of opioid-related side effects [146–148]. The intramuscular and subcutaneous routes are less preferred in the context of surgery since they can be associated with pain on administration as well as erratic and unreliable levels of absorption of corresponding analgesics.

Transmucosal and Transdermal Routes

The transmucosal (TM) and transdermal (TD) routes of administration have been described to provide analgesia after surgery. Fentanyl can be delivered through both routes but the transmucosal route is not preferred and not recommended in the postoperative period. On the other hand, an iontophoretic transdermal system (ITS) has been recently released in the market and shows to be as efficacious and cause less opioid-related adverse effects as compared to morphine IVPCA [149, 150]. This new technology employs the use of a micro electric current (170 μA) to deliver 40 μg of fentanyl upon patient's request (patient-controlled analgesia). Although the first initial serum concentrations of fentanyl are lower using ITS when compared to the intravenous route, the subsequent systemic concentrations increase over time until they are comparable to those achieved by intravenous administration [151].

(2) ***Regional Anesthesia Techniques***

(a) **Overview**

When possible, regional anesthesia should be considered as one of the primary techniques for providing adequate postoperative analgesia. Regional anesthesia is not only superior in terms of management of postoperative pain and providing improved patient satisfaction when compared to intravenous analgesic control, but also can improve other clinical outcomes in appropriately selected patients, including lower the risk of cardiovascular and pulmonary complications [152–154]. The concept of patient-controlled analgesia (PCA) is also applicable for regional anesthetic techniques where a catheter is in place for purposes of continuous analgesia (Table 30.4). Patient-controlled epidural analgesia is one of the most commonly used forms of PCA in this context and is used to manage postoperative pain after both abdominal and thoracic surgery.

The choice of a regional anesthesia technique should be based on several factors, including patient age and comorbidities, anatomic location of the surgical incision, projected postoperative pain trajectory, and overall patient expectations [155]. In a study of patients undergoing major orthopedic/spine, thoracic, and abdominal surgery, a series of five distinct pain trajectory groups was established based on similar postoperative pain scores and opioid requirements over the course of 7 postoperative days. More than half of the evaluated patients qualified as part of the moderate-to-high or high-pain group, indicating that most major surgeries will necessitate appropriate techniques for extended analgesia [156] Another factor that needs to be considered with regional anesthesia interventions is the presence and timing of administration of antiplatelet medications or systemic anticoagulation. Recommendations related to regional anesthesia (neuraxial, PNBs) procedures in this context are dictated by the American Society of Regional Anesthesia (ASRA) guidelines to diminish the risk of hematoma formation.

A variety of regional anesthesia techniques can be utilized successfully for perioperative multimodal pain management, including neuraxial anesthesia (spinal, epidural, or combined spinal-epidural), peripheral nerve blocks, fascial plane blocks, local wound infiltration, field blocks, and intra- or periarticular local anesthetic infiltrations [157]. In addition, the use of specific local anesthetic formulations, additives to local anesthetics, delayed-release formulations, and continuous catheter systems each have an impact on the analgesic effect provided by a particular regional anesthesia intervention.

(b) **Neuraxial Anesthesia**

Neuraxial analgesia can be used for thoracic/chest wall, abdominal, or lower extremity surgery. However, a variety of side effects can be associated with the use of neuraxial anesthesia, including hypotension, urinary retention, motor weakness, and opioid-induced respiratory depression, especially with higher concentrations of local anesthetics and opioids [158]. The administration of opioids in the epidural or intrathecal space should also be approached with caution in patients at risk of respiratory depression, in particular with the use of hydromorphone or morphine. In addition, based on the intended duration and extent of analgesic effect, various combinations of local anesthetic concentrations and volume can be used in conjunction with a specific neuraxial technique (spinal vs epidural, with or without a catheter system) to achieve a desired outcome.

In addition to neuraxial anesthesia, there are alternative regional anesthesia techniques that can be used to achieve similar effective and widespread analgesia of the chest wall and/or abdomen. These include the paravertebral block (PVB) as well as erector spinae plane block (ESPB). Both techniques allow the option of providing unilateral and segmental analgesic coverage. The erector spinae plane block (ESPB) was initially described for management of thoracic neuropathic pain, but has since been shown to provide analgesic benefit for major thoracic, spine, abdominal, and orthopedic surgeries [159]. In addition, ESPB has the added benefit of being regarded as a more superficial interfascial plane block, thus allowing it to serve as a potential option in patients who otherwise would not be candidates for neuraxial anesthesia or PVB in the setting of systemic anticoagulation or coagulopathy.

Table 30.4 Recommended doses of commonly used non-opioid analgesics

Route	Name	Dose	Adverse effects/comments
Intravenous	Acetaminophen	1 g every 6–8 h	Liver failure
	Ketorolac	15–30 mg every 6–8 h	Renal impairment, bleeding and gastric erosion/PUD*
	Diclofenac sodium	18.75–50 mg every 6–8 h	Renal impairment, bleeding*
	Ibuprofen	800 mg every 6 h	Renal impairment, bleeding*
Oral	Naproxen	250–500 mg every 6–12 h	Renal impairment, bleeding*/Delayed onset of effect
	Ibuprofen	200–400 mg every 6 h	Renal impairment, bleeding*
	Ketorolac	15–30 mg every 8 h	Renal impairment, bleeding*
	Celecoxib	200 mg every 12 h	Anastomotic leak
	Pregabalin	75–150 mg every 12 h	Sedation, confusion, dizziness
	Gabapentin	100–300 mg every 8 h	Sedation, confusion, dizziness

Doses of NSAIDs and other analgesics should be administered considering patients' expectations, comorbidities, and type of surgery. * The short-term use of NSAIDs has demonstrated no serious gastrointestinal outcomes such as bleeding or perforation or cardiovascular events
PUD Peptic ulcer disease

When epidural analgesia and paravertebral blocks are contraindicated, intrapleural (IB), extrapleural (EB), and intercostal nerve blocks (INB) can be considered for postoperative pain relief after thoracic or upper abdominal surgery [160, 161]. Although IB and INB are superior to intravenous analgesia, they do not provide similar quality of analgesia when compared to epidural or paravertebral blocks [162]. EB consists of creating a space between the parietal pleura and thoracic wall followed by placement of a catheter that will be used to administer a solution of local anesthetic after completion of the thoracotomy. INB can be done by direct visualization during thoracotomy or percutaneously. Two to 5 mL of local anesthetic is injected inferior to the rib, to avoid intravascular injection, over the span of two to three intercostal spaces above and below the incision [163]. Single or intermittent boluses or continuous administration of local anesthetics through the catheters can be used for IB and INB. Although the rate of complications of IB and INB are low, both blocks have a risk of local anesthetic toxicity and pneumothorax [160, 161].

(c) **Peripheral Nerve Blocks (PNBs)**

Nerve plexus or selective peripheral nerve blockade hase become a cornerstone piece in multimodal analgesia regimens, with the use of ultrasound-guided techniques providing improved efficacy and safety of these interventions [154]. Peripheral nerve blocks (PNBs) can be used for purposes of serving as the primary anesthetic technique, or to supplement other modes of anesthetic management. Benefits of regional anesthesia include effective postoperative analgesia, reduced pain and opioid consumption, reduced opioid-related side effects (nausea, vomiting, sedation), and improved recovery timeline following surgery [164].

For analgesia of the upper extremity, a series of brachial plexus blocks (interscalene, supraclavicular, infraclavicular, and axillary) can be utilized, each anesthetizing a different level of the brachial plexus [164]. For analgesic coverage of the shoulder and posterior aspect of the arm, the interscalene block (ISB) is best utilized for optimal analgesia. However, this block has the highest risk of hemidiaphragmatic paresis from unilateral phrenic nerve blockade, and thus should be used with caution in patients with preexisting respiratory depression or chronic pulmonary comorbidities. In addition, the ISB frequently omits analgesic coverage of the lower nerve roots, thus not useful for some aspects of the distal arm and hand. The supraclavicular brachial plexus block provides extensive upper limb anesthesia and is associated with risks of intravascular injection, pneumothorax, and diaphragmatic hemiparesis (up to 50% of patients). The infraclavicular and axillary brachial plexus blocks provide analgesic coverage to the distal two-thirds of the arm extending to the forearm and hand. The infraclavicular brachial plexus block does not provide analgesic coverage of the axillary nerve (innervates deltoid and skin over deltoid) and is associated with potential risks of intravascular injection, pneumothorax, and phrenic nerve blockade (up to 25% of patients). The axillary brachial plexus block omits the musculocutaneous nerve, and thus this nerve would need to be blocked separately to provide analgesic coverage of the lateral forearm. Of note, the axilla and medial portion of the upper arm are innervated by the intercostobrachial nerve of the T2 nerve root (not part of brachial plexus). Therefore, a separate subcutaneous "field" injection distal to the axillary crease needs to be performed to provide analgesic coverage for surgical incision or tourniquet-related pain.

For analgesia of the lower extremity, a subset of blocks can be utilized to target nerves originating from the lumbar and sacral plexus. Blockade of nerves originating from the lumbar plexus (femoral, lateral femoral cutaneous, obturator nerve) as well as sacral plexus (sciatic nerve) provides analgesia following surgery of the lower extremity, including hip, knee, femoral shaft, tibia, and ankle. For instance, the femoral nerve block (L2–L4) provides analgesic coverage over the anterior compartment of the thigh, knee, and medial aspect of the lower extremity below the knee extending to the medial ankle. Femoral nerve blockade is also associated with motor blockade of the quadricep and results in 80% reduction in quadricep strength. More recently, the fascia iliaca block has been utilized as a compartment block of the lumbar plexus to target the femoral and lateral femoral cutaneous nerves, with potential for providing analgesic coverage of obturator nerve with larger volumes of local anesthetic formulations [165]. On the other hand, in order to provide coverage of the posterior compartment of the leg and posterolateral aspect of the lower leg and ankle, the sciatic nerve is targeted at both proximal (subgluteal) and distal (lateral popliteal) locations. The sciatic nerve block is useful for surgery involving the posterior aspect of the knee, the tibia, and lateral ankle. The sciatic nerve receives contributions from both the lumbar and sacral plexus and splits into the tibial and common peroneal nerves proximal to the posterior aspect of the knee.

(d) **Fascial Plane Blocks**

Traditionally, regional anesthesia of the abdominal wall and trunk was primarily focused on the use of epidural analgesia. However, with the more prevalent use of postoperative anticoagulation and emphasis on early ambulation, the focus has shifted to abdominal wall fascial plane blocks as an alternative method for achieving effective analgesia. These techniques include the transversus abdominis plane (TAP) block, rectus sheath block, and quadratus lumborum (QL) block. Each of these fascial plane blocks targets the anterior and/or lateral cutaneous branches of the thoracoabdominal nerves that originate from the low thoracic spinal nerves (T6–T12) [166]. The TAP block and rectus sheath block provide sensory cutaneous analgesia of the abdominal wall, while the QL block has the added benefit of providing visceral analgesia through spread of the local anesthetic to the paravertebral space, especially with the posterior QL block approach.

Initially, regional anesthesia of the chest wall was primarily focused on the use of thoracic epidural analgesia, PVB, and intercostal nerve blocks. However, similar in progression to abdominal wall blocks, the development of fascial plane blocks for the chest wall created a shift toward these alternative techniques for achieving chest wall analgesia that is both effective and safe [167]. These fascial plane blocks include the pectoral nerve type-1 (PECS1, interpectoral plane) block, pectoral nerve type-2 (PECS2, pectoserratus plane) block, the serratus anterior plane block, and parasternal intercostal plane blocks. This group of blocks targets the anterior and lateral cutaneous branches of T2–T6 spinal nerves. The PECS1 (interpectoral plane) block additionally targets the pectoral nerves that originate from the brachial plexus and innervate the pectoralis major and minor muscles. These various fascial plane blocks can be utilized to provide effective analgesia for breast surgery, thoracotomy, sternotomy, and treatment of rib fractures.

(e) **Regional Techniques for Extended Analgesia**

Catheter-based techniques in regional anesthesia consist of the continuous infusion of local anesthetic formulations with the goal of providing prolonged analgesia (Table 30.4) [168]. Catheters are placed, most often with ultrasound guidance, in the proximity of nerve groups or in fascial planes, and can be maintained for several days following surgical intervention, even in the ambulatory setting [169]. Catheter dislodgment and infection are the common concerns associated with the use of catheters [170]. However, benefits of a continuous catheter system include increased duration of analgesia, opioid-sparing analgesic benefit, and overall patient satisfaction. With the introduction of novel block techniques, including a variety of peripheral nerve blocks and fascial plane blocks, the use of catheters has shown to be a valuable alternative to more "traditional" regional anesthetic techniques, such as epidural analgesia, when the goal is to achieve prolonged analgesia in the postoperative setting [171–173].

As a potential option for extended analgesia, liposomal bupivacaine became clinically available in more recent years, with a theoretical analgesic effectiveness of 72 h following initial injection through the slow, continuous release of bupivacaine over an extended period of time. This local anesthetic formulation initially gained significant interest and was approved for surgical site local infiltration, but has since expanded its indication to use in TAP blocks and ISB for shoulder surgery [174]. Although initial findings from studies were positive, in more recent evaluations, liposomal bupivacaine has not exhibited convincing evidence in support of its use for surgical site infiltration or peripheral nerve blocks. For instance, infiltration with liposomal bupivacaine showed no superior analgesic benefit when compared to peripheral nerve blocks in knee and shoulder surgery [174]. Studies evaluating the analgesic effectiveness of perineural liposomal bupivacaine in peripheral nerve blocks have provided inconsistent results, with a more recent meta-analysis concluding that perineural liposomal bupivacaine provides no clinical benefit in comparison to plain local anesthetic [175].

Therefore, for purposes of extending the duration and quality of analgesia, strategies should focus on the use of long-acting local anesthetics (i.e., ropivacaine and bupivacaine) in combination with adjuncts such as ketorolac, buprenorphine, dexamethasone, clonidine or dexmedetomidine and/or epinephrine for peripheral nerve blocks, intra-articular injections, or wound infiltrations [56, 176–178].

Of note, a single-dose extended-release formulation of morphine is also commercially available. The epidural administration of this liposomal-based formulation results in a sustained release of morphine. Extended release epidural morphine (EREM™) has been used in the context of multimodal analgesia with good clinical results [179].

(3) ***Other Techniques***

There is a growing interest in investigating alternative therapeutic approaches to provide analgesia and reducing opioid consumption in patients with acute surgical pain. Cryotherapy, acupuncture, transcutaneous electrical nerve stimulation (TENS), and hypnosis are the most commonly employed techniques in this area.

Cryotherapy (cryoanalgesia or cryoneurolysis) involves the direct application of cold temperatures (-20 to -100 degrees Celsius) using a probe that generates a cooling effect at the site of application for the purpose of causing reversible neuronal injury [180]. This technique results in Wallerian degeneration, characterized by inhibition of nerve signal transmission distal to the site of injury [181]. Due to the reversible nature of this injury, the affected nerve regenerates over the course of weeks to months [182]. Cryoneurolysis has been used extensively in the treatment of chronic pain conditions (postherpetic and occipital neuralgia, phantom limb pain), and more recently has been implicated as a potential analgesic tool in the acute pain setting for purposes of providing extended analgesia when there is an anticipation of prolonged postoperative pain. Of note, several studies have identified the benefit of utilizing intercostal cryoneurolysis following thoracotomy, especially in providing opioid-sparing analgesia, improving pulmonary function outcomes, and decreasing hospital length of stay [183]. However, cryoneurolysis has also been associated with postoperative persistent pain formation after its application on neural structures [184–188].

Acupuncture is a medical treatment that originated in Asia and has been used in the perioperative period to treat postoperative nausea and vomiting and to provide analgesic benefit [189]. The mechanism of acupuncture-induced analgesia is still unknown but several theories have been speculated including the release of enkephalin, β-endorphin, endomorphin, endocannabinoids and modulation of the autonomic system [190]. Several acupoints such as ST34 (knee), ST36 (knee), KI6 (ankle), LI4 (hand), and P6 (forearm), as well as modes of stimulation including manual (traditional), and electric have been used to provide analgesia [189, 191]. Among those modalities, electrical stimulation appears to be more effective than manual [189]. Although the results of clinical trials are conflicting, the evidence suggests that the opioid- and anesthetic-sparing effects of acupuncture are clinically relevant when this technique is used before induction of anesthesia with an onset of effect after approximately 15 to 30 min [189, 192].

TENS (transcutaneous electrical nerve stimulation) is a non-invasive technique used to provide postoperative analgesia. Its mechanism of action is based on the gate theory of pain. Thus, it is postulated that electrical stimulation through the skin inhibits the transmission of pain impulses through the spinal cord and the release of endogenous opioids, such as endorphins, by the brain or the spinal cord [193]. TENS has been shown to provide analgesia and reduce analgesic consumption after cardiac surgery, cholecystectomy, and neck surgery, but has not been found to be effective following thoracotomy and bone marrow aspiration [194–199].

30.3 Conclusion

Pain management serves as a vital component of perioperative clinical care in patients undergoing surgical and invasive interventions. Given the multitude of factors that contribute to pain transmission as well as the variable components of surgical pain, it is essential to utilize a multimodal analgesic technique in managing perioperative pain. This approach includes a variety of pharmacologic interventions that each target individual components of the pain transmission pathway, in addition to regional anesthesia techniques such as neuraxial anesthesia and peripheral nerve blockade. More recently, the incorporation of ultrasound-guided fascial plane blocks has provided alternative methods of achieving abdominal and chest wall analgesia while at the same time improving the overall safety profile of these interventions. Advances in novel analgesic techniques as well as pharmacological formulations continue to improve the extent and duration of analgesic benefit provided to patients in the perioperative period.

In summary, perioperative pain management and the use of multimodal modalities serve as an important aspect of improving pain control, limiting cumulative side effects of monotherapy, optimizing patient recovery, and reducing the potential for development of persistent postoperative pain.

Summary Questions (Choose the Most Appropriate Answer)

1. Mechanisms necessary for pain formation and discrimination are the following, except:
   a. Transduction
   b. Transmission
   c. Perception
   d. **Convection**
   ***Convection** is heat transfer by mass motion of a fluid such as air or water when the heated fluid is caused to move away from the source of heat, carrying energy with it.*
2. Peripheral sensitization is responsible for:
   a. Primary hyperalgesia
   b. Secondary hyperalgesia
   c. Tertiary hyperalgesia
   d. Hyperacusis
   Peripheral sensitization occurs when inflammatory mediators stimulate polymodal nociceptors in which they cause a drop in the excitatory thresholds. As a result of peripheral sensitization, noxious stimuli evoke a stronger response at nociceptors.
3. Central sensitization is responsible for:
   a. Primary hyperalgesia
   b. **Secondary hyperalgesia**
   c. Referred hyperalgesia
   d. Hyperosmia
   Central sensitization can occur after inflammation or nerve damage. Neurons in the dorsal horn of the spinal cord undergo significant changes including expansion of the receptive fields, increased responses (wind-up), and lowering of the thresholds.
4. Adequate planning for postoperative pain management should include the following considerations:
   a. Type and location of surgery
   b. Patient's comorbidities
   c. Patient's social and psychological perception of pain
   d. **All of the above**
   Postoperative pain management involves multidimensional and multidisciplinary care. Understanding of surgical approach (minimally invasive versus open), patient's comorbidities (advanced age, obesity, or obstructive sleep apnea) and psychological factors (anxiety, depression, alexithymia) are crucial to decide and plan appropriate multimodal pain strategies.
5. Multimodal analgesic therapy involves:
   a. The administration of intravenous analgesic only
   b. The use of regional analgesia only
   c. The use of hypnosis and acupuncture only
   d. **The use of pharmacological and non-pharmacological therapies**
   Multimodal analgesia refers to the use of a variety of pharmacological and non-pharmacological therapies with the objective of minimizing trauma and decreasing nociceptive signals from injured tissues, spinal cord and supraspinal sites of the nervous system.
6. Regional anesthesia is indicated for:
   a. Abdominal surgery only
   b. Thoracic surgery only
   c. Orthopedic procedures only
   d. **It is indicated in a wide variety of surgical procedures**
   Different techniques including neuraxial procedures, peripheral nerve and fascial plane blocks, wound infiltration, and use of continuous infusions of local anesthetic solutions have been utilized to provide postoperative analgesia to surgical patients.
7. Intravenous opioids analgesics are:
   a. The only analgesic that can be used for postoperative pain management
   b. The most effective analgesic for postoperative pain
   c. Associated with few adverse events
   d. **Recommended as part of a multimodal analgesic regimen**
   Intravenous, neuraxial, and oral opioids are commonly used intra- or postoperatively to provide analgesia. However, their use has been associated with side effects including respiratory depression, nausea and vomiting, ileus, drowsiness, urinary retention, confusion, and hyperalgesia. Therefore, the judicious use of these drugs is recommended in the perioperative period.
8. COX inhibitors are recommended:
   a. As part of a multimodal analgesic technique
   b. Only for minimally invasive surgical procedures
   c. In patients with recent history of renal failure
   d. In patients with recent history of peptic ulcer disease
   ***Non-steroidal anti-inflammatory drugs** are adjuvant analgesics with proven efficacy in the context of multimodal analgesia for surgery. Overall, NSAIDs can be administered safely in the perioperative period. However, their use (in particular ketorolac) should be limited to short periods of time and avoided in patients with coagulopathy, renal failure, or history of peptic ulcer.*
9. A healthy 48 year-old woman is scheduled for open pancreatic surgery. An effective multimodal analgesic strategy should include:
   a. Only intravenous and neuraxial opioids
   b. Only epidural analgesia

c. A continuous infusion of intravenous opioids plus preoperative COX-inhibitors
d. **Patient controlled-epidural analgesia (low concentration of local anesthetic and opioid additive) plus perioperative use of COX-inhibitors and/or acetaminophen. Breakthrough pain can be rescued with intravenous opioids.**
A multimodal analgesic regimen is recommended in the management of this patient to avoid the cumulative adverse effect of each individual drug and decrease nociceptive signals from injured tissues, spinal cord and supraspinal sites of the nervous system.

10. A 55 year-old man with history of severe obstructive sleep apnea is scheduled for a thoracotomy. The following analgesic strategies can be used effectively and safely ***except:***
a. Patient controlled epidural analgesia in addition to 1 gm of acetaminophen (every 6 h) and 75 mg of pregabalin preoperatively
b. Paravertebral block in addition to 30 mg of intravenous ketorolac (every 8 h) and 1 gm of acetaminophen (every 6 h)
c. **Continuous intravenous opioid analgesia (50 μg of fentanyl/hour)**
d. Intercostal block in addition to 30 mg of intravenous ketorolac (every 8 h) plus 1 gm of acetaminophen (every 6 h) and patient controlled intravenous fentanyl analgesia (10 μg every 10–15 min, no basal rate)
Epidural, paravertebral block and intercostal nerve blocks can be considered for postoperative pain relief after thoracic surgery in combination with COX-inhibitors, acetaminophen and opioid intravenous patient control analgesia. Continuous infusion of opioids in patients with history of sleep apnea is not recommended because of an increased risk of respiratory depression.

References

1. Apfelbaum JL, Chen C, Mehta SS, Gan TJ. Postoperative pain experience: results from a national survey suggest postoperative pain continues to be undermanaged. Anesth Analg. 2003;97(2):534–40.
2. Kehlet H, Jensen TS, Woolf CJ. Persistent postsurgical pain: risk factors and prevention. Lancet. 2006;367(9522):1618–25.
3. Mathiesen O, Wetterslev J, Kontinen VK, Pommergaard HC, Nikolajsen L, Rosenberg J, et al. Adverse effects of perioperative paracetamol, NSAIDs, glucocorticoids, gabapentinoids and their combinations: a topical review. Acta Anaesthesiol Scand. 2014;58(10):1182–98.
4. Senard M, Deflandre EP, Ledoux D, Roediger L, Hubert BM, Radermecker M, et al. Effect of celecoxib combined with thoracic epidural analgesia on pain after thoracotomy. Br J Anaesth. 2010;105(2):196–200.
5. Ng A, Hall F, Atkinson A, Kong KL, Hahn A. Bridging the analgesic gap. Acute Pain. 2000;3:1–6.
6. Koizumi S, Fujishita K, Inoue K, Shigemoto-Mogami Y, Tsuda M. Ca2+ waves in keratinocytes are transmitted to sensory neurons: the involvement of extracellular ATP and P2Y2 receptor activation. Biochem J. 2004;380(Pt 2):329–38.
7. Julius D, Basbaum AI. Molecular mechanisms of nociception. Nature. 2001;413(6852):203–10.
8. Ulmann L, Hirbec H, Rassendren F. P2X4 receptors mediate PGE2 release by tissue-resident macrophages and initiate inflammatory pain. EMBO J. 2010;29(14):2290–300.
9. Mork H, Ashina M, Bendtsen L, Olesen J, Jensen R. Experimental muscle pain and tenderness following infusion of endogenous substances in humans. Eur J Pain. 2003;7(2):145–53.
10. Rotto DM, Hill JM, Schultz HD, Kaufman MP. Cyclooxygenase blockade attenuates responses of group IV muscle afferents to static contraction. Am J Physiol. 1990;259(3 Pt 2):H745–50.
11. Cao YQ, Mantyh PW, Carlson EJ, Gillespie AM, Epstein CJ, Basbaum AI. Primary afferent tachykinins are required to experience moderate to intense pain. Nature. 1998;392(6674):390–4.
12. Leonard PA, Arunkumar R, Brennan TJ. Bradykinin antagonists have no analgesic effect on incisional pain. Anesth Analg. 2004;99(4):1166–72.
13. Basbaum AI, Bautista DM, Scherrer G, Julius D. Cellular and molecular mechanisms of pain. Cell. 2009;139(2):267–84.
14. Lirk P, Picardi S, Hollmann MW. Local anaesthetics: 10 essentials. Eur J Anaesthesiol. 2014;31(11):575–85.
15. Habib AS, Gan TJ. Role of analgesic adjuncts in postoperative pain management. Anesthesiol Clin North Am. 2005;23(1):85–107.
16. Herrero JF, Laird JM, Lopez-Garcia JA. Wind-up of spinal cord neurones and pain sensation: much ado about something? Prog Neurobiol. 2000;61(2):169–203.
17. Cairns BE, Svensson P, Wang K, Hupfeld S, Graven-Nielsen T, Sessle BJ, et al. Activation of peripheral NMDA receptors contributes to human pain and rat afferent discharges evoked by injection of glutamate into the masseter muscle. J Neurophysiol. 2003;90(4):2098–105.
18. McCarthy RJ, Kroin JS, Tuman KJ, Penn RD, Ivankovich AD. Antinociceptive potentiation and attenuation of tolerance by intrathecal co-infusion of magnesium sulfate and morphine in rats. Anesth Analg. 1998;86(4):830–6.
19. Gorman AL, Elliott KJ, Inturrisi CE. The d- and l-isomers of methadone bind to the non-competitive site on the N-methyl-D-aspartate (NMDA) receptor in rat forebrain and spinal cord. Neurosci Lett. 1997;223(1):5–8.
20. Park J, Yu YP, Zhou CY, Li KW, Wang D, Chang E, et al. Central mechanisms mediating thrombospondin-4 induced pain states. J Biol Chem. 2016;291(25):13335–48.
21. Willis WD Jr. The somatosensory system, with emphasis on structures important for pain. Brain Res Rev. 2007;55(2):297–313.
22. Loggia ML, Juneau M, Bushnell MC. Autonomic responses to heat pain: heart rate, skin conductance, and their relation to verbal ratings and stimulus intensity. Pain. 2011;152(3):592–8.
23. Perlaki G, Orsi G, Schwarcz A, Bodi P, Plozer E, Biczo K, et al. Pain-related autonomic response is modulated by the medial prefrontal cortex: An ECG-fMRI study in men. J Neurol Sci. 2015;349(1–2):202–8.
24. Nielsen R, Nikolajsen L, Kroner K, Molgaard H, Vase L, Jensen TS, et al. Pre-operative baroreflex sensitivity and efferent cardiac parasympathetic activity are correlated with post-operative pain. Acta Anaesthesiol Scand. 2015;59(4):475–85.
25. Bruehl S, Chung OY. Interactions between the cardiovascular and pain regulatory systems: an updated review of mechanisms

and possible alterations in chronic pain. Neurosci Biobehav Rev. 2004;28(4):395–414.
26. Kumar N, Thapa D, Gombar S, Ahuja V, Gupta R. Analgesic efficacy of pre-operative stellate ganglion block on postoperative pain relief: a randomised controlled trial. Anaesthesia. 2014;69 (9):954–660.
27. Hulata DF, Le-Wendling L, Boezaart AP, Hurley RW. Stellate ganglion local anesthetic blockade and neurolysis for the treatment of refractory ventricular fibrillation. A A Case Rep. 2015;4(5):49–51.
28. Grundy D. Neuroanatomy of visceral nociception: vagal and splanchnic afferent. Gut. 2002;51(Suppl 1):i2-5.
29. Blackshaw LA. Transient receptor potential cation channels in visceral sensory pathways. Br J Pharmacol. 2014;171(10):2528–36.
30. Hockley JR, Boundouki G, Cibert-Goton V, McGuire C, Yip PK, Chan C, et al. Multiple roles for NaV.19 in the activation of visceral afferents by noxious inflammatory, mechanical, and human disease-derived stimuli. Pain. 2014;155(10):1962–75.
31. Randich A, Gebhart GF. Vagal afferent modulation of nociception. Brain Res Brain Res Rev. 1992;17(2):77–99.
32. Baudic S, Jayr C, Albi-Freldzer A, Fermanian J, Masselin-Dubois A, Bouhassira D, et al. Impact of alexithymia and emotional repression on postsurgical pain in women with breast cancer: a prospective longitudinal 12 months study. J Pain. 2015;17(1):90–100.
33. Kim YS, Do H, Lee JW, Jeong J, Shin YW, Yi K, et al. Patient reporting pain intensity immediately after surgery can be associated with underlying depression in women with breast cancer. Psychooncology. 2015;25(3):308–15.
34. Carroll IR, Hah JM, Barelka PL, Wang CK, Wang BM, Gillespie MJ, et al. Pain duration and resolution following surgery: an inception cohort study. Pain Med. 2015;16(12):2386–96.
35. Higuchi D. Prognostic value of preoperative coping strategies for pain in patients with residual neuropathic pain after laminoplasty for compressive cervical myelopathy. Asian Spine J. 2015;9 (5):675–82.
36. Van Damme S, Crombez G, Bijttebier P, Goubert L, Van Houdenhove B. A confirmatory factor analysis of the pain catastrophizing scale: invariant factor structure across clinical and non-clinical populations. Pain. 2002;96(3):319–24.
37. Archer KR, Heins SE, Abraham CM, Obremskey WT, Wegener ST, Castillo RC. Clinical significance of pain at hospital discharge following traumatic orthopaedic injury: general health, depression, and PTSD outcomes at 1 Year. Clin J Pain. 2015;32(3):196–202.
38. Pope D, El-Othmani MM, Manning BT, Sepula M, Markwell SJ, Saleh KJ. Impact of age, gender and anesthesia modality on post-operative pain in total knee arthroplasty patients. Iowa Orthop J. 2015;35:92–8.
39. Pereira MP, Pogatzki-Zahn E. Gender aspects in postoperative pain. Curr Opin Anaesthesiol. 2015;28(5):546–58.
40. Hallen M, Sevonius D, Westerdahl J, Gunnarsson U, Sandblom G. Risk factors for reoperation due to chronic groin postherniorrhaphy pain. Hernia: J Hernias Abdom Wall Surg. 2015;19(6):863–9.
41. Cho CH, Ye HU, Jung JW, Lee YK. Gender affects early postoperative outcomes of rotator cuff repair. Clin Orthop Surg. 2015;7(2):234–40.
42. Racine M, Tousignant-Laflamme Y, Kloda LA, Dion D, Dupuis G, Choiniere M. A systematic literature review of 10 years of research on sex/gender and pain perception—part 2: do biopsychosocial factors alter pain sensitivity differently in women and men? Pain. 2012;153(3):619–35.
43. Racine M, Tousignant-Laflamme Y, Kloda LA, Dion D, Dupuis G, Choiniere M. A systematic literature review of 10 years of research on sex/gender and experimental pain perception - part 1: are there really differences between women and men? Pain. 2012;153(3):602–18.
44. Kehlet H, Edwards RR, Buvanendran A. Persistent postoperative pain: Pathogenic mechanisms and preventive strategies. In: Tracey I, editor. Pain 2012 - Refresher Courses: 14th World Congress on Pain. Seatle: International Association for the Study of Pain/IASP Press; 2012. p. 133–43.
45. Wildgaard K, Ringsted TK, Hansen HJ, Petersen RH, Kehlet H. Persistent postsurgical pain after video-assisted thoracic surgery - an observational study. Acta Anaesthesiol Scand. 2016;60 (5):650–8.
46. Guimaraes-Pereira L, Valdoleiros I, Reis P, Abelha F. Evaluating persistent postoperative pain in one tertiary hospital: incidence, quality of life, associated factors, and treatment. Anesth Pain Med. 2016;6(2): e36461.
47. Puolakka PA, Rorarius MG, Roviola M, Puolakka TJ, Nordhausen K, Lindgren L. Persistent pain following knee arthroplasty. Eur J Anaesthesiol. 2010;27(5):455–60.
48. Lewis GN, Rice DA, McNair PJ, Kluger M. Predictors of persistent pain after total knee arthroplasty: a systematic review and meta-analysis. Br J Anaesth. 2015;114(4):551–61.
49. Glare P, Aubrey KR, Myles PS. Transition from acute to chronic pain after surgery. Lancet. 2019;393(10180):1537–46.
50. Richebe P, Capdevila X, Rivat C. Persistent postsurgical pain: pathophysiology and preventative pharmacologic considerations. Anesthesiology. 2018;129(3):590–607.
51. Bayman EO, Brennan TJ. Incidence and severity of chronic pain at 3 and 6 months after thoracotomy: meta-analysis. J Pain. 2014;15(9):887–97.
52. Carley ME, Chaparro LE, Choiniere M, Kehlet H, Moore RA, Van Den Kerkhof E, et al. Pharmacotherapy for the prevention of chronic pain after surgery in adults: an updated systematic review and meta-analysis. Anesthesiology. 2021;135(2):304–25.
53. Andreae MH, Andreae DA. Regional anaesthesia to prevent chronic pain after surgery: a Cochrane systematic review and meta-analysis. Br J Anaesth. 2013;111(5):711–20.
54. Chaparro LE, Smith SA, Moore RA, Wiffen PJ, Gilron I. Pharmacotherapy for the prevention of chronic pain after surgery in adults. Cochrane Database Syst Rev. 2013;7:CD008307.
55. Chen YK, Boden KA, Schreiber KL. The role of regional anaesthesia and multimodal analgesia in the prevention of chronic postoperative pain: a narrative review. Anaesthesia. 2021;76 (Suppl 1):8–17.
56. Cummings KC 3rd, Napierkowski DE, Parra-Sanchez I, Kurz A, Dalton JE, Brems JJ, et al. Effect of dexamethasone on the duration of interscalene nerve blocks with ropivacaine or bupivacaine. Br J Anaesth. 2011;107(3):446–53.
57. Lavand'homme P. Rebound pain after regional anesthesia in the ambulatory patient. Curr Opin Anaesthesiol. 2018;31(6):679–84.
58. Barry GS, Bailey JG, Sardinha J, Brousseau P, Uppal V. Factors associated with rebound pain after peripheral nerve block for ambulatory surgery. Br J Anaesth. 2021;126(4):862–71.
59. Woo JH, Lee HJ, Oh HW, Lee JW, Baik HJ, Kim YJ. Perineural dexamethasone reduces rebound pain after ropivacaine single injection interscalene block for arthroscopic shoulder surgery: a randomized controlled trial. Reg Anesth Pain Med. 2021;46 (11):965–70.
60. Fang J, Shi Y, Du F, Xue Z, Cang J, Miao C, et al. The effect of perineural dexamethasone on rebound pain after ropivacaine single-injection nerve block: a randomized controlled trial. BMC Anesthesiol. 2021;21(1):47.

61. Marino J, Russo J, Kenny M, Herenstein R, Livote E, Chelly JE. Continuous lumbar plexus block for postoperative pain control after total hip arthroplasty. A randomized controlled trial. J Bone Jt Surg Am Vol. 2009;91(1):29–37.
62. Lee HJ, Yeomans DC. Opioid induced hyperalgesia in anesthetic settings. Korean J Anesthesiol. 2014;67(5):299–304.
63. Dahan A, Aarts L, Smith TW. Incidence, reversal, and prevention of opioid-induced respiratory depression. Anesthesiology. 2010;112(1):226–38.
64. Pang W, Liu YC, Maboudou E, Chen TX, Chois JM, Liao CC, et al. Metoclopramide improves the quality of tramadol PCA indistinguishable to morphine PCA: a prospective, randomized, double blind clinical comparison. Pain Med. 2013;14(9):1426–34.
65. Gan TJ, Wase L. Oliceridine, a G protein-selective ligand at the mu-opioid receptor, for the management of moderate to severe acute pain. Drugs Today. 2020;56(4):269–86.
66. DeWire SM, Yamashita DS, Rominger DH, Liu G, Cowan CL, Graczyk TM, et al. A G protein-biased ligand at the μ-opioid receptor is potently analgesic with reduced gastrointestinal and respiratory dysfunction compared with morphine. J Pharmacol Exp Ther. 2013;344(3):708–17.
67. Murphy GS, Szokol JW. Intraoperative methadone in surgical patients: a review of clinical investigations. Anesthesiology. 2019;131(3):678–92.
68. Gottschalk A, Durieux ME, Nemergut EC. Intraoperative methadone improves postoperative pain control in patients undergoing complex spine surgery. Anesth Analg. 2011;112(1):218–23.
69. Murphy GS, Szokol JW, Avram MJ, Greenberg SB, Marymont JH, Shear T, et al. Intraoperative methadone for the prevention of postoperative pain: a randomized, double-blinded clinical trial in cardiac surgical patients. Anesthesiology. 2015;122(5):1112–22.
70. Yadeau JT, Paroli L, Kahn RL, Jules-Elysee KM, Lasala VR, Liu SS, et al. Addition of pregabalin to multimodal analgesic therapy following ankle surgery: a randomized double-blind, placebo-controlled trial. Reg Anesth Pain Med. 2012;37(3):302–7.
71. Zhang J, Ho KY, Wang Y. Efficacy of pregabalin in acute postoperative pain: a meta-analysis. Br J Anaesth. 2011;106(4):454–62.
72. Eroglu C, Allen NJ, Susman MW, O'Rourke NA, Park CY, Ozkan E, et al. Gabapentin receptor alpha2delta-1 is a neuronal thrombospondin receptor responsible for excitatory CNS synaptogenesis. Cell. 2009;139(2):380–92.
73. Verret M, Lauzier F, Zarychanski R, Perron C, Savard X, Pinard AM, et al. Perioperative use of gabapentinoids for the management of postoperative acute pain: a systematic review and meta-analysis. Anesthesiology. 2020;133(2):265–79.
74. Mariano ER, Dickerson DM, Szokol JW, Harned M, Mueller JT, Philip BK, et al. A multisociety organizational consensus process to define guiding principles for acute perioperative pain management. Reg Anesth Pain Med. 2022;47(2):118–27.
75. Myles PS, Corcoran T. Benefits and risks of dexamethasone in noncardiac surgery. Anesthesiology. 2021;135(5):895–903.
76. Gu X, Peng L, Yang D, Ma Q, Zheng Y, Liu C, et al. The respective and interaction effects of spinal GRs and MRs on radicular pain induced by chronic compression of the dorsal root ganglion in the rat. Brain Res. 2011;1396:88–95.
77. Hirata F, Schiffmann E, Venkatasubramanian K, Salomon D, Axelrod J. A phospholipase A2 inhibitory protein in rabbit neutrophils induced by glucocorticoids. Proc Natl Acad Sci U S A. 1980;77(5):2533–6.
78. Kardash KJ, Sarrazin F, Tessler MJ, Velly AM. Single-dose dexamethasone reduces dynamic pain after total hip arthroplasty. Anesth Analg. 2008;106(4):1253–7.
79. Bergeron SG, Kardash KJ, Huk OL, Zukor DJ, Antoniou J. Perioperative dexamethasone does not affect functional outcome in total hip arthroplasty. Clin Orthop Relat Res. 2009;467(6):1463–7.
80. De Oliveira GS, Bialek JM, Turan A, McCarthy RJ, Sessler DI. Perioperative dexamethasone and the development of chronic postmastectomy pain: a single-center observational cohort study. Reg Anesth Pain Med. 2015;40(5):539–44.
81. Abdallah FW, Johnson J, Chan V, Murgatroyd H, Ghafari M, Ami N, et al. Intravenous dexamethasone and perineural dexamethasone similarly prolong the duration of analgesia after supraclavicular brachial plexus block: a randomized, triple-arm, double-blind, placebo-controlled trial. Reg Anesth Pain Med. 2015;40(2):125–32.
82. YaDeau JT, Paroli L, Fields KG, Kahn RL, LaSala VR, Jules-Elysee KM, et al. Addition of dexamethasone and buprenorphine to bupivacaine sciatic nerve block: a randomized controlled trial. Reg Anesth Pain Med. 2015;40(4):321–9.
83. Desai N, Kirkham KR, Albrecht E. Local anaesthetic adjuncts for peripheral regional anaesthesia: a narrative review. Anaesthesia. 2021;76(Suppl 1):100–9.
84. Bell RF, Dahl JB, Moore RA, Kalso E. Peri-operative ketamine for acute post-operative pain: a quantitative and qualitative systematic review (Cochrane review). Acta Anaesthesiol Scand. 2005;49(10):1405–28.
85. McNicol ED, Schumann R, Haroutounian S. A systematic review and meta-analysis of ketamine for the prevention of persistent post-surgical pain. Acta Anaesthesiol Scand. 2014;58(10):1199–213.
86. Roth GJ, Stanford N, Majerus PW. Acetylation of prostaglandin synthase by aspirin. Proc Natl Acad Sci U S A. 1975;72(8):3073–6.
87. Lee P, McAuliffe N, Dunlop C, Palanisamy M, Shorten G. A comparison of the effects of two analgesic regimens on the development of persistent post-surgical pain (PPSP) after breast surgery. J Anaesth Intensiv Care. 2013;20(2):83–93.
88. Liu ZF, Chai XQ, Chen KZ. Flurbiprofen axetil enhances analgesic effect of fentanyl associated with increase in beta-endorphin levels. J. 2011;25(5):679–84.
89. Danelich IM, Wright SS, Lose JM, Tefft BJ, Cicci JD, Reed BN. Safety of nonsteroidal antiinflammatory drugs in patients with cardiovascular disease. Pharmacotherapy. 2015;35(5):520–35.
90. Warner TD, Giuliano F, Vojnovic I, Bukasa A, Mitchell JA, Vane JR. Nonsteroid drug selectivities for cyclo-oxygenase-1 rather than cyclo-oxygenase-2 are associated with human gastrointestinal toxicity: a full in vitro analysis. Proc Natl Acad Sci USA. 1999;96(13):7563–8.
91. Oliveri L, Jerzewski K, Kulik A. Black box warning: is ketorolac safe for use after cardiac surgery? J Cardiothorac Vasc Anesth. 2014;28(2):274–9.
92. Tunali Y, Akcil EF, Dilmen OK, Tutuncu AC, Koksal GM, Akbas S, et al. Efficacy of intravenous paracetamol and dexketoprofen on postoperative pain and morphine consumption after a lumbar disk surgery. J Neurosurg Anesthesiol. 2013;25(2):143–7.
93. Lin X, Zhang R, Xing J, Gao X, Chang P, Li W. Flurbiprofen axetil reduces postoperative sufentanil consumption and enhances postoperative analgesic effects in patients with colorectal cancer surgery. Int J Clin Exp Med. 2014;7(12):4887–96.
94. Gan TJ, Candiotti K, Turan A, Buvanendran A, Philip BK, Viscusi ER, et al. The shortened infusion time of intravenous ibuprofen, part 2: a multicenter, open-label, surgical surveillance trial to evaluate safety. Clin Ther. 2015;37(2):368–75.

95. Mowafi HA, Elmakarim EA, Ismail S, Al-Mahdy M, El-Saflan AE, Elsaid AS. Intravenous lornoxicam is more effective than paracetamol as a supplemental analgesic after lower abdominal surgery: a randomized controlled trial. World J Surg. 2012;36 (9):2039–44.
96. Hakkarainen TW, Steele SR, Bastaworous A, Dellinger EP, Farrokhi E, Farjah F, et al. Nonsteroidal anti-inflammatory drugs and the risk for anastomotic failure: a report from Washington state's surgical care and outcomes assessment program (SCOAP). JAMA Surg. 2015;150(3):223–8.
97. Jahr JS, Breitmeyer JB, Pan C, Royal MA, Ang RY. Safety and efficacy of intravenous acetaminophen in the elderly after major orthopedic surgery: subset data analysis from 3, randomized, placebo-controlled trials. Am J Ther. 2012;19(2):66–75.
98. Wickerts L, Warren Stomberg M, Brattwall M, Jakobsson J. Coxibs: is there a benefit when compared to traditional non-selective NSAIDs in postoperative pain management? Minerva Anestesiol. 2011;77(11):1084–98.
99. Nussmeier NA, Whelton AA, Brown MT, Langford RM, Hoeft A, Parlow JL, et al. Complications of the COX-2 inhibitors parecoxib and valdecoxib after cardiac surgery. N Engl J Med. 2005;352(11):1081–91.
100. Klein M, Gogenur I, Rosenberg J. Postoperative use of non-steroidal anti-inflammatory drugs in patients with anastomotic leakage requiring reoperation after colorectal resection: cohort study based on prospective data. BMJ. 2012;345: e6166.
101. Ferrari RA, Ward SJ, Zobre CM, Van Liew DK, Perrone MH, Connell MJ, et al. Estimation of the in vivo effect of cyclooxygenase inhibitors on prostaglandin E2 levels in mouse brain. Eur J Pharmacol. 1990;179(1–2):25–34.
102. Pelissier T, Alloui A, Caussade F, Dubray C, Cloarec A, Lavarenne J, et al. Paracetamol exerts a spinal antinociceptive effect involving an indirect interaction with 5-hydroxytryptamine3 receptors: in vivo and in vitro evidence. J Pharmacol Exp Ther. 1996;278(1):8–14.
103. Alloui A, Pelissier T, Dubray C, Lavarenne J, Eschalier A. Tropisetron inhibits the antinociceptive effect of intrathecally administered paracetamol and serotonin. Fundam Clin Pharmacol. 1996;10(4):406–7.
104. Apfel CC, Turan A, Souza K, Pergolizzi J, Hornuss C. Intravenous acetaminophen reduces postoperative nausea and vomiting: a systematic review and meta-analysis. Pain. 2013;154(5):677–89.
105. Remy C, Marret E, Bonnet F. Effects of acetaminophen on morphine side-effects and consumption after major surgery: meta-analysis of randomized controlled trials. Br J Anaesth. 2005;94(4):505–13.
106. Hyllested M, Jones S, Pedersen JL, Kehlet H. Comparative effect of paracetamol, NSAIDs or their combination in postoperative pain management: a qualitative review. Br J Anaesth. 2002;88 (2):199–214.
107. Sinatra RS, Jahr JS, Reynolds LW, Viscusi ER, Groudine SB, Payen-Champenois C. Efficacy and safety of single and repeated administration of 1 gram intravenous acetaminophen injection (paracetamol) for pain management after major orthopedic surgery. Anesthesiology. 2005;102(4):822–31.
108. Singla NK, Parulan C, Samson R, Hutchinson J, Bushnell R, Beja EG, et al. Plasma and cerebrospinal fluid pharmacokinetic parameters after single-dose administration of intravenous, oral, or rectal acetaminophen. Pain Pract. 2012;12(7):523–32.
109. Wasserman I, Poeran J, Zubizarreta N, Babby J, Serban S, Goldberg AT, et al. Impact of intravenous acetaminophen on perioperative opioid utilization and outcomes in open colectomies: a claims database analysis. Anesthesiology. 2018;129 (1):77–88.
110. Teng Y, Zhang Y, Li B. Intravenous versus oral acetaminophen as an adjunct on pain and recovery after total knee arthroplasty: a systematic review and meta-analysis. Medicine. 2020;99(50): e23515.
111. Jibril F, Sharaby S, Mohamed A, Wilby KJ. Intravenous versus Oral acetaminophen for pain: systematic review of XE "Current" current evidence to support clinical decision-making. Can J Hosp Pharm. 2015;68(3):238–47.
112. Khan JS, Yousuf M, Victor JC, Sharma A, Siddiqui N. An estimation for an appropriate end time for an intraoperative intravenous lidocaine infusion in bowel surgery: a comparative meta-analysis. J Clin Anesth. 2015;28:95–104.
113. Sun Y, Li T, Wang N, Yun Y, Gan TJ. Perioperative systemic lidocaine for postoperative analgesia and recovery after abdominal surgery: a meta-analysis of randomized controlled trials. Dis Colon Rectum. 2012;55(11):1183–94.
114. Wuethrich PY, Romero J, Burkhard FC, Curatolo M. No benefit from perioperative intravenous lidocaine in laparoscopic renal surgery: a randomised, placebo-controlled study. Eur J Anaesthesiol. 2012;29(11):537–43.
115. Terkawi AS, Sharma S, Durieux ME, Thammishetti S, Brenin D, Tiouririne M. Perioperative lidocaine infusion reduces the incidence of post-mastectomy chronic pain: a double-blind, placebo-controlled randomized trial. Pain Physician. 2015;18(2): E139–46.
116. Dhir R, Singh MR, Kaul TK, Tewari A, Oberoi R. Effect of intravenous esmolol on analgesic requirements in laparoscopic cholecystectomy. J Anaesthesiol Clin Pharmacol. 2015;31 (3):375–9.
117. Haghighi M, Sedighinejad A, Mirbolook A, Naderi Nabi B, Farahmand M, Kazemnezhad Leili E, et al. Effect of intravenous intraoperative esmolol on pain management following lower limb orthopedic surgery. Korean J Pain. 2015;28(3):198–202.
118. Hageluken A, Grunbaum L, Nurnberg B, Harhammer R, Schunack W, Seifert R. Lipophilic beta-adrenoceptor antagonists and local anesthetics are effective direct activators of G-proteins. Biochem Pharmacol. 1994;47(10):1789–95.
119. Albrecht E, Kirkham KR, Liu SS, Brull R. Peri-operative intravenous administration of magnesium sulphate and postoperative pain: a meta-analysis. Anaesthesia. 2013;68(1):79–90.
120. Banihashem N, Hasannasab B, Esmaeili A, Hasannasab B. Addition of intrathecal magnesium sulfate to bupivacaine for spinal anesthesia in Cesarean section. Anesth Pain Med. 2015;5 (3): e22798.
121. Khalili G, Janghorbani M, Sajedi P, Ahmadi G. Effects of adjunct intrathecal magnesium sulfate to bupivacaine for spinal anesthesia: a randomized, double-blind trial in patients undergoing lower extremity surgery. J Anesth. 2011;25(6):892–7.
122. Malleeswaran S, Panda N, Mathew P, Bagga R. A randomised study of magnesium sulphate as an adjuvant to intrathecal bupivacaine in patients with mild preeclampsia undergoing caesarean section. Int J Obstet Anesth. 2010;19(2):161–6.
123. Shukla D, Verma A, Agarwal A, Pandey HD, Tyagi C. Comparative study of intrathecal dexmedetomidine with intrathecal magnesium sulfate used as adjuvants to bupivacaine. J Anaesthesiol Clin Pharmacol. 2011;27(4):495–9.
124. Farag E, Argalious M, Abd-Elsayed A, Ebrahim Z, Doyle DJ. The use of dexmedetomidine in anesthesia and intensive care: a review. Curr Pharm Des. 2012;18(38):6257–65.
125. Kaur H, Singh G, Rani S, Gupta KK, Kumar M, Rajpal AS, et al. Effect of dexmedetomidine as an adjuvant to levobupivacaine in supraclavicular brachial plexus block: a randomized double-blind prospective study. J Anaesthesiol Clin Pharmacol. 2015;31 (3):333–8.

126. Nethra SS, Sathesha M, Dixit A, Dongare PA, Harsoor SS, Devikarani D. Intrathecal dexmedetomidine as adjuvant for spinal anaesthesia for perianal ambulatory surgeries: a randomised double-blind controlled study. Indian J Anaesth. 2015;59(3): 177–81.
127. Mohamed SA, Fares KM, Mohamed AA, Alieldin NH. Dexmedetomidine as an adjunctive analgesic with bupivacaine in paravertebral analgesia for breast cancer surgery. Pain Phys. 2014;17(5):E589–98.
128. Zeng XZ, Xu YM, Cui XG, Guo YP, Li WZ. Low-dose epidural dexmedetomidine improves thoracic epidural anaesthesia for nephrectomy. Anaesth Intensive Care. 2014;42(2):185–90.
129. Nakayama M, Ichinose H, Nakabayashi K, Satoh O, Yamamoto S, Namiki A. Analgesic effect of epidural neostigmine after abdominal hysterectomy. J Clin Anesth. 2001;13(2):86–9.
130. Kida K, Ohtani N, Shoji K, Yasui Y, Masaki E. Postoperative pain status after intraoperative systemic dexmedetomidine and epidural neostigmine in patients undergoing lower abdominal surgery. Eur J Anaesthesiol. 2008;25(11):869–75.
131. Lauretti GR, Hood DD, Eisenach JC, Pfeifer BL. A multi-center study of intrathecal neostigmine for analgesia following vaginal hysterectomy. Anesthesiology. 1998;89(4):913–8.
132. Jain A, Jain K, Bhardawaj N. Analgesic efficacy of low-dose intrathecal neostigmine in combination with fentanyl and bupivacaine for total knee replacement surgery. J Anaesthesiol Clin Pharmacol. 2012;28(4):486–90.
133. Lauretti GR, Mattos AL, Reis MP, Pereira NL. Combined intrathecal fentanyl and neostigmine: therapy for postoperative abdominal hysterectomy pain relief. J Clin Anesth. 1998;10 (4):291–6.
134. Zhong QS, Ge SJ, Wang B, Xue ZG. Optimal single-dose epidural neostigmine for postoperative analgesia after partial hepatectomy. Indian J Pharmacol. 2014;46(6):613–6.
135. Chen SR, Pan HL. Activation of muscarinic receptors inhibits spinal dorsal horn projection neurons: role of GABAB receptors. Neuroscience. 2004;125(1):141–8.
136. Kim MH, Lee YM. Intrathecal midazolam increases the analgesic effects of spinal blockade with bupivacaine in patients undergoing haemorrhoidectomy. Br J Anaesth. 2001;86(1):77–9.
137. Prakash S, Joshi N, Gogia AR, Prakash S, Singh R. Analgesic efficacy of two doses of intrathecal midazolam with bupivacaine in patients undergoing cesarean delivery. Reg Anesth Pain Med. 2006;31(3):221–6.
138. Salimi A, Nejad RA, Safari F, Mohajaerani SA, Naghade RJ, Mottaghi K. Reduction in labor pain by intrathecal midazolam as an adjunct to sufentanil. Korean J Anesthesiol. 2014;66(3):204–9.
139. Lim J, Lim G, Sung B, Wang S, Mao J. Intrathecal midazolam regulates spinal AMPA receptor expression and function after nerve injury in rats. Brain Res. 2006;1123(1):80–8.
140. Cox RF, Collins MA. The effects of benzodiazepines on human opioid receptor binding and function. Anesth Analg. 2001;93 (2):354–8.
141. Goodchild CS, Guo Z, Musgreave A, Gent JP. Antinociception by intrathecal midazolam involves endogenous neurotransmitters acting at spinal cord delta opioid receptors. Br J Anaesth. 1996;77 (6):758–63.
142. Crawford ME, Jensen FM, Toftdahl DB, Madsen JB. Direct spinal effect of intrathecal and extradural midazolam on visceral noxious stimulation in rabbits. Br J Anaesth. 1993;70(6):642–6.
143. Abdollahpour A, Azadi R, Bandari R, Mirmohammadkhani M. Effects of adding midazolam and sufentanil to intrathecal bupivacaine on analgesia quality and postoperative complications in elective cesarean section. Anesth Pain Med. 2015;5(4): e23565.
144. Samantaray A, Hemanth N, Gunnampati K, Pasupuleti H, Mukkara M, Rao MH. Comparison of the effects of adding dexmedetomidine versus midazolam to intrathecal bupivacaine on postoperative analgesia. Pain Physician. 2015;18(1):71–7.
145. Wong K, Phelan R, Kalso E, Galvin I, Goldstein D, Raja S, et al. Antidepressant drugs for prevention of acute and chronic postsurgical pain: early evidence and recommended future directions. Anesthesiology. 2014;121(3):591–608.
146. Day AR, Smith RV, Scott MJ, Fawcett WJ, Rockall TA. Randomized clinical trial investigating the stress response from two different methods of analgesia after laparoscopic colorectal surgery. Br J Surg. 2015;102(12):1473–9.
147. Cata JP, Noguera EM, Parke E, Ebrahim Z, Kurz A, Kalfas I, et al. Patient-controlled epidural analgesia (PCEA) for postoperative pain control after lumbar spine surgery. J Neurosurg Anesthesiol. 2008;20(4):256–60.
148. Schenk MR, Putzier M, Kugler B, Tohtz S, Voigt K, Schink T, et al. Postoperative analgesia after major spine surgery: patient-controlled epidural analgesia versus patient-controlled intravenous analgesia. Anesth Analg. 2006;103(5):1311–7.
149. Viscusi ER, Grond S, Ding L, Danesi H, Jones JB, Sinatra RS. A comparison of opioid-related adverse events with fentanyl iontophoretic transdermal system versus morphine intravenous patient-controlled analgesia in acute postoperative pain. Pain Manag. 2015;6(1):19–24.
150. Sinatra RS, Viscusi ER, Ding L, Danesi H, Jones JB, Grond S. Meta-analysis of the efficacy of the fentanyl iontophoretic transdermal system versus intravenous patient-controlled analgesia in postoperative pain management. Expert Opin Pharmacother. 2015;16(11):1607–13.
151. Minkowitz HS, Danesi H, Ding L, Jones JB. Development of the fentanyl iontophoretic transdermal system (ITS) for patient-controlled analgesia of postoperative pain management. Pain Manag. 2015;5(5):327–37.
152. Helwani MA, Avidan MS, Ben Abdallah A, Kaiser DJ, Clohisy JC, Hall BL, et al. Effects of regional versus general anesthesia on outcomes after total hip arthroplasty: a retrospective propensity-matched cohort study. J Bone Joint Surg Am. 2015;97 (3):186–93.
153. Hausman MS Jr, Jewell ES, Engoren M. Regional versus general anesthesia in surgical patients with chronic obstructive pulmonary disease: does avoiding general anesthesia reduce the risk of postoperative complications? Anesth Analg. 2015;120 (6):1405–12.
154. Ilfeld BM. Continuous peripheral nerve blocks: a review of the published evidence. Anesth Analg. 2011;113(4):904–25.
155. Neal JM, Barrington MJ, Brull R, Hadzic A, Hebl JR, Horlocker TT, et al. The second ASRA practice advisory on neurologic complications associated with regional Anesthesia and pain medicine: executive summary 2015. Reg Anesth Pain Med. 2015;40(5):401–30.
156. Vasilopoulos T, Wardhan R, Rashidi P, Fillingim RB, Wallace MR, Crispen PL, et al. Patient and procedural determinants of postoperative pain trajectories. Anesthesiology. 2021;134 (3):421–34.
157. Boezaart AP, Davis G, Le-Wendling L. Recovery after orthopedic surgery: techniques to increase duration of pain control. Curr Opin Anaesthesiol. 2012;25(6):665–72.
158. Popping DM, Elia N, Van Aken HK, Marret E, Schug SA, Kranke P, et al. Impact of epidural analgesia on mortality and morbidity after surgery: systematic review and meta-analysis of randomized controlled trials. Ann Surg. 2014;259(6):1056–67.
159. Forero M, Adhikary SD, Lopez H, Tsui C, Chin KJ. The erector spinae plane block: a novel analgesic technique in thoracic neuropathic pain. Reg Anesth Pain Med. 2016;41(5):621–7.
160. Dravid RM, Paul RE. Interpleural block—part 2. Anaesthesia. 2007;62(11):1143–53.

161. Dravid RM, Paul RE. Interpleural block—part 1. Anaesthesia. 2007;62(10):1039–49.
162. Steinthorsdottir KJ, Wildgaard L, Hansen HJ, Petersen RH, Wildgaard K. Regional analgesia for video-assisted thoracic surgery: a systematic review. Eur J Cardiothorac Surg. 2014;45 (6):959–66.
163. Detterbeck FC. Efficacy of methods of intercostal nerve blockade for pain relief after thoracotomy. Ann Thorac Surg. 2005;80 (4):1550–9.
164. Jones MR, Novitch MB, Sen S, Hernandez N, De Haan JB, Budish RA, et al. Upper extremity regional anesthesia techniques: a comprehensive review for clinical anesthesiologists. Best Pract Res Clin Anaesthesiol. 2020;34(1):e13–29.
165. Jones MR, Novitch MB, Hall OM, Bourgeois AP, Jeha GM, Kaye RJ, et al. Fascia iliaca block, history, technique, and efficacy in clinical practice. Best Pract Res Clin Anaesthesiol. 2019;33(4):407–13.
166. Chin KJ, McDonnell JG, Carvalho B, Sharkey A, Pawa A, Gadsden J. Essentials of our current XE "Current" understanding: abdominal wall blocks. Reg Anesth Pain Med. 2017;42(2):133–83.
167. Chin KJ, Versyck B, Pawa A. Ultrasound-guided fascial plane blocks of the chest wall: a state-of-the-art review. Anaesthesia. 2021;76(Suppl 1):110–26.
168. Mariano ER, Sandhu NS, Loland VJ, Bishop ML, Madison SJ, Abrams RA, et al. A randomized comparison of infraclavicular and supraclavicular continuous peripheral nerve blocks for postoperative analgesia. Reg Anesth Pain Med. 2011;36(1):26–31.
169. Ilfeld BM, Enneking FK. Continuous peripheral nerve blocks at home: a review. Anesth Analg. 2005;100(6):1822–33.
170. Stathellis A, Fitz W, Schnurr C, Koeck FX, Gebauer M, Huth J, et al. Periarticular injections with continuous perfusion of local anaesthetics provide better pain relief and better function compared to femoral and sciatic blocks after TKA: a randomized clinical trial. Knee Surg Sports Traumatol Arthrosc. 2015;25:2702–7.
171. Niraj G, Kelkar A, Hart E, Horst C, Malik D, Yeow C, et al. Comparison of analgesic efficacy of four-quadrant transversus abdominis plane (TAP) block and continuous posterior TAP analgesia with epidural analgesia in patients undergoing laparoscopic colorectal surgery: an open-label, randomised, non-inferiority trial. Anaesthesia. 2014;69(4):348–55.
172. Niraj G, Kelkar A, Jeyapalan I, Graff-Baker P, Williams O, Darbar A, et al. Comparison of analgesic efficacy of subcostal transversus abdominis plane blocks with epidural analgesia following upper abdominal surgery. Anaesthesia. 2011;66 (6):465–71.
173. Bashandy GM, Abbas DN. Pectoral nerves I and II blocks in multimodal analgesia for breast cancer surgery: a randomized clinical trial. Reg Anesth Pain Med. 2015;40(1):68–74.
174. Ilfeld BM, Eisenach JC, Gabriel RA. Clinical effectiveness of liposomal bupivacaine administered by infiltration or peripheral nerve block to treat postoperative pain. Anesthesiology. 2021;134 (2):283–344.
175. Hussain N, Brull R, Sheehy B, Essandoh MK, Stahl DL, Weaver TE, et al. Perineural liposomal bupivacaine is not superior to nonliposomal bupivacaine for peripheral nerve block analgesia. Anesthesiology. 2021;134(2):147–64.
176. Kehlet H, Andersen LO. Local infiltration analgesia in joint replacement: the evidence and recommendations for clinical practice. Acta Anaesthesiol Scand. 2011;55(7):778–84.
177. YaDeau JT, LaSala VR, Paroli L, Kahn RL, Jules-Elysee KM, Levine DS, et al. Clonidine and analgesic duration after popliteal fossa nerve blockade: randomized, double-blind, placebo-controlled study. Anesth Analg. 2008;106(6):1916–20.
178. Candido KD, Franco CD, Khan MA, Winnie AP, Raja DS. Buprenorphine added to the local anesthetic for brachial plexus block to provide postoperative analgesia in outpatients. Reg Anesth Pain Med. 2001;26(4):352–6.
179. Peravali R, Brock R, Bright E, Mills P, Petty D, Alberts J. Enhancing the Enhanced Recovery Program in Colorectal Surgery - Use of Extended-Release Epidural Morphine (DepoDur(R)). Ann Coloproctol. 2014;30(4):186–91.
180. Evans PJ, Lloyd JW, Green CJ. Cryoanalgesia: the response to alterations in freeze cycle and temperature. Br J Anaesth. 1981;53 (11):1121–7.
181. Ilfeld BM, Preciado J, Trescot AM. Novel cryoneurolysis device for the treatment of sensory and motor peripheral nerves. Expert Rev Med Devices. 2016;13(8):713–25.
182. Ilfeld BM, Gabriel RA, Trescot AM. Ultrasound-guided percutaneous cryoneurolysis for treatment of acute pain: could cryoanalgesia replace continuous peripheral nerve blocks? Br J Anaesth. 2017;119(4):703–6.
183. Ilfeld BM, Finneran JJ. Cryoneurolysis and percutaneous peripheral nerve stimulation to treat acute pain. Anesthesiology. 2020;133(5):1127–49.
184. Miguel R, Hubbell D. Pain management and spirometry following thoracotomy: a prospective, randomized study of four techniques. J Cardiothorac Vasc Anesth. 1993;7(5):529–34.
185. Sepsas E, Misthos P, Anagnostopulu M, Toparlaki O, Voyagis G, Kakaris S. The role of intercostal cryoanalgesia in post-thoracotomy analgesia. Interact Cardiovasc Thorac Surg. 2013;16(6):814–8.
186. Mustola ST, Lempinen J, Saimanen E, Vilkko P. Efficacy of thoracic epidural analgesia with or without intercostal nerve cryoanalgesia for postthoracotomy pain. Ann Thorac Surg. 2011;91(3):869–73.
187. Lu Q, Han Y, Cao W, Lei J, Wan Y, Zhao F, et al. Comparison of non-divided intercostal muscle flap and intercostal nerve cryoanalgesia treatments for post-oesophagectomy neuropathic pain control. Eur J Cardiothorac Surg. 2013;43(3):e64-70.
188. Robinson SR, Purdie GL. Reducing post-tonsillectomy pain with cryoanalgesia: a randomized controlled trial. Laryngoscope. 2000;110(7):1128–31.
189. Lu Z, Dong H, Wang Q, Xiong L. Perioperative acupuncture modulation: more than anaesthesia. Br J Anaesth. 2015;115 (2):183–93.
190. Sun Y, Gan TJ, Dubose JW, Habib AS. Acupuncture and related techniques for postoperative pain: a systematic review of randomized controlled trials. Br J Anaesth. 2008;101(2):151–60.
191. Zhang Q, Gao Z, Wang H, Ma L, Guo F, Zhong H, et al. The effect of pre-treatment with transcutaneous electrical acupoint stimulation on the quality of recovery after ambulatory breast surgery: a prospective, randomised controlled trial. Anaesthesia. 2014;69(8):832–9.
192. Cho HK, Park IJ, Jeong YM, Lee YJ, Hwang SH. Can perioperative acupuncture reduce the pain and vomiting experienced after tonsillectomy? A meta-analysis. Laryngoscope. 2015;126:608–15.
193. Sluka KA, Vance CG, Lisi TL. High-frequency, but not low-frequency, transcutaneous electrical nerve stimulation reduces aspartate and glutamate release in the spinal cord dorsal horn. J Neurochem. 2005;95(6):1794–801.
194. Solak O, Emmiler M, Ela Y, Dundar U, Kocoiullari CU, Eren N, et al. Comparison of continuous and intermittent transcutaneous electrical nerve stimulation in postoperative pain management after coronary artery bypass grafting: a randomized,

placebo-controlled prospective study. Heart Surg Forum. 2009;12 (5):E266–71.
195. Silva MB, de Melo PR, de Oliveira NM, Crema E, Fernandes LF. Analgesic effect of transcutaneous electrical nerve stimulation after laparoscopic cholecystectomy. Am J Phys Med Rehabil. 2012;91(8):652–7.
196. Bjordal JM, Johnson MI, Ljunggreen AE. Transcutaneous electrical nerve stimulation (TENS) can reduce postoperative analgesic consumption. A meta-analysis with assessment of optimal treatment parameters for postoperative pain. Eur J Pain. 2003;7(2):181–8.
197. Park C, Choi JB, Lee YS, Chang HS, Shin CS, Kim S, et al. The effect of intra-operative transcutaneous electrical nerve stimulation on posterior neck pain following thyroidectomy. Anaesthesia. 2015;70(4):434–9.
198. Engen DJ, Carns PE, Allen MS, Bauer BA, Loehrer LL, Cha SS, et al. Evaluating efficacy and feasibility of transcutaneous electrical nerve stimulation for postoperative pain after video-assisted thoracoscopic surgery: a randomized pilot trial. Complement Ther Clin Pract. 2015;23:141–8.
199. Tucker DL, Rockett M, Hasan M, Poplar S, Rule SA. Does transcutaneous electrical nerve stimulation (TENS) alleviate the pain experienced during bone marrow sampling in addition to standard techniques? A randomised, double-blinded, controlled trial. J Clin Pathol. 2015;68(6):479–83.

Special Problems in Anesthesia

31

Sam D. Gumbert

Abstract

Professional conduct embodies the treatment of patients, family members, and coworkers with dignity and kindness. These values underscore physicians' unique position in society as healers and the vital importance of acknowledging diversity with sensitivity and compassion. The practice of medicine requires the highest standards of professionalism during clinical practice, education, and research. Modern medical bioethics is a framework composed of four pillars: patient autonomy, beneficence, nonmaleficence, and social justice. Physician impairment is the inability to safely fulfill these obligations of patient care secondary to substance use disorder, fatigue, or aging.

Keywords

Anesthesia • Substance abuse • Fatigue • Aging • Disability • Ethics • Practice management • Medicolegal issues • Do-not-resuscitate • Jehovah's Witness • Informed consent • Patient safety • Medication errors

Key Points

- **Substance Abuse**—Substance use disorder (SUD) is diagnosed at higher rates in the specialty of anesthesiology. It encompasses a spectrum of substances, including alcohol, illicit street drugs, and pharmaceuticals. The cause of substance use disorder is multifactorial and diagnosed across the spectrum of anesthesia providers.

  Self-reporting is uncommon, with death often the first presentation of addiction. The detection of impaired physicians can be challenging, with practitioners frequently demonstrating only subtle changes in performance. Prevention strategies include education, auditing, verification of drug wastage, and pharmaceutical tracking systems. Rehabilitation often encompasses extended inpatient treatment with medical practice reentry challenged with high rates of relapse and death. The use of random drug testing is controversial and utilized with varying degrees of success.

- **Fatigue**—Fatigue influences both cognitive and motor components of clinical care. Sleep deprivation is comparable to intoxication after 24 h of continuous clinical service, with decreased provider performance and increased risk of error.
- **Aging**—Aging can impact professional performance, including providers' stamina, cognition, and technical skills. In partnership with the individual, practice accommodations such as reduced call burden, or weekly service hours, should be considered to extend physician longevity.
- **Disability**—The 1990 Americans with Disabilities Act (ADA) and the Individuals with Disabilities Education Act (IDEA) are federal civil rights laws prohibiting discrimination against people with disabilities. The ADA restricts employment discrimination and educational intolerance of "qualified individuals with disabilities." Title II of the ADA applies specifically to educational institutions, which require equal access to educational opportunities, extracurricular activities, and facilities regardless of physical or mental disability. These laws maintain that reasonable modifications of policies, practices, and procedures are mandated to preserve equal educational opportunity. In anesthesiology, an otherwise qualified individual with a

S. D. Gumbert (✉)
Department of General Anesthesia, Anesthesiology Institute, Cleveland Clinic, Cleveland Clinic Lerner College of Medicine of Case Western Reserve University, Cleveland, OH, USA
e-mail: Gumbers@ccf.org

M. Argalious et al. (eds.), *Basic Sciences in Anesthesia*,
https://doi.org/10.1007/978-3-031-60203-0_31

physical or mental impairment will be allowed the opportunity to complete a residency program with appropriate accommodation.
- **Professionalism**—Professional conduct embodies the treatment of patients, family members, and coworkers with dignity and kindness. These values underscore physicians' unique position in society as healers and the vital importance of acknowledging diversity with sensitivity and compassion.
- **Ethics**—Hospitals have recognized the relevance of bioethics by establishing ethics committees to be consulted in challenging ethical clinical situations. Modern medical bioethics is a framework of four pillars: patient autonomy, beneficence, nonmaleficence, and social justice that serve as a helpful foundation for considering moral behavior in medicine.
- **Patient Safety**—Patient Safety Achieving a New Standard for Care, the Institute of Medicine identified five core competencies that all physicians should be able to exemplify. These competencies include patient-centered care, the capability to work in interdisciplinary teams, engagement of evidence-based practices, application of quality improvement concepts, and utilization of informatics. Safety curricula competencies relate to how students view patient safety while transforming attitudes and skills within a broader healthcare culture.
- **Competencies**—Graduate Medical Education (GME) resident evaluation is a competency-based assessment system. Residents are assessed in 6-month intervals on performance and behavioral milestones, with developmental feedback on their practice independent of their level of training. Milestone evaluation delivers concrete benchmarks of progress and aspirational goals across anesthesia practice. Developmental benchmarks determine residency advancement instead of the historical reference of training duration.

31.1 Impairment

31.1.1 Substance Abuse

Prior to 2000, the statistical prevalence of SUD in physicians was similar to the general population [1–3]. However, recent evidence suggests the prevalence of physician SUD has increased in the past two decades. The cause of substance use disorder is multifactorial and diagnosed across the spectrum of healthcare providers. Environmental and hereditary elements influence the likelihood of substance abuse and its course [4]. Statistically, SUD in medical professionals varies by gender, age, and inherent risk factors. Approximately 15.4% of physicians will develop a substance use disorder (SUD) during their careers, a slightly higher prevalence than the general population (12.6%) [5] . Dermatology (OR = 1.902; $p = 0.0080$) and Orthopedic Surgery (OR = 2.071; $p = 0.0008$) currently have the highest reported rates of SUD [5]. Unfortunately, rates for SUD in anesthesiology remain in the top five medical specialties [5].

31.1.2 Risk Factors of SUD in Physicians

Several risk factors are independently associated with SUD among physicians, including years of practice, gender, and relationship status. Dependence rates are highest in married, female, and younger, less experienced physician subgroups [5–7]. Female physicians are almost twice as likely to have SUD compared to male peers [6]. Finally, statistics further show a higher rate of SUD in physician subgroups that are dissatisfied with their marriage or partnership [5]. Increased rates of SUD correlate with higher rates of suicidal ideation, diminished quality of life, and career dissatisfaction [5].

The development of SUD among anesthesiology residents remains largely enigmatic. Historical factors traditionally thought to increase the risk of SUD in anesthesia residents differ statistically from other areas of medicine and include male sex, psychiatric history, and family history of SUD [8]. Table 31.1 examines SUD in anesthesiology and illustrates common themes of addiction and factors unique to the specialty (Table 31.1) [9].

31.1.3 Incidence of SUD in Anesthesia

Alcohol is the primary substance of misuse by physicians [10]. Physicians' abuse of prescription medications, pharmaceuticals, or illicit street drugs is relatively rare [10]. The most commonly abused alternative is cannabis (2.7%), followed by opiates (1.3%). When examining SUD in anesthesia training programs, the estimated incidence of substance abuse is approximately 1% annually per year of training [4]. In a survey of anesthesia residency programs between 2007 and 2017, 3.7% of residents and 1.16% of faculty were diagnosed with SUD [11]. Anesthesiology residents most commonly abused opioids (39%), followed by propofol (20.3%) and alcohol (15.2%) [4, 11]. These statistics mirror a 2015 Canadian analysis by Boulis et al. that found rates of residents with SUD (1.6%) with opioids the highest substance of reported abuse [12].

Similar to other medical specialties, attending anesthesiologists were most likely to self-report alcohol abuse (50%)

Table 31.1 Substance use disorders risk factors in anesthesia

General risk factors
1. Family history of substance abuse 2. Childhood abuse—physical, emotional, or sexual 3. Dysfunctional support network 4. Mental health disorder 5. Male 6. Experimenting with drugs/alcohol at a young age 7. Peers with SUD 8. Tendency for doctors to self-medicate 9. Sense of professional immunity from addiction
Additional risk factors specific to anesthesiologists
1. Frequent exposure to opiates and sedatives 2. Accessibility and administration of anesthesia drugs, including opiates, ketamine, benzodiazepines, propofol, and inhaled agents 3. Perioperative administration of small doses of controlled substances facilitates ease of diversion 4. Prior history of SUD may be drawn to specialty because of potential drug access 5. Expert parenteral skills allow for self-medication

as the primary substance of misuse, followed by opioids (23.7%) [4]. Interestingly, studies analyzing referrals for treatment of SUD, instead of self-reporting, report lower rates of substance abuse (0.86 to 1.6%) but much higher rates of opioid addiction. Likely, physicians who abuse alcohol do not seek treatment in a formal program at the rates of those who misuse illicit drugs. Notably, by restricting the analysis to confirmed substance abuse cases, these studies potentially underestimate the true prevalence of SUD in anesthesiologists [4].

The rates of resident SUD have nearly doubled compared to the previous interval of survey statistics [4, 11, 13, 14]. The profound upsurge of propofol abuse in resident and faculty cohorts is equally concerning. Wischmeyer et al. and Fry et al. published findings that show propofol is now the most commonly abused anesthetic agent in Australia and New Zealand by anesthesia providers [10, 15]. The increase in the prevalence of nonopioid abuse of anesthetic drugs such as propofol, benzodiazepines, ketamine, and inhaled agents is an area for growing educational need and vigilance [16–19].

31.1.4 Detection of SUD

Although physicians' elevated social status brings many tangible and intangible rewards, it also has an isolating effect when confronted with a disease such as addiction [16, 20]. Physicians tend to protect their workplace performance and professional image well beyond the deterioration of their private life. This isolation and delay in intervention can lead to disastrous physical and professional consequences. Despite considerable resources and educational measures committed to preventing and treating substance abuse, the statistical prevalence of SUDs continues to rise [16, 20].

31.1.5 Consequence of SUD

Detection of SUD is challenging. Physicians often fear that disclosing an addictive illness could cause loss of standing within the medical community, their license to practice medicine, the capacity to complete their training program, or ultimately their ability to earn a living. Unfortunately, this contributes to higher suicide and accidental death rates than self-reporting rates.

In physicians, the fear and isolation created by SUD often end tragically in a coma, near death, or death in 5–10% of initial presentations [4] . Further, the consequence of SUD in medical practice increases the risk of self-reported medical errors ($p = 0.0011$), with SUD impacting the quality of delivered health care [5], [21].

Less than half of the resident physicians with SUD will finish their training program, and 43% will relapse over a 30-year career [4]. For those residents who developed SUD, a risk of unfavorable outcomes existed, including failure to complete a residency (odds ratio 14.9; 95% CI 9–24.6), obtaining board certification (odds ratio 10.4; 95% CI 7–15.5), or completing subspecialty certification (odds ratio 34.6; 95% CI 12–100) [22]. Professional actions such as loss or restriction of their medical license were also significantly increased (hazard ratio 6.8; 95% CI 3.8–12.2) [22].

31.1.6 Treatment of SUD

While there is no cure for SUD, lifelong recovery is the goal of monitoring and treatment programs [23]. Substance abuse is a treatable medical condition with an excellent prognosis, especially for physicians [19, 24, 25]. Treatment modalities frequently include behavioral counseling, cognitive behavioral therapy, and medication-assisted treatment, which utilizes medicines such as methadone or buprenorphine to control the physiologic symptoms of SUD [26–28]. Five-year relapse rates, though high, are 1/3 those of the general population [25]. These statistics reflect the numerous provisions, oversight, and resources set forth by credentialing and state medical boards for comprehensive rehabilitation for physicians. These plans often include mandatory inpatient rehabilitation, followed by extended outpatient therapy, and mandatory substance abuse monitoring by state Physician Health Programs (PHP) [23]. Physician Health Programs offer a confidential resource for physicians suffering from addictive, psychiatric, medical, or other impairing disorders to coordinate and document compliance with treatment recommendations. Referrals may come from colleagues, medical boards, medical staff, medical schools, family members, or self-referrals.

Comprehensive recovery is challenging. Physicians must overcome the stigma of addiction and establish a new social support system, develop healthy life skills and treat underlying medical comorbidities. Physicians' treatment is complex and best provided at a site specializing in physician intervention with knowledge of the Physician Health Program (PHP) and state medical surveillance programs. Sobriety is a lifelong challenge. With adequate vigilance and treatment, physicians have successfully reentered clinical practice.

31.1.7 Reentry to Practice

Reentry to the specialty after treatment of SUD is controversial. The Physician Health Programs (PHP) affords a pathway to supervised return to medical practice; however, the relapse rate is high and has a reported 5–10% mortality rate [29]. The controversy of practice reentry is even more conspicuous in residents with implications for training completion, treatment cost, and future employment status. Once identified, only 55% of programs allow for reentry following the successful completion of a treatment program [11]. Of those identified with SUD, 72% of training programs guaranteed treatment, but only 52% of programs offered to pay for the initial evaluation [11]. Efforts to improve identification and reduce dependence among anesthesiologists have existed for as long as physicians have self-administered anesthetic agents.

31.1.8 Prevention of SUD

Healthcare systems have implemented monitoring and preventive measures to identify SUD. Anesthesia trainees now receive required education early in their residency careers about the hazards of SUD and at-risk symptoms of addiction for identifying dependency in their peers. Measures taken by pharmacies to reduce the risk of diversion and substance abuse by personnel include electronic tracking systems to alert for questionable transactions, statistical analysis of provider dispensing/ordering, random testing of waste solutions, and random provider drug testing. Interestingly, few civilian hospitals perform random medical staff screenings, more commonly opting for pre-employment or for-cause drug screening. Randomized drug screening increases system costs and has the potential to interfere with clinical workflow.

Medical education is not protective against developing SUD. The rigorous training, emotional stress, and heightened expectations that physicians experience place physicians at an increased risk. Work-related stress, burnout, depression, and anxiety are intertwined with addiction, increasing the possibility of harm to the practitioner and those around them [4]. Although many theories have been suggested to explain the relatively high rates of addiction among physicians, the clinical reality is that it is simply a high-risk population for SUDs [25]. Rehabilitation programs designed to treat physicians with SUD reduce the risk for relapse; however, the consequences of relapse are tragic, with death commonly the earliest symptom.

31.1.9 Fatigue

Due to extended work hours and circadian disruption, fatigue has long been regarded as the "Achilles heel" for patient safety in medical training and health care [30]. Considerable laboratory data demonstrates that fatigue degrades cognitive and motor performance [32]. These potential effects are most acute for inexperienced residents in training, but the effects of fatigue are pervasive among all healthcare practitioners [32]. Fa [33, 34] After 24 h of continual wakefulness, cognitive and motor performance decline, producing functional deficits comparable to a blood alcohol concentration of 0.10 percent or narcolepsy [35, 36].

31.1.10 Effects of Fatigue

Fatigue influences clinical tasks such as hand–eye coordination, speed, and accuracy, with mistakes of omission being the most common cognitive mistake related to fatigue [37], In anesthesia training, fatigue reduces laryngoscopy efficiency, the quality of pre-anesthesia assessment, and increased rates of needle sticks and wet taps [38–41]. These risks are highest during the low point of human circadian rhythms, between 01:00 and 07:00 A.M [42].

In addition to affecting performance and functionality, sleep deprivation can lead to depression and social isolation [43]. Sustained fatigue reduces immune function, increases irritable bowel syndrome and depression rates, and increases the risk of personal safety and trauma [44]. Strategies to reduce the impact of fatigue include napping, caffeine, and breaks from clinical work [45].

However, despite many anecdotes about medical errors, a definitive study has not demonstrated widespread systemic harm in health care due to fatigue. Even when fatigue was deemed causative for a specific medical catastrophe, though tragic, these isolated events fail to show wider statistical causation of patient harm [46].

31.1.11 ACGME Duty Hours and Supervision Reform

In 1984, the Libby Zion legal case triggered the formation of a commission to examine resident physicians' supervision and work hours in New York [47]. The commission recommended that New York hospitals adopt regulations that limit consecutive duty hours while increasing the quality and availability of staff supervision. These proposals formed the framework for graduate education policy for work hours and resident supervision. The primary oversight of these policies remains under the Accreditation Council for Graduate Medical Education (ACGME), which sets standards for residency training via 27 residency-review boards [48]. Common requirements specify that programs are responsible for educating faculty and residents to recognize symptoms of fatigue while ensuring adequate sleep facilities and safe resident transportation.

Several factors established the need for common duty hour standards within health care: increased patient acuity and occupational demands of residents, scientific understanding of the adverse performance consequences of fatigue, and growing public pressure for reform [48]. In late 2001, this culminated in legislation to regulate excessive duty hours as a workplace health hazard [49].

In 2003, ACGME implemented national duty hour limits, setting a maximum 80 h workweek and reducing shift lengths to less than 30 consecutive hours [50]. Implemented rules further restricted "on-call" shifts to no more than every third night and required an average of one day off per week. The ACGME revised duty hour regulations in July 2011 for junior postgraduate year-1 (PGY-1) residents. The consensus was that junior learners would benefit from further work hour restrictions and a regulated learning environment. The consecutive permitted duty hours for a single shift were reduced from a maximum of 30 h to 16 h for PGY1 residents. Senior residents with more clinical experience and knowledge were allowed to care for patients for 24 h and beyond if continuity of care was warranted.

Duty hour statutes have engendered considerable debate since their implementation. A systematic examination found that while resident well-being improved after implementing the 2003 and 2011 duty hour regulations, there was no apparent effect on patient clinical outcomes. Research failed to reveal a significant difference in mortality, hospital readmission rates, patient safety indicators, or length of stay since implemented 2003 and 2011 reforms [51–57] . A 2015 review of 27 studies found that concentrating on-duty hours alone failed to improve patient care or resident wellness [58]. In 2014, JAMA analyzed 30-day mortality rates and 30-day-all-cause readmission rates among Medicare beneficiaries, demonstrating no significant differences in outcomes with duty hour reforms [59]. The reasons for the lack of effect on safety outcomes are unclear. Resident supervision has improved, which may minimize trainee discontinuity; however, safety reductions may be attenuated by an increased number of transitions of care. Finally, despite reduced duty hours, burnout and fatigue remain common hazards among residents.

Further, evidence suggests that these reforms intended to improve well-being may have an untended negative impact on education and clinical experience. Surveys of faculty and residents determined that clinical experience and dedicated education time may have declined, although residents' quality of life improved. After implementing duty hour reform, a 2014 systemic review discovered that surgical residents performed fewer cases and scored lower on certification exams [60]. Despite this, patient outcomes and physician competency were similar before and after reform implementation [61].

As a result of this emerging data, the ACGME has increased the length of each shift of PGY-1 residents from 16 to 24 h and allows for an additional 4 h of service time to manage transitions in care, allowing for the promotion of professionalism, empathy, and commitment. First-year residents continue to have an 80-h weekly cap on service hours and must have an average of one day off per week. Call responsibilities are limited to a maximum of one call every three nights. These new regulations went into effect in July 2017.

31.1.12 Aging

The percentage of active members older than 65 in the American Society of Anesthesiologists increases annually [62]. Physicians entering into the later stages of their career can offer robust benefits to their practice and health care.

There are physiologic and cognitive changes that commonly occur with aging that pose unique challenges for older anesthesiologists. These changes can affect the aging physicians' practice by enriching skills such as wisdom and experience while diminishing others, like cognitive function, motor, and fine dexterity. It is important to note that age-related transformations affect practitioners in unique ways.

The senior physician may wish to remain clinically active, and the workplace can benefit from their experience. Practice groups should establish policies to address issues surrounding this growing subset of senior anesthesiologists. For example, limiting overnight calls, shift duration, or shift frequency may extend the career of the anesthesiologist while improving job satisfaction and patient safety. Alternatively, the senior physician may add value to education, research, or administrative leadership. Modifying a staff schedule or expanding alternative leadership affords career longevity and professional satisfaction.

Currently, there is no universally accepted consensus on the function of cognitive testing to evaluate professional competency in an aging physician. Local policies guiding the evaluation of an individual anesthesiologist's qualifications are more suitable than compulsory retirement age or testing provisions. To create a transparent pathway with constituent input, tools to manage an aging workforce should be established within an organization. Such a framework would manage worker expectations and establish resources for physicians in their late careers. Consultation with the senior physician, human resources, institution, and practice leadership should occur humanely before any practice modification.

31.1.13 Disability and the Americans with Disabilities Act

The 1990 Americans with Disabilities Act (ADA) and the Individuals with Disabilities Education Act (IDEA) are federal civil rights laws prohibiting discrimination against people with disabilities [63, 64]. The ADA restricts employment discrimination and educational intolerance of "qualified individuals with disabilities." Title II of the ADA applies notably to educational institutions, which mandate equal access to educational opportunities, extracurricular activities, and facilities regardless of physical or mental disability. These laws maintain that reasonable modifications of policies, practices, and procedures are required to preserve equal opportunities.

ACGME mandates that qualified individuals have the same opportunity, with appropriate accommodations, to complete a residency training program. A disability—physical or mental—cannot be the sole reason to discriminate against a candidate [65]. An accommodation is a reasonable adjustment or modification of the work environment enabling a disabled qualified applicant to perform essential job functions [63 64]. For example, mechanical orthopedic devices or a wheelchair have successfully permitted individuals to practice clinically. Likewise, issues with senses such as hearing or vision loss have been overcome with cochlear implants, hearing aids, or glasses. Diagnosis of mental health conditions can be managed successfully with medications, counseling, and routine clinical supervision.

It is critical to note that employers or residency training programs are not required to lower quality or quantity standards to make an accommodation [66]. Ultimately, the individual must be able to complete the primary mental and physical responsibilities of the practice of anesthesiology. Candidates with a disability not mitigated by reasonable accommodation and pose a "direct threat to health and safety" are not protected under the ADA [66]. Eligibility for credentialing, licensure, and board certification, occurs after reviewing a candidate's academic clinical performance, letters of recommendation, and medical records. Incorporating historical practice accommodations and critical training reviews ensures public safety.

31.2 ACGME Core Competencies

31.2.1 The Six ACGME Core Competencies [67]

Practice-Based Learning and Improvement
Patient Care and Procedural Skills
Systems-Based Practice
Medical Knowledge
Interpersonal and Communication Skills
Professionalism

The traditional model of evaluation of graduate medical education (G.M.E.) has been global evaluation by faculty accompanied by high-stakes written and oral benchmark examinations. In 2001 and again in 2018, the ACGME revised the education and evaluation of physicians through the Outcomes Project and produced six core competencies of medical education practice, their definitions, and tools for evaluating mastery. Competency-based training is a progression of mastery of specific knowledge and skills through learner-centered milestone competencies [67]. These competencies are.

31.2.2 Patient Care

Residents must be able to provide patient care that is benevolent, appropriate, and efficacious for treating health problems and advancing health care.

31.2.3 Medical Knowledge

Residents should exhibit an understanding of established and evolving biomedical, clinical, epidemiological, and social-behavioral sciences and their application to patient care.

31.2.4 Interpersonal and Communication Skills

Residents must display interpersonal and communication aptitude to effectively exchange information and collaboration with patients, families, and other health professionals. Residents should:

- communicate effectively across socioeconomic and cultural backgrounds
- communicate effectively with health professionals and health-related agencies
- effectively work as a partner or leader of a healthcare team
- act in a consultative role to other physicians and health professionals
- maintain comprehensive, timely, and legible medical records

31.2.5 Practice-Based Learning and Improvement

Trainees must exhibit the capacity to examine and assess their patient care, evaluate and incorporate scientific evidence-based literature, and demonstrate self-evaluation and lifelong learning. In the course of their training, residents should satisfy the following objectives:

- self-assessment of strengths, shortcomings, and knowledge gaps
- establish learning and improvement objectives
- implement changes with the goal of practice improvement using quality improvement (QI) methods
- integrate constructive evaluation feedback into everyday practice
- application of evidence-based medicine from scientific literature to patient's health concerns
- optimize and promote learning via information technology
- educate patients and their families, learners, and members of the healthcare team

31.2.6 Systems-Based Practice

Residents should exhibit knowledge and responsiveness to the healthcare system and incorporate other resources within the system to deliver optimal care. Residents must demonstrate an ability to:

- effectively work in an assortment of healthcare delivery environments
- coordinate patient care associated with their clinical specialty
- regard cost awareness and risk–benefit analysis for both inpatient and population-based care
- encourage quality patient and systems-based care
- work inter-professionally to enhance safety and care quality
- Recognize healthcare system errors and implement potential creative solutions.

31.2.7 Professionalism

Residents must exhibit a dedication to professional responsibility and adhere to ethical doctrines. Residents should demonstrate:

- empathy, integrity, and consideration for others
- place the needs of patients before their own
- respect autonomy and patient privacy
- be accountable to the medical profession, their patients, and society
- sensitive to patient diversity, including gender, age, culture, race, religion, disabilities, and sexual orientation

31.2.8 Next Accreditation System (NAS) and Clinical Compliance Committee (CCC)

Further, the Outcome Project established a new approach to the accreditation of GME programs. The Next Accreditation System (NAS) contains a behaviorally-based set of standards for each competency and tool for assessing milestone achievement launched in 2009 and implemented entirely in 2015 [67, 68]. A residency program maintains a Clinical Compliance Committee (CCC) that reviews resident milestone progress every six months [67]. Program accreditation is based on annual self-assessment and reporting with periodic in-person site visits as warranted for program evaluation.

31.3 Professionalism, Ethics, Practice Management, Medicolegal Issues

31.3.1 Professionalism

Physicians maintain a contract with patients and society to comport themselves professionally. At the core of professionalism is the root word profession. In a professional culture, individuals share a commitment to self-regulate and adhere to lofty standards of conduct and ethics. Physicians regulate themselves through national societies, board certification, state medical agencies, hospital credentialing, and peer review. In 1999, the ACGME established six core competencies for evaluation and education during residency and fellowship training. One of these core pillars of education is Professionalism.

Professional conduct embodies the treatment of patients, family members, and coworkers with dignity and kindness. These values underscore physicians' unique position in society as healers and the vital importance of acknowledging diversity with sensitivity and compassion. Professionalism and the ethics surrounding medical practice personify many behaviors demonstrated in ACGME Core Competencies [69].

31.3.1.1 Professionalism Sub-competencies

Sub-competencies allow for granular analysis of a resident's Professionalism Competence [69]. These include:

- Demonstrating Professional Conduct and Accountability
- Demonstrating Humanism and Cultural Proficiency
- Maintaining Emotional, Physical, and Mental Health
- Pursuing Continual Personal and Professional Growth

The ACGME Professionalism sub-competencies highlight the standards of physician conduct. These competencies include placing their patient's needs above their own, aspiring for lifelong learning, assuming responsibility, and treating individuals with respect and dignity. The delivery of safe, efficacious, and efficient health care demands technical ability and enduring culture of respect for the medical profession.

31.3.1.2 Demonstrating Professional Conduct and Accountability

How physicians present themselves can instantly influence the perceived quality of care they deliver. Professional conduct includes being prepared and appropriately dressed for clinical service and encompasses completing medical records honestly and in a timely fashion. Good citizenship includes advocating for their patients' interests, being accountable and acknowledging errors, and seeking the guidance of colleagues and mentors when faced with challenges. Medicine requires an awareness of one's limitations through constant self-assessment while pursuing a lifelong desire for self-improvement and learning.

31.3.1.3 Demonstrating Humanism and Cultural Proficiency

Humanism seeks to deliver health care with honesty, empathy, benevolence, and regard for the dignity and opinions of each patient and their families. Observing a person's inherent value involves shaking hands, acknowledging all stakeholders, and openly and humanely addressing patient concerns. Maintaining confidentiality and patient privacy is fundamental to trust in the physician–patient relationship.

A resident can also show Professionalism and Competency by demonstrating a philosophy of altruism and advocacy. Physicians should exhibit unselfish regard for the interest of patients and their families while advocating for their welfare and healthcare needs. Finally, empathy is an understanding of the unique qualities of each patient, including gender, age, ethnicity, disability, and sexual orientation. Residents should be mindful of how these attributes affect the delivery of patient care and well-being. By acknowledging and understanding the uniqueness of each patient, the physician can foster a better patient-physician relationship and offer better medical care.

31.3.1.4 Maintaining Emotional, Physical, and Mental Health and Pursues Continual Personal and Professional Growth

Professionalism mandates continual development and evolution of knowledge and technical skills throughout the lifespan of a career in medicine. Lifelong learning—continues well after residency or fellowship training has finished. Educational opportunities include regular participation in departmental, national, and state conferences, simulation, online continuing education modules or questions, and hands-on workshops. Anesthesiologists should enhance their knowledge through participation in the Maintenance of Certification in Anesthesiology (MOCA) program. MOCA is a web-based platform that guides lifelong learning through an interactive assessment tool for educational and quality initiatives that support the acquisition of up-to-date medical knowledge and outcomes research to improve patient safety. Medicine continuously evolves with new information, changing technology, and practice guidelines. Physicians must maintain proficiency for safe and ethical practice.

31.3.2 Ethics

31.3.2.1 Why Ethics?

Bioethics is a standard element of medical education. Learners often face ethical decisions in medical school and residency training. In a self-reporting study of internal medicine residents, greater than 80% of respondents acknowledged an ethical dilemma involving the American College of Physicians Ethics Manual [70]. Infractions included failing to clarify resuscitation preferences, acting as a personal physician to friends and loved ones, or being influenced by corporate incentives. Likewise, ethical setbacks in anesthesiology are similarly prevalent [71]. In a review of training records of anesthesia residents, greater than 20% of residents received at least one critique of unprofessional conduct [72].

The teaching of ethics in medical education should not inspire people to be good; truthfully, the opposite holds. Moral integrity is selected for and should be an inherent virtue of a physician. So why teach medical ethics? Exceptional moral logic can improve ethical behavior by giving learners tools to resolve complicated conflicts [71].

31.3.2.2 Ethical Theory

Conventionally, ethics encompasses the moral judgment of right and wrong. Two classic theories, Consequentialism and Deontology, define right or wrong in absolute terms. Consequentialism ethical doctrine holds that morality is an act conditionally based upon its outcome. A more straightforward way to express this is the "ends justify the means.“ If an act has an overall benefit, it does not matter about the act itself. Utilitarianism, a type of consequentialism, advocates for actions promoting happiness and opposes acts resulting in unhappiness. Utilitarianism is an effort to answer the pragmatic question, "What should a person do?" This theory maintains that the best action is the one that brings about the most significant benefit. Utilitarianism is generally regarded on a societal scale, considering the moral effects on a community and not just the individual patient.

In contrast, Deontology is an ethical theory that emphasizes the relationship between duty and the morality of human acts. Deontology is also known as "duty-based ethics.“ This ideology is dependent on the physician's duty and obligation and that some actions are morally compulsory regardless of their consequences for human welfare.

31.3.2.3 Modern Medical Bioethics

Modern medical bioethics is a framework of four pillars: patient autonomy, beneficence, nonmaleficence, and social justice that serve as a helpful foundation for considering moral behavior in medicine [73]. The pillars offer a framework that explores the most appropriate action in a particular moral dilemma.

31.3.2.4 Patient Autonomy

Autonomy maintains that each individual with capacity has the right to make their own decisions, and providers have an ethical responsibility to respect this independence. In the physician–patient relationship, patients are notably vulnerable, leading to potential moral conflict. Autonomy requires a patient to be informed and understand treatment options (including no intervention) and the inherent risks of each. Autonomy maintains that a patient should be free from external influence and informed throughout the decision-making process.

Compromising patient autonomy can result in moral injury, irrespective of a genuine transgression. For example, a child presenting for surgery may explicitly express a desire not to get an IV. Although consent by a lawful guardian supersedes the child's wishes, autonomy may be compromised, resulting in moral injury if placed without consideration of the child's wishes. The best practice would be to get permission from the child's legal guardian and assent from the minor to maintain autonomy whenever possible [74].

31.3.2.5 Nonmaleficence

The Latin maxim, "primum non-nocere," captures the principle of nonmaleficence: "above all, do no harm." Recent studies estimate that medical errors may account for as many as 251,000 deaths annually in the United States, making medical errors the third leading cause of death [75].

With the expansion of medical treatment capacity, an increased opportunity for patient harm naturally increases. By being aware of these statistics, physicians should undertake ongoing efforts to participate in morbidity and mortality conferences, root cause analysis processes, and quality improvement initiatives to reduce the incidence of iatrogenic harm.

31.3.2.6 Beneficence

The commitment to healing is fundamental to medical practice, which directs the doctrine of beneficence. There must be a net benefit of a diagnostic pathway, treatment plan, or societal healthcare policy balanced against the relative risk of harm. For example, pharmaceutical pricing is a familiar cause of this moral concession. Patients with atrial fibrillation may benefit from a newer, more expensive direct oral anticoagulant than warfarin. The principle of beneficence is compromised when a patient cannot take the best medication because of financial limitations.

31.3.2.7 Social Justice

The final pillar of bioethics is social justice. Justice demands that limited resources be equitably accessible across society. Care should not depend upon demographic variables such as race, religion, socioeconomic status, gender, sexual orientation, age, or cultural background.

31.3.2.8 Ethics Summary

Contemporary ethics differ from traditional theories of Consequentialism and Deontology, utilizing case-based precedents, which operate more like legal precedents to establish ethical standing. Education in ethics aims to give physicians tools to help resolve these unavoidable dilemmas. The difficulty of weighing one's obligation to the individual versus society can be a daily problem for anesthesiologists, and establishing ethical precedent to guide decision-making is invaluable.

Hospitals have recognized the relevance of bioethics by establishing ethics committees to be consulted in challenging ethical clinical situations. In concert with the patient and healthcare provider, bioethics committees help educate and construct a framework to help resolve moral dilemmas. Additionally, there is a medicolegal benefit when appropriate bioethical panel documents a framework of precedents to support a judgment.

31.3.2.9 Practice Management and Ethics

The atmosphere in which physicians practice and patients obtain care continues to evolve. Increasingly employment models, shifts in practice design, new regulatory requirements, and market influences affect the practice of medicine. These changes may prioritize the business of medicine instead of the delivery of health care. Physicians must consider the effect the practice environment has on their ethical and professional responsibilities.

All healthcare delivery arrangements have inherent advantages and disadvantages. Physicians should ensure governing bodies and affiliated practices are structured to acknowledge and sustain a commitment to the profession of medicine and patient-centered care. Most states prohibit the "corporate practice of medicine," restricting the commercialization of medical practice, interference with physician clinical judgment, or undue influence on physicians' self-regulation of medical practice [76]. These statutes minimize the potential corporate financial conflict with shareholders that may contradict physicians' obligation to patient care. Regulation and enforcement vary; however, the underlying principle is that an individual or organization cannot regulate or define state medical practice without a medical license.

Business practices can challenge the ethics and professionalism of individual physicians and the social mission of institutions. It is the collective responsibility of the medical profession to adhere to these ethical boundaries. Physicians must be mindful of how business practices, employment language, and contracts influence medicine. If a practice or policy has the potential to compromise patient care, a physician is obligated to object and refer to the appropriate regulatory agency.

Healthcare delivery contracts come with advantages, and disadvantages, with salient problems for professionalism and ethics. Recently health care has pivoted from a volume-based fee-for-service model to a value-based system to improve population health, reduce health expenditures, and improve healthcare inequities.

The 2010 Affordable Care Act passage has led to the introduction of value-based care in the United States. Value-based health care is a healthcare delivery framework that incentivizes the quality of care provided instead of quantity. Under a value-based healthcare model, providers are reimbursed based on healthcare outcomes. When aligned with medical ethics, professionalism, and evidence-based care, value-based care inducements have supported high-quality health care [77].

Choosing the least expensive option is compelling but must be undertaken within the context of patient care outcomes. Efficiency and productivity are essential, but patient care should remain the intrinsic motivation of service, professionalism, and clinical integrity.

31.3.2.10 Do-Not-Resuscitate

Advance directives in health care establish a framework for patients to delineate how and under what circumstances they will receive treatment, such as a do-not-resuscitate (DNR) or do-not-intubate (DNI). Advance directives respect the ethical principle of patient autonomy [78, 79].

On December 6, 1989, the Supreme Court affirmed that Cruzan vs. Missouri was permissible with "clear and convincing evidence" to sustain a patient's wishes to remove life support. Consequently, on December 1, 1991, the Patient Self-Determination Act (PSDA) became the foundation for advanced written directives [79]. The PSDA facilitates a dialogue between physicians, patients, and family members. The PSDA requires that healthcare institutions receiving Medicare or Medicaid funds advise patients of state regulations of a living will and appointment of a medical power of attorney [79]. Advance directives guide healthcare providers to openly discuss their wishes, including CPR, DNR, and DNI.

Advance directives pose distinct challenges during the perioperative period and warrant further clarification by providers. The inherent risk of anesthesia and associated surgical complications differ significantly from other clinical settings. Within the perioperative window, care that an advance directive would suspend would otherwise be routine [80].

In 2001, 2008, 2013, and 2018 the American Society of Anesthesiologists (ASA) published guidelines for the ethical care of patients with advanced care directives during the perioperative period [81]. These guidelines address anesthesia in elective and emergent circumstances for competent and incompetent patients [81].

Documented communication of the patient's wishes is critical for perioperative care for patients with DNR orders and limiting treatment directives. Institutional policies that automatically suspend advanced directives prior to anesthetic care may not sufficiently address a patient's rights to self-determination and should be revised [81]. The administration of anesthesia necessarily involves practices considered "resuscitation" in other clinical settings. Prior to anesthesia, any existing directives to limit care, such as a

DNR, should be reviewed with the patient or designated medical power of attorney so that the status is clarified or modified based on the patient's preferences [81]. The medical chart should document the specific modifications and timing of resuscitation preferences. Advanced directives should respect the patient's autonomy and provide a satisfactory outcome during the perioperative setting. Potential options include [81]:

- Complete Resuscitation: A complete suspension of advanced directives with a return to standard resuscitation measures
- Limited Attempt with Selected Resuscitation Measures: The patient specifies specific resuscitation procedures they are willing to suspend during the perioperative period. For example, a patient may be agreeable to a pharmacological resuscitation with tracheal intubation but decline defibrillation and CPR.
- Limited Attempt at Resuscitation Defined by Patient's Goals and Values: The care team's clinical judgment determines which resuscitation procedures are appropriate within the context of the stated values of a patient. For example, some patients may desire full resuscitation efforts to manage adverse but reversible clinical events; however, they refrain from treatment in situations that would result in permanent sequelae, such as dependence upon life-sustaining technology. In such cases, the anesthesiologist should document the discussion with particular attention to the stated goals and wishes of the patient.

Modification of advanced directives should also clearly indicate the timing of reinstatement of preexisting advance directives; this commonly occurs when the patient leaves the post-anesthesia care unit or has recovered from the acute effects of anesthesia [81]. It is necessary to discuss and document whether there are any exceptions to the injunction against intervention under a recognized complication of the surgical procedure or anesthetic (i.e., treatment of anaphylaxis) [81]. The healthcare team members, including the primary care physician of record, should be included in this process and updated via the medical record.

If a conflict arises, the following resolution processes may be helpful. If an anesthesiologist finds a decision morally irreconcilable, they should withdraw and arrange alternative care [81]. However, if an intervention conflicts with accepted norms of care, ethics, or policy, the case should be referred to an institutional review committee [81]. If alternatives are not promptly available, the American Medical Association's Principles of Medical Ethics states that care should proceed with adherence to the patient's known intended directives in compliance with their plans and values [81]. A hospital committee should be established with anesthesiology, nursing, ethics, legal, and surgery representatives, allowing for case review, discussion, and ethical policy application to these moral challenges.

31.3.2.11 Anesthesia and the Jehovah's Witness

The Jehovah's Witness religion is a Christian movement established in the United States in the 1870s, with over six million members worldwide. The Jehovah's Witness believe in the literal interpretation of the Bible, which prohibits the 'consumption' of blood-related products as outlined in the Old Testament. Jehovah's Witness also believes blood is "unclean" once withdrawn from the body, prohibiting donating or storing blood components (i.e., cell savor or fractionated blood products) [82]. Jehovah's Witnesses are generally familiar with their rights, treatment options, and the potential outcome of transfusion refusal. Elders of the Jehovah's community or Hospital Liaison Committee may act in an advisory capacity and serve as an excellent resource for the care team. Case law is now unambiguous, protecting the autonomy of Jehovah's Witness right of transfusion refusal [82, 83].

Respect for a patient's autonomy requires the acceptance of a patient's right to refuse transfusion, even if contrary to the physician's belief system [84]. The physician is obligated to value the expression of a patient's beliefs, even if the result is death. Most hospitals have developed consent forms for Jehovah's Witnesses detailing explicit exclusions. When obtaining restricted consent, the risks and benefits of blood therapy require a detailed, witnessed discussion [84]. If the patient stays steadfast in their refusal, the specific restrictions are documented and signed by all parties. A revised witnessed consent is updated in the medical record if consent is changed [83].

31.3.2.12 Emergencies

When a patient's Jehovah's Witness status is unknown, a physician is obligated to treat a patient, including transfusion of blood components, if necessary, in an emergency [83]. If informed by relatives or friends of a patient's Jehovah's Witness status, a written advance directive is required to withhold therapy in a life-threatening circumstance [83].

31.3.2.13 Minors

Jehovah's Witness children present special legal considerations. A candid discussion should occur among the surgeon, anesthesiologist, parents, and child (if old enough) of the likelihood of perioperative blood loss and transfusion risk. Most parents will accept that consideration will be made to avoid transfusion; however, ethically, a doctor is obligated to transfuse a minor in a life-saving circumstance [83]. Children under 16 can legally give consent if they comprehend the risks and benefits under Gillick Competence [83].

Nonetheless, courts have established a willingness to overrule a child's refusal in specific medical circumstances.

If the parents refuse consent, but a transfusion is in the child's best interest, an appeal for a 'specific issue order' can be made to the court to remove the parental authority and allow for a blood transfusion. A hospital ethics committee can assist in coordinating such a measure. Blood should be administered in time-sensitive scenarios that do not allow for such a legal petition [83]. Failure to provide life-saving therapy to a child could induce negligent criminal prosecution [83].

31.3.2.14 Preoperative Consideration

The Jehovah's Witnesses patients require preoperative optimization to reduce hemorrhage risk and maximize the potential for a successful surgery. Preoperative assessment of hematologic factors, clotting studies, medications (e.g., anticoagulants, antiplatelet drugs, and supplements), and optimization of nutritional status with supplemental enteral feeding or total parenteral nutrition should be undertaken [83]. Preoperative anemia and clotting derangements should be corrected pharmacologically with iron, folate, B12, and erythropoietin to enhance blood cell production and clotting derangements with vitamin K [83].

31.3.2.15 Ethics in Research

Beauchamp and Childress's four principles, autonomy, nonmaleficence, beneficence, and justice, are fundamental to ethical biomedical research. Sound scientific research is impartial with rigorous research methodology, diverse subject recruitment, and ethical and humane treatment of subjects and animals [85]. The Declaration of Helsinki and the Belmont Report set research standards for the treatment of human subjects, including: [86, 87]

- The benefits of a proposed research trial should outweigh the inherent risk to the individual research subject, supporting the ethical principles of beneficence and nonmaleficence. Vulnerable classes (juveniles, incarcerated, mentally impaired, economically impoverished) need appropriate protection.
- Individual research participants are treated with fairness and respect with an equal appropriation of benefits across subjects, reinforcing the ethical principle of justice.
- Individual privacy is protected, participants' is well-being sustained, and the ethical principle of autonomy is honored without consequence [85].

Research must include explicit statements of permission granted by an Institutional Review Board (IRB) with documentation of informed consent prior to data collection. The disclosure of findings should incorporate appropriate authorship, consideration for intellectual property, and be free of monetary influence [88, 85]. Research must disclose possible conflicts of interest and financial support. Data and methodology, including research design and statistical analysis, should allow for transparent scientific validation and replication [85, 88]. Finally, the dissemination of research is often fraught with ethical issues, including plagiarism, data manipulation, duplicative submission or publication, and figure manipulation, which requires meaningful ethical adherence [85, 88].

31.4 Medical Informed Consent

Medical informed consent is the ethical and legal premise of patient autonomy [89]. Every individual has the right to make decisions affecting their health care when informed of the risks, benefits, and alternatives of medical intervention. There are four principles of informed consent [89, 90]:

- Capacity (or capability) to make the decision.
- Appropriate disclosure of the expected benefits and risks with the disclosure of the probability that the benefits or risks may occur.
- Patient comprehension of pertinent information.
- A willingness to freely provide consent without coercion or duress.

Medical informed consent is vital to the physician's ability to diagnose and treat while preserving the individual's right to autonomy. An *informed medical choice* is an educational process that emphasizes the possible risks, benefits, and alternatives of medical intervention. Ethically, physicians are responsible for identifying the most appropriate intervention based on available scientific medical evidence and clinical experience that meets or exceeds the standard of care [89]. This dialogue is the foundation of a patient-physician relationship and mutually benefits both parties. It encourages collaborative, informed decision-making between partners, and enhances patient wellness, understanding, and satisfaction. Informed consent also allows for shared decision-making authority and accountability for outcomes. Medical informed consent is an integral part of the fiduciary responsibility of physicians.

Informed consent statutes mandate the disclosure of the relative dangers of a proposed medical plan and the possible alternatives to encourage a knowledgeable decision-making process. A patient's comprehension and understanding of the potential risks are necessary to support the standard of informed consent [89]. Early law statutes surrounding medical consent developed from the tort of battery, performing a treatment without the patient's consent, conducting a substantially different procedure than discussed, exceeding the scope of the proposed consent, or an alternate physician not named in the consent performing the procedure. The legal analysis of informed medical consent has evolved from an allegation of battery to negligence; the physician fails to meet the standard of care, with a causal connection between a physician's oversight to perform a duty that causes harm.

The professional standard of informed medical consent requires that a physician disclose information in a fashion consistent with physicians with similar training in a comparable medical practice, *Canterbury v Spence* [89]. The second method is the materiality or "prudent patient" approach, which allows a jury to decide if other information would have been considered essential for disclosure by a reasonable patient, *Cowman v Hornaday*, 1983 [89] . Courts acknowledge situations when nondisclosure is justified, including circumstances of patient's cognitive incompetence, medical emergencies, and the privileged therapeutic exception [89]. Physicians are not required to disclose risks if a patient is already aware of risks or generally considered common knowledge, *Kissinger v Lofgren*, 1987 [89]. Individual state laws define which policies and exceptions apply to individual physicians' practice.

31.4.1 Patient Safety

In the 1990s, international studies began to examine healthcare safety, outcomes, and quality metrics [91]. A startling statistic by the World Health Organization (WHO) found that in high-income countries, one in ten hospitalized patients suffers a preventable adverse event [92]. There has been a notable increase in engagement by healthcare systems, with measures to improve healthcare safety and provider education. However, the statistical scale remains daunting. A WHO study reports that seven types of adverse events yield 43 million preventable injuries a year, making medical harm one of the most common causes of preventable morbidity and mortality annually [93]. In practice, studies have found that education, an improved safety culture, and an atmosphere of teamwork all contribute to decreased rates of patient harm and hospital mortality [94–96].

31.4.2 Core Competencies and Patient Safety

The groundbreaking Institute of Medicine's report *To Err Is Human* influenced the worldwide initiative to advance safer healthcare and safety education [97] . The development of integrated competencies over content has transformed health professionals' view of their role in patient safety and quality improvement. In its report Patient Safety Achieving a New Standard for Care, the Institute of Medicine identified five core competencies that all physicians should be able to exemplify [98 99]. These included the requirement of patient-centered care, the capability to work in interdisciplinary teams, engagement of evidence-based practices, application of quality improvement concepts, and utilization of informatics.

There is growing evidence that education can enhance healthcare quality and patient safety. New patient safety curricula include competencies related to how students view patient safety while transforming attitudes and skills within a broader healthcare culture. Medical schools have begun introducing patient safety training into the curriculum, including lectures, problem-based learning, hands-on experiences, and improved knowledge and systems-based thinking [67].

Learners now analyze individual safety problems through a systematic lens of quality improvement, identifying and testing potential solutions.

However, there are challenges associated with integrating patient safety into education and resident training. There are barriers of embarrassment, guilt, blame, and denial surrounding medical errors that hinder safety and educational improvement. Medical education and healthcare organizations must value and instill a transparent culture of patient safety and quality improvement.

31.4.3 Medication Errors

Human error poses a significant risk for hospitalized patients causing an estimated 100,000 to 400,000 deaths in the United States annually [100]. Medical error constitutes the third leading cause of mortality in the United States, with medication complications making up almost 20% of events [91, 101]. Five percent of medications administered during surgery are medically administered in error [100]. A recent 2022 study evaluating 4000 medication errors determined that the most frequent types of mistakes were incorrect dose 29.4% (miscalculation of dose, concentration, or infusion rate), substitution errors 28.1% (syringe or ampule/vial swap), and incorrect route of administration (7.6%). Eighty-nine percent of medication errors were considered preventable, with 38% causing moderate or severe patient harm [102].

Errors in the administration of medications in the perioperative arena occur in an exceptionally complicated work environment. The anesthesia provider is commonly the only practitioner involved in prescribing, formulating, dispensing, and administering diverse medications without safeguards commonly utilized in other hospital environments [103] . Further, the administration of medications is in a high-stakes and high-stress environment. Efforts to improve medication administration safety (Table 31.2) include standardization of

Table 31.2 Medication safety strategies

Patient information and documentation	– Medication reconciliation completed in EMR – Standardized documentation of medication administration across perioperative period – Verified patient identification, dosing weight, allergies – Preoperative time out to verify required antibiotics, and unique medications for procedures with dose and schedule
Anesthesia information systems and cognitive aids	– Automatic electronic reminders of medication dose, timing, drug interactions, and patient allergies – Weight-based dose guidelines – Infusion pumps with medication dosing guardrails – Checklists, rescue protocols, and common infusion rate charts
Automated medication dispensing systems and medication tray organization	– Standardized layout across all anesthesia locations – Clearly labeled division and modular organization of medications – Management of medication flow including stocking and distribution by pharmacy – Eliminate uncommon drugs from typical locations – Designate a special medication slot or drawer for unique medications specific to a service area or case – Preferential use of single vial medications -If a multi-dose vial is required unused portion is discarded at the conclusion of the anesthetic – Formulary designed to avoid the purchase of look-alike medications-Avoidance of storing similar appearing medications in proximity – Add alert labels for look-alike medications
Management of medication administration and dangerous drug management	Administration – Every medication labeled with name, date, and concentration, – Barcode system use with audible and visual cues – Preprinted, color-coded labels – Discard unlabeled syringes – Minimize provider prepared syringes Use prefilled syringes, compounded or diluted medications prepared by pharmacy – Read and verify every vial, ampoule, and syringe label before administration – Verify high-risk medications (e.g., heparin and insulin), dilutions, and weight-based doses with two people – Limit provider access to concentrated drug formulations instead rely on pharmacy preparation (e.g., insulin, heparin) – Standardize medication concentrations across healthcare system – Alert label on concentrated or high-risk drugs – Smart pump for all medication infusions-Standardized smart pumps across hospital units -Incorporate pumps with drug libraries, guardrails, and alarms – IV solutions (i.e., glucose, heparin, hypertonic saline, sterile water) stored separately from standard IV crystalloid solutions
Clearly identify the route of administration:	– Designate specific route of administration on order sets (epidural, IV, etc.) – Labels on every infusion line and port – No ports on epidural/intrathecal lines
Specialized carts	– Designated carts with detailed protocols and medications for malignant hyperthermia, cardiac arrest, regional anesthesia, and OB
Transitions of care, communication, safety culture, and education	– Transitions of care require protocol-driven review of allergies, drugs administered, and dose/timing of future required medications – Verbal medication orders are verified by repeating the dose and drug, announcing when it is administered, and properly documenting the administration in the EMR – Discard or return all unused medications at the end of each case – Establish written policies for medication safety – Establish a culture of respect and collaboration that endorses patient safety and compliance including a QA system for incident reporting, analysis, and process improvement – Provide adequate supervision and education for learners – Designated pharmacist for operating room operations and educational support – Changes in supplied medications (new labels, concentrations, etc.) should trigger alerts to staff and alert labels

drug treys, adopting barcode and syringe color-coded systems, limiting "look-alike" vials, and requiring infusions on pumps with guardrails and alerts [100].

31.4.4 Disclosure of Error

Most providers and patients acknowledge that healthcare services are potentially hazardous and that errors occur despite the best efforts of individuals and institutions [104]. Patients expect to be informed when exposed to an injury, especially when it occurs in error [105]. Ample evidences in health law, medicine, and the social sciences confirm that the open disclosure of an adverse event is ethically warranted and demonstrates exemplary practice [106].

It is also unmistakable how disclosure impacts the patient, family, the physician–patient relationship, the provider's second victim effect, and the healthcare institution itself [107]. In the United States, health state and federal regulatory agencies, specialty medical boards, and credentialing entities endorse the practice of medical error disclosure [106]. Physicians should disclose detailed information, regardless of whether the patient asks, using a direct statement that a medical mistake occurred. A description of the error, the reasons it occurred, and how it will be potentially prevented in the future should be presented as part of the discussion. Finally, a thoughtful apology should be made to the patient and the family for the adverse event [107]. Many states have specific laws that allow the treatment team to disclose details of medical events without the risk of a legal admission of liability.

Questions (Choose the Most Appropriate Answer)

1. Substance use disorder (SUD) in anesthesiology:
   a. Is more common in staff than residents
   b. The cause of substance use disorder is multifactorial
   c. SUD is easily detected by peers and colleagues
2. Which of the following is a true statement about fatigue and medical care:
   a. With sleep deprivation greater than 24 h, impairment is equivalent to that associated with legal intoxication with alcohol
   b. Fatigue is not associated with an increased risk of medical errors or omission
   c. Fatigue impairs cognitive tasks more than procedural tasks
3. Aging influences performance:
   a. In a predictable manner
   b. Can be accommodated with scheduling alterations to extend the career of senior physicians
   c. Mandates national standards for retirement
4. A DNR order requires that:
   a. Always requires the complete suspension of advanced directives to return to standard resuscitation measures in the perioperative period
   b. The patient can specify specific resuscitation procedures they are willing to suspend during the perioperative period
   c. The care team's clinical judgment only determines which resuscitation procedures are appropriate
5. Which of the following is a correct statement about medication errors:
   a. Syringe swaps are rare
   b. Unlabeled syringes should be used if the medication is expensive
   c. Frequently occurs because of similarity in the size or color of vials
6. The 1990 Americans with Disabilities Act (ADA) and the Individuals with disabilities education Act (IDEA) are federal civil rights laws prohibiting discrimination against:
   a. Employment discrimination and educational intolerance of "qualified individuals with disabilities."
   b. These laws maintain that reasonable modifications of policies, practices, and procedures are mandated to preserve equal educational opportunity.
   c. In anesthesiology, an otherwise qualified individual with a physical or mental impairment will be allowed the opportunity to complete a residency program with appropriate accommodation.
   d. All of the above.
7. Autonomy maintains that
   a. Each individual with capacity has the right to make their own decisions, and providers have an ethical responsibility to respect this independence
   b. A net benefit of a diagnostic pathway, treatment plan, or societal healthcare policy balanced against the relative risk of harm
   c. Care should not depend upon demographic variables such as race, religion, socioeconomic status, gender, sexual orientation, age, or cultural background
8. The five core competencies and Patient Safety include the following subcomponents:
   a. Patient-centered care
   b. Capability to work in interdisciplinary team
   c. Utilization of informatics for quality improvement
   d. All of the above
9. Jehovah's Witness right to refuse a blood transfusion is protected under the ethical principle of:

   a. a. Autonomy
   b. b. Beneficence
   c. c. Nonmaleficence
10. When disclosing a medical error
    a. Physicians should disclose detailed information, regardless of whether the patient asks
    b. Use a direct statement that a medical mistake occurred
    c. A description of the error, the reasons it occurred, and how it will be potentially prevented in the future should be presented as part of the discussion
    d. A thoughtful apology should be made to the patient and the family for the adverse event
    e. e. All of the above

Answers

1. D. substance abuse in anesthesiology is a prevalent occupational risk in anesthesia with an incidence of about 1% per year of training. Although addiction to anesthesia drugs is deadly, self-reporting is rare, and detection is often difficult. The causes of chemical dependence of anesthesiologists are multifactorial. While there is no cure for SUD, lifelong recovery is the goal of monitoring and treatment programs.
2. A. fatigue is universally acknowledged to be associated with medical error. when sleep deprivation exceeds 24 h, impairment is equivalent to that associated with legal intoxication or narcolepsy. Fatigue affects cognitive and motor performance and can lead to depression and social isolation.
3. B. Aging influences clinical performance gradually, but not in a predictable manner. Any abrupt changes in performance usually have another explanation besides the impact of aging. Accommodation for the aging physician can be successful, including reducing call frequency or duration. The ASA does not have requirements for cognitive testing or retirement age.
4. B. The patient can specify which resuscitation procedures they want to suspend during the perioperative period. For example, a patient may be agreeable to a pharmacological resuscitation with tracheal intubation but decline defibrillation and CPR.
   Institutional policies that automatically suspend advanced directives prior to anesthetic care may not sufficiently address a patient's rights to self-determination and should be revised.
5. C. Errors in administering medications in the perioperative arena occur within a complicated work environment. The most frequent mistakes were incorrect medication dosing (miscalculation of dose, concentration, or infusion rate) and substitution errors (syringe or ampule/vial swap). Human error poses a significant risk for hospitalized patients causing an estimated 100,000 to 400,000 deaths in the United States annually.
6. D. The 1990 Americans with Disabilities Act (ADA) and the Individuals with Disabilities Education Act (IDEA) are federal civil rights laws that protect Employment discrimination and educational intolerance of "qualified individuals with disabilities." These laws maintain that reasonable modifications of policies, practices, and procedures are mandated to preserve equal educational opportunity to an otherwise qualified individual with a physical or mental impairment. For example, in anesthesia residency training, mechanical orthopedic devices or a wheelchair have successfully permitted individuals to practice clinically. Likewise, issues with senses such as hearing or vision loss have been overcome with cochlear implants, hearing aids, or glasses. Diagnosis of mental health conditions can be managed successfully with medications, counseling, and routine clinical supervision.
7. A. autonomy maintains that each individual with capacity has the right to make their own decisions, and providers have an ethical responsibility to respect this independence.
8. D. The development of integrated competencies over content has transformed health professionals' view of their role in patient safety and quality improvement. In its report, Patient Safety Achieving a New Standard for Care, the Institute of Medicine identified five core competencies that all physicians should be able to exemplify. [98 99] These included the requirement of patient-centered care, the capability to work in interdisciplinary teams, engagement of evidence-based practices, application of quality improvement concepts, and utilization of informatics.
9. A. Respect for a patient's autonomy requires the acceptance of a Jehovah Witness patient's right to refuse transfusion, even if contrary to the physician's own belief system. The commitment to healing is fundamental to medical practice, which directs the doctrine of beneficence. Finally, The Latin maxim, "primum non-nocere," captures the principle of nonmaleficence: or "above all, do no harm."
10. E. In the United States, health state and federal regulatory agencies, specialty medical boards, and credentialing entities endorse the practice of medical error disclosure. Physicians should disclose detailed information, regardless of whether the patient asks, using a direct statement that a medical mistake occurred. A description of the error, the reasons it occurred, and how it will be potentially prevented in the future should be presented as part of the discussion. Finally, a

thoughtful apology should be made to the patient and the family for the adverse event.

Notes

Philibert [41]

References

1. McAuliffe WE, Rohman M, Breer P, Wyshak G, Santangelo S, Magnuson E. Alcohol use and abuse in random samples of physicians and medical students. Am J Public Health. 1991;81:177–82.
2. Hughes PH, Brandenburg N, Baldwin DC Jr, et al. Prevalence of substance use among US physicians. JAMA. 1992;267:2333–9.
3. Paris RT, Canavan DI. Physician substance abuse impairment: anesthesiologists vs. other specialties. J Addict Dis. 1999;18:1–7.
4. Bryson EO. The opioid epidemic and the current prevalence of substance use disorder in anesthesiologists. Curr Opin Anaesthesiol. 2018;31:388–92.
5. Oreskovich MR, Shanafelt T, Dyrbye LN, et al. The prevalence of substance use disorders in American physicians. Am J Addict. 2015;24:30–8.
6. Dyrbye LN, Shanafelt TD, Balch CM, Satele D, Sloan J, Freischlag J. Relationship between work-home conflicts and burnout among American surgeons: a comparison by sex. Arch Surg. 2011;146:211–7.
7. Dyrbye LN, Shanafelt TD, Balch CM, Satele D, Freischlag J. Physicians married or partnered to physicians: a comparative study in the American College of Surgeons. J Am Coll Surg. 2010;211:663–71.
8. Bryson EO, Silverstein JH. Addiction and substance abuse in anesthesiology. Anesthesiology. 2008;109:905–17.
9. Mayall R. Substance abuse in anaesthetists. Bja Education. 2016;16:236–41.
10. Fry RA, Fry LE, Weeks A. Substance use disorder amongst Australian and New Zealand anaesthetic trainees: an analysis of 30 years of data. Anaesth Intensive Care. 2015;43:530.
11. Allison C, Malley MD, Elizabeth M. O'Brien MD, Yinghui Low MD (2018) Substance use disorder among physicians: 2017 survey of ACGME-accredited academic anesthesiology programs. American society of Anesthesiologsits Annual Meeting San Fransico2018
12. Boulis S, Khanduja PK, Downey K, Friedman Z. Substance abuse: a national survey of Canadian residency program directors and site chiefs at university-affiliated anesthesia departments. Can J Anaesth. 2015;62:964–71.
13. Warner DO, Berge K, Sun H, Harman A, Hanson A, Schroeder DR. Substance use disorder among anesthesiology residents, 1975–2009. JAMA. 2013;310:2289–96.
14. Booth JV, Grossman D, Moore J, et al. Substance abuse among physicians: a survey of academic anesthesiology programs. Anesth Analg. 2002;95:1024–30.
15. Wischmeyer PE, Johnson BR, Wilson JE, et al. A survey of propofol abuse in academic anesthesia programs. Anesth Analg. 2007;105:1066–71.
16. Iwersen-Bergmann S, Rösner P, Kühnau H, Junge M, Schmoldt A. Death after excessive propofol abuse. Int J Legal Med. 2001;114:248–51.
17. Zacny JP, Lichtor JL, Thompson W, Apfelbaum JL. Propofol at a subanesthetic dose may have abuse potential in healthy volunteers. Anesth Analg. 1993;77:544–52.
18. Zuleta-Alarcon A, Coffman JC, Soghomonyan S, Papadimos TJ, Bergese SD, Moran KR. Non-opioid anesthetic drug abuse among anesthesia care providers: a narrative review. Can J Anaesth. 2017;64:169–84.
19. McLellan AT, Skipper GS, Campbell M, DuPont RL. Five year outcomes in a cohort study of physicians treated for substance use disorders in the United States. BMJ. 2008;337:a2038.
20. Berge KH, Seppala MD, Schipper AM. Chemical dependency and the physician. Mayo Clin Proc. 2009;84:625–31.
21. West CP, Huschka MM, Novotny PJ, et al. Association of perceived medical errors with resident distress and empathy: a prospective longitudinal study. JAMA. 2006;296:1071–8.
22. Warner DO, Berge K, Sun H, Harman A, Hanson A, Schroeder DR. Risk and outcomes of substance use disorder among anesthesiology residents: a matched cohort analysis. Anesthesiology. 2015;123:929–36.
23. DuPont RL, Merlo LJ. Physician health programs: a model for treating substance use disorders. Judges J. 2018;57:32.
24. Volkow ND, Koob GF, McLellan AT. Neurobiologic advances from the brain disease model of addiction. N Engl J Med. 2016;374:363–71.
25. DuPont RL, McLellan AT, White WL, Merlo LJ, Gold MS. Setting the standard for recovery: physicians' health programs. J Subst Abuse Treat. 2009;36:159–71.
26. Kampman K, Jarvis M. American society of addiction medicine (ASAM) national practice guideline for the use of medications in the treatment of addiction involving opioid use. J Addict Med. 2015;9:358–67.
27. Buckley DN, Ibrahim M. Brief review: obstetric care and perioperative analgesic management of the addicted patient. Can J Anaesth. 2014;61:154–63.
28. Domino KB, Hornbein TF, Polissar NL, et al. Risk factors for relapse in health care professionals with substance use disorders. JAMA. 2005;293:1453–60.
29. Samuelson ST, Bryson EO. The impaired anesthesiologist: what you should know about substance abuse. Can J Anaesth. 2017;64:219–35.
30. Leach DC. Residents' work hours: the Achilles heel of the profession? Acad Med. 2000;75:1156–7.
31. Arnedt JT, Owens J, Crouch M, Stahl J, Carskadon MA. Neurobehavioral performance of residents after heavy night call vs after alcohol ingestion. JAMA. 2005;294:1025–33.
32. Dinges DF, Pack F, Williams K, et al. Cumulative sleepiness, mood disturbance, and psychomotor vigilance performance decrements during a week of sleep restricted to 4–5 hours per night. Sleep. 1997;20:267–77.
33. Kahol K, Leyba MJ, Deka M, et al. Effect of fatigue on psychomotor and cognitive skills. Am J Surg. 2008;195:195–204.
34. Gaba DM, Howard SK. Fatigue among clinicians and the safety of patients. N Engl J Med. 2002;347:1249–55.
35. Howard SK, Gaba DM, Rosekind MR, Zarcone VP. The risks and implications of excessive daytime sleepiness in resident physicians. Acad Med. 2002;77:1019–25.
36. Dawson D, Reid K. Fatigue, alcohol and performance impairment. Nature. 1997;388:235.
37. Ritchie K. Sleep deprivation and performance of residents. JAMA. 1989;261:859–60.
38. Weinger M, Vora SH, CN H, et al. (1998) Evaluation of the effects of fatigue and sleepiness on clinical performance in on-call anesthesia residents during actual nighttime cases and simulated cases. Evaluating Patient Safety and Reducing Errors in Health Care
39. Ayas NT, Barger LK, Cade BE, et al. Extended work duration and the risk of self-reported percutaneous injuries in interns. JAMA. 2006;296:1055–62.

40. Nurok M, Czeisler CA, Lehmann LS. Sleep deprivation, elective surgical procedures, and informed consent. N Engl J Med. 2010;363:2577–9.
41. Philibert I. Sleep loss and performance in residents and non-physicians: a meta-analytic examination. Sleep. 2005;28:1392–402.
42. Macias DJ, Hafner J 2nd, Brillman JC, Tandberg D. Effect of time of day and duration into shift on hazardous exposures to biological fluids. Acad Emerg Med. 1996;3:605–10.
43. Ben Simon E, Walker MP. Sleep loss causes social withdrawal and loneliness. Nat Commun. 2018;9:3146.
44. Barger LK, Cade BE, Ayas NT, et al. Extended work shifts and the risk of motor vehicle crashes among interns. N Engl J Med. 2005;352:125–34.
45. Arora V, Dunphy C, Chang VY, Ahmad F, Humphrey HJ, Meltzer D. The effects of on-duty napping on intern sleep time and fatigue. Ann Intern Med. 2006;144:792–8.
46. Glickman RM. House-staff training–the need for careful reform. N Engl J Med. 1988;318:780–2.
47. Leape LL. The girl who died twice: every patient's nightmare: the libby zion case and the hidden hazards of hospitals. JAMA. 1996;275:1031.
48. Wallack MK, Chao L. Resident work hours: the evolution of a revolution. Arch Surg. 2001;136:1426–32.
49. Ehlers TB. Patient and physician safety and protection act: crucial federal legislation to improve the lives of residents and patients. Conn Pub Int LJ. 2004;4:1.
50. Kohn LT, Corrigan JM, Donaldson MS, McKay T, Pike K (2000) To err is human. building a safer health system 600: 2000
51. Volpp KG, Rosen AK, Rosenbaum PR, et al. Mortality among hospitalized Medicare beneficiaries in the first 2 years following ACGME resident duty hour reform. JAMA. 2007;298:975–83.
52. Volpp KG, Rosen AK, Rosenbaum PR, et al. Mortality among patients in VA hospitals in the first 2 years following ACGME resident duty hour reform. JAMA. 2007;298:984–92.
53. Volpp KG, Rosen AK, Rosenbaum PR, et al. Did duty hour reform lead to better outcomes among the highest risk patients? J Gen Intern Med. 2009;24:1149–55.
54. Volpp KG, Small DS, Romano PS, et al. Teaching hospital five-year mortality trends in the wake of duty hour reforms. J Gen Intern Med. 2013;28:1048–55.
55. Press MJ, Silber JH, Rosen AK, et al. The impact of resident duty hour reform on hospital readmission rates among Medicare beneficiaries. J Gen Intern Med. 2011;26:405–11.
56. Rosen AK, Loveland SA, Romano PS, et al. Effects of resident duty hour reform on surgical and procedural patient safety indicators among hospitalized Veterans Health Administration and Medicare patients. Med Care. 2009;47:723–31.
57. Silber JH, Rosenbaum PR, Rosen AK, et al. Prolonged hospital stay and the resident duty hour rules of 2003. Med Care. 2009;47:1191–200.
58. Bolster L, Rourke L. The effect of restricting residents' duty hours on patient safety, resident well-being, and resident education: an updated systematic review. J Grad Med Educ. 2015;7:349–63.
59. Patel MS, Volpp KG, Small DS, et al. Association of the 2011 ACGME resident duty hour reforms with mortality and readmissions among hospitalized Medicare patients. JAMA. 2014;312:2364–73.
60. Ahmed N, Devitt KS, Keshet I, et al. A systematic review of the effects of resident duty hour restrictions in surgery: impact on resident wellness, training, and patient outcomes. Ann Surg. 2014;259:1041–53.
61. Jena AB, Schoemaker L, Bhattacharya J. Exposing physicians to reduced residency work hours did not adversely affect patient outcomes after residency. Health Aff. 2014;33:1832–40.
62. Health ASoACoO. Statement on the aging anesthesiologist 2018.
63. Americans with disabilities Act PLN-, 104 Stat. 327 (1990), 42 U.S.C. § 12101 et seq.
64. Americans with disabilities act amendments act PLN-, 122 Stat. 3553 (2008), 42 U.S.C. § 12101 et seq.
65. Education ACfGM (2018) Program director guide to the common program requirements; 2012
66. Field MJ, Jette AM, (2007) America IoMCoDi. The Americans with disabilities act in a health care context. The Future of Disability in America: National Academies Press (US)
67. Edgar LM, Hogan S, Hamstra S, Holmboe E (2020) The milestones guidebook. Accreditation council for graduate medical education 2020: 1–36
68. Mainiero MB, Lourenco AP. The ACGME core competencies: changing the way we educate and evaluate residents. R I Med J. 2011;94:164.
69. TEam NK (2017) Exploring the ACGME core copetencies: professionalism. N Engl J Med Knowl
70. Green MJ, Mitchell G, Stocking CB, Cassel CK, Siegler M. Do actions reported by physicians in training conflict with consensus guidelines on ethics? Arch Intern Med. 1996;156:298–304.
71. Waisel DB, Truog RD. An introduction to ethics. Anesthesiology. 1997;87:411–7.
72. Rhoton MF. Professionalism and clinical excellence among anesthesiology residents. Acad Med. 1994;69:313–5.
73. Beauchamp TL. The 'four principles' approach to health care ethics. Princ Health Care Ethics. 2007;29:3–10.
74. Tait AR, Hutchinson RJ. Informed consent training in pediatrics-are we doing enough? JAMA Pediatr. 2018;172:211–2.
75. Anderson JG, Abrahamson K. Your health care may kill you: medical errors. Stud Health Technol Inform. 2017;234:13–7.
76. DeCamp M, Snyder Sulmasy L. American College of Physicians Ethics P, Human Rights C Ethical and professionalism implications of physician employment and health care business practices: a policy paper from the American college of physicians. Ann Intern Med. 2021;174:844–51.
77. Emanuel EJ, Ubel PA, Kessler JB, et al. Using behavioral economics to design physician incentives that deliver high-value care. Ann Intern Med. 2016;164:114–9.
78. Koch KA. Patient self-determination act. J Fla Med Assoc. 1992;79:240–3.
79. Sumrall WD, Mahanna E, Sabharwal V, Marshall T. Do not resuscitate, Anesthesia, and perioperative care: a not so clear order. Ochsner J. 2016;16:176–9.
80. Clemency MV, Thompson NJ. Do not resuscitate orders in the perioperative period: patient perspectives. Anesth Analg. 1997;84:859–64.
81. Ethics ASoACo. (2001) Ethical guidelines for the Anesthesia care of patients with Do-Not-resuscitate orders or other directives that limit treatment. American Society of Anesthesiologsits; Reaffirmed: October 17, 2018 (original approval) pp 1–3
82. Benson KT. The Jehovah's witness patient: considerations for the anesthesiologist. Anesth Analg. 1989;69:647–56.
83. Milligan LJ, Bellamy MC. Anaesthesia and critical care of Jehovah's witnesses. Continuing education in Anaesthesia. Crital Care Pain. 2004;4:35–9.
84. Smith ML. Ethical perspectives on Jehovah's Witnesses' refusal of blood. Cleve Clin J Med. 1997;64:475–81.
85. Navalta JW, Stone WJ, Lyons TS. Ethical issues relating to scientific discovery in exercise science. Int J Exerc Sci. 2019;12:1–8.
86. Beauchamp TL (2008) The belmont report. The Oxford textbook of clinical research ethics pp 149–55

87. Association WM. World medical association declaration of Helsinki. Ethical principles for medical research involving human subjects. Bull World Health Organ. 2001;79:373.
88. Avasthi A, Ghosh A, Sarkar S, Grover S. Ethics in medical research: general principles with special reference to psychiatry research. Indian J Psychiatry. 2013;55:86–91.
89. Paterick TJ, Carson GV, Allen MC, Paterick TE. Medical informed consent: general considerations for physicians. Mayo Clin Proc. 2008;83:313–9.
90. Richard A Wagner M (2020) PhD Informed consent form and important. emedicinehealth. www.emedicinehealth.com/informed_consent/article_em.htm: emedicinehealth
91. Leape LL, Brennan TA, Laird N, et al. The nature of adverse events in hospitalized patients. Results of the Harvard Medical Practice Study II. N Engl J Med. 1991;324:377–84.
92. Donaldson LJ, Fletcher MG. The WHO world alliance for patient safety: towards the years of living less dangerously. Med J Aust. 2006;184:S69-72.
93. Jha AK, Larizgoitia I, Audera-Lopez C, Prasopa-Plaizier N, Waters H, Bates DW. The global burden of unsafe medical care: analytic modelling of observational studies. BMJ Qual Saf. 2013;22:809–15.
94. Aiken LH, Clarke SP, Cheung RB, Sloane DM, Silber JH. Educational levels of hospital nurses and surgical patient mortality. JAMA. 2003;290:1617–23.
95. Aiken LH, Cimiotti JP, Sloane DM, Smith HL, Flynn L, Neff DF. Effects of nurse staffing and nurse education on patient deaths in hospitals with different nurse work environments. Med Care. 2011;49:1047–53.
96. Berry JC, Davis JT, Bartman T, et al. Improved safety culture and teamwork climate are associated with decreases in patient harm and hospital mortality across a hospital system. J Patient Saf. 2020;16:130–6.
97. Kohn L, Corrigan J, Donaldson M. To Err is Human: Building a Safer Health System (Institute of Medicine). Washington: National Academy Press; 1999.
98. Knebel E, Greiner AC (2003) Health professions education: a bridge to quality
99. Wu AW, Busch IM (2019) Patient safety: a new basic science for professional education. GMS J Med Educ 36
100. Wahr JA, Abernathy JH 3rd, Lazarra EH, et al. Medication safety in the operating room: literature and expert-based recommendations. Br J Anaesth. 2017;118:32–43.
101. Makary MA, Daniel M. Medical error-the third leading cause of death in the US. BMJ. 2016;353: i2139.
102. Kim JY, Moore MR, Culwick MD, Hannam JA, Webster CS, Merry AF. Analysis of medication errors during anaesthesia in the first 4000 incidents reported to webAIRS. Anaesth Intensive Care. 2022;50:204–19.
103. Eichhorn JH. APSF hosts medication safety conference Consensus group defines challenges and opportunities for improved practice. APSF Newsletter. 2010;25:1–8.
104. Blendon RJ, DesRoches CM, Brodie M, et al. Views of practicing physicians and the public on medical errors. N Engl J Med. 2002;347:1933–40.
105. Mazor KM, Simon SR, Yood RA, et al. Health plan members' views about disclosure of medical errors. Ann Intern Med. 2004;140:409–18.
106. Hannawa AF, Beckman H, Mazor KM, Paul N, Ramsey JV. Building bridges: future directions for medical error disclosure research. Patient Educ Couns. 2013;92:319–27.
107. Gallagher TH, Waterman AD, Ebers AG, Fraser VJ, Levinson W. Patients' and physicians' attitudes regarding the disclosure of medical errors. JAMA. 2003;289:1001–7.

Part V
Physics in Anesthesia and Other Special Topics

Contents

The Anesthesia Machine

32

Crystal Manohar and Ehab Farag

Abstract

This chapter delves into the intricacies of anesthesia delivery systems, detailing the three primary circuits—high pressure, intermediate pressure, and low-pressure circuits—each with distinct roles and mechanisms. It emphasizes the regulation of oxygen and nitrous oxide pressures, highlighting safety mechanisms such as fail-safe valves to prevent hazards in case of pressure fluctuations. Essential components like flow control valves and proportioning systems are elucidated for their critical functions in regulating gas flow and maintaining proper gas concentrations. Safety devices like fail-safe valves and oxygen flush valves are discussed, along with their roles in ensuring patient safety during anesthesia delivery. Moreover, the chapter touches upon the significance of filters and heat and moisture exchangers in preventing cross-contamination and maintaining optimal conditions within the anesthesia breathing circuit, emphasizing their relevance in infection control, particularly in the context of the COVID-19 pandemic.

Keywords

Anesthesia machine • Pin index safety system • Diameter index safety system • Pipeline • Cylinder • Flow tube • Vaporizer • Check valve • Fail-safe • Flow meter • Waste gas scavenging

Key Points

1. There are 3 pressure systems in the anesthesia machine.
2. The cylinder is attached to the anesthesia machine via Pin Index Safety System.
3. The pipelines are attached to the anesthesia machine via Diameter Index Safety System.
4. Chain link and proportionating systems are safety systems to avoid delivering hypoxic mixtures.
5. The oxygen analyzer is the key feature in the anesthesia machine to avoid delivering hypoxic mixture.
6. The vaporizers' outputs are temperature-dependent and not affected by ambient pressure except for Tec 6 vaporizer (GE Healthcare, Chicago, IL) for desflurane.
7. The contemporary vaporizers incorporate a temperature compensation device in the form of a bimetallic strip device.
8. The contemporary anesthesia machines incorporate the open interface of the scavenging system to avoid developing barotrauma to the patient.
9. The oxygen flush valve delivers 35 L/min with pressure of 45 pounds per square inch gauge (psig).
10. The Aladin vaporizers (GE Healthcare, Chicago, IL) use magnetic strips for liquid anesthetic identification.

C. Manohar
Anesthesiology and Critical Care Medicine, Department of Anesthesiology, University of Texas Health San Antonio, San Antonio, TX, USA
e-mail: manohar@uthscsa.edu

E. Farag (✉)
Anesthesiology, Department of General Anesthesiology, Cleveland Clinic Lerner College of Medicine, Case Western University, Cleveland, OH 44195, USA
e-mail: farage@ccf.org

E. Farag
Departments of General Anesthesia and Outcomes Research, Cleveland Clinic, Cleveland, OH, USA

M. Argalious et al. (eds.), *Basic Sciences in Anesthesia*,
https://doi.org/10.1007/978-3-031-60203-0_32

11. Standards for Anesthesia Machines and Work Stations:
    - 5 2000: American Society for Testing and Materials (ASTM) F 1850-00, recommends the following standards for newly manufactured anesthesia machines—they must have monitors that measure the following parameters:
      - 5 Continuous breathing system pressure
      - 5 Exhaled tidal volume
      - 5 Ventilatory carbon dioxide concentration
      - 5 Anesthetic vapor concentration
      - 5 Inspired O_2 concentration
      - 5 O_2 supply pressure
      - 5 Arterial hemoglobin O_2 saturation
      - 5 Arterial blood pressure
      - 5 Continuous electrocardiogram (ECG)

The anesthesia workstation must have a prioritized alarm system.

32.1 Generic Anesthesia Machine

The pressures within the anesthesia machine can be divided into 3 circuits: a high pressure, an intermediate pressure, and a low-pressure circuit. The high-pressure circuit is confined to the cylinders and the cylinders' primary pressure regulators. For oxygen, the pressure range of the high-pressure circuit extends from a high of 2200 pounds per square inch gauge (psig) to 45 psig, which is the regulated cylinder pressure. For nitrous oxide (N_2O), the high-pressure circuit pressures range from a high of 750 psig in the cylinder to a low of 45 psig. The intermediate pressure circuit begins at the regulated cylinder supply sources at 45 psig, includes the pipeline sources at 50–55 psig, and extends to the flow control valves. Second-stage pressure regulatory may be used to decrease the pipeline supply pressures to the flow control valves, to even lower pressures, such as 14 or 26 psig within the intermediate pressure circuit. This regulator ensures a constant supply pressure to O_2 flow control valve. Thus, even if the O_2 supply pressure to the machine decreases to less than 45–50 psig, the flow set on the O_2 flow meter will be maintained as long as it exceeds 14 psig. The low-pressure circuit extends from the flow control valves to the common gas outlet. The low-pressure circuit includes the flow tubes, the vaporizers, and a one-way check valve on most Datex-Ohmeda machines (GE Healthcare, Chicago, IL).

The hospital piping system provides gases to the machine at approximately 50 psig, which is the normal working pressure of most machines. The O_2 cylinder source is regulated from 2200 psig to approximately 45 psig, and N_2O cylinder is regulated from 745 to 45 psig. A safety device, fail-safe valve, is located downstream from the N_2O supply. This valve shuts off or proportionally decreases the supply of N_2O or other gases if the O_2 supply pressure decreases.

The flow control valves represent an important landmark because they separate the intermediate pressure circuit from the low-pressure circuit. The low-pressure circuit is the part of the machine that is downstream from the flow control valves. A one-way check valve is usually present in many Datex-Ohmeda anesthesia machines; its purpose is to prevent back flow into the vaporizer during positive-pressure ventilation, thereby minimizing the effects of downstream intermittent pressure fluctuations on the inhaled anesthetic concentration. The O_2 flush valve connects the pipeline directly to the common gas outlet.

32.2 Pipeline Supply Sources

The pipeline supply source is the primary gas source for the anesthesia machine. In most hospitals, the O_2 pipeline is supplied from a bulk liquid source. The pipeline inlet fittings are gas-specific, Diameter Index Safety System (DISS), threaded body fittings (◉ Fig. 32.1). The DISS provides threaded, non-interchangeable connections for medical gas lines, which minimize the risk of misconnection. A check valve is located downstream from the inlet. It prevents reverse flow of gases from the machine to the pipeline or the atmosphere (◉ Fig. 32.2).

32.3 Cylinder Supply Source

Anesthesia machines have reserve *E* cylinders if a pipeline supply source is not available or if the pipeline fails. O_2 tanks are fitted at the factory to a pressure of approximately 2000 psig at room temperature. A full *E* cylinder of O_2 (internal volume of approximately 4.8 L) at a pressure of 2000 psig will produce approximately 660 of gaseous O_2 at atmospheric pressure. The cylinder attaches to the machine through the hanger-yoke assembly. The hanger-yoke assembly orients and supports the cylinder, provides a gas-like seal, and ensures a unidirectional flow of gases into the machine. Each hanger yoke is equipped with a Pin Index Safety System (PISS). The PISS is a safeguard introduced to eliminate cylinder interchanging. Each gas or combination of gases has a specific pin arrangement. A check valve is located downstream from each cylinder. The check valve has several functions. First, it minimizes gas transfer from a cylinder at a high pressure to one with lower pressure. Second, it allows an empty cylinder to be exchanged for a full one while gas flow continues from the other cylinder into the machine with minimal loss of gas.

Fig. 32.1 Diameter index safety system (DISS) (reprinted with permission from Brockwell and Andrews [1])

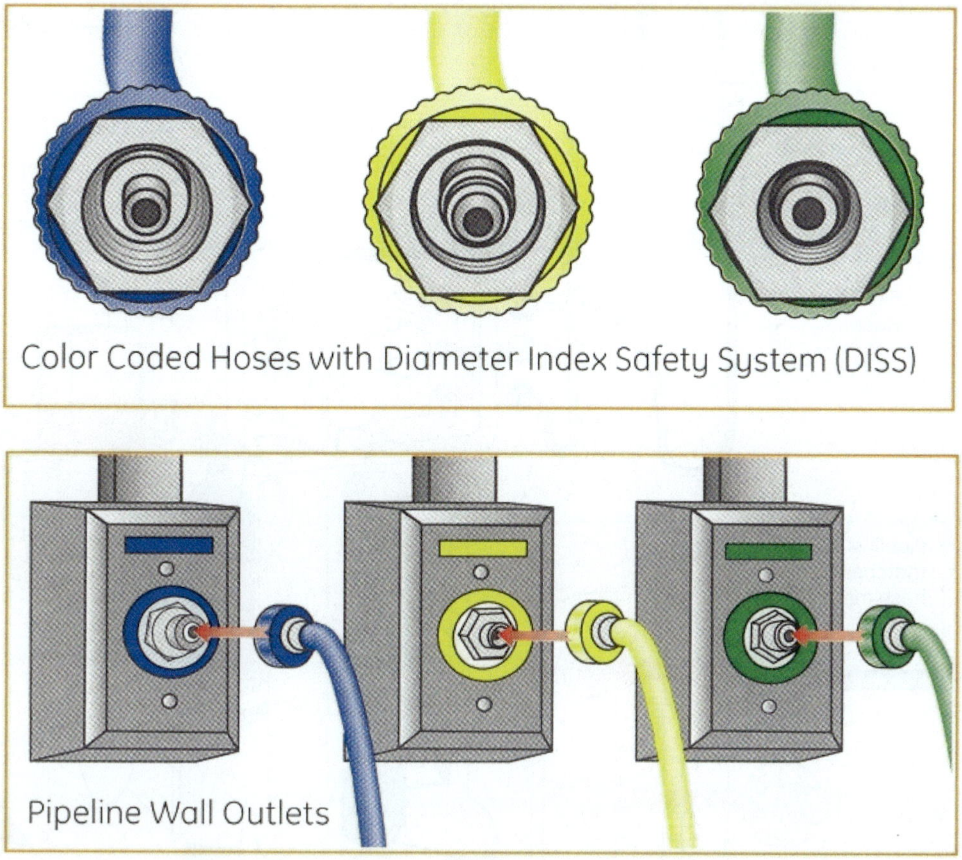

Third, it minimizes leakage from an open cylinder to the atmospheres if one cylinder is absent. The check valves may leak; therefore, if a yoke does not have a tank hanging on it, a yoke plug should be inserted. This prevents leakage of gas in the event of an incompetent check valve, which might otherwise cause depletion of the O_2 tank. The high input pressure of the cylinder is reduced to 45 psig by the oxygen pressure regulator. Failure of the pressure reduction function of a regulator can transmit excessively high pressure (up to 2200 psig) to the machine's low-pressure system. To protect against such occurrences, the regulator incorporates a pressure relief valve in the low-pressure chamber in which excess pressures are vented to the atmosphere. The cylinders should be turned off except during the preoperative machine checking period or when pipeline source is unavailable, to avoid depletion of the cylinder (◉ Figs. 32.3, 32.4, and 32.5).

32.4 Safety Devices of Oxygen Supply Pressure Failure

The 2000 ASTM F 1850-00 standard states, "The anesthesia gas supply device shall be designed so that whenever O_2 supply pressure is reduced to below the manufacturer specific minimum, the delivered O_2 concentration shall not decrease below 19% at the common gas outlet." If the oxygen pressure in the high-pressure system decreases (usually to <30 psig), an oxygen supply alarm is activated within 5 s.

32.5 Fail-Safe Valve

In Datex-Ohmeda machines, when the oxygen pressure in the machine's high-pressure system falls below 20 psig, the flow of N_2O and all other gases to their flow control valves is interrupted. This valve is an all-or-nothing valve; it opens at oxygen pressures of 20 psig or more and is closed at pressures less than 20 psig (◉ Fig. 32.6). The fail-safe valve in the North American Dräger Narkomed machines (Dräger, Lübeck, Germany) is called the oxygen failure protection device (OFPD). There is 1 OFPD for each of the gases supplied to the machine. As the oxygen supply pressure decreases, the OFPD proportionately reduces the supply pressure of each of the other gases to their flow control valves. The supply of N_2O and other gases is completely interrupted when O_2 supply pressure falls below 12 ± 4 psig (◉ Fig. 32.7).

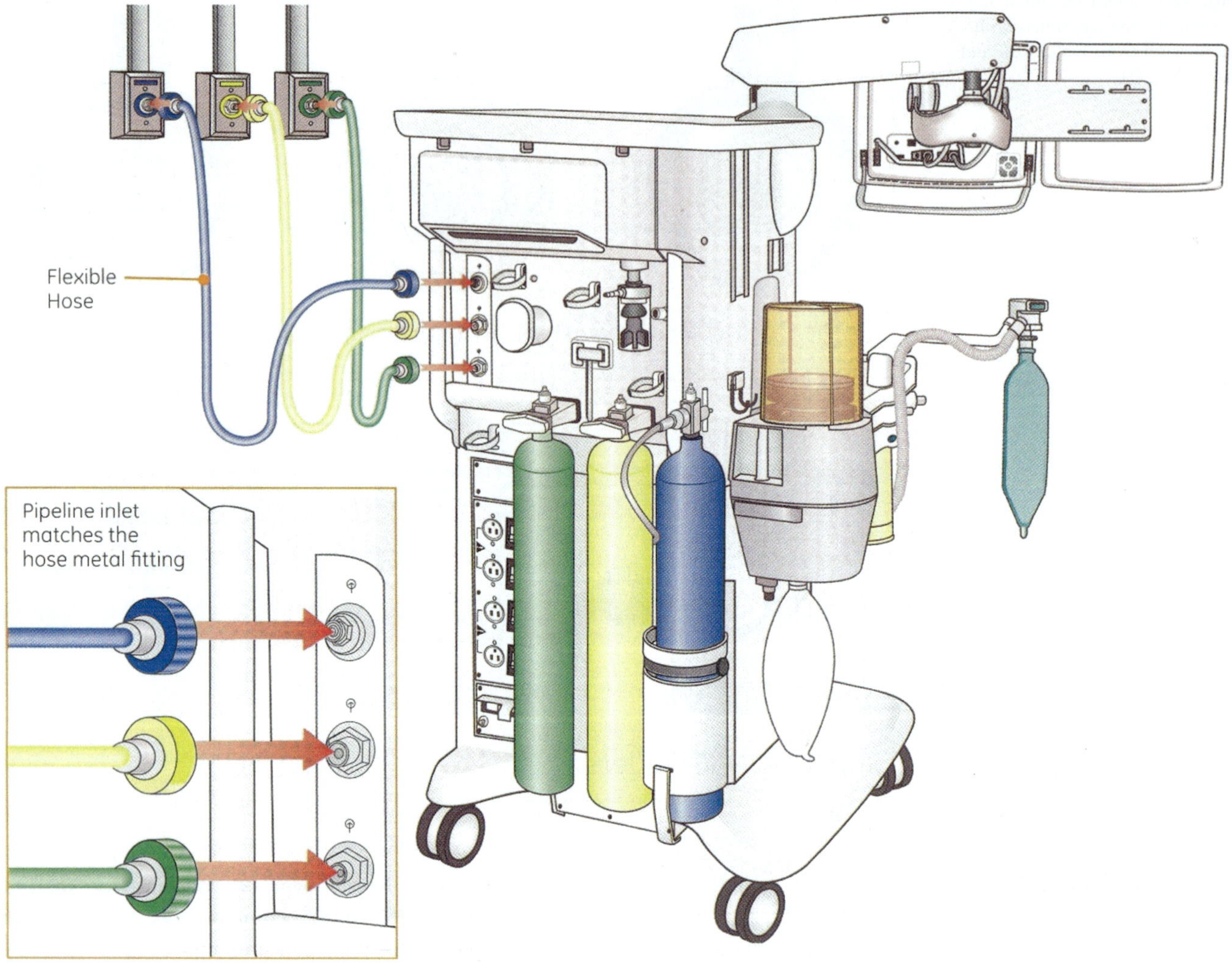

Fig. 32.2 Pipeline supply connections (reprinted with permission from Brockwell and Andrews [1])

32.6 Flow Meter Assemblies

With traditional glass flow meter assemblies, the flow control valve regulates the amount of flow that enters a tapered, transparent flow tube known as a Thorpe tube.

32.6.1 Physical Principles of Conventional Flow Meters

Flow tubes are tapered, with the smallest diameter at the bottom of the tube and the largest at the top. The term "variable orifice" designates this type of unit because the annular space between the float and the inner wall of the flow tube varies with the position of the float. The annular space is tubular (diameter of the space is shorter than its length) at low flow rates, laminar flow is present, and viscosity determines the gas flow rate (Hagen–Poiseuille Equation). The annular space (its diameter of the orifice is almost equal to its length) simulates an orifice at high flow rates, and turbulent gas flow then depends predominately on the density of the gas (Graham's Law). Of, note the oxygen flow meter can be used for helium at low flow rates as they have the same viscosity (◉ Fig. 32.8). Similarly, the nitrous oxide flow meter can be used for carbon dioxide at high flows as they have the same density.

32.6.2 Components of Flow Meter Assemblies

32.6.2.1 Flow Control Valve Assembly

The assembly of the flow control valve is composed of a flow control knob, a needle valve, a valve seat, and a pair of valve steps. The assembly can receive its pneumatic input directly from the pipeline source (50 psig) or from a second-stage

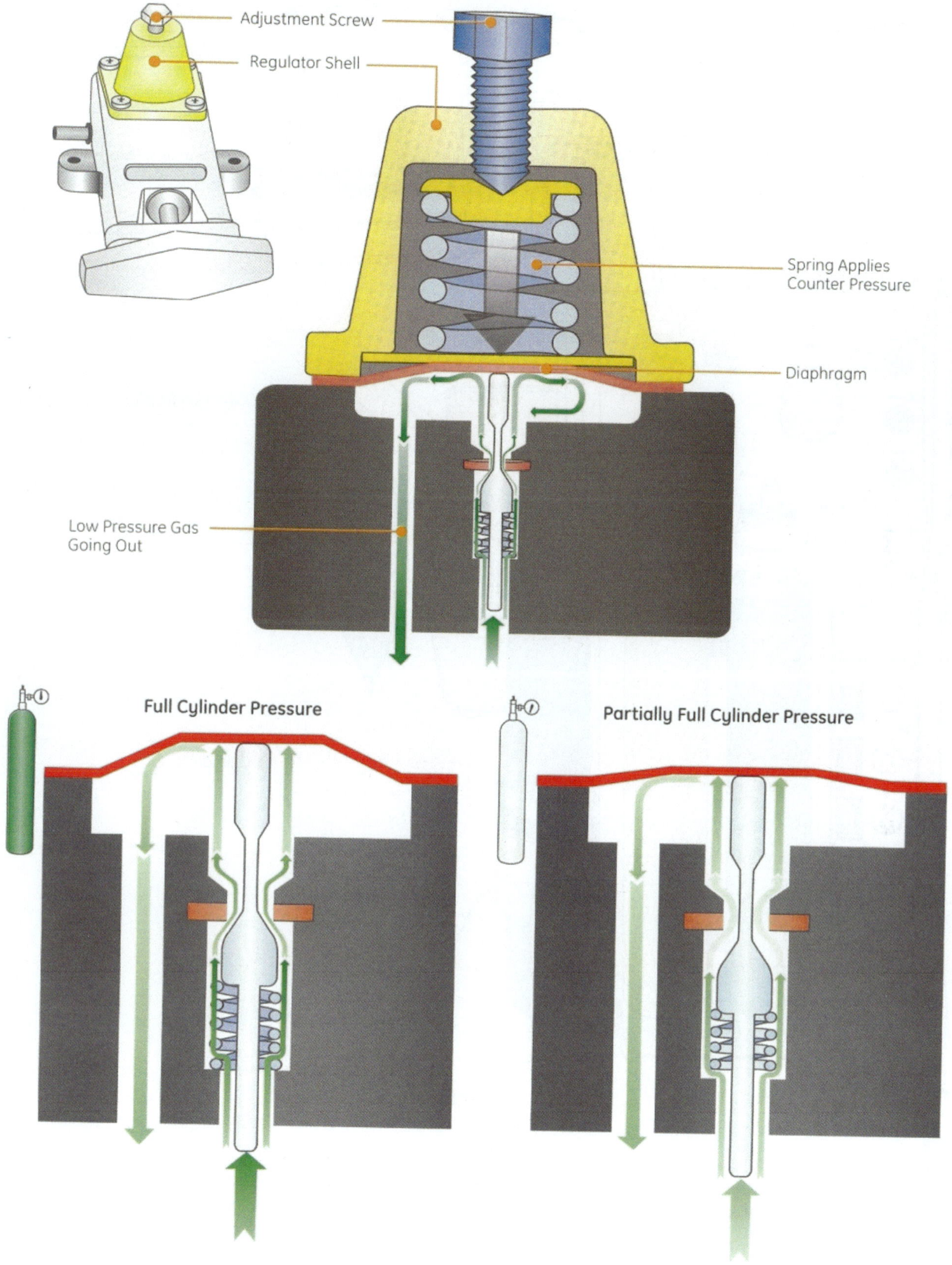

Fig. 32.3 Yolk system assembly (reprinted with permission from Brockwell and Andrews [1])

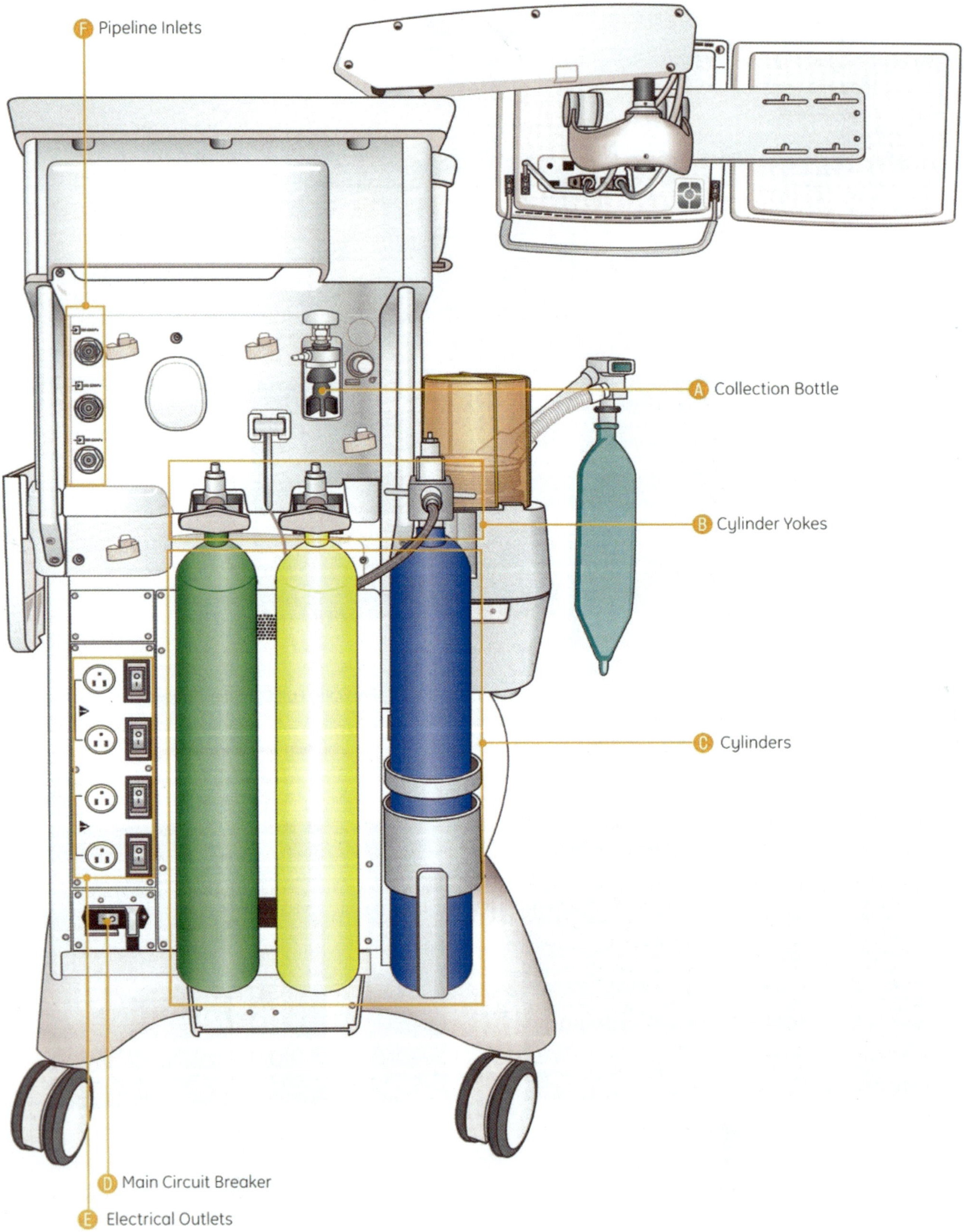

Fig. 32.4 Cylinder attachment to anesthesia machine (reprinted with permission from Brockwell and Andrews [1])

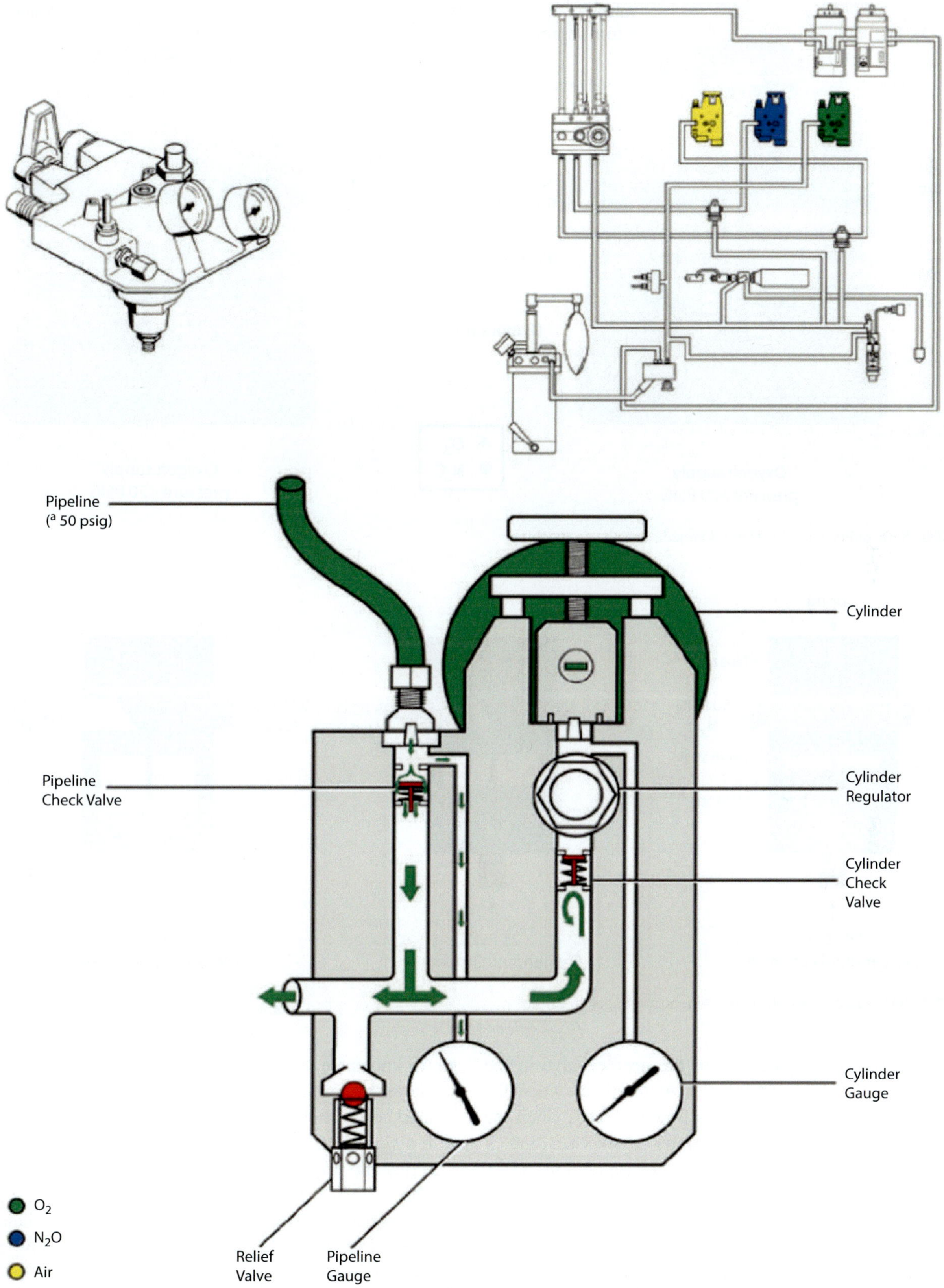

Fig. 32.5 Pipeline and cylinder systems attachment to the anesthesia machine. Pipeline pressure is a nominal 50 psi. As gas enters the gas supply module the pressure is reflected on the pipeline gauge located on the front panel of the machine. A check valve on the cylinder side prevents gas from flowing out the cylinder connection when the pipeline gas supply is being used; and a check valve on the pipeline side when the cylinder is being used. The regulator will regulate the pressure from the cylinder to 45 PSI for O_2. (© GE HealthCare. Reprinted by permission)

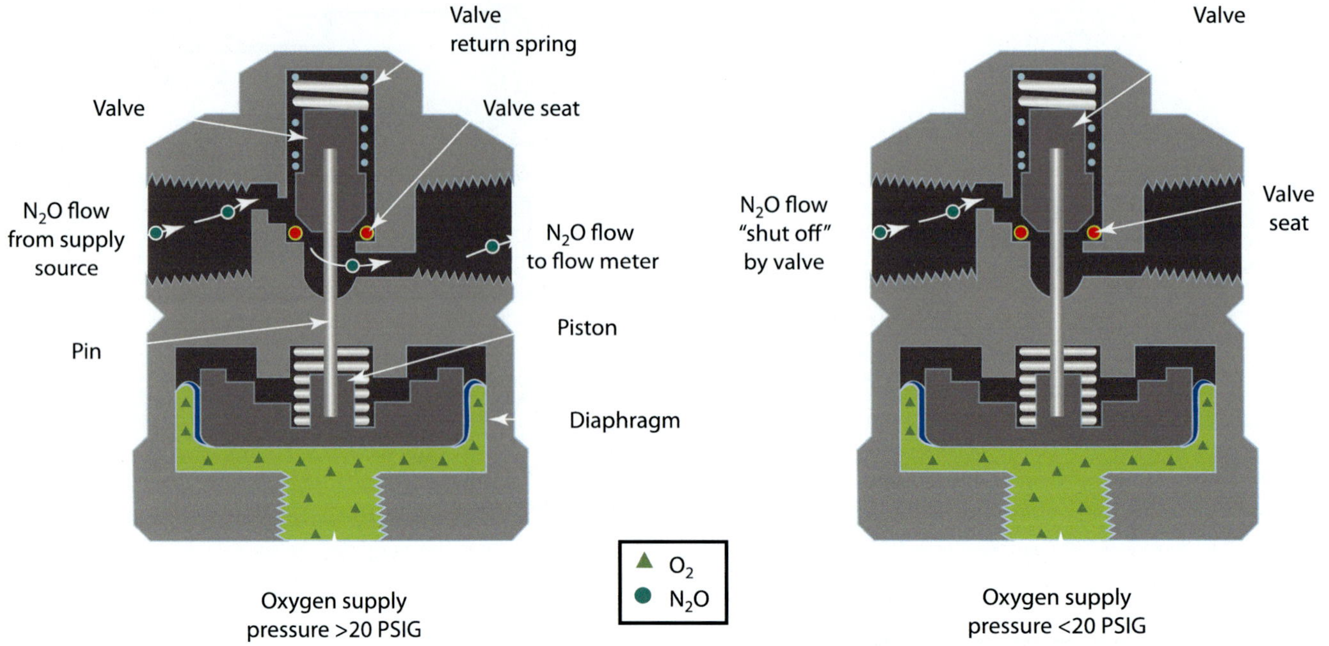

Fig. 32.6 Safe safety valve in Datex-Ohmeda anesthesia machine

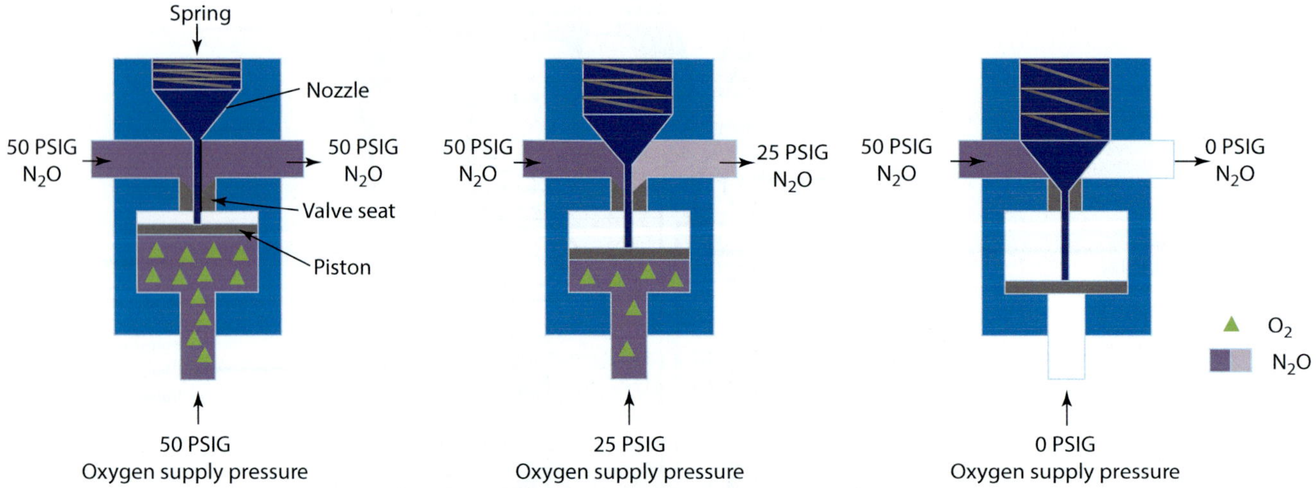

Fig. 32.7 Safe safety valve in North American Dräger machine

pressure regulator. The location of the needle valve in the valve seat changes to establish different orifices when the flow control valve is adjusted. Gas flow increases when the flow control valve is turned counter clockwise, and it decreases when the valve is turned clockwise (◉ Fig. 32.9).

32.6.2.2 Safety Features

- The O_2 flow control knob is larger and physically distinguishable from other gas knobs.
- All knobs are color coded for the appropriate gas, and the chemical formula or name of the gas is permanently marked on each.
- If a single gas has 2 flow tubes, the tubes are arranged in series and are controlled by a single flow control valve.
- The oxygen flow meter should be downstream (close to the patient) to other flow meters to avoid delivering hypoxic mixture in case of leak of the flow meters (◉ Fig. 32.10).

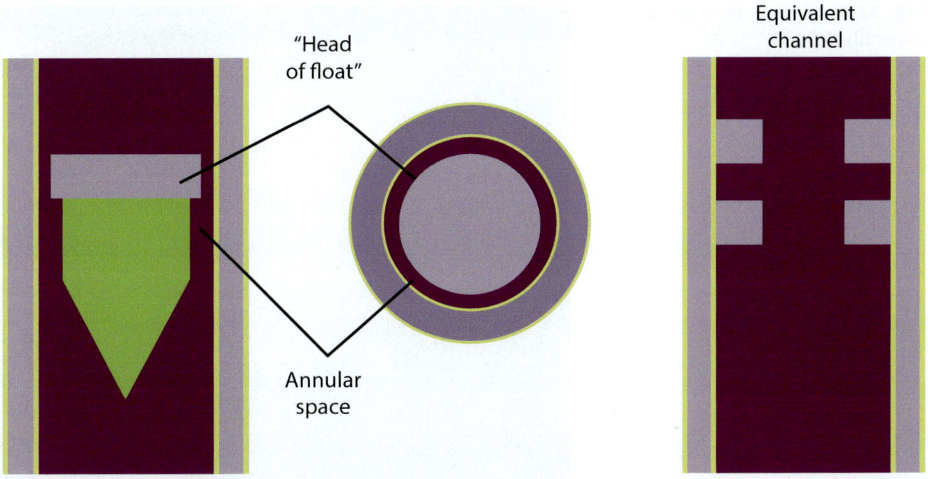

Fig. 32.8 Annular space between the float and the inner wall of the flow tube. Note the annular space resembles the shape of tube at low flow rates and orifice at high flow rates

Contemporary anesthesia machines use several different types of bobbins or floats including plumb-bob floats, rotating, skirted floats, and ball floats. Flow is read at the top of plumb-bob and skirted floats and at the center of the ball on the ball-type floats.

Flow tubes are equipped with float stops at the top and bottom of the tube. The upper step stop prevents the float from ascending to the top of the tube and plugging the outlet. It also ensures that the float is visible at maximum flows instead of being hidden in the manifold. The bottom float stop provides a control foundation for the indicator when the flow control valve is turned off. Rib guides are used with ball-type floats. The triangular thickening of the inside of the tube keeps the ball centered. The flow meters are calibrated at atmospheric pressure (760 mmHg) at room temperature (20 °C). Variations in temperature as a rule are slight and do not produce significant changes. Pressure variations affect the flow according to the following equation:

$$F_1 = F_0 x (d_0/d_1),$$

where F_1 is the real flow at new pressure, F_0 is the flow at sea-level atmospheric pressure, d_0 is the density of the gas at sea-level atmospheric pressure, and d_1 is the density of the gas at the new pressure. So according to this equation, the flow recorded at the flow meters in hyperbaric chamber is lower than the real flow and vice versa at low-pressure settings in high altitudes.

Hot Wire Anemometer for Flow Sensors

Flow sensors are used in respiratory gas monitoring to measure the flow rate and volume of gas delivered to the patient. Flow sensors can be placed in close proximity to the patient to measure inhaled and exhaled gases or they can be placed near the expiratory valve to measure the expired gas mixture.

Hot wire anemometry (HWA) is a type of flow sensor that utilizes the concept of heat transfer. HWA has a fine electrical wire that is heated to an ambient temperature. Gas flows around the HWA and causes the heated wired to cool and thus reduces the wire resistance proportionally. Monitoring the change in resistance of the heated wire as the temperature changes allows the gas flow to be determined.

HWA can be further classified as constant current anemometers or constant temperature anemometers, which are more commonly used. In constant current anemometers, a constant current is passed through the sensing wire. As gas flows in the anemometer, heat transfers from the sensing wire to the flowing gas causing the temperature and resistance of the sensing wire to be reduced. This change in resistance is proportional to the gas flow.

In constant temperature anemometers (CTA), the sensing wire resistance is kept constant. As gas flows through the HWA, heat is dissipated and causes a reduction in wire resistance. This is offset by a voltmeter which adjusts the change in resistance. Consequently, the temperature of the hot sensing wire is maintained at a constant level. Flow rate is thus proportional to the current needed to maintain the temperature of the hot wire. HWA is the basic component for measuring the gas flow rate in the modern digital flowmeters.

32.7 Proportioning Systems

Nitrous oxide and oxygen are interfaced mechanically or pneumatically so that the minimum oxygen concentration at the common gas outlet is between 23 and 25%, depending on the manufacturer.

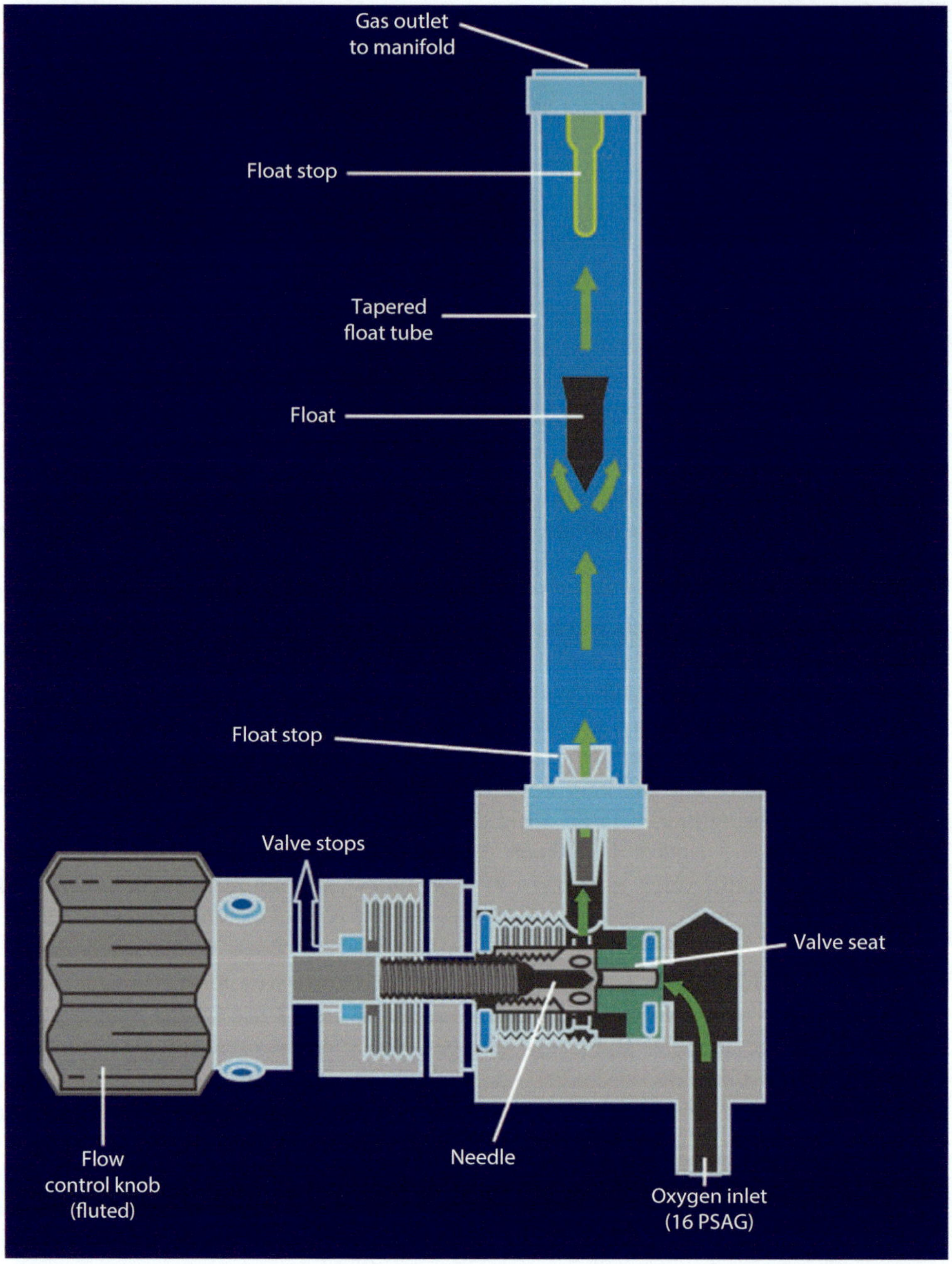

Fig. 32.9 Oxygen flow meter assembly

32.7.1 Datex-Ohmeda Link-25 Proportion Limiting Control System

In this Datex-Ohmeda system, there is a 14-tooth sprocket on the nitrous oxide flow control valve and a 29-tooth sprocket on the oxygen flow control valve. A pin on the O_2 sprocket engages a pin on the O_2 flow control knob if the flow control valves are adjusted so that 25% concentration of O_2 is reached. This causes the O_2 and N_2O flow control valves to turn together to maintain a minimum of 25% O_2. The proportioning of N_2O to O_2 (75–25%) is completed because the N_2O flow control valve is supplied from a second-stage regulator that reduces N_2O pressure to 26 psig before it reaches the flow control valve. The O_2 flow control is supplied at a pressure of 14 psig from a second-stage O_2 regulator. This minimum O_2 ratio device permits independent control of each gas as long as the percentage of O_2 is above the minimum. It should be rated that these devices only link 2 gases: nitrous oxide and oxygen (◉ Fig. 32.11). Administrations of a third gas such as helium can result in a hypoxic mixture.

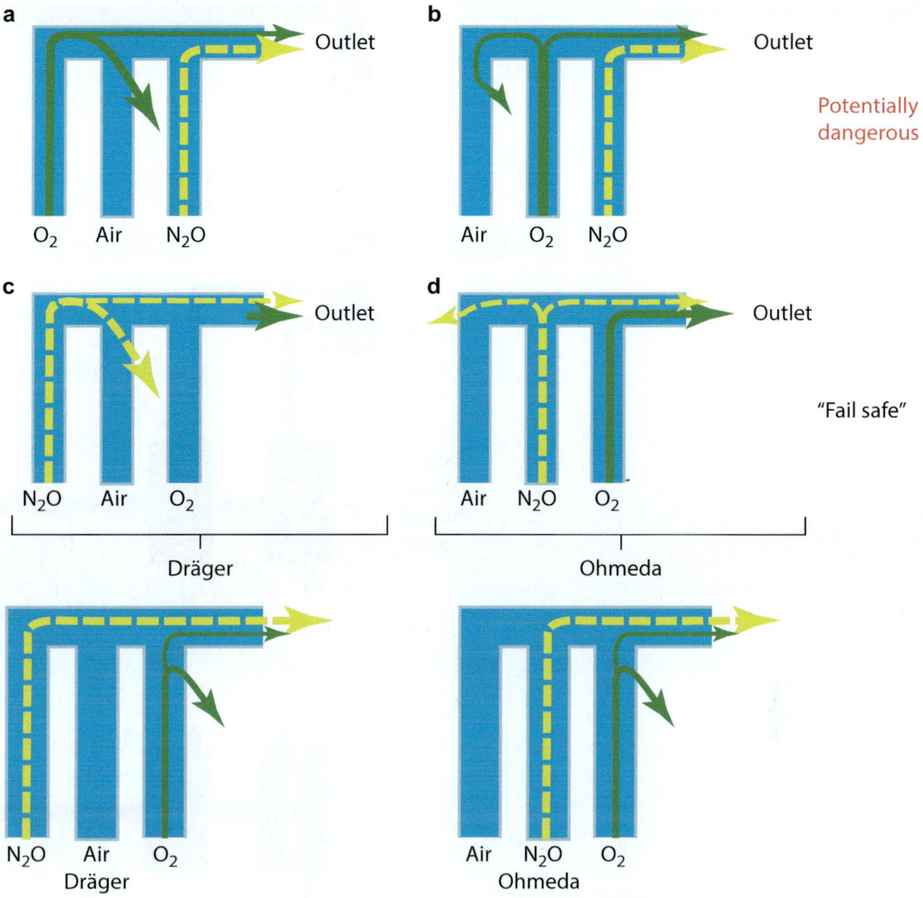

Fig. 32.10 Position of flow meters to avoid delivering hypoxic mixture

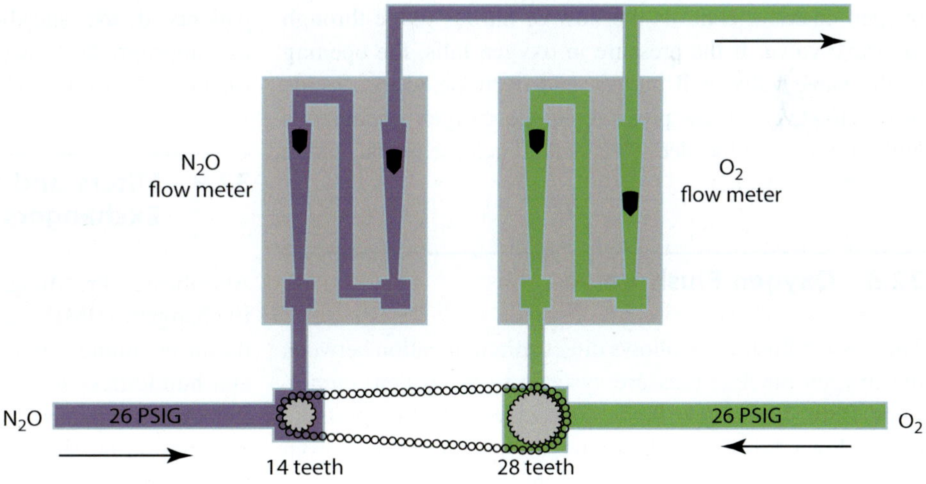

Fig. 32.11 Datex-Ohmeda Link 25-proportion limiting control system

32.7.2 North American Dräger Oxygen Ratio Monitor Controller

North American Drägers' proportioning system, the oxygen ratio monitor controller (ORMC) is used in the North American Dräger machine. The ORMC is a pneumatic oxygen-nitrous oxide interlock system designed to maintain fresh gas O_2 concentration of at least $25 \pm 3\%$. ORMC controls the fresh gas oxygen concentration to levels substantially higher than 25% at oxygen flow rates of less than 1 L/min. ORMC limits nitrous oxide flow to prevent delivery of a hypoxic mixture. In this system, the pressure of the

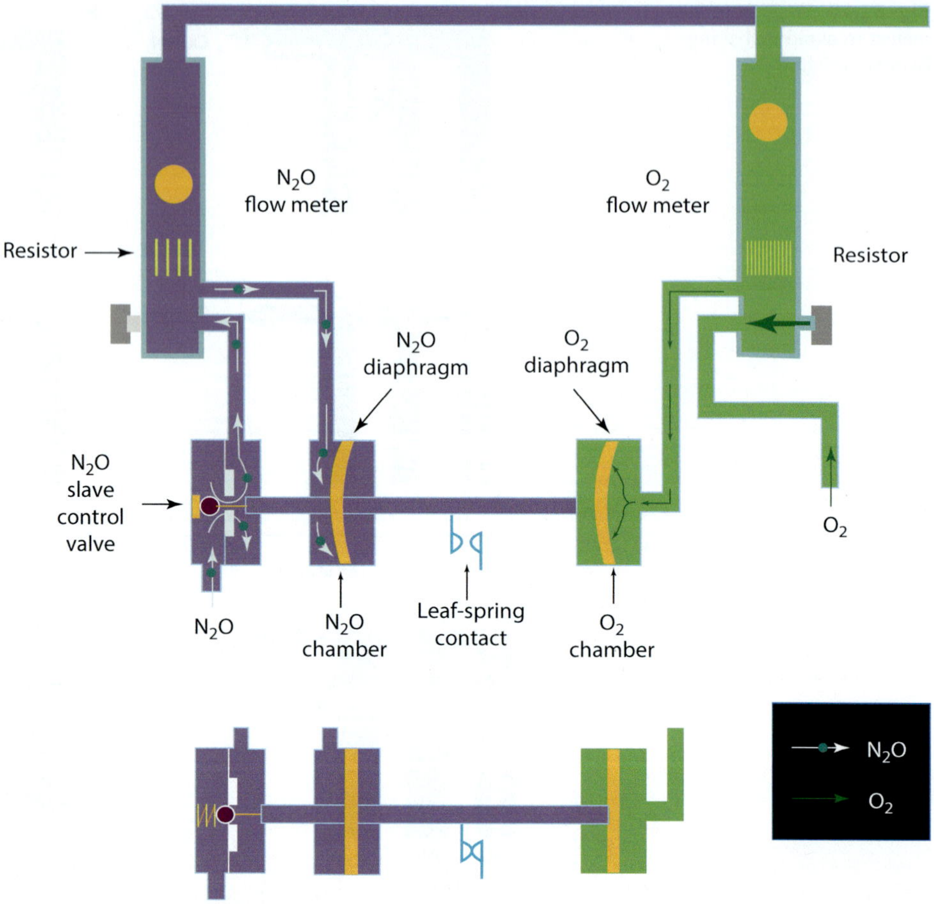

Fig. 32.12 North American Dräger pneumatic proportion linkage system

oxygen chamber controls the flow of nitrous oxide through the slave valve. If the pressure in oxygen falls, the opening in the slave valve will narrow and decrease nitrous oxide flow. However, if the pressure in the oxygen chamber is high, it will open the sleeve valve and increase nitrous oxide flow (◉ Fig. 32.12).

32.8 Oxygen Flush Valve

The oxygen flush valve allows direct communication between the oxygen pipeline-pressure systems to the patient circuit. Flow from the oxygen flush valve enters the low-pressure circuit downstream from the vaporizers and downstream from the Datex-Ohmeda machine outlet check valve.

Actuation of the valve delivers 100% oxygen at a rate of 35–75 L/min to the breathing circuit. The oxygen flush valve is associated with several hazards. A defective or damaged valve can stick in a fully open position, resulting in barotraumas. A valve sticking in a partially open position can result in awareness by the patient because the oxygen flow from the incompetent valve dilutes the inhaled anesthetic. Oxygen flushing during the inspiratory phase of positive-pressure ventilation can produce barotrauma in patients if the anesthesia machine does not incorporate an appropriately adjusted inspiratory pressure limiter (◉ Figs. 32.13 and 32.14).

32.9 Filters and Heat and Moisture Exchangers

Anesthesia breathing filters and Heat and Moisture Exchangers (HMEs) are commonly employed in the anesthesia breathing circuit. The upper airway normally warms and humidifies air as it goes into the lower airway, but this function is typically bypassed with an artificial airway during anesthesia. HMEs replace this function.

Anesthesia breathing filters provide an effective barrier to prevent cross-contamination between patients, breathing systems, respiratory and anesthetic equipment, and the clinical environment. Breathing system filters became increasingly used in 1990’s after reports of cross-infection with hepatitis C became evident and were attributed to contaminated anesthesia breathing systems. With the COVID 2019 pandemic and concern of viral transmission, there has been increased interest and use of breathing system filters.

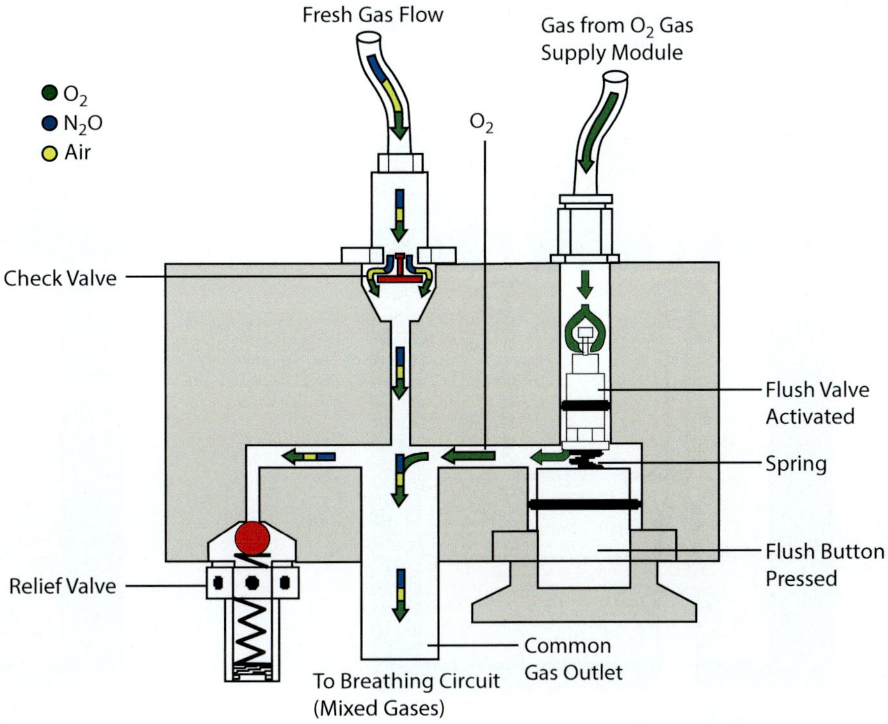

Fig. 32.13 North American Dräger pneumatic proportion linkage system

Filters work via multiple mechanisms. For large particles, they function as sieves. Filters utilize inertial impaction, interception, diffusion, and electrostatic attraction mechanisms to remove small particles (<2 μm).

There are four types of filters used in anesthesia breathing systems: pleated mechanical filters, electrostatic filters, heat and moisture exchange filters (HMEF), and membrane filters. Pleated mechanical filters have a thick sheet of tightly packed hydrophobic fibers that capture particulates within the depth of the filter. The filter's pleated material contributes to its very high filtration efficiency and may provide some heat and moisture exchange when placed near the airway. Electrostatic filters contain a thin sheet of less tightly woven electrostatic fibers and have a 1000-fold lower filtration efficiency than pleated mechanical filters. HMEs that have an electrostatic or pleated mechanical filter are called heat and moisture exchange filters (HMEF). HMEs and HMEFs are only effective for humidification when placed close to the airway. Membrane filters have ultra-small pores and channels that prevent particle passage by acting as a sieve. Membrane filters are not classified as breathing system filters, but are hydrophobic and are commonly used in water traps.

There is no one single standard for testing the filtration efficiency of breathing system filters. The salt test method is often used to quantify the number of 0.1–0.3-μm airborne sodium chloride particles that pass through the filter during a short-term challenge at airflow rates similar to those encountered at intended rates. This method does not assess the filtration performance for droplets or aerosols and does not test the filtration performance for microorganisms. The salt (NaCl) filtration efficiency is often reported as a percentage, where a higher percentage is better.

Breathing system filters often contain statements about bacterial and/or viral filtration efficiency. There is no standard test for determining the bacterial and/or viral efficiency of these filters. In general, higher percentages of bacterial and viral filtration efficiency is better.

Anesthesia providers should also note manufacturer specifications regarding resistance to flow through filter (lower is better), humidification, and internal volume.

Importantly, it must be recognized that use of breathing system filters is not without risk. Filters add dead space which can increase carbon dioxide rebreathing, and slow inhalational induction and emergence. Filters can become obstructed and lead to hypoventilation and barotrauma. The

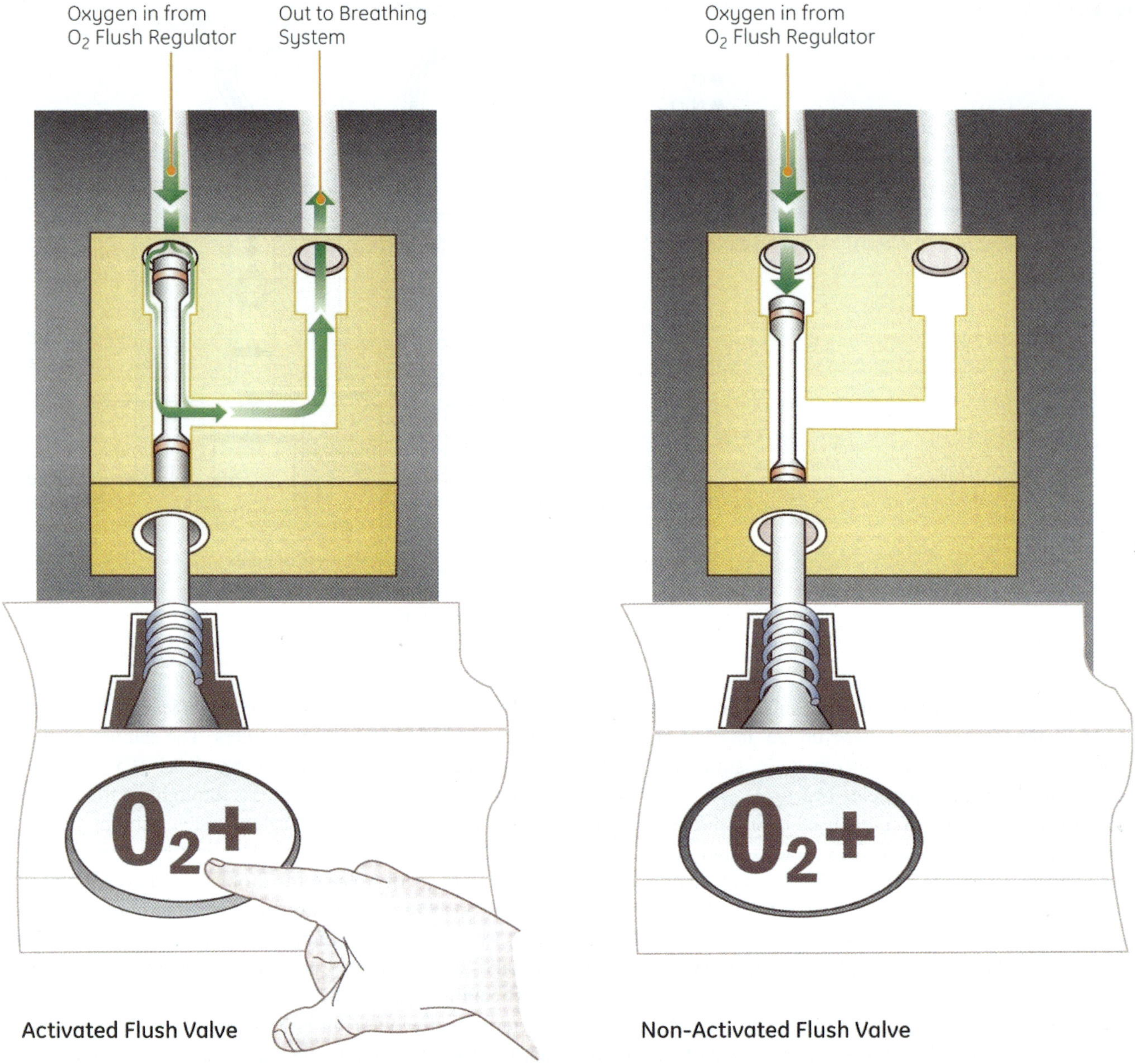

Fig. 32.14 Oxygen flush valve (Reprinted with permission from Brockwell and Andrews [1])

added weight of filters to the breathing circuit may increase the risk of accidental disconnection. Filters also add resistance to the inspiratory and/or expiratory flow which in turn increases work during spontaneous breathing and affects pulmonary mechanics.

Currently, there is no regulation to use breathing system filters on anesthesia machines. However, the APSF and ASA recommend using breathing system filters to avoid cross-contamination, especially in light of the coronavirus pandemic.

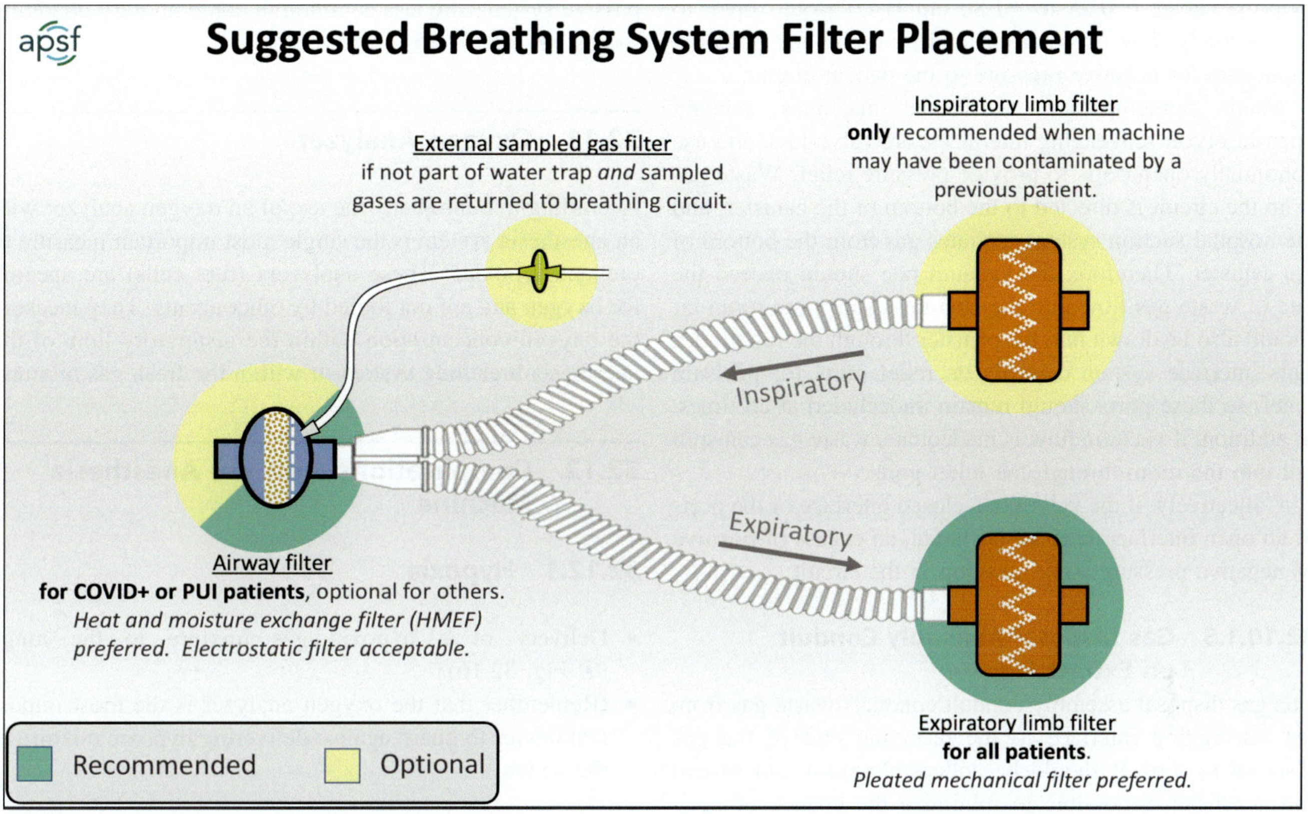

32.10 Waste-Gas Scavenging Systems

The tubing for the scavenging systems has an internal diameter of either 19 or 30 mm, compared with the 22-mm anesthesia circuit and ventilator tubing and the 15-mm common gas outlet and tracheal connectors. The scavenging system interfaces with the hospital suction system to remove gas flow from the patient circuit.

32.10.1 Scavenging Systems

32.10.1.1 Components

Scavenging systems classically have 5 components:

1. The gas-collecting assembly.
2. The transfer tubing.
3. The scavenging interface.
4. The gas disposal assembly tubing.
5. An active or passive disposal system.

32.10.1.2 Gas-Collecting Assembly

The gas-collecting assemblies are the points of waste gas exit from the breathing circuit to the transfer tubing. Waste anesthetic gases are vented from the anesthesia system either through the adjustable pressure-limiting (APL) valve (pop-off valve) or through ventilator relief valve.

32.10.1.3 Transfer Tubing

The transfer tubing carries excess gas from the gas-collecting assembly to the scavenging interface. The tubing must have 30-mm connectors on either end, which are distinct from the 22-mm connectors on the breathing system tubing. The tubing must be sufficiently rigid to prevent kinking to minimize the chance of occlusion, or it must contain pressure relief in case of occlusion. Occlusion or kinking can increase the pressure in the breathing circuit and barotrauma.

32.10.1.4 Scavenging Interface

Closed anesthesia systems use spring-loaded valves to ensure that excessively high or low pressures are not applied to the patient circuit. Thus, if the systems are not connected to negative pressure (suction), excess pressure in the interface caused by gas entering it from the circuit would first cause distension of the interface reservoir bag, then the excess would be vented via the position pressure-relief valve at about +5 cm H_2O. In the event that excessive suction might be applied to the circuit, the reservoir bag would first be sucked empty, and then 1 (Ohmeda interface) or 2 (North American Dräger closed interface) negative pressure-relief (pop-in) valves (−0.25 to −1.80 cm H_2O) would open to preferentially draw in room air and minimize the potential application of negative pressure to the patient circuit.

Many contemporary anesthesia machines contain open-reservoir scavenging interfaces, are valve-less, and use continually open ports to provide pressure relief. Waste gas from the circuit is directed to the bottom of the canister, and the hospital suction system aspirates gas from the bottom of the canister. Therefore, the vacuum rate should exceed the rate of waste gas flow into the chamber, and some room air should also be drawn into the canister through the relief port. This interface system depends on relief ports for pressure relief, so these ports should remain unoccluded at all times. In addition, if vacuum flow is inadequate, waste gas can spill out into the room through the relief ports.

Collectively, if the valves in a closed interface or the ports in an open interface become occluded, an excess of positive or negative pressure could develop in the circuit.

32.10.1.5 Gas Disposal Assembly Conduit on Extract Flow

The gas disposal assembly conduit conducts waste gas from the scavenging interface to the receiving end of the gas disposal system. It should be collapsible-proof and should run overhead if possible to minimize the chance of accidental occlusion.

32.10.1.6 An Active or Passive Disposal System

An active system relies on a hospital central evacuating system to remove gas from the scavenging system. A passive system simply vents the gas into a nonrecirculating heating, ventilation, and air conditioning system or simply through a hose to the building's exterior through the wall. Of note, passive systems are less common in contemporary operating rooms (◉ Fig. 32.15).

32.11 Oxygen Analyzer

According to Schreiber, "the use of an oxygen analyzer with an anesthesia system is the single most important measure to prevent hypoxia." These analyzers (fuel cells) are specific for oxygen and are not fooled by other agents. They measure the oxygen concentration within the inspiratory limb of the anesthesia breathing system or within the fresh gas mixture.

32.12 Complications with the Anesthesia Machine

32.12.1 Hypoxia

- Delivery of a hypoxic gas mixture to the lungs (◉ Fig. 32.16).
- (Remember that the oxygen analyzer is the most important device to guard against delivering hypoxic mixture to the patient)

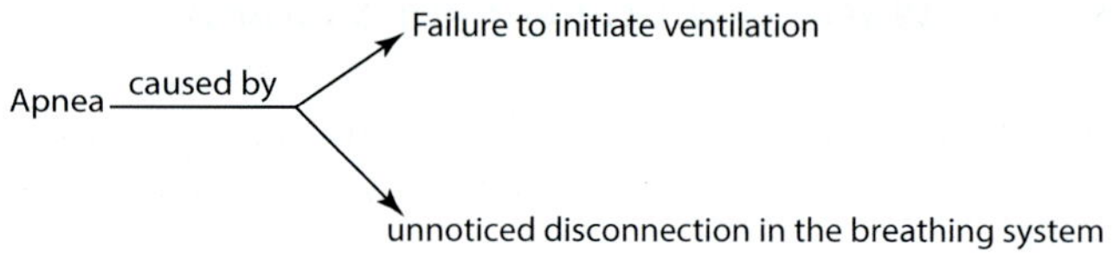

Fig. 32.16 Causes of hypoxia

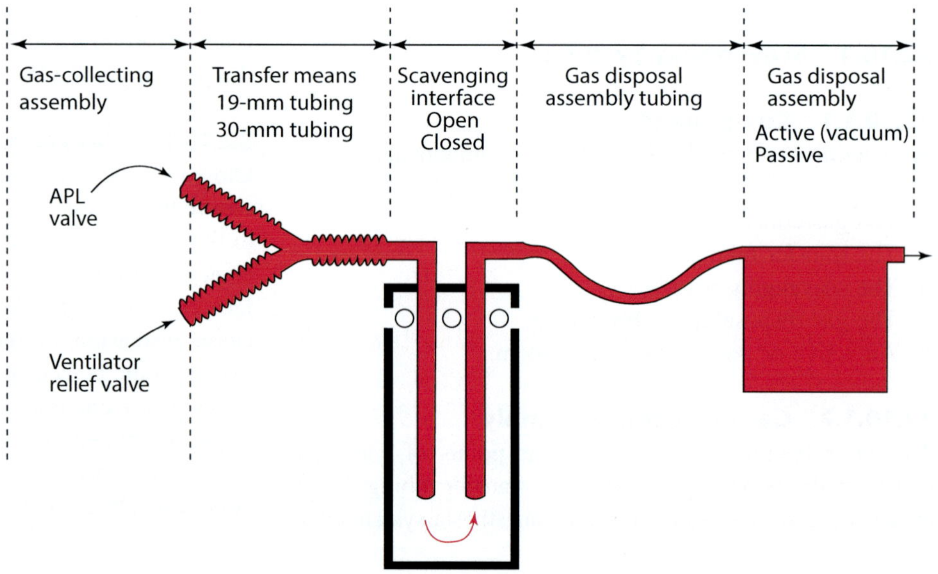

Fig. 32.15 Scavenging system: note the open interface in contemporary anesthesia machines (reprinted with permission from Brockwell and Andrews [1])

- Crossed pipe lines either before entering the machine or within the machine
- The oxygen flow control valve or O_2 piping system in the machine may be obstructed, preventing the flow of O_2 to the flow control valve.
- The flow control valve bobbin or flow meter may become stuck because of static electricity, girt or dirt, and it may appear that gas is flowing from the O_2 flow control valve even when it is not
- Excessive leak inside the machine, which results in loss of the O_2 before it reaches the common gas outlet (remember the permissible limit leak: 150 ml/min inside the intermediate pressure system, and 30 ml/min in the low pressure system).

32.12.2 Hyperoxia

- A leak in a hanging-bellow ventilator → entrainment or injection of driving gas from the bellows housing → inspired O_2 concentration.

32.12.3 Hypoxia

- When nitrous oxide is located in the downstream position of the flowmeters and there is a flowmeter leak, a hypoxic mixture can be created as oxygen flow passes primarily through the leak in the air flow tube, allowing nitrous oxide to be largely directed to the common gas outlet. Placing the oxygen flowmeter in the downstream position helps prevents delivery of hypoxic mixtures.

32.12.4 Hypercarbia and Incompetent Valves

- Possible if exhausted soda lime not recognized and replaced.
- Incompetent inspiratory and expiratory valves in the breathing system may lead to rebreathing of CO_2 and subsequent hypercapnia. Valve incompetence is usually due to a warped disk or seat irregularity.
- During inhalation, the inspiratory valve opens and allows the patient to breath a mixture of fresh and exhaled gas that passed through the CO_2 absorber. Normally, CO_2 measured at sample line is washed into the patient by fresh gas, but with an incompetent inspiratory valve this does not occur and the measured CO_2 is washed back into the inspiratory limb. This allows the measured CO_2 to remain elevated and results in a delayed downslope in the inspiratory portion of the capnogram.
- With an incompetent expiratory valve, previously exhaled gas enters the expiratory limb resulting in rebreathing at the Y piece and leads to an increased in inspired CO_2 on the capnogram. Without correction, over time the end tidal CO_2 will also increase.
- Flow from the anesthesia machine → inadequate ventilation and hypercarbia (◉ Fig. 32.17a, b)

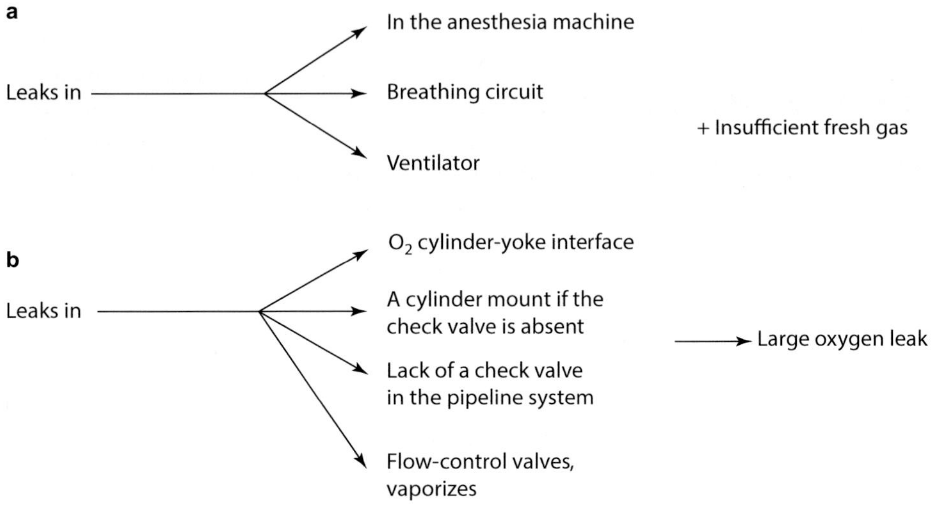

Fig. 32.17 a, b Causes of hypercarbia

32.12.5 Electrical Failures

- The newer anesthesia machines are equipped with a power cord and accept an electrical input of 90–130 V at 50–60 Hz. There are 4 electrical outlets on the anesthesia machine into which additional equipment can be plugged. There is also a battery backup system consisting of a 12-V rechargeable battery. If AC power fails, the backup battery provides power only to the ventilator control circuits, the monitors built into the machine, and the alarm system. This backup system is only effective for 30 min.
- Part of the pre-anesthesia/machine checklist should include confirmation and function of both AC and battery power daily. Ensure that the anesthesia machine is running off AC power, not battery power. The first obvious sign of power failure can be a complete shutdown when the system is running off batteries (not AC power) that become exhausted.

32.12.6 Barotrauma

- The oxygen flush valve allows 100% oxygen to be delivered manually to the patient via high flow rates (35–75 L/min) to overcome circuit leaks or to quickly increase the inspired oxygen concentration. Damaged, defective or exuberant use of the oxygen flush valve can result in barotrauma to patient lungs and dilute inhaled anesthetic agent concentration placing patients at risk for intraoperative awareness.

32.13 Vaporizers

32.13.1 Variable Bypass Vaporizers

When volatile anesthetics evaporate, their resultant saturated gas concentrations exceed the safety clinical standards. Therefore, concentrations should be diluted to safe ranges.

Variable bypass refers to carefully regulating the concentration of vaporizer output by diluting gas after it is fully saturated with anesthetic agent with a larger flow of gas. The vaporizer's output concentration determined by the concentration control dial is the product of the ratio of the gas that flows through the bypass chamber and the vaporizing chamber, and a temperature-compensating device further adjusts that ratio. Vaporizer concentration control dials are labeled to set vaporizer output in terms of volume percent (v/v%), and the vaporizers are calibrated at sea level.

The presence of a wicking system in the vaporizing chamber helps to saturate the fresh gas that is diverted to the chamber. The fresh gas is flowing over the liquid agent therefore it is called **flow-over** vaporizer. Of note, the vaporizer is **agent-specific** as the physical properties and clinical concentrations of each agent are unique; therefore, the concentration-specific diverting ratios are agent-specific. The modern vaporizers are calibrated at 20 °C. Most of the modern variable bypass vaporizers are **out-of-circuit** as their output is introduced into the patient's breathing circuit through the fresh gas, whereas if the vaporizers are located within the patient's breathing circuit, they are designated as in-**circuit** or **draw-over**.

The evaporation of liquid anesthetic requires energy, which is referred to as the **latent** heat, which is the number of calories required to change 1 g of liquid into vapor without change in temperature. This energy loss can lead to significant decreases in temperature within the remaining liquid, which will reduce vapor pressure and subsequent vaporization. Therefore, vaporizers are constructed of metals that have relatively high thermal conductivity, which helps them maintain a uniform internal temperature during evaporation by allowing them to absorb environmental heat more effectively. The modern vaporizers are **temperature compensating**; therefore, they are equipped with an automatic temperature-compensating device that helps maintain constant vaporizer output over a wide range of operating temperatures by automatically altering the ratio of gas flowing to the bypass and vaporizing champers. When temperature increases, the valve in the bypass opens wider to create a higher splitting ratio (see Appendix) so that more gas flows through and less gas enters the vaporizing chamber. A smaller volume of a higher concentration of vapor emerges from the vaporizing chamber; this vapor, when mixed with an increased bypass gas flow, maintains the vaporizer's output at a reasonable rate when temperature changes are not extreme.

Some older vaporizers had the temperature sensitive valve in the form of a gas-filled bellows linked to a valve in the bypass gas flow. As the temperature increased, the bellows expanded, causing the valve to open more the bypass channel. Contemporary vaporizers use a bimetallic strip for temperature compensation that is incorporated into a flap valve in the bypass machine. This metallic strip is composed of 2 metals with different *coefficients of expansion* or change of unit length per unit change of temperature. Nickel and brass have been used in bimetallic strip valves because brass has a greater *coefficient of expansion* than nickel. As temperature increases, one surface of the flap expands more than the other, causing the flap to bend in a manner that opens the valve orifice wider, increasing the bypass flow.

32.13.2 Factors that Influence Variable Bypass Vaporizer Output

ASTM standards state that the average output should not deviate from the concentration set by +30 or −20% or more than +7.5 or −5% of the maximum setting.

32.13.2.1 Impact of Gas Flow Rate

Vaporizer output can vary with the extreme rates of gas flowing through the vaporizer. The output of variable bypass vaporizers tends to be slightly less than the dial setting at low flow rates (<250 mL/min) to advance the vapor molecules upwardly because of the relatively high density of inhaled anesthetic agents. At extremely high flow rates, such as 15 L/min, the output is less than the dial setting at high anesthetic concentrations. This effect is mainly due to cooling during rapid evaporation, incomplete mixing, failure to saturate the carrier gas in the vaporizing chamber, and increased resistance to high gas flow.

32.13.2.2 Impact of Temperature Change

Automatic temperature-compensating mechanisms in the bypass chamber maintain constant vaporizer output with varying temperature. Therefore, manufactures' published operating temperatures range from 10 to 40 °C.

32.13.2.3 Impact of Intermittent Backpressure

The intermittent backpressure that results from either the inspiratory phase of positive-pressure ventilation or use of the oxygen flush valve may lead to higher than expected vaporizer output due to retrograde transmission of pressure from the patient's circuit to the vaporizer. Therefore, gas molecules are compressed in both the bypass and vaporizing chambers. However, when the backpressure builds suddenly during the expiratory phase of positive-pressure ventilation, vapor exits the vaporizing chamber through both its inlet and outlet, thereby enhancing the vapor output concentration. This effect is called the **pumping effect**, which is more pronounced at low flow rates, low dial settings, and low levels of liquid anesthetic in the vaporizing chamber. Moreover, the pumping effect is enhanced by rapid respiratory rates, high peak inspired pressures, and the rapid drops in pressure during expiration.

The pumping effect can be reduced by the following design modifications in modern vaporizers:

1. Small vaporizing chambers reduce the vapor volumes that can be discharged from the vaporizing chamber into the bypass chamber during the expiratory phase.
2. Some vaporizers have a long spiral tube or labyrinth that serves as the inlet to the vaporizing chamber. Therefore, when the pressure in the vaporizing chamber is released the vapor does not enter the bypass channel because of the tube length.
3. Some vaporizers contain a baffle system in the vaporizing chamber.
4. Some machines include a one-way check valve before the breathing circuit inlet to minimize the pumping effect.

32.13.2.4 Impact of Carrier Gas Composition

Variable bypass vaporizer output can be influenced by the composition of the fresh gas as a result of differences in solubility of anesthetic vapors specially using nitrous oxide. Nitrous oxide is more soluble than oxygen in the halogenated liquid that results in reducing the carrier gas flow rate vaporizer output. However, once the anesthetic liquid becomes saturated with nitrous oxide, vaporizing chamber output increases, and a new steady state is established.

32.13.2.5 Impact of Barometric Pressure Changes

Hypobaric Conditions

Vapor pressure is temperature-dependent but influenced by barometric pressure. Therefore, as altitude increases and the barometric pressure declines, the partial pressure of the anesthetic agent in the variable bypass-vaporizing chamber remains constant despite a decline in the partial pressures of other constituent breathing gases and the total ambient pressure. This situation results in significantly increased volume percent concentration of anesthetic agent within the vaporizing chamber and at the outlet of the vaporizer. However, the partial pressure output of a variable bypass vaporizer changes proportionally less than the volume percent concentrations altitude increases. Because anesthetic partial pressure is the main factor to determine the anesthetic depth, there is no need to adjust the dial to a lower setting at higher altitude.

Hyperbaric Conditions

Under hyperbaric conditions, there will be a significant decrease in anesthetic concentration (v/v%) and mild decrease in partial pressure output. However, the partial pressure of halothane increases slightly with increasing barometric pressure. This effect can be explained by increased atmospheric density on the flow of gas through the vaporizer and the increased thermal conductivity of air at higher pressure.

32.13.2.6 Safety Features

Modern variable vaporizers incorporate many features that have minimized or eliminated many hazards with using the vaporizers:

1. Agent-specific, keyed filling devices help prevent filling a vaporizer with the wrong agent.
2. Vaporizers are firmly secured to a vaporizer manifold on the anesthesia workstation, thus reducing the vaporizer tipping and spillage of the liquid anesthetic to the bypass chamber.
3. Interlock systems prevent the administration of more than one inhaled anesthetic agent.

32.13.3 Desflurane Vaporizer

The vapor pressure of desflurane is 3–4 times that of other contemporary inhaled anesthetics agents (669 mmHg at 20 ° C), and it boils at 22.8 °C, which is basically room temperature. Therefore, it needs a special Tec 6 desflurane vaporizer.

1. At room temperature, the vapor pressure of desflurane is almost 1 atm. Therefore, tremendous gas flow rates would be required to dilute the vaporizing chamber output to clinical concentrations. At 1 atm and 20 degree Celsius, 100 ml/min passing through the vaporizing chamber would entrain 735mL/min of desflurane (as compared with 29, 46, and 47 mL/min of enflurane, isoflurane, and halothane, respectively). To produce a 1% desflurane output, the amount of bypass flow required to dilute the large volume of desflurane-saturated anesthetic vapor would approximately 73 L/min in contrast to 5 L/min or less for the other three inhalation anesthetics.
2. Desflurane high rate of evaporation would cause substantial anesthetic cooling.
3. Desflurane is more likely to boil at room temperature. Therefore, the output would be uncontrollable.

32.13.4 Tec 6 Vaporizer

The principle of operation of the Tec 6 is that liquid desflurane is heated in chamber, or sump, to 39 °C to produce vapor under pressure (~1500 mmHg, or 2 atm absolute pressure). The vapor leaves the sump via a variable pressure-regulating valve, the opening of which is continuously adjusted based on the output from a pressure transducer so that the pressure of the desflurane vapor entering the rotary valve in the user-controlled concentration dial is the same as the pressure difference generated by the fresh gas inflow from the anesthesia machine flow meters into a fixed restrictor (10 cm/H_2O/L/min). Therefore, according to Poiseuille's law for laminar flow, the flow will be proportional to the pressure difference across the resistance. The concentration dial and rotary valve control the quantity of desflurane vapor added to the fresh gas flow so that what emerges from the vaporizer outlet is the dialed-in concentration of desflurane. In the Tec 6, unlike other vaporizers, no fresh gas enters the desflurane sump. Tec 6 is probably more accurately described as a dual-gas blender than as a vaporizer. The manufacturer calibrates the Tec 6 with 100% oxygen as fresh gas. When a carrier gas other than 100% oxygen is at low flow rates, a clear trend toward reduction in vaporizer output emerges. This reduction correlates with the decrease in viscosity of the carrier gas. Nitrous oxide is less viscous than oxygen and generates lower backpressure upstream. As a result, the working pressure is reduced. At low flow rates with nitrous oxide as the carrier gas, vaporizer output is approximately 20% less than the dial setting.

32.13.4.1 Effects of Changes in Altitude on Output

At high altitude, if ambient pressure is 500, 7% desflurane (1 MAC) creates partial pressure of only 35 mmHg in contrast to 53 mmHg at sea level, which is only 0.66 of the minimum alveolar concentration (MAC) partial pressure (P_{MAC1}). The P_{MAC1} is the partial pressure exerted by the MAC volume concentration, which is the main determinant factor for the depth of anesthesia. Therefore, at higher altitude for this decrease in potency output, a higher concentration (10.4%) of 500 mmHg renders a desflurane partial pressure of 52 mmHg. Conversely, at higher ambient pressures, a lower concentration dial setting would be indicated to create the same potency output.

Safety Features

Because desflurane's vapor pressure is nearly 1 atm, misfiling a variable bypass vaporizer with desflurane could theoretically result in both overdose and creation a hypoxic gas mixture. The desflurane vaporizer has a unique, anesthetic specific filling system to minimize this potential hazard. Each desflurane bottle has a "SAF-T-Fill" adaptor indented to prevent use with traditional vaporizers. The SAF-T-Fill system helps prevent both misfiling of variable bypass vaporizers and leakage of desflurane to the atmosphere. The shut-off valve located downstream from the desflurane sump closes and terminates the output if any of the following conditions occur: (1) the anesthetic level decrease to less than 20 mL, (2) the vaporizer is tilted, (3) a power failure occurs, or (4) the pressure difference between the vapor and fresh gas circuits exceeds a specific tolerance.

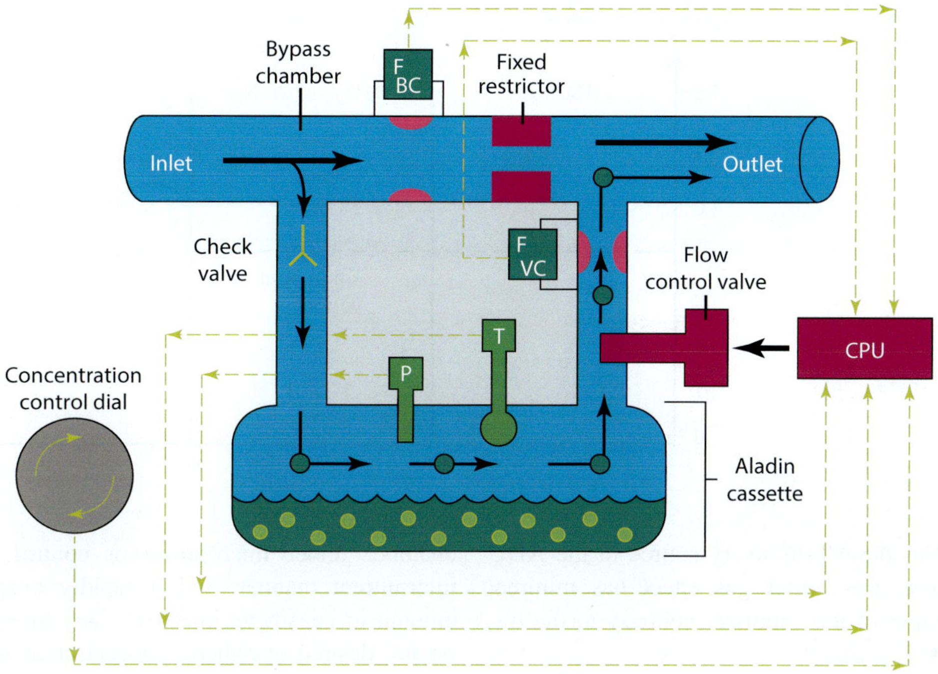

Fig. 32.18 Aladin cassette vaporizer

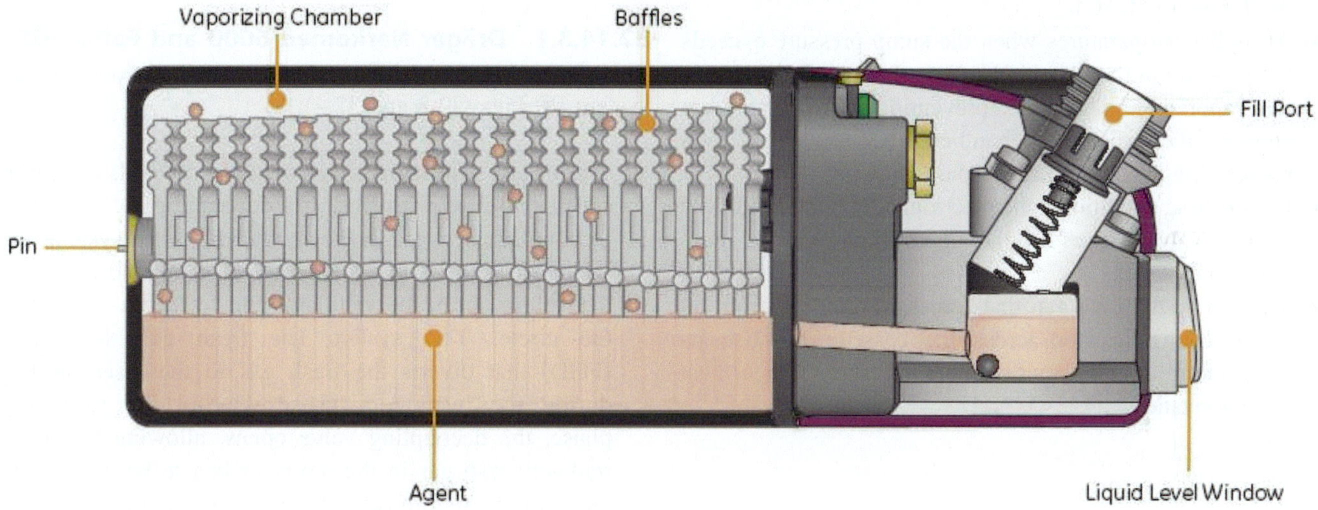

Fig. 32.19 Aladin cassette vaporizer (Reprinted with permission from Brockwell and Andrews [1])

32.14 New Advances in the Vaporizers and Circuits

32.14.1 Datex-Ohmeda Aladin Cassette Vaporizer

- The Aladin™ cassette system is unique and electronically controlled. The vaporizer consists of a permanent internal control unit housed within the anesthesia delivery unit (ADU) and interchangeable Aladin agent cassette that contains anesthetic liquid.
- The cassettes are color coded for each anesthetic agent. They are also magnetically coded so that the ADU can identify which anesthetic cassette has been inserted.
- The heat of the S/5 ADU cassette vaporizer is the electronically controlled flow control valve located in the vaporizing chamber outlet. This valve is controlled by a central processing unit (CPU) (◉ Figs. 32.18 and 32.19).

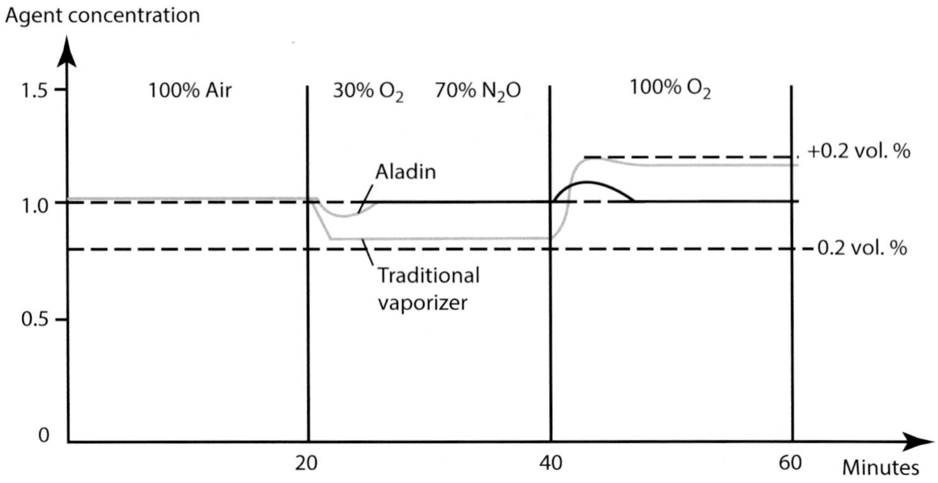

Fig. 32.20 Aladin cassette vaporizer performance. It is minimally affected by carrier gas contrary to the traditional ones

- The CPU receives input from every source in the ADU system. Therefore, the carrier gas effect has minimal effect on the output of the vaporizer contrary to the traditional ones (◉ Fig. 32.20).
- The one-way check valve protects against backflow of agent into the bypass chamber.
- Vaporization of desflurane is a challenging task if the room temperature is greater than the boiling point of desflurane (22.8 °C).
- At higher temperatures when the sump pressure exceeds the pressure in the bypass chamber, the one-way valve in the vaporizing inlet shuts, preventing carrier gas from entering the vaporizing chamber. The carrier gas then passes straight through the bypass chamber.
- Under these conditions, the electronically controlled flow control valve meters in the appropriate flow of pure desflurane vapor.
- The S/5 ADU has a fan that forces warmed air from an agent-heating resistor across the cassette to raise its temperature to counteract the heat loss due to latent heat of vaporization.

32.14.2 Maquet Injection-Type Vaporizer

The Maquet vaporizer (Maquet Critical Care AB, Solna, Sweden) is an electronically controlled, injection-type vaporizer that is used exclusively with Maquet Flow-in anesthesia workstations. Gas from the anesthesia machine is used to pressurize an anesthetic liquid storage container. Pressurization of the reservoir provides the force to drive liquid anesthetic agent through the vaporizer injector and minimizes evaporation of the agent within the chamber. Liquid anesthetic agent is injected into a heated vaporizing chamber under microprocessor control in a pulsed and intermittent manner, and it rapidly evaporates. The total amount of anesthetic injected at any given interval is based on the desired anesthetic concentration and the fresh flow through the vaporizer.

32.14.3 The New Circle System Designs

32.14.3.1 Dräger Narkomed 6000 and Fabius GS

This system has many differences from the traditional Dräger system (◉ Figs. 32.3 and 32.4):

1. The piston ventilator is electrically powered, electronically controlled with fresh gas decoupling.
2. Decoupling system: In the traditional circle system, the tidal volume delivered to the patient's lung is the sum of the volume from the ventilator and fresh gas that enters the circle. This system has fresh gas decoupling (FGD) that diverts the fresh gas to the reservoir bag during the inspiratory phase. During the expiratory phase, the decoupling valve opens, allowing the accumulated fresh gas in the reservoir bag to be drawn into the circle system to refill the piston ventilator's chamber or descending bellows.

The advantage of circle system FGD is the decreased risk of barotraumas because the system isolates the fresh gas from coming into the system from the patient while the ventilator's exhaust valve is closed (◉ Figs. 32.21 and 32.22).

The disadvantages include:

1. The bellows or piston of circle system with FGD refills under shift negative pressure, so it might create negative

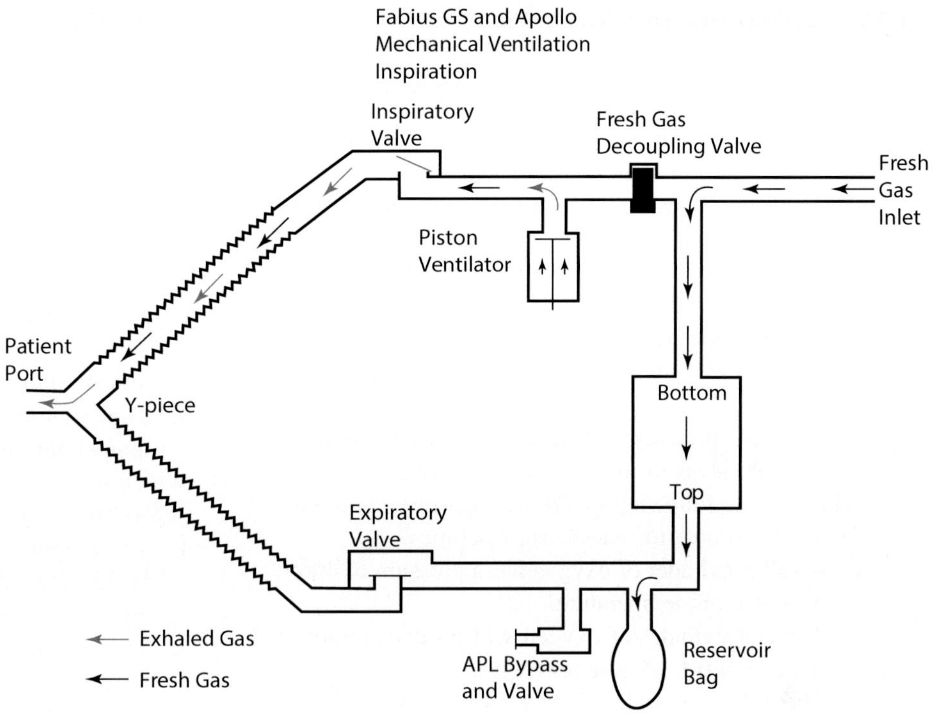

Fig. 32.21 Fabius GS and Apollo breathing system performance during inspiratory phase of mechanical ventilation. Fabius GS and Apollo breathing systems during mechanical inspiration. APL—adjustable pressure limiting (reprinted with permission from Dorsch and Dorsch [2])

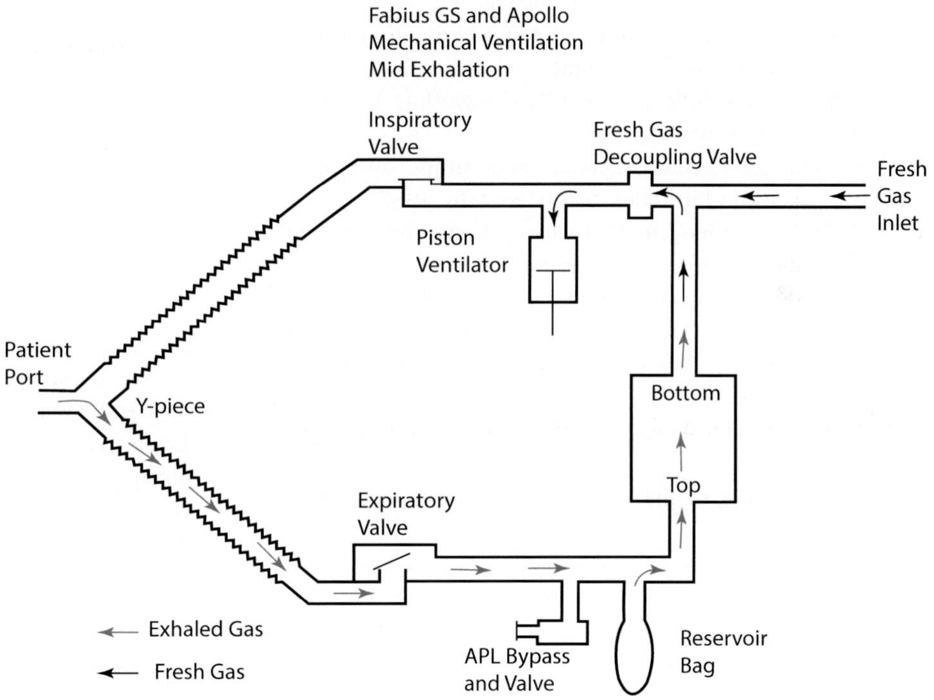

Fig. 32.22 Fabius GS and Apollo breathing system performance during expiratory phase of mechanical ventilation. Fabius GS and Apollo breathing systems during mechanical mid exhalation. APL—adjustable pressure limiting (reprinted with permission from Dorsch and Dorsch [2])

pressure in a patient's airways. To solve this problem, a relief valve that opens below a preset value, such as −2 cmH_2O, to entrain room air into the patient's circuit. If this goes undetected, the entrained atmospheric gases can lead to awareness or hypoxia due to dilution of inhalation anesthetic or lowering of enriched oxygen concentration.

2. If the reservoir bag is removed or has a significant leak, room air may enter the breathing circuit that can lead to awareness or hypoxia.
3. Significant pollution of the operating room can occur due to the escape of inhalation anesthetics or nitrous oxide from an ill-fitted or leaking reservoir bag [3–16].

32.15 Questions and Answers

Questions (Choose the Most Appropriate Answer)

1. Which of the following is FALSE regarding the pressures within the anesthesia machine?
   1. There are 3 circuits: a high pressure, intermediate and a low-pressure circuit.
   2. The pressure range in the high-pressure circuit for oxygen extends from a high of 2200 to 45 psig.
   3. The pressure range in the high-pressure circuit for nitrous oxide ranges from a high of 1500 to 45 psig.
   4. The low pressure circuit extends from the flow control valves to the common gas outlet
2. Which of the following is TRUE regarding the cylinder supply source for anesthesia machines?
   1. A full E cylinder of oxygen has a pressure of 4000 psig at room temperature.
   2. A full E cylinder of oxygen will produce approximately 660 L of gaseous oxygen.
   3. The Diameter Index Safety System (DISS) prevents cylinder interchanging.
   4. The cylinder attaches to the machine through the hanger-yoke assembly allowing bidirectional flow of gases into the machine.
3. Which of the following is TRUE regarding the pipeline supply sources?
   1. The gas-specific pipeline inlet fitting system is called the Pin Index Safety System (PISS).
   2. The pipeline supply source is the backup gas source for the anesthesia machine.
   3. The gas pressure in the pipeline source is 50 psig.
   4. There is a check valve downstream from the inlet preventing flow of gases from the pipeline to the machine.
4. Which of the following is TRUE regarding the oxygen flush valve?
   1. Actuation of the valve delivers 100% oxygen at 15 L/min.
   2. It allows direct communication between the oxygen pipeline-pressure system to the patient circuit.
   3. Oxygen flushing during the expiratory phase of positive pressure ventilation can produce barotrauma.
   4. A valve sticking in the closed position can result in awareness under anesthesia.
5. What is the oxygen pressure required to keep the fail-safe valve open?
   1. 10 psig
   2. 20 psig
   3. 50 psig
   4. 100 psig
6. Which of the following is TRUE of modern temperature compensating vaporizers?
   1. Vaporizers are constructed of metals with low thermal conductivity in order to maintain a uniform internal temperature.
   2. The bypass valve closes smaller as temperature increases.
   3. Energy gained during the evaporation of liquid anesthetic can lead to significant increases in temperature within the remaining liquid.
   4. The vaporizer can compensate for changes in temperature over the range of 10–40 °C.
7. Which of the following is true of very low flow rates (<250 mL/min) and very high flow rates (>15 L/min)?
   1. The output of variable bypass vaporizers tends to be less than the dial setting at very low flow rates and very high flow rates.
   2. The output of variable bypass vaporizers tends to be greater than the dial setting at very low flow rates and at very high flow rates.
   3. The output of variable bypass vaporizers tends to be greater than the dial setting at very low flow rates and less than the dial setting at very high flow rates.
   4. The output of variable bypass vaporizers tends to be less than the dial setting at very low flow rates and greater than the dial setting at very high flow rates.
8. Why does desflurane require a special vaporizer compared to isoflurane and sevoflurane?
   1. Desflurane vaporizes very slowly.
   2. Desflurane cools rapidly with vaporization.
   3. Desflurane has a high boiling point.
   4. Desflurane has low potency.
9. Under which condition is the “pumping effect,” or the change of pressure affecting the output of the vaporizer, enhanced?
   1. High flow rates
   2. Low amount of liquid anesthetic in the vaporizing chamber
   3. Low peak inspiratory pressures
   4. High dial settings
10. In a variable bypass vaporizer, the splitting ratio (R) is dependent on which of the following?
    1. Minimum alveolar concentration of the agent
    2. Saturated vapor concentration of the agent
    3. Concentration of oxygen
    4. Fresh gas flow

Answers

1. **C**. The pressures within the anesthesia machine can be divided into 3 circuits: a high pressure, an intermediate pressure, and a low-pressure circuit (answer A). The high-pressure circuit is confined to the cylinders and the cylinders' primary pressure regulators. For oxygen, the pressure range of the high-pressure circuit extends from a high of 2200 pounds per square inch gauge (psig) to 45 psig, which is the regulated cylinder pressure (answer B). For nitrous oxide (N_2O), the high-pressure circuit pressures range from a high of 750 psig, *not 1500 psig,* in the cylinder to a low of 45 psig (answer C). The intermediate pressure circuit begins at the regulated cylinder pressure sources at 45 psig, includes the pipeline sources at 50–55 psig, and extends to the flow control valves. The low-pressure circuit extends from the *flow control valves* to the common gas outlet (answer D). The low-pressure circuit includes the flow tubes, the vaporizers, and a one-way check valve on most Datex-Ohmeda machines.
2. **B**. A full E cylinder of oxygen is approximately 2000 psig at room temperature (answer A) and will produce approximately 660 L of gaseous oxygen (answer B.). The cylinder attaches to the machine through the hanger-yoke assembly. Each hanger yoke is equipped with a Pin Index Safety System (PISS), which prevents cylinder interchanging, not the DISS (answer C.). The hanger-yoke assembly also supports the cylinder, provides a gas-like seal, and ensures a *unidirectional* flow of gases into the machine (answer D.)
3. **C**. The hospital piping system provides gases to the machine at approximately 50–55 psig, which is the normal working pressure of most machines. The pipeline inlet fittings are gas-specific, Diameter Index Safety System (DISS), threaded body fittings, not PISS (answer A). The pipeline supply source is the primary gas source for the anesthesia machine (answer B). The gas cylinder source functions as the backup gas source should the pipeline fail. The check valve downstream from the pipeline inlet functions to prevent reversal of flow from the machine to the pipeline or the atmosphere (answer D).
4. **B**. The oxygen flush valve allows direct communication between the oxygen pipeline-pressure system to the patient circuit. Actuation of the valve delivers 100% oxygen at a rate of 35–75 L/min to the breathing circuit (answer A). The oxygen valve is associated with several hazards. A defective or damaged valve stuck in a fully open position will result in barotrauma. A valve sticking in a *partially open position* can result in awareness under anesthesia due to the oxygen flow from the incompetent valve dilute the inhaled anesthetic agent (answer D). Oxygen flushing during the *inspiratory* phase of positive pressure ventilation can produce barotraumas if the anesthesia machine does not incorporate an appropriately adjusted inspiratory pressure limiter (answer C).
5. **B**. The fail-safe valve opens at oxygen pressure of 20 psig or more and is closed at pressures less than 20 psig. The fail-safe valve is synonymous to a pressure-sensor shut off valve. In the North American Dräger Narkomed machines, it is called the oxygen failure protection device (OFPD). It is an all-or-nothing valve that interrupts the flow of N2O and all other gases when the oxygen pressure falls below 20 psig.
6. **D**. Answer A is false: Vaporizers are constructed of metals with *high* thermal conductivity in order to maintain a uniform internal temperature. Answer B is false: The bypass valve *opens wider* as temperature increases. Answer C is false: Energy is *lost* during the evaporation of liquid anesthetic, which leads to a *decrease* in temperature of the remaining liquid (this is the concept of latent heat of vaporization).
7. **A**. At very low flow rates, there is not enough turbulence to advance the vapor molecules upward because of the relatively high density of inhaled anesthetic agents. At very high flow rates, there may be cooling during rapid evaporation, incomplete mixing, failure to saturate the carrier gas in the vaporizing chamber, and increased resistance to high gas flow, all of which lead to a less than expected concentration of vapor.
8. **B**. Desflurane has a very high vapor pressure (669 mmHg) at room temperature compared to isoflurane (238 mmHg) and sevoflurane (157 mmHg), which causes it to vaporize quickly (answer A). Desflurane has a high latent heat of vaporization; therefore, it cools rapidly as it is evaporated (answer B). Desflurane has a low boiling point (22.8 °C) at atmospheric pressure compared to isoflurane (48.5 °C) and sevoflurane (58.5 °C) (answer C). Desflurane is less potent than isoflurane and desflurane, but this has no role of influence on the construction of the vaporizer (answer D).
9. **B**. The "pumping effect" is more pronounced at *low* flow rates (answer A), low levels of liquid anesthetic in the vaporizing chamber (answer B), high peak inspiratory pressures (answer C), *low* dial settings (answer D), rapid respiratory rates, and rapid drops in pressure during expiration.
10. **B**. When fresh gas enters a variable bypass vaporizer, the flow is directed into the vaporizing chamber and the bypass channel. The ratio of flow between these 2 paths is the splitting ratio (R). It is equal to [(*S*/

$F) - 1]/1 - S$, where S is the saturated vapor concentration of the agent, and F is the fractional concentration of the agent.

Appendix

Splitting Ratios

Leigh has published a mathematical derivation of the splitting ratio (R) and a formula for calculating the splitting ratio for a given fractional concentration (F) of agent:

$$R = [(S/F) - 1]/1 - S,$$

where S is the saturated vapor concentration of the agent (as a fractional concentration).

Thus, for 1% isoflurane:

$$F = 0.01, S = 0.31, \text{and}$$

$$R = [(0.31/0.01) - 1]/1 - 0.31 = 30/0.069 = 44 : 1$$

The fractional concentration of agent (F) produced by a given splitting ratio (R) is as follows:

$$F = S/[R(1 - S) + 1]$$

Thus, for sevoflurane (S = 0.21) in a vaporizer set to a splitting ratio of 12:1:

$$F = 0.21/[12(1 - 0.21) + 1]$$
$$= 0.21/[12 \times 0.79) + 1] = 0.21/10.48 = 0.02 \text{ or } 2\%$$

Anesthesia Machine/Workstation Checklist ~ Preanesthesia Checkout (PAC) 2008

The anesthesia workstation should be evaluated prior to administration of anesthesia. The checklist should be completed daily in all locations where anesthesia is to be administered. Refer to appropriate operator manuals for specific procedures and precautions.

1. Emergency Ventilation Equipment:
   - Verify Self-inflating Manual Ventilation Device (e.g., AMBU bag) available and functioning.
2. Verify O_2 Cylinder Supply:
   - Verify Auxiliary Oxygen Cylinder (should be at least half full ~1000 psi) with regulator available and ability to open cylinder valve. Close valve after checking.
   - Check central oxygen pipeline supply; hoses should be connected, and pipeline gauges read ≥ 50 psi.
3. Verify patient suction is available and functioning to clear the airway*.
4. Turn on anesthesia delivery system and confirm that AC Power is available.
   - Verify visual indicators of power source show both AC and battery power.
   - Ensure connection of power cord to a functional AC power source.
5. Verify availability of required monitors and check alarms.*
   - Verify appropriate monitoring supplies (BP cuff, oximetry probes, EKG leads, capnography, etc.) are available.
   - Verify visual and audible alarm systems functioning for each monitor device.
6. Verify that vaporizers are adequately filled and filler ports are tightly closed.*
7. Verify no leaks exist in gas supply lines between flowmeters and the common gas outlet.
   - Perform a thorough leak test by turning on each vaporizer individually to check for leaks at the vaporizer mount(s) or inside the vaporizer.
   - A negative pressure test may be necessary to check for leaks between the flowmeter and common gas outlet.
8. Calibrate O_2 Monitor:
   - Ensure monitor reads 21% O_2 in room air.
   - Very low O_2 alarm is enabled and functioning.
   - Reinstall O_2 sensor in circuit and flush breathing system with O_2. Verify monitor now reads >90% O_2.
9. Check Scavenging System:
   - Verify proper connections between scavenging system and both APL (pop-off) valve and ventilator relief valve.
   - Ensure positive and negative pressure relief is functioning properly.
   - Ensure (waste-gas) vacuum level is adequate.
10. Verify Carbon Dioxide Absorbent is not exhausted.*
    - Absorbent should be replaced if characteristic color change is present or inspired CO_2 is greater than zero indicating rebreathing of CO_2.
11. Breathing system pressure and leak testing:*
    - Ensure breathing circuit is complete, undamaged and unobstructed. Test should be performed with circuit in configuration to be used for delivery of anesthesia.
    - Install breathing circuit accessory equipment (humidifier, PEEP valve, filter, etc.) to be during the anesthetic.
    - Perform leak check per manufacturer's recommendation. Proper testing will show that pressure can be developed in breathing system during both manual and mechanical ventilation and pressure can be relieved during manual ventilation by opening the APL valve.

12. Verify gas flows properly through the breathing circuit during both inspiration and exhalation.*
    - Use a test lung or second reservoir bag to confirm flow through circuit is not impeded. Test should be completed in manual and mechanical ventilation modes.
    - *Manual Mode Test:* ventilate manually and ensure inflation and deflation of artificial lungs and correct feel of system resistance and compliance.
    - *Mechanical Ventilation Test:* Verify that ventilator bellows and artificial lungs fill and empty appropriately without sustained pressure at end expiration.
    - Complete regular valve competence tests. Presence of carbon dioxide in inspired gases can help detect an incompetent valve.
13. Document completion of anesthesia workstation checkout procedures.*

*To be completed prior to each anesthetic use.

References

1. Brockwell RC, Andrews JJ. Inhaled anesthetic delivery systems. In: Miller RD, Cucchiara RF, Miller ED, editors. Miller's anesthesia. 6th ed. Philadelphia: Churchill Livingstone; 2005. p. 273–314.
2. Dorsch JA, Dorsch SE. Chapter 5. The anesthesia machine. In: Dorsch JA, Dorsch SE, editors. Understanding anesthesia equipment. 5th ed. Philadelphia: Lippincott Williams & Wilkins; 2008.
3. American Society for Testing and Materials. Standard specification for particular requirements for anesthesia workstations and their components (ASTMF 1850–00). West Conshohocken: American Society for Testing and Materials; 2000.
4. Dorsch JA, Dorsch SE. The anesthesia machine. In: Dorsch JA, Dorsch SE, editors. Understanding anesthesia equipment. 4th ed. Baltimore: Williams & Wilkins; 1999. p. 75–118.
5. Schreiber PJ. Safety guidelines for anesthesia systems. Telford: North American Dräger; 1985.
6. Eisenkraft JB, Sommer RM. Equipment failure: anesthesia delivery systems. In: Benumof JL, Saidman LJ, editors. Anesthesia and perioperative complications. 2nd ed. St. Louis: Mosby; 1999. p. 112–60.
7. Eisenkraft JB. Chapter 2. The anesthesia machine and workstation. In: Ehrenwerth J, Eisenkraft JB, Berry JM, editors. Anesthesia equipment: principles and applications. 2nd ed. Philadelphia: Elsevier Saunders; 2013.
8. Venticinque SG, Andrews JJ. Chapter 29. Inhaled anesthetics: delivery systems. In: Miller RD, Cohen NH, Eriksson LI, Fleisher LA, Wiener-Kronish JP, Young WL, editors. Miller's anesthesia. 8th ed. Philadelphia: Elsevier Saunders; 2015.
9. Subrahmanyam M, Mohan S. Safety features in anaesthesia machine. Indian J Anaesth. 2013;57:472–80.
10. Guidelines for Pre-Anesthesia Checkout Procedures. Sub-Committee of ASA Committee on Equipment and Facilities. 2008.
11. Feldman, J, Loeb, R, Philip, J. FAQ on Anesthesia Machine Use, Protection, and Decontamination during the COVID 19 Pandemic. Last updated February 19, 2021. https://www.apsf.org/faq-on-anesthesia-machine-use-protection-and-decontamination-during-the-covid-19-pandemic/
12. Urdaneta F, Loeb R. HEPA filters. Do we really know enough? Breathing system filters in the era of COVID 19. APSF Newslett. 2021;36(1):11–4.
13. Tham R, Oberle M. How Do Flow Sensors Work? APSF Newslett. 2008;23(1):10–2.
14. Garg R, Gupta RC. Analysis of oxygen, anaesthesia agent and flows in anaesthesia machine. Indian J Anaesth. 2013;57:481.
15. Mondonedo J, et al. Comparison of pneumotachography and anemometry for flow measurement for mechanical ventilation with volatile anesthetics. J Clin Monit Comput. 2017;31(6):1263–71. https://doi.org/10.1007/s10877-016-9956-z.
16. Bokoch MP, Weston SD. Inhaled anesthetic delivery systems. In: Gropper MA, Miller RD, Cohen NH, Eriksson LI, Fleisher LA, Leslie K, Wiener-Kronish JP, editors. Miller's anesthesia. 9th ed. Elsevier: Inc; 2020. p. 594–6.

Physical Measurements in Anesthesia

33

D. John Doyle and Anthony Cartwright

Abstract

The aim of this chapter is to understand the physical measurements of anesthesia. This chapters delves into the applications of kinetic theory of gases, vapor pressure, Boyle's law, and the Doppler principle, among others, in clinical medicine.

Keywords

Anaesthesia • Kinetic theory • Vapor pressure • Boyle's law • Charles' law • Dalton's law • Henry's law • Fick's law • Van der Walls effect • Laplace's law

Key Points

1. Pressure = force/area. This may be measured by electronic and non-electronic means and forms the basis of many measurements in anesthesia.
2. Dalton's Law of Partial Pressures states that in a mixture of non-reacting gases, the total pressure exerted is equal to the sum of the partial pressures of the individual gases.
3. The ideal gas laws describe the relationship between pressure, temperature, and volume of an ideal gas. The ideal gas laws may be combined into the ideal gas equation, which may be written as PV = nRT, where P = pressure, V = volume, n = number of moles, R = ideal gas constant, and T = temperature.
4. Medical gas cylinders come in standard sizes and have a color nomenclature that denotes the contents of the cylinder. Gas from a medical gas cylinder is usually delivered via pressure-reducing valves in order to reduce the cylinder pressure from, for oxygen, around 2000 pounds per square inch (PSI) to a safer and more usable 50 PSI.
5. Temperature is a measure of heat energy and reflects whether an object may transfer heat to or from another object. Temperature may be measured via electronic or non-electronic means.
6. Different inhalational anesthetic agents have different solubilities. This varies with temperature and pressure, which is why anesthetic vaporizers are designed to maintain a constant temperature and pressure. This solubility affects their speed of onset, offset, and potency.
7. Laminar gas and fluid flow is governed by the Hagen–Poiseuille equation. A change in conditions or surroundings may alter the flow making it turbulent, which is much less efficient.
8. The humidification of inspired gases is extremely important and may be achieved in a number of ways in the intubated patient.
9. Doppler shift of sound is used in a variety of medical applications, including ultrasound. The principle states that the frequency of an emitted sound will change if the origin of the sound moves in relation to the observer.
10. Newer medical alarm systems are becoming "smarter," and will trigger based on a number of preset variables resulting in context-sensitive warnings or even the ability to integrate with other systems to generate a response; e.g., page the attending physician.

33.1 Goals and Objectives

The principal goals and objective of this chapter are to understand the following concepts and their application to anesthesiology and clinical medicine:

D. J. Doyle (✉)
Department of General Anesthesiology, Cleveland Clinic, Cleveland, OH, USA
e-mail: djdoyle@hotmail.com

A. Cartwright
Practice Plus Group, The University of Sheffield, Plymouth, UK
e-mail: tony_cartwright@me.com

M. Argalious et al. (eds.), *Basic Sciences in Anesthesia*,
https://doi.org/10.1007/978-3-031-60203-0_33

- The kinetic theory of gases
- Pressure and its measurement
- Units of pressure measurement and their conversion
- Vapor pressure
- The ideal gas law
- Boyle's law
- Charles' Law
- Dalton's law
- Henry's law
- Fick's law of diffusion
- The van der Walls effect
- Laplace's law
- The Bernoulli effect
- Venturi devices
- Relationship between pressure, flow, and resistance
- Hagen–Poiseuille's law
- Laminar versus turbulent gas flow
- Helium/oxygen mixtures
- Flowmeter design
- The Doppler principle and its clinical application

33.2 Pressure

33.2.1 Definition

Pressure is force per unit area, and in the case of gases is the result of the kinetic properties of gas molecules as they strike the walls of their container or as they strike the sensor of a measuring device. The SI unit of pressure is the Pascal (Pa). The Pascal is defined as a pressure of 1 Newton (N) acting over an area of 1 square meter. The Newton is defined as the force that will cause an object of 1 kg to accelerate at a rate of 1 m per second per second.

$$N = kg\ m^{-1}s^{-2}$$

Gravity will cause a 1 kg object to accelerate in a vacuum, where there is no resistance from air, at a rate of 9.81 kg m^{-1} s^{-2}, making the force of gravity on a 1 kg object to be 9.81 N. This is referred to as a kilogram weight. 1 Newton is therefore equal to 1/9.81 kg weight, which is 102 g weight, corresponding to a force of 102 g m^{-2}. This is a very small amount of pressure, so the unit of pressure commonly used is the kilopascal (kPa), rather than the pascal.

Discussions about pressure in anesthesia may be confusing because of various different units used in the clinical literature:

- Atmospheres (atm)
- bar
- mmHg
- cmH_20
- pascals (Pa)
- PSI (pounds per square inch)
- N/m^2
- $dynes/cm^2$

In order for the reader to relate to these different units, atmospheric pressure at sea level may be written as:

1 atm = 1.01 bar = 760 mmHg = 1033 cmH_2O = 101 kPa = 14.7 psi = 101,325 N/m^2 = 1,013,250 $dynes/cm^2$.

American engineers often use PSI units. Scientists often use Pascal units (SI). Clinicians use mmHg for blood pressures, and cmH_2O for airway pressures and sometimes for CVP measurements.

33.2.2 Pressure Measurement

Historically, pressure (Fig. 33.1) has commonly been measured using a column of liquid. Your more venerable colleagues are likely familiar with using a manometer tube to measure central venous pressure. This consisted of a flexible tube, which was filled with saline before being attached to a central venous line. The other end was attached to the bottom of an open-topped glass tube, again filled with saline. The glass tube, or manometer had gradations of centimeters marked on the side and when the '0' was placed at the height of the heart, the central venous pressure could be measured off the side of the manometer (Fig. 33.2).

A similar mechanism may be used to measure higher pressures, and mercury would often be used for this range of pressure, as mercury is 13.6 times denser than water. It is therefore easy to see that a 100 cm column of water could be represented by a 7.36 cm column of mercury, a more manageable height. One atmosphere would be represented by 760 mm of mercury, and this was put to good use in early barometers (Fig. 33.3).

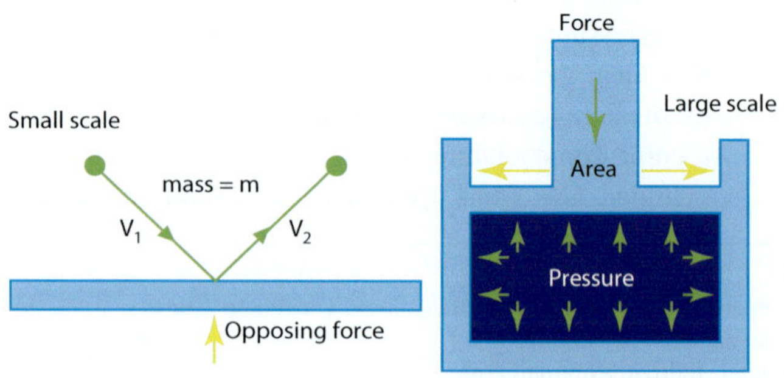

Fig. 33.1 The concept of pressure illustrated on microscopic (left) and macroscopic (right) scales

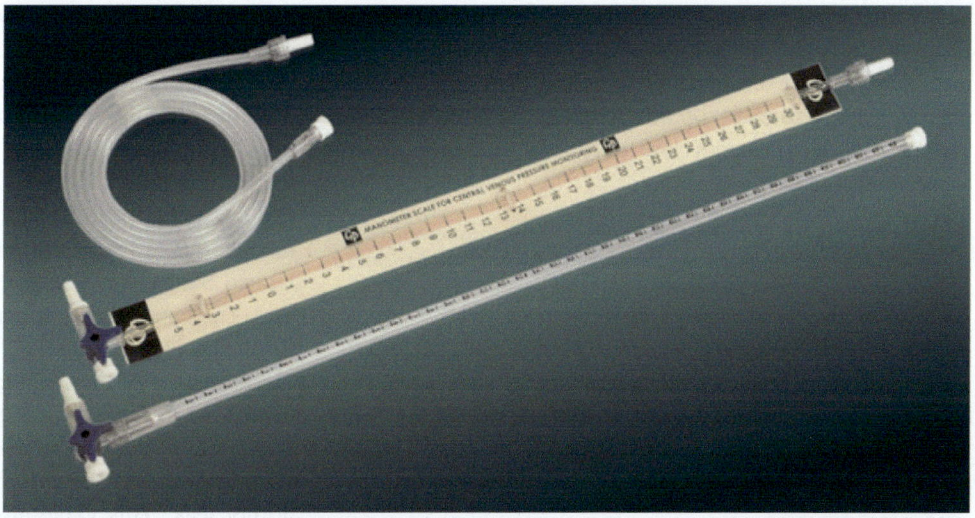

Fig. 33.2 A glass manometer

An alternative to a column of fluid is the Bourdon gauge which is an aneroid gauge (from the Greek aneros, meaning without liquid). This type of aneroid gauge is based on the principle of a curved metallic tube uncoiling when the pressure inside the tube increases. The end of the tube is connected to a series of levers and gears which then moved a needle (Fig. 33.4).

A pressure measurement may be displayed in a variety of ways and the following are all common within medicine and anesthesia:

- **Absolute pressure** is "zero-referenced" with respect to a perfect vacuum, and thus is equal to gauge pressure plus atmospheric pressure.

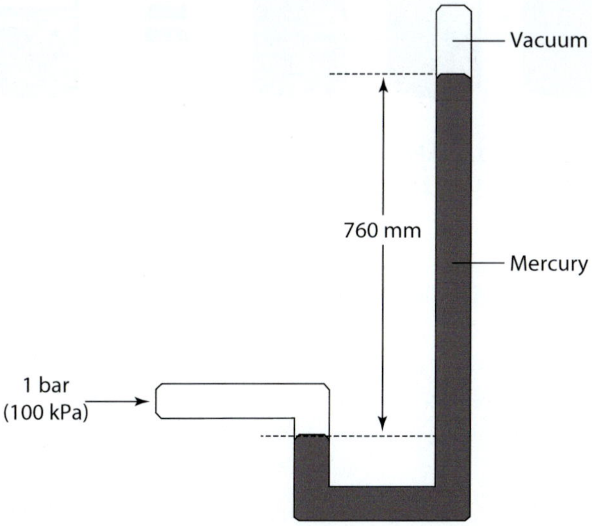

Fig. 33.3 An early barometer

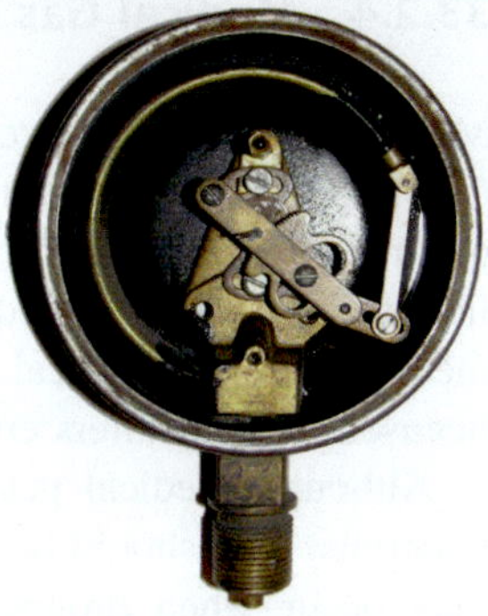

Fig. 33.4 The internal construction of a bourdon tube gauge (dial and indicator needle removed). Note the curved brass tube that slightly straightens out with pressurization, eventually rotating the indicator needle. *source* Yegor Chernyshev at English Wikipedia. Image licensed under CC BY-SA 3.0 via Creative Commons

- **Gauge pressure** is "zero-referenced" with respect to ambient air pressure (atmospheric pressure), and thus is to absolute pressure minus atmospheric pressure.
- **Differential pressure** is the difference in pressure between two measurements.

For the most part, anesthesiologists can disregard atmospheric pressure and use gauge pressure readings that are relative to atmospheric pressure. Gas cylinder, blood pressure, and ventilator pressure readings are all gauge pressure readings.

To look at these readings in the clinical context, a full oxygen cylinder typically has a gauge pressure reading of 137 bar. Atmospheric pressure is approximately 1 bar, so the absolute pressure is the sum of gauge pressure and atmospheric pressure or 138 bar.

33.2.3 Dalton's Law of Partial Pressures

When a mixture of non-reacting, pure gases are placed in a sealed container, the pressure that each exerts on the walls of the container is proportional to the percentage that that gas makes of the whole mixture. For example, if a cylinder of Entonox (50% O_2 and 50% N_2O) is at a pressure of 100 kPa, the oxygen will exert a partial pressure of 50 kPa and the nitrous oxide also exert a partial pressure of 50 kPa. This is summarized by Dalton's law of partial pressures which states that:

> *In a mixture of non-reacting gases, the total pressure exerted is equal to the sum of the partial pressures of the individual gases.*

The formulaic representation of this law is:

$$P_{\text{total}} = P_{\text{a}} + P_{\text{b}} + P_{\text{c}} + P_{\text{d}} + \ldots + P_{\text{n}}$$

Figure 33.5 provides a good representation of this equation to see how Dalton's law of Partial Pressures applies to air.

33.2.4 Medical Gas Cylinders

Medical gases are delivered in cylinders of various sizes (Table 33.1) made of aluminum, stainless steel, or another non-reactive material. Oxygen may also be delivered in liquid form to be stored in a storage tank at any large medical facility. Medical gases are produced by stringently licensed manufacturers ensuring 99.995% purity.

Although medical gas cylinders are made from strong materials, they should be handled with care as an explosion may occur when dropped on a concrete floor. Cylinders should be stored at a constant temperature, upright, indoors, and protected from the weather. Manufacturers regularly evaluate cylinders using an endoscope and other tools to ensure that faulty cylinders are withdrawn from service.

Color coding is used to identify the contents of gas cylinders, although color coding varies throughout the world. An International Organization for Standardization (ISO) standard, ISO 32, covers colors of cylinders for medical gases but not all countries use this standard. In the United States, for example, color coding is not regulated by law. The common color codes for medical gas cylinders are displayed in Table 33.2.

On the top of the cylinder is an identification label giving details of contents, pressures, volumes, and any hazard warnings. Seated in the neck of the cylinder is the cylinder valve that closes the cylinder and ensures that the contents do not leak. This valve also allows a secure fit for refilling and for attachment to the yolk that delivers oxygen directly to the patient or to the anesthesia machine.

On the face of the cylinder valve is a series of small holes below the outlet for the gas (Fig. 33.6). These accept a reciprocal pin system, called the Pin Index Safety System, on the yolk (Fig. 33.6, top). The position of the holes and matching pins are specific to a particular gas cylinder, thereby helping to ensure that the correct gas is connected to the correct yolk.

On larger cylinders, a bull nose connection system (Fig. 33.6, bottom) is used with a variety of male and female connections as well as right- and left-hand threads to reduce the possibility of incorrect connections.

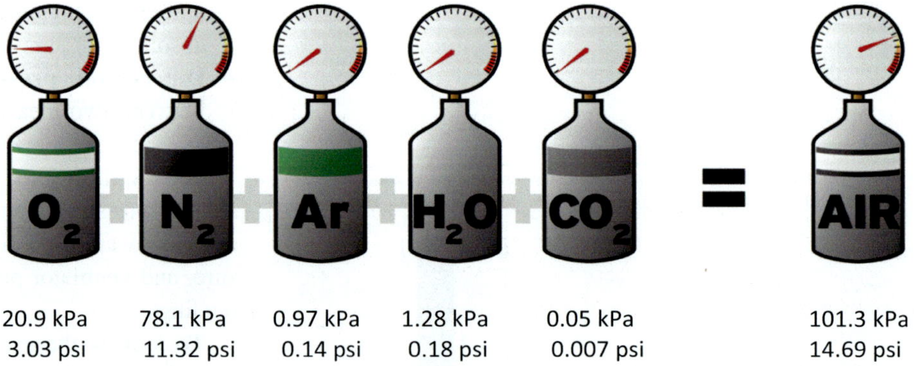

Fig. 33.5 A representation of how Dalton's law of partial pressures applies to air

Table 33.1 Sizes of commonly used medical gas cylinders

Size	Capacity (L)	Pressure (psi)	Tare wt (kg)	Valve type
B	200	1900	2.27	Pin index
D	400	1900	3.4	Pin index
E	660	1900	5.4	Pin index
F	1360	1900	14.5	Bull nose
G	3400	1900	34.5	Bull nose
H	6900	2200	53.2	Bull nose
M	3450	2200	29.0	Bull nose

Table 33.2 Color coding of USA and ISO medical gases

Gas	USA	ISO
Oxygen (O_2)	Green	White
Air	Yellow	White / Black
Carbon dioxide (CO_2)	Gray	Gray
CO_2 and O_2	Gray / Green	Gray / White
Helium (He)	Brown	Brown
He and O_2	Brown / Green	Brown / White
Nitrous Oxide (N_2O)	Blue	Blue
Cyclopropane (C_3H_6)	Orange	Orange
Ethylene (C_2H_4)	Red	Violet
Nitrogen	Black	Black

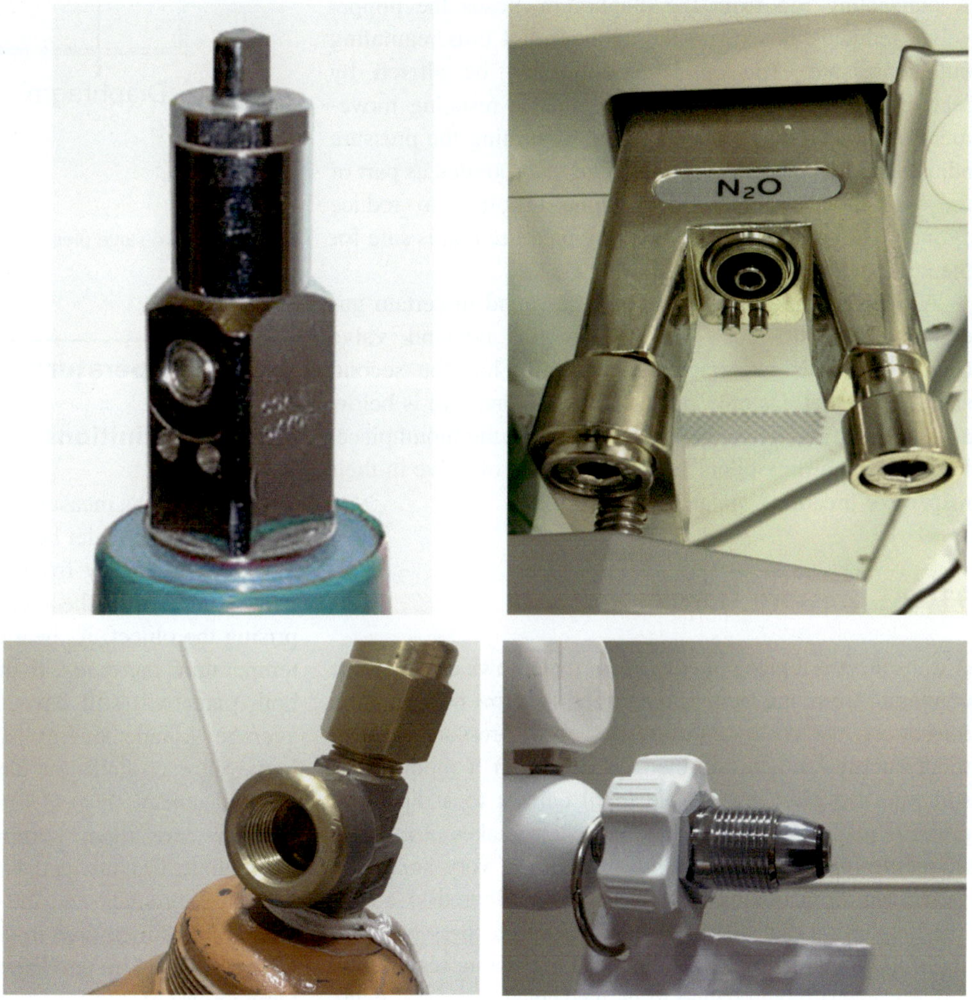

Fig. 33.6 Top: Cylinder valve and receiving yoke showing pin index system. Bottom: Bull nose connection system used on larger cylinders

33.2.5 Pressure-Reducing Valve

A pressure-reducing valve is used to control the pressure to which a patient or piece of medical equipment is exposed when connected to a medical gas cylinder. The most common type of pressure-reducing valve in anesthesia is the single-stage-reducing valve (Fig. 33.7). In this valve, the inlet gauge is measuring the gauge pressure of the cylinder, which in the case of oxygen is 137 bar when full. This pressure places a force on the diaphragm, displacing it.

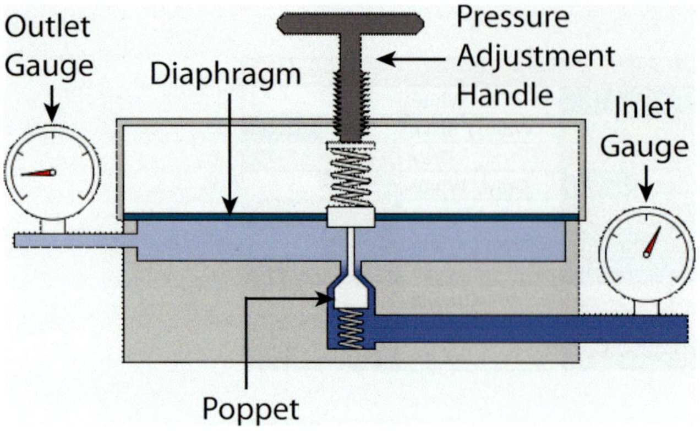

Fig. 33.7 Single-stage pressure reducing valve

A connecting rod from the diaphragm closes the poppet valve, reducing flow from the cylinder and thus regulating outlet pressure. The outlet pressure can be altered by relaxing or compressing the spring that is resisting movement of the diaphragm; this is done by turning the pressure adjustment handle. This valve is often incorporated as part of the yolk of the anesthesia machine in order to reduce cylinder gauge pressure to a working pressure that is safe for the equipment.

A two-stage reducing valve may be found in certain gas delivery systems, such as an Entonox demand valve (Fig. 33.8). This two-stage valve usually has the second stage set so that gas only passes when the pressure is below atmospheric, i.e., when the patient draws on the mouthpiece. Firemen and airline pilots also use this type of valve in their respective breathing apparatus.

33.2.6 Pressure Transducers

A transducer is a piece of equipment that allows energy to be converted from one form into another. In terms of a pressure transducer, the energy is converted from pressure to electrical energy, and this is then displayed on a monitor via software that converts the electrical current to a displayed pressure reading. The conversion of energy takes place most frequently using a strain gauge, which is a very small foil pattern on an insulating flexible backing, adhered to a flexible diaphragm that distorts when exposed to pressure. The strain gauge is therefore also distorted, and this results in a tiny but measurable change in its resistance measured using a circuit called a Wheatstone Bridge.

One of the more common uses of a pressure transducer in clinical practice is the measurement of invasive arterial blood pressure. The transducer is part of the arterial line and is exposed to the arterial pressure waveform via saline-filled tubing. The resulting waveform and blood pressure values are displayed on a digital monitor.

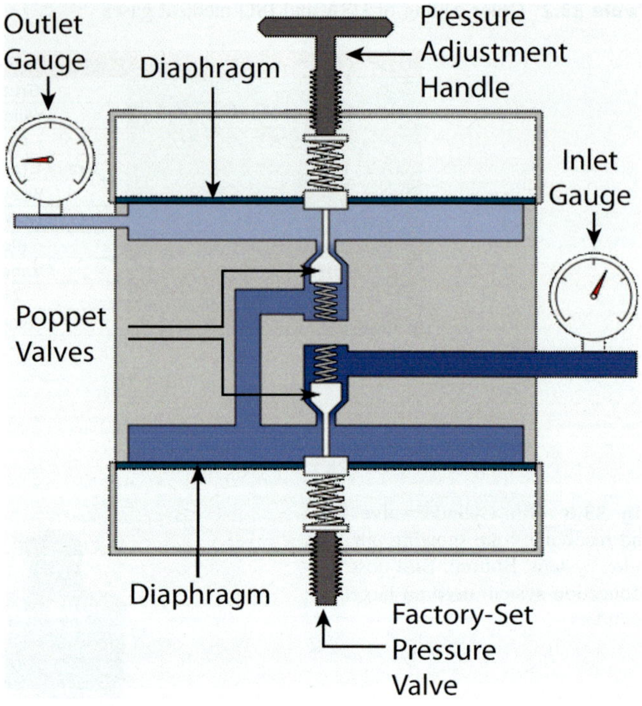

Fig. 33.8 Two-stage pressure reducing valve

33.3 Temperature

33.3.1 Definitions

Temperature is a measure of heat energy and defines whether an object will transfer heat to another object or, alternatively, receive heat energy from another object. Heat is generated by an increase in the mean energy of the molecules comprising the object. As heat energy is applied to an object, its temperature increases. If the object is then divided in two, both parts will still have the same temperature (the same average kinetic energy of its constituent components), however, each half now has half of the heat capacity of the original object.

There are three commonly used temperature scales: Fahrenheit, Celsius, and Kelvin. Americans and Europeans use the Fahrenheit and the Celsius scales respectively, with temperatures measured in degrees Fahrenheit (°F) or degrees Celsius (°C). On the Fahrenheit scale, water freezes at a temperature of 32 °F and boils at 212 °F (at one atmosphere pressure). Absolute zero on this scale is not at 0 °F, but at − 459 °F. Using the Celsius scale the freezing point of water is 0 °C and the boiling point is 100 °C, while, Absolute Zero corresponds to a temperature of − 273.15 °C. The degree Kelvin (°K) is the SI unit of temperature and is used by the scientific community. The Kelvin scale is an absolute, thermodynamic temperature scale using as its null point absolute zero, the temperature at which all thermal motion ceases in the classical description of thermodynamics.

The relationship between the different scales is as follows:

- °C = 5/9 x (°F–32)
- °F = 9/5°C + 32
- °C = °K–273.15
- °K = °C + 273.15

33.3.2 Temperature Measurement

Many methods are available for measuring temperature and the best way of classifying them is to divide them into those that use non-electrical methods and those that use electrical methods of measurement. Those that use non-electrical methods include the mercury, or alcohol-filled glass thermometer, the bimetallic strip thermometer, and the Bourdon gauge thermometer. Electrical methods use one of three basic principles; the resistance thermometer, the thermistor, and the thermocouple. Infrared thermometers are also commonly used on the floor and in the community. All the electrical methods produce extremely small changes in current or voltage and employ a Wheatstone Bridge circuit to make these small changes measurable.

The **glass thermometer** consists of a glass tube filled with mercury or some other liquid where temperature increase causes the liquid to expand. The reading is then taken from the maximum point that the fluid has reached. A maximum reading thermometer has a small metal marker above the level of mercury. Once the mercury has cooled and therefore contracted back down the thermometer, the metal marker indicates the maximum temperature reached. Mercury has historically been used in medical practice, however this has almost been completely removed due to its toxicity. Alcohol sometimes replaces mercury in thermometers for measuring very low temperatures due to mercury solidifying at − 39 °C. Alcohol, however, boils at 78.5 °C, so cannot be used in the higher ranges that mercury may be used.

A **bimetallic strip thermometer** uses two metals whose coefficients of linear expansion are different and are fixed together such that the composite bimetal assembly bends in proportion to temperature. If this is placed in a coil design, the deflection is amplified and a needle may be placed at the distal end of the strip causing a deflection on a scale.

A **Bourdon gauge thermometer** uses the principle of expansion of gases with increasing temperature. A Bourdon gauge measures the pressure within a sealed, gas-filled tube. As the temperature within the tube increases, the pressure also increases resulting in a movement of the needle in the gauge. The scale displays temperature but is truly measuring pressure.

The **resistance thermometer** consists of a length of fine coiled wire, frequently platinum, whose resistance increases linearly with temperature (Fig. 33.9).

A **thermistor** ("thermal resistor") is an electrical resistor whose resistance varies inversely with temperature (Fig. 33.9). It is usually based on a bead of a metal oxide.

A **thermocouple** consists of two dissimilar conductors in contact and is based on the principle that a junction of dissimilar metals will produce a temperature-dependent electric potential, a phenomenon known as the thermoelectric, or Seebeck, effect (Fig. 33.10).

Temperature sensing chips (integrated circuit sensors) are popular in many applications because of their low-cost, high degree of linearity, and relatively high voltage outputs.

Infrared thermometers determine the temperature of an object from a portion of the thermal radiation ("blackbody radiation") emitted by the object. Contact with the object is not needed.

33.4 Gas Physics

33.4.1 Kinetic Theory of Gases

On the microscopic scale, gases are modeled by the **kinetic theory of gases**. This model assumes that the molecules have very small sizes relative to the distance between them and that the molecules are in constant, random motion (Fig. 33.11) related to their **kinetic energy**, which is given by $\mathbf{e = ½mv^2}$, where m is the mass of the molecules and v is its velocity.

The molecules frequently collide with each other and with the walls of the container holding the gas molecules. Like all molecules, gas molecules have physical properties of mass, velocity, momentum, and energy. At the macroscopic level, these properties are related to properties of density, pressure, and temperature. In the case of temperature, the temperature of a gas is related to the mean kinetic energy of the gas; the higher the temperature, the greater the molecular motion.

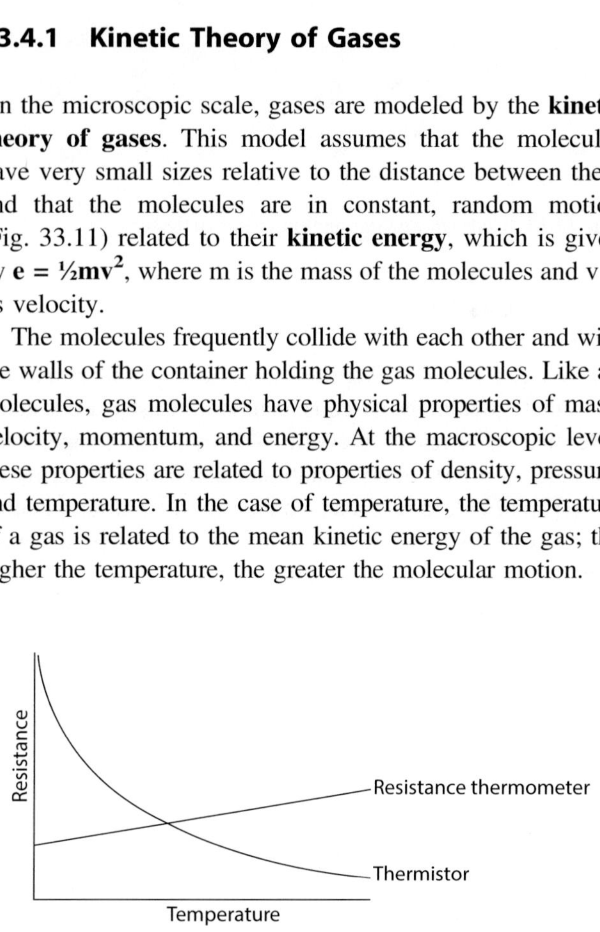

Fig. 33.9 Resistance changes based on temperature

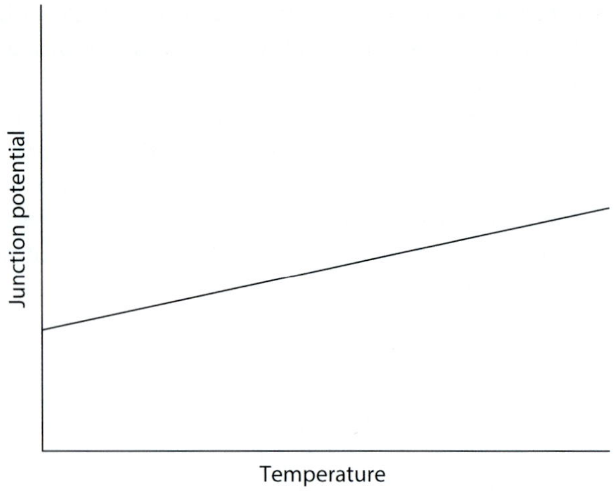

Fig. 33.10 The seebeck effect

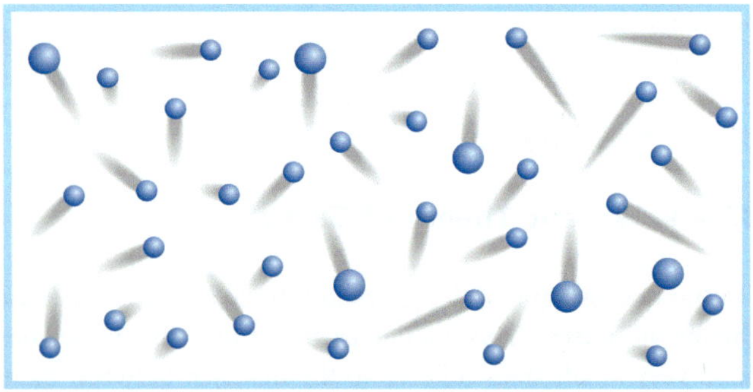

Fig. 33.11 Constant random motion of gas molecules

33.4.2 Gas Laws

Air is a gas, and it is therefore important to understand the laws that govern its gaseous behavior. Gases are usually described in terms of pressure, volume, and temperature. Pressure is most often quantified clinically in terms of mmHg, cmH_2O, kPa, or bar, volume in ml, and temperature in degrees Celsius or degrees Fahrenheit. Perhaps the most important law of gas flow in airways is the Ideal (or Perfect) Gas Law, which can be written as:

$$PV = nRT$$

where P = pressure of gas (Pascals or mm Hg),

V = volume of gas (m^3 or cm^3 or ml)

n = number of moles of the gas in volume V,

R = gas constant (8.3143 J g-mol^{-1} K^{-1}, assuming P in Pascals, V in m^3)

T = absolute temperature (in Kelvins or K, 273.16 K = 0 ° C).

The ideal gas law is the equation of state of a hypothetical ideal gas. It is a good approximation to the behavior of many gases under many conditions and is derived from Avagadro's Law, Boyle's Law, and Charles' Law.

Avogadro's Law. Avogadro stated that equal volumes of all ideal gases at the same temperature and pressure contain the same number of molecules. One mole is the quantity of a substance containing the same number of particles as there are in 0.012 kg of ^{12}C. This number is 6.023×10^{23} molecules and is called **Avogadro's number**. One mole of an ideal gas takes up 22.4 L at standard temperature and pressure (STP). STP may be defined as a temperature of 273.16 K at 1 atmosphere (760 mm Hg).

Boyle's law, which is the First Ideal Gas Law, states that, at a constant temperature, the product of pressure and volume is equal to a constant (Fig. 33.12), that is, P × V = Constant (at constant T). Hence, P is proportional to 1/V. Gases do not obey Boyle's law at temperatures approaching their point of liquefaction (the state where the gas becomes a liquid). A simple application of Boyle's Law is the calculation concerning the contents of a cylinder of oxygen. If a 10 L cylinder of oxygen is at a pressure of 137 bar (13,700 kPa), then this same quantity of gas at atmospheric pressure (100 kPa) will occupy 1370 L.

Charles' law states that, at a constant pressure, volume is proportional to temperature, that is, V is proportional to T (at constant P). See Fig. 33.13.

Gay-Lussac's law states that, at a constant volume, pressure is proportional to temperature, so that

$$P/T = k_3$$

When a gas obeys both Charles' law and Boyle's law, it is said to be an ideal gas and obeys the ideal gas law, PV = *n*RT, as previously described.

The above laws mandate the input or removal of heat energy to the system. However, the state of a gas can be altered without adding energy into the system. This is called an Adiabatic Process and is defined as a thermodynamic process during which no energy is transferred as heat across the boundaries of the system. An example of this is the rapid compression of a gas. This will cause a rise in temperature, sometimes requiring cooling. This is particularly relevant with respect to anesthesia. When an oxygen cylinder connected to the back of an anesthetic machine is turned on rapidly, the rapid compression of the gases in the connecting pipes and gauges causes an increase in temperature.

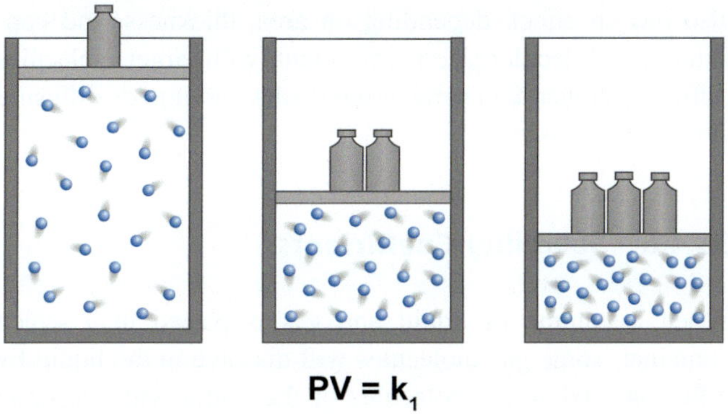

Fig. 33.12 Boyle's law

We may also make use of this Adiabatic Process with an instrument called the Cryoprobe. This is an instrument that has an extremely cold tip, as low as − 70 °C and is used in dermatology, gynecology, and ophthalmic surgery in order to rapidly freeze tissues. The principle of the Cryoprobe is to allow the release and therefore rapid expansion of a gas, typically nitrous oxide or carbon dioxide, in the tip of a handheld probe. The rapid expansion of the gas causes a large fall in temperature as the energy to overcome the attraction between the molecules of the gas has to come from the kinetic energy of the molecules themselves.

33.4.3 Non-ideal Gases: The Van Der Waals Effect

Ideal gases are assumed to have no forces of interaction. Real gases, however, have intermolecular attraction, resulting in a weak force of attraction. This is called a Van Der Waals Force and requires that the ideal gas law be written as:

$$\left[P + \frac{an^2}{v^2}\right](V - nb) = nRT$$

where

P = pressure of gas (Pascals or mm Hg),

V = volume of gas (m^3 or cm^3 or ml)

n = number of moles of the gas in volume V,

R = gas constant (8.3143 J g-mol^{-1} K^{-1} assuming P in Pascals, V in m^3)

T = absolute temperature (K),

a, b = physical constants for a given gas

The terms a and b for a given gas may be found in physical chemistry textbooks and other sources. This formulation, provided by van der Waals, accounts for intermolecular forces fairly well.

33.4.4 Critical Temperature and Critical Pressure

Critical temperature is defined as the temperature above which a gas cannot be liquefied, regardless of the pressure applied to the gas.

Fig. 33.13 Charles' law

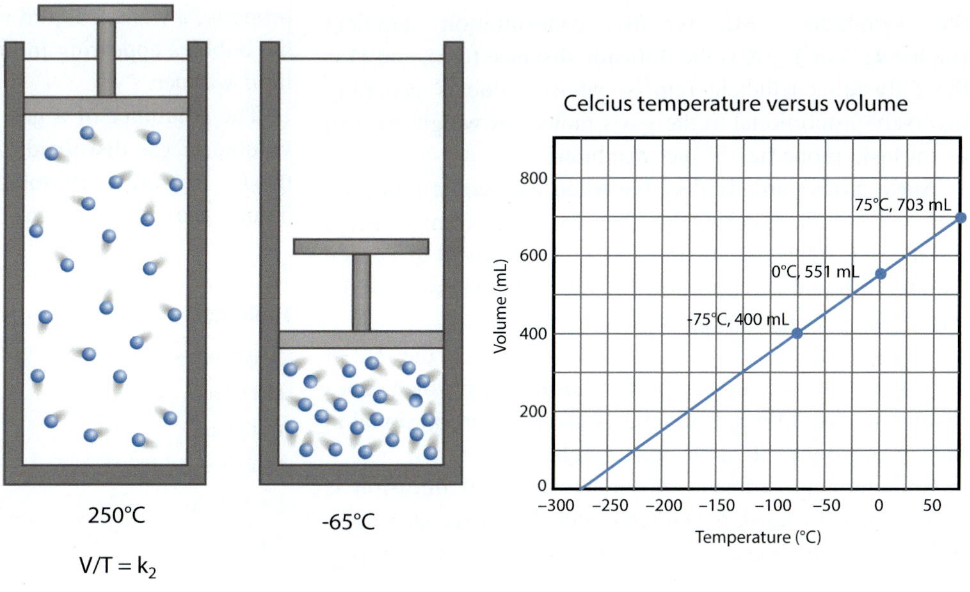

For example, when preparing medical gases, oxygen will always be a gas at room temperature as its critical temperature is − 119 °C. However, when a nitrous oxide cylinder is filled, there is a pressure at which the nitrous oxide is liquefied at room temperature as the critical temperature of nitrous oxide is 36.5 °C.

The **critical pressure** of a gas is the vapor pressure exerted by a substance at its critical temperature.

The terms critical temperature and critical pressure apply to a single gas. When there is a mixture of gases, there is a temperature at which the gases may separate into their constituent components. This is termed the **pseudocritical temperature**. This is clinically important as Entonox may separate into Oxygen and Nitrous Oxide at a cylinder temperature of − 5.5 °C, which when opened, may deliver a hypoxic mix to a patient. The pseudocritical temperature of Entonox at pipeline pressure (59 psi) is − 30 °C, therefore it normally has no risk of separation in hospital pipelines.

33.4.5 Diffusion of Gases

Diffusion describes the process of the movement of molecules through a layer or surface. Clinically, diffusing of gases through a membrane is most applicable to gas flow across alveolar membranes. The most used relation to govern diffusion is **Fick's first law of diffusion**, which states that the rate of diffusion of a gas across a barrier is proportional to the concentration gradient for the gas. Fick's law may be expressed mathematically as:

$$\text{Flux} = -D\frac{\Delta C}{\Delta X}$$

where the Flux is the number of molecules/cm^2/s crossing the membrane, ΔC is the concentration gradient (molecules/cm^3), ΔX is the diffusion distance (cm), and D is the diffusion coefficient (cm^2/s) whose value is generally inversely proportional to the gas's molecular weight as well as intrinsic properties of the membrane.

Since gases partially dissolve when they come into contact with liquid, **Henry's law** becomes important in some instances. It states that the mass of a gas dissolved in a given amount of liquid is proportional to the partial pressure of the gas in the gas phase at constant temperature.

The varying size of gas molecules also affects the rate of diffusion. This is described by **Graham's Law** which states that the rate of diffusion of a gas is inversely proportional to the square root of its molecular weight.

Summarizing diffusion, it can be said that diffusion is proportional to tension gradients and therefore, also solubility. The membrane across which diffusion is occurring also has an effect, depending on area, thickness, and constituents. Molecular size is important, with larger molecules diffusing slower than smaller molecules and liquids diffusing slower than gases.

33.4.6 Solubility Coefficients

When a volume of liquid and gas is placed in a sealed container, some gas molecules will dissolve in the liquid by diffusion, and some molecules of the liquid will evaporate into the gas to form a vapor. Evaporation is the process whereby atoms or molecules in a liquid state gain sufficient kinetic energy to overcome the surface tension and become a gas. Eventually, this will reach a state of equilibrium, where there is the maximum amount of gas dissolved and maximum amount of liquid evaporated, at a constant temperature. At this point, the solution is termed a saturated solution and the partial pressure exerted by the vapor is termed the saturated vapor pressure.

Vapor pressure describes the partial pressure contributed by various liquids. When a liquid's vapor pressure equals atmospheric pressure, a liquid boils. The concept of vapor pressure is important in the design of anesthetic vaporizers. The vapor pressure of a liquid increases with its temperature (Table 33.3).

Temperature and pressure both have direct effects on the amount of gas dissolved in a liquid. If the pressure of the gas above the liquid doubles then, at equilibrium, there will be twice the amount of gas molecules dissolved in the liquid. This is defined by Henry's Law, which states that at a constant temperature, the amount of a given gas dissolved in a given liquid is directly proportional to the partial pressure of the gas in equilibrium with the liquid. As a general property, a warmer liquid will hold less dissolved gas, hence the bubbles appearing in line of saline after going through a fluid warmer.

The solubility of a gas is also described in terms of the volume of gas dissolved in 1 L of solvent at STP. In anesthesia, the Ostwald Solubility Coefficient is used which defines the volume of gas that dissolves in 1 unit volume of

Table 33.3 Saturated vapor pressure of various anesthetic agents

Vapor pressure (kPa) at 20 °C	
Halothane	32.3
Isoflurane	33.2
Sevoflurane	22.7
Desflurane	89.2
N_2O	5200

the liquid at the temperature concerned. Because this solubility coefficient is independent of pressure, it takes into account the fact that while there is twice the amount of molecules of gas dissolved if the pressure of the gas is doubled, the volume that that amount of dissolved gas would occupy is the same at that pressure, due to Boyle's Law. Hence 0.01 L of nitrogen dissolved at atmospheric pressure (100 kPa) will occupy 0.05 L at 200 kPa. This is a problem for divers as the pressure of their inspired air increases by 1 atmosphere for approximately every 10 m of depth. If the diver resurfaces too quickly, the nitrogen dissolved in their blood and tissues at above atmospheric pressure can form bubbles as it expands with decreasing pressure causing pain, confusion, seizures, coma, and death if seriously affected.

33.4.7 Pressure, Flow, and Resistance

The laws of fluid mechanics dictate an intricate relationship among pressure, flow, and resistance. Pressure is defined as a force per unit area and as mentioned previously, is usually measured clinically as mmHg or cmH_2O. However, it is commonly measured scientifically in Pascals (Newtons force per square meter).

Flow (or the rate of flow) is equal to the change in pressure (pressure drop or pressure difference) divided by the resistance experienced by the fluid. For example, if the flow is 100 ml/s at a pressure difference of 100 mmHg, the resistance is 100 mmHg/100 ml/s = 1 mmHg/ml/s. In *laminar* flow systems only, the resistance is constant, independent of the flow rate.

An important relation that quantifies the relationship of pressure, flow, and resistance in laminar flow systems (Fig. 33.14), is given by the Hagen–Poiseuille (or simply, Poiseuille) equation. Poiseuille's law states that the fluid flow rate through a horizontal straight tube of uniform bore is proportional to the pressure gradient and the fourth power of the radius and is related inversely to the viscosity of the gas and the length of the tube. This law, *which is valid for laminar flow only*, may thus be stated as:

$$\Delta P = \frac{8\mu L}{\pi r^4} \times \text{Flow}$$

where μ is the fluid viscosity (poise [g/cm · s]) and L is the length of the tube (cm).

When the flow rate exceeds a *critical velocity* (the flow velocity below which flow is laminar), the flow loses its laminar velocity profile, becomes disorderly, and is termed *turbulent* (Fig. 33.15). The point at which this occurs may be calculated using Reynold's Number. This is a dimensionless number that helps predict when fluid flow becomes turbulent. The formula may be written as:

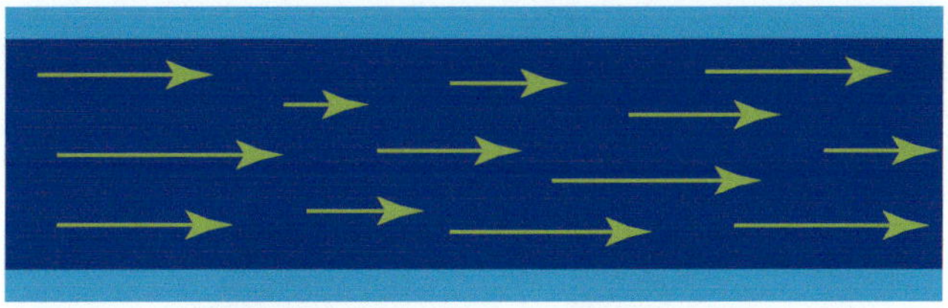

Fig. 33.14 Laminar flow

$$\text{Reynold's Number(Re)} = \frac{\text{Density} \times \text{Velocity} \times \text{Diameter of tube}}{\text{Viscosity}}$$

When Re < 2000, laminar flow is more likely and when Re > 2000, turbulent flow is more likely. When turbulent flow exists, the relationship between pressure drop and flow is no longer governed by the Hagen–Poiseuille equation. Instead, the pressure gradient required (or the resistance encountered) during turbulent flow varies as the square of the flow rate.

Laminar Flow. When flow is low velocity and through long narrow tubes, it tends to be more orderly and streamlined and to flow in a straight line. This type of flow is called laminar flow. Laminar flow is directly proportional to the driving pressure. During quiet breathing, laminar flow exists from the medium-sized bronchi down to the level of the bronchioles. During exercise, when the airflow is more rapid, laminar flow may be confined to the smallest airways.

Turbulent Flow. When air flows at higher velocities, especially through an airway with irregular walls, flow is generally disorganized, even chaotic, and tends to form eddies. This turbulent flow is found mainly in the largest airways, like the trachea (Fig. 33.16).

33.4.8 Flow Through an Orifice

Flow through an orifice (defined as a tube whose length is smaller than its radius) is always somewhat turbulent. Clinically, airway-obstructing conditions such as epiglottitis or swallowed obstructions are often best viewed as breathing through an orifice. Under such conditions, the approximate

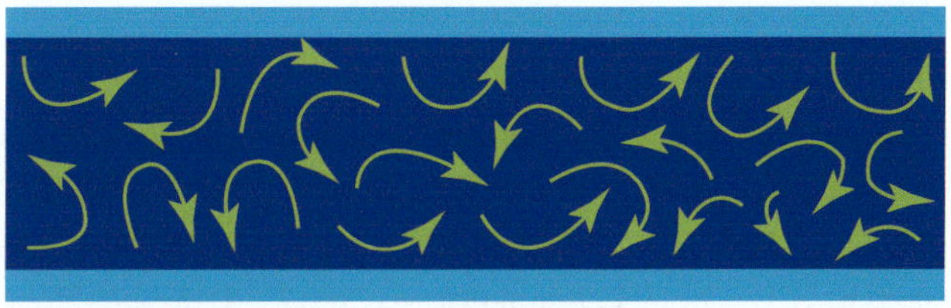

Fig. 33.15 Turbulent flow

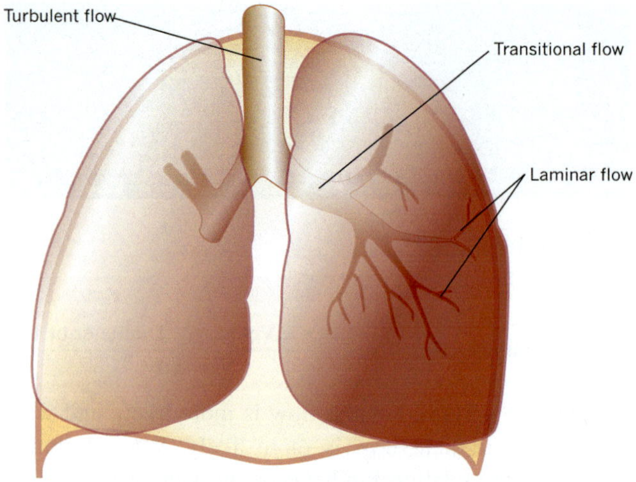

Fig. 33.16 Types of flow under relaxed breathing conditions

flow across the orifice varies inversely with the square root of the gas **density**. This is in contrast to laminar flow conditions, where gas flow varies inversely with gas **viscosity**. The viscosity values for helium and oxygen are similar, but their densities are very different (Table 33.4). Table 33.5 provides useful data to allow comparison of gas flow rates through an orifice.

33.4.8.1 Helium–oxygen Mixtures

The low density of helium allows it to play a significant clinical role in the management of some forms of airway obstruction. The usual available mixtures of helium and oxygen are 20% O_2: 80% He and 30% O_2: 70% He and are usually administered by a non-rebreathing face mask in patients who face an increased work-of-breathing effort because of the presence of airway pathology (e.g., edema) but in whom endotracheal intubation is preferably withheld at this time.

33.4.8.2 Clinical Vignette

Rudow et al. provide the following story (*Rudow M, Hill AB, Thompson NW* et al.: *Helium–oxygen mixtures in airway obstruction due to thyroid carcinoma, Canadian Anaesthestists' Society Journal 33:498, 1986.*) A 78-year-old woman with both breast cancer and ophthalmic melanoma developed airway obstruction from a thyroid carcinoma that extended into her mediastinum and compressed her trachea. She had a 2-month history of worsening dyspnea, especially when positioned supine. On examination, inspiratory and expiratory stridor was present. Noted on the chest x-ray were a large superior mediastinal mass and pulmonary metastases. A solid mass was identified on a thyroid ultrasound scan. Computed tomography revealed a large mass at the thoracic inlet and extending caudally. Clinically, the patient was exhausted and in respiratory distress.

Almost instant relief was obtained by giving the patient a mixture of 78% He: 22% O_2, with improvements in measured tidal volume and oxygenation. Later, a thyroidectomy was carried out to relieve the obstruction. Here, anesthesia was conducted by applying topical anesthesia to the airway with awake laryngoscopy and intubation performed in the sitting position. Once the airway was secured using an armored tube, the patient was given a general anesthetic with an intravenous induction. Following the surgery, extubation occurred without complication.

Table 33.4 Viscosity and density differences of anesthetic gases

	Viscosity@ 300 K	Density@ 20 °C
Air	18.6 μ(mu)Pa × s	1.293 g/L
Nitrogen	17.9 μ(mu)Pa × s	1.250 g/L
Nitrous oxide	15.0 μ(mu)Pa × s	1.965 g/L
Helium	20.0 μ(mu)Pa × s	0.178 g/L
Oxygen	20.8 μ(mu)Pa × s	1.429 g/L

Table 33.5 Relative gas flow rates through an orifice. Adapted from [1]

	%	Density (g/L)	Relative flow
Air	100	1.293	1.0
Oxygen	100	1.429	0.96
Helium (He)	100	0.179	2.68
He-oxygen	20/80	1.178	1.048
He-oxygen	60/40	0.678	1.381
He-oxygen	80/20	0.429	1.73

33.4.9 Laplace's Law

One consideration that is important in anesthesia is Laplace's law for a sphere. It states that, for a sphere with one air–liquid interface (e.g., an alveolus), the equation relating the transmural pressure difference, surface tension, and sphere radius is:

$$P = \frac{2T}{R}$$

where

P = transmural pressure difference (dynes/cm^2) [1 dyne/cm^2 = 0.1 Pa = 0.000 751 torr],

T = surface tension (dynes/cm)

R = sphere radius (cm)

The key point in Laplace's law is that the smaller the sphere radius, the higher the transmural pressure. However, real (in vivo) alveoli do *not* obey Laplace's law because of the action of pulmonary surfactant, which acts to decrease the surface tension disproportionately than that which is predicted using physical principles. When pulmonary surfactant is missing from the lungs, the lungs take on the behavior described by Laplace's law, making the alveoli collapse on themselves and then being almost impossible to reinflate. This is why surfactant is so important clinically.

33.4.10 The Bernoulli Effect and the Venturi Principle

The fall in pressure at points of flow constriction (where the flow velocity is higher) is known as the Bernoulli effect and is due to an increase in kinetic energy across the narrowing. As the kinetic energy increases, the potential energy must fall as the total energy of the system must remain constant. Consequently, pressure falls, as illustrated in Fig. 33.17. In essence, passing a fluid through a narrow orifice will lead to a pressure reduction along with an increase in the fluid velocity.

This phenomenon is used in apparatus employing the Venturi principle, for example, gas nebulizers, Venturi flowmeters, and some oxygen face masks. If an opening is placed at the narrowing, the lower pressure due to the Bernoulli effect sucks in (entrains) air to mix with oxygen. It can also be used as a source of laboratory suction.

33.4.11 Flowmeters

Many flowmeters are just disguised pressure gauges employing a flow restrictor or orifice with a known resistance (Fig. 33.18). Flow is determined from pressure using the following relationship:

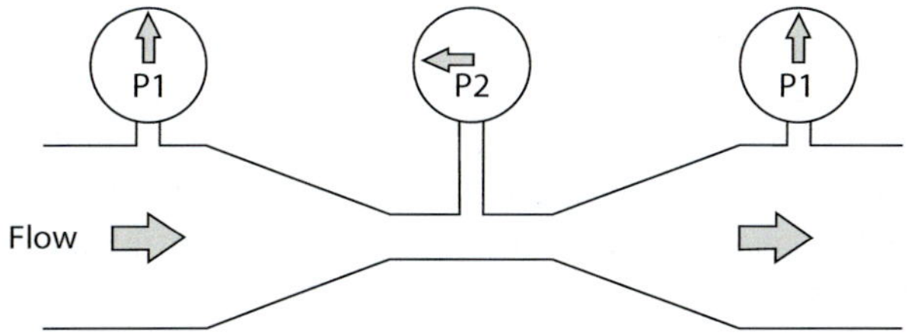

Fig. 33.17 The Venturi principle

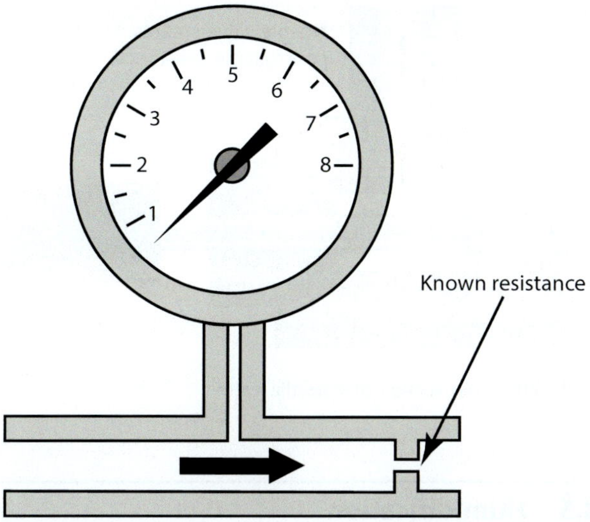

Fig. 33.18 A pressure gauge calibrated to display flow

$$\text{Flow} = \text{Pressure} \times \text{Resistance}$$

Modern anesthesia machines that display flow rates as a figure on a screen may also employ this relationship between pressure and flow – the flow may be derived using a pressure transducer measuring the pressure in a tube with a fixed, known resistance.

Flowmeters in many older anesthesia machines and current floor oxygen delivery systems employ a sapphire ball or similar indicator in a Thorpe tube, which is wider at the top than at the bottom. The higher the flow, the higher the ball rises. Flow is read at the center of the ball (Fig. 33.19).

The flow is controlled using a needle valve, which creates a variable resistance that may be adjusted by the user (Fig. 33.20).

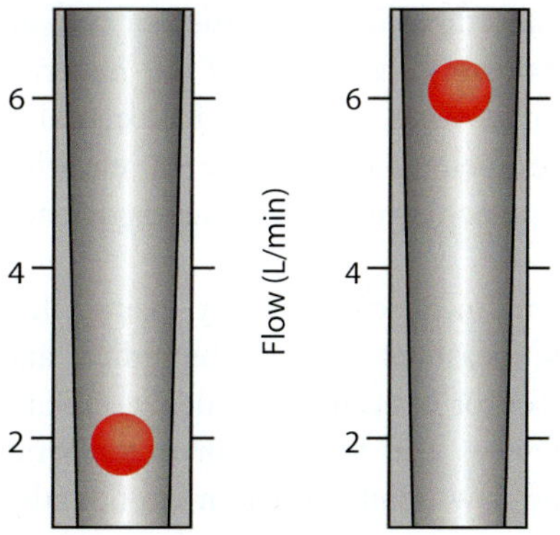

Fig. 33.19 Design of a standard flowmeter

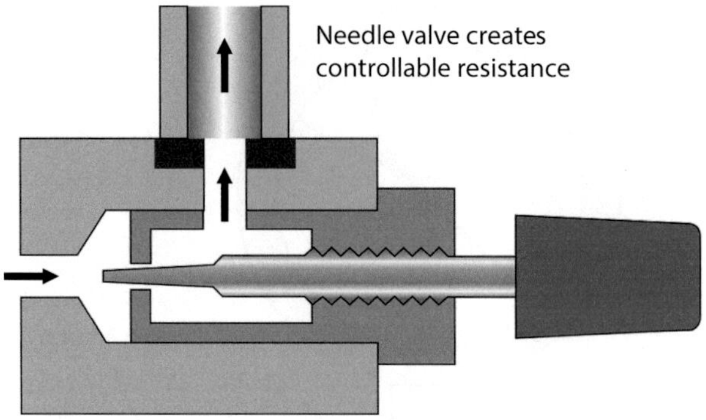

Fig. 33.20 Cross section of a needle valve

33.5 Humidification

33.5.1 Definitions

Humidity describes the amount of water vapor (the gaseous state of water) in the air. There are two measurements of humidity of interest to clinicians: absolute humidity and relative humidity.

Absolute humidity is the absolute water content of air at a given temperature expressed in grams per cubic meter. **Relative humidity**, conventionally expressed as a percent, describes the existing absolute humidity in relation to the maximum possible for that temperature. Note that humid air is less dense than dry air because a molecule of water (MW = 18) has less mass than either a molecule of nitrogen (MW = 28) or a molecule of oxygen (MW = 32).

33.5.2 Measurement

Humidity is measured using a hygrometer, which has several designs and principles. In the metal-paper coil type hygrometer water vapor is absorbed onto a salt-impregnated paper strip attached to a metal coil, causing the coil to change shape. In capacitive hygrometers, the effect of humidity on the dielectric properties of a material is measured, i.e., reflecting the ability of the material to store an electrical charge when used in an electrical capacitor. In resistive hygrometers, the change in electrical resistance (rather than capacitance) of a material due to humidity is measured.

The measurement of humidity using these electrical devices only measures absolute humidity, and a separate temperature sensor is needed to calculate relative humidity. Yet other devices use the measured temperature of condensation (the dew point) to determine humidity.

33.5.3 Clinical Uses

When breathing, the upper respiratory tract naturally humidifies air to a humidity of 34 g/m^3. If this process is bypassed, by for example an endotracheal tube, then dry air will desiccate the lower airways resulting in dry and tenacious sputum forming plugs that may block bronchi.

In order to humidify the gases in an anesthetized patient a heat and moisture exchange (HME) filter is commonly used. This small filter is attached at the patient end of the circle and contains a small block of paper, sponge, foam, or similar material that is impregnated with a hygroscopic substance. When warm, moist air passes through this filter during expiration, the air is cooled and moisture forms on the filter. This moisture then evaporates and is returned to the patient during inspiration.

Physiotherapists use humidification to treat patients. This is often done by using a water bath which heats saline causing evaporation. The patient then breathes in this humidified gas via a delivery system. A much greater level of humidity may be achieved using an ultrasonic plate which vibrates causing the release of very fine droplets as a vapor when either a liquid is dropped onto the plate, or the plate vibrates under the surface of a liquid.

33.6 The Principle of Doppler Ultrasound

The Doppler Effect describes how the frequency of a sound, and therefore perceived pitch, changes as the origin of the sound passes the observer. This occurs due to the manner in which sound is propagated. Sound waves are regions of high and low pressure that are generated by a source and that travel through air at STP at a fixed speed (approximately 340 m/s). If the source moves toward the observer of the sound, then the distance between the high-pressure points in the sound wave will reduce, reducing the wavelength, which results in a perceived increase in frequency. The reciprocal is true as the sound source moves away from the observer, resulting in an increased wavelength, and lower frequency.

This principle is used in Doppler Ultrasound. This is commonly used as an ultrasonic blood flow detector in vascular medicine. A vibrating crystal in a handheld probe is placed on the skin over an artery. The crystal produces very high-frequency ultrasound waves. The movement of red blood cells toward the probe head causes the reflection of the ultrasound waves and a slight change in pitch of the reflected wave. While no quantitative values can be measured, the change in pitch is converted to an audible sound that the observer can then use to make an assessment of blood flow within the artery.

33.7 Medical Alarms

Microcomputer technology has revolutionized the design of patient monitors for use in modern hospital Operating Rooms (ORs) and Intensive Care Units (ICUs). Until recent years, separate monitors existed for tracking blood pressure, the electrocardiogram (EKG), arterial oxygen levels, etc. Each monitor had its own alarm system with its own default alarms conventions, but all alarms tended to sound the same, as manufacturers all used similar piezoelectric acoustical devices to provide audio warning signals. The result was an unintegrated, awkward system of monitors often designed such that when an alarm sounded the user had to visually scan all the monitors to establish the source of the alarm.

Aware of these difficulties, manufacturers of anesthesia machines and patient monitors set about to design integrated patient monitoring systems, where all alarms are routed through a common operator interface to facilitate alarm recognition and management. A number of exciting developments such as redundant signal methods or "smart alarms" have now been introduced either commercially or experimentally, with considerable potential to improve patient safety.

Despite all these developments, many anesthesiologists working in the "clinical trenches" have become quite cynical about many of the developments in clinical alarm technology, regarding them as more nuisances to deal with rather than as contributions to patient care. For example, many anesthesiologists note that because they are usually more-or-less permanently situated near the patient's head, they are able to keep an eye on the patient on a moment-to-moment basis, so that they are usually aware of any clinical deterioration before an alarm sounds, with the result that when the alarm does sound, dealing with the alarm (e.g. silencing it, etc.) may distract the anesthesiologist from his or her efforts to treat the patient (e.g. administering drugs to restore the patient's blood pressure into the normal range).

Of course, an important counter-argument to this line of thought is that anesthesiologists do not always maintain 100% vigilance, especially when fatigued or distracted, so that alarms may notify him or her of any life-threatening conditions that may have escaped their notice. This argument may be especially true in the ICU setting, where a physician will be caring for many patients.

The potential value of alarms notwithstanding, a high level of frustration exists among healthcare workers about clinical alarm designs. Of all the complaints presented by clinicians about current alarm technology, unquestionably the high rate of false alarms would be first on their list. For example, even small amounts of patient movement can introduce artifacts into the patient's electrocardiogram, pulse oximeter signal, blood pressure signal, and other monitored variables. Quite often the artifact is not recognized to be garbage by the alarm management software, resulting in the false annunciation of some alarm condition. So common and so frustrating is this situation that many of my colleagues globally disable all alarms to allow them to focus on caring for the patient rather than dealing with false alarms.

(Note that the "alarm policy engine" in some advanced alarm designs may not allow some alarms to be disabled under ANY circumstances. A good example is an alarm signaling a low concentration of oxygen in the gas mixture with which the patient's lungs are being ventilated. This would be an appropriate alarm policy setting since false alarms are rare for the oxygen concentration signal and since low oxygen levels can quickly lead to brain damage).

Edworthy and Meredith [1] reviewed many of the issues of alarm design from the perspective of cognitive psychology, with an emphasis on the construction of effective alarm sounds. They point out that there may be circumstances where excessive use of auditory warnings may be counter-productive, while the principle of "urgency mapping" (involving a graded series of alarms with increasing perceived urgency levels) may be helpful to produce ergonomically sensible alarm systems.

In a study by Kestin et al. [2], 50 patients undergoing anesthesia were monitored to determine the frequency of false alarms. They found that 75% of all the alarms overall were spurious, 22% represented a change above the upper alarms limits, but only 3% corresponded to patient risk situations. With electrocardiogram (ECG) alarms the situation was worse, with 81% of the alarms being spurious, 19% representing a change above the upper alarm limits, and 0% representing a patient risk situation. Similar results were obtained with blood pressure alarms, and heart rate alarms from pulse oximeters.

A similar study by Lawless [3] reviewed the false alarm problem in a pediatric ICU. During a seven-day period, ICU staff recorded the type and number of alarms, categorizing them as false, significant, or due to staff manipulations. Of 2176 alarm soundings, 68% were false, 26.5% were due to staff manipulations, while only 5.5% were significant. Of interest, the pulse oximeter was the largest alarm source (44%), with ventilators (31%), and electrocardiograms (24%) being other common alarm sources. By contrast, only 1% of alarms were from the capnometer, a device that measures expired carbon dioxide levels from the lung.

As already noted, not infrequently, anesthesiologists disable alarms at the beginning of a case to avoid false alarms and other alarm-related difficulties. McIntyre [4] conducted a retrospective study in which he asked the question "Have you ever deliberately deactivated an audible alarm device at the start of a case?". The majority (57%) of respondents replied "Yes".

These and other studies tend to support two points. First, most alarms (fortunately) do not signify a potentially critical medical event. (In fact, in a study by O'Carroll [5] only eight of 1455 alarms related to such events while Kestin et al. [2] found that only 3% of alarms represented life-threatening events.) Secondly, poorly performing alarm systems may hinder, rather than help, the delivery of clinical care [1, 6], especially in environments where noise pollution may be problematic [7].

33.7.1 "Smart" Alarm Systems in Computerized Medical Equipment

In recent years, a number of developments in clinical alarm technology have been introduced commercially or experimentally with considerable potential to improve patient safety. These developments have been influenced by new concepts in ergonomics and cognitive engineering, as well as on comments from real-world practitioners. Examples of important developments include:

1. **Prioritized alarms** e.g., low, medium, and high priority alarms with associated audio and video characteristics designed to convey a sense of urgency).
2. **Cascading alarms** - alarms that increase in severity over time if the original problem is not fixed.
3. **Psychoacoustically optimized auditory alarms** that are nonstartling but convey a sense of how urgent the alarm is.
4. **"Smart" alarms** (knowledge-based alarms) that combine expert systems' techniques with alarm technology either to provide more informative alarms or to reduce the frequency of false alarms, or to provide clinicians initial suggestions about how to deal with the problem behind the alarm.
5. **"Integrated" alarm systems**, where monitoring devices are all connected to a central alarm management system that controls both the audio alarm pattern, and any information displayed (usually on a video display).

33.7.2 Integrated Alarms

One problem with the addition of numerous separate patient monitoring devices in the Operating Room is the existence of a variety of different alarm devices, all with similar audio characteristics that may make it difficult to readily determine the alarm source. This and related problems have been a motivating factor in the development of so-called "integrated" alarm systems. The key idea behind integrated alarms is that all monitoring devices are connected to a central alarm management system that controls both the audio alarm pattern and any information displayed (usually on electronic display). The alarm characteristics (sound intensity, sound pattern, etc.) in turn depend on the assigned alarm priority (high, medium, low) based on national, and/or international standards (eg. ISO 9703).

Without doubt, the development of integrated monitoring systems is a significant clinical development, and as such continues to be the result of important standards efforts across the globe. Nevertheless, some limitations of such integrated alarm systems have become apparent, at least with some designs. Two case reports illustrate the point.

Jones et al. [8] describe a critical anesthetic accident related to the use of an integrated alarm system where a patient accidentally received a hypoxic gas mixture (one too low in oxygen concentration), but the problem was not immediately recognized because of the existence of a single audible alarm sounding to signal the existence of three alarm conditions, one being of primary importance (low oxygen concentration) and the other two being a result of the first condition (low patient oxygen levels and high heart rate). The authors make suggestions to improve the design of integrated alarm systems and note that "A hierarchical system of sound pattern, and repetition may convey an appropriate degree of urgency and minimize the obtrusiveness of alarms that are less serious".

A similar case report was presented by Chui and Gin [9] where an anesthetic circuit disconnect was not immediately recognized because of the nature of the integrated alarm system in handling multiple alarm conditions. The following commentary by the authors is noteworthy:

> "We think that the integrated alarm system .... contributed partly to the mishap. After the sounding of a warning alarm, the system will not provide further audible signals despite triggering by other monitors.... We believe that certain modifications to the alarm system may be desirable. The warning system should change either its pitch, or its loudness to warn against continuous sounding of the alarm. The integrated alarm system should also either change the prevailing audible signals if there is further triggering of the warning alarms. Anesthesiologists should be aware that allowing the audible warming system to sound continuously has the same effect as disabling all the audible alarms."

33.7.3 Smart Alarms

Active consideration of so-called "smart alarms" has arisen in recent times by clinicians, manufacturers, and standards bodies, all of whom are interested in providing meaningful alarm systems with increased reliability. Such alarms may be capable of making decisions without operator intervention by utilizing a priori knowledge (and are thus sometimes called "knowledge-based alarms"). Such alarm designs, for example, may offer the ability to change alarm priority with elapsed time ("cascading" alarms) or to suppress secondary alarms that are the consequence of a primary alarm condition. Yet other smart alarm designs may suggest either a diagnosis (or diagnostic list) compatible with a set of variables or suggest an operator intervention to learn more about how to handle the situation.

With respect to making management suggestions, some experimental smart alarm systems offer a context-sensitive display triggered by an alarm. For instance, if a patient's heart rate goes too low, say under 30 or 35 beats per minute, it might suggest giving atropine, calling for the crash cart, and checking for low oxygen levels in the patient. It could even page the responsible physician to inform him that one of his patients is in trouble. Note, however, that if the information offered is off-base, this hurts rather than helps the situation. (Such problems have been known to occur with smart alarm systems in the aviation environment.)

Technical developments in progress at the moment are leading to the eventual complete interconnection and computer control of ICU and Operating Room devices such as the anesthesia workstation, the patient monitor, the pulse oximeter, and even drug infusion pumps. Most of these efforts are centered on the so-called "Medical Information Bus" (IEEE Standard 1073). In particular, the ability to regulate infusion pumps from a central control point offers obvious potential advantages when many infusion pumps are used, as is common in the ICU or cardiac surgery environment. However, a less appreciated potential benefit of such an arrangement is that it may allow for automatic initial management of certain hazardous clinical conditions. For example, it is commonplace to use infusions of dopamine (a drug which raises blood pressure), and sodium nitroprusside (a drug which lowers blood pressure) during and after cardiac surgery. However, not infrequently the anesthesiologist may momentarily forget that a drug infusion is running, and may forget to turn off an existing nitroprusside infusion as their first response to the management of a hypotensive (low blood pressure) episode, or forget to discontinue an existing dopamine infusion in order to treat an episode of hypertension (excessive blood pressure). The ability to control infusion pumps from a central controlling station offers the potential to provide early warning about such events.

For example, as noted above, this arrangement might allow for "smart" alarms to suggest to the anesthesiologist, for example, to discontinue a nitroprusside infusion when a low blood pressure alarm has been triggered. It would even be possible to automatically discontinue the offending infusion if no manual response was detected within a given time period. Indeed, the concept of "smart alarms" could even be extended, for example, to have automatic initiation of a drug to support the blood pressure should the crisis not be resolved in a timely manner. Along the same lines, smart alarms could even be designed to automatically "call for help" should certain clinical crises not be resolved in an acceptable time period.

As exciting as these concepts are, however, experience with complex systems suggests that skepticism and even paranoia remain appropriate. Designers must remember that automatic computer interventions can occur in error.

33.7.4 Alarm Glossary

Alarm A signal indicating the occurrence of a condition (new onset or duration beyond a maximum time limit) that requires an intervention by the operator.

Threshold alarms An alarm that triggers when a variable exceeds (or drops below) a fixed threshold.

Redundant alarms An alarm arrangement that uses collateral information.

Collateral information A second source of information that can serve to reduce the frequency of false alarms in a monitored variable (such as heart rate) by introducing redundancy into the system.

Integrated alarms An arrangement that connects together a number of separate alarm systems into a common information display arrangement with alarm prioritization and visual and auditory enunciators.

Cascading alarms An alarm arrangement where the severity of an alarm condition increases over time when the precipitating event is not eliminated.

"Smart" alarms (knowledge-based alarms) Alarm systems that are capable of decision-making, for example, to allow for context-sensitive alarm prioritization or to suppress alarms which are the consequence of a primary alarm.

Low priority alarm A signal indicating the need for operator awareness.

Medium priority alarm A signal indicating that a prompt operator response is required.

High priority alarm A signal indicating that an immediate operator response is required.

Questions to MCQs

1. **Identify the true statement regarding pressure:**
   a. The pressure within a full medical gas cylinder may be safely applied directly to a patient
   b. Airway pressures are commonly quoted in kPa or bar
   c. Absolute pressure is gauge pressure minus atmospheric pressure
   d. A pressure transducer creates a large (>3V) voltage when exposed to pressure e.A two-stage pressure reducing valve may be used in patient

demand inhalational device, e.g. for Entonox delivery

2. **Identify the false statement concerning Dalton's Law of Partial Pressures:**
   a. Dalton's Law of Partial Pressure applies to all gases, regardless of their physical or chemical properties
   b. In a cylinder of Entonox (50% O_2 and 50% N_2O), the partial pressure exerted by each of the 2 constituent gases is equal
   c. The partial pressure of O2 in air at STP is approximately 21 kPa (156 mm Hg)
   d. For the law to be true, the gases must be non-reacting
   e. The sum of all of the partial pressures will equal the total pressure of the gas
3. **Identify the false statement concerning the Ideal Gas Law:**
   a. Boyle's Law states that pressure is proportional to volume
   b. The volume of gaseous oxygen in a compressed cylinder may be calculated using Boyle's law
   c. Charles' law states that, at a constant pressure, volume is proportional to temperature
   d. At a constant volume, pressure is proportional to temperature e.The Ideal Gas Law applies only to ideal gases; corrections when intermolecular forces and other factors come into play may sometimes be needed
4. **Identify the true statement regarding medical gas cylinders:**

   a. An oxygen cylinder valve must be greased before attaching to an anesthetic machine
   b. All cylinders are endoscoped by the manufacturer at each filling
   c. Medical gas cylinders should never be taken into an MRI scanner
   d. The pressure in a full nitrous oxide cylinder is 138 bar
   e. Oxygen cylinders in the United States are painted green despite white being the color designated by the International Standards Organization (ISO 32:1977)
5. **Which if the following is true regarding temperature:**

   a. A glass thermometer can only be filled with mercury
   b. Absolute zero (−273.15 °C) is the lowest possible temperature
   c. A typical thermistor's resistance increases linearly with temperature
   d. Infrared thermometers are used to measure a patient's rectal temperature
   e. Tympanic membrane temperature measurements require contact with the tympanic membrane
6. **Which if the following is true regarding solubility:**

   a. At 20 °C, desflurane has a higher saturated vapor pressure than halothane
   b. Temperature and pressure have no effect on the amount of gas dissolved in a liquid
   c. As a general principle, a warmer liquid will hold more dissolved gas
   d. When a diver undergoes decompression, the dissolved oxygen forms bubbles which can cause the symptoms of 'the bends'
   e. When a liquid's vapor pressure equals atmospheric pressure, the liquid freezes
7. **Which if the following is false regarding rate of diffusion of a gas across a membrane:**

   a. Graham's law may be applied to the process that occurs in the lung alveoli
   b. It is proportional to the tension gradient (difference in partial pressure of the gas across the membrane)
   c. It is inversely proportional to the thickness of the membrane the gas passes through.
   d. It is proportional to its solubility and inversely proportional to the square root of its molecular weight (Graham's Law)
   e. Graham's law describes the rate at which a dissolved gas diffuses across a membrane given certain properties of the membrane such as membrane thickness and membrane surface area
8. **The Venturi principle may be used in the following except:**

   a. Internal operation of ventilators (pneumatic control systems)
   b. Suction generators
   c. Defibrillator operation
   d. Waste gas scavenging
   e. Venturi-type oxygen masks
9. **Which of the following is true of humidifiers:**

   a. A heat-moisture exchanger (HME) uses an active process for humidifying expired air
   b. Some HMEs are designed to reduce patient exposure to pathogens
   c. A cold water bath can provide humidification greater than that seen in the normal upper trachea

   d. Use of ultrasonic nebulizers to deliver asthma medications are far more effective than metered-dose inhalers used with spacers
   e. Normal humidity in the upper trachea is 90 g/m^3

10. **Which of the following is true concerning the Doppler shift principle:**

    a. When the wavelength of a sound wave shortens, the perceived pitch will decrease
    b. The Doppler shift is due to a change in the velocity of the sound
    c. Ultrasound waves can be heard
    d. An ultrasonic blood flow detector can quantify blood flow (volume over time)
    e. This principle is commonly used to monitor fetal wellbeing

Answers TO MCQs

1. **E**—The pressure in a full gas cylinder is very high indeed (wwell over 500 psi) and would cause severe barotrauma if applied directly to a patient. Airway pressures are usually quoted in cm H_2O, however other units may be applied. Absolute pressure is the sum of gauge and atmospheric pressure. Pressure transducers do not create a voltage. They work by altering their resistance or capacitance under pressure. A two stage pressure reducing valve is exactly the process for delivery of a cylinder stored gas to a patient. The same system is used to deliver oxygen to firefighters and pilots.
2. **A**—Dalton's Law of Partial Pressures only applies to an ideal gas and this gas should have components that are non-reacting. The partial pressure of each component is calculated by taking the percentage of that component of the total pressure exerted by the gas. So a 50/50 mix of 2 gases will exert the same partial pressure as each component will exert 50% of the total pressure. Oxygen will exert a partial pressure of 20.8kPa at STP as a component of room air.
3. **A**—Boyle's Law states that pressure is inversely proportional to volume, i.e. the greater the pressure, the less the volume. This gas law may be used to calculate total volume of a compressed gas, ie a size E O_2 cylinder containing 4.78 litres of gas at a pressure of 138 bar will expand to fill 660 litres of volume at atmospheric pressure (1 bar). The ideal gas law tends to fail at lower temperatures or higher pressures, when intermolecular forces and molecular size become important.
4. **E**—Exposing grease or oil to high pressure oxygen is a fire risk and may produce an explosion. Medical gas cylinders are endoscoped at testing, usually at intervals of every 5–10 years. Some gas cylinders are made from aluminum and are therefore MRI compatible (not being ferromagnetic); however, this should always be checked prior to entering an MRI room. A full nitrous oxide cylinder will have an internal pressure of 44 bar until the tank is almost empty. This is due to nitrous oxide being a liquid under pressure as it is usually stored below its critical temperature. In the US, O_2 cylinders are painted green despite white being the color designated by the International Standards Organization (ISO 32:1977)
5. **B**—A glass thermometer may also contain alcohol; this is commonly used to measure lower scale temperatures in the laboratory. Absolute zero is indeed the lowest possible temperature. A thermistor's resistance decreases in a non-linear fashion with increasing temperature. Infrared thermometers can be used to measure temperature rapidly and non-invasively but not in the rectal area. Rectal thermometry is often poorly tolerated, especially in children, since the thermometer is inserted just over 1 cm into the rectum and left in place for approximately 10 s. Tympanic membrane temperature measurements do not require contact with the tympanic membrane; they sense (transduce) the infrared radiation coming from the ear drum.
6. **A**—At 20 °C, desflurane has a higher saturated vapor pressure (669 mm Hg) than halothane (243), sevoflurane (157), isoflurane (238) or enflurane (172). As a result of its high vapor pressure, desflurane boils at a mere 22.8 °C. Temperature and pressure have a direct effect on the amount of gas dissolved in a liquid. A warmer liquid will generally hold less dissolved gas. This can be demonstrated by looking at the IV fluid leaving a line warmer. The symptoms of the 'bends' is caused by bubbles of nitrogen (not oxygen) coming out of solution during rapid decompression and lodging in blood vessels. When a liquid's vapor pressure equals atmospheric pressure, the liquid boils (not freezes).
7. **E**—Graham's law may indeed be applied to the process that occurs in the lung alveoli. According to Fick's Law, the diffusion rate of a gas across a membrane is proportional to the difference in partial pressure, proportional to the area of the membrane and inversely proportional to the thickness of the membrane. Graham's Law states that the rate of diffusion of

a gas is inversely proportional to the square root of its molecular weight and proportional to its solubility. Fick's Law (not Graham's law) describes the rate at which a dissolved gas diffuses across a membrane given properties of the membrane such as membrane thickness and membrane surface area.

8. **C**—All of these devices except the defibrillator may use the vacuum created by a Venturi to allow them to work.
9. **B**—A HME passively (not actively) humidifies inspired air using the moisture deposited on a membrane during expiration. Some HMEs are indeed designed to reduce patient exposure to pathogens, such as with the use of bactericidal membranes. A cold-water bath produces an absolute humidity of 33 g/m^3, compared to the normal humidity of the upper trachea, which is 44 g/m^3. Ultrasonic nebulizers use high frequency vibration to produce extremely small, highly stable droplets. but recent data suggest that metered-dose inhalers with spacers may be as efficacious as nebulizers for asthma treatment.
10. **E**—When the wavelength of a sound shortens, the frequency, and therefore perceived pitch will increase. This is due to the speed of sound being constant in a set medium, ie in air at stp the speed of sound is ~340 m/s. Human ears cannot hear ultrasound waves. An ultrasonic blood flow detector converts the reflected ultrasound signal into an audible sound which can be appreciated by the user. This is qualitative, not quantitative. A fetal heart monitor commonly uses the same technology to assess fetal heart rate during pregnancy and labor.

References

1. Edworthy J, Meredith CS. Cognitive psychology and the design of alarm sounds. Med Eng Phys. 1994;16:445–9.
2. Kestin IG, Miller BR, Lockhart CH. Auditory alarms during anesthesia monitoring. Anesthesiology. 1988;69:106–9.
3. Lawless ST. Crying wolf: false alarms in pediatric intensive care unit. Crit Care Med. 1994;22:981–5.
4. McIntyre JW. Ergonomics: anaesthetist's use of auditory alarms in the operating room. Int J Clin Monit Comput. 1985;2(1):47–55.
5. O'Carroll TM. Survey of alarms in an intensive therapy unit. Anaesthesia. 1986;41:724–34.
6. Momtahan K, Hetu R, Tansley B. Audibility and identification of auditory alarms in operating rooms and an intensive care unit. Ergonomics. 1993;36:1159–76.
7. Kam PCA, Kam AC, Thompson JF. Noise pollution in the anaesthetic and intensive care environment. Anaesthesia. 1994;49:982–6.
8. Jones D, Lawson A, Holland R. Integrated monitor alarms and "alarm overload." Anaesth Intensive Care. 1991;19:101–2.
9. Chui PT, Gin T. False alarms and the integrated alarm system: report of a potential hazard. Anesth Analg. 1994;79:192–3.

More Information

10. John Doyle D, Grady KO (1995) Physics and biomechanics of the airway. In: Benumof JL (eds.) Airway Management: Principles and Practice. C.V. Mosby
11. Davis PD, Kenny GNC (2003) Basic physics and measurement in Anaesthesia. Butterworth-Heinemann; 5th edition
12. Dorsch JA, Dorsch SE (1999) Understanding anesthesia equipment. Lippincott Williams & Wilkins; 4th edition
13. Yentis SM, Hirsch NP, Smith GB (2013) Anaesthesia and intensive care A-Z. Elsevier, Butterworth-Heinemann; 5th Edition
14. Hutton P, Cooper GM, James FM III, Butterworth JF IV. Fundamental principles and practice of Anaesthesia. Dunitz; 2002

Breathing Systems

34

Jack Buckley and Myroslav Figura

Abstract

Breathing systems were originally developed in 1907 to deliver nitrous oxide for anesthesia. An ideal breathing system would reliably deliver a set concentration of oxygen, effectively remove carbon dioxide, have low resistance to breathing with minimal dead space, be portable, have efficient use of gases, and conserve heat and humidity. Mapleson systems achieve most of the objectives with the exception of conservation of gases, heat, and humidity. Circle systems are significantly more complex, but by allowing rebreathing of exhaled gases, it leads to the conservation of gases, heat, and humidity. This increase in complexity requires frequent maintenance and limits the portability of the system. The rebreathing of the gases also increases the production of potentially harmful substances including compound A and carbon monoxide.

Keywords

Breathing systems • Mapleson circuits • Circle systems • Carbon dioxide absorber • Adjustable pressure relief valve • Dead space • Compound A • Carbon monoxide

Key Points

– Ideal features for a breathing system include reliable delivery of various concentrations of oxygen, effective removal of carbon dioxide, low resistance to breathing with minimal dead space, efficient use of gases, and conservation of heat and humidity in the airways.
– Mapleson circuits have the advantage of being able to provide positive pressure ventilation with a relatively simple and portable design. The disadvantages of Mapleson circuits include poor conservation of gases, heat, and humidity.
– The circle system improves the shortcomings of the Mapleson system with significant improvements in the ability to conserve gases, heat, and humidity. This comes at the expense of making a significantly more complex system that is not portable.
– The carbon dioxide absorber converts carbon dioxide into calcium carbonate. This allows the rebreathing of gases in the circle system.
– Compound A is produced when the strong base in the carbon dioxide absorber removes hydrogen fluoride from sevoflurane. It is a nephrotoxin in rats and has unclear clinical significance in humans.
– Carbon monoxide is produced by desiccated carbon dioxide absorbers. The risk is greatest with desflurane and first-start cases Monday morning. This occurs since the anesthesia machine is less likely to be used during the weekend and the carbon dioxide absorber can dry out when not in use.

34.1 Introduction

One of the first breathing systems was developed by Barth in 1907 for the use of nitrous oxide to provide anesthesia. It consisted of a nitrous oxide cylinder, a valve, and a reservoir bag. The valve could be adjusted to allow complete rebreathing from the reservoir bag to breathing completely from the atmosphere, or somewhere in between. This system allowed some degree of control of the amount of nitrous oxide and oxygen delivered to the patient. The next

J. Buckley (✉) · M. Figura
Department of Anesthesiology, UCLA Medical Center, Los Angeles, CA, USA
e-mail: jcbuckley@mednet.ucla.edu

M. Figura
e-mail: mfigura@mednet.ucla.edu

M. Argalious et al. (eds.), *Basic Sciences in Anesthesia*,
https://doi.org/10.1007/978-3-031-60203-0_34

step in the development of breathing systems occurred when Magill and Rowbothom designed a single lumen endotracheal tube. This led to the development of the "Magill's circuit" (Mapleson A circuit). Additional breathing systems were developed with the goal of designing one that was reliable and efficient for both spontaneous and controlled ventilation.

Requirements for breathing systems:

- Delivery of oxygen can be reliably delivered to the patient at the desired concentration and easily adjusted
- Effectively removes carbon dioxide
- Low resistance to breathing
- Minimal amount of dead space.

Desirable features:

- Efficient use of gases
- Humidification of gases
- Conservation of heat
- Portable
- Simple, sturdy, and compact design that allows easy testing and troubleshooting of the components
- Ability to remove waste anesthesia gases to prevent pollution of the operating room

Even with today's modern anesthesia machine, no breathing system is able to achieve all of the desirable features listed above and for this reason different breathing systems are used for different settings.

34.2 Classification of Breathing Systems

As more breathing systems were designed, multiple authors tried to develop classification systems based on the amount of rebreathing, presence of a carbon dioxide absorber, and the presence or absence of unidirectional valves. A common and relatively simple classification system is shown in ◘ ◉ Table 34.1.

Table 34.1 Classification of breathing systems

	Reservoir	Rebreathing	Example
Open	No	No	Open drop
Semi-open	Yes	No	Non-rebreather circuit
Semi-closed	Yes	Partial	Circle system with flows of 2 L/min
Closed	Yes	Complete	Circle system with flows just sufficient to replace uptake of Oxygen

34.3 Non-rebreathing Systems

34.3.1 Insufflation

The term insufflation refers to a breathing system that is not in contact with the patient but instead blows oxygen and the anesthesia gases across a patient's face. There are 2 common methods where insufflation is used in modern practice. The first is in pediatric patients who will not allow the placement of an intravenous line or the application of an oxygen face mask to their face. In this case, the oxygen mask is held near the patient's face and when they breath in, they inhale the oxygen and the anesthesia gases that are supplied by the mask. The other example of insufflation is during cataract surgery and procedures performed typically under conscious sedation or monitored anesthesia care (MAC) when the patient's face is fully covered with the surgical drapes. Frequently oxygen tubing is then placed under the drapes to blow oxygen at high flows near the patient's face to minimize the rebreathing of carbon dioxide. The disadvantage of insufflation is positive pressure ventilation cannot be done and the concentration of oxygen delivered is variable even at high flow rates.

34.3.2 Open-Drop Anesthesia Systems

In modern medicine, open-drop anesthesia systems are no longer in use, but since they were one of the earliest methods for providing anesthesia, they deserve a brief description. These were the primary methods for administering ether or chloroform anesthesia to patients. They consisted of a face mask with a gauze-covered opening where a highly volatile anesthetic was then dripped onto the gauze. When the patient inhaled, the flow of air through the gauze caused the liquid volatile anesthetic to become a gas. The depth of anesthesia was controlled by the amount of volatile anesthetic liquid applied to the gauze. The major disadvantage of this system is the patient had to be breathing spontaneously and there was no way to monitor the concentration of volatile anesthetic the patient was inspiring.

34.3.3 Mapleson Circuits

The development of the Mapleson circuits attempted to overcome the major shortcomings of the insufflation and open-drop systems. Compared to previous breathing systems, the Mapleson circuits had the following advantages:

- Ability to deliver a reliable concentration of oxygen and volatile anesthetics
- Provide positive pressure ventilation

- Ability to scavenge waste gases
- Portable and relatively simple design

Since there are no unidirectional valves or CO_2 absorbers, the CO_2 is eliminated by fresh gas flows that flush the CO_2 into the atmosphere or scavenger via the pop-off valve. The Mapleson circuits are classified based on the location of the following parts as seen in ◉ Fig. 34.1:

- **Fresh gas inlet** – Supplies oxygen, air, and volatile anesthetics to the system
- **Reservoir bag** – Acts as a reservoir for the gases and a method for creating positive pressure
- **Pop-off valve/Adjustable pressure relief valve** – Allows the release of excess gases from the system. Closing of the valve allows increasing levels of pressure to be achieved
- **Face mask**

Although the Mapleson circuits all have the same components, the comparison of the circuits and the amount of CO_2 rebreathing that occurs can be complex. Rebreathing that occurs for each circuit is affected by the position of the pop-off valve in relationship to the fresh gas input and the reservoir tubing and bag. Each type of Mapleson system has different levels of fresh gas flows required to prevent rebreathing. In addition, each class of circuit responds differently to spontaneous versus controlled ventilation in relation to the fresh gas flows required to prevent rebreathing.

Mapleson A (see ◉ Fig. 34.1) is considered the most efficient circuit for spontaneous ventilation but is not recommended for controlled ventilation due to the need for unpredictably high fresh gas flows required to prevent rebreathing. By changing the position of the pop-off valve and the fresh gas inlet, the system becomes a Mapleson D (see ◉ Fig. 34.1), which is significantly more efficient for controlled ventilation. This is because the fresh gas flushes the exhaled gases away from the patient and toward the pop-off valve. The Bain circuit is a modified Mapleson D system that incorporates the fresh gas inlet tubing inside the larger corrugated breathing tube. This decreases the size of the system and allows warming of the inspired gases by the exhaled gases. A major disadvantage of Bain circuit is if the fresh gas inlet tubing is disconnected or kinked, this will lead to significant rebreathing of exhaled gases.

34.3.3.1 Efficiency of Mapleson Circuits

Spontaneous Ventilation A > DFE > CB.

Controlled Ventilation DFE > BC > A.

(Refer to ◉ Fig. 1.1 for the different Mapleson circuits by letter.)

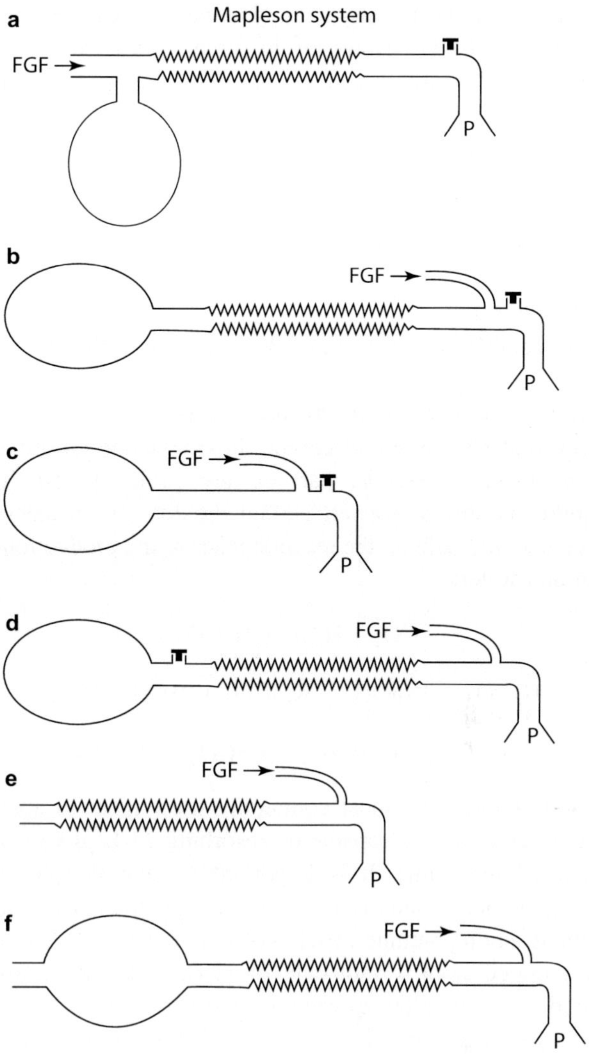

Fig. 34.1 a–f Mapleson system. *FGF* fresh gas flow, *P* patient

While the Mapleson systems were a significant improvement from previous breathing systems, the major disadvantage remained to be poor conservation of heat and humidity. In addition, the minimum flows required to prevent rebreathing are typically 5–10 L/min for an adult.

34.3.4 The Circle System

The circle system was designed to overcome some of the limitations of the Mapleson circuits. Through the rebreathing of exhaled gases, humidity and heat are maintained. Since the exhaled gases are rebreathed, this leads to a conservation of volatile anesthetics, oxygen, and air. These advantages have resulted in the circle system being the ventilation system used in all modern anesthesia machines. While the oxygen, nitrogen, and the volatile anesthetics are rebreathed,

CO_2 absorbers chemically neutralize the CO_2 so there is no rebreathing of CO_2. However, to achieve these results, the complexity of the breathing system was substantially increased. As shown in ◉ Fig. 34.2, the necessary components of a circle system include:

1. CO_2 absorber
2. Unidirectional valves
3. Fresh gas inlet
4. Y-connector
5. Adjustable pressure relief valve ("pop-off valve")

34.3.4.1 Carbon Dioxide Absorber

To prevent rebreathing of carbon dioxide, a carbon dioxide absorber is an essential part of any circle system. The absorber is able to convert carbon dioxide gas to calcium carbonate. In addition, the reaction leads to the production of heat and water:

$$CO_2 + H_2O \rightarrow H_2CO_3$$

$$H_2CO_3 + 2NaOH \rightarrow Na_2CO_3 + 2H_2O + \text{Heat}$$

$$Na_2CO_3 + Ca(OH)_2 \rightarrow CaCO_3 + 2NaOH$$

Soda lime is the most commonly used agent to absorb carbon dioxide. It is capable of absorbing 23 L of CO_2 per 100 g of soda lime. It is important to note that for the reaction to occur water is necessary to begin the reaction, but as the reaction continues, each molecule of CO_2 leads to the net production of 1 molecule of H_2O. Since the carbon dioxide absorber requires water to start the reaction, they are packaged by the manufacturer with 14–19% water content.

As the absorber is exhausted, hydrogen ions accumulate. To monitor the pH, an indicator dye (ethyl violet) is added to the absorber granules, which causes the white absorber granules to turn purple as they are exhausted. If an exhausted carbon dioxide absorber is not used for a time, the granules may return to the original white color. However, the absorber is still exhausted and cannot absorb additional carbon dioxide. All modern anesthesia machines monitor the inspired and expired carbon dioxide. With a properly functioning carbon dioxide absorber, inspired carbon dioxide should be zero and the absorber should be changed once the inspired carbon dioxide is present. If it is not possible to replace the carbon dioxide absorber, high flows (> 5 L/min) can effectively wash out the carbon dioxide from the system.

The absorber granules are capable of absorbing and releasing volatile anesthetic gases. This is clinically relevant when the absorber canisters are changed during a surgical case. When this occurs, the new absorber canister will absorb the volatile anesthetic in the anesthesia machine and the depth of anesthesia will decrease temporarily. The other clinically significant scenario is in patients at risk of malignant hyperthermia. In these patients if an anesthesia machine is used that had previously been used with volatile anesthetics, then the patient may be exposed to volatile anesthetics. Since this could trigger an episode of malignant hyperthermia, a new carbon dioxide absorber should be used.

34.3.4.2 Unidirectional Valves

In a circle system, unidirectional valves are essential to maintain the flow of gases in the correct direction. This is important to prevent rebreathing of the expired gases with carbon dioxide present. There are 2 valves in the system.

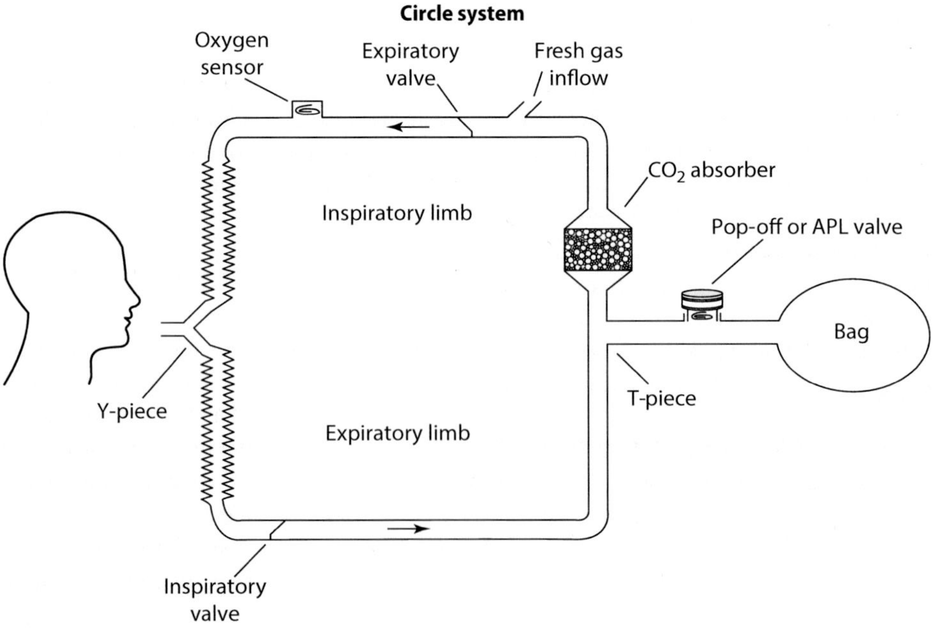

Fig. 34.2 Circle system

During inspiration, the inspiratory valve opens and the expiratory valve closes. During expiration, the expiratory valve opens and the inspiratory valve closes. The most common malfunction of the unidirectional valves is incomplete closure—usually due to a warped valve. If this occurs, then rebreathing of carbon dioxide is possible and hypercapnia can result.

34.3.4.3 Fresh Gas Inlet

One of the advantages of the circle system is the rebreathing of oxygen and volatile anesthetic gases. However, due to the uptake of oxygen and volatile gases by the patient, there must be continuous addition of oxygen and volatile gases to the circle system. This occurs via the fresh gas inlet. When adding gases to the system, it is important to remember that gases from the fresh gas inlet will be diluted by the gases already in the circuit. For example, a typical circle system in a modern anesthesia machine will have a volume of 7 L. If the fresh gas inlet is at low flows (< 1 L/min), there can be a significant difference between the concentration of volatile gases coming from the vaporizer via the fresh gas inlet and the concentration delivered to the patient. This is most apparent during induction and emergence from anesthesia. To compensate for the dilution effect, a high flow rate (> 5 L/min) can be used.

34.3.4.4 Adjustable Pressure Relief Valve ("Pop-Off Valve")

As previously mentioned, higher fresh gas flows can be used to speed changes in the concentration of volatile anesthetics in the circuit. The adjustable pressure relief valve will vent off the excess gases from the circle system to maintain a set volume. The adjustable pressure relief valve is also used to adjust the pressure in the system during positive pressure ventilation. During spontaneous ventilation, the adjustable pressure relief valve should be fully open to minimize the pressure to which the patient is exposed.

34.3.4.5 Order of Components in the Circle System

To optimize the efficiency of the circle system, the components of the circle system are arranged in the following order, starting from the patient during expiration:

- Expiratory limb of circuit going to the expiratory unidirectional valve.
- After the expiratory unidirectional valve, the adjustable pressure relief valve is next and it is positioned before the carbon dioxide absorber. The result is the excess exhaled gas is vented away before it goes through the absorber. This conserves the absorber since the excess gas does not need to have the carbon dioxide removed.
- After the carbon dioxide absorber is the fresh gas inlet. This positioning allows the newly supplied gas to bypass the adjustable pressure relief valve and the carbon dioxide absorber. Therefore, all of the new gases are directly supplied to the patient.
- The inspiratory unidirectional valve is next, and then gas moves through the inspiratory limb of the circuit where it delivers gases to the patient.

34.3.4.6 Dead Space

Dead space is defined as ventilation that does not reach the alveoli and therefore is not effective in exchanging oxygen and carbon dioxide. As the dead space increases, the tidal volumes must increase to maintain a given carbon dioxide. Due to the unidirectional valves in the circle system, the dead space begins at the Y-piece where the inspiratory limb joins with the expiratory limb. Therefore, increasing the length of the circle system does not increase the amount of dead space.

34.3.4.7 Disadvantages of the Circle System

While the circle system has many advantages compared to the Mapleson breathing system, there are a few disadvantages:

- **Complexity**—The circle system is more complicated and it requires frequent maintenance and daily machine checks to ensure the essential components are functioning properly.
- **Size**—The circle system is significantly larger and less portable.
- **Breathing Resistance**—Due to the unidirectional valves and the carbon dioxide absorber, there is more resistance. However, even in a premature infant, a circle system can be used.

34.3.4.8 Circle System with High Versus Low Flows

One of the significant advantages of the circle system is the ability to run low fresh gas flows due to the rebreathing of exhaled gases. The rebreathing of exhaled gases can lead to significant differences in the concentration of volatile anesthetic between the fresh gas inlet and the gas delivered to the patient. One example where this is clinically significant is during induction of anesthesia. During this time, there is rapid uptake of volatile anesthetics and the expired gases have minimal amounts of volatile anesthetics. If low fresh gas flows are used, then even if high concentrations of volatile gases are delivered via the fresh gas inlet, the gases will be significantly diluted by the larger volume of exhaled gases from the patient. This will result in a delay in induction of anesthesia. The same is true during emergence from anesthesia. If low flows are used, then the expired volatile anesthetics will continue to circulate in the breathing system even if volatile anesthetics are no longer being delivered via the fresh gas inlet. Therefore, to speed induction and emergence from anesthesia, high flows (> 5 L/min) are typically used.

With low fresh gas flows, it is also essential to monitor the concentration of the inspired oxygen concentration that is delivered to the patient. This is because with low flows the majority of the gases will be rebreathed. During ventilation, the oxygen is absorbed while the nitrogen is not. With time the concentration of nitrogen will increase and potentially a hypoxic mixture of gases can be delivered to the patient. With higher flows, this does not occur because the excess volume of gas is vented from the system via the pop-off valve and the concentration of the inspired gases more closely matches the gases from the fresh gas inlet. This also applies to nitrous oxide. Initially during induction, the nitrous oxide is absorbed and the concentration of oxygen is maintained. However, as the absorption of nitrous oxide slows, the nitrous oxide will accumulate in low fresh gas flows and a hypoxic mixture can also be delivered. For these reasons, it is essential to monitor the concentration of oxygen and anesthetics that are being delivered to the patient with a gas analyzer when using a circle system.

34.3.5 Closed Circle System

In a closed circle system, the fresh gas flows of oxygen are matched with the uptake of oxygen by the patient. If done correctly, then no excess gases are vented via the pop-off valve. A closed circle system maximizes the advantages of the circle system, which include conservation of gases, humidity, and heat. However, a closed circle system exacerbates the problems listed previously for low fresh gas flows. Delivery of volatile anesthetics is particularly difficult with a closed circle system due to the changing uptake of the volatile anesthetics as the patient progresses from induction to maintenance of anesthesia. Due to the extremely low fresh gas flows (0.2–0.3 L/min), it is difficult to rapidly change the concentration of oxygen or volatile anesthetics in the breathing circuit. For these reasons, closed circle systems are not frequently used in clinical practice.

34.3.6 Use of Circle Systems in Neonates

Several adaptations have been made to the circle system to decrease the work of breathing for neonates. For adult circuits, the dead space begins at the y-piece, which joins the inspiratory and expiratory limbs of the circuit. The dead space consists of the Y-piece, the endotracheal tube, and the airways down to the level of the alveoli. In an adult, the total amount of dead space represents only a small amount of the total tidal volume. However, in pediatrics, and especially neonates, the dead space can represent a significant portion of the tidal volume. To minimize the dead space, a septum can be added to the y-piece and then the volume of the y-piece is no longer part of the dead space. The pediatric circuit also consists of narrower and more rigid corrugated tubing to minimize the compliance of the system.

34.3.7 Potential Complications with the Circle System

34.3.7.1 Compound A

The carbon dioxide absorber consists of a strong base that can lead to the removal of hydrogen fluoride from the volatile anesthetics. With sevoflurane this can lead to the production of compound A. In rats, it has been shown to be a nephrotoxin, but in humans, it has an unclear significance. After a prolonged exposure of high levels of compound A in otherwise healthy volunteers, there is a transient albuminuria. To minimize exposure to compound A, it is recommended to use a minimum fresh gas flow of 2 L/min. This will allow a continuous washout of compound A from the circle system.

34.3.7.2 Production of Carbon Monoxide

The use of desiccated soda lime in the carbon dioxide absorber can lead to the production of significant quantities of carbon monoxide. The risk of carbon monoxide production varies for the different agents:

$$\text{desflurane} > \text{isoflurane} > > \text{sevoflurane}$$

Since this only occurs with desiccated soda lime, there is a higher incidence of carbon monoxide production with the use of old soda lime during the first case of the day. As the soda lime is used to remove carbon dioxide, water is produced by the reaction. This rehydrates the desiccated soda lime and subsequent surgical cases have a lower incidence of carbon monoxide exposure. The highest risk is on Monday morning after the anesthesia machines were not used over the weekend. For the same reason, anesthesia machines at offsite locations where the anesthesia machines are only used infrequently also have a high risk of exposure to carbon monoxide. Any time the fresh gas flows are left on at high flows and the machine is not connected to a patient, there is a risk of drying out the soda lime. If the fresh gas flows are left on overnight when the anesthesia machine was not in use, the soda lime should be replaced. If carbon monoxide is produced, then the use of low fresh gas flows will lead to an accumulation of carbon dioxide in the system. The risk of carbon monoxide production with new soda lime is low because it arrives pre-hydrated from the manufacturer.

34.3.7.3 Malfunction of Unidirectional Valves

The valves consist of a horizontal ceramic disc that rests on the valve seat. As gas flows through, the disc is lifted up. When the flow reverses, the disk is pushed down and it seals the valve and prevents reversal of flow. The most common malfunction of the valve is due to warping of the disc or improper seating of the disc. When this happens to either valve, the result is rebreathing of exhaled gases and potentially hypercapnia. The expiratory valve is exposed to the moisture in the exhaled gases and is the most common valve to malfunction.

34.3.8 Manual Resuscitator Bag "Ambu Bag"

Common uses for the Ambu bag, which is shown in ◉ Fig. 34.3, include transport of patients and emergency ventilation when a ventilator is not available or is not functioning properly. The advantages include a small and easily portable ventilation system. It has few moving parts and is extremely reliable. Components of an Ambu bag include a self-expanding bag, reservoir tubing, oxygen source, and a non-rebreather valve.

The Ambu bag can be either connected to an endotracheal tube or used with a face mask to provide positive pressure ventilation. The self-expanding bag is used to create positive pressure. Since it is a self-expanding bag, it can be used without an oxygen source, unlike the Mapleson circuits that require compressed gas to expand the reservoir bag. With the use of high flow oxygen (> 8 L/min) close to 100% oxygen can be delivered to the patient. Unlike the circle system, there is no rebreathing of gases, and therefore, it has similar disadvantages to the Mapleson circuits.

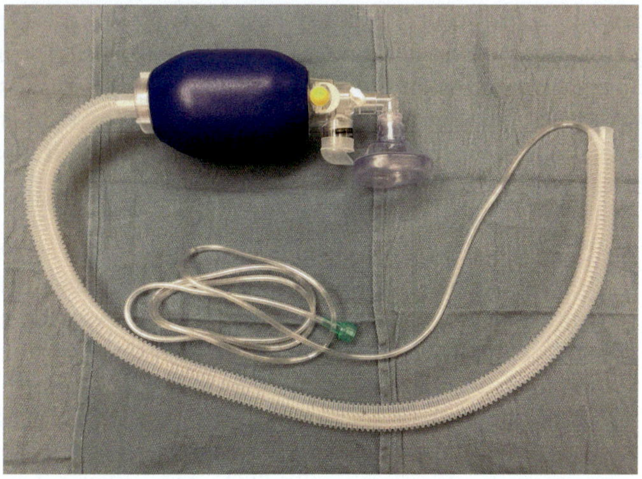

Fig. 34.3 Ambu bag

34.4 Conclusion

Breathing systems have come a long way since the creation of open-drop anesthesia. An optimal breathing system would include a simple, reliable, portable system that can also make efficient use of the gases with conservation of heat and moisture. So far, no current breathing systems have been able to achieve all the desired characteristics. The Mapleson systems are primarily used where a portable breathing system is required or in locations where a circle system is not available. A circle system is typically the optimum system, assuming portability is not needed. However, with all the advantages of the circle system comes a significant increase in complexity. This leads to the need for more frequent maintenance and constant monitoring of the inspired gases to ensure a safe delivery of the desired gases to the patient.

34.5 Questions and Answers

Questions (Choose the Most Appropriate Answer)

1. The following are all characteristics of Mapleson circuits EXCEPT:
   A. Ability to provide positive pressure ventilation
   B. Ability to scavenge waste gases
   C. Portable
   D. Contains a carbon dioxide absorber
2. A disadvantage of the Mapleson system is:
   A. Complex design
   B. Poor conservation of heat
   C. High level of resistance during expiration
   D. Unable to provide high concentrations of oxygen
3. All are necessary components of a circle system except:
   A. Carbon dioxide absorber
   B. Self-inflating reservoir bag
   C. Unidirectional valves
   D. Adjustable pressure relief valve
4. For the carbon dioxide absorber to work, the following are necessary:
   A. Water
   B. Heat
   C. Hydrochloric acid
   D. Sodium hydroxide
5. The following can occur after the carbon dioxide absorber is changed:
   A. Increase in concentration of carbon dioxide
   B. Decrease in concentration of oxygen
   C. Decrease in concentration of volatile anesthetics
   D. Decrease in concentration of water content

6. If the unidirectional valves malfunction in the circle system the following can occur:
   A. Hypercapnia
   B. Hypocapnia
   C. Hypoxia
   D. Increased concentration of volatile agents
7. Increasing the length of the circuit tubing in a circuit system will increase the amount of dead space
   A. True
   B. False
8. Which of the following are NOT TRUE about compound A?
   A. Produced by the removal of hydrogen fluoride from sevoflurane
   B. Is a nephrotoxin in rats
   C. With sevoflurane fresh gas flows of at least 1 L/min are recommended
   D. Prolonged exposure in humans leads to transient albuminuria
9. The following is true about the production of carbon monoxide by the soda lime carbon dioxide absorber:
   A. Sevoflurane is more likely to produce carbon monoxide compared to desflurane.
   B. It is most likely to occur during surgeries lasting greater than 6 h.
   C. It occurs when the soda lime is exhausted and cannot absorb additional carbon dioxide.
   D. It is most likely to occur during the first case of the day.
10. All of the following breathing circuits require compressed gas (typically oxygen) to function properly except:
   A. Ambu bag
   B. Circle system
   C. Mapleson circuit
   D. Insufflation

Answers

1. **D**. The essential components of a Mapleson circuit include a fresh gas inlet, reservoir bag, pop-off valve, and a face mask. This provides the ability to provide positive pressure ventilation. The pop-off valve is where the exhaled gases are vented and this allows a scavenger system to be connected to the circuit. This is done if the Mapleson circuit is used with volatile anesthetics to prevent the contamination of the patient care area. Since the Mapleson system consists of only a few lightweight components, it is highly portable. A carbon dioxide absorber is not included in the components of a Mapleson system but is instead found in the circle system.
2. **B**. The advantages of the Mapleson system include a relatively simple and portable design. Compared to other ventilation systems, including the circle system, a Mapleson system has very low resistance during exhalation. If pure oxygen is supplied to the system in adequate flows (> 5 L/min), then the patient will receive close to 100% oxygen. Since the Mapleson system does not recirculate the exhaled gases as occurs in the circle system, this leads to a loss of heat and moisture.
3. **B**. The following are all necessary components of a circle system including: carbon dioxide absorber, unidirectional valves, fresh gas inlet, reservoir bag, and adjustable pressure relief valves. In the circle system, the reservoir bag is soft plastic and only expands if the pressure relief valve is closed and gas fills the bag. An example of a self-inflating reservoir bag occurs in an Ambu bag.
4. **A**. For absorption to take place the following reaction occurs:

$$CO_2 + H_2O \rightarrow H_2CO_3$$

$$H_2CO_3 + 2NaOH \rightarrow Na_2CO_3 + 2H_2O + \text{Heat}$$

$$Na_2CO_3 + Ca(OH)_2 \rightarrow CaCO_3 + 2NaOH$$

The first step in the reaction is the combination of carbon dioxide with water. For this reason when the carbon dioxide absorber is packaged by the manufacturer, it includes 14–19% water. This allows the absorber to immediately start working once it is placed in the circle system. Once the reaction is underway, for every molecule of carbon dioxide that combines with a molecule of water, the end result is the production of 2 molecules of water. This allows water to be available for the next reaction to occur. The most likely reason that water is not present is if the fresh gas flows were left on overnight when a patient is not connected to the circle system. The fresh gas flows have no water present, and if exposed to the absorber for several hours, this can lead to the depletion of water. If this occurs, then the absorber should be replaced.

5. **C**. When the carbon dioxide absorber is replaced, it begins working immediately so the concentration of carbon dioxide will be either unchanged or it will begin to decrease if the previous absorber was exhausted. The absorber does not absorb oxygen so the oxygen concentration will be unchanged. Since the absorber is saturated with water from the manufacturer, the water content in the circuit will likely be unchanged or increase slightly. When the absorber is replaced, it will absorb the volatile anesthetics if present and the depth of anesthesia for the patient will decrease temporarily.

The absorber quickly becomes saturated with volatile anesthetics, and then the depth of anesthetics will remain constant.

6. **A**. The purpose of the unidirectional valves is to ensure that the gases move through the circuit in only 1 direction. When there is a malfunction in 1 of the valves, it allows the gases to move in both directions. This will lead to rebreathing of the exhaled gases and hypercapnia will develop. Hypoxia would be unlikely because the exhaled gases still have oxygen present and even with rebreathing the patient will still receive sufficient oxygen. Malfunctioning valves will have no impact on the concentration of the volatile agents.
7. **B**. False. Due to the unidirectional valves in the circle system, the gases are only able to move in 1 direction. Therefore, no matter how long the circuit is, the dead space begins at the y-piece that joins the expiratory limb and the inspiratory limb with the endotracheal tube.
8. **C**. Compound A is produced by the removal of hydrogen fluoride from sevoflurane by the carbon dioxide absorber. Rats exposed to compound A show signs of renal injury and healthy humans develop a transient albuminuria. Due to the potential for renal injury in humans, it is recommended to run fresh gas flows of at least 2 L/min to minimize the buildup of compound A in the circle system.
9. **D**. The production of carbon monoxide is greatest with desflurane than isoflurane and sevoflurane has the lowest risk. It occurs when the soda lime is desiccated. As soda lime removes carbon dioxide, it leads to the production of water. So longer surgeries have a lower risk of carbon monoxide production. An exhausted absorber does not produce carbon monoxide. The first case of the day has the highest risk of having desiccated soda lime, especially if the fresh gas flows were left on when the anesthesia machine was not in use. This leads to the first case of the day having the highest risk of carbon dioxide production.
10. **A**. The circle system and the Mapleson circuit both require a compressed gas source to fill the reservoir bag since the bag is not self-expanding. For insufflation, there is nothing in contact with the patient, but it works by blowing oxygen toward the patient's face. The Ambu bag is the only system with a self-inflating reservoir bag; this allows it to be used with or without a compressed gas source.

References

1. Barash PG, Cullen BF, Stoelting RK, Cahalan MK, Stock MC, editors. Clinical anesthesia. 6th ed. Philadelphia: Lippincott Williams & Wilkins; 2009. p. 649–80.
2. Miller RD, Eriksson LI, Fleisher LA, Wiener-Kronish JP, Young WL. Miller's anesthesia. 7th ed. Philadelphia: Elsevier; 2009. p. 692–702.

Physics of Instrumentation

35

Verghese T. Cherian and Arne O. Budde

Abstract

It is important for the anesthesiologist to be familiar with the physics of instrumentation to be able to effectively use the information provided by various monitors in the operating room. The basic physical principles of some of the commonly used monitors and equipment are explained here.

Keywords

Monitors • Physical principles • Working of monitoring equipment • Gas analyzers • Arterial pressure monitoring • Pulse oximeter • Blood pressure monitoring • Body warmers • Thermometers • Defibrillator

Key Points

- It is crucial to understand the physical principles and functioning of the monitoring devices, in order to interpret the results and know their limitations.
- Solubility of all gases increases with a fall in temperature of the solvent and thus lowers its partial pressure.
- Oxygen, because of its unpaired electron in the outer orbit, is "paramagnetic" or attracted toward a magnetic field, while most other gases used in anesthesia are "diamagnetic" or repelled from a magnetic field.
- Molecules with two or more dissimilar atoms absorb infrared (IR) radiation, and different molecules have distinct IR absorption spectra.
- Although the transducer must be set at the level of the heart (fourth intercostal space, mid-axillary line) to measure the blood pressure accurately, it is not crucial for zeroing the transducer.
- The amount of heat energy required to humidify the inspired gas is five times greater than that needed to warm it to body temperature.
- A capacitor is an electrical component that can store energy, and it is the most important component of a defibrillator.

35.1 Introduction

As an anesthesiologist, one is surrounded by equipment that monitors vital signs, measures blood gases and anesthetic agents, and devices that are used to keep our patients safe. It is crucial to understand the physical principles and functioning of these devices, in order to interpret the results and know their limitations.

35.2 Blood Gas Measurement

During "blood gas" analysis, the parameters that are directly measured are pH, PO_2, and PCO_2, while the bicarbonate level is calculated from the pH and the PCO_2 using the Siggaard-Andersen nomogram.

35.2.1 Electrodes

The **polarographic (Clark) oxygen electrode** can measure partial pressure of oxygen in blood or a gas sample. It

V. T. Cherian (✉) · A. O. Budde
Department of Anesthesiology and Perioperative Medicine, Penn State Health, Milton S. Hershey Medical Center, Hershey, PA, USA
e-mail: vcherian@pennstatehealth.psu.edu

A. O. Budde
e-mail: abudde@pennstatehealth.psu.edu

M. Argalious et al. (eds.), *Basic Sciences in Anesthesia*,
https://doi.org/10.1007/978-3-031-60203-0_35

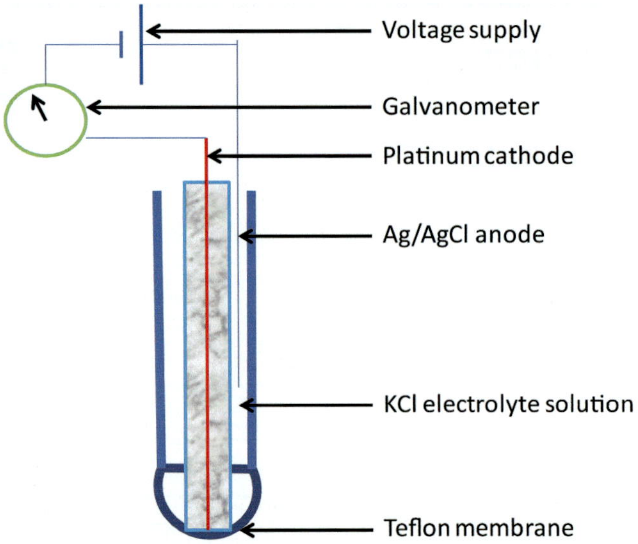

Fig. 35.1 Clark-type oxygen electrode

consists of a platinum cathode and a silver/silver chloride anode immersed in a potassium chloride solution and separated from the blood sample by an oxygen-permeable Teflon membrane, which allows the oxygen tension in the blood to equilibrate with the electrolyte solution. The electrode is maintained at 37 °C (Fig. 35.1).

When a voltage of 700 mV is applied across the electrodes the following reactions occur:

- **Cathode**: $O_2 + 2H_2O + 4e^- = 4OH^-$
- **Electrolyte**: $KCl + OH^- = KOH + Cl^-$
- **Anode**: $Ag + Cl^- = AgCl + e^-$

The amount of electrons that are taken up at the cathode is proportional to the oxygen tension, and this current can be processed and displayed as PO_2.

The **pH (Sanz) electrode** works on the principle that an electrical potential develops across a glass membrane, which is proportional to the pH difference across it. The pH electrode consists of 2 "half" cells: a glass electrode and a reference electrode. The glass electrode is an Ag/AgCl electrode system enclosed in a glass membrane and maintaining a constant pH within itself, while the reference electrode is a Hg/HgCl electrode, which comes in contact with the blood sample through a semipermeable membrane. The chloride solution acts as the bridge between the two electrodes. The whole system is maintained at 37 °C. Current flows from the reference electrode through the semipermeable membrane through the sample in the measuring chamber and to the glass electrode. Depending on the pH of the sample, the potential will develop across the glass membrane, which will be displayed in pH units. The potential output is 60 mV per pH unit (Fig. 35.2).

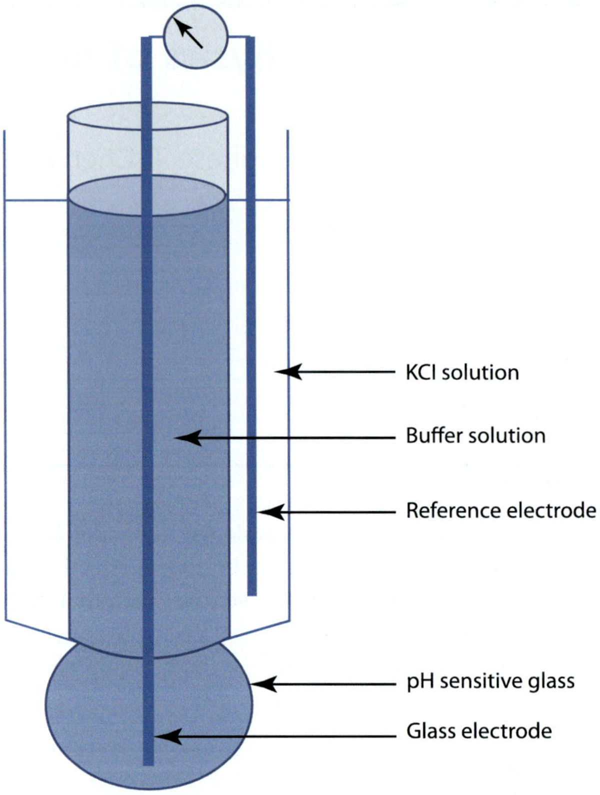

Fig. 35.2 pH (Sanz) electrode

The $\mathbf{CO_2}$ **(Severinghaus) electrode** is similar to the pH electrode with the electrode in contact with a sodium bicarbonate solution and separated from the blood sample by a Teflon semipermeable membrane. CO_2 from the blood sample diffuses across the membrane and reacts with the bicarbonate solution to form H^+, which is measured by the pH electrode:

$$CO_2 + H_2O \rightleftharpoons H_2CO_3 \rightleftharpoons H^+ + HCO^{3-}$$

The amount of H + produced is proportional to the PCO_2 in the blood. Similar to the pH electrode, the whole system is maintained at 37 °C.

35.2.2 Hypothermia and Blood Gas

Solubility of all gases increases with a fall in temperature of the solvent and thus lowers its partial pressure. Therefore, hypothermia increases the solubility of O_2 and CO_2 and consequently lowers the PO_2 and PCO_2. The PCO_2 decreases by approximately 2 mmHg and PO_2 decreases by approximately 5 mmHg per °C below 37 C. Hypothermia also changes the pH; for every °C drop in temperature, the pH increases by 0.015 units.

Since, the analysis of the blood sample from a hypothermic patient occurs at 37 °C, the PO_2 and PCO_2 values would be artificially high. The result can be corrected for the patient's temperature. This becomes especially important in significantly hypothermic patients, such as during cold cardiopulmonary bypass or deep hypothermic circulatory arrest.

35.2.2.1 pH–STAT

Historically, it was thought that in a hypothermic patient undergoing cardiopulmonary bypass, a reduced PCO_2 would result in cerebral vasoconstriction and ischemia. Therefore, CO_2 was added to the oxygenator to maintain a temperature-corrected PCO_2 of 40 mmHg (5.3 kPA) and a pH of 7.4. The advantage of this was increased cerebral blood flow allowing better oxygen delivery. However, there was concern that it could lead to micro-embolization and loss of autoregulation.

35.2.2.2 α(Alpha)-STAT

Hypothermia reduces the efficacy of the bicarbonate and the phosphate buffers, and the amino acids (alpha imidazole ring of histidine) become the primary buffer. During hypothermia, pH increases because of low H^+ (decreased dissociation), but electro-neutrality is maintained as there is less available OH^-. This is more physiological. The advantages are maintenance of cerebral autoregulation and normal cellular transmembrane electro-neutrality. The resultant alkalosis better preserves protein function and enzyme activity. Therefore, proponents of α(alpha)-stat maintain uncorrected PCO_2 and pH at normal levels. The α(alpha)-stat method is the more acceptable and standard approach.

35.3 Respiratory and Anesthetic Gas Measurement

35.3.1 Paramagnetic Oxygen Analyzer

Oxygen, because of its unpaired electron in the outer orbit, is "paramagnetic" or attracted towards a magnetic field, while most other gases used in anesthesia are "diamagnetic" or repel from a magnetic field. Historically, two spheres, connected together to look like a dumbbell, filled with nitrogen (a diamagnetic gas) were suspended in a magnetic field. In the resting stage, the dumbbell would try to move away from the magnetic field. However, when oxygen-containing gas was passed around it, the oxygen being attracted to the magnetic field would move the dumbbell towards the magnetic field. This displacement, depends on the concentration of oxygen and could be electronically extrapolated as the concentration of oxygen. However, the construction of modern analyzers has fewer moving parts, but still uses the same principle (Fig. 35.3). A highly sensitive pressure transducer measures the pressure difference between two streams of gas: the "sample" and the "reference." Further downstream to the transducer, both the gases pass through a common channel, across which a "pulsed" electromagnetic field is generated at around 100 Hz. When the magnetic field is applied, oxygen molecules are attracted toward it, causing a low pressure upstream. The pressure difference between the two streams, which is measured by the transducer, would be proportional to the difference in oxygen concentration. The electric output from the transducer displays it as volume percentage of oxygen in the sample gas. Of all the gases the anesthesiologists encounter, nitric oxide is the only other gas that is also paramagnetic.

35.3.2 Fuel Cell (Galvanic Cell)

The fuel cell is similar to the Clark polarographic electrode except that it generates its own voltage without any external power source. It consists of a gold cathode and a lead anode immersed in potassium hydroxide solution. Oxygen from the gas sample is reduced at the cathode to form OH^-, which moves to the anode to form electrons, thus generating a potential difference. The current generated is proportional to the concentration of oxygen in the sample:

- **Cathode**: $O_2 + 2H_2O + 4e^- \rightarrow 4\ OH^-$
- **Anode**: $2Pb + 4(OH^-) \rightarrow 2PbO + 2H_2O + 4e^-$

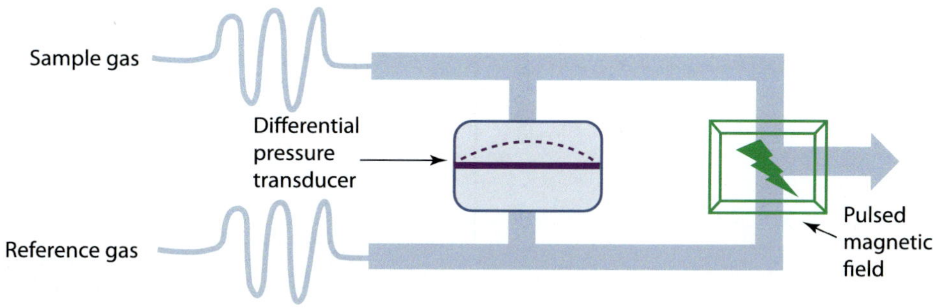

Fig. 35.3 Pulsed-field paramagnetic oxygen analyzer

35.3.3 Infrared Spectrophotometry

Absorption spectroscopy is the fundamental principle used in capnography, pulse oximeter, and most anesthetics gas monitors. Molecules with *two or more dissimilar atoms* absorb infrared (IR) radiation, and different molecules have distinct IR absorption spectra. The absorbance peaks of CO_2 and N_2O are between 4 and 5 μm and that of the anesthetic gases are between 8 and 13 μm. According to the Beer–Lambert law, the amount of IR radiation absorbed is directly proportional to the concentration of the molecule and the distance traveled in the medium.

In a gas analyzer, a source emits IR radiation, which is passed through a chamber containing the sample gas and also a reference chamber and focused on an IR photo sensor. The amount of absorbed radiation is proportional to the concentration of the gas. Numerous readings per minute provide a continuous waveform of gas concentration during the respiratory cycle. There are two types of IR technology available today: (1) the "blackbody radiation," which produces a broad spectrum of IR radiation and filters are used to obtain specific wavelengths of radiation and (2) the "microstream," which generates IR emissions at specific wavelength that matches the absorption spectrum of the gas to be monitored.

35.3.3.1 Limitations of Infrared Spectroscopy

Oxygen, nitrogen, helium, xenon, and argon do not absorb IR radiation and cannot be measured by this technique. The absorption spectra of CO_2 and N_2O overlap, and the presence of N_2O broadens the CO_2 absorption spectrum (collision broadening), leading to a falsely elevated value. Water vapor absorbs IR and can interfere with measurement of CO_2 and anesthetic agents. Hydro-fluoro-alkanes, used as propellants in inhalers, have an absorption spectrum similar to halothane and can interfere with measurement of volatile agents.

35.3.4 Pulse Oximeter

The conventional pulse oximeter consists of two light-emitting diodes: a photocell detector and a microprocessor with a visual display unit. The light-emitting diodes emit light at wavelengths of 660 nm (red) and 940 nm (infrared), since these give a better separation of absorbance. At 940 nm, the light absorbance of oxyhemoglobin is one-and-a-half times more than that of deoxyhemoglobin, while at 660 nm, the deoxyhemoglobin absorbs 10 times as much as oxyhemoglobin (Fig. 35.4). At 805 nm, both the deoxyhemoglobin and the oxyhemoglobin absorb equally and this is called the "isosbestic" point. The ratio (R) of absorbance at 660 and 940 nm bears a linear relationship to oxygen saturation. At high O_2 saturations, this ratio is less than 1. At approximately 85% saturation, this ratio is equal to 1. The values for R can be mathematically calculated down to saturations of 0%, but these are not accurate clinically.

The main purpose of the pulse oximeter is to detect the amount of HbO in the arterial blood. However, at the fingertip, light is also absorbed by tissues and venous blood. An ingenious concept is incorporated into modern pulse oximeters. With each pulse, there is a surge of arterial blood across the measuring point and the amount of light absorbed would increase, cyclically. The pulse oximeter emits and analyzes light signals at a very rapid rate (400–600/s), and this can detect the peaks and troughs of the arterial pulse wave. If the light absorption at the trough (which includes all the tissue absorbers) is subtracted from the light absorption at the peak, then in theory the remaining is the absorption due to the added volume of arterial blood only. The ratio of the absorbance of the pulsatile to that of the non-pulsatile at both the wavelengths is calculated.

Even though traces of carboxyhemoglobin (COHb) and methemoglobin (MethHB) may be present normally, the

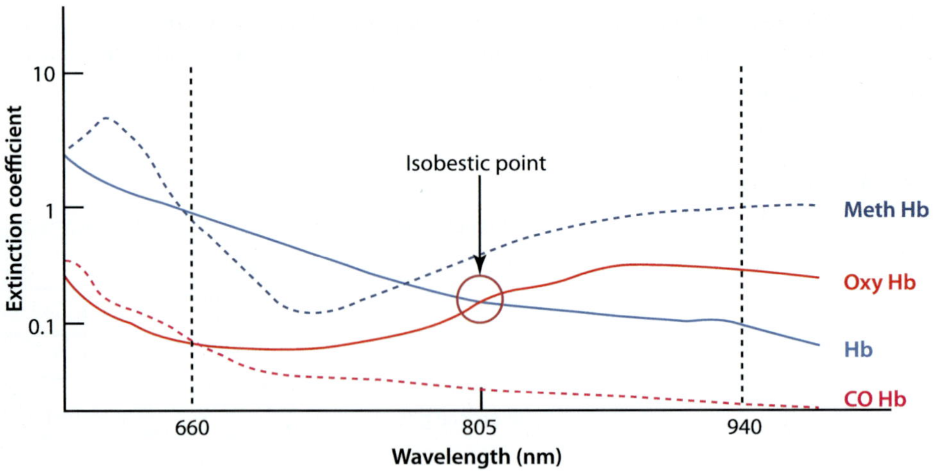

Fig. 35.4 Absorption spectrum of different forms of hemoglobin, according to wavelength of light

pulse oximeter assumes the presence of only oxyhemoglobin and reduced hemoglobin. Significant levels of COHb or MethHB can cause error in pulse oximeter readings. Since the COHb absorbs the red light very similarly to HbO and does not absorb the infrared, the pulse oximeter tends to read higher values in the presence of COHb. Methemoglobin absorbs both red and infrared waves equally, and therefore, the absorbance ratio, R, is 1. Therefore, the pulse oximeter tends to shift the SpO_2 toward 85%. Other factors that interfere with the pulse oximetry reading are dark-colored nail polishes, dyes (methylene blue and indigo-cyanine green), high bilirubin levels, tremors or movement of the hand, vasoconstriction, and ambient light. If the signals from the finger are low, alternative sites—such as ear lobe, ala of the nostril, or, in neonates, the foot or the palm—could be used. Pulse oximeter probes used during magnetic resonance imaging (MRI) have a fiber-optic system as the wires in a standard probe would generate heat in the radio-frequency environment and can cause burns.

35.3.4.1 Co-oximeter

A co-oximeter is a device that measures the blood concentration of carboxyhemoglobin (COHb), methemoglobin (MethHb), oxyhemoglobin (HbO_2), and reduced hemoglobin (HHb) using a sample of the arterial blood. A noninvasive co-oximeter (Masimo Rainbow® Pulse Co-oximeter; Masimo Corp., Irvine, CA), which looks similar to the usual pulse oximeter, is currently available. It uses multiple frequencies of light to calculate the saturation of carboxyhemoglobin, methemoglobin, oxyhemoglobin (SpO_2), and total hemoglobin. It also measures the oxygen content (SpOC), the perfusion index, and the pleth variability index:5

- **Fractional Saturation**: HbO/(Hb + HbO + MethHb + COHb) (needs a co-oximeter)
- **Functional Saturation**: HbO/(Hb + HbO) (pulse oximeter)

35.3.5 Mass Spectrometry

The concentration of a gas in a mixture can be measured by its mass–charge ratio. The sample of gas is passed through an ionizing chamber where an electron gun ionizes the molecules. These charged molecules are then accelerated through a magnetic field before striking a detector plate. The charged gas molecules are deflected by the magnetic field depending on their mass and create a series of peaks on the detector plate. The position of these peaks identifies the gas, and their height corresponds to the concentration. The mass spectrometer is very accurate but tedious and expensive and is mainly used for research or monitoring ambient gas levels from operating rooms. The gas sample cannot be returned to the patient as the molecules are ionized.

35.3.6 Raman Scattering

When an electromagnetic radiation collides with a gas molecule, it normally scatters with the same energy, and this is known as *Rayleigh scattering*. This is how we see things even though they do not emit light of their own. However, occasionally collision of electromagnetic wave energizes the molecule, and when it returns to its resting state, it emits the energy at a wavelength characteristic of the particular molecule. This is known as *Raman scattering*. This scattered light can be filtered out from the Rayleigh scattering and analyzed to identify the specific gas and its concentration. An intense beam of laser is passed through a sample chamber, and the Raman scattering is measured on a photodetector. This technique is fast and accurate and can be used to measure a number of gases. This technique is used to identify gases on distant planets.

35.3.7 Piezoelectric Absorption

Quartz crystal when placed in an electric field oscillates at a characteristic natural frequency. However, when such crystals are coated with oil, volatile anesthetic would dissolve in the lipid layer and increase the mass of the crystal, altering the frequency of oscillation. The change in frequency reflects the change in mass, which is proportional to the concentration of gas in the sample. The response time is fast, but it cannot differentiate between the gases.

35.4 Intra-Arterial Blood Pressure Monitoring

The intra-arterial blood pressure (IABP) measurement system consists of a column of fluid connecting the arterial system to a pressure transducer. The arterial pressure wave transmits through the fluid column and vibrates the diaphragm of the transducer, which then converts it into an electrical signal.

35.4.1 Sine Wave

A wave is the movement of energy through a medium. Sine wave is the simplest waveform and can be considered as the path taken by a point around a circle and mathematically defined by function $y = \sin x$. It is described by its

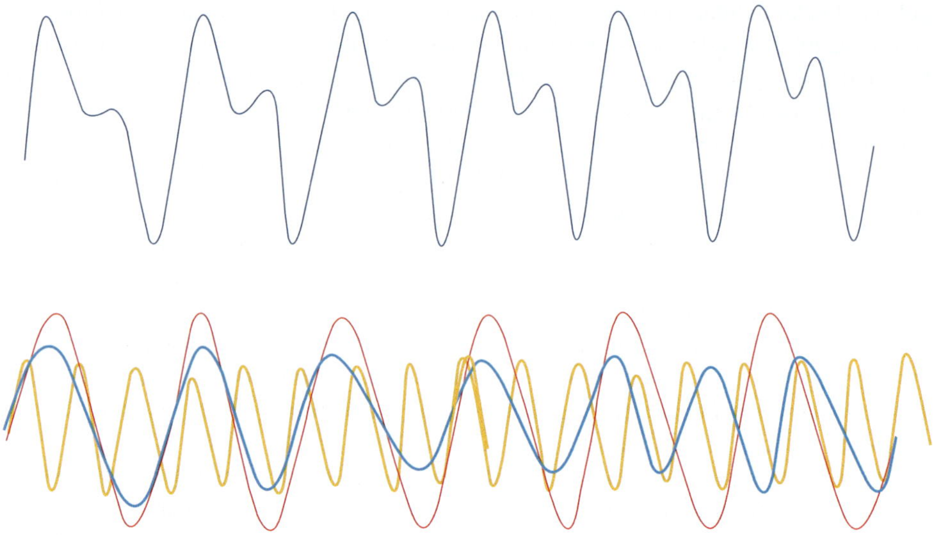

Fig. 35.5 A complex "arterial" waveform, which can be broken down into multiple, component sine waves (fundamental and harmonic). This analysis is known as Fourier analysis

"amplitude"—maximum displacement; and its "frequency"—number of cycles per second. Sine waves of differing amplitude and frequency can combine to form a complex wave. Conversely, a complex wave like the arterial pressure wave can be broken down into multiple component waves. The arterial pressure wave would have a "fundamental" wave, with a frequency equal to the pulse rate (1–3 Hz) and a series of "harmonic" waves, with frequencies in multiples (up to 8–10 times) of the fundamental frequency ($\sim$24 Hz). The process of analyzing a complex wave into its constituent sine waves is known as Fourier analysis (Fig. 35.5).

35.4.2 Natural Frequency and Resonance

Every material when struck, oscillates at its "natural" frequency, and this depends on physical properties of the material, such as density and thickness and also of the adjacent material. If an external force or a wave, with a frequency similar to the natural frequency, is applied, the material would oscillate at its maximal amplitude, and this is known as "resonance." Therefore, if the natural frequency of the IABP monitoring system is close to the frequency of any of the components of an arterial waveform, it would vibrate excessively and distort the signal. Since the range of pulse rate usually seen clinically is 60–180/min or 1–3 Hz, the natural frequency of the arterial pressure transducer should be greater than 8–10 times this fundamental frequency. Most commercially available systems have a natural frequency of around 200 Hz. However, the natural frequency of the system can be reduced by the addition of three-way taps, long tubing, the presence of air bubbles and clots, and it is increased by using shorter and wider arterial cannula and tubing.

35.4.3 Damping

The arterial pressure monitor, in addition to having a high natural frequency, also needs an appropriate damping coefficient (zeta or ζ). Damping can be construed as the force that brings the transducer system back to its resting stage after the oscillation in order to detect the next wave. Therefore, a critical damping is essential for proper functioning of the system, and overdamping or underdamping would adversely affect the measurement. Underdamping leads to large amplitude oscillations and factitiously high systolic and low diastolic pressure readings, although the mean arterial pressure may be accurate. On the contrary, in an overdamped system, the oscillations are subdued and blunted and it reads an erroneously low systolic and a high diastolic pressure, while the mean pressure reading would remain unchanged. In an IABP measuring system, damping is increased by factors that impede fluid flow in the system, namely density of the fluid, a compliant tubing and narrowing (kinks, vasospasm) or obstruction (clots, air bubbles), which are very similar to the factors that lower the natural frequency. The optimal damping coefficient of 0.7 provides the balance between rapid response and accuracy.

35.4.4 "Fast Flush" Test

The IABP monitoring system uses a flushing system, wherein a bag of saline, pressurized to 300 mmHg, infuses at 2–4 ml/h through the fluid-filled tubing to maintain the patency of the cannula. This system can also be used to perform the "fast flush" test to calculate the natural

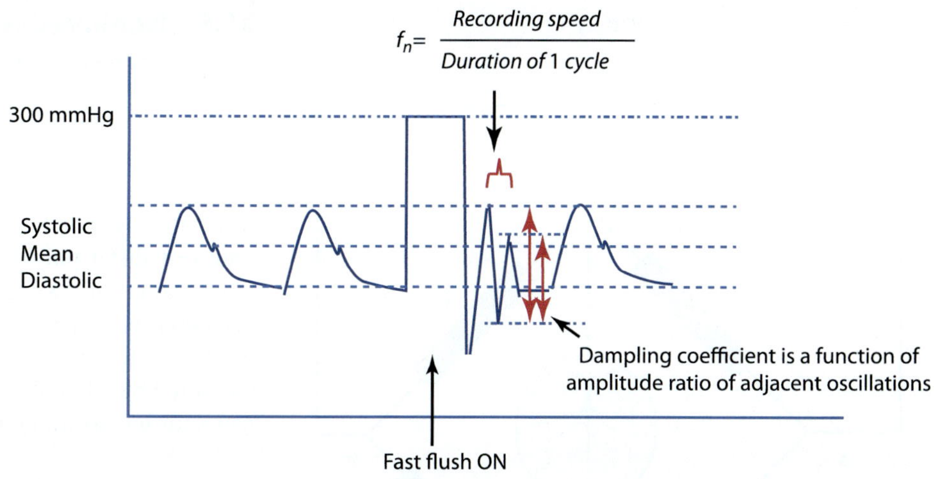

Fig. 35.6 Fast flush test

frequency and the damping coefficient of the system. A short burst of flush is applied, and the pressure waves on the monitor are analyzed. The square wave corresponds to the exposure of the transducer to the 300 mmHg pressure of the flushing system. This is followed by sharp waves oscillating at the natural frequency of the system, and it can be calculated by dividing the screen speed by the wavelength of the resonant waves. Therefore, the closer the oscillation cycles, the higher the natural frequency. Similarly, the ratio of the amplitudes of the second to the first post-flush waves (amplitude ratio) can be used to derive the damping coefficient from standard nomograms. A low-amplitude ratio corresponds to a high damping coefficient, or the system comes to rest quickly (Fig. 35.6).

35.4.4.1 Clinical Significance

Although the desired technical requirements for arterial pressure monitoring are a natural frequency greater than 25 Hz and a damping coefficient of 0.7, these conditions are rarely met in routine clinical practice. Most catheter-tubing transducer systems are underdamped (damping coefficient of 0.15–0.45) and have an acceptable natural frequency of 12–25 Hz. If the fn of the system is less than 7 Hz, it is unacceptable, and if the fn is greater than 24 Hz, damping will have minimal effect on the arterial wave recording.

35.4.5 Transducer

Transducers convert one form of energy into another, and the pressure transducers used for IABP monitoring convert pressure into electrical signal that can be measured and displayed. The arterial pressure wave transmits down the fluid column and displaces the diaphragm of the transducer. This displacement is measured using a strain gauge, which is based on the physical principle that the resistance of a wire increases when it is stretched and decreases when compressed. Therefore, the pressure exerted by the arterial pulse wave on the diaphragm would compress and stretch the wire attached to the diaphragm, and the change in resistance of the wire can be measured precisely by incorporating it as one of the limbs of a "Wheatstone bridge."

35.4.5.1 Wheatstone Bridge

Wheatstone bridge is a circuit designed to measure an unknown resistance. Current is passed through two parallel circuits, each with two resistances in series. A galvanometer connects the two circuits in the middle to detect any flow of current between the circuits (Fig. 35.7). The resistances can be adjusted so that no current flows through the galvanometer and the bridge is said to be balanced, and at this stage, the ratio of the resistances is:

$$R1/R2 = R3/Rx$$

So, if Rx is the resistance attached to the diaphragm and it changes with oscillation of the diaphragm, the adjustable resistance $R2$ can be electronically tuned to balance the bridge and the change in resistance required would reflect the change in pressure and can be electronically displayed.

35.4.5.2 Practical Points

- **Zeroing**—The transducer must be exposed to the atmosphere and calibrated to read zero before it is exposed to the arterial pressure. Note that the level of the transducer is not crucial for zeroing.
- **Leveling**—The transducer must be set at the level of the heart (fourth intercostal space, mid-axillary line) to measure the blood pressure accurately. This is the "phlebostatic" axis (Fig. 35.8). If not, the hydrostatic pressure of the column of blood would cause error. A 10 cm error in

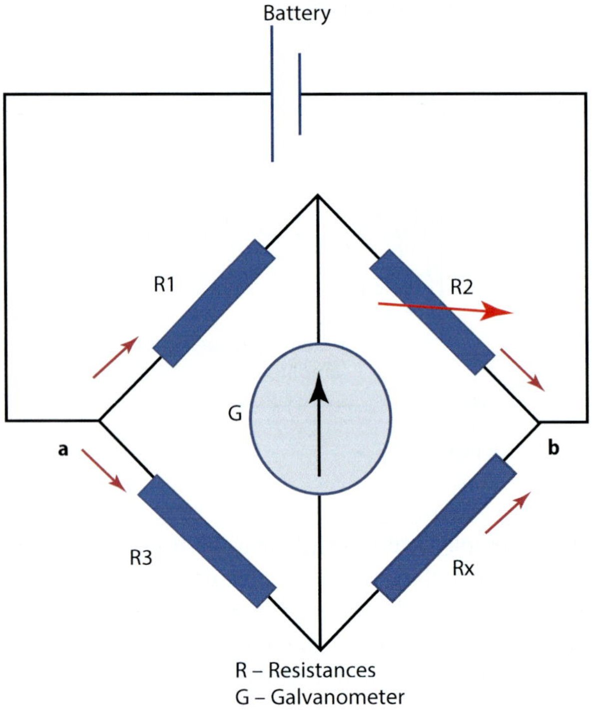

Fig. 35.7 The Wheatstone bridge. Current passes from point "a" to point "b" through two parallel circuits: (1) *R*1 and *R*2 and (2) *R*3 and *R*x. A galvanometer (*G*) connects these circuits in the middle. The resistances can be adjusted so that no current flows through *G*, at which point the bridge is said to be balanced. When the bridge is balanced, then $R1/R2 = R3/Rx$. If *Rx* (resistance attached to the diaphragm) changes, the adjustable resistance *R*2 can be electronically tuned to balance the bridge, which would indicate the change in *Rx*

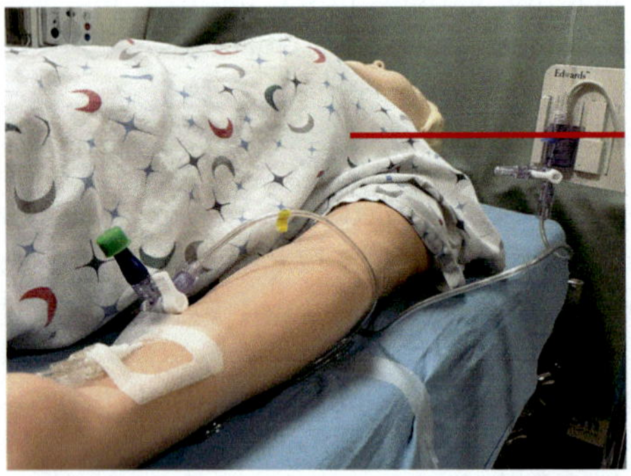

Fig. 35.8 The transducer should be at the level of the heart (phlebostatic axis)

level would result in 7.5 mmHg difference in pressure. However, if one is interested in monitoring the pressure of the cerebral circulation (e.g., in a patient undergoing shoulder surgery in beach-chair position or cervical spine surgery/sub-occipital craniotomy in sitting position), the transducer should be placed at the level of the tragus.

35.5 Noninvasive Blood Pressure Measurement

The basic tenet of noninvasive blood pressure (NIBP) measurement is occlusion of an artery (usually brachial) using a pneumatic cuff and recording the return of pulse distal to it when the pressure in the cuff is released. The return of distal pulse can be detected by digital palpation, auscultation of "Korotkoff" sounds using a stethoscope, detection by Doppler ultrasound probe or automatically by oscillometric principles. The pressure in the cuff can be measured by a liquid (mercury) filled manometer, an aneroid gauge or an electronic pressure transducer.

35.5.1 Korotkoff Sounds

When a sphygmomanometer cuff applied over the upper arm is inflated and gradually deflated, a series of five distinct sounds can be auscultation over the brachial artery, as described by Nikolai Korotkoff in 1905. The first clear snapping sound coincides with the systolic pressure, which increases in intensity (second sound) to a crescendo (third sound) before becoming muffled (fourth sound) and finally disappears (5th sound) when the cuff pressure falls below the diastolic pressure.

35.5.2 Oscillometry

In an automatic NIBP monitor, a microprocessor inflates the pneumatic cuff to occlude the artery and then deflates it in a stepwise manner. As the pneumatic cuff deflates and the arterial flow returns, the vessel wall starts to vibrate and this is detected by the sensors on the cuff. The mean arterial pressure is the point of maximum oscillation and is most accurately measured. The systolic and the diastolic pressures are calculated as the rapid rise and fall of the oscillations, respectively.

Although, these devices are simple and convenient to operate, inappropriate cuff size (over-reading with small cuff), limb movement, external pressure over the cuff, and arrhythmias can lead to inaccuracies in measurement.

35.6 Continuous Noninvasive Arterial Pressure (CNAP)

Continuous measurement of the arterial pressure, using a tiny pneumatic cuff to wrap around a finger and an infrared plethysmography to measure blood volume and flow in the finger, was first described by Jan Penaz, a Czech physiologist, in 1973.

35.6.1 Vascular Unloading Technique

An infrared plethysmography technology can be used to measure the flow and volume of blood in the finger, which changes with each pulsation (increasing during systole and decreasing during diastole). However, if a cyclical, external pressure is applied to the finger, then the blood flow and volume in the artery can be kept constant. This is the basic principle of "vascular unloading" or volume clamp technique (Fig. 35.9). The cuff pressure, which mirrors the pressure inside the artery, can be displayed as the arterial pulse pressure. The added advantage of this technique is the analysis of the pulse pressure variation, which is used for "goal-directed" fluid management. This technique provides a continuous reliable measurement of arterial pressure, but it needs repeated calibration. The arterial pressure varies with the changes in vascular tone, which is dependent on the sympathetic tone and use of vasoactive drugs, and also there is a physiological difference between the pressures measured from more proximal arteries.

35.6.2 Arterial Tonometry

A pressure transducer, placed over a superficial artery (radial), senses the pressure exerted by the pulse and displays it as an arterial wave form.

35.7 Cardiac Output (CO)

Cardiac output (CO) or the volume of blood ejected by each ventricle per minute mathematically equals the product of stroke volume (SV) and the heart rate (HR). The factors that can modify the CO are the heart rate, the cardiac rhythm, the preload, the contractility, and the afterload of the ventricles and their proclivity to ischemia. CO provides a measure of systemic oxygen delivery and global tissue perfusion.

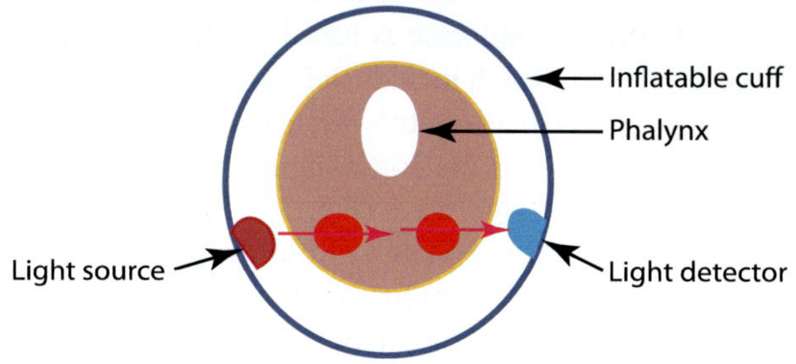

Fig. 35.9 Continuous noninvasive arterial pressure monitoring by volume clamp method. Cross-sectional view of the inflatable cuff around the finger. The cuff pressure is adjusted 1000 times each second to keep the diameter of the finger arteries constant (volume clamping). Continuous recording of the cuff pressure results in real-time finger pressure waveform

Adolph Fick (1829–1901), in 1870, was the first to describe the method to estimate the cardiac output. He suggested that if the amount of a marker taken up by an organ is known, then the blood flow to an organ can be calculated by measuring the concentration of the marker in the arterial supply and the venous drainage of that organ. Applying this principle, if the oxygen consumption (VO_2) of a person is measured by a spirometer using a closed rebreathing circuit with a CO_2 absorber, and the oxygen content of the arterial (Ca) and the mixed venous blood (Cv) is measured, then the CO can be calculated.

$$VO_2 = (CO \times Ca) - (CO \times Cv); \quad CO = VO_2/(Ca - Cv)$$

E.g., Cardiac output = (250 ml O_2/minute)/(200 ml O_2/L − 150 ml O_2/L) = 5 L/minute.

The various techniques that can be used to measure CO are the indicator dilution method, the arterial pulse waveform analysis, ultrasonography, and the bioimpedance method.

35.7.1 Indicator Dilution Technique

An indicator is injected into a vein and is then sampled over time, in either the pulmonary artery or a systemic artery. The concentration of the indicator would display a rapid rise followed by a logarithmic decay. The volume of blood the indicator gets diluted in determines the rate of decay. The Stewart–Hamilton equation states that if a known amount of a substance is injected upstream, the change in its concentration downstream is related to the flow (Fig. 35.10). The flow (volume over time) in this situation is the cardiac output. The indicators used could be thermodilution of a cold or warm thermal bolus, or lithium.

Pulmonary artery catheter (PAC) was initially developed to measure the pressure in the various chambers of the heart and was later modified by Jeremy Swan and William Ganz, to measure the central filling pressures and the CO.

The PAC is a multi-channel catheter, about 110 cm long, that is inserted through the internal jugular or the subclavian vein into the right atrium. It is then gently "floated," aided by an inflatable balloon at the tip, through the right ventricle into the pulmonary artery (Fig. 35.11). This passage of the PAC can be guided by transducing the channel that opens at the tip of the PAC and observing the pressure waves at the different locations. The aim is to site the tip of the catheter in the middle branch of the left or right pulmonary artery to measure the pressure in the pulmonary artery. In that position, if the terminal balloon is inflated, the flow through that arteriole is blocked and the tip is "wedged" and displays the blood pressure distal to it. This pulmonary artery wedge pressure correlates to the left ventricular end-diastolic

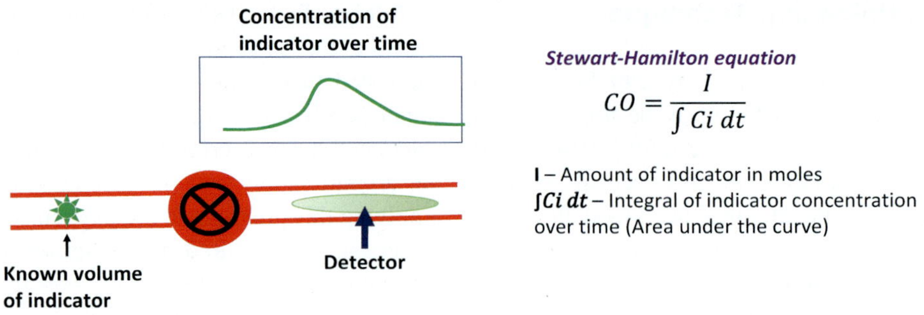

Fig. 35.10 An indicator is injected upstream and measured by a detector downstream. The integral of its concentration over time can be used to measure the cardiac output using the Stewart–Hamilton equation

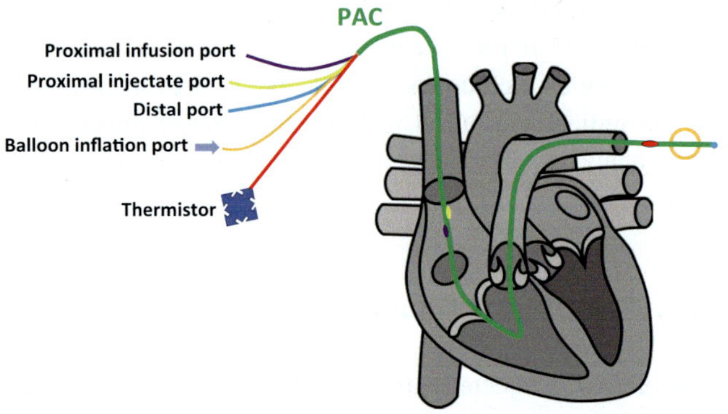

Fig. 35.11 The pulmonary artery catheter (PAC) is a multi-lumen catheter, which is gently 'floated' through the right ventricle into the pulmonary artery

pressure or the preload. One of the channels of the PAC opens into the right atrium and reflects the central venous pressure. A rapid response thermistor, to measure the temperature of the blood, is located at the tip of the catheter.

The PAC is the gold standard of CO measurement against which other methods are compared. A 10 ml bolus of cold (~0 °C) saline or isotonic dextrose solution is injected into the right atrium, and the temperature of the blood in the pulmonary artery is measured continuously by the thermistor. The initial decrease in temperature would be followed by a slow return to the baseline. The rate of return depends on the flow of blood that dilutes the bolus of cold saline. The area under the "temperature" curve represents the change in temperature over time which would be inversely proportional to the CO.

A continuous CO monitoring PAC uses the same thermodilution principle, but instead of a bolus of cold injectate, an electric filament located along the proximal part of the catheter emits pulses of thermal energy and the change in the blood temperature is recorded by the thermistor at the tip of the PAC. Another advance in PAC construction is the incorporation of a tiny light source near the catheter tip which can measure the oxygen saturation of the surrounding blood, using reflectance oximetry. When the catheter is in the appropriate position, it measures the mixed venous oxygen saturation (SvO_2).

35.7.2 Arterial Pressure Waveform Analysis:

"Windkessel" effect: When the left ventricle (LV) contracts, it ejects a stroke volume (≈70 ml) under (systolic) pressure (≈120 mmHg). The elastic wall of the aorta distends to accommodate the stroke volume and subsequently recoils to push this volume forward at (diastolic) pressure (≈80 mmHg). Otto Frank, the German physiologist who first described this phenomenon, wherein a cyclical ventricular contraction generates a constant flow through the blood vessels, called it the "Windkessel" effect. The fire engines of those times used an air chamber (Windkessel chamber) that converted the sinusoidal pressure generated by the rotatory pump into a constant water stream.

Mathematical Analysis: The general principle of the arterial pressure waveform analysis is that the systolic pressure–time integral (SPI) or the area under the systolic part of the arterial curve is directly proportional to the stroke volume and inversely proportional to the total arterial compliance. The estimate of aortic compliance is based on the three-element Windkessel model, which include the compliance of the great arteries (C), the resistance of the vascular system, principally in the arterioles (R) and the aortic impedance (Z) due to the elastic, reflective pressure wave (Fig. 35.12).

Therefore, to measure the CO from the arterial pressure waveform, the arterial compliance should be known. This can either be estimated based on the patient's biometric values such as gender, age, height, and weight (uncalibrated technique), or calculating it by first measuring the CO using the Fick's principle (calibrated technique).

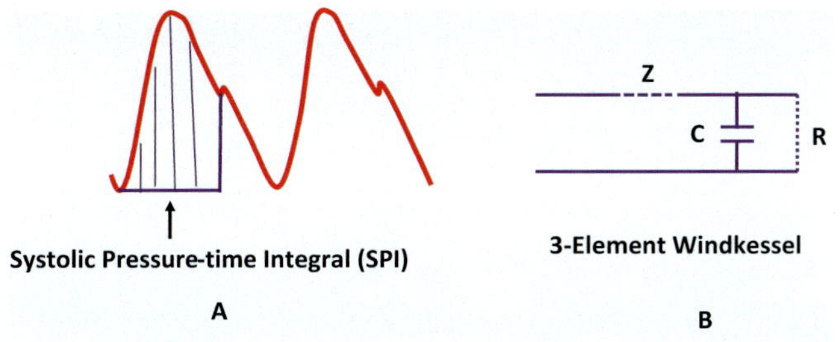

Fig. 35.12 The systolic pressure–time integral (SPI) or the area under the systolic part of the arterial curve (A), is directly proportional to the stroke volume and inversely to the arterial compliance. The estimate of aortic compliance is based on the three-element Windkessel model (B). [Z—impedance, C—capacitor, R—resistor]

- FloTrac/Vigileo: The FloTrac sensor is attached to a standard arterial line. The monitor analyzes the arterial waveform and calculates the CO by incorporating the value of aortic compliance based on the population demographics (e.g., age, weight, height, and gender). A newer model (Clear-Sight®) generates the arterial waveform by using a finger cuff and vascular unloading technique.
- Pulse Index Continuous Cardiac Output (PiCCO): This system uses a transpulmonary thermodilution method to calibrate its algorithm. It requires a standard central line and a thermistor-tipped arterial cannula which is placed within the femoral or the brachial artery. Cold saline is injected into the central line, and the temperature change is measured at the arterial cannula. The CO is measured using the Stewart–Hamilton equation. This information is then used to calibrate the program that analyzes the pulse pressure waveform.
- Lithium Dilution Cardiac Output (LiDCO): This system uses a lithium dilution method to calibrate its algorithm and requires only a standard arterial cannulation. Lithium chloride is injected into a central or even a peripheral vein, and the change in concentration is measured by an electrode sampling at the arterial cannula site.

35.7.3 Ultrasonography

Although ultrasound are sound waves greater than 20,000 Hz (Hz), the frequency used for medical imaging is 2–20 MHz. The speed of ultrasound through soft tissue is 1540 m/s. Echocardiography uses ultrasound to delineate the structure and function of the heart, and the ultrasound probe can be placed either on the chest wall, known as the transthoracic echocardiography (TTE), or inserted into the esophagus, the trans-esophageal echocardiography (TEE).

Doppler Principle: When an ultrasound wave strikes a moving object, some of it gets reflected with a change in its frequency. The reflected waves are at a higher frequency if the object is moving toward the probe and lower if it is moving away. The shift in frequency is proportional to the velocity of the moving object. The frequency of the reflected wave can be detected by the ultrasound probe and using the Doppler frequency shift equation, and the velocity of the reflector can be calculated.

$$\text{Frequency(received)} = \frac{2 \times \text{Frequency(transmitted)} \times \text{Velocity of reflector} \times \text{Cos}\theta}{\text{Speed of sound in tissue}}$$

Θ—Angle of insonation.

The basic premise of using ultrasonography to calculate the CO is to measure the cross-sectional area of the left ventricular outflow tract (LVOT) and the velocity of blood expelled through it using the Doppler principle (Fig. 35.13).

The diameter of the LVOT, about 1 cm from the aortic valve, is measured by specific orientation of the ultrasound probe, namely the mid-esophageal long-axis (TEE) or the parasternal long-axis (TTE) view. Assuming the LVOT to be circular, the area is calculated using the formula for area of a circle ($A = \pi r^2$). Using a deep trans-gastric (TEE) or the apical five-chamber (TTE) view, a pulsed-wave Doppler is used to measure the velocity of the red cells at the LVOT. Care should be taken to measure it at the same location the LVOT diameter was measured. The area under the curve of this spectral Doppler profile is known as the velocity time integral (VTI). This depicts the distance a red cell travels per beat or the stroke distance, which when multiplied by the estimated cross-sectional area of the aorta, gives the stroke volume. As evident in Fig. 35.13, most echocardiogram machines are programed to calculate the LVOT area and the stroke volume, and the accuracy of the measurement depends on the expertise of the proceduralists to attain the appropriate view.

35.7.4 Bioimpedance and Bioreactance

The human body is able to conduct electrical current because of the presence of charged ions within the body fluids. According to Ohm's law ($I = V/R$), the current passing through a substance is inversely proportional to the resistance it offers to the potential difference. This resistance is termed "impedance" when it is an alternating current. Impedance can be defined as a combination of Ohmic resistance and reactance, or resistance to an alternating current, and is denoted as Z. The "bioimpedance" varies between different tissues, e.g., blood (150 Ω/cm), plasma (63 Ω/cm), lungs (1275 Ω/cm), and fat (2500 Ω/cm).

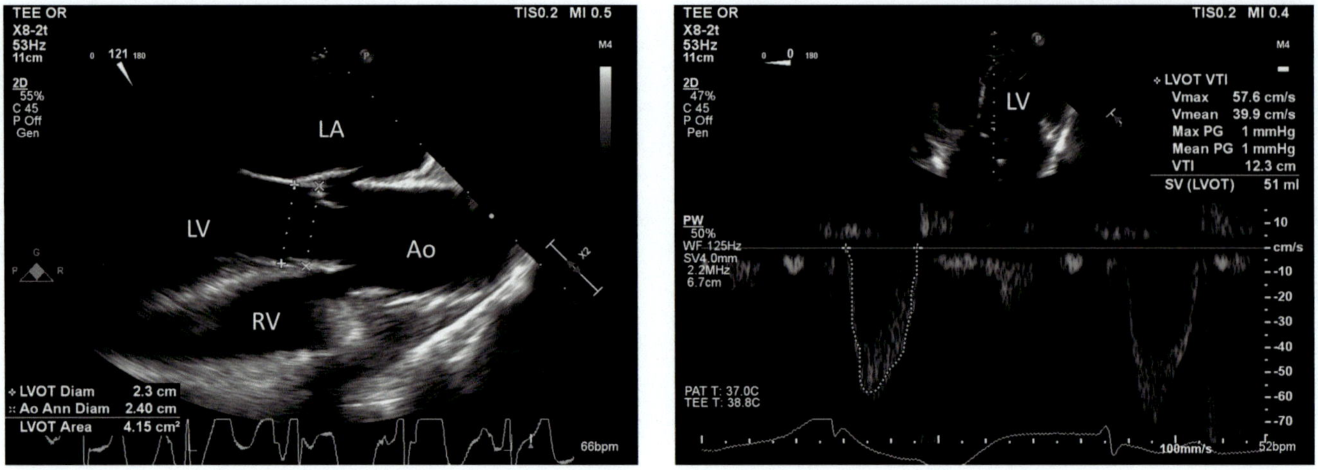

A B

Fig. 35.13 Trans-esophageal Echocardiographic (TEE) views showing (A) the diameter at the left ventricular outlet tract, and (B) measuring the Velocity Time integral (VTI) using the pulsed-wave Doppler and calculating the stroke volume (SV)

The basic principle of the **bioimpedance** cardiography is that thorax is viewed as two concentric cylinders, a low impedance, inner one containing blood and a higher impedance, outer one constituting the lung and other body tissues. Since the volume of blood increases with each systole, the bioimpedance decreases during the ejection phase and returns to baseline (Zo) during diastole. Electrodes are applied at the base of the neck (thoracic inlet) and the costal margins (thoracic outlet), and a high-frequency, low-amplitude current (1.4–1.8 mA at 30–75 kHz) is transmitted between these electrodes and the change in their amplitude is measured (Fig. 35.14). This information can be used to calculate the rate of the change of Z ($\Delta Z/\Delta t$), which correlates to the flow of blood into the aorta, during systole.

The stroke volume is proportional to the product of $\Delta Z/\Delta t$, the ventricular ejection time (VET), and the volume of electrically participating tissue (VEPT), which is essentially

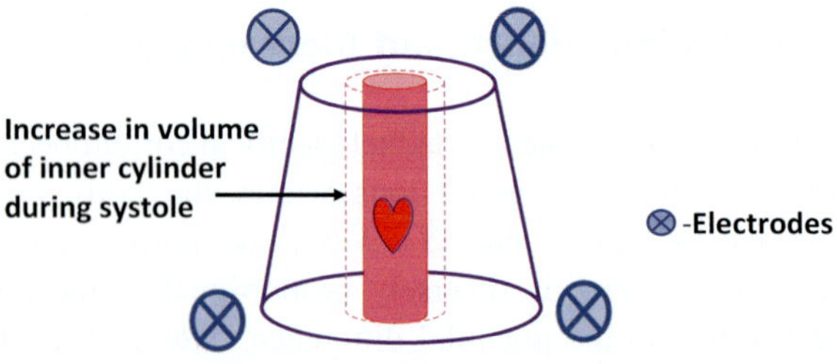

Fig. 35.14 The bioimpedance model views the chest as two concentric cylinders, a low impedance, inner one containing blood, and a higher impedance, outer one constituting the lung and other thoracic tissues. The volume of the inner cylinder increases during systole. The electrodes are applied at the base of the neck (thoracic inlet) and the costal margins (thoracic outlet), and a high-frequency (30–75 kHz), low-amplitude current (1.4–1.8 mA) is transmitted between them

the thoracic volume. The VET is calculated from the R–R interval on the ECG, and the VEPT is predicted from the height, weight, and gender of the subject.

$$\mathrm{SV} = \frac{\Delta Z}{\Delta t} \times \mathrm{VET} \times \mathrm{VEPT}$$

Although this technique of measuring CO was originally used in astronauts, in the 1960s, several modifications have been incorporated over the years. Two significant modifications are substituting the cylindrical model of the chest to a truncated cone and use of the formula that accounts for deviation from ideal body weight in calculating the thoracic volume. The bioimpedance technique is unreliable during arrhythmias (VET is measured from the R–R interval), acute changes in tissue water (pulmonary edema or pleural effusion would alter the bioimpedance), changes in temperature and humidity (impact on the electric conductivity between the electrodes and the skin), and mechanical factors such as noise from electrocautery, mechanical ventilation, and surgical manipulation.

Bioreactance is an improved technology which analyzes the relative phase shifts in the voltage of the alternating currents. According to bioreactance, the human thorax is considered an electric circuit with resistors (R) and capacitors (C), which together generate the two components of thoracic impedance (Zo), namely amplitude and phase (phi, ϕ). The pulsatile ejection of blood from the heart modifies the value of R and of C, leading to instantaneous changes in the amplitude and the phase of Zo. Since phase shifts can occur only because of pulsatile flow, and the overwhelming component of thoracic pulsatility stems from the aorta, the bioreactance signal is strongly correlated with aortic flow. This is impacted less by movement artifact, patient body variance, and thoracic fluid which would be relatively static.

The bioreactance device is made up of a high-frequency (75-kHz) sine wave generator and four dual electrodes to establish electrical contact with the body. Each electrode sticker contains one electrode that transmits the high-frequency sine wave into the body, while the other electrode is used by the voltage input amplifier. The signal processing unit detects the relative phase shift ($\Delta\phi$) of the input signal. The peak rate of change in phase ($\Delta\phi/\mathrm{d}t$) is proportional to the peak aortic flow.

$$\mathrm{SV} = K \times \mathrm{VET} \times \frac{\Delta\phi}{\mathrm{d}t}$$

K is a constant of proportionality which is determined by bioreactance.

35.8 Autotransfusion Devices

The technique of transfusing patients with their own blood has reduced the need for allogenic blood transfusion and thus reduces its associated risks. This is achieved by either perioperative donation or blood salvage during surgery.

35.8.1 Preoperative Autologous Donation

Patients can donate a unit of their blood weekly, up to three or more times, prior to surgery depending on their physical status and hematocrit. Anemia, which limits donation, can be corrected by erythropoietin or iron supplements. The donated blood is stored similar to other donated blood.

35.8.2 Acute Normovolemic Hemodilution

During the early stage of the intraoperative period, 2–4 units of blood can be withdrawn from the patient and replaced with an equivalent volume of crystalloids. The goal is to dilute the hematocrit to 27–30%, depending on the patient's medical status. The donated blood is stored in the operating room in normal blood donation bags with anticoagulant and transfused back into the patient at the end of the surgery.

35.8.3 Intraoperative Blood Salvage

The technique of collecting blood lost during surgery, processing it, and transfusing it back to the patient can be considered during surgery with significant blood loss (liver transplantation, spinal instrumentation, major trauma, and cardiac surgery). It is contraindicated if contamination with pus, feces, amniotic fluid, or malignant cells is suspected. The Cell Saver® (Haemonetics Corp., Braintree, MA) collects the blood via suction and mixes it with anticoagulant. This is then centrifuged to separate the red cells, which are then washed with saline and collected in bags ready to be transfused back into the patient. The potential problem is dilutional coagulopathy as platelet and clotting factors are removed during the process. Some surgeries (cardiac and orthopedic) are associated with more blood loss postoperatively than during the operative period and could benefit by using this technique in the postoperative period.

35.9 Body Warming Devices

Loss of body heat occurs in the perioperative period irrespective of the type of anesthesia. There are several mechanisms by which heat transfers from a warmer body to its surroundings, causing hypothermia.

35.9.1 Mechanism of Heat Loss

1. **Redistribution**—During the initial operative period, there is redistribution of heat from the core to the surface, depending on the temperature gradient, room temperature, body exposure, and extent of vasodilatation due to loss of sympathetic tone and vasodilatory effect of anesthetics.
2. **Radiation**—Heat transfers by infrared radiation between two objects that are not in contact. This is the mechanism of maximum heat loss during the perioperative setting.
3. **Convection**—Convection is the transfer of heat from the body to moving air or liquid, and it depends on the speed of the moving fluid and the difference between the body and the ambient temperature.
4. **Conduction**—Transfer of heat between bodies in contact occurs by conduction, and it depends on the temperature difference and the area of contact between the two.
5. **Evaporation**—Conversion of water into vapor needs energy, even though there is no rise in temperature, and the amount of energy needed depends upon the temperature of water. This energy is known as latent heat of vaporization ("massic enthalpy of evaporation") and is taken from the body surface, thereby decreasing the temperature of the body. This type of heat loss occurs from the skin, the respiratory tract, and the open wounds. The amount of vaporization is inversely proportional to the relative humidity of the gas in contact with the surface and the area of exposure.

35.9.2 Strategies to Minimize Heat Loss

Perioperative hypothermia is associated with increased postoperative morbidity, and the various strategies that are used to minimize loss of body heat could be divided into three broad categories:

35.9.2.1 Insulation

Stagnant air is a good insulator and can be trapped next to the patient's body by using insulating covers such as surgical drapes, cotton blankets, and conductive plastic sheets. Since heat loss is proportional to the exposed skin surface, this passive insulation can limit heat loss. Care should be taken not to use material that can develop static electricity, such as wool or ordinary plastic.

35.9.2.2 Active Warming Devices

Heat can be supplied to the patient by different devices. Although very efficient in maintaining the body temperature, it may be associated with potential problems such as skin burns, increased heat loss through radiation, and possibility of infection.

a. *Forced Air Warmers*—These are the most commonly used devices, wherein an electric heater blows warm air through an air blanket that is draped over the patient's exposed body surface. A thermostat controls the temperature of the air. These devices can increase the body temperature by approximately 0.75 °C/h.
b. *Heating Mattress*—An underbody mattress that is electrically heated, or has circulating warm water or air, has the advantage that it can cover a large area irrespective of the operative site. However, in a lean or an emaciated patient, the contact may happen only over bony prominences with compression of the cutaneous vessels. At these points, there is potential for burns as the poor circulation may delay the dissipation of heat. Underbody forced air warmers are effective in neonatal and pediatric patients.
c. *Radiant Heaters*—Overhead infrared radiant heaters are effective in maintaining body temperature in certain situations where whole body exposure is needed, such as in the trauma bay and neonatal resuscitation. Although it has a thermostat controlled by a temperature probe placed over the patient, care should be taken to maintain the recommended distance from the patient. Another disadvantage is discomfort to the operating team.

35.9.2.3 Internal Warming Devices

Warming of intravenous fluids and blood and ventilation with warm and humidified gases is an effective way to decrease perioperative hypothermia.

a. *Fluid Warmer*—Infusion of 1 L of crystalloid at 20 °C can decrease the body temperature by 0.25 °C. Thermostat-controlled water baths circulate warm water through the outer channel of coaxial intravenous (IV) infusion tubing with the IV fluid going through the inner channel.
b. *Humidification of the Inspired Gas Mixture*—Use of advanced airway devices reduces the surface area available to warm and humidify the inspired gas mixture. Since the inhaled anesthetic gases are cold and dry, heat is needed to warm and humidify them. The amount of heat energy required to humidify the inspired gas is five times greater than that needed to warm it to body temperature.

- Heat loss from warming 1 L of inspired gas (20–37 °C):

$$\text{Volume} \times \text{Specific heat} \times \text{Temperature}$$
$$1 \times 1.2\ \mathrm{J/L/^{\circ}C} \times 17\,^{\circ}\mathrm{C} = 20.4\ \mathrm{J}$$

- Heat loss from humidifying 1 L of inspired gas at 37 °C:

$$\text{Volume} \times \text{Water required} \times \text{specific heat}$$
$$1 \times 44\ \mathrm{mg/L} \times 2.4\ \mathrm{MJ/Kg} = 105.6\ \mathrm{J}$$

Humidification can be achieved by ultrasonic heated humidifiers that actively add water vapor into inspired gases or the passive heat and moisture exchange (HME) filters. The active humidifiers are more commonly used in intensive care units during prolonged ventilation, while HME filters are the ones commonly used during the intraoperative period. HMEs are made from hygroscopic paper filter encased in a plastic case. The other advantage of humidifying the inspired gases is reduction of bronchial mucosal drying and preservation of ciliary function.

35.10 Temperature Measurement

Significant changes in body temperature occur in an anesthetized patient, and this could be due to anesthetic-induced cutaneous vasodilatation, infusion of large volumes of cold fluids, loss of body heat due to exposure, alteration of thermoregulatory mechanism, or induced hypothermia. Measurement of body temperature forms part of the standard American Society of Anesthesiologists (ASA) monitoring.

There are a variety of technologies available to measure temperature. These are based on changes in property of material due to changes in temperature:

1. **Thermistor**—The resistance to passage of current through a metal oxide increases exponentially as the temperature decreases and this change in resistance can be measured and presented as temperature. A thermistor consists of a small bead of metal (manganese, nickel, iron) oxide that is fused into a wire with a source of current and a means to measure this current. The advantage of a thermistor is small size, rapid response, sensitivity, and relatively inexpensive.
2. **Thermocouple**—At the junction of two dissimilar metals (thermocouple), there is a potential difference that depends on the temperature of the junction. This is the principle of Seebeck effect. The change in current due to the change in potential difference would indicate the change in temperature. A thermocouple thermometer consists of two dissimilar metals (copper and constantan) attached to each other at both ends: One end is kept at a constant reference temperature, and the other end acts as the temperature measuring probe. The advantage is that this probe can be in form of a needle (similar to ones used to measure the temperature of cooked poultry in an oven).
3. **Platinum Wire**—The electrical resistance of a wire increases with temperature, and for platinum, it is found to be almost linear. Whenever a change in resistance is to be measured, it is incorporated into a Wheatstone bridge (Fig. 35.7).
4. **Liquid Crystal**—Certain organic crystals when heated transition through an intermediate state before they liquefy. During this phase, they are optically active and emit different colors depending on the temperature. These thermochromic crystals can be incorporated into a plastic strip and when applied to the patient's forehead will display the color according to the temperature.
5. **Infrared**—Infrared radiation emitted by any object is proportional to its temperature. Therefore, small handheld devices that measure IR from the skin or tympanic membrane can be used to measure body temperature.
6. **Mercury**—The classic mercury thermometer uses the principle that the volume of a liquid is proportional to its temperature. Mercury thermometer are rarely use in clinical anesthesia for safety issues such as injury by broken glass and infection.

35.11 Defibrillator

Arrhythmia can lead to inefficient myocardial function (atrial fibrillation, ventricular tachycardia) or no function at all (ventricular fibrillation). A defibrillator is a device that can be used to pass a direct current (DC) through the heart to reset the electrical activity with the hope that it restarts with a normal rhythm. It was invented by Kouwenhoven in 1932.

35.11.1 Capacitor

A capacitor is an electrical component that can store energy, and it forms the most important component of a defibrillator. It consists of two conductive plates separated by an insulator (dielectric). The amount of energy stored depends on the charge and potential difference:

$$\text{Energy}(\text{Joules} - J) = \text{Charge}(C) \times \text{Potential}(V)$$

One coulomb (C) is the amount of electric charge (6.24×10^{18} electrons) that passes when 1 A (A) of current flows over 1 s. Capacitance is the amount of electric charge that a capacitor can store; 1 F (F) is the capacitance when a potential of 1 V (V) is applied across a capacitor with a charge of 1 C.

When the power source is connected to the capacitor (during "charging"), electrons flow to one of the plates of the capacitor and electrons from the other plate flow back to the power source. This creates a potential difference between the plates. The buildup of charge, and thus the potential difference, is exponential (Fig. 35.15). The amount of energy stored in the capacitor is given by the equation:

$$\left[J = 1/2FV^2\right]$$

To store up to 400 J in a capacitor with a capacitance of 32 μ(mu)F, a voltage of 5000 V is needed:

$$\left[J = 1/2 \times 32 \times 10^{-6} \times 5000^2 = 400\text{J}\right]$$

35.11.2 Power Source

Previously, inbuilt step-up transformers were used to convert 110/220 V alternating current (AC) to 5000 AC, which was then converted to 5000 DC by a rectifier. However, modern defibrillators have a rechargeable battery that provides DC. This DC has to be first converted to AC using an inverter

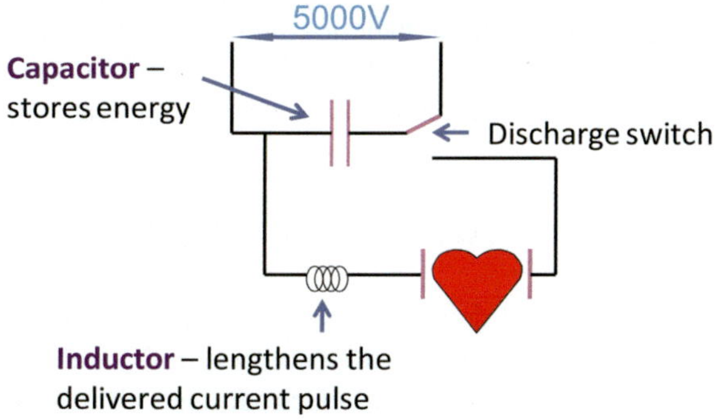

Fig. 35.15 The physical principle of a defibrillator

before it can be amplified and rectified to 5000 DC. The step-up transformer can provide variable output, thus allowing the clinician the flexibility to select the amount of charge.

35.11.3 Discharge

The stored energy is then discharged through the paddles/pads placed over the patient's chest. The amount of current that passes through the heart is about 35 A, but it depends on the impedance of the skin, chest wall, and other tissues, which is usually about 50–150 Ω (ohm) with good contact and electrode gel. The defibrillating current, to be effective, must be sustained for several milliseconds, but the energy from a capacitor discharges rapidly. Therefore, incorporated into the paddle circuit is an inductor—a coil of wire that produces a magnetic field when current passes through it. This magnetic field produces a current in the direction opposite to the original current, thus prolonging the current decay. Henry is the unit of inductance.

35.11.4 Waveform

The older models of defibrillator use a monophasic waveform, where the current flows in one direction only. However, most modern ones employ biphasic waveform, wherein the initial direction of current flow is reversed half way, by reversing the polarity of the paddles. The biphasic waveform is more efficient and requires lower energy, which reduces the myocardial damage.

35.11.5 Implantable Cardioverter-Defibrillator (ICD)

These devices continuously monitor the cardiac rhythm and can automatically treat life-threatening arrhythmias. These implantable devices have miniature capacitors (Al/Al_2O_3) and long-lasting lithium batteries and can deliver pacing pulse or a 5–40 J DC directly to the myocardium through electrodes. The newer versions are MRI conditional.

35.11.6 Automated External Defibrillators

Automated external defibrillators (AEDs) are now available in many public buildings, airports, and train stations. It consists of a battery pack and electrode pads. It can detect cardiac rhythm, analyze them, and inform the rescuer if a shock is advised and deliver it appropriately.

35.12 Questions and Answers

Questions (Choose the Most Appropriate Answer)

1. Which of the following is NOT TRUE of the infrared gas analyzer?
   A. Water vapor interferes with the measurement.
   B. The sampled gas cannot be added back to the breathing circuit.
   C. It is based on Beer-Lambert's law.
   D. Gases such as helium and xenon cannot be measured.
2. The pulse oximeter is based on which physical principle?
   A. Boyle's law
   B. Avogadro's law
   C. Beer-Lambert law
   D. Bernoulli principle
3. Oxygen in a gas mixture can be measured by all the following EXCEPT
   A. Paramagnetic analyzer
   B. Galvanic Cell analyzer
   C. Polarographic analyzer
   D. Infrared gas analyzer
4. A 20 G arterial line is placed and connected to a transducer that is located 10 cm below the level of the heart. The system is zeroed at the stopcock located at the wrist while the patient's arm is stretched on the arm board. How will the arterial line pressure compare with the true blood pressure? It would be …
   A. 10 mmHg higher
   B. 7.5 mmHg higher
   C. Same
   D. 7.5 mmHg lower
   E. 10 mmHg lower
5. A 70-year-old is to undergo right hip arthroplasty. A 20 G A-line is inserted into the right radial artery and zeroed with the transducer at the level of the heart. On positioning in left decubitus position, the right arm is placed on a pillow such that the right wrist is 20 cm above the heart, while the transducer is positioned at the level of the sternum. The BP reads 120/80. The actual pressure would be…
   A. 105/65 mmHg
   B. 100/60 mmHg
   C. 120/80 mmHg
   D. 135/95 mmHg
   E. 140/100 mmHg
6. In ◘ Fig. 35.16 showing the arterial pressure recording, what do the arrows in the figure denote?
   A. Respiratory variations
   B. Atrial fibrillation
   C. Under-damped waveform

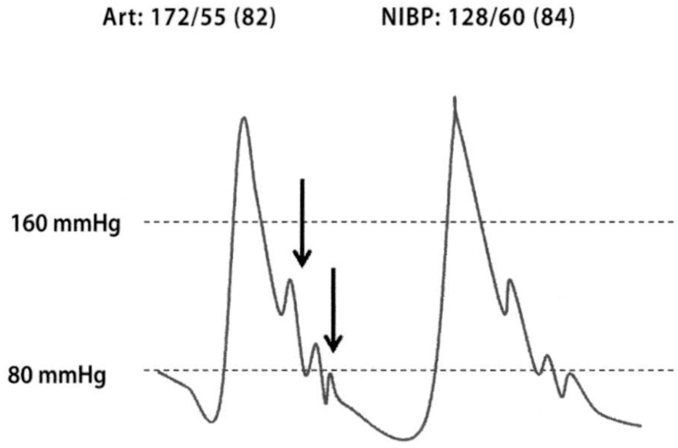

Fig. 35.16 Arterial pressure recording

D. Over-damped waveform
E. Stroke volume variation

7. Which statement about mass spectrometry is true?
   A. The analyzing chambers operate at atmospheric pressure.
   B. The ions are accelerated by an anode plate.
   C. Mass spectrometry requires tiny amounts of gas to analyze.
   D. The sample from a mass spectrometer can be returned to a circle system to allow low flow anesthesia.
   E. Mass spectrometry is less accurate than infrared absorption spectrometry.
8. Compared with use of alpha-stat blood gas management in a patient undergoing cardiopulmonary bypass, use of pH stat management is associated with:
   A. Decreased carbon dioxide content in blood
   B. Decreased P50
   C. Improved myocardial preservation
   D. Increased cerebral blood flow
9. Which of the following is true regarding a defibrillator?
   A. A high-voltage AC current is passed through the chest to defibrillate.
   B. A capacitor is a segment of wire with high resistance that can store energy.
   C. The amount of current that passes through the chest is about 200 amperes.
   D. An inductor is used to prolong the duration of defibrillating current.
   E. A 360 Joules monophasic current is more efficient than 200 Joules biphasic current.
10. Which of the following physical principles is NOT used to measure patient body temperature?
    A. Rise in temperature increases electrical resistance through a wire.
    B. Rise in temperature increases pressure within a chamber containing gas.
    C. As temperature decreases the resistance of current through a metal oxide increases.
    D. The potential difference in a thermocouple is proportional to the temperature.
    E. Infrared radiation from a body is proportional to its temperature.

Answers

1. **B**. Molecules with two or more dissimilar atoms absorb infrared (IR) radiation, and different molecules have distinct IR absorption spectra. The sample of gas aspirated can be returned to the circuit after analysis. The amount of gas aspirated for sample varies from 60 to 200 ml/min.
2. **C.**
   - 5 *Boyle's Law* – Pressure and volume of a gas have an inverse relationship, when temperature is held constant.
   - 5 *Avogadro's Law* – Equal volumes of all gases, at the same temperature and pressure, have the same number of molecules.
   - 5 *Lambert's law* stated that absorbance of a material sample is directly proportional to its thickness (path length). *Beer*'s law stated that absorbance is proportional to the concentrations of the attenuating material.
   - 5 *Bernoulli principle* – An increase in velocity is accompanied by a decrease in density and/or pressure.
   - **D**. Molecules with two or more dissimilar atoms absorb infrared (IR) radiation, and different molecules have distinct IR absorption spectra. Oxygen, nitrogen, helium, xenon, and argon do not absorb IR radiation and cannot be measured by this technique.
   - **C**. It is important to zero the electromechanical transducer system with the reference point at the approximate level of the heart (phlebostatic axis). This will eliminate the effect of the fluid column of the transducer system on the arterial BP reading of the system.

In this question, the system was zeroed at the stopcock, which was located at the patient's wrist (approximate level of the ventricle). Blood pressure expressed by the arterial line will, therefore, be accurate, provided the distance between the patient's wrist and the stopcock remains the same. Would the system have been zeroed at the transducer stopcock, the arterial pressure would have been off by

13.6 mmHg (conversion factor of 1.36 from cmH_2O to mmHg).

5. **C**. The system should be zeroed with the reference point of the transducer at the approximate level of the aortic root, eliminating the effect of the fluid column of the system on arterial BP readings. Since the transducer is at the level of the heart, the BP would be accurate.
6. **C**. The displayed signal reflects the actual pressure as well as distortions from the measuring system (i.e., the catheter, tubing, stopcocks, or amplifier). In an underdamped signal, as in this case, exaggerated readings are noted (widened pulse pressure). In an over-damped signal, readings are diminished (narrowed pulse pressure). Note however the mean BP tends to correlate with the noninvasive blood pressure.
7. **C**. Mass spectrometry:
   - 5 Highly accurate, needs tiny amount and can differentiate different gases
   - 5 Mainly for research and environment analysis
   - 5 Needs high vacuum
   - 5 Gases cannot be returned to the patient, due to ionic degradation
   - 5 Long delay time
8. **D**. Solubility of all gases, including CO_2 and O_2, in blood increases with a fall in temperature. Thus, hypothermia causes the PO_2 and PCO_2 to fall and the pH to rise. Analysis of a sample taken from a hypothermic patient occurs at 37 °C, and the PO_2 and PCO_2 results are artificially high. The result can be corrected to represent the pH, PO_2, and PCO_2 at the patient's temperature. In practice such correction is unnecessary.

When cardiopulmonary bypass was developed, it was thought that the reduction in $PaCO_2$ during hypothermia would result in cerebral vasoconstriction. In pH stat management, CO_2 was added to the oxygenator to maintain a temperature-corrected $PaCO_2$ of 5.3 kPa and a pH of 7.4. The alternative and now standard strategy is that of alpha-stat in which a non-temperature-corrected $PaCO_2$ of 5.3 kPa and a pH of 7.4 is maintained. The true value of $PaCO_2$ is lower than this, but the associated alkalosis is thought to aid enzyme function during hypothermia.

9. **D**. A direct current is used for defibrillation.

A capacitor is an electrical component that can store energy, and it forms the most important component of a defibrillator. It consists of two conductive plates separated by an insulator (dielectric).

The amount of current that passes through the heart is about 35A, but it depends on the impedance of the skin, chest wall, and other tissues, which is usually about 50–150 Ω(ohm) with good contact and electrode gel. The defibrillating current, to be effective, must be sustained for several milliseconds, but the energy from a capacitor discharges rapidly. Therefore, incorporated into the paddle circuit is an inductor—a coil of wire that produces a magnetic field when current passes through it. This magnetic field produces a current in the direction opposite to the original current, thus prolonging the current decay.

The biphasic waveform is more efficient and requires lower energy, which reduces the myocardial damage.

10. **B**. Although rise in temperature increases pressure within a chamber containing gas, this principle is not used to measure temperature.

Electric resistance through a wire increases linearly with rise in temperature. A thermistor works on the principle that the resistance to passage of current through a metal oxide increases exponentially as the temperature decreases. At the junction of two dissimilar metals (thermocouple), there is a potential difference that depends on the temperature of the junction. This is the principle of Seebeck effect.

Small handheld devices that measure temperature from the skin or tympanic membrane are based on the principle that infrared radiation emitted by any object is proportional to its temperature.

The classic mercury thermometer uses the principle that the volume of a liquid is proportional to its temperature.

Further Reading

1. Westerhof N, Lankhaar J-W, Westerho BE. The arterial Windkessel. Med Biol Eng Comput. 2009;47:131–41. https://doi.org/10.1007/s11517-008-0359-2.
2. Davis PD, Kenny GNC. Basic physics and measurement in anaesthesia. 5th ed. New Delhi: Butterworth-Heinemann; 2005.

Electrical and Fire Safety in the Operating Room

36

D. John Doyle

Abstract

This chapter explores essential aspects of electrical and fire safety in operating rooms. It delves into technical concepts like Ohm's law and the distinction between AC and DC currents, emphasizing the importance of electrical grounding, isolation transformers, and monitoring systems like the line isolation monitor. Physiological effects of electrical shocks are categorized into macroshock and microshock, with attention to their impact on the body. Fire safety considerations encompass identifying fuel sources, oxidizers, and ignition sources within the fire triangle framework, alongside management strategies for operating room fires, including preventive measures, appropriate fire extinguisher selection, and compliance with standards. Principles of fire safety are outlined, such as understanding intraoperative fire dynamics and the significance of fire drills in fostering preparedness among operating room personnel.

Keywords

Anaesthesia • Fire safety • Electrical safety • Operating room • Fire safety education • Fire prevention • Ignition sources

Key Points: Electrical Safety

- If the electron flow or current flow is always in the same direction, it is referred to as *direct current* (DC); if the electron flow reverses direction at a regular interval, it is termed *alternating current* (AC).
- The current that passes through an electrical resistor when a voltage difference is applied across it is governed by Ohm's law.
- The electrical power consumed by an electrical device is measured in watts and is the product of the voltage applied to the device and the electrical current that passes through the device.
- Capacitors are a key component in the design of cardiac defibrillators, where they serve as an energy storage device.
- When an electrical shock occurs, damage can occur in one of two ways: (1) Electrical current can disrupt the normal physiological function of cells or (2) the electrical current may raise the temperature of the tissue sufficiently to produce a burn.
- The severity of an electrical shock is determined by the amount of current (amperes), its path through the body, and the duration of the current flow.

Key Points: Fire Safety

- All fires require three items: a fuel source, an oxidizing agent (usually oxygen), and a source of ignition (the "fire triangle").
- Potential fuel sources found in the operating room include alcohol prep solutions and flammable surgical drapes.
- Common oxidizer sources include oxygen delivered by face mask or nasal cannula as well as nitrous oxide.
- Common sources of ignition include electrocautery, lasers, defibrillators, and even fiber optic light sources.
- The ASA has published an algorithm for use in the event of an operating room fire.

36.1 Introduction

36.1.1 Electrical Safety

Electrical safety in the operating room depends first on an understanding of a number of technical concepts such as Ohm's law (voltage equals current times resistance) and the

D. J. Doyle (✉)
Department of General Anesthesiology, Cleveland Clinic, Cleveland, OH, USA
e-mail: djdoyle@hotmail.com

M. Argalious et al. (eds.), *Basic Sciences in Anesthesia*,
https://doi.org/10.1007/978-3-031-60203-0_36

difference between AC and DC current. In addition, one must understand the use of electrical grounding, electrical isolation transformers, and other protection devices. The performance of electrical isolation transformers are monitored using a line isolation monitor. The effect of electrical current passing through the body is determined by the amount of current (amperes), its path through the body, and the duration of the current flow. Should an electrical shock occur, damage can occur via the disruption of the normal physiological function of cells or raising the temperature of the tissue sufficiently to produce a burn. Macroshock refers to large amounts of current flowing through a person, which can cause harm or death. Microshock refers to very small amounts of current (in the microampere and milliampere range) and applies only to the electrically susceptible patient, such as an individual who has an external conduit that is in direct contact with the heart.

36.1.2 Fire Safety

Operating room fires continue to be a sporadic problem in the United States and around the world. These include non-airway fires (e.g., surgical drapes ignited by high-intensity light cords used for surgical headlights) as well as often deadly airway fires (e.g., endotracheal tracheal tube inadvertently ignited during tracheostomy surgery). A fire requires three elements (fire triangle or triad): a fuel source, an oxidizer, and an ignition source. Potential fuel sources include alcohol-containing prep solutions, surgical drapes, surgical sponges, and gauzes, as well as plastic airway devices. Oxidizers include oxygen and nitrous oxide. Ignition sources include electrosurgical devices, and lasers as well as other sources. Management of operating rooms fires are best handled via prevention, having a carbon dioxide fire extinguisher near the entrance of every OR and by following the ASA algorithm for managing OR fires.

Keywords: Electrical Safety

- Alternating current
- Capacitance
- Conductors
- Current
- Direct current
- Electrocautery
- Electrocution
- Electromagnetic interference
- Ground-fault circuit interrupter
- Insulators
- Joules
- Line isolation monitor
- Macroshock
- Microshock
- Ohm's law
- Power
- Resistance
- Safety
- Semiconductors
- Voltage
- Watts

Keywords: Fire Safety

- Airway fires
- ASA operating room fire algorithm
- Classes of fire extinguishers
- Fire drills
- Fire safety
- Fuel sources
- Fire standards and guidelines
- Fire triangle
- Ignition sources
- Oxidizers
- Oxygen use precautions
- OR fire safety guidelines

Chapter Outline

- Static electricity
- Conductors, semiconductors, and insulators
- Direct and alternating currents
- Electrical resistance
- Electrical energy
- Capacitance
- Electrical shock hazards
- Grounding
- The line isolation monitor
- Ground-fault circuit interrupters
- Electromagnetic interference (EMI)
- Implanted defibrillators
- Electrocautery
- Understanding intraoperative fires
- Fire extinguisher choice and location
- Managing an or fire
- Fire drills

36.2 Principles of Electricity

36.2.1 Static Electricity

Static electricity discharges can produce sparks that give you a mild but unpleasant shock, but more ominously have produced deadly operating room explosions in the days when explosive anesthetic agents such as cyclopropane or diethyl ether were in common use [4]. For this reason, in the past, many operating rooms utilized a number of special safety precautions to prevent explosions from static electricity (e.g., conductive flooring and footwear, conductive patient face masks and patient breathing circuits containing embedded carbon granules, restrictions on operating room apparel, such as forbidding personnel from wearing nylon or Dacron garments)

36.2.2 Conductors, Semiconductors, and Insulators

A conductor is any substance that permits the flow of electrons (or electric current). Copper, gold, and silver are examples of excellent conductors of electricity. Glass, plastic, rubber, and ceramics cannot conduct electricity and are called (electrical) *insulators*. Note that some electrical insulators (e.g., diamonds) may still be good conductors of heat.

Semiconductors conduct electricity under some conditions but not others, making them useful for the control of electrical current. For example, semiconductor diodes conduct electricity in one direction only, having low (ideally zero) resistance to the flow of electrical current (electron flow) in one direction, and high (ideally infinite) resistance to the flow of electrons in the other. Diodes are useful in converting alternating current to direct current (*vide infra*).

In SI units, a coulomb is one ampere-second. That is, an electrical current of 1 ampere flowing for one second represents 1 coulomb of electrons. Expressed differently, one coulomb is the amount of electrical charge held by 6.24×10^{18} electrons.

36.2.3 Direct and Alternating Currents

If the electron flow or current flow is always in the same direction, it is referred to as *direct current* (DC) (see Fig. 36.1). However, if the electron flow reverses direction at a regular interval, it is termed *alternating current* (AC) (see Fig. 36.2). Alternating current usually takes on a sinusoidal form. The alternating current from the wall that we use every day in North America completes 60 cycles per second (60 Hz); in Europe, the frequency is 50 Hz. The voltage supplied is usually 120 volts (but often 220 volts in Europe).

36.2.4 Electrical Resistance

Some materials are not perfect conductors of electricity; that is, they display electrical resistance. In fact, one can think of

Direct Current

Current flows in one direction only.

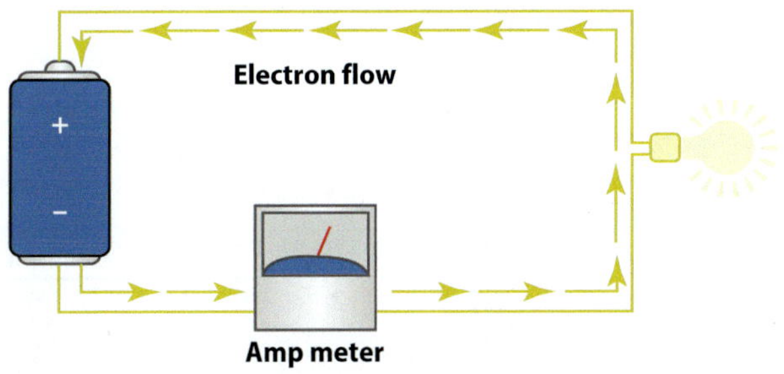

Fig. 36.1 If the electron flow or current flow is always in the same direction, it is referred to as *direct current* (DC). In this case the electrons travel from the negative terminal of the battery, through the amp meter and light bulb (or other load) and return to the battery through the positive terminal. By contrast, the "conventional current" is said to go in the opposite direction, from the positive terminal of the battery to the negative terminal of the battery. Used with permission, The Cleveland clinic center for medical art and photography © 2016. All rights reserved

a conductor as a material having very low (ideally zero) resistance while insulators can be thought of having very high (ideally infinite) resistance to the flow of electrons. The current that passes through an electrical resistor when a voltage difference is applied across it is given by Ohm's law:

$$V = I \times R,$$

where

- V is the electromotive force (in volts)
- I is current (in amperes)
- R is resistance (in ohms)

Example 1 What resistance across a 100-volt source would produce a current of 100 ma (= 0.1 amp)?

Answer

From Ohm's law, $R = V/I$ = 100 volts/0.1 amp = 1000 ohms. ◀

Example 2 If a 200-volt pulse from a nerve stimulator results in a current flow of 50 ma, what is the skin resistance?

Answer

From Ohm's law, $R = V/I$ = 200 volts/0.05 amp = 4000 ohms. ◀

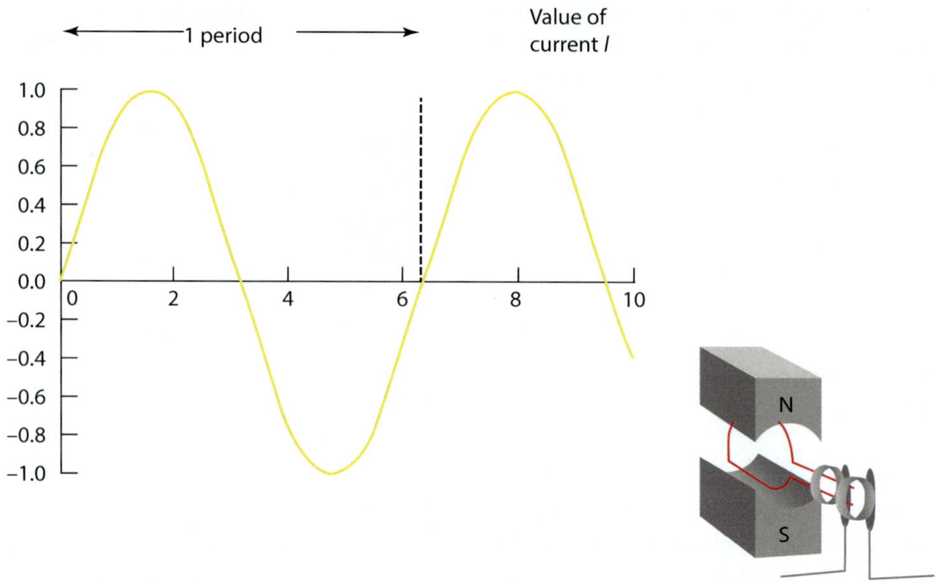

Fig. 36.2 Alternating current usually takes on a sinusoidal form, often the result of a wire assembly rotating past a magnet assembly (note the North and South poles) as illustrated schematically on the lower right. The alternating current from the wall that we use every day in North America completes 60 cycles per second (60 Hz); in Europe the frequency is 50 Hz. The voltage supplied is usually 120 volts (usually 220 volts in Europe). Used with permission, The Cleveland clinic center for medical art and photography © 2016. All rights reserved

Note that Ohm's law ($V = I \times R$) is analogous to the physiologic equation describing systemic blood pressure:

$$(\text{MAP}-\text{RAP}) = \text{CO} \times \text{SVR}$$

That is, the difference between the mean blood pressure and the right atrial pressure is equal to the cardiac output (CO) times the systemic vascular resistance (SVR), where SVR is in Woods units. Finally, to convert vascular resistance in Woods units to the more commonly used dyn s cm^{-5} units, multiply by 80:

$$\text{SVR} = [(\text{MAP}-\text{RAP})/\text{CO}] \times 80\left(\text{dyn s cm}^{-5}\right)$$

36.2.5 Electrical Power

The electrical power (W) consumed by an electrical device is measured in watts:

$$W = V \times I$$

Here, V is the voltage applied to the device, and I is the electrical current that passes through the device.

Example 1 What is the power consumed by a patient warmer which draws 10 amperes when plugged into a 110 volt source?

Answer

From $W = V \times I$, the power consumed is 110 volts × 10 amperes = 1100 watts. ◀

Example 2 If a 200 volt pulse from a nerve stimulator results in a current flow of 50 ma, what is the power delivered to the patient?

Answer

From $W = V \times I$, the power delivered is 200 volts × 0.05 amp = 10 watts. ◀

36.2.6 Electrical Energy

The watt-second (or joule, J) is commonly used to denote electrical energy expended in doing work. The energy produced by a cardiac defibrillator is measured in watt-seconds (or joules), while the kilowatt-hour is frequently used to measure larger quantities of electrical energy. As an example, electrical utility companies charge their customers on the basis of kilowatt-hours of electricity consumed. The formula to use here is $J = W \times T$ where W is the power consumed in watts and T is the time in seconds over which the power is consumed. Note that a kilowatt-hour (kWh) is equivalent to 3,600,000 watt-seconds or joules.

Example 1 What is the energy consumed by a 100 W fluid warmer when operated for 1 h?

Answer

From $J = W \times T$, the energy consumed is 100 W × 60 min × 60 s/min = 360,000 J. ◀

Example 2 What is the answer to example 1 kWh?

Answer

The power consumed is 0.1 kW × 1 h = 0.1 kWh. ◀

36.2.7 Capacitance

A *capacitor* consists of any two conductors (such as parallel plates) that are separated by an insulator. A capacitor stores charge (electrons). In a DC circuit, the capacitor plates are charged by a voltage source (i.e., a battery) and there is only a momentary current flow as the capacitor charges. No further current can then flow unless a resistance is connected between the two plates and the capacitor is subsequently discharged. In contrast to DC circuits, a capacitor in an AC circuit permits current flow, depending on the *impedance* presented by the capacitor at a given frequency of alternating current.

Capacitors are a key component in the design of cardiac defibrillators (Figs. 36.3 and 36.4), where they serve as an energy storage device according to the formula $E = ½\, C\, V^2$, where E is the energy in joules (J), C is the capacitance in farads, and V is the voltage in volts. For example, if the capacitance of the capacitor is 1000 μF (microfarad) and the voltage applied to it is 1000 V, then the stored energy is 500 J based on the following calculation:

$$E = 1/2CV^2 = 1/2\left(1000 \times 10^{-6}\right)\left(1000^2\right) = 500\ \text{J}.$$

Note that the energy delivered during an initial monophasic defibrillation is usually 200 J, with less energy typically used for biphasic defibrillation.

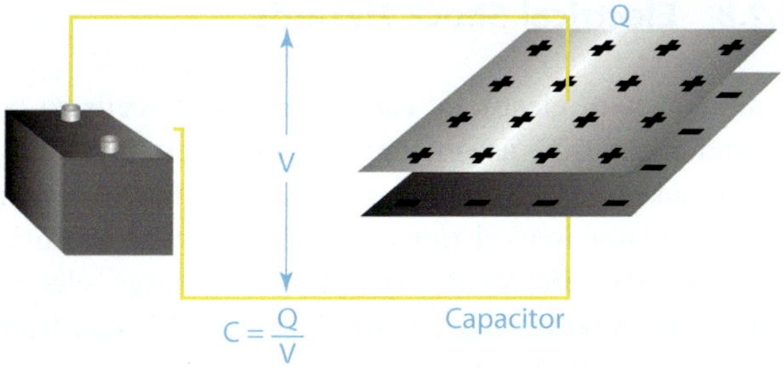

Fig. 36.3 A *capacitor* consists of any two conductors (such as parallel plates) that are separated by an insulator. A capacitor stores charge (electrons). Used with permission, The Cleveland clinic center for medical art and photography © 2016. All rights reserved

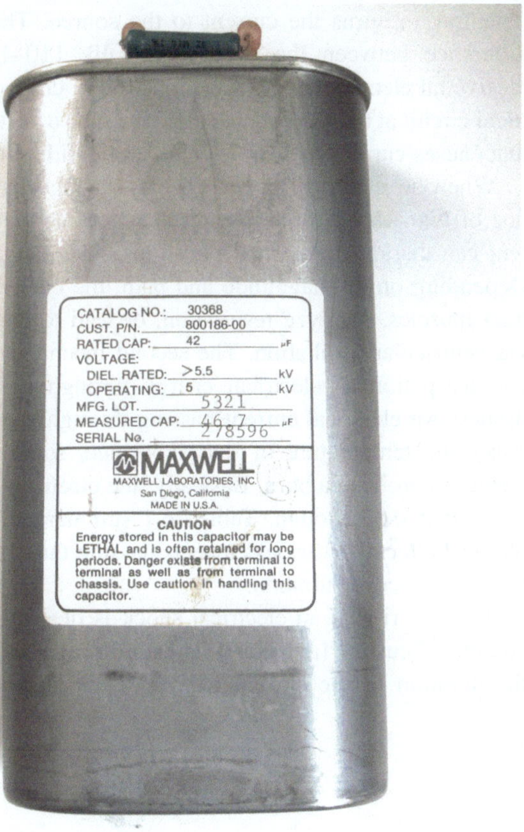

Fig. 36.4 A high-energy capacitor used on a cardiac defibrillator. The capacitor is rated 42 microfarad at 5000 volts. Using the formula $E = ½\, C\, V^2$ the energy stored in the capacitor becomes = ½ (42 × 10^{-6}) (5000^2) = 525 J. Image from Wikipedia: https://upload.wikimedia.org/wikipedia/commons/3/34/High-energy_capacitor_from_a_defibrillator_42_MFD_%40_5000_VDC.jpg (Image made available under the creative commons CC0 1.0 universal public domain dedication)

36.2.8 Electrical Shock Hazards

Stimulation with electricity can cause muscle cells to contract and can thus be used therapeutically in equipment such as pacemakers or defibrillators or diagnostically when a nerve stimulator is used to assess the degree of neuromuscular blockade. However, contact with a large electrical voltage (like a power line), whether AC or DC, can lead to injury or even death, often as a result of ventricular fibrillation. It takes approximately three times as much DC current as AC current to cause ventricular fibrillation.

Figure 36.5 illustrates a typical AC electrical power arrangement in schematic form. A typical electrical outlet consists of two wires ("hot" and "neutral") in conjunction with a third "ground" connection (Fig. 36.6). The wire designated as "hot" carries the current to the load while the other ("neutral") returns the current to the source. The potential difference between the two is typically 110–120 V. To receive an electrical shock, one must be in contact the electrical circuit at two points, and there must be a voltage supply that causes current to flow through an individual (Fig. 36.7).

When an electrical shock occurs, damage can occur in one of two ways. In the first mechanism, the electrical current can disrupt the normal physiological function of cells. Depending on its magnitude and path, the current can contract muscles, paralyze respiration, or lead to cardiac arrest via ventricular fibrillation. The second mechanism involves the dissipation of electrical energy throughout the body's tissues: An electrical current passing through any resistance raises the temperature of that substance, sometimes sufficiently to produce a burn. Basically, the electricity cooks the tissue it passes through. Table 36.1 summarizes the physiological effects of various currents passing through the body for a one-second duration.

The severity of an electrical shock is determined by the amount of current (amperes), its path through the body, and the duration of the current flow. For the purposes of this discussion, it is helpful to divide electrical shocks into two categories. Macroshock refers to large amounts of current flowing through a person, which can cause harm or death. Microshock refers to very small amounts of current (in the microampere and milliampere range) and applies only to the electrically susceptible patient, such as an individual who has an external conduit that is in direct contact with the heart. This can be a pacing wire or a saline-filled catheter such as a central venous or pulmonary artery catheter. In the case of an electrically susceptible patient, even minute amounts of current (microshock) may cause ventricular fibrillation.

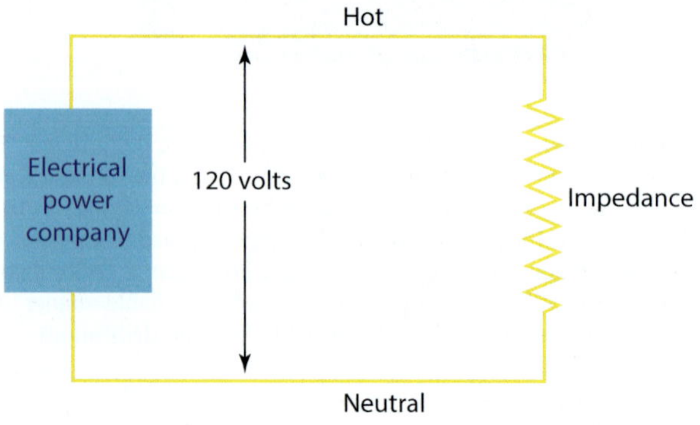

Fig. 36.5 Schematic illustration of a typical AC electrical power arrangement. Used with permission, The Cleveland clinic center for medical art and photography © 2016. All rights reserved

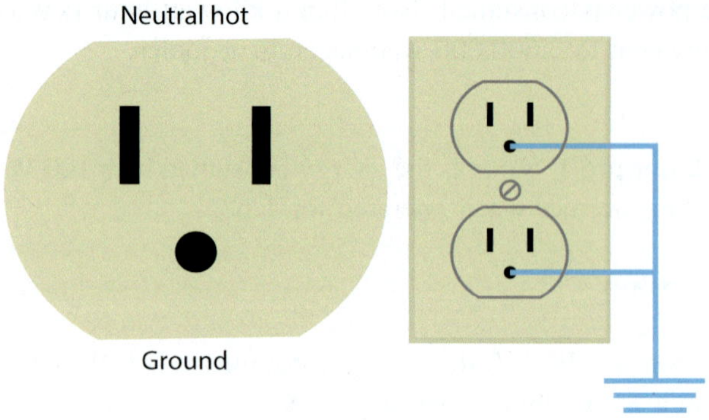

Fig. 36.6 A typical electrical outlet consists of two wires ("hot" and "neutral") in conjunction with a third "ground" connection. The wire designated as "hot" carries the current to the load while the other ("neutral"), returns the current to the source. The potential difference between the two is typically 110–120 V. Used with permission, the Cleveland clinic center for medical art and photography © 2016. All rights reserved

In the electrically susceptible patient, ventricular fibrillation can be produced by a current that is below the threshold of human perception. The exact amount of current necessary to cause ventricular fibrillation in this type of patient is unknown (the experiments would be unethical) but based on animal experiments is believed to be as little as 20 μA.

36.2.9 Grounding

Ground connections on electrical plugs are used to help prevent electric shocks. An electrical shock may occur when an individual gets connected between the hot and neutral connectsions in a circuit, either directly as shown in Fig. 36.7, or via a frayed wire that has resulted in a short circuit producing a "hot case," as illustrated in Fig. 36.8.

Note, however, that if a three-pronged plug is employed so that the case is grounded, any short circuit current from a frayed wire or similar problem will safely return any current to the ground instead of travellng through the victim. This is illustrated in Fig. 36.9.

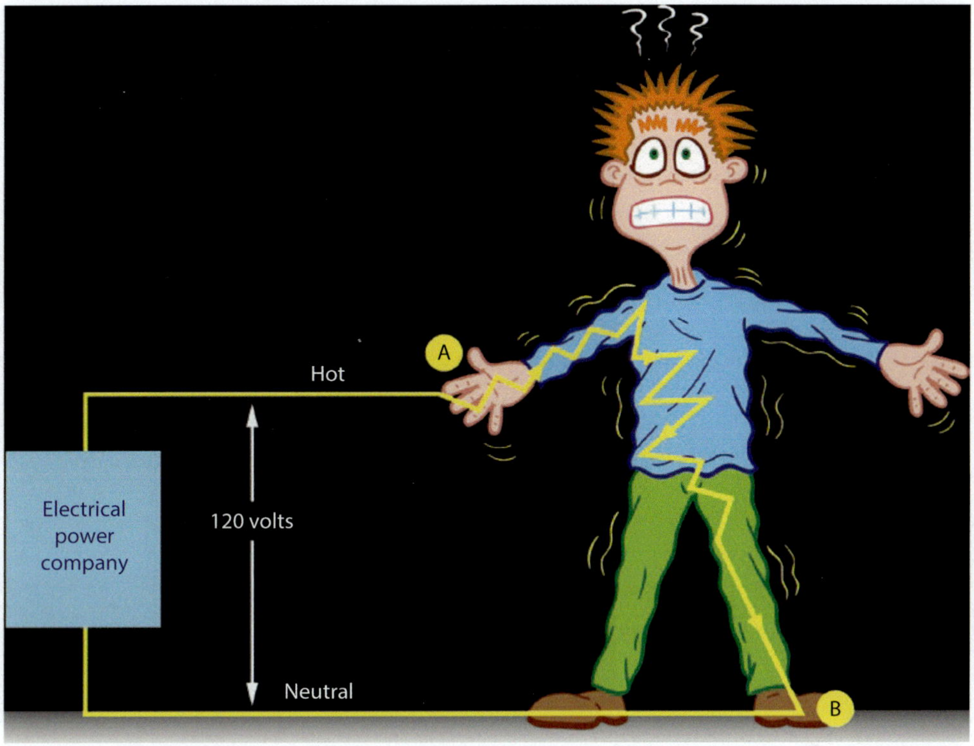

Fig. 36.7 To receive an electrical shock, one must be in contact an active electrical circuit at two points. Used with permission, The Cleveland clinic center for medical art and photography © 2016. All rights reserved

Table 36.1 Physiological effects of various degrees of electrical current

Electric current (1 s contact)	Physiological effect
20 μA	Can possibly cause ventricular fibrillation in a "microshock" setting
1–5 mA	Threshold of feeling, tingling sensation.
10–20 mA	"Can't let go!" current - onset of sustained muscular contraction.
100–300 mA	Ventricular fibrillation in "macroshock" setting

36.2.10 The Line Isolation Monitor

Isolated power systems are frequently used in operarting rooms. Such systems use an **isolation transformer** system so that neither of the two output lines powering the operarting room equipment offers any voltage with respect to ground (Figs. 36.10, 36.11, 36.12, and 36.13). This helps eliminate the shock hazard associated with working in wet environments like the operarting room.

However, this safety system only works reliably if the isolation transformer and the things connected to it are working properly. To check that the isolation system is working correctly, a line isolation monitor (LIM) is used. The LIM monitors the isolated power system to ensure that it is fully isolated from ground, and has an indicator that indirectly displays the impedance to ground of each side of the isolated power system. The LIM meter will indicate the total amount of leakage current in the system resulting from AC capacitance effects, and from any equipment plugged into the system. The reading on the LIM meter does not mean that an actual current is flowing; rather, it tells us how much current would flow in the event of a **first fault**. The LIM is usually set to alarm at 2–5 mA, depending on the system. Once this limit is reached, alarms are triggered. This does not necessarily mean that there is a hazardous situation, but only that the system is no longer totally isolated from ground. It would require a **second fault** to create a dangerous situation. For example, if the LIM were set to alarm at 2 mA, using Ohm's law, the lowest allowable impedance for either side of the isolated power system would be 60,000 ohms, since by Ohm's law $R = 120/0.002 = 60,000$ ohms. Therefore, if either side of the isolated power system had less than 60,000 ohms impedance to ground, the LIM would trigger an alarm. Figure 36.13 provides a sample LIM policy used in hospitals.

36.2.11 Ground-Fault Circuit Interrupters

Activities carried using electrical equipment in wet areas such as bathrooms are especially hazardous. The use of ground-fault circuit interrupter (GFCI) devices or isolated

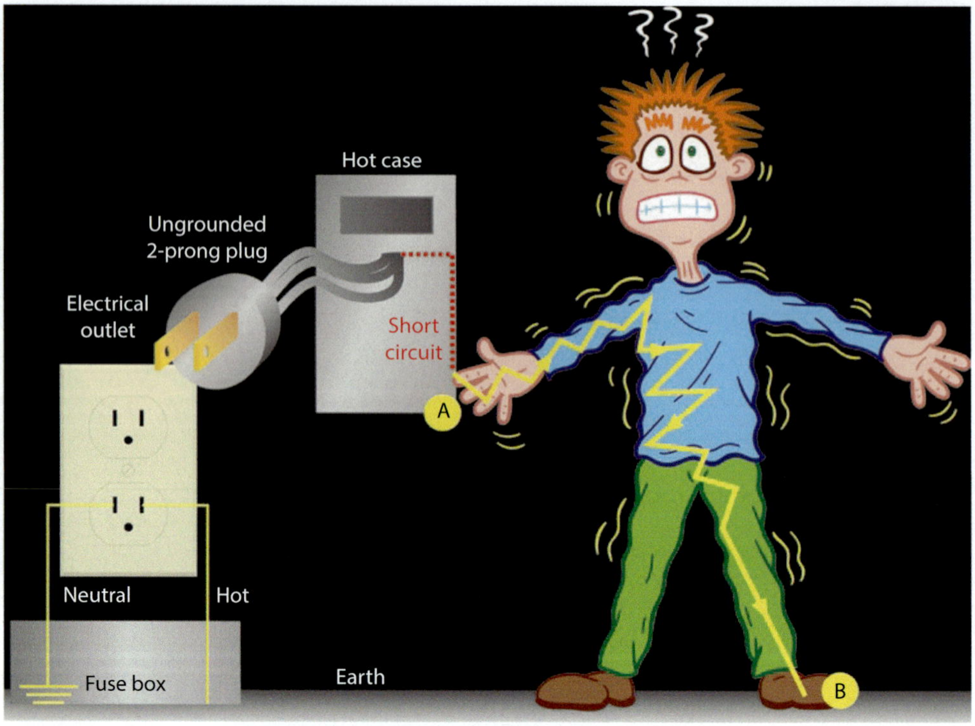

Fig. 36.8 In the absence of an electrical grounding system, a frayed wire or other problem may result in a short circuit, producing a "hot case" that could electrocute anyone that touches it. Used with permission, The Cleveland clinic center for medical art and photography © 2016. All rights reserved

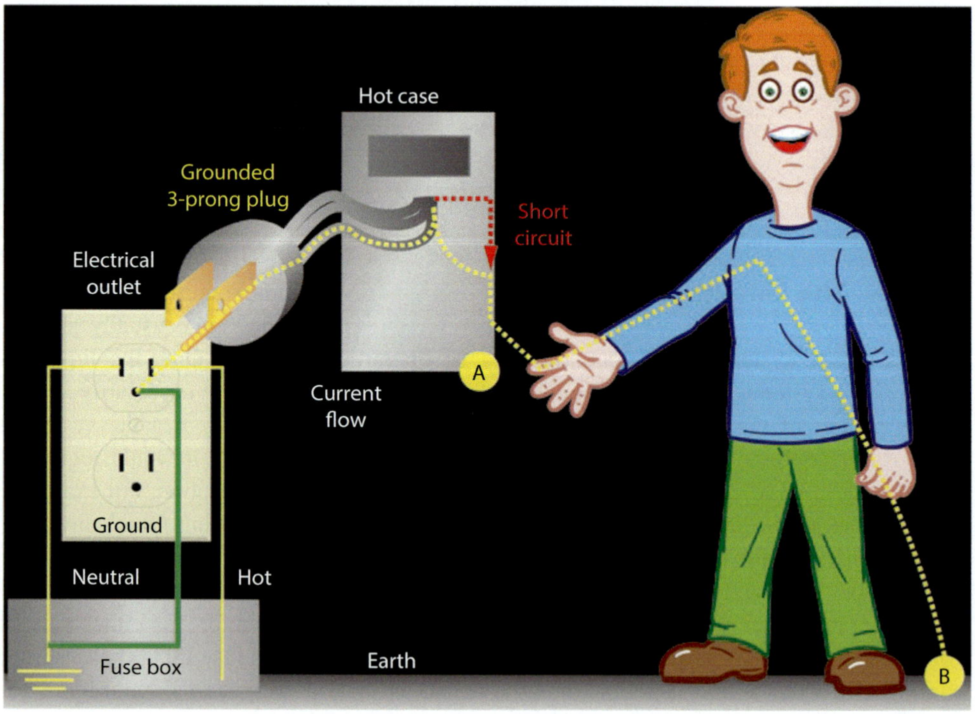

Fig. 36.9 When an electrical grounding system is used, any frayed wire that would ordinarily result in a short circuit and a "hot case" instead results in electricity passing through the ground wire rather than through anyone who might be in contact with the "hot case." Used with permission, The Cleveland clinic center for medical art and photography© 2016. All rights reserved

power systems can be helpful in reducing the hazards involved. The ground-fault circuit interrupter (GFCI) (illustrated in Figs. 36.14 and 36.15) is another device to help prevent individuals from receiving an electrical shock in a grounded power system. Electrical codes for most new construction require that a GFCI circuit be present in potentially hazardous (*e.g.,* wet) areas such as outdoor electrical outlets. Ordinarily, the current in both the hot and neutral wires in a power outlet is equal. The GFCI monitors both sides of the circuit for the equality of current flow; if a difference is detected, the power is immediately interrupted. If an individual should contact a faulty piece of equipment

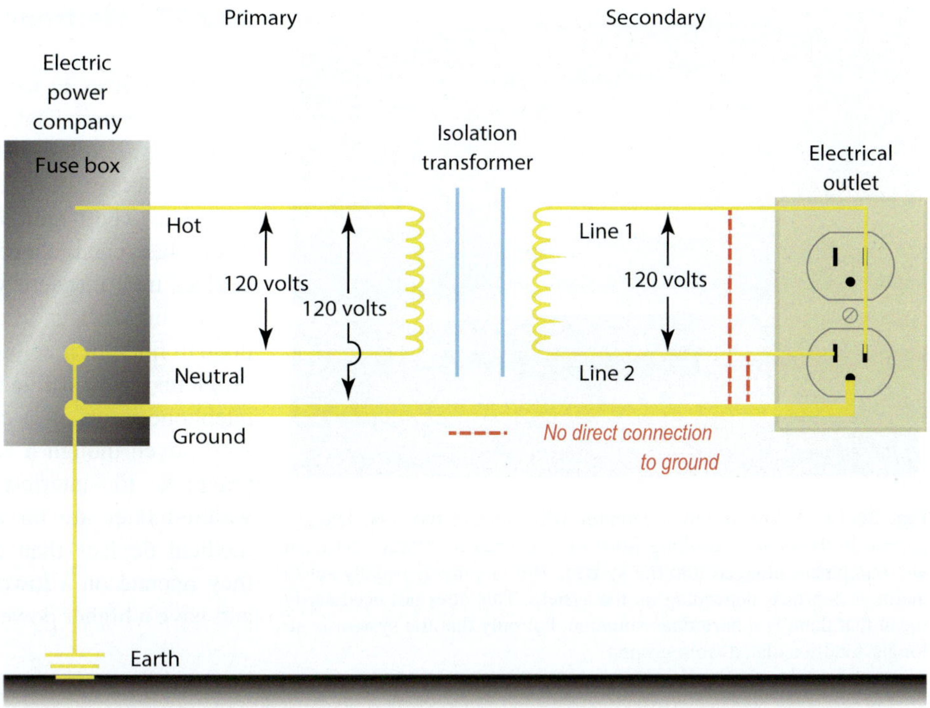

Fig. 36.10 Isolated power systems are frequently used in operarting rooms. Such systems use an isolation transformer system so that neither of the two output lines powering the operarting room equipment offers any voltage with respect to ground. Used with permission, the Cleveland clinic center for medical art and photography© 2016. All rights reserved

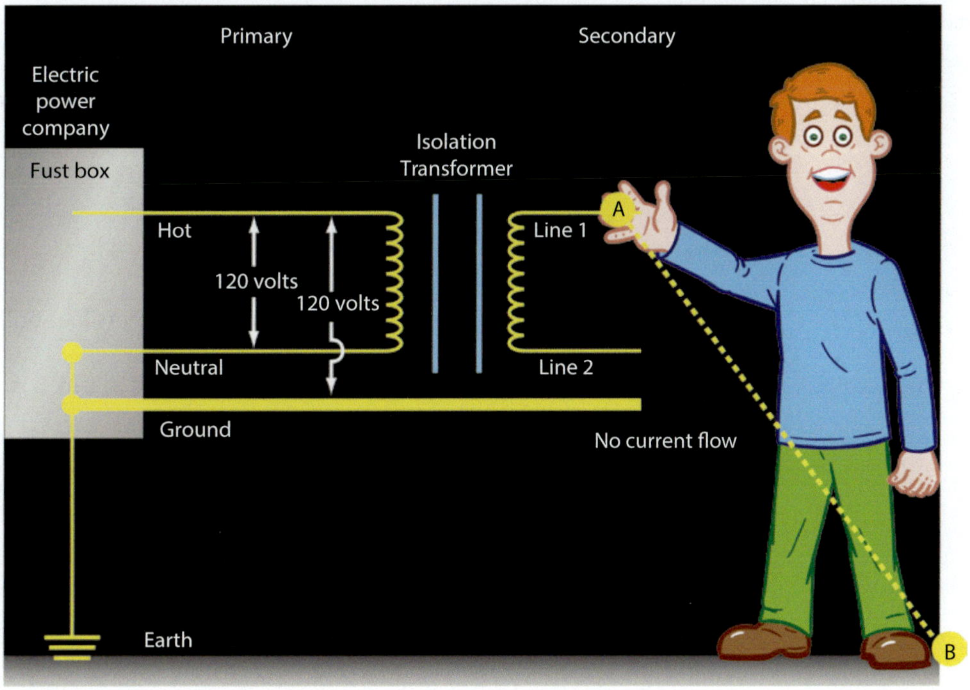

Fig. 36.11 When an isolated electrical power systems is used, since neither of the two output lines offers any voltage difference with respect to ground, no shock hazard is offered to anyone who comes into contact with either one of the two outputs of the isolation transformer. Used with permission, the Cleveland clinic center for medical art and photography© 2016. All rights reserved

such that current flowed through the person, an imbalance between the two sides of the circuit would be created, which would be detected by the system. Because the GFCI can detect very small current differences (in the range of 5 mA), the GFCI will open the circuit in a few milliseconds, thereby interrupting the current flow before a significant shock occurs. Thus, the GFCI provides a high level of protection at a very modest cost. The disadvantage of using a GFCI in the operating room is that it interrupts the power without warning. A defective piece of equipment could no longer be used, which might be a problem if it were of a life-support nature, whereas if the same faulty piece of equipment were plugged into an isolated power system, the LIM would alarm, but the equipment could still be used.

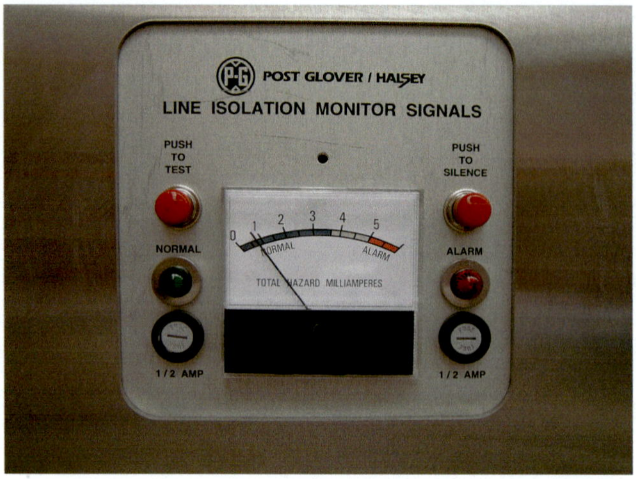

Fig. 36.12 A line isolation monitor will indicate the total leakage current in the system resulting from AC capacitance effects, and from any equipment plugged into the system. The monitor is usually set to alarm at 2–5 mA, depending on the system. This does not necessarily mean that there is a hazardous situation, but only that the system is no longer totally isolated from ground

36.2.12 Electromagnetic Interference (EMI)

Rapid advances in technology have led to an explosion in wireless communication devices. These include cellular telephones, cordless telephones, walkie-talkies, and wireless Internet access devices. All of these have something in common: They emit electromagnetic interference (EMI). There has been concern that the EMI emitted by these devices may interfere with pacemakers or various types of monitoring devices in critical care areas. Studies have been done to find out if cellular telephones or walkie-talkies cause problems with cardiac pacemakers. Any time a cellular telephone is on, it is communicating with the cellular network, even though a call is not in progress. Therefore, the potential to interfere with devices exists. However, walkie-talkies are far more likely to cause problems with medical devices than cellular telephones. This is because they operate on a lower frequency than cellular telephones and have a higher power output. The ECRI recommends that

Fig. 36.13 A sample hospital policy pertaining to line isolation monitor (LIM) alarms

SAMPLE HOSPITAL POLICY

LINE ISOLATION MONITOR ALARM

BACKGROUND

Line isolation monitor (LIM) alarms help protect both patient and clinician against electrical shocks. Whenever these devices alarm, a potentially unsafe electrical condition exists.

PROCEDURE

When a LIM alarm sounds, the cause is often due to a defective electrical device. The user should silence the alarm and unplug the last piece of equipment plugged in before the alarm sounded. If the alarm clears after unplugging the last item connected, it is safe to proceed as long as the item is not plugged in again.

If the alarm continues to sound, call Clinical Engineering.

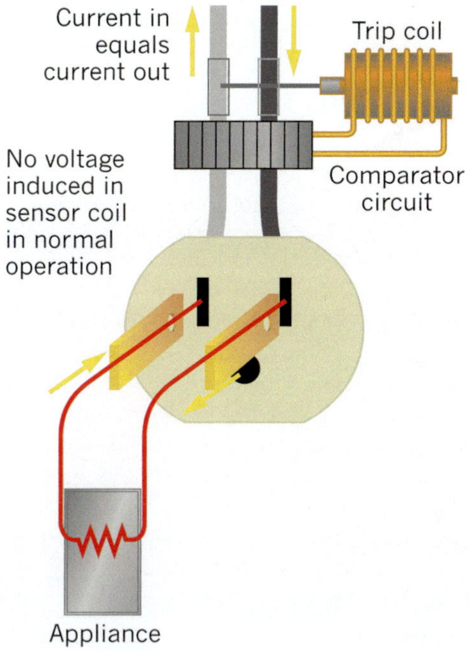

Fig. 36.14 A ground fault circuit interrupter (GFCI) monitors both sides of a circuit for the equality of current flow; if a difference is detected, the power is immediately interrupted. Used with permission, the Cleveland clinic center for medical art and photography© 2016. All rights reserved

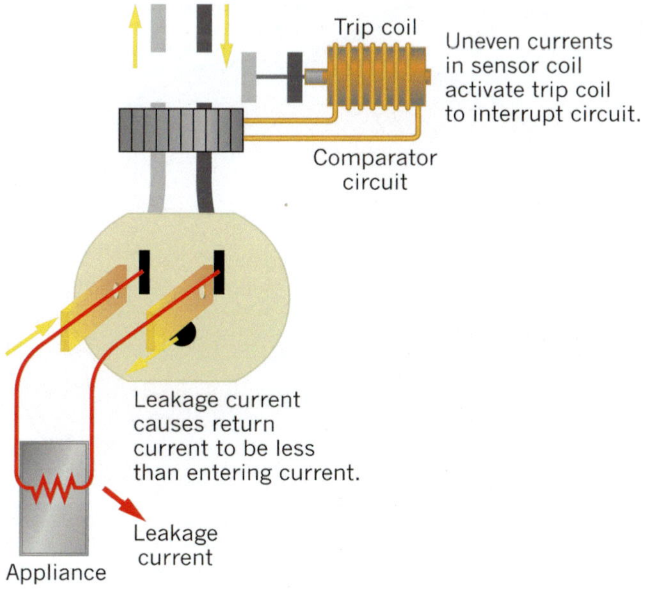

Fig. 36.15 When a leakage current that might cause an electrical shock is detected by a ground fault circuit interrupter (based on a detecting differences in current), the power is immediately interrupted via the trip coil. Used with permission, the Cleveland clinic center for medical art and photography© 2016. All rights reserved

cellular telephones be maintained at a distance of 1 m from medical devices while walkie-talkies be kept at a distance of 6–8 m.

36.2.13 Implanted Defibrillators

Automatic implantable cardioverter-defibrillators (AICDs) are capable of sensing ventricular tachycardia (VT) and ventricular fibrillation (VF) and then automatically defibrillating the patient using their internal energy source [2]. It is important to be aware that the use of a unipolar cautery may cause electrical interference that could be interpreted by the AICD as VT or VF. This would trigger a defibrillation pulse that might itself cause an episode of VT or VF. Patients with an AICD are also at risk during electroconvulsive therapy. In both cases, the AICD should be disabled. Although most AICDs can be disabled with a magnet, some require a special programming device to turn it off. The device is later reactivated at the end of surgery. It is always best to consult with the AICD/pacemaker service before starting surgery. Finally, an external defibrillator and a noninvasive pacemaker should be readily available whenever a patient with an AICD is anesthetized.

36.2.14 Electrocautery

Electrocautery can be used to cut or to coagulate tissue using radiofrequency electrical energy. This electrical energy does not produce shock effects (like VT or VF) because it is high in frequency, in the megahertz region. Special attention should be directed at placement of the electrocautery return pad (sometimes erroneously called a “ground plate”) to avoid electrical burns to the patient (see Figs. 36.16 and 36.17).

36.3 Principles of Fire Safety

36.3.1 Understanding Intraoperative Fires

All fires require three items: a fuel source, an oxidizing agent (usually oxygen), and a source of ignition, as illustrated in Fig. 36.18 (Fire Triangle). Potential fuel sources for operating room fires include alcohol-based antiseptic solutions, patient drapes, surgical gauzes and sponges, the patient’s own hair, and even endotracheal tubes ignited by a laser beam. Even intestinal methane gas can be a fuel source, as occurred in a 1981 case when a colon was opened by electrocautery, followed by “a loud explosion, producing a 10-cm rent in the serosa of the colon.” [3].

Normally oxygen is the oxidizing agent involved in fires, but nitrous oxide is also an effective oxidizing agent, as evidenced by its occasional use in racing cars and high-performance aircraft. Be aware that open oxygen delivery systems, such as nasal cannulas or Venturi face

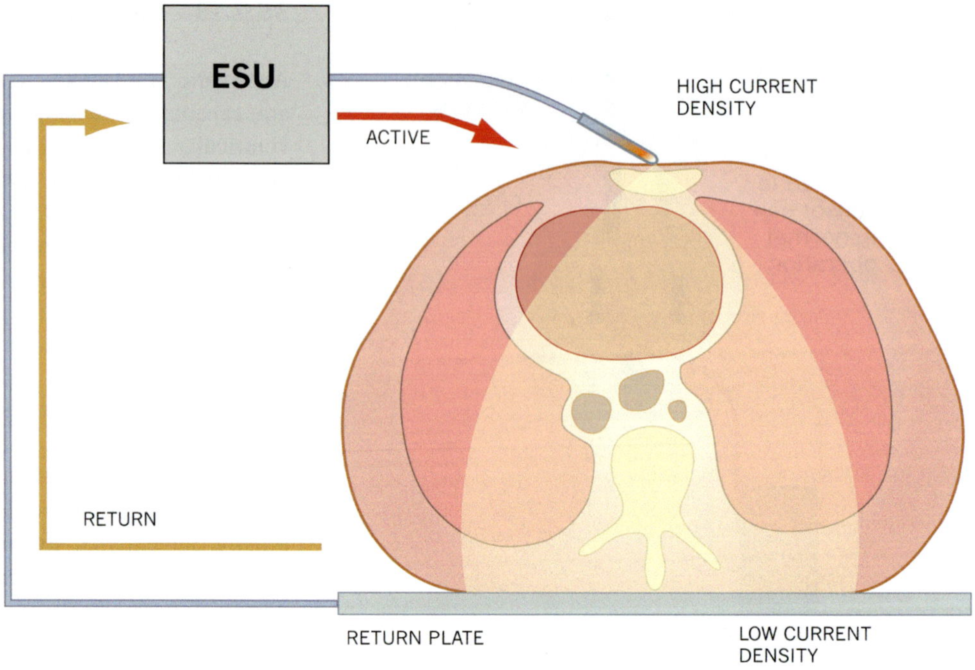

Fig. 36.16 Typical setup for electrocautery. Special attention should be directed at placement of the electrocautery return pad (sometimes erroneously called a "ground plate") to avoid electrical burns to the patient. Used with permission, the Cleveland clinic center for medical art and photography© 2016. All rights reserved

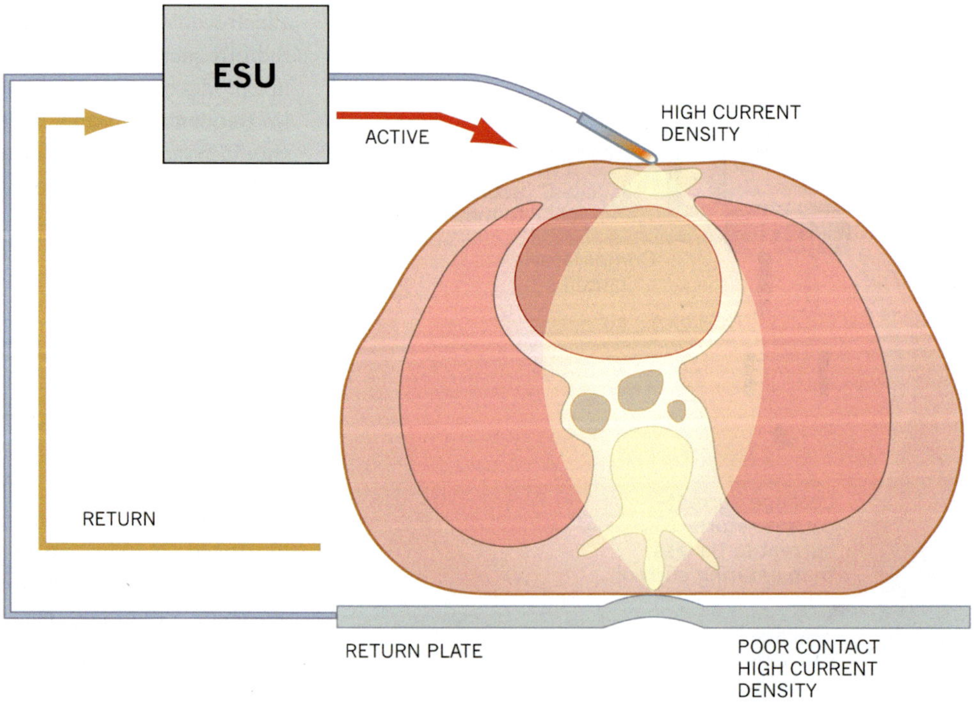

Fig. 36.17 Poor placement of an electrocautery return pad may result in electrical burns to the patient by virtue of excessive current density. Used with permission, the Cleveland clinic center for medical art and photography© 2016. All rights reserved

masks, present a greater fire risk compared to closed delivery systems such as an endotracheal tube or supraglottic airway. That said, ordinary endotracheal tubes are easily ignited by a laser when high levels of oxygen are employed.

The three most common ignition sources involved in operating room fires today are lasers, the electrosurgical unit ("Bovie," cautery, diathermy), and the high-intensity light cords used for surgical headlights. In the past, sparks from nylon or similar garments would occasionally ignite cyclopropane or ether used as anesthetics. Further details are available in the recent literature [1, 5–7].

Tips on fire risk management are presented in Table 36.2. Foremost among these is known the fire risk class to which the patient belongs (Table 36.3).

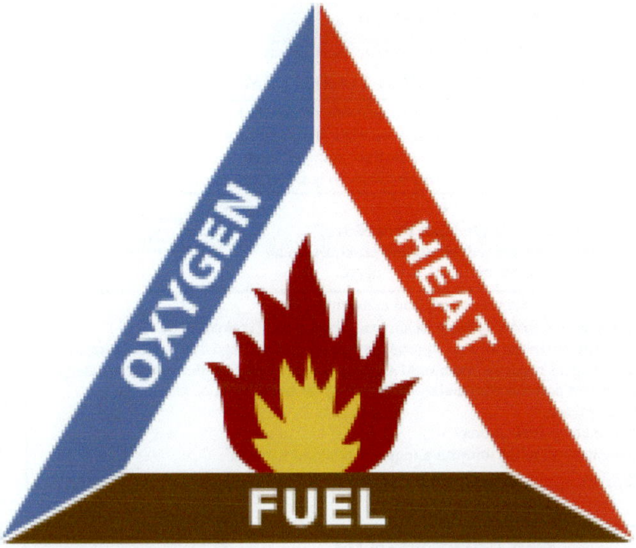

Fig. 36.18 The fire triangle is a simple conceptual model for understanding the necessary ingredients for ordinary fires. Three elements are needed for a fire to occur: heat (ignition), fuel, and an oxidizing agent (normally oxygen). Fire extinguishers put out fires by taking away one or more elements of the fire triangle; for example, covering a fire with a layer of CO_2 from a CO_2 fire extinguisher blocks the fire's access to oxygen. *Image credit* Wikipedia image used under the creative commons attribution-share alike 3.0 unported license

Table 36.2 OR fire safety tips and guidelines

• Conduct OR fire drills annually or more often
• Know the fire risk score (1, 2 or 3) for your patient (Table 36.3)
• Keep a CO_2 fire extinguisher in each operating room
• Use fire-retardant surgical drapes
• With unintubated patients, avoid tenting of the surgical drapes to prevent oxygen accumulation; use the minimum necessary oxygen
• In fire risk cases, keep a basin of sterile saline on the OR field for ready use
• Keep the electrocautery tip in its holster when it is not being used
• Power high-intensity light sources only when they are being used

Table 36.3 Fire risk score for surgical patients

Add one point for each if the following:
(1) Surgical site or incision above the xiphoid
(2) Patient receiving oxygen via face mask or nasal cannula (open oxygen source)
(3) Available ignition source (e.g., electrosurgery unit, laser, light cable)
Patients with 3 points are at high-risk, necessitating special attention to the fire prevention and management techniques described in this chapter.
Reference: OR Manager Vol. 22 No. 1 January 2006 https://www.ormanager.com/wp-content/uploads/2012/06/ORMVol22No1scoringFireRisk.pdf

36.3.2 Fire Extinguisher Choice and Location

Fire extinguishers put out fires by taking away one or more elements of the fire triangle. As an example, covering a fire with a layer of CO_2 from a CO_2 fire extinguisher reduces the fire's oxygen supply via gas displacement. In many facilities, a 5 lb. CO_2 extinguisher is wall mounted just inside the entrance of each operating room or procedure room. The advantages of CO_2 extinguishers are that they can be used in Class B fires (flammable liquids) and Class C (electrical) fires, and to lesser extent on Class A (textile, wood, and paper) fires. Also, CO_2 extinguishers leave no residue. Note that water mist type fire extinguishers may not be appropriate for operating room use due to infection control concerns. However, a bowl of sterile water or saline in conjunction with a soaked sterile sponge would also be suitable to quench a surgical site fire.

36.3.3 National Fire Protection Association (NFPA) Standards

The National Fire Protection Association (NFPA) has published document *NFPA 99: Health Care Facilities Code* for guidance in fire and explosion prevention in the operating room and other hospital areas. This document "establishes criteria for levels of healthcare services or systems based on risk to the patients, staff, or visitors in healthcare facilities to minimize the hazards of fire, explosion, and electricity." Another important document published by the same association is *NFPA 110: Emergency and Standby Power Systems,* which is mostly concerned with providing "alternate sources of electrical power in buildings and facilities in the event that the normal electrical power source fails."

36.3.4 Managing an OR Fire

In ordinary non-OR fires, the RACE acronym is a reminder to Rescue, Alarm, Confine, and Extinguish fires. In the OR, the situation is more complex, since if the fire occurs on the patient (e.g., drape ignition), the main concern is extinguishing the fire and/or removing the burning material from the patient. Here, a preexisting basin of saline located on the OR table can be used to help quench the fire while the burning drapes are pulled off and fully extinguished using the nearby fire extinguisher. Particular reference should be made to the operating room fire algorithm developed by the American Society of Anesthesiologists Task Force on Operating Room Fires [1], as illustrated in Fig. 36.19. If a fire occurs in an area in which oxygen is in use, the zone valve(s) controlling that area must be closed. Naturally, affected patients must be immediately rescued.

Fig. 36.19 Operating room fires algorithm (2013 edition) published by the American Society of Anesthesiologists. Used with permission from Apfelbaum et al. [1]

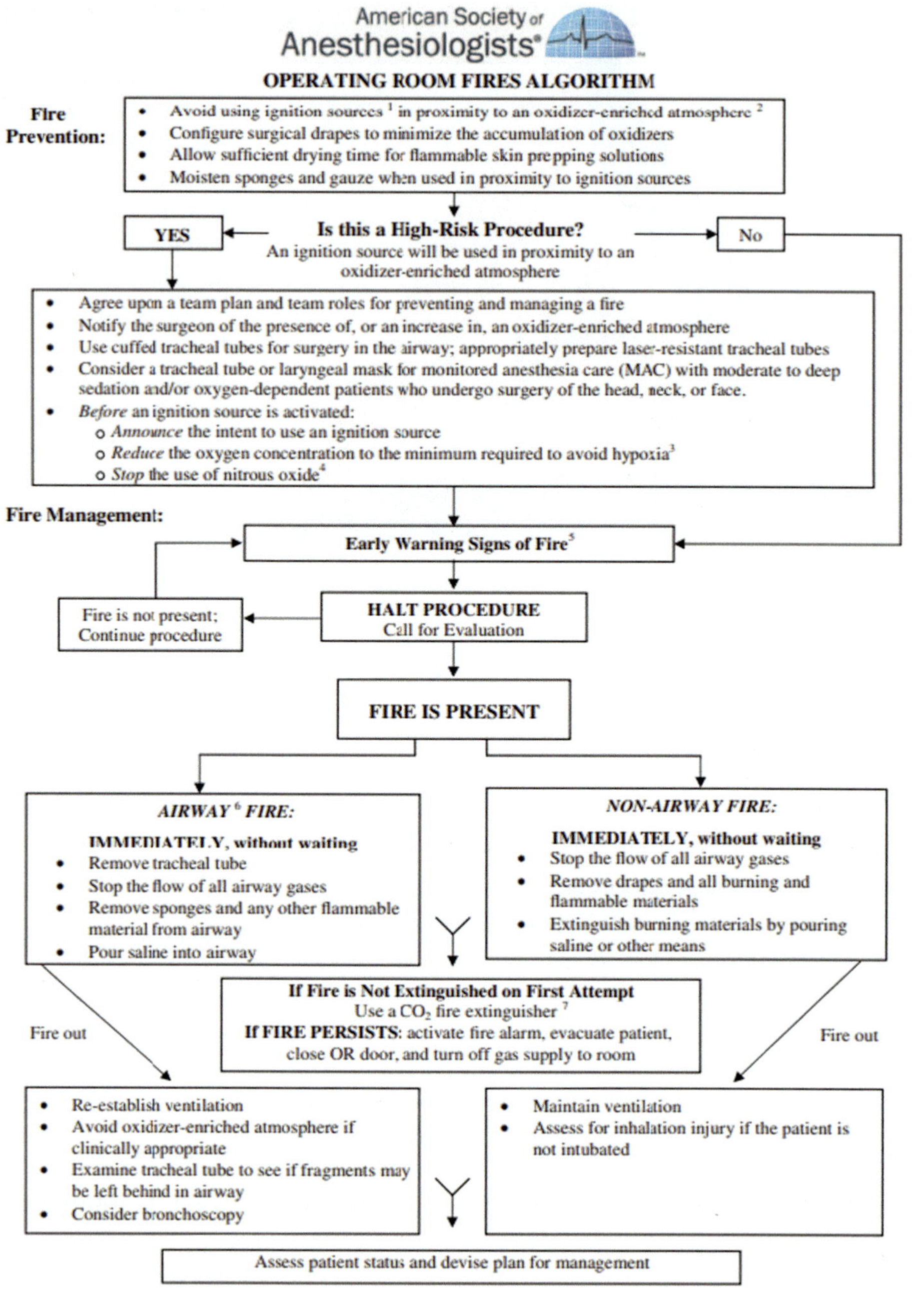

1 Ignition sources include but are not limited to electrosurgery or electrocautery units and lasers.

2 An oxidizer-enriched atmosphere occurs when there is any increase in oxygen concentration above room air level, and/or the presence of any concentration of nitrous oxide.

3 After minimizing delivered oxygen, wait a period of time (*e.g.*, 1-3 min) before using an ignition source. For oxygen dependent patients, *reduce* supplemental oxygen delivery to the minimum required to avoid hypoxia. Monitor oxygenation with pulse oximetry, and if feasible, inspired, exhaled, and/or delivered oxygen concentration.

4 After stopping the delivery of nitrous oxide, wait a period of time (*e.g.*, 1-3 min) before using an ignition source.

5 Unexpected flash, flame, smoke or heat, unusual sounds (*e.g.*, a "pop," snap or "foomp") or odors, unexpected movement of drapes, discoloration of drapes or breathing circuit, unexpected patient movement or complaint.

6 In this algorithm, airway fire refers to a fire in the airway or breathing circuit.

7 A CO_2 fire extinguisher may be used on the patient if necessary.

36.3.5 Fire Drills

Prevention recommendations from the Anesthesia Patient Safety Foundation (APSF), including an educational video, can be found on the APSF Web site at https://www.apsf.org/videos/or-fire-safety-video/. Fire drills are an important means to prepare operating room and surgical suite personnel in the event of a fire. These drills are usually conducted annually (or more frequently) and serve as important opportunities for improvement as equipment and system problems are identified.

36.4 Questions and Answers

Questions

1. You discover the electrical cord on a fluid warmer has been damaged and some of the cord's insulation is missing. Which is the best course of action?

   A. Wrap tape around the damaged spot to prevent electrical shocks.
   B. Check to see if the warmer still works.
   C. Tag the warmer with an "out of service" tag and notify the department responsible for equipment maintenance.
   D. Make sure that the cord does not come in contact with the floor.
2. Which of the following is the least important in determining the effect of an electrical shock on the body:

   A. Intensity of the current.
   B. Path through the body.
   C. Duration of the current.
   D. Body mass index (BMI).
3. Which of the following is a poor conductor of electricity?

   A. Copper
   B. Silver
   C. Gold
   D. Rubber
4. What is the proper way to unplug operating room electrical devices from a power strip?

   A. Simply pull on the cord until the plug comes out.
   B. Put your foot on the power strip to hold it steady while you pull the cord loose.
   C. Use your hand to remove the plug, being careful not to pull on the cord itself.
   D. Request assistance from the Clinical Engineering department.
5. Identify the false statement:

   A. A line isolation monitor (LIM) measures the total hazard current (THC) in an isolated power system.
   B. It takes approximately three times as much DC current as AC current to cause ventricular fibrillation.
   C. Cellular telephones communicate with their cellular network only when a call is in progress, and so only produce electromagnetic interference (EMI) when a call is made.
   D. To receive an electrical shock, one must be in contact the electrical circuit at two points, and there must be a voltage supply that causes current to flow through an individual.
   E. When an electrical shock occurs, damage can occur either via an induced physiological effect or by directly burning the victim.
6. The SI unit of electrical current is ____________.

   A. ampere
   B. watt
   C. volt
   D. joule
7. Ohm's law relates voltage with __________.

   A. Power
   B. Energy
   C. Current
   D. Capacitance
8. The electrical current flowing through a wire ______________.

   A. Depends only on the voltage difference applied.
   B. Depends only on the resistance of the wire.
   C. Depends on both the wire's resistance and voltage difference applied.
   D. Does not depend on resistance and voltage difference applied.
9. The SI unit of power is ____________.

   A. ampere
   B. watt
   C. volt
   D. joule
10. Which of the following is a good conductor of heat but a poor conductor of electricity?

    A. Copper
    B. Silver

C. Cooper
D. Diamond

11. Wood, fabric and paper fires are classified:

A. Class A
B. Class B
C. Class C
D. Class D

12. Which is not a component of the fire triangle?

A. Fuel
B. Nitrogen
C. Ignition / heat
D. Oxidizer / oxygen

13. Where should one aim a fire extinguisher nozzle when extinguishing a fire?

A. At the top of the fire
B. At the middle of the fire
C. At the base of the fire
D. Aim for all the above

Answers

1. **C**

The best course of action is to tag the warmer with an "out-of-service" tag and notify the department responsible for equipment maintenance. Typically, the department responsible for equipment maintenance will be the Clinical Engineering department. It would be wrong to simply wrap tape around the damaged spot to prevent electrical shocks and reintroduce the unit into clinical service, as this would not be a professional repair. Checking to see whether the warmer still works would expose the user to an electrical shock hazard and would be unwise. Making sure that the cord does not come in contact with the floor is not important as long as the fluid warmer is not plugged in and is an insufficient safety precaution if it is.

2. **D**

The effect of an electrical shock on the body is determined by the intensity of the current, the path the current takes through the body (especially if the current passes through the heart), and the time duration of the current. Body mass index (BMI) is relatively unimportant in determining the effect of an electric shock in comparison with the other three factors.

3. **D**

Electrical conductivity is a measure of how well electricity will flow through a particular material. Metals are good conductors of both electricity and heat. Since copper, silver, and gold are metals, they are all good conductors of electricity. Rubber is a poor conductor of electricity, which is why it is sometimes used to insulate electrical wires.

Note that some metals are way better conductors of electricity than others. For instance, copper conducts electricity about 40 times better than stainless steel. Electrical conductivity in metals is good because metals form a crystal lattice where the outer shell electrons are shared and easily move through the lattice. In stainless steel, an alloy of iron and chromium, the chromium atoms disrupt this lattice and produce collisions among moving electrons that decrease conductivity.

4. **C**

If you simply pull on the cord until the plug comes out, you risk avulsing the cord from the plug; this is true even if you put your foot on the power strip to hold it steady while you pull the cord loose. If you request assistance from the Clinical Engineering department, they will likely oblige you and then talk among themselves about what a moron you are for the next few weeks. The correct answer is to use your hand to remove the plug, being careful not to pull on the cord itself to avoid avulsing the cord from the plug.

5. **C**

All of the above statements are true except for the statement concerning cellular telephones. A cellular telephone is a portable electronic device used for mobile communication that utilizes a network of specialized base stations. Cellular telephones come in GSM and CDMA types, with the GSM type usually requiring a SIM card. Cellular telephones communicate with their cellular network both when a call is in progress as well as when they are in standby mode, awaiting a call.

6. **A**

See the table below for an explanation.

Symbol	Name	SI unit	
I	Electric current	Ampere	A
Q	Electric charge	Coulomb	C
E, V	Electromotive force	Volt	V
R	Electric resistance	Ohm	Ω
P	Electric power	Watt	W
C	Capacitance	Farad	F

7. **C**

Recall that Ohm's law is V = I × R, where

- *V* is the electromotive force (in volts)
- *I* is current (in amperes)
- *R* is resistance (in ohms)

Thus Ohm's law relates voltage with current, and not power, energy, or capacitance.

8. **C**

From Ohm's law, we know that the electrical current flowing through a wire depends on both the wire's resistance and the voltage difference applied. The other answers are incorrect because they are not compatible with Ohm's law.

9. **B**

See the table below for an explanation.

Symbol	Name	SI unit	
I	Electric current	Ampere	A
Q	Electric charge	Coulomb	C
E, V	Electromotive force	Volt	V
R	Electric resistance	Ohm	Ω
P	Electric power	Watt	W
C	Capacitance	Farad	F

10. **D**

Metals are good conductors of both electricity and heat. Since copper, silver, and gold are metals, they are all good conductors of both electricity and heat. Diamonds are poor electrical conductors, but are a good conductor of heat, because of "strong covalent bonding and low phonon scattering." In fact, the thermal conductivity of diamond is about five times that of copper.

Here are more details. Electrical conductivity requires the ability to transport electrons, but the electrons in diamonds are tightly bound (strong covalent bonding), so it does not conduct electricity well. The conduction of heat, however, only requires the ability to transmit the mechanical energy of molecular motions, which diamonds do well because the atoms in its crystal lattice are "strongly coupled."

11. **A**

Wood, fabric, and paper are common sources of **Class A** fires. This kind of fire is encountered across several different industries, with trash fires being a common example.

12. **B**

A fire triangle (Fig. 36.18) is a conceptual model for understanding the necessary elements for starting a fire. Nitrogen does not support combustion.

13. **C**

When using a fire extinguisher, one should aim at the base of the fire. If you aim higher up at the flames, the extinguishing agent will pass right through the fire and be far less effective.

References

1. Apfelbaum JL, Caplan RA, Barker SJ, Connis RT, Cowles C, Ehrenwerth J, Nickinovich DG, Pritchard D, Roberson DW, Caplan RA, Barker SJ, et al. Practice advisory for the prevention and management of operating room fires XE "Operating room fire" : an updated report by the American society of anesthesiologists task force on operating room fires. Anesthesiology. 2013;118(2):271–90.
2. Epstein AE, DiMarco JP, Ellenbogen KA, et al. ACC/AHA/HRS 2008 guidelines for device-based therapy of cardiac rhythm abnormalities. J Am Coll Cardiol. 2008;51(21):e1-62.
3. Freund PR, Radke HM. Intraoperative explosion: methane gas and diet. Anesthesiology. 1981;55(6):700–1.
4. Franco A, Diz JC, Cortés J, Alvarez J. Fires and explosions with anaesthetics. Br J Anaesth. 1995;75(6):821–8222.
5. Jones TS, Black IH, Robinson TN, Jones EL. Operating room fires. Anesthesiology. 2019;130(3):492–501. https://doi.org/10.1097/ALN.0000000000002598.
6. Kaye AD, Kolinsky D, Urman RD. Management of a fire in the operating room. J Anesth. 2014;28(2):279–87. https://doi.org/10.1007/s00540-013-1705-6.
7. Watson DS. New recommendations for prevention of surgical fires. AORN J. 2010;91(4):463–9. https://doi.org/10.1016/j.aorn.2009.12.023.

Need More Information? Some Suggested Readings

8. Barker SJ, Doyle DJ. Electrical safety in the operating room: dry versus wet. Anesth Analg. 2010;110(6):1517–8.
9. Buczko GB, McKay WP. Electrical safety in the operating room. Can J Anaesth. 1987;34(3):315–22.
10. Hull CJ. "Electrocution" hazards in the operating theatre. Br J Anaesth. 1978;50(7):647–57.
11. Kerr DR, Malhotra IV. Electrical design and safety in the operating room and intensive care unit. Int Anesthesiol Clin. 1981;19(2):27–48.
12. Litt L, Ehrenwerth J. Electrical safety in the operating room: important old wine, disguised new bottles. Anesth Analg. 1994;78(3):417–9.
13. Wills JH, Ehrenwerth J, Rogers D. Electrical injury to a nurse due to conductive fluid in an operating room designated as a dry location. Anesth Analg. 2010;110(6):1647–9.

Mechanical Ventilation

37

Aaron J. Douglas

Abstract

The use of mechanical ventilation is a common intervention in both the operating room and intensive care units worldwide. Often the goal is merely to facilitate a patient undergoing major surgery, other times it is to prevent life-threatening deterioration in a critically ill patient. It needs to be remembered that mechanical ventilation is a supportive therapy, and it rarely treats the underlying disease process. With this sentiment in mind, much of the focus of positive pressure ventilation is aimed at preventing its negative effects such as lung injury, infection, and hypotension. There are numerous ways that mechanical ventilation may damage the body. The various types of lung damage caused by ventilators are collectively known as ventilator-induced lung injury (VILI). Specific examples of VILI that mechanical ventilation may induce include parenchymal air leaks, also known as barotrauma, and diffuse alveolar over-distension that causes a volutrauma injury to the lung. Another mechanism of injury is due to the cyclic opening and closing of the alveoli, and this is termed atelectrauma.

Keywords

Mechanical ventilation • Volume control ventilation • Pressure control ventilation • Inverse ratio ventilation • Airway pressure release ventilation • High-frequency ventilation • Recruitment maneuvers • Sigh breaths • Continuous positive airway pressure (CPAP) • Positive end-expiratory pressure (PEEP) • Assist control ventilation (ACV) • Intermittent mandatory ventilation (IMV) • Synchronized intermittent mandatory ventilation (SIMV) • Pressure support ventilation (PSV) • Bilevel positive airway pressure (BPAP or BiPAP) • High-flow oxygen therapy

Key Points

1. Mechanical ventilation can cause volutrauma, atelectrauma, and biotrauma, especially when used inappropriately. Operating a ventilator within what is known as the lung "safe zone" minimizes its damaging effects.
2. There are four phases of the respiratory cycle: (1) the change from expiration to inspiration, (2) inspiration, (3) the change from inspiration to expiration, and (4) expiration. These are the control points that form the basis to help classify mechanical ventilators.
3. Ventilators are best classified by phase variables (trigger, cycle, limit) and control variables (pressure, volume, flow, time).
4. In volume control ventilation (VCV) the lungs are inflated at a constant inspiratory flow rate to a preset tidal volume. The advantage of VCV is the ability to deliver a constant tidal volume, and hence minute ventilation (if at a constant respiratory rate).
5. In pressure control ventilation (PCV) a pressure target is selected on the ventilator. Both tidal volume and inspiratory time may vary from breath to breath during a pressure-controlled breath.
6. Tidal volume is not guaranteed with PCV. The major benefit during PCV is the ability to control the peak alveolar pressure, and possibly reduce the incidence of ventilator-induced lung injury (VILI).
7. A normal I:E ratio during mechanical ventilation is usually set at 1:2 or below (for example 1:2.5) in an adult patient. Reversing the normal I:E ratio results in higher airway and alveolar pressures, and is called inverse ratio ventilation (IRV).
8. Airway Pressure Release Ventilation (APRV) is a form of IRV. It may be thought of as the application of two

A. J. Douglas (✉)
Department of Anesthesiology, Saint Luke's Health System, Kansas City, MO, USA
e-mail: adouglas@saint-lukes.org

M. Argalious et al. (eds.), *Basic Sciences in Anesthesia*,
https://doi.org/10.1007/978-3-031-60203-0_37

alternating levels of continuous positive airway pressure (CPAP) that are applied for set periods of time. The patient is allowed to breathe spontaneously during APRV. APRV improves oxygenation through higher mean airway pressures that recruit alveoli.
9. High frequency ventilation (HFV) is a collection of ventilator modes combining very high respiratory rates and very low tidal volumes.
10. Recruitment maneuvers (RM), also sometimes called "sighs" or "sigh breaths", are transient increases in transpulmonary pressure designed to open up collapsed alveoli. RMs can be performed on an anesthesia machine, a conventional ventilator, or a high frequency oscillation device.

37.1 Introduction

Mechanical ventilation (MV) is a common intervention in both operating rooms (OR) and intensive care units (ICUs) worldwide. Goals of mechanical ventilation range from facilitating a patient undergoing major surgery to preventing life-threatening deterioration in a critically ill patient. This support maintains (and often improves) oxygenation, ventilation, and unloading of the respiratory muscles. There are four main reasons to institute mechanical ventilation:

1. Failure of respiratory drive (neurologic disorders, severe muscular weakness, overdose, etc.)
2. Failure of Oxygenation (inadequate PaO_2)
3. Failure of Ventilation (excessive PCO_2)
4. As an adjunct to support the periprocedural or perioperative period

Recognizing when to institute mechanical ventilation is a vital skill. Varying criteria have often been published, but its implementation takes clinical experience and judgement. Cited intubation criteria are published in Table 37.1. The main indications are respiratory failure, altered mental status, and inability to protect one's airway.

37.2 Adverse Effects of Mechanical Ventilation on the Lung

A crucial concept is that mechanical ventilation is mostly a supportive therapy and often does not treat the underlying disease process. For example, a patient with severe pneumonia is supported with mechanical ventilation while being treated with antibiotics. Perhaps you are supporting an intubated patient with a myasthenic crisis who is undergoing

Table 37.1 Criteria for instituting mechanical ventilation

Respiratory rate >35 or <5 breaths per minute
pH < 7.25
Excessive work or breathing or impending muscle failure
Hypoxia (commonly PaO_2 < 60 mmHg)
Hypercarbia (typically PCO_2 > 60 mmHg)
Worsening or poor mental status
Inability to protect airway and/or excessive secretions
Airway control during major surgery or trauma

plasmapheresis. With this sentiment in mind, much of the focus of positive pressure ventilation is aimed at preventing patient harm including lung injury, infection, hypotension, and excessive work of breathing.

There are numerous mechanisms by which mechanical ventilation may damage the lungs and body. The various types of lung damage caused by ventilators are collectively known as ventilator-induced lung injury (VILI). Specific types of VILI include barotrauma, volutrauma, and biotrauma. Barotrauma (parenchymal air leak) is alveolar rupture from positive pressure ventilation. The escaped air tracks along the bronchovascular spaces into the lung parenchyma. This extra-alveolar gas may then lead to subcutaneous emphysema, pneumomediastinum, or rupture through the pleural space leading to a pneumothorax. Another common ventilator injury is volutrauma. Volutrauma is also called diffuse alveolar over-distension and is the overstretching of lung parenchyma. Overstretching of the alveolar units leads to edema and worsening gas exchange. Atelectrauma is the term used for the cyclic opening and closing of collapsed alveoli especially at low lung volumes. The repeated opening and closing of the alveolus leads to increased shear stress, loss of surfactant, and microvascular injury [1]. All of the aforementioned ventilator injuries (barotrauma, volutrauma, and atelectrauma) lead to the widespread release of inflammatory mediators. The release of these mediators is called biotrauma [2]. In fact, this biotrauma not only further exacerbates lung injury, but also has been implicated as a cause of multiple organ dysfunction by causing inflammation at distal organ sites [3].

To help prevent injury, mechanical ventilators should operate within what is known as the lung "safe zone" (◉). The concept of the "safe zone" (Figure 37.1) avoids low lung volumes where the alveoli have cyclic closing (atelectrauma), and avoids lung over-distention (volutrauma). Using this strategy is a rational approach to help minimize the biotraumatic injury of mechanical ventilation [4]. Preventing adverse consequences can therefore be mitigated by using a mode that opens alveoli and prevents their

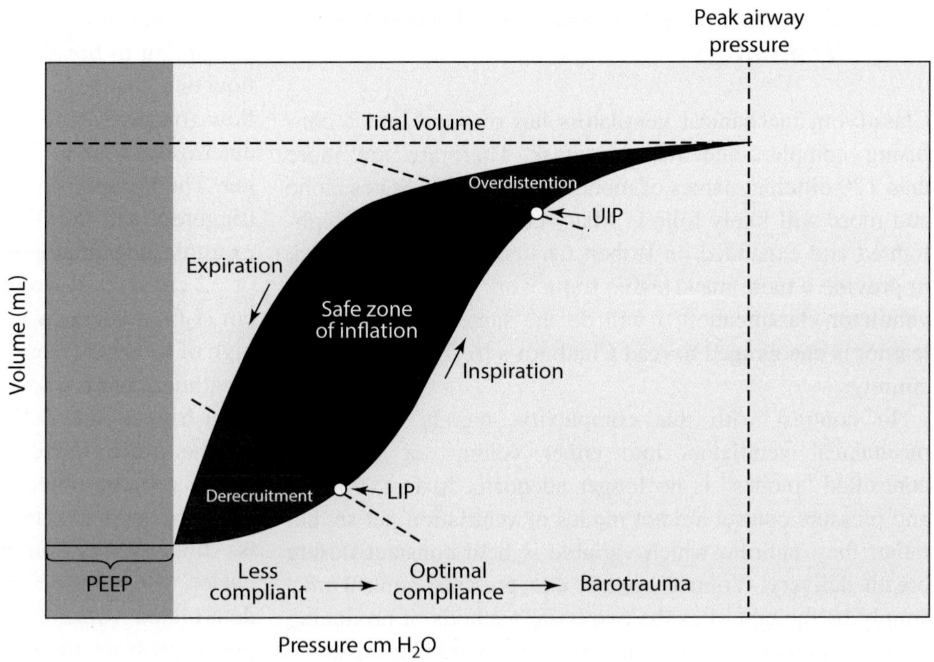

Fig. 37.1 Pressure volume loop of mechanical ventilation safe zone

collapse. This is the "open lung concept" of mechanical ventilation. To say it best, "Open up the lung and keep it open" [5].

The safe zone of mechanical ventilation. LIP, lower inflection point; UIP, upper inflection point.

37.2.1 The Effect of Mechanical Ventilation on Organ Systems

Besides the direct lung effects of mechanical ventilation outlined in the opening paragraphs, MV affects almost every organ system. Patients who are mechanically ventilated (especially for long durations) are at an increased risk of both critical illness polyneuropathy and polymyopathy. Both can lead to severe weakness. Positive pressure ventilation when combined with dyssynchrony of the ventilator may also lead to a ventilator-induced diaphragmatic dysfunction and further difficulty in weaning. The endotracheal tube (ETT) in and of itself may also lead to complications. Bypassing the body's natural physical defenses (the larynx and vocal cords), may lead to ventilator-associated pneumonia (VAP), laryngeal edema, weakness of the swallowing muscles, and tracheomalachia. Patients needing mechanical ventilation beyond 3–4 weeks usually require a tracheostomy to help avoid some of these problems.

Mechanical Ventilation especially with high positive end-expiratory pressure (PEEP) levels can may cause venous outflow obstruction of the head and may raise intracranial pressure (ICP). Hypoventilation leads to elevated PCO_2, acidosis, and cerebral vasodilation which also raises ICP and will exacerbate this problem. Conversely, hyperventilation decreases cerebral blood flow and increases the affinity of hemoglobin for oxygen which will impair O_2 delivery.

The effects of MV on the cardiovascular system are complex. In normal spontaneously breathing persons intrathoracic pressure is lowest (about −5 cm H_2O) during inhalation. During this time of low intrathoracic pressure, venous return to the heart is at its maximum. This phenomenon is reversed during MV. Positive pressure breathe delivery increases intrathoracic pressure, and this impedes venous return. Positive pressure also decreases the afterload on the left ventricle. To summarize, positive pressure breath delivery decreases preload to the heart and decreases LV afterload. This effect is magnified in volume-depleted individuals, and severe hypotension may be seen when initiating MV. MV also increases pulmonary vascular resistance and afterload on the right ventricle (especially when combined with high PEEP). For this reason, caution must be exercised in patients with RV failure.

The decrease in cardiac output along with elevations in antidiuretic hormone (ADH) also leads to decreased urine output. Both invasive and noninvasive MV may cause gastric distention that creates an aspiration risk. Gastric stress ulcers are also common when patients are on a ventilator longer than 48 h. Finally, MV is uncomfortable and can lead to high sedation needs. This leads to further deconditioning, delirium, and often a delay in starting enteral nutrition.

37.3 Classification Systems for Mechanical Ventilators

Classifying mechanical ventilators has evolved into a confusing, complex, and frustrating task. There are now more than 170 different names of modes in the United States alone and more will likely follow. Many current texts have highlighted and expanded on Robert Chatburn's excellent work to provide a more manageable framework on which to learn ventilator classification. I will do the same. The interested learner is encouraged to read Chatburn's [6, 7] work in their entirety.

In contrast with this complexity, merely classifying mechanical ventilators into either volume or pressure-controlled "modes" is no longer adequate. In fact, volume and pressure control are not modes of ventilation per se, but rather they indicate which variable is held constant during breath delivery. Volume control and pressure control may simply be thought of as the two basic methods of producing positive pressure lung inflation. To complicate matters, many newer ventilators use microprocessor control to regulate BOTH pressure and volume. These control systems are termed "dual control modes." A common example of a dual control mode is pressure-regulated volume control (PRVC) ventilation which has become common on ventilators and anesthesia machines. The following paragraphs outline how ventilator modes are constructed.

37.4 Control and Phase Variables

The most modern approach (and simplest method) is to classify ventilators based on control variables, phase variables, and the breath pattern. Ventilator modes are defined by these three parameters. The control variable is the primary variable that is manipulated by the ventilator to generate a breath. Control variables include pressure, volume, or flow. Mechanical ventilators also control one or more of the four "phases" of the respiratory cycle and hence are called phase variables. The four phases of the respiratory cycle are (1) the change from expiration to inspiration, (2) inspiration, (3) the end of inspiration, (4) exhalation. Ventilation phase variables describe how a ventilator starts, sustains, and terminates a breath at one of these breakpoints. The phase variables are named the trigger, the cycle, and the limit.

The *trigger* variable describes how the breath begins (starts inspiration). The ventilator may be triggered by time, flow, pressure, or volume. If the ventilator starts the breath (because the patient is not breathing), the trigger is time. For example, if the respiratory rate is set at 12 breaths per minute, the ventilator will trigger (initiate) a breath every 5 s regardless of patient effort. Ventilator modes may also use a flow trigger or a pressure trigger. For example, if a patient is attempting to breathe, the ventilator may detect a change in flow or a change in pressure within the circuit. The change in flow (or pressure) will lead the ventilator to deliver a predetermined breath. This is known as a flow or pressure trigger. The term *sensitivity* refers to how easily a breath may be triggered, and this feature is adjusted by the clinician. For example, a ventilator breath may have a trigger of −1 cm H_2O or −2 cm H_2O. It would take more patient effort to create −2 cm H_2O to trigger a ventilator breath than −1 cm H_2O. Too high of a trigger (more negative) will greatly increase work of breathing, and too low a trigger (close to zero) may create a "hair trigger" and deliver unintended breaths.

The *cycle* defines what ends the breath. A ventilator breath may be time, flow, or pressure cycled. If the inspiratory period ends after a predetermined time, then the breath is "time-cycled." In a flow-cycled breath, the ventilator cycles to expiration once the flow has decreased to a predetermined value. Conversely, when inspiration ends at a preset pressure threshold, the breath is said to be pressure cycled.

The final phase variable is the *limit (also sometimes called "target")*. The limit describes the variable that controls the size of the breath. The limit is the maximum value a variable (pressure, volume, flow, or time) may reach. An example is a pressure-limited breath. During a pressure-limited breath, a maximum pressure limit is set by the clinician and this value is never exceeded. The following pages highlight basic modes, and hopefully, these somewhat confusing terms will begin to make more sense.

37.5 Targeting Volume or Pressure

As previously discussed, conventional modes of mechanical ventilation deliver positive pressure by controlling either volume or pressure. Modes that use volume control or pressure control are also sometimes called "volume targeted" or "pressure targeted", respectively.

With volume control ventilation (VCV) the lungs are inflated at a constant inspiratory flow rate to a preset tidal volume. There continues to be airflow at the end of inspiration with VCV, and for this reason, peak airway pressures tend to be higher than in pressure control modes. The advantage of modes that use volume control is the ability to deliver a constant tidal volume, and hence minute ventilation (if at a constant respiratory frequency). In the event of increased airway resistance (or decreased compliance), the ventilator will simply increase the inflation pressure to deliver the preset volume. The exception is if the pressure exceeds the high-pressure alarm (adjustable by the user), then the breath will terminate early and the TV may not be achieved.

In pressure-controlled ventilation (PCV), a pressure target is selected on the ventilator by the physician. The delivered inspiratory flow rate is not constant, but rather gas flow is provided rapidly at first and then exponentially decelerates. This variable and decaying nature of the flow velocity profile often reduces work of breathing and airflow hunger. With PCV the inspiratory flow rate falls to zero at the end of inspiration. This results in a lower peak airway pressure compared to VCV. Both tidal volume and inspiratory time may vary from breath to breath during a pressure-controlled breath. For example, in the face of increased airway pressures (e.g., bronchospasm, worsening compliance), the TV will be variable and the delivered minute ventilation may not be adequate. Table 37.2 highlights basic user settings and considerations on volume, pressure, and dual control modes.

The major benefit during PCV is the ability to control the peak alveolar pressure, and possibly reduce the incidence of VILI. It should be noted, however, that the greatest contribution to lung damage is not from elevated peak alveolar pressures, but from elevated mean airway pressures. While the benefits of PCV sound enticing it has not shown clear superiority compared to VCV modes.

37.6 Essential Modes of Ventilation

There are three broad categories of modes in mechanical ventilation: conventional modes, unconventional modes (including biphasic modes), and adaptive modes. All use the concepts of volume or pressure targeted. Conventional modes of mechanical ventilation are the most commonly used, and operate according to the user's input settings (inspiratory pressure, tidal volume, FiO_2, etc.). Adaptive modes are learning modes of mechanical ventilation, wherein the control settings are automatically regulated by a microprocessor. For example, an adaptive mode may automatically adjust FiO_2 and pressure as the patient begins to successfully wean. Biphasic modes include BiPAP and Airway Pressure Release Ventilation (APRV). Alternative modes and techniques include inverse ratio ventilation, and high frequency modes. All are discussed later in this chapter.

37.7 Conventional Modes

The conventional modes (and terms) that are most critical for the anesthesiologist to understand include Continuous Mandatory Ventilation (CMV), assist control ventilation (ACV), synchronized intermittent mandatory ventilation (SIMV), and pressure support ventilation (PSV or PS). Table 37.2 highlights similarities and differences.

Assist control ventilation (AC) (◉ Fig. 37.2) is a time-triggered and/or patient-triggered mode of mechanical ventilation. It is also called *Continuous Mandatory Ventilation* (CMV). The breaths may either be volume-cycled or pressure-cycled (i.e., AC-VCV or AC-PCV). The physician sets either the TV (for AC-VCV) or the pressure and inspiratory time (AC-PCV). The key feature is that the

Table 37.2 Comparison of mechanical ventilation targets

Target	Mode examples	User settings	Notes
PCV	Pressure A/C Pressure SIMV Pressure support (PS)	**Inspiratory pressure** Inspiratory time (I:E) Respiratory rate FiO_2 PEEP	As respiratory system compliance worsens, TV may decrease As respiratory system compliance improves, TV may increase TV is NOT guaranteed and will be variable
VCV	Volume A/C Volume SIMV	**Tidal volume** Inspiratory flow Respiratory rate FiO_2 PEEP	Able to deliver a consistent TV If respiratory compliance worsens, Ventilator will increase pressure to deliver constant TV- this may be damaging Constant airflow at end inspiration, and hence higher peak airway pressures compared to PCV
Dual control	PRVC	**Tidal volume** **Min–Max pressure** Inspiratory time Respiratory rate FiO_2 PEEP	PRVC is a pressure controlled and volume targeted mode. A TV is selected, for example 500 mL. A maximum pressure is also selected, for example 30 cm H_2O. The algorithm will gradually increase or decrease the delivered pressure to meet the target TV. The ventilator will use the lowest pressure to target the specified TV. This is a form of adaptive ventilation

A/C—assist control; PEEP—positive end expiratory pressure; PCV—pressure control ventilation; VCV—volume control ventilation, PRVC—pressure regulated volume control; SIMV—synchronized intermittent mandatory ventilation

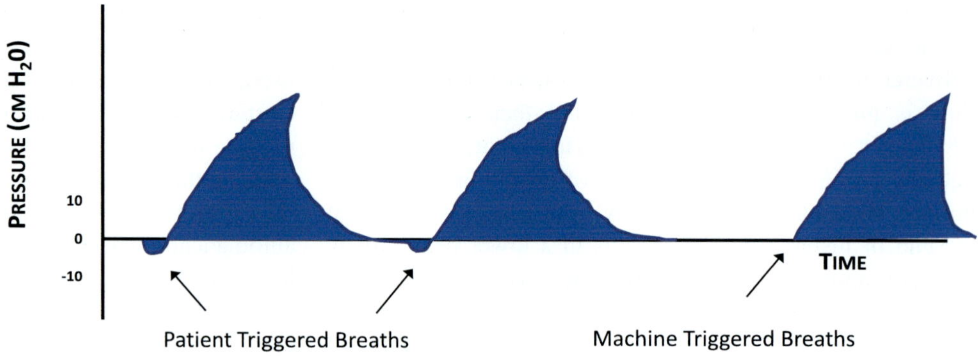

Fig. 37.2 Assist control—pressure control mode. Assist control, pressure control mode. *Note* The first two breaths dip below baseline signaling that they are patient triggered. The third breath is machine triggered

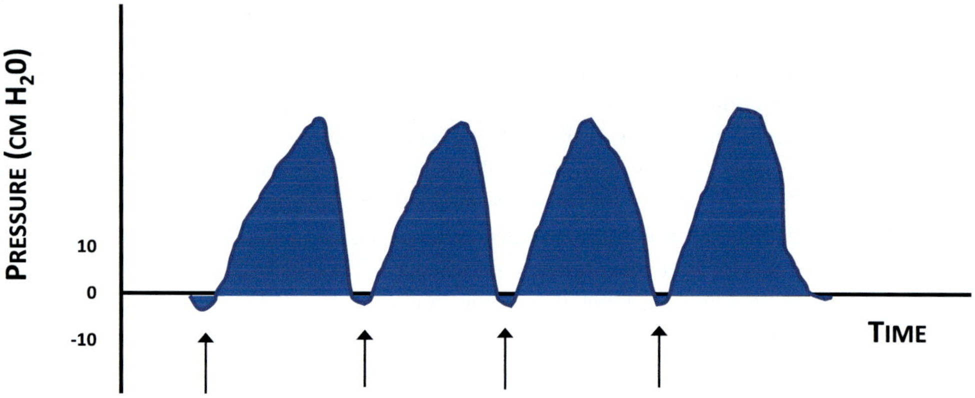

Fig. 37.3 Assist control—pressure control mode—rapid triggering. Rapid patient triggered breaths in assist control. The arrows denote a decrease in pressure (by the patient attempting to breath) leading to a machine triggered breath

ventilator delivers the set tidal volume or inspiratory pressure every time a breath is triggered by the patient. The two negative deflections (below the baseline) in ◉ Fig. 37.2 demonstrate two patient-triggered breaths, followed by a machine-triggered breath. If the patient is not breathing spontaneously the ventilator will deliver breaths (at the set tidal volume) at the set minimal respiratory rate (time triggered). In A/C a patient may inadvertently hyperventilate and be able to rapidly trigger the ventilator (Fig 37.3). In addition to very high minute ventilation, rapid firing of ACV can lead to breath stacking with insufficient time for exhalation. Such patients typically need an increase in sedation.

Synchronized Intermittent mandatory ventilation (SIMV) (◉ Fig 37.4) is designed to allow spontaneous unassisted breathing between ventilator breaths. Similar to ACV, a set number of mandatory breaths are selected. The patient may breathe spontaneously between breaths without ventilator support. The tidal volume and frequency are determined by the patient's respiratory drive and strength. Positive end-expiratory pressure (PEEP) has been added to the patient in ◉ Fig 37.5; notice how this shifts the baseline airway pressure upward. If PEEP is applied, the baseline airway pressure never returns to zero. *Synchronous intermittent mandatory ventilation* was developed with the intent to combat patient and ventilator asynchrony. SIMV senses patient inspiratory effort and enables a patient to receive a synchronized patient-triggered breath. SIMV prevents delivery of larger than intended tidal volumes (breath stacking) by synchronizing patient-triggered breaths with mandatory breaths. SIMV is used in the operating room facilitating emergence from anesthesia as patients transition from controlled to spontaneous respirations.

Pressure Support Ventilation (PSV) are patient-triggered breaths that are supported by gas flow (this is also called inspiratory flow). The preset pressures are typically in the 5–20 cm H_2O range. For instance, 5 cm H_2O provides less support than 20 cm H_2O. The graphical display of PSV is shown in ◉ Fig 37.6. Work of breathing is inversely related to the level of PS; the higher the PS the easier it is for the patient to breathe. The ventilator's inspiratory flow terminates when a certain threshold flow has been reached—typically 25% of the peak flow rate. All breaths are patient-initiated, and all breaths are supported. Because the ventilator delivers support only when a patient triggers a breath, appropriate apnea alarms must be present. Most ventilators offer a "backup" rate in case a patient stops breathing. Should over-sedation or prolonged apnea occur, most ventilators will automatically switch modes to control respiration (CMV for example). PSV is a very interactive mode that allows the patient to determine both the tidal volume and duration of inspiration. PSV is frequently combined with continuous positive airway pressure (CPAP) to increase the functional residual capacity. PSV trials are often used to facilitate patient weaning from mechanical ventilation.

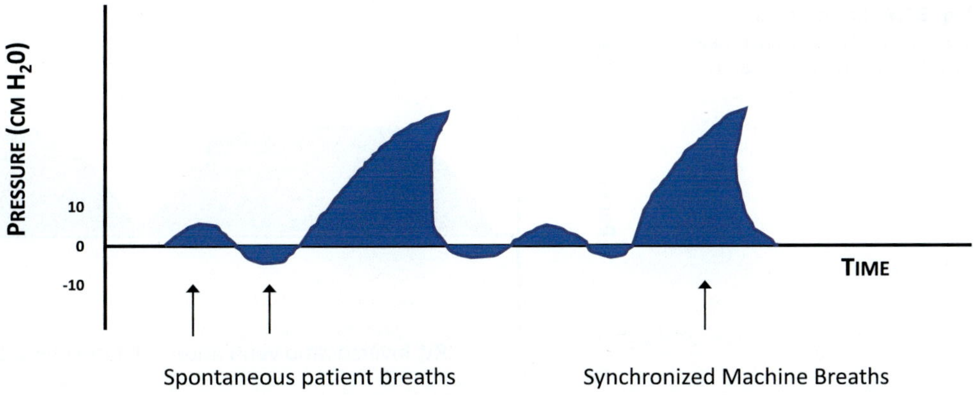

Fig. 37.4 Synchronized intermittent mandatory ventilation (SIMV)

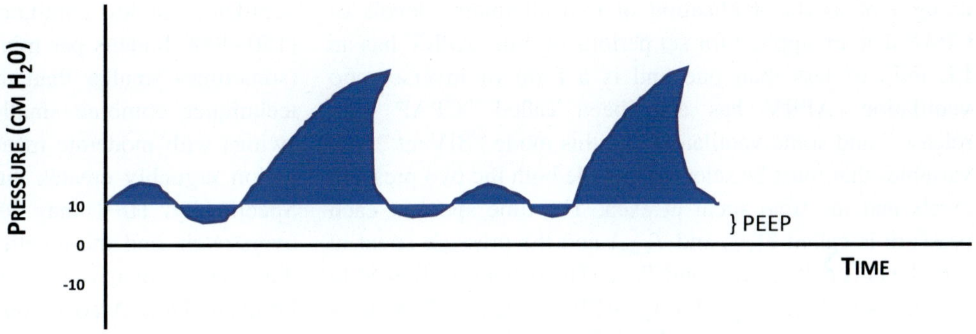

Fig. 37.5 Synchronized intermittent mandatory ventilation (SIMV) with PEEP application

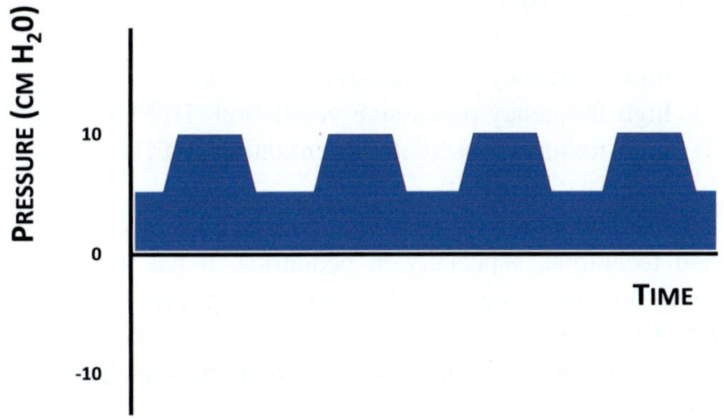

Fig. 37.6 Pressure support ventilation. PSV—pressure support ventilation. Spontaneous breathing mode. This waveform has an approximate PEEP level of 5 cm H_2O and a Pressure Support of approximately 10 cm H_2O

37.7.1 Unconventional Modes

Numerous alternative modes of mechanical ventilation exist, and the following few deserve mention. Arguably, the most important include Inverse ratio ventilation (IRV), Airway Pressure Release Ventilation (APRV), High frequency ventilation, and BiPAP/CPAP. The following paragraphs highlight their importance.

A normal inspiratory to expiratory ratio (abbreviated as I:E) is normally less than one. In an adult patient undergoing mechanical ventilation, it is usually set at 1:2 or below (for example 1:2.5). An I:E ratio of 1:2 represents 1 s spent in inhalation and 2 s spent in exhalation. A shorter inspiratory time encourages lung emptying (because more time will be spent in exhalation), while a longer inspiratory time improves oxygenation. Reversing the normal I:E ratio results in higher airway and alveolar pressures, and is called *inverse ratio ventilation* (IRV) [8]. Inverse ratio ventilation (◉ Fig 37.7) is defined as an I:E ratio of >1:1. IRV is not a mode per se, but rather a ventilatory strategy. Inverse ratio ventilation may be either volume cycled (VC-IRV) or pressure cycled (PC-IRV). PC-IRV is used much more commonly and can be describes as a pressure-controlled, time triggered, pressure limited, and a time-cycled mode of ventilation. IRV appears to improve oxygenation (primarily through an increase in mean airway pressure), ventilation/perfusion (V/Q) matching, decreased shunting, and reduced dead space (through recruitment of collapsed alveoli) [9].

IRV is uncomfortable and deep sedation or paralysis is often needed unless the IRV mode also allows spontaneous breathing (as in airway pressure release ventilation [APRV]). APRV is addressed later in this chapter. IRV may also lead to air trapping and may result in barotrauma secondary to increased mean airway pressures and auto-PEEP. The higher mean airway pressures seen in IRV may also lead to decreased venous return and decreased cardiac output. The use of inverse ratio ventilation is almost extinct as safer and more accepted methods of mechanical ventilation have prevailed.

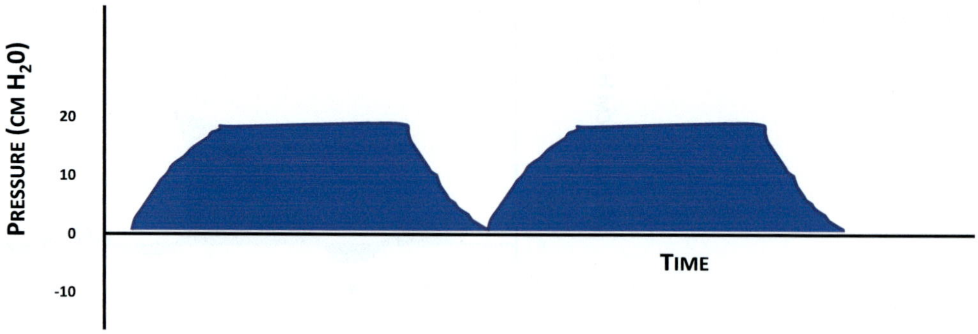

Fig. 37.7 Inverse ratio ventilation. IRV—inverse ratio ventilation. I:E ratio of <1:1

Airway Pressure Release Ventilation (APRV) may be thought of as the application of two alternating levels of CPAP that are applied for set periods of time. APRV has an I:E ratio of less than one and is a form of inverse ratio ventilation. APRV has also been called "CPAP with release," and some ventilators call this mode "BiVent." The variables that must be selected include both the two pressure levels and the time spent at each. The time spent at each pressure is called T_{High} and T_{Low}, and the pressure spent at each level is called P_{High} and P_{Low}. The patient is allowed to breathe spontaneously during APRV. Figure 37.8 is a graphical representation of APRV. Theoretical advantages of APRV include a near-complete recruitment of collapsed alveoli and improved oxygenation. The improved oxygenation is accomplished through relatively high mean airway pressures. Recruitment and improved oxygenation are not instantaneous, and quick results should not be expected with this mode of mechanical ventilation. Improvement with APRV may take up to 24 h. Contraindications include severe chronic obstructive pulmonary disease (COPD) and asthma, as APRV allows for very little lung emptying time. Use of APRV under these conditions makes patients susceptible to hyperinflation and volutrauma [10].

High frequency ventilation (HFV) is a collection of ventilator modes combining very high respiratory rates (150–3000 breaths per minute) and very low tidal volumes (sometimes smaller than the anatomic dead space). These techniques combine smaller tidal pressure (and volume) swings with moderate mean airway pressures. This combination arguably creates the ideal lung protective strategy. Specifically, HFV may lead to reductions in both lung overstretch, and the repetitive closing and opening injuries that conventional ventilation may cause. The United States Food and Drug Association (FDA) defines high frequency as any mode that uses >150 breaths per minute. There are three main types of HFV:

(1) high frequency jet ventilation (HFJV),
(2) high frequency percussive ventilation (HFPV),
(3) high frequency oscillatory ventilation (HFOV).

High frequency jet ventilation (HFJV) is a commonly used technique, especially in pediatrics. It has similarities but is not the same as a ***Low Frequency Jet Ventilation (LFJV)*** in the operating room. *LFJV* uses a handheld device connected to the high-pressure O_2 line on the wall. The O_2 is

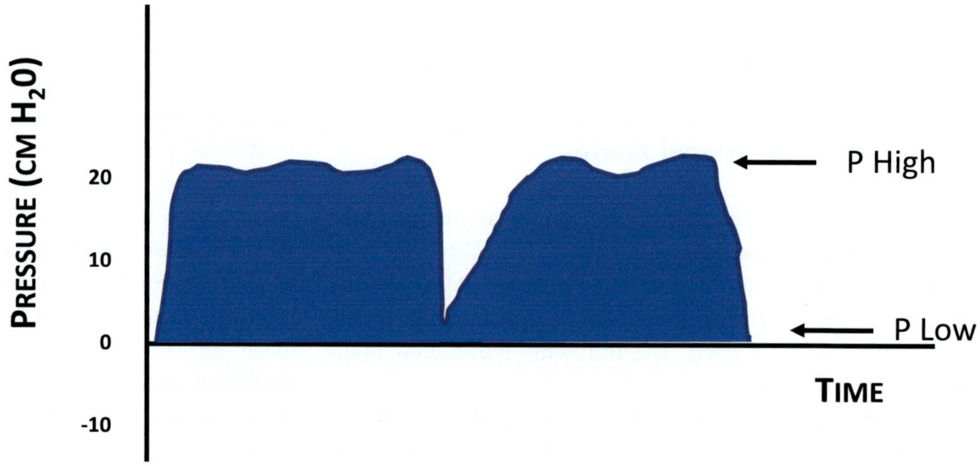

Fig. 37.8 Airway pressure release ventilation (APRV). APRV—airway pressure release ventilation. The oscillating pattern (at P_{High}) represents the patient spontaneously breathing. The P_{High} is approximately 20 cm H_2O, and the P_{Low} is near 0 cm H_2O

passed through a pressure-reducing valve and regulator (that is adjustable). LFJV has been used in airway surgery, bronchoscopy, and plays a role in the management of the difficult airway (through a cricothyroidotomy cannula). Breaths (also called pulses) are delivered via a cannula (similar to an IV cannula), or through tubing that is attached to the side port of a rigid bronchoscope. The nozzle or cannula should ideally be aligned along the long axis of the airway to be most effective. LFJV typically uses 8–10 (but can be up to 30) breaths per minutes administered as pulses. Insufflation should be for approximately 1 s followed by 3–4 s of expiration. In adults, the starting pressure is 20 psi, and is gradually increased until chest rise is visible. Pressures should not exceed 50 psi to avoid barotrauma. Because LFJV is often employed thorough a cannula or an open circuit during airway surgery, it may be difficult to monitor elevations in $PaCO_2$. End-tidal CO_2, transcutaneous CO_2 devices ($TcCO_2$), and serial arterial blood gases have all been used for monitoring of CO_2. LFJV can result in barotrauma, airway trauma (if the cannula becomes malpositioned), severe acidosis from CO_2 retention, and gastric distention.

As mentioned, LFJV is not the same as *High Frequency Jet Ventilation (HFJV)*. HFJV uses a jet ventilator, and in conjunction with a conventional mechanical ventilator. HFJV utilizes a cannula (typically 14 or 16 gauge) inserted into a standard endotracheal tube or a special triple-lumen endotracheal tube. A high frequency gas is pulsed through a nozzle at high frequencies. The velocity of the expelled gas creates a drag effect to entrain gases along a jet stream. Expiration is passive through lung recoil. Initial settings are a pressure of approximately 35 psi, respiratory rate of 100–150 breaths per minute, and an inspiratory fraction of 20–40%. The inspiratory fraction is the inspiratory time divided by the respiratory cycle time, and should not exceed 40%. An arterial blood gas should be measured after approximately 15 min to determine if settings should be adjusted. If the $PaCO_2$ is elevated, steps taken should include increasing the driving pressure in 5 psi increments to a maximum of 50 psi, and increasing the inspiratory fraction by 5% (not to exceed 40%). Low PaO_2 can be remedied by adding PEEP in 3–5 cm H_2O increments and increasing the driving pressure. HFJV is used most commonly in the intraoperative setting for upper airway surgery and tracheal reconstructions.

High frequency oscillatory ventilation (HFOV), as the name implies, uses high frequency low volume oscillations. HFOV is the most common mode of high frequency ventilation. Very small tidal volumes are used (1–2 mL). A proprietary machine is needed, and such machines are frequently referred to as “oscillators”. The ventilator piston pump oscillates between 3 and 15 Hz (up to 900 breaths per minute) against a diaphragm that is actively driven both ways. The oscillations create a higher mean airway pressure leading to alveolar recruitment and improved gas exchange. The respiratory rate is so fast the airway pressure is simply oscillating around a constant mean airway pressure. Because the diaphragm has a “to and fro” movement during oscillation, inspiration, and expiration are both active components. The active expiration separates HFOV apart from other modes of HFV. The active expiration component is advantageous in controlling $PaCO_2$ and in preventing hyperinflation. The technique HFOV is very effective in recruiting alveolar units. HFOV improves $PaO_2{:}FiO_2$ ratio but does not improve outcomes in ARDS.

High frequency percussive ventilation (HFPV) is a hybrid mode that combines HFV and a conventional mechanical ventilator. A gas-driven piston is fitted to the end of an endotracheal tube and generates pressure oscillations of 3–10 Hz. These pressure oscillations are combined in conjunction with a typical pressure-targeted breath. There is some data showing improved mucokinesis, potentially improving pulmonary toilet and reducing the requirements for endotracheal suctioning [11]. HFPV has been used most commonly in patients with trauma, burns, and inhalational injuries.

37.7.2 Adaptive and Learning Modes

Newer and more exciting modes of mechanical ventilation include adaptive and learning modes. Ventilator modes with the ability to adapt and “learn” are becoming more commonplace. There are two major reasons for advancement in this technology, the first of these is asynchrony. Patient-ventilator asynchrony is a major problem in mechanical ventilation. It is caused by a disconnect between patient effort and ventilator breath delivery leading to “fighting the vent”. Asynchrony causes significant patient discomfort, poor sleep, VILI, and difficulty weaning from the ventilator. The second reason is the tremendous human resources needed to monitor lung injury and readiness of weaning. With an aging population and increased use of mechanical ventilation, it is difficult for respiratory therapists and physicians to actively manage a high number of ventilators.

Adaptive Ventilation are mode of ventilation that are closed-loop controlled and regulated by a microprocessor. *Adaptive Support Ventilation© (AVS)* (Hamilton Medical, Switzerland) is one such example. ASV is programmed to automatically adjust based on the patient’s lung mechanics. For example, the ventilator may automatically switch to PSV when the patient meets certain weaning requirements, or to apply lung protective strategies. By adapting to the patient’s demands it is thought that ASV may decrease weaning times. Both advanced programming and artificial intelligence are likely to make these the modes of the future.

A second adaptive principle is phrenic nerve monitoring. It has been known since the 1960s that there is an electrical correlation between phrenic nerve activity and diaphragmatic activity [12]. Neurally Adjusted Ventilator Assist (NAVA) (Maquet Inc., Wayne, NJ) harnesses this physiologic principle. NAVA delivers assisted ventilation in proportion to, and in synchrony with, the patient's own respiratory efforts. A catheter (called an Edi catheter) is inserted either orally or nasogastrically. The Edi catheter contains embedded electrodes that measure electrical activity from inside the esophagus and from the stomach. The catheter measures the electrical signal (called "EAdi") from both above and below the diaphragm. This electrical potential can then be used to trigger a ventilator breath or be used to identify the degree of ventilator asynchrony. In essence, NAVA is using patient effort as a ventilator controller. Conveniently, many Edi catheters also contain a lumen that may be used to deliver both medications and nutrition.

37.8 Noninvasive Ventilation

Noninvasive positive pressure ventilation (NPPV) provides ventilator assistance without an artificial airway in place (i.e., endotracheal tube). NPPV alleviates many complications of invasive ventilation including trauma (hemorrhage or laceration), infections due to bypassing the airway, and patient discomfort that leads to impaired swallowing and speaking. NPPV is delivered via a tight-fitting facemask (either partial or full) or via a nasal apparatus. NPPV may be attached to either a critical care ventilator or a portable positive pressure ventilator designed mainly for use in the home. There are three basic modes of NPPV: continuous positive airway pressure (CPAP), pressure support ventilation (PSV), and bilevel positive airway pressure. Bilevel positive airway pressure (BPAP) is frequently called "BiPAP". BiPAP is a trademarked device by Respironics Incorporated, headquartered in Murrysville, Pennsylvania. Although these modes are generally referred to as noninvasive, any mode of mechanical ventilation can be applied through a noninvasive facemask. Pressure support ventilation was discussed previously in this chapter.

The CPAP mode provides continuous airway pressure to a spontaneously breathing patient. The pressure is applied to the airways throughout the respiratory cycle (inhalation and exhalation). This pressure stents open large airways and helps prevent alveolar collapse. The principal effect is to increase the functional residual capacity and to increase oxygenation (PaO_2 and/or SpO_2). CPAP does not augment the tidal volume (or minute ventilation) and therefore has a limited role in patients with hypercarbic respiratory failure. CPAP is an excellent and frequent choice for patients with cardiogenic pulmonary edema. CPAP is typically set at 5–15 cm H_2O.

Bilevel positive airway pressure is closely related to the APRV mode discussed earlier in this chapter. BPAP is essentially CPAP that alternates between two varying pressure levels (a high and a low pressure). The high-pressure level is termed the inspiratory positive airway pressure (IPAP), and the lower pressure level is termed the expiratory positive airway pressure (EPAP). EPAP is equivalent to positive end-expiratory pressure (PEEP). During inhalation in BPAP, the device imparts a higher IPAP pressure to the airways and this directly augments the tidal volumes. BPAP results in a higher mean airway pressure compared to CPAP and this translates to more alveolar recruitment. The increased lung recruitment improves lung compliance and enhances tidal volumes. A key difference between BPAP and APRV is one is applied invasively (APRV) and one is applied non-invasively (BPAP). Another difference is during BPAP mode most of the respiratory cycle time is spent at the lower pressure level, and in APRV most time is spent at the higher pressure level.

Several contraindications and complications o NPPV exist. Complications include skin breakdown and ulceration from the tight-fitting mask, gastric distension (rarely reported with peak pressures less than 20 cm H_2O), and patient intolerance. There are many contraindications to NPPV and including respiratory arrest, poor mental status, inability to clear secretions, untreated pneumothorax, marked hemodynamic instability, patients who are high aspiration risk, and recent esophageal anastomosis. Indications for NPPV include COPD and asthma exacerbations (especially with hypercarbia), cardiogenic pulmonary edema, chest wall deformities, neuromuscular diseases, and possibly hypoxemic respiratory failure (conflicting evidence). In patients who do not require emergent intubation a trial of NPPV is worthwhile assuming they have a disease known to respond to noninvasive ventilation [13].

37.9 The Role of Recruitment Maneuvers (Sigh Breaths)

Infiltrative lung disease produces severe dysfunction through alveolar flooding (with cells, debris, microorganisms, etc.) and collapse. In many disease processes collapsed alveoli can be reopened (recruited) through positive pressure ventilation. Three techniques to enhance alveolar recruitment have been described: the application of PEEP, prolonging the inspiratory time (because this increases the mean airway pressure), and recruitment maneuvers. Recruitment maneuvers (RM), also sometimes called "sighs" or "sigh breaths" are transient increases in transpulmonary pressure designed to open up collapsed alveoli. RMs can be performed on an anesthesia machine, a conventional ventilator, or a high-frequency oscillation device. RMs reduce atelectasis partly through release of surfactant as well as the act of physical distension on the alveoli [13]. There is no standardized way to perform a recruitment maneuver, and multiple methods have been described and named: sighs, extended sighs, and sustained inflations. Other methods may exist.

1. Sigh breaths have been described as three consecutive breaths set at 45 cm H_2O pressure [14].
2. Extended sighs have been described as a stepwise increase in PEEP and decrease in tidal volume over the course of 2 min with a goal PEEP of 30 cm H_2O for a duration of 30 s [15].
3. A sustained inflation has also been described as increasing pressures to a peak pressure of 40 cm H_2O and held for 30 s [16]. Of note, hemodynamics tend to worsen the longer the sustained inflation is held. The sustained inflation technique is probably the most commonly performed RM by anesthesiologists in the operating room.

After a recruitment maneuver is performed the level of PEEP should be increased, as this helps to prevent decruitment. Signs of a successful recruitment maneuver include an increase in SpO_2 or PaO_2, and a reduction in $PaCO_2$. The inspired fraction of oxygen may affect lung recruitment secondary to absorption atelectasis. RM's are frequently performed with 100% oxygen, but this may theoretically lead to the recruitment maneuver being unsustained [17]. While it is easy to describe the various methods of RM's, indications are less clear. Atelectasis beginning with the induction of general anesthesia is a well-described phenomenon and reversing derecruited lung makes physiologic rationale. Sigh maneuvers (or sustained inflations) can easily be performed intraoperatively by "squeezing the bag" and sustaining positive pressure by adjusting the airway pressure limiting valve present on the anesthesia machine. Like all recruitment maneuvers, excessive pressure may lead to hypotension secondary to decreased preload, barotrauma, or even a pneumothorax. Sigh breaths in the setting of ARDS on the other hand are very controversial. ARDS typically leads to alveolar flooding and consolidation of the parenchyma. Recruiting lungs in this scenario makes little physiologic sense, and in fact RM's may lead to over-distension and damage of normal lung parenchyma. Although recruitment maneuvers may transiently improve oxygenation, in randomized studies there has been no proven outcome [18].

37.10 High-Flow Oxygen Therapy

Mechanical ventilation (MV) is a labor-intensive and cumbersome endeavor, not to mention it may lead to patient injury. Avoiding MV is an ideal solution, and the advent of high-flow oxygen therapy is a strategy that deserves mention. The use of high-flow nasal cannula (HFNC) has greatly increased in popularity over the past decade and for good reason. Conventional oxygen therapy (COT) by nasal cannula (typically 1–15 L of flow) has significant drawbacks. COT has poor patient tolerance due to drying of nasal passages which is typically seen at flow rates >5 L/min. In addition, COT delivers a notoriously inaccurate FiO_2. Patients in respiratory distress often have high inspiratory flow rates, sometimes in excess of 100L. This high inspiratory flow rate easily outstrips and entrains room air oxygen (21%). Oxygen therapy must therefore meet or exceed a patient's inspiratory flow to deliver a stable FiO_2 to the alveolus [19]. Intermediate flow devices such as Venturi masks are more predictable but still suffer from this phenomenon. High-Flow systems are able to combat this problem to precisely deliver FiO_2 of 21–100% and at flow rates of up to 60 L/min. The gas from HFNC is heated, humidified, and then administered through soft widebore nasal prongs. This has multiple physiological benefits including the following:

1) Improved oxygenation
2) Decreased work of breathing
3) Generation of low levels of CPAP (the high-flow adds pressure to the nasopharynx and trachea)
4) Decreased dead space
5) High patient compliance due to improved comfort
6) Improved secretion clearance (secretions are gradually humidified making their mobilization easier)

The ability of Hi-Flow nasal cannula to mildly pressurize the upper airway does lead to lung recruitment and an increase in end-expiratory lung volumes, especially in obese patients [20]. Theoretically, every 10 L of flow generates approximately 1cm H_2O of PEEP [21]. This effect is blunted in patients with an open mouth ("mouth breathers").

Uses of HFNC are several and include:

1) Preoxygenation before laryngoscopy
2) Acute hypoxemic respiratory failure
3) Hypercapnic respiratory failure
4) Post-operative respiratory failure
5) Pulmonary edema, especially from heart failure
6) OSA
7) Patients with Do Not Intubate orders
8) Patients unable to tolerate noninvasive ventilation (due to claustrophobia, skin breakdown, etc.)

Patients with respiratory failure without hypercapnia are commonly started at FiO_2 of 100% and a flow rate of 5–60 L/min (most are started out >30 L of flow). FiO_2 should then be adjusted to maintain SpO_2 of >90%, while the flow rate should remain unchanged. After weaning the FiO_2 to 40% patients may then be transitioned to standard nasal cannula. Patients must be monitored closely for typical signs of worsening respiratory failure: increase work of breathing, worsening oxygenation, etc.

37.11 Monitoring the Patient and Ventilator

Alarms on a ventilator may be visual, such as flashing lights, or audible, such as a bell, but most frequently they are both. The obvious goal of any alarm is to warn of potential safety events that may result in patient harm. Physicians who use a mechanical ventilator are encouraged to be familiar with the manual supplied by the manufacturer to fully understand a device's alarm features. The graphical display of a ventilator is rich in information, and further study of lung mechanics is required for accurate interpretation. Ventilators are typically able to display both loops (flow, volume, etc.) and waveforms. The waveforms on a ventilator are known as scalars. Loops and scalars are beyond the scope of this chapter. A brief synopsis of common ventilator alarms follows.

Most ventilators have a loss of electric power alarm. The alarm is activated in the event of electrical power disconnection (i.e., disconnecting the power cord). Modern ventilators almost always have some sort of battery backup that will power the ventilator for a few minutes to a few hours. This battery backup is crucial not only for inadvertent power cord interruption but also for transporting patients from one area of the hospital to another. Apnea alarms are another mandatory monitor to ensure the patient has not stopped breathing (in a spontaneous breathing mode). The highest accepted apnea period is 20 s. If the apnea alarm is triggered, there is usually an audible and visual alarm on the ventilator. Most modern ventilators revert to a backup mode that automatically provides full ventilator support in cases of apnea. For safety reasons, an apnea alarm must never be disabled on an ICU ventilator or an anesthesia machine.

All modern positive pressure ventilators include airway pressure monitors. Low-pressure alarms help identify both circuit leaks and unintended patient disconnections. Low-pressure alarms are typically set approximately 10 cm H_2O below the peak inspiratory pressure (PIP), which will be discussed in the next paragraph. The high-pressure alarm alerts the clinician of an over-pressurized ventilator circuit. Common reasons for the high-pressure alarm to trigger include patient dyssynchrony, coughing, decreased lung compliance, and kinking of the endotracheal tube. High-pressure alarms are usually set at approximately 10 cm H_2O above the PIP.

An understanding of peak and plateau pressures isan important concept. Their exact calculation will vary depending on how the breath is delivered (square waveform, decelerating, etc.), and is beyond the scope of this chapter. In

Table 37.3 Initial ventilator settings

User settings	Notes
Respiratory rate Breaths per minute (bpm)	A normal RR is 12–20. Most operating room patients will fall into this category of need Patients with COPD may need between 8 and 15 to avoid auto PEEP due to dynamic obstruction Patients with ARDS often need 20–25 bpm. They frequently have a very high minute ventilation Raising the RR will elevate the mean airway pressure
Tidal volume	Normal pulmonary mechanics: 6–8 mL/kg of predicted body weight (PBW) Patients with ARDS: 4–6 mL/kg of PBW Patients with COPD: 4–8 mL/kg of PBW Pplat should be kept <28 cm H_2O to avoid lung injury, especially in ARDS. Some sources argue for <30 cm H_2O, but the more conservative <28 cm H_2O is ideal. The term "Driving Pressure" refers to Pplat—PEEP. It should be kept <15 cm H_2O if possible. The inspiratory pressure on PCV is often incorrectly referred to as the driving pressure
Minute ventilation	Minute ventilation equals tidal volume × respiratory rate Minute ventilation is not a direct setting, but rather the product of 2 variables Typical minute ventilation is 3.5–10 L per minute Critically ill patients may have a very elevated drive, exceeding 15 L/min
PEEP	Typically set 5–10 cm H_2O, can be >20 cm H_2O in patients with ARDS PEEP decreases both preload and afterload and may worsen hemodynamics The term "best PEEP" refers to the PEEP level where in compliance and PaO_2 are optimal. Information from flow/volume loops and serial ABGs are used to determine the best PEEP
FiO_2	Recommended to start at 1.0, and titrate to keep PaO_2 >55 mmHg and SPO_2 88–92% Note Oxygen toxicity is thought to occur at FiO_2 >60%. This is time dependent (longer time at high FiO_2 is worse). Toxicity is likely an oxidative injury. Use lowest FiO_2 necessary
Trigger sensitivity	Use the lowest triggering possible that does not cause auto-triggering A pressure trigger is typically −1 or −2 cm H_2O, or a flow trigger of 1 or 2 L/min

ABG—arterial blood gases; COPD—chronic obstructive pulmonary disease; PEEP—positive end expiratory pressure; Pplat—plateau pressure; PCV—pressure control ventilation general, the peak inspiratory pressure (PIP) represents airway resistance in the main airways (proximal airways). Normal PIP is preferably <35 cm H_2O, and is abnormal if >40 cm H_2O. Endotracheal tube kinking, mucus plugs, and severe bronchospasm or asthma result in increased PIP and an unchanged plateau pressure. The plateau pressure (Pplat) is a measurement of compliance of the entire lung (alveoli, parenchyma, and chest wall). In normal lungs the plateau pressure is usually slightly less than the PIP. A rising plateau pressure signal worsening compliance. Causes of elevated plateau include tension pneumothorax, endobronchial intubation, acute respiratory distress syndrome (ARDS), congestive heart failure (CHF), pulmonary edema, pleural effusions, and chest wall restriction either from extrinsic compression or deformity. Plateau pressure should be kept <30 cm H_2O to avoid ventilator-induced lung injury. Table 37.3 outlines basic considerations for initial ventilator settings that are a safe and good starting point for both critically ill patients and those undergoing major surgery.

Questions (Choose the Most Appropriate Answer)

1. When choosing Pressure Control Ventilation the clinician can control all of the following EXCEPT:
   A. I:E ratio
   B. PEEP
   C. Respiratory rate
   D. Tidal volume
2. Which mode of ventilation results in the same tidal volume being delivered regardless if the breath is patient-triggered or delivered by the ventilator?
   A. Pressure support ventilation (PSV)
   B. Assist control ventilation (ACV)
   C. Synchronized intermittent mandatory ventilation (SIMV)
   D. Pressure control ventilation (PCV)
3. An increased peak AND plateau pressures are consistent with which patient condition?
   A. Endotracheal tube in right mainstem bronchus
   B. Mucus plugging
   C. Endotracheal tube kink
   D. Bronchospasm
4. The term trigger is used to describe how a mechanical ventilator:
   A. Starts inspiration
   B. Sustains inspiration
   C. Terminates the breath
   D. Regulates flow acceleration
5. You have a patient with a traumatic brain injury that needs tight control of $PaCO_2$. Which method of mechanical ventilation would best ensure a patient's $PaCO_2$ remains constant?
   A. Pressure control ventilation (PCV)
   B. Synchronized intermittent mandatory ventilation (SIMV)
   C. Volume control ventilation (VCV)
   D. Airway pressure release ventilation (APRV)
6. The following ventilator graphic (Fig. 37.5) is most consistent with which mode of mechanical ventilation?
   A. High frequency oscillatory ventilation
   B. Assist control ventilation
   C. Intermittent mandatory ventilation
   D. Airway pressure release ventilation
7. Which mode prevents a patient from spontaneously taking a breath?
   A. Synchronous intermittent mandatory ventilation (SIMV)
   B. Controlled mandatory ventilation (CMV)
   C. Pressure control mode (PCV)
   D. Assist control ventilation (ACV)
8. Which one of the following modes may lead to respiratory alkalosis?
   A. Synchronous intermittent mandatory ventilation (SIMV)
   B. Controlled mandatory ventilation (CMV)
   C. Pressure control mode (PCV)
   D. Assist control ventilation (ACV)
9. Which mode of high frequency ventilation has an active expiratory component?
   A. High frequency jet ventilation (HFJV)
   B. High frequency percussive ventilation (HFPV)
   C. High frequency positive pressure ventilation (HFPPV)
   D. High frequency oscillatory ventilation (HFOV)
10. Which patient below is the best candidate for non-invasive ventilation?
    A. 35-year-old in sudden acute respiratory arrest
    B. 63-year-old with a COPD exacerbation
    C. 47-year-old obtunded man with pneumonia
    D. 57-year-old with a small pneumothorax and severe asthma exacerbation

Answers

1. **D**, Tidal volume. In a pressure-controlled mode, the breaths are generated by holding the pressure constant, and the tidal volume delivered will therefore be variable. During a pressure control breath, the physician sets the peak inspiratory pressure, inspiratory time, and respiratory rate.
2. **B**, Assist control ventilation. ACV is a mode in which mandatory breaths or patient-triggered breaths are delivered at a set frequency, pressure (or volume), and inspiratory flow. All ventilator breaths will therefore be the same whether or not the breath was patient triggered or machine triggered.

3. **A**, Right mainstem intubation. An increased PIP along with an increased Pplat signal decreased lung compliance (ARDS, pulmonary edema, pleural effusion, endobronchial intubation, Trendelenburg position, and abdominal insufflation). An isolated increase in PIP with an unchanged Pplat indicates increased airway resistance (kinked ET tube, mucus plug, and bronchospasm).
4. **A**, Starts inspiration. Phase variables describe how a ventilator starts, sustains, and terminates an inspiration. Phase variables include trigger, limit, and cycle. The trigger describes how the breath begins (starts inspiration). The cycle describes how the machine ends inspiration.
5. **C**, Volume control ventilation. In VCV the lungs are inflated at a constant inspiratory flow rate to a preset tidal volume. VCV delivers a constant tidal volume, and therefore minute ventilation. This mode would help target a goal $PaCO_2$.
6. **D**, Airway pressure release ventilation (APRV). Note the alternating levels of pressure. The pressure is never allowed to fully return to baseline. Also note the majority of the breath cycle is spent at the higher pressure (P high), with brief releases down to the low pressure (P low). The notching at the higher pressure (approximately 40 cm H_2O on the graph) denotes the patient spontaneously breathing.
7. **B**, CMV. In controlled mandatory ventilation the minute ventilation is entirely determined by the preset respiratory rate and tidal volume. The patient is not able to initiate additional breaths above the set ventilator rate. This mode frequently needs deep patient sedation. The patient may initiate a breath in the other listed modes of mechanical ventilation.
8. **D**, ACV. In assist control, all ventilator breaths are the same whether or not the breath was patient triggered or machine triggered (i.e., constant tidal volume). A patient may rapidly trigger the ventilator leading to a markedly increased minute ventilation and potentially a respiratory alkalosis.
9. **D**, High frequency oscillatory ventilation (HFOV). HFOV is the most common mode of high frequency ventilation. The oscillations create a higher mean airway pressure leading to alveolar recruitment and improved gas exchange. Very small tidal volumes are used (1–2 mL). The ventilator piston pump oscillates against a diaphragm that is actively driven both ways. Since the diaphragm has a "to and fro" movement during oscillation, inspiration, and expiration are both active components. The active expiration component is advantageous in controlling $PaCO_2$ and in preventing hyperinflation.
10. **B**, COPD exacerbation. Patient selection is a key to successful noninvasive ventilation. Contraindications include respiratory arrest, poor mental status, inability to clear secretions, untreated pneumothorax, marked hemodynamic instability, patient who is a high aspiration risk, and recent esophageal anastomosis. Indications for NPPV include COPD and asthma exacerbations (especially with hypercarbia), cardiogenic pulmonary edema, chest wall deformities, or neuromuscular diseases.

References

1. Chiumello D, Prostine G, Slutsky AS. Mechanical Ventilation affects local and systemic cytokines in an animal model of acute respiratory distress syndrome. Am J Respir Crit Care Med. 1999;160:109–16.
2. Imai Y, Parodo J, Kajikawa O, de Perrot M, Fischer S, Edwards V, et al. Injurious mechanical ventilation and end-organ epithelial cell apoptosis and organ dysfunction in an experimental model of acute respiratory distress syndrome. JAMA. 2003;289(16):2104–12.
3. Slutsky AS, Tremblay LN. Multiple system organ failure. Is mechanical ventilation a contributing factor? Am J Respir Crit Care Med. 1998;157:1721–5.
4. Ranieri VM, Suter PM, Tortorella C, De Tullio R, Dayer JM, Brienza A, et al. Effect of mechanical ventilation on imflammatory mediators in patients with acute respiratory distress syndrome: a randomized controlled trial. JAMA. 1999;282(1):54–61.
5. Lachmann B. Open up the lung and keep the lung open. Intensive Care Med. 1992;18:319–3121.
6. Chatburn RL. Fundamentals of mechanical ventilation. Cleveland Heights, OH: Mandu Press Ltd.; 2003.
7. Chatburn RL. Classification of ventilator modes: update and proposal for implementation. Respir Care. 2007;52(3):301–23.
8. Reynolds EO. Effect of alterations in mechanical ventilator settings on pulmonary gas exchange in hyaline membrane disease. Arch Dis Child. 1971;46(246):152–9.
9. Mercat A, Gaïni L, Teboul JL, Lenique F, Richard C. Cardiorespiratory effects of pressure-controlled ventilation with and without inverse ratio in the adult respiratory distress syndrome. Chest. 1993;104(3):871.
10. Stawicki SP, Goyal M, Sarini B. High-frequency oscillatory ventilation (HFOV) and airway pressure release ventilation (APRV): a practical guide. J Intens Care Med. 2009;24:215–29.
11. Freitag L, Long WM, Kim CS, Wanner A. Removal of excessive bronchial secretions by asymmetric high-frequency oscillations. J Appl Physiol. 1989;67(2):614–9.
12. Lourenço RV, Cherniack NS, Malm JR, Fishman AP. Nervous output from the respiratory center during obstructed breathing. J Appl Physiol. 1966;21(2):527–33.
13. Celikel T, Sungur M, Ceyhan B, Karakurt S. Comparison of noninvasive positive pressure ventilation with standard medical therapy in hypercapnic acute respiratory failure. Chest. 1998;114:1636.
14. Pelosi P, Cadringer P, Bottino N, Panigada M, Carrieri F, Riva E, et al. Sigh in acute respiratory distress syndrome. Am J Respir Crit Care Med. 1999;159:872–80.

15. Lim CM, Koh Y, Park W, Chin JY, Shim TS, Lee SD, et al. Mechanistic scheme and effect of "extended sigh" as a recruitment maneuver in patients with acute respiratory distress syndrome: a preliminary study. Crit Care Med. 2001;29:1255–60.
16. Arnal JM, Paquet J, Wysocki M, Demory D, Donati S, Granier I, et al. Optimal duration of a sustained inflation recruitment maneuver in ARDS patients. Intensive Care Med. 2011;37 (10):188–94.
17. Rothen HU, Sporre B, Engberg G, Wegenius G, Hogman M, Hedenstiema G. Influence of gas composition on recurrence of atelectasis after a reexansion maneuver during general anesthesia. Anesthesiology. 1995;82:832–42.
18. Brower RG, Lanken PN, MacIntyre NR, Matthay MA, Morris A, Ancukiewicz M, et al. The national heart, lung, and blood institute ARDS clinical trials network. Higher versus lower positive end-expiratory pressures in patients with the acute respiratory distress syndrome. N Engl J Med. 2004;351(4):327–36.
19. Chanques G, Riboulet F, Molinari N, et al. Comparison of three high flow oxygen therapy delivery devices: a clinical physiological cross-over study. Minerva Anesthesiol. 2013;79:1344–55.
20. Corley A, Caruana LR, Barnett AG, Tronstad O, et al. Oxygen delivery through high-flow nasal cannulae increase end-expiratory lung volume and reduce respiratory rate in post-cardiac surgical patients. Br J Anaesth. 2011;107:998–1004.
21. Groves N, Tobin A. High flow nasal oxygen generated positive airway pressure in adult volunteers. Aust Crit Care. 2007;20: 126–31.

Statistics Made Simple: Introduction to Biostatistics and Research Design for the Anesthesiologist

38

Edward J. Mascha

Abstract

This chapter aims to help the reader understand types of data and how to use descriptive statistics, as well as normal distribution, measures of location, and variability. It also seeks to explain hypothesis testing, statistical errors, confidence interval, *P*-value, and familiarise readers with common study designs, and some of their pros and cons. Finally, this chapter will aid readers in understanding which statistical test to use in basic research situations.

Keywords

Biostatistics • Research design • Normal distribution • Standard deviation • Mean deviation • Hypothesis testing • Standard error • Confidence interval • Signal-to-noise ratio • *P*-value • Central limit theorem • Data dredging • Study design • Statistical tests • Univariable analysis • Multivariable analysis

Key Points

- **Research should be focused** on a small set of pre-defined exposure and outcome variables. Such focus improves the quality of research and also helps reduce false-positive results.
- **Plot** your data; true trends should be seen there.
- **Know** your statistics program; consult a statistician regularly if doing your own analyses.
- **Check assumptions** (e.g., normality) of data before assuming it.
- **Standard deviation (SD)** gives variability for individuals; **standard error (SE)** for means (include N [entire sample size]).
- **Multivariable** analysis always needed in retrospective studies to reduce confounding on *the* association of interest. **Randomized** study is best way to minimize selection bias.
- **Negative test/study** does ***not*** mean no true association.
- ***P*-value** is probability of a result as extreme as the one observed if the null hypothesis were true.
- **Confidence intervals are key.** Always accompany the estimated treatment effect and *P*-value with a 95% confidence interval.
- **Central limit theorem** means that the sampling distribution of any statistic (e.g., the sample mean) has a normal distribution, and this allows statistical inference from a sample to the population of interest.
- **Sample size justification** is a key element in study design, and should be included in each research protocol as well as each published report.

E. J. Mascha (✉)
Section of Biostatistics, Full Staff Biostatistician, Department of Quantitative Health Sciences, Cleveland Clinic, Cleveland, OH, USA
e-mail: maschae@ccf.org

E. J. Mascha
Anesthesiology, Cleveland Clinic Lerner College of Medicine at Case Western Reserve University, Cleveland, OH, USA

38.1 Introduction

The role of the field of statistics, a specific branch of mathematics, is to help in the design, analysis, and reporting of the results of experiments in order to make inferences about a population of interest from a study sample. Real problems faced by the clinician or clinician scientist who wishes to understand and use statistical methodology in research are the complexity of statistical methods, which are considerably beyond university-level calculus, and also the constant and rapid growth of the field. Due to the sophisticated algorithms involved in most methodologies, nearly all statistical analysis is done nowadays using computer

M. Argalious et al. (eds.), *Basic Sciences in Anesthesia*,
https://doi.org/10.1007/978-3-031-60203-0_38

software, as opposed to by hand. However, although statistical software is widely available, it is quite easy to misuse it. Common mistakes by the non-statistician user are application of the wrong statistical method for the research question at hand, and not assessing the data assumptions inherent in the chosen statistical method. Such mistakes can easily lead to the wrong conclusion.

It is the goal of this chapter to explain the basic terms (◉ Table 38.1) and concepts of statistical design and analysis, so that the clinical reader can better appreciate some of the subtleties likely to be encountered—either in reading medical research literature or when engaging in one's own research with the collaboration of a trained biostatistician. With this brief introduction to statistical methods we do not intend to enable the reader to function as a para-statistician, but rather to provide a basic understanding of the key concepts inherent in most research designs and analyses. A key goal is to enable the reader to better appreciate, understand, and critique the statistical portions of papers encountered in the medical literature.

Table 38.1 Glossary of statistical terms

Term	Definition
Agreement studies	Studies assessing how well different methods of measuring the same underlying quantity agree with each other. Typical analyses are Bland-Altman methods (see Bland-Altman) including plotting differences versus the average of each pair and calculating limits of agreement
Alpha	Probability of rejecting the null hypothesis when the null is true in the population; probability of making a false-positive conclusion when conducting 1 or more tests; equal to the significance level or type I error
Alternative hypothesis	The hypothesis that one wishes to claim; the opposite of the null hypothesis
Analysis of variance (ANOVA)	Statistical method used to compare 2 or more groups on the mean of the outcome variable; equivalent to a 2-sample t-test if only 2 groups
Association	A relationship between 2 variables; assessed in many ways, depending on study design and type of variables
Beta	Probability of not rejecting the null hypothesis when it is false; probability of making a false-negative conclusion; type II error; 1 minus power
Bell-shaped curve	See normal distribution
Bland-Altman analysis	Bland-Altman method of assessing agreement between 2 methods of measurement; for example, includes plotting the difference between methods on the outcome versus the average of each pair, and calculating limits of agreement. Limits of agreement are the mean difference ± SD of the difference
Bonferroni correction	Method used to maintain an overall type I error (or alpha), say at 0.05, by setting the significance criterion for particular tests to alpha divided by number of tests
Case-control study	Study assessing the association between exposure and outcome that is designed by first identifying subjects with and without the outcome and then assessing whether or not they had the exposure
Categorical variable	A variable that is categorized, either ordinal (e.g., Likert scale) or nominal (e.g., gender, blood type)
Causal inference	Making conclusions that one variable causes the outcomes in another, as opposed to the variables simply being associated
Central limit theorem	Key statistical theorem that states that the mean of repeated samples from a population will approximately equal the mean of the population, and the sampling distribution of the mean will have a normal distribution (bell-shaped curve)
Chi-square test	T-test used to compare 2 or more groups on a binary outcome variable
Cohort study	A prospective study following a group or groups of patients over time
Confidence interval (95%)	Interval defined as an estimate or estimated effect ±1.96 × standard errors; 95% of such intervals contains the true estimate or estimated effect
Continuous variable	A variable, such as blood pressure or body mass index (BMI), that is measured on a continuum
Confounding	Means "distortion". A variable that is associated with both the exposure and the outcome, and that should therefore be adjusted for when assessing association between exposure and outcome to prevent distortion of the effect of interest
Correlation coefficient	A measure of the linear relationship between 2 variables
Cox proportional hazards regression model	Regression method used to compare groups on time to an event, especially when all patients do not have the event during follow-up. Main assumption is that the hazard functions (function defined by percent having event over) are parallel for the groups being compared. A hazard ratio is estimated to compare groups on survival

(continued)

Table 38.1 (continued)

Term	Definition
Cross-sectional study	Association between 2 variables at a fixed moment in time
Data dredging	Practice of conducting many tests in a single dataset with the rather unfocused goal of searching for something that will be significant
Dependent data	Data that is not independent, and often represents repeated measurements on the same subjects or units
Dependent variable	The outcome variable in a regression model
Diagnostic accuracy	Measures that assess how well a variable of interest can discriminate the truth, and measured by sensitivity, specificity, positive and negative predictive value, as well as the area under the receiver operating characteristic curve (for continuous or ordinal predictor)
Discrete variable	Variable that represents counts, such as number of infections for a subject
Dispersion	Variability; the degree to which units differ from each other on some outcome
Effect size	The true difference or effect divided by its standard deviation
Estimation/estimate	A quantity measured in a sample that tries to capture the truth in the given population
Evidence-based medicine	Medical practice which allows itself to be informed by rigorous research results
Explanatory variable	The independent variable of interest, and which a researcher desires to associate with an outcome
Histogram	Display of data that bins patients into equal-sized bars based on an outcome of interest and graphs the bars either horizontally or vertically
Independent data	Data that are not correlated with each other—typically from different subjects
Independent variable	Explanatory variable in a model, also sometimes called the predictor variable or exposure variable
Inference	Making a decision about an association of treatment effect in a population of interest from data on a sample from that population
Interquartile range	Difference between the 3rd and 1st quartiles (75th and 25th percentiles) of a variable
Interval scaled variable	The quantitative variable for which a common distance between any 2 values has the same meaning
Interaction	An interaction is present if the relationship between 2 variables (say exposure A and outcome B) is different for different levels of a third variable (interacting variables C)
Linear regression	Statistical model with continuous dependent variable
Kaplan-Meier curve	Method used to display survival or failure curves for time-to-event data and compare curves using log-rank or Wilcoxon tests
Kruskal-Wallis test	Generalization of the Wilcoxon Rank-Sum test to more than 2 groups
Limits of agreement (95%)	Mean bias (or difference) between 2 methods of measurement $\pm 1.96 \times$ standard deviation of the difference. Shows where 95% of differences are expected to fall
Logistic regression	Statistical model with binary dependent variable
Log-rank test	Test used to compare 2 or more survival curves (see Kaplan-Meier)
McNemar's test	Test used to compare 2 paired or correlated proportions
Mean	Average of a set of data points; equal to the sum of the values divided by the sample size
Median	Middle value among a set of data values sorted from smallest to largest. For an even number of observations, the median is the average of the 2 middle points
Meta-analysis	Quantitative synthesis of results of more than 1 research study on the same topic
Mode	Most common value in a sample
Multiple comparisons procedures	Method used to control the type I error at a nominal level (usually 5%) when multiple comparisons are performed or multiple outcomes are assessed in the same study
Multiple testing problem	The phenomenon that repeated testing increases the chance of false-positive findings
Multivariable model	A statistical model that contains more than 1 independent or explanatory variable
Multivariate analysis	A statistical model that contains more than 1 dependent or outcome variable, such as in a repeated measures model
Negative predictive value	The probability of the true disease status being negative given that the test result or predictor is negative
Nominal variable	A type of variable that is not continuous, discrete, or ordinal—but only a name and without any inherent ordering, such as gender or blood type

(continued)

Table 38.1 (continued)

Term	Definition
Non-normally distributed data	Data that does not follow a bell-shaped or Gaussian curve distribution
Normally distributed data	Data that does have a bell-shaped or Gaussian distribution
Normal distribution	A bell-shaped or Gaussian distribution defined by a mean and standard deviation
Null hypothesis	The research hypothesis that researchers want to reject, and typically represents no association for the research question of interest
Observational study	A study in which the independent variable or exposure variable is not under the control of the researcher
Odds ratio	The ratio of the odds of an outcome in one group versus another. An odds ratio expresses the association between an exposure variable and an outcome variable, but does not imply causal inference between the 2 variables
Ordinal variable	A data variable that consists of a limited number of ordered categories, such as ASA physical status or a Likert scale
P-value	Probability value. A *P*-value gives the probability of observing a result as extreme or more extreme than the one observed in a research study if the hypothesis were, in fact, true
Paired *t*-test	A statistical test used to compare to dependent samples on a continuous outcome. Oftentimes the dependent samples represent measurements of the same patients under 2 different scenarios, such as before and after an intervention
Pearson correlation	A measure of the linear association between 2 continuous or ordinal variables. The square of the Pearson correlation (R-squared) represents the proportion of variance in one variable explained by the other
Population	The group of subjects or units that are the target of a research study; i.e., the subjects, or units that one wishes to generalize to
Positive predictive value	The probability that the true status is positive given that the test or predictor value is positive
Power of a test	The probability of rejecting the null hypothesis for a given statistical method under a particular alternative hypothesis treatment effect
Prediction model	A statistical model built particularly for the purpose of predicting individual patient values, and typically assessed for model fit (calibration) and how well the model can discriminate among the outcome values or explain the variance in the outcome
Propensity score methods	Statistical methods used to control confounding by first modeling the probability of having the exposure as a function of potentially confounding variables, and then either matching exposed versus unexposed on that risk score (the propensity score) or weighting inversely on it when assessing the association between exposure and outcome
Proportion	A measure of central location defined as the number of events divided by the number of patients who are subjects. Equivalent to the mean of a binary variable with values 0 and 1
Quartiles	The data values corresponding to the 25th and 75th percentiles of a sample are referred to as the first and third quartiles
Randomized trial	Research design in which the experimental units are randomly assigned to receive 1 of the 2 or more interventions being assessed, thus removing confounding or selection bias
Range	The difference between the largest and smallest data value in a sample
Rejecting the null	The decision to disavow the null hypothesis (typically of no association) based on a statistical test that gives a small *P*-value, or else based on a confidence interval for the association of interest that does not contain the null hypothesis value
Relative risk	The ratio of 2 proportions, typically estimated in a randomized study when comparing 2 groups on the outcome of interest
Research hypothesis	The scientific hypothesis upon which researchers build a research study
Repeated measures ANOVA	A statistical method that includes repeated measurements on the same subjects, or units, and accounts for the likely correlation within those subjects or units when either comparing times or comparing groups over time
R-squared	The statistic that estimates the proportion of the variance in the outcome variable, which is explained by 1 or more predictor variables in a linear regression, and is equal to the square of the Pearson correlation for simple linear regression
Sample	The particular set of subjects, or units, that are measured in a research study; we make inferences on the population of interest from the data in the sample

(continued)

Table 38.1 (continued)

Term	Definition
Sample size calculation/justification	The calculation gives either the number of required subjects or the power to detect a difference in a research study. Components needed to calculate a sample size are the treatment effect of interest, estimated variability of the primary outcome, significance level, and power
Scatterplot	A graph plotting 2 continuous variables—one on the vertical axis and the other on the horizontal axis—to visually assess their association
Sensitivity	The probability that truly diseased patients will test positive
Significance criterion	The *P*-value criterion used to indicate whether the null hypothesis will be rejected or not
Significance level	The type I error or probability of at least 1 false-positive finding in a research hypothesis or set of hypotheses
Spearman correlation	A method to assess association between 2 quantitative variables using the rankings of the data values as opposed to the actual data values
Specificity	The probability of truly non-diseased patients testing negative
Standard deviation	Roughly speaking, the average deviation from the mean in a sample; the square root of the variance
Standard error of the mean	The estimated variability of the mean of a group or of the difference between groups. For a single group, the standard error is equal to the standard deviation divided by the square root of N
Statistic	A quantitative measurement on a sample whose goal is to estimate the same quantity in the population of interest
Statistical errors	Alpha (type I error) and beta (type II error)
t-test	Statistical method used to compare independent samples on a continuous outcome, or else to compare the single mean to a constant
Test statistic	The signal-to-noise ratio used in every statistical test, such as the difference in means divided by the standard error of the difference
Treatment effect	The difference between groups or the association of interest. Can be defined in many ways
Variance	In a sample, the measurement of how much the individual units differ from each other on an outcome of interest
Wilcoxon rank-sum test	Mann-Whitney or Wilcoxon-Mann-Whitney test: compares groups on the ranks of the data. Equivalent to a t-test on the ranks. Does not directly compare medians
Wilcoxon signed ranks test	A nonparametric test used to compare dependent samples on a continuous or ordinal outcome variable using the ranks of the differences instead of the actual values

38.2 Types of Data

Appreciation of the various types of data is an important step in understanding which statistical test would be most appropriate for a given situation [1]. The main types of data are **interval** or **continuous**, such as creatinine or blood pressure; **ordinal** or **ranked** data, such as American Society of Anesthesiologists (ASA) class (I, II, III, IV) or a Likert scale response (e.g., satisfaction with care from low to high as 1, 2, 3, 4, 5); and **categorical** or nominal, such as male/female, alive/dead, or red/white/blue/green. Categorical data with two categories (male/female) is also called **binary** data. It is always a loss of information and therefore a less powerful analysis to make a continuous variable (say, age) into a binary variable (say, <50, ≥ 50), although it is occasionally the best way to answer a specific research question. Counts such as number of children in a family or number of postoperative infections are called **discrete** measurements, and can often be analyzed using the same statistical methods as truly continuous data.

38.3 Descriptive Statistics

Summary statistics such as mean (standard deviation) for "normally distributed" data and median (25th%, 75th%) for non-normally distributed data are very useful ways to report study results. But any statistical analysis should also include plots of the data to visualize the relationship(s) that a statistical model is trying to express. It is a good rule of thumb that one should not report statistical results that cannot be visualized to some degree in a graphical display. A boxplot showing median, mean, quartiles, and range of data is an excellent way to display continuous data, and much better than simply plotting the mean and standard deviation

(SD) (or standard error of the mean [SEM]) with a so-called "detonator" plot. In addition, if the data set is quite small, it is good to report a listing of the data points for each observation.

38.4 Normal Distribution

The frequency distribution of many variables is naturally a bell-shaped curve; symmetrically distributed with higher concentration of data near the central value, and less data moving away from the center (◉ Fig. 38.1). Examples are age, body mass index (BMI), blood pressure, height, weight, log-transformed length of stay (actual LOS is non-symmetrically shaped—skewed to the right). Gaussian distribution is another name for the "normal" distribution. Data following a true normal distribution has specific properties: it is defined by two parameters, a mean and standard deviation (SD); data are symmetrically distributed around a mean; ~68% of data points lie within 1 SD of the mean; mean = median.

One main benefit of having data that follow the normal distribution is that many common statistical methods assume normal distribution, including independent and paired t-tests, analysis of variance, and linear regression. One can assess if data are normally distributed by: (1) making a histogram (frequency polygon) of the data and check if bell-shaped, symmetric; and (2) statistically test whether variable is normally distributed (Shapiro Wilks test, Kolmogorov-Smirnov test, and others).

Statistical methods that assume a particular distribution (and the associated "parameters", such as mean and SD) for the data are called parametric tests, while those that do not assume a distribution are called non-parametric. Parametric tests include t-tests, linear regression, and analysis of variance, for example. Continuous data that is not normally distributed (and cannot be transformed to be so) must be analyzed by statistical methods that do not assume normality; i.e., by a non-parametric test. For example, comparing groups on length of stay (LOS) or blood loss data is best done with the non-parametric Wilcoxon rank-sum test as opposed to the parametric t-test because these data are typically not normally distributed. The Wilcoxon rank-sum (also called Mann-Whitney or Wilcoxon-Mann-Whitney) test simply compares the groups on the average rankings and is analogous to a t-test on the rankings of the data.

38.5 Measures of Central Tendency

When describing data it is always important to give some idea of the average value or central tendency of the data, as well as the amount of dispersion or variability (see next topic). For categorical data with 2 (binary) or more values, the central tendency is described by the proportion of observations in each category, where proportion = number of events divided by entire sample size N (i.e., #events/N). For continuous data, central tendency is best described by the mean (sum of individual values divided by N) for **normally** distributed data, and by the median, or middle value, for **non-normally** distributed data. The median is equal to the middle value or median if N is odd, and is equal to the mean of the middle 2 values if N is even. For example, median LOS of (2, 4, 5, 5, 12) is 5, and median LOS of (2, 4, 5, 12) is 4.5. The mode is the most common value; e.g., mode LOS of (2, 4, 5, 5, 12) is 5.

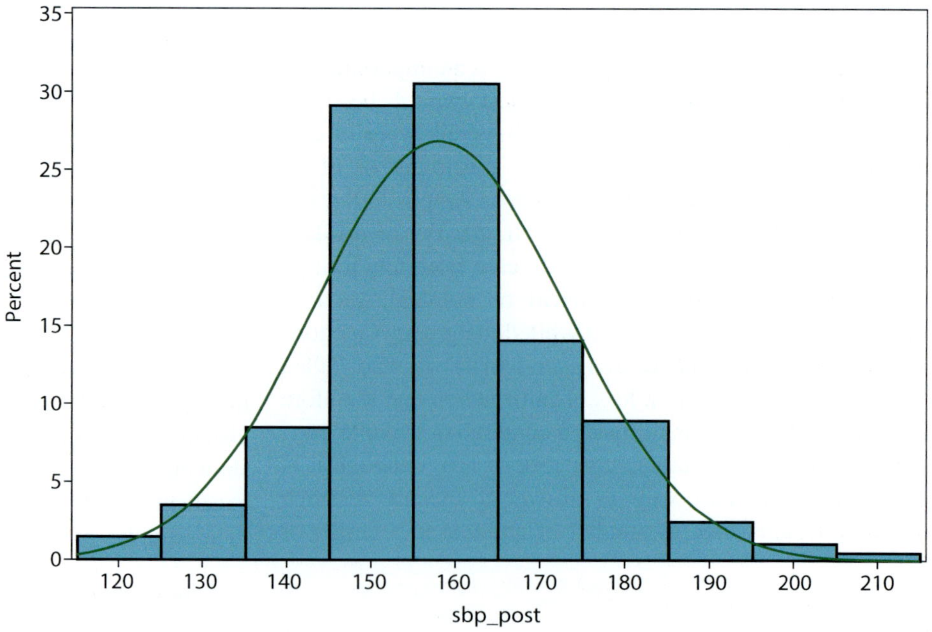

Fig. 38.1 Example of a *bell-shaped curve*

38.6 Measures of Dispersion

Along with an appropriate measure of central tendency, we should always report the amount of dispersion or variability between units of observation (patients, measurements, etc.). For continuous data, the SD is the most common measure of dispersion for individual data points. The SD is roughly the average deviation from mean, and is calculated as the square root of the sum of squared deviations from the mean, divided by $N - 1$. Example:

$$\begin{aligned} &\text{SD of } (2,4,5,5,12) \\ &= \frac{\text{sqrt}[(2-5.6)2+(4-5.6)2+(5-5.6)2+(5-5.6)2+(12-5.6)2]}{N-1} \\ &= \text{sqrt}(57.2/4) \\ &= 3.78 \end{aligned}$$

Note that the SD is not an appropriate measure of dispersion when the data are not normally distributed (such as length of stay, any time-to-event or duration data, and blood loss). In that case, one should report the median and the quartiles of the data (25th, 75th percentiles) instead of the mean (SD). The reason is that when data are highly skewed or contain outliers, those more extreme values may unduly affect the mean and standard deviation, whereas they would have much less effect on the median and quartiles.

In research, we are also interested in the variability of the mean of a variable, which is actually a random variable. When reporting a mean, we want to know how precise our estimate is. For example, what would be the amount of variability if the mean were observed over and over for numerous studies? We estimate this variability of the mean by the standard error, sometimes call the standard error of the mean (SEM), which is actually an estimate of the SD of the mean if it were observed over and over. It is estimated as SD divided by the square root of *N*. In general, which is better to report along with a mean: the SD or the SEM? A rule of thumb is that we report the SD when we are describing individuals, as in a table giving baseline characteristics of a sample being studied. The SD does not depend on *N*, so usually better to report. However, the SEM is helpful when comparing groups on the mean, as long as the *N* is reported as well.

38.7 Hypothesis Testing

Nearly all research involves formulating and then testing a research hypothesis. In this section we will discuss the following topics regarding hypothesis testing and how they relate to statistics:

- Posing a research question (null, alternative hypotheses)
- Inference: from sample to population
- Statistical errors: alpha, beta (power); negative studies
- Estimating treatment effect
- Confidence interval (CI); *P*-value (probability value)
- Data dredging; multiple comparison problem

38.7.1 The Research Question (Null, Alternative Hypotheses)

It is very important when conducting research to pose a *single* research question, a priori. Example: Does chlorhexidine rinse (CR) used twice a day reduce incidence of VAP (ventilator-associated pneumonia) versus standard care (SC) in patients ventilated $\geq$48 h?

The **null hypothesis (Ho)** is what you want to refute. For example:

- Ho: proportion with VAP using CR = proportion with VAP using SC.

The **alternative hypothesis (Ha)** is what you hope to find! For example:

- Ha: proportion getting VAP using CR $\neq$ proportion using SC.

Note: How is the treatment effect assessed in this example? In this example, it would be by estimating the relative risk. Relative risk of VAP = proportion VAP on CR/ proportion VAP on SC. A relative risk of 1.0 means no difference between groups.

38.7.2 Inference: From Sample to Population

The purpose of statistics, and research in general, is to generalize and make inferences from a sample to a target population. That is the reason we use the word "estimate", since we are trying to estimate a population parameter from a sample, be it 15 or 1500 patients. Whenever reporting results it is important to qualify them by the word "estimate" instead of implying that we are reporting a known parameter from the population.

38.7.3 Testing the Research Question

If we have a statistically significant result, such that we have enough evidence against the null hypothesis (say, if $P < 0.05$), we "reject the null" and conclude that there is some treatment effect (in the population). We would conclude in our example that the relative risk (RR) $\neq$ 1.0, and that equivalently, the difference between groups in VAP proportion $\neq$ 0: we claim a "statistically significant difference".

If we have a non-statistically-significant result ("negative" study), it means that there is not clear evidence against the null (say, $P > 0.05$), so we do NOT "reject the null" and do NOT conclude there is a treatment effect. We conclude that there is no reason to reject that RR $\neq$ 1.0, but we DO NOT "accept the null" and claim no treatment effect. Rather, we say "no evidence" to reject the null. It is possible that the study is underpowered (small N) to detect the true treatment effect, or that really is no treatment effect. We do not know. For example, relative risk estimate (95% CI) = 0.85 (0.68, 1.04); $P = 0.08$. Conclusion: Do not reject the null hypothesis that relative risk = 1.0.

38.7.4 Decision-Making and Statistical Errors: Alpha and Beta

After performing a statistical analysis we either reject the null hypothesis (if $P < 0.05$) or do not reject the null (if $P > 0.05$). Since we only have a sample, and not the population, what is the chance that we make the wrong decision? The significance level (alpha, or Type I error) is the probability of rejecting the null when the null is actually true (in the population). This is the false-positive rate and is typically set at 0.05. Beta is the probability of not rejecting the null when we should have; i.e., when it was false (there was some treatment effect). Power is 1 minus beta, and is the probability of rejecting the null when we should; i.e., when the null is false (and thus the alternative is true). Study design goals are to minimize the false-positive probability (alpha, significance level) and to minimize the false-negative probability (beta = 0.10 or 0.20 usually), so the power of a test is 0.90 or 0.80 (1 minus beta).

38.7.5 Estimating the Treatment Effect or Association of Interest

After collecting data for a study, we summarize the association of interest [2]. Whether comparing groups or assessing an association between one factor and another, a research study often has a treatment effect of association of interest that is being estimated, and which directly corresponds to the hypothesis of interest. When comparing 2 group on the mean of the outcome of interest we usually estimate the difference between means and its confidence interval (see later for more detailed discussion of confidence intervals). However, if the data are consistent with the log-normal distribution (e.g., if the distribution of the logarithm of the outcome appears to be normally distributed and similar variance between groups), the ratio of the mean of the log-transformed data can be estimated and is called the ratio of geometric means. When comparing 2 proportions we estimate the difference between them, or else the ratio of proportions (i.e., p1/p2 = relative risk, typically in a randomized clinical trial) or the odds ratio (i.e., [p1/[1 − p1]/p2 [1 − p2], typically in non-randomized studies). When comparing 2 groups on a time-to-event such as survival, we estimate either the hazards ratio from a Cox proportional hazards model,[1] or else the difference between median survival times from Kaplan-Meier survival analyses, for example.

38.7.6 Confidence Intervals

Accompanying any assessment of treatment effect or association should be a confidence interval (CI). Confidence intervals tell us the precision with which we are estimating the mean (or proportion), difference in means, relative risk, etc. A 95% CI is constructed so that 95% of the time the true difference in means or effect of interest falls between the lower and upper limit. We should always report the confidence interval and/or SE, and never just a point estimate, where a point estimate is the statistic of interest you estimate from your sample (see previous section). A 95% CI is point estimate ± 1.96 standard errors. Why does the formula use 1.96? In the normal distribution, 95% of data are inside 1.96 SE of mean. So 1.96 corresponds to a type I error of 5%.

What affects the width of a confidence interval? The sample size, so that higher N will decrease width; the level of confidence/significance (lower confidence decreases width); the variability of the estimate (lower SD decreases width); adjusting for covariates (usually decreases width). A narrower CI width gives more accurate estimate of treatment effect.

38.7.7 Signal-to-Noise Ratio

In order to test the hypothesis of interest we typically construct an observed signal-to-noise ratio and compare it to what we would expect under the null hypothesis. If the observed signal-to-noise ratio is much larger than what we expect under the null (corresponding to a small P-value), we reject the null hypothesis and claim evidence of an association or difference. The signal-to-noise ratio is constructed as the ratio of the estimated treatment effect (see previous section) to the standard error of the estimated treatment effect or association. This ratio is usually called the test statistic, and is usually

[1] Refer to Cox DR. Regression Models and Life-Tables. London, UK: Imperial College. 1972.

either a *t*-statistic or *z*-statistic, depending on the test being used. We compare the observed statistic to what we would observe (under repeated sampling) if the null hypothesis were true. The cutoff value for determining if we have a statistically significant result depends on what we have a priori set as the alpha level (see previous section: Decision-Making and Statistical Errors: Alpha and Beta). For example, if we had chosen the traditional 0.05 alpha level in the design phase, we would claim a statistically significant result if the signal-to-noise ratio (z-statistic) were greater than approximately 1.96 or less than −1.96, assuming a 2-tailed test. For a 2-tailed test, the cutoff or critical value for significance (say, 1.96) is the value of the test statistic under the null hypothesis that allows 1/2 of alpha on the left and 1/2 of alpha on the right, assuming that the entire area is 1.0.

38.7.8 *P*-Value

The *P*-value (or probability value), is the probability that a signal-to-noise ratio as large as the one found in the study would occur if the null hypothesis were true. In other words, it is the probability of observing a result as extreme or more extreme than the observed one **if** the null hypothesis were **true**. If the probability (*P*-value) is very small (usually if $P < 0.05$), we conclude that the null hypothesis is false, and choose the alternative. If *P*-value is significant at 0.05, the 95% CI will not overlap the null hypothesis effect (which often is 0). For example: if *P*-value = 0.045, 95% CI for difference in 2 means will not cross zero (maybe 95% CI for difference in means = [1, 9]).

The *P*-value is NOT the same as the significance level. Note that the significance level is set before the study begins, and represents the amount of false-positive error one is willing to suffer, while the *P*-value is calculated by comparing the observed data to the null hypothesis distribution. A significant *P*-value is one that falls below the accepted false-positive rate.

38.7.9 Central Limit Theorem

The central limit theorem is a key statistical theorem, which says that with large enough sample size (usually over 30) the *mean* of any variable has a *normal* distribution. This is true even if individual values are not at all normally distributed, and it is quite a cool natural phenomenon. It is also true for statistics other than the mean, such as difference means. Why does this matter? The fact that the mean of normally distributed and even non-normally distributed variables have a normal sampling distribution is the main reason why statisticians can conduct statistical tests. For example, whenever we formulate a test statistic such as z = mean/SE, and refer it to a normal distribution (mean 0, SD 1) to obtain a meaningful *P*-value, we rely heavily on the central limit theorem.

38.7.10 Data Dredging

Assessing multiple outcomes in a single research study is often called "data dredging" or "fishing" because the investigation is not focused. It is important to choose **one** hypothesis to test—choose a *single* primary outcome and *single* exposure of interest. If assessing >1 variable for association, we must list all of them in the publication, whether significant or not. The problem with multiple testing is that it leads to greatly increased type I errors, and thus false-positive results. Multiple comparisons (e.g., 10 ways to compare 5 groups) greatly increase type I error. We use a Bonferroni correction to maintain type I error at 0.05 by setting the significance criterion for a particular test to 0.05/# tests. For example, if there are 10 tests, each one is significant if $P < 0.005$ (not 0.05).

38.8 Study Designs

Although there are many options, most research designs can be classified as being either randomized or non-randomized [3–5]. The randomized controlled trial (RCT) is the only design that can truly discuss cause-effect relationships. Non-randomized studies can discuss "association" but not cause-effect, because of potential confounders and assignment bias. Other important study designs are agreement/reliability studies, diagnostic testing, survey, and estimation studies (e.g., prevalence of a disease).

38.8.1 Randomized Controlled Trial

A randomized controlled trial is by far the best way to assess effect of an intervention, and it is the only design that can cleanly estimate the average causal effect of one treatment versus another. This is true because in an RCT there is no selection bias and no assignment bias. Therefore, in an RCT the randomized groups are usually well-balanced on baseline factors, and the only systematic difference is due to the intervention (if there is an effect). It would be difficult to have a true **confounding** variable in an RCT. Why? Because a **confounder** is a variable that is associated with both the outcome and intervention, and because of the randomization there will typically be no difference between groups on baseline factors, and therefore no association between the baseline and intervention groups. However, it is important to note that adjusting for baseline variables in an RCT can increase the treatment effect precision, and can thus be helpful. Randomized studies usually follow the intention-to-treat principle in which all patients who are randomized are included in the primary analysis.

Design options for the RCT include interim analyses for futility (no effect), efficacy (some effect), and safety; stratifying the randomization on factors known to influence outcome; factorial designs where more than 1 factor is assessed in the same study (example: effect of glucose monitoring [versus standard care] and effect of BIS monitoring [low versus high]; cross-over designs, where each patient receives each treatment in random order (lots of limitations to these, but can be done well given the correct conditions).

38.8.2 Non-randomized Studies

Non-randomized studies often seek to assess the relationship or association between an exposure and an outcome. None of these can estimate the mean causal effect as in a randomized study. These studies need multivariable analysis to adjust for potential confounders.

38.8.3 Case-Control Study

A case-control study is a non-randomized study especially helpful with rare diseases or illnesses that take many years to develop, making the RCT impractical. In a case-control study, diseased patients (cases) are matched with non-diseased (controls) on important predictors of disease; the cases and controls are then compared on exposure of interest by a measure of association called an odds ratio. An odds ratio is the estimated odds of disease in the exposed versus non-exposed. Case-control example: the association between smoking and lung cancer.

38.8.4 Cohort Study

In a cohort study, we follow a group of patients over time to observe the outcome(s) of interest, typically comparing patients with 2 or more different exposures and assessing relationships with the outcome(s); the exposure groups are not randomized. The Framingham Heart Study is a good example of a cohort study.

38.8.5 Cross-Sectional Study

A cross-sectional is a study that assesses the association between outcome and predictor in a snapshot of time. For example, we might research whether patients having higher BMI are more likely to have longer hospital stays.

38.8.6 Other Types of Studies

Other important study designs include agreement studies, diagnostic testing studies, estimation studies, surveys, and meta-analyses. **Agreement/reliability** studies may assess how well 2 or more methods or raters agree on their designation of either a categorical or continuous outcome. Special statistical methods are required. For continuous variables, the Bland-Altman method is very useful: plotting the inter-rater differences by the mean of 2 measures. In agreement studies, the intraclass correlation coefficient, or better, Linn's concordance correlation coefficient, can be used to summarize the level of within-subject agreement in relation to the between-subject agreement (but the usual Pearson correlation coefficient is not appropriate).

Diagnostic Testing

Studies typically assess the accuracy of a medical test or procedure in relation to the true disease or condition. Several summaries of the data are useful: sensitivity is the proportion of cases that test positive; specificity is the proportion of non-cases that test negative; positive predictive value is the true positives out of the positive tests; and negative predictive value is the true negatives out of the negative tests. Accuracy with a continuous predictor is calculated as the area under a receiver operating characteristic curve, which plots the sensitivity and 1 minus specificity over the range of the predictor. [Add Ref #10. Vetter, Thomas R. MD, MPH[*]; Schober, Patrick MD, PhD, MMedStat[†]; Mascha, Edward J. PhD[‡,§]. Diagnostic Testing and Decision-Making: Beauty Is Not Just in the Eye of the Beholder. Anesthesia & Analgesia 127(4):1085–1091, 2018.|https://doi.org/10.1213/ANE.0000000000003698]

Estimation Studies

Simply seek to estimate a population parameter, either continuous or binary. An example would be estimating the prevalence of a disease. No testing or power analysis is needed. Since the goal is to obtain a point estimate and CI for parameter of interest, sample size is based on the desired amount of precision, measured by the standard error and desired width of the CI.

Surveys

Are conducted for many reasons, and typically involve taking a random sample of observations from the population of interest. Vigorous follow-up on those sampled is crucial. Response bias (are those who responded representative of the whole population?) is an issue to deal with so that good follow-up from a small sample is much better than poor follow-up from a big sample.

Meta-Analysis

Is the process or technique of synthesizing research results by using various statistical methods to retrieve, select, and combine results from previous separate but related studies. A proper meta-analysis does a thorough literature search on the topic of interest and strives to report unpublished as well as published studies since publication bias is a large issue in meta-analysis.

38.8.7 Sample Size Calculations

Sample size is usually determined in the design phase of a study, and depends on 4 parameters: the magnitude of the effect of interest (e.g., difference between groups), the variability of the primary outcome, the chosen alpha level, and the chosen beta level (1 minus power). Increased variability or power will increase sample size while increasing alpha or the treatment effect of interest will decrease sample size. Likewise, power increases as variability decreases or the effect of interest increases. Sample size justification should be included in each research protocol and also in each published manuscript. There are many freely available sample size programs on the Internet, but calculations should be either done by a professional statistician or reviewed by one. [Add Ref #11 Mascha, Edward J. PhD[*]; Vetter, Thomas R. MD, MPH[†]. Significance, Errors, Power, and Sample Size: The Blocking and Tackling of Statistics. Anesthesia & Analgesia 126(2):691–698, 2018.| https://doi.org/10.1213/ANE.0000000000002741]

38.9 Choice of Statistical Test

A summary of basic and most commonly used statistical tests is given in Table 38.2 [1, 6–9].

38.9.1 Comparing Groups

If the outcome of interest is normally distributed, we would use a **2-sample t-test** if there are 2 independent groups, and analysis of variance (**ANOVA**) if more than 2 groups. A **paired t-test** is used if data are matched, or for before-after designs. If a continuous variable is non-normally distributed (including skewed, ordinal), we use **Mann-Whitney** or **Wilcoxon** (2 independent groups) or **Kruskal-Wallis** (3 or more) groups. For ordinal paired data we use **Friedman's test** (for 3 or more groups or times) or **Wilcoxon Signed Rank test** (2 groups or times).

It is therefore quite important to understand one's design (paired or unpaired). Groups are considered paired whenever they represent measurements on the same patients, or even when they represent 2 or more related or matched samples.

For 2 categorical/nominal factors, we would use **chi-square test** for association for a univariable analysis and **logistic regression** for two-level outcome and multiple nominal or continuous predictors.

Survival data has a time-to-event outcome and are analyzed with special methods that account for the varying lengths of follow-up (cannot use a chi-square): **Kaplan-Meier analysis** for univariable; **Cox proportional hazards regression** for multivariable [1].

Table 38.2 Common statistical tests based on given independent and dependent variable

	Outcome: "Dependent" variable data type			
Explanatory "independent" variable	Normal/continuous	Non-normal/ordinal	Categorical	Time to event
Independent groups: 2	2-sample *t*-test	Mann-Whitney	Chi-square test	Kaplan-Meier log-rank test or Cox proportional hazards regression
Independent groups: >2	ANOVA (analysis of variance)	Kruskal-Wallis	Chi-square test	
Dependent groups (# groups)	Paired *t*-test (2)	Wilcoxon signed rank (2) @@Friedman's test (>2)	McNemar's test (2)	
Continuous predictor	Pearson correlation coefficient; linear regression	Spearman correlation	Logistic regression	Cox proportional hazards regression

38.9.2 Correlation/Regression (Relationship Between 2 Continuous or Ordinal Variables)

Pearson correlation is used if both variables are continuous; **Spearman correlation** if at least 1 of the 2 variables is ordinal or highly non-normal.

Linear regression is used to model relationships between a normally distributed continuous outcome and any combination of nominal, continuous, or ordinal predictors. The R-squared from linear regression tells what proportion of the variance in the outcome is explained by the set of predictors used.

38.10 Univariable Versus Multivariable Analyses

Univariable analysis usually means we are assessing the relationship between 2 factors, often called an outcome factor and a predictor factor. When we assess the relationship between an outcome and more than 1 predictor at a time, such as in multiple linear regression, it is called a multivariable (MV) analysis. Although not addressed in detail here, when there is more than 1 outcome variable, such as in factor analysis or repeated measures ANOVA, it is called a multivariate (not multivariable) analysis due to the multiple responses per patient. This distinction is not always made clear in the medical literature.

38.10.1 Randomized Studies

In randomized studies, a multivariable analysis is not usually needed because of baseline balance. However, adjusting for baseline factors that are correlated with the outcome will improve power as a direct result of the decrease in the standard error of the treatment effect. Randomized studies usually follow the intention-to-treat principle in which all patients who are randomized are included in the primary analysis.

38.10.2 Non-randomized Studies

In non-randomized studies, an MV analysis is crucial because groups being compared, say 2 different treatments, are not balanced on important predictors of outcome. MV analysis on all baseline factors that might be remotely related to outcome or group assignment is needed in order to adjust for selection bias, assignment bias, and confounding (as stated earlier, a confounder is a variable related to both the exposure/intervention and the outcome).

Another common method to adjust for confounding in a non-randomized study is to use propensity score analysis. In propensity score analysis, first, a logistic regression model is fit with the exposure of interest as the outcome variable and considering all potentially confounding variables of interest as the predictors. From this model a propensity score for each patient is estimated, indicating the probability that this patient received the exposure (even though researchers know whether it was received or not). The exposures of interest are then compared on the outcome of interest using an appropriate statistical test either after first matching exposed and unexposed patients on the propensity score or by inversely weighting each observation by a function of the propensity score in the appropriate test. [Add reference # 12 here: Schulte PJ, Mascha EJ. Propensity Score Methods: Theory and Practice for Anesthesia Research. *Anesth Analg* 2018;127(4):1074–1084. https://doi.org/10.1213/ANE.0000000000002920 [published Online First: 2018/05/12]

An **independent predictor of the outcome** is one that is still significant after adjusting for other factors associated with the outcome. Caution: if 2 very related factors (e.g., BMI and weight) are included in the model-building process (i.e., considered for the model), it is very possible that only 1 may show up in the model even though both are highly related to outcome in the univariable analysis. Statistical analysts oftentimes try to obtain the most parsimonious (i.e., efficient) model, striking a balance between how much of the variance in the outcome is explained and the complexity of the model.

38.11 Conclusion

Evidence-based medicine means guiding medical practice by evidence from good research. Hopefully, this chapter's summary of major research designs, concepts, and methods will encourage and enable the reader to be an evidence-based practitioner.

38.12 Questions and Answers

Questions (Choose the Most Appropriate Answer)

1. Which of the following is true?
   A. Confidence intervals give basically the same information as *P*-values.
   B. *P*-values and 95% confidence intervals give different conclusions about 5% of the time.
   C. 95% confidence intervals contain the "truth" about 95% of the time.
   D. 95% confidence intervals always contain some of the "truth".

E. None of the above.

2. A statistic **not** needed for a boxplot is:
   A. Mean
   B. Median
   C. Standard deviation
   D. 1st quartile
   E. 3rd quartile
   F. Minimum and maximum
3. Which 2 modifications to the experimental design will increase power?
   A. Increase the effect size
   B. Increase the Type I error rate, say from 0.05 to 0.10
   C. Decrease the sample size
   D. Increased variability of the outcomes (e.g., standard deviation)
   E. A and B
   F. A and C
   G. A and D
   H. B and C
4. In diagnostic accuracy studies, sensitivity is the proportion of?
   A. Truly diseased patients who test positive on the test.
   B. The proportion of positively tested patients who truly have the disease.
   C. The proportion of non-diseased patients who test negative.
   D. None of the above.
5. Confounding due to a given baseline variable is a concern when:
   A. The baseline variable is related to the exposure.
   B. The baseline variable is related to the outcome.
   C. Only A or B.
   D. Both A and B.
6. The false-positive probability in a research design is also the:
   A. Power of the test
   B. False-negative probability
   C. *P*-value
   D. Type I error
   E. None of the above
7. Which one of the following can best be concluded from a negative study?
   A. No treatment effect
   B. Study was underpowered
   C. Groups are equivalent
   D. Not sufficient evidence to reject null
   E. More data will give significant result
8. The repeated samples of a mean or median from the same population would have a normal (bell-shaped) distribution:
   A. Only if individual patient data are normal
   B. Only if individual patient data are almost normal
   C. Always
   D. Always, as long as large samples are taken
   E. Never
9. The best test to compare 2 independent groups on a continuous normally distributed outcome would be?
   A. Chi-square test
   B. T-test
   C. Wilcoxon rank-sum test
   D. Kaplan-Meier analysis
   E. Pearson correlation
10. The best test to compare 2 groups on a yes/no (binary) outcome is?
    A. Chi-square test
    B. T-test
    C. Wilcoxon rank-sum test
    D. Kaplan-Meier analysis
    E. Linear regression
11. Simple linear regression would NOT be appropriate when?
    A. The outcome variable (Y) is continuous.
    B. The outcome variable (Y) is binary.
    C. The independent variable (X) is continuous.
    D. The independent variable (X) is binary.
    E. None of the above.

Answers

1. **C**. 95% confidence intervals contain the "truth" about 95% of the time.
2. **C**. Standard deviation is not needed for a boxplot.
3. **E**. Both answers A (increase the effect size) and B (increase the type 1 error rate) will increase power.
4. **A**. In diagnostic accuracy studies, sensitivity is the proportion of truly diseased patients who test positive on the test.
5. **D**. Confounding due to a given baseline variable is a concern for both A (the baseline variable is related to the exposure) and B (the baseline variable is related to the outcome).
6. **D**. The false-positive probability is also the type 1 error.
7. **D**. In a negative study there is not sufficient evidence to reject the null hypothesis.
8. **C**. The repeated samples of a mean or median from the same population would **always** have a normal (bell-shaped) distribution.
9. **B**. The t-test is best for comparing 2 independent groups with a continuous normally distributed outcome.
10. **A**. The Chi-square test is the best test to compare 2 groups on a yes/no (binary) outcome.
11. **B**. When the outcome variable (Y) is binary, simple linear regression would not be appropriate.

References

1. Motulsky H. Intuitive biostatistics. New York, NY: Oxford University Press Inc; 1995. http://www.graphpad.com/www/Book/Choose.htm
2. Lang T, Secic M. How to report statistics in medicine. 2nd ed. New York: American College of Physicians; 2006.
3. Clancy MJ. Overview of research designs. Emerg Med J. 2002;19(6):546–9.
4. Davis DW. Types of research designs. Neonatal Netw. 2003;22(5):65–7.
5. Hully S, Cummings S, Browner W, Grady D, Hearst N, Newman T. Designing clinical research. 2nd ed. Philadelphia, PA: Lippincott Williams & Wilkins; 2001.
6. Bland M. An introduction to medical statistics. 3rd ed. Oxford: Oxford University Press; 2000.
7. Streiner N. PDQ statistics. Toronto: B.C. Decker Inc.; 1986.
8. Rosenbaum SH. Ch 23. Outcomes and statistics in anesthesia. In: Miller RD, Cucchiara RF, Miller ED, editors. Miller's Anesthesia. Volume 1, 6th ed. London: Elsevier. 2004. p. 881–90.
9. Glanz S. Primer of biostatistics. New York, NY: McGraw-Hill; 2001.

39 Infection Prevention in Anesthesiology

Srdjan Jelacic and Andrew Bowdle

Abstract

This chapter provides a focused review of healthcare-associated pathogens, their modes of transmission, and their sources in the operating room which include patients, operating room staff, surfaces, and air. We also discuss infection prevention measures that have been shown to prevent pathogen transmission in the operating room and are intended to protect both the providers and patients.

Keywords

Operating room • Anesthesia • Environmental contamination • Patient contamination • Hand contamination • Air contamination • Infection prevention

Key Points

1. Healthcare-associated pathogens include bacteria, viruses, and fungi. Some of the most concerning pathogens include multi-drug resistant bacteria, novel coronaviruses, influenza viruses, and *Candida auris*.
2. Pathogen transmission can occur via four major modes including direct contact with infected persons, contact with infected objects (fomites), larger respiratory particles, often called droplets, and smaller respiratory particles, which may be airborne.
3. The sources of operating room pathogens include patients, operating room staff, and the operating room environment (surfaces, equipment, and air).
4. Infection prevention measures should address all pathogen sources in the operating room (patients, providers, surfaces, and air) and their modes of transmission (direct and indirect contact, droplet, and airborne).
5. Patients—utilize optimal decolonization procedures and antibiotic prophylaxis targeted to individual patients and procedures.
6. Providers—encourage frequent hand hygiene which is optimally provided by wearable gel dispensers.
7. Surfaces—operating room surfaces should be subjected to more thorough decontamination, especially in the anesthesia work area. Consideration should be given to evidence-based practices such as the use of closed injection ports covered by alcohol-containing caps and covering equipment that is difficult to clean with disposable plastic covers. Reusable laryngoscopes and videolaryngoscopes should be subjected to high-level disinfection or sterilization; alternatively, single-use products can be considered.
8. Only sterilization reliably destroys some of the most resistant pathogen to disinfectants including *Clostridium difficile* spores, Mycobacteria, non-enveloped viruses such as norovirus and fungi.
9. Air—although high air exchange with filtered air provides some protection in the operating room, the presence of airway and surgical aerosols, surgical smoke, and constant close contact between providers for long periods of time introduces risks for airborne infection. Surgical smoke evacuation and the routine use of respiratory protection (e.g., N-95 respirators or similar) should be considered.

39.1 Healthcare-Associated Pathogens

39.1.1 Bacteria

Bacteria are the most commonly encountered pathogens in healthcare setting. Bacteria are the main cause of nosocomial infections also known as healthcare-associated infections

S. Jelacic · A. Bowdle (✉)
Department of Anesthesiology, University of Washington, 1959 NE Pacific Street, Seattle, WA 98195, USA
e-mail: bowdle@uw.edu

S. Jelacic
e-mail: sjelacic@uw.edu

M. Argalious et al. (eds.), *Basic Sciences in Anesthesia*,
https://doi.org/10.1007/978-3-031-60203-0_39

(HAIs) which include central line-associated bloodstream infections (CLABSI), catheter-associated urinary tract infections (CAUTI), surgical site infections (SSI), and ventilator associated pneumonia (VAP). Although there are innumerable bacterial species, the 2015–2017 National Healthcare Safety Network data summary estimates that majority of HAIs (83%) are caused by only 13 bacterial species.

Bacteria are classified using a multistep Gram staining method named after Danish bacteriologist Hans Christian Gram. Gram staining yields results more quickly than culturing which makes it a useful technique when rapid diagnosis is essential for initiation of treatment. The Gram staining of bacteria also reveals the shape of bacterial cells which can be used to further divide bacteria into bacilli (rod-shaped) and cocci (sphere-shaped). Table 39.1 lists common healthcare-associated bacteria that can be identified with Gram staining. Some bacteria exhibit a gram-variable pattern with a mix of cells that stain both as gram-positive and gram-negative while some bacteria cannot be predictably stained and are referred to as gram-indeterminate bacteria.

The most concerning group of bacteria are the multi-drug resistant bacteria which are a substantial healthcare burden. Examples of multi-drug resistant bacteria include methicillin-resistant *S. aureus* (MRSA), vancomycin-intermediate *S. aureus* (VISA) and vancomycin-resistant *S. aureus* (VRSA), *Enterobacteriaceae* with extended-spectrum cephalosporin resistance consistent with extended-spectrum beta-lactamase (ESBL) production, vancomycin-resistant *Enterococcus* (VRE), carbapenem-resistant *Enterobacteriaceae* and *Acinetobacter* species, and *Pseudomonas aeruginosa*.

39.1.2 Fungi

Fungal pathogens are the second most common pathogen encountered in the healthcare setting. Fungal infections are usually related to indwelling devices such as central lines or urinary catheters, immunosuppression, and a contaminated environment. Fungal pathogens can be broadly divided into yeasts and molds. *Candida* species such as *Candida albicans* is an example of yeast and is associated with CLABSI. *Candida auris* is an emerging multi-drug resistant fungus associated with nosocomial outbreaks [1]. Of particular concern is its ability to survive in the hospital environment and its resistance to commonly used ammonium-based disinfectants due to a formidable ability to form biofilm. *Candida auris* is commonly found on hospital floors, sinks and other high-touch surfaces [2]. Contact transmission via healthcare workers as a vector has been implicated as major source of nosocomial surface contamination. While *C. auris* is difficult to eradicate from surfaces, it is susceptible to alcohol-based hand gel.

Aspergillus species from environmental sources are a well-known example of a mold associated with infections in severely immunocompromised patients. Although several hospital outbreaks due to airborne fungal pathogens have been reported, most of the *Aspergillus* infections are sporadic.

Table 39.1 Classification and examples of healthcare-associated Gram staining bacteria

	Cocci	Bacilli
Gram-positive bacteria	Coagulase+ *Staphylococcus aureus** Coagulase *Staphylococcus epidermidis* *Staphylococcus saprophyticus* α-hemolytic *Streptococcus pneumoniae* β-hemolytic *Streptococcus pyogenes* *Streptococcus agalactiae* γ-hemolytic *Enterococcus faecalis* *Enterococcus faecium*	Spore forming *Clostridioides difficile** *Clostridium sordellii**
Gram-negative bacteria	*Neisseria meningitidis* *Haemophilus influenzae*	*Acinetobacter baumanii** *Bacteroides* species *Burkholderia cepacian** *Enterobacter* species *(E. cloacae)* *Escherichia coli** *Klebsiella oxytoca** *Klebsiella pneumoniae** *Pseudomonas aeruginosa** *Proteus* species *(P. mirabilis)* *Serratia marcescens*

*Included on Centers for Disease Control and Prevention list or organism in healthcare settings. https://www.cdc.gov/hai/organisms/organisms.html

39.1.3 Viruses

Viral pathogens are the least reported source of HAIs. Until recently, the main concern for viral infections was blood-borne viruses such as hepatitis A, B, and C and human immunodeficiency virus (HIV). However, respiratory viral infections are emerging as a significant source of nosocomial viral infections. Although some human coronaviruses cause common colds, novel coronaviruses emerging from zoonotic reservoirs can cause severe respiratory disease.

The first epidemic of the twenty-first century to be caused by coronavirus was the severe acute respiratory syndrome (SARS) epidemic in 2002–2003, responsible for significant nosocomial outbreaks in Singapore and Toronto, with 10% mortality rate. In 2012, another novel coronavirus epidemic emerged on the Arabian Peninsula, termed Middle East Respiratory Syndrome (MERS), with 34% mortality rate. MERS coronavirus was also responsible for multiple nosocomial outbreaks with a significant number of infections among healthcare workers. The coronavirus disease 2019 (COVID-19) pandemic, still ongoing, was caused by the severe acute respiratory syndrome coronavirus 2 (SARS-CoV-2). As of writing this chapter, there are globally over 750 million confirmed cases and over 6.9 million deaths according to the World Health Organization (https://covid19.who.int) with an estimated 1% mortality rate. With continually emerging variants of concern and sub-variants, SARS-CoV-2 remains a constant threat to the public and healthcare system.

Other notable respiratory viruses include seasonal influenza and novel influenza viruses, responsible for 4 major pandemics in 1918–1919 (H1N1), 1957–1958 (H2N2), 1968–1969 (H3N2), and 2009 (H1N1). Two novel and highly pathogenic avian influenza A viruses (H5N1 and H7N9) emerged in 1997 and 2013, respectively, with mortality rate ranging from 39 to 53%. These avian influenza infections are currently rare due to mass immunization of Chinese poultry in 2017. Other less pathogenic nosocomial respiratory viruses include respiratory syncytial virus, adenovirus, norovirus, parainfluenza virus, rhinovirus and human metapneumovirus.

39.2 Modes of Pathogen Transmission

Pathogen transmission can occur via four major modes including direct contact with infected persons, contact with infected objects (fomites), larger respiratory particles, often called droplets, and smaller respiratory particles, which may be airborne (Fig. 39.1). The success of pathogen transmission depends on the infectivity of the pathogen, host susceptibility and environmental factors. Traditionally, a single mode of transmission was used to explain a successful transmission event but growing evidence suggests that these events are complex and involve multiple modes of transmission occurring either independently or simultaneously. This has also led to confusion about the terminology used for different modes of transmission which has yet to be settled. Proving the existence and relative importance of various modes of transmission for a particular pathogen may be challenging.

For example, "direct contact" commonly refers to direct physical contact between the source (infectious individual) and susceptible host, but respiratory droplet transmission may sometimes be considered as a form of contact transmission, since respiratory droplet transmission occurs over a relatively short distance, usually less than 2 m. The term "droplet contact" has been used to refer to transmission via droplets while some use "direct contact" or "close contact" to refer to transmission via both physical contact and exposure to droplets. The World Health Organization (WHO) uses terms such as "direct", "indirect", and "close" contact when describing SARS-CoV-2 transmission but fails to clarify if "close contact" means respiratory droplets only or both physical contact and respiratory droplets.[1] Transmission by respiratory particles is discussed in more detail below.

Clear understanding and interpretation of different modes of transmission is important since the Centers for Disease Control and Prevention (CDC) and WHO base their advice about infection prevention precautions (contact, droplet, and airborne precautions) on the presumed modes of transmission.[2]

Transmission of pathogens in the operating room is poorly understood (see below). Only bacterial transmission by direct and indirect contact in the operating room has been well studied, such as studies by Loftus et al. describing the transmission of *S. aureus* [3], *Enterococcus* [4], and Gram-negative bacteria [5].

39.2.1 Contact

Pathogen transmission via contact includes direct and indirect contact between the infectious individual and susceptible host. Direct contact transmission occurs when an infectious individual is in direct physical contact with the susceptible individual without an intermediate object. Indirect contact requires a contaminated intermediate object, also known as a fomite. Transmission by fomites is affected by

[1] WHO Scientific Brief "Transmission of SARS-CoV-2: implications for infection prevention precautions" available at https://www.who.int/news-room/commentaries/detail/transmission-of-sars-cov-2-implications-for-infection-prevention-precautions.

[2] CDC Transmission-Based Precautions are available at https://www.cdc.gov/infectioncontrol/basics/transmission-based-precautions.html.

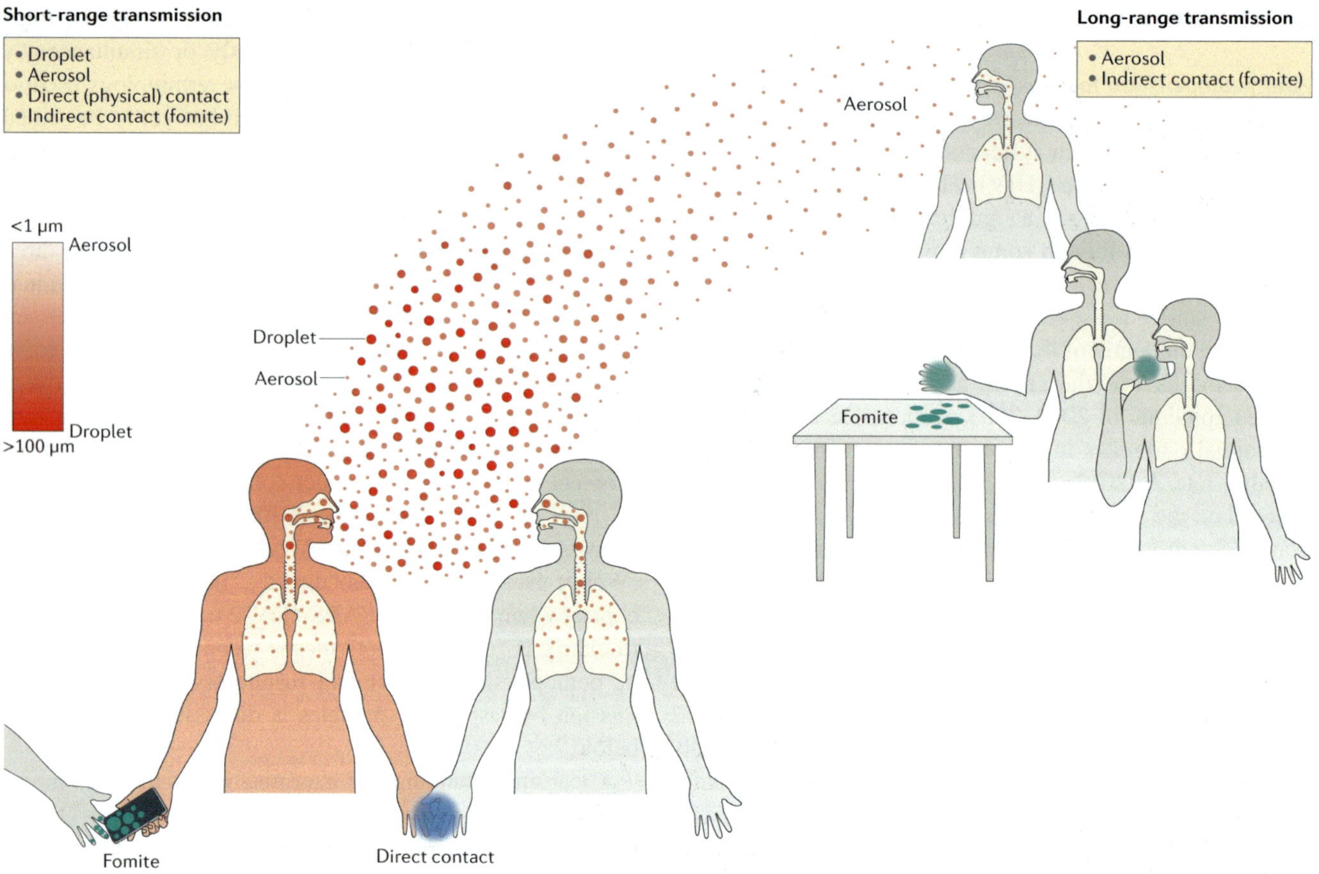

Fig. 39.1 Modes of pathogen transmission including direct and indirect contact, droplet and airborne (reproduced with permission from Leung NHL. Transmissibility and transmission of respiratory viruses. Nat Rev Microbiol. 2021; 19(8):528–545, Copyright 2023, Springer Nature)

Table 39.2 Survival times on environmental surface and infectious dose for common nosocomial pathogens

Pathogen	Survival time	Infectious dose
Klebsiella	Up to 30 months	~100 CFU
Escherichia coli	Up to 16 months	~100 CFU
Methicillin-resistant *S. aureus*	Up to 7 months	4 CFU
Acinetobacter	Up to 5 months	250 CFU
Clostridium difficile	Up to 5 months	5 spores
Vancomycin-resistant *Enterococcus*	Up to 4 months	~100 CFU
Norovirus	Up to 7 days	20 virions

CFU—colony forming units

Adapted from Dancer SJ. Controlling hospital-acquired infection: focus on the role of the environment and new technologies for decontamination. Clin Microbiol Rev. 2014 Oct;27(4):665–690

the pathogens' ability to survive on environmental surfaces as given in Table 39.2.

39.2.2 Droplet

Droplet transmission involves large respiratory particles (droplets) traveling through air from the respiratory tract of the infectious individual to mucosal surfaces of susceptible individual over short distances, of approximately 2 m or less. Larger respiratory particles move toward the ground faster than smaller particles due to gravitational force. Respiratory particles with a wide range of sizes are generated when breathing, talking, coughing, or sneezing. Historically, respiratory particles have been distinguished by size, with a size of 5 μm often used to distinguish droplets, which are larger respiratory particles, from airborne particles (sometimes referred to as "aerosols"), which are smaller. Airborne particles can remain suspended in the air for long periods of time and travel long distances. Rather than using an arbitrary size cut-off, a more modern concept recognizes a spectrum of respiratory particle sizes that can sometimes travel long distances depending on the conditions of both the ambient and the exhaled air such as temperature, humidity, and airflow. The term "aerosol" transmission is sometimes used to describe the entire size spectrum of respiratory particles, from larger droplet to smaller airborne particles or used interchangeably with airborne as in "aerosol-generating procedure".

39.2.3 Airborne

Airborne transmission involves smaller respiratory particles which may remain suspended in air for prolonged periods of time and travel over longer distances. A spectrum of small respiratory particles is generated by breathing, talking, coughing, or sneezing as well as by the process of liquid evaporation from larger respiratory particles. While airborne transmission was once thought to be restricted to a few specific pathogens, such as tuberculosis, measles and chickenpox, airborne transmission of other pathogens is likely, especially respiratory viruses, including SARS-CoV-2 and influenza. Early in the COVID-19 pandemic, transmission of SARS-CoV-2 was thought to be limited to droplets, but airborne transmission was soon recognized as the most likely route of transmission. When dealing with a novel respiratory virus, a prudent approach is to assume the presence of airborne transmission unless proven otherwise.

39.3 Sources of Pathogens

Operating room pathogens come from a variety of sources including the patient's own flora, cross infections from operating room staff, cross infections from patient to patient, and the operating room environment which includes surfaces, equipment, and air. The operating room is a busy, frequently noisy, and chaotic environment with multiple patient contacts and a high burden of soiled surfaces. Although the surgical field, which includes the draped patient, scrub table, and any draped equipment, is sterile, the remaining areas of the operating room should be considered as contaminated despite environmental cleaning and disinfection. A concept of "fecal patina" was previously developed and proposed as a model for pathogen spread in the operating room [6]. The proposed model involves an interplay among patients, provider hands and environmental surfaces (Fig. 39.2). Each element of this model is discussed below along with additional consideration of airborne pathogens and their role.

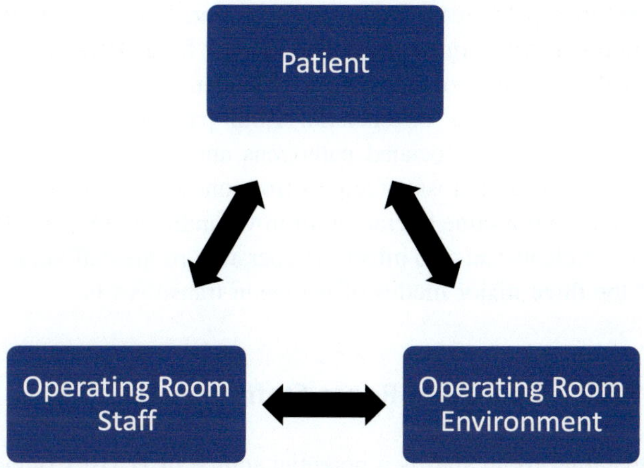

Fig. 39.2 Sources of pathogens in the operating room (adapted from Munoz-Price LS, Weinstein RA. Fecal patina in the anesthesia work area. Anesth Analg. 2015;120(4):703–705)

Several studies by Loftus et al. provided evidence for environmental contamination in the operating room and, particularly, the anesthesia work area [3–5, 7, 8]. In their initial study, they found that the anesthesia machine adjustable pressure-limiting valve and intravenous stopcocks were highly contaminated at the end of surgery with mostly skin organisms, but MRSA, VRE, and *Enterobacter cloacae* were also isolated [7]. In a subsequent study, all three bacterial sources contributed to between-case and within-case transmission and intravenous stopcock contamination, with the environment (adjustable pressure-limiting valve and agent dial) being a significantly more frequent source of contamination than providers' hands or patients' nasopharynx and axillae [8]. With the exception of one *Pseudomonas* and one *Serratia* organism, the majority of isolates were skin flora such as *S. aureus* and *S. epidermidis*. A subsequent multicenter study described the transmission of S. *aureus* [3], *Enterococcus* [4], and Gram-negative rods [5] in the operating room. Highly transmissible *S. aureus* originating from patients' nasopharynx and axillae, and providers' hands accounted for the majority of operating room transmission events. The majority of *Enterococcus* phenotypes were isolated from providers' hands. Gram-negative rods were predominantly isolated from providers' hands but also from patients and the environmental surfaces.

39.3.1 Patients

Patient colonization with healthcare-associated pathogens is a significant risk factor for developing SSI and other HAIs. The majority of postoperative *S. aureus* HAIs originate from the patients' own flora [9–11]. Published studies have mainly focused on colonization with *S. aureus* and skin flora but other pathogens should be considered, especially the Gram-negative organisms found in gut flora. Patients can also be a source of respiratory pathogens if infected with respiratory viruses or bacteria. Both patient colonization with healthcare-associated pathogens and respiratory infections can lead to cross infections from one surgical patient to another in the same operating room via indirect contact. The same patients can also infect the operating room staff via any of the three major modes of pathogen transmission.

39.3.2 Operating Room Staff

Operating room staff is a potential source of HAIs. Contact transmission is of particular concern, since during a procedure, anesthesia providers and nursing staff have hundreds of contacts with environmental and patient body surfaces. The flow and frequency of these interactions make hand hygiene challenging especially during critical periods such as intubation and extubation, which can further increase the contamination of the operating room environment. Operating room staff can also be a source of airborne pathogens especially if infected with respiratory viruses or bacteria. There is strong evidence to support airborne transmission of certain bacteria including *Bordetella pertussis*, *S. pyogenes*, and *S. aureus* by healthcare workers to patients [12]. A term "cloud" healthcare worker has been suggested to describe the phenomenon of some healthcare workers' ability to transmit bacteria via airborne route, especially when a viral upper respiratory infection is superimposed on nasal colonization by a bacterial pathogen.

39.3.3 Operating Room Environment

The operating room environment, which includes many different surfaces and operating room air, is a unique source of healthcare-associated pathogens. Since multiple patients may undergo procedures in a single operating room during a single day, environmental cleaning and disinfection between each procedure is a significant challenge, especially given the presence of multiple pieces of equipment along with constant pressure for faster room turnovers.

While Loftus et al. focused on high-touch surfaces such as the anesthesia machine adjustable pressure-limiting valve and anesthetic vaporizer dial, the operating room floor is a surface that is often overlooked since it is rarely touched. Healthcare-associated pathogens including *C. difficile* spores and multi-drug-resistant organisms have been cultured from hospital floors [13]. Fomites such as shoe covers, socks, and wheelchairs have been identified as a potential mechanism for not only introducing floor contamination but also disseminating contaminants from the floor to other hospital surfaces [14]. A non-pathogenic virus deliberately inoculated onto hospital room floors was shown to rapidly disseminate to high-touch surfaces inside and outside the room [15]. According to a national survey, hospital floors are infrequently cleaned with antimicrobial disinfectants [16]. There is also evidence that the operating room floor can be contaminated by either dirty footwear or bacterial sedimentation from the air and can remain contaminated despite cleaning [17]. Dirty footwear worn by operating room staff can lead to significant floor contamination regardless of the type of footwear used (street shoes, clean shoes, or shoe covers). Floor contamination in the operating room is concerning since many items are in frequent contact with the floor and placed back on the patients' body surfaces [18], including intravenous tubing and injection ports, monitoring cables, drapes, operating room bed safety belts, and other equipment. However, at this time, the relevance of the operating room floor to pathogen transmission and HAIs is unclear.

Another often overlooked environmental source of pathogens is air. Operating rooms have a high airflow (recommended minimal air exchange is 15 times per hour), are filtered by high-efficiency particulate air (HEPA) rated or similar filters and have slightly positive pressure inside the room when the doors are closed. The positive pressure hypothetically reduces the likelihood of bacterial contamination of the surgical field by moving the contaminated air away from the surgical field and out of the room. Although this may protect the surgical field, it may pose a risk to operating room staff inside the room as well as those outside the room. Aerosol particles may originate from various sources in the operating room including staff and patients, smoke from surgical cautery or lasers, and tissue aerosols from cutting tools such as saws. The prolonged close proximity of operating room staff to each other, particularly in the anesthesia work area, also raises the concern for transmission of respiratory infections between staff.

Airborne pathogen transmission in the operating room has not been extensively studied. Some evidence for the association between airborne bacterial contamination and SSI came from a series of studies performed in the 1980s which showed that "ultraclean air" (arbitrarily defined as air containing less than 10 bacteria-carrying particles per m^3) significantly reduced the rate of joint prosthesis infections [19]. There is also some experience converting positive pressure operating rooms to negative pressure to protect staff from patients with transmissible airborne respiratory infections [20, 21]; whether this is advisable and whether it increases the risk for SSI is unknown.

Smoke is a byproduct of energy-based instruments used in the operating room such as mono- and bipolar diathermy (electrocautery), ultrasonic scalpels, and lasers [22]. Although some studies have found viral DNA in the smoke generated by laser and electrocoagulation, to the best of our knowledge, the presence of the live virus in surgical smoke has not been demonstrated. However, the CDC recommends the routine use of smoke scavenging for surgical electrocautery.[3]

Airway management can also generate aerosols and is thought to play a role in respiratory virus transmissions [23–25]. Traditionally, airway management has been considered an aerosol-generating procedure. However, the amount of aerosol generated by intubation or extubation may in fact be less than the amount of aerosol generated by coughing and sneezing [26]. Therefore, patients who are under monitored anesthesia care should be considered as a potential source of respiratory aerosols, in a manner similar to patients undergoing general anesthesia.

39.4 Infection Prevention

The infection prevention measures in the operating room have mainly focused on optimizing patient risk factors, antimicrobial prophylaxis, ensuring proper surgical staff hand cleaning, maintaining sterility of the surgical field, and environmental surface cleaning and disinfection. The updated 2017 CDC SSI prevention guidelines emphasized intraoperative glycemic control, normothermia, and increased oxygenation [27], although increased oxygenation has subsequently been challenged because of the possibility that it could activate aerobic bacteria in the patient's microbiome [28]. Adherence to these infection control measures in the operating room is important but only represents the tip of the iceberg of infection control issues that need to be addressed. Traditionally, the SSI prevention measures were focused on the surgeon and the patient, but more recently, growing evidence demonstrates that the anesthesia provider is an important vector in pathogen transmission and the anesthesia work area surfaces are an important reservoir of pathogens [29].

39.4.1 Antimicrobial Prophylaxis

Antimicrobial prophylaxis has played an important role in reducing SSIs since guidelines were first published in 1992 with subsequent revisions in 1999 and 2013 [30]. Clean procedures do not necessarily require prophylactic antibiotics. Antibiotic prophylaxis is indicated in patients undergoing clean-contaminated and contaminated procedures associated with a high rate of infections (Appendix). It is also indicated in clean procedures when there are significant consequences to infection (e.g., prosthetic implants). The use of antibiotics in dirty procedures or in established infections is considered treatment rather than prophylaxis. The most recent guidelines emphasize optimal preoperative antimicrobial timing (within 60 min before incision), dose adjustment for obese patients, and intraoperative redosing (if procedure duration exceeds 2 half-lives of the antimicrobial or there is excessive blood loss). Although antimicrobial prophylaxis is important, other factors also play a role in SSI including the surgeon's experience and technique, the duration of the procedure, hospital and operating room environments, instrument-sterilization issues, preoperative preparation (e.g., surgical scrub, skin antisepsis, appropriate hair removal), perioperative management (temperature and glycemic control), and the underlying medical condition of the patient.

When colonization with MRSA is not suspected, cefazolin is usually considered adequate coverage for skin flora. When MRSA is suspected, vancomycin should be administered in addition to cefazolin. Because vancomycin is ineffective against Gram-negative bacteria, and cefazolin is superior to vancomycin in effectiveness against methicillin-susceptible *S. aureus* (MSSA), vancomycin should be administered along with, not instead of cefazolin [28]. Patients with a history of minor penicillin allergy such as a rash can safely receive cephalosporins. Only when there is a history of a serious reaction to penicillin, such as anaphylaxis, should cephalosporins be withheld. Because cephalosporins are considerably more effective against MSSA than the antibiotics which are used as substitutes, cephalosporins should not be withheld because of a minor reaction to penicillin [28].

39.4.2 Patient Decolonization

Patient decolonization serves as an adjuvant to antimicrobial prophylaxis for reducing the risk of SSI. Patient colonization with healthcare-associated pathogens is a significant risk factor for developing SSI and other HAIs. Two different patient decolonization strategies have been explored including universal decolonization (performed on every patient) and targeted decolonization (performed only in patients who test positive for *S. aureus* on a screening test). The benefit of screening surgical patients includes both the ability to identify candidates for decolonization and to optimize antimicrobial prophylaxis by adding vancomycin for those patients colonized with MRSA. However, the screening of surgical patients has been controversial due to the need for significant resources to perform screening and issues with false negative results [31].

The two common strategies for the decolonization of patients who test positive for *S. aureus* are mupirocin

[3] CDC National Institute for Occupational Safety and Health: Health and Safety Practices Survey of Healthcare Workers—Surgical Smoke available at https://www.cdc.gov/niosh/topics/healthcarehsps/smoke.html.

ointment for nasal decolonization and chlorhexidine wash for skin decolonization [32]. Patient decolonization appears to be effective in reducing postoperative infections in patients who are carriers of MSSA or MRSA. However, nasal mupirocin treatment is difficult to administer due to patient non-compliance with multi-day treatment. Another concern with mupirocin treatment is development of *S. aureus* resistance to mupirocin. Alternative decolonization treatment regimens that are easier to administer are needed. Due to these concerns, nasal povidone iodine was identified as an effective alternative for patients undergoing orthopedic procedures [33].

Furthermore, a more individualized approach to perioperative decolonization and antimicrobial prophylaxis are needed. Targeting gram-positive organisms by *S. aureus* screening, nasal decolonization, and cephalosporin-based antibiotic prophylaxis appeared to be inadequate in a study of the organisms causing SSI in spine fusions [34]. The skin of the inferior regions of the back, particularly the sacroiliac region, contained predominantly Gram-negative organisms with a high degree of cefazolin resistance. This indicates that a patient and procedure-specific approach to perioperative decolonization and antimicrobial prophylaxis is needed. The spectrum of antimicrobial prophylactic activity should be matched to the microbiology of the patient's skin flora at the surgical site.

39.4.3 Hand Hygiene

The WHO five moments for hand hygiene is an established recommendation for performing hand hygiene when interacting with patients in healthcare setting. The five moments of hand hygiene guideline recommend performing hand hygiene before touching a patient, before a procedure, after a procedure or body fluid exposure risk, after touching a patient, and after touching a patient's surroundings. Several studies have confirmed low compliance with hand hygiene by anesthesia providers [35–37]. Despite the relative simplicity of the WHO recommendations, compliance is virtually impossible to achieve in the operating room especially during busy times such as induction and emergence, because of the frequency of contacts between the patient, anesthesia providers and the surrounding environment. While hand hygiene in the operating room is often synonymous with alcohol-based gel, it is important to remember that not all pathogens are susceptible to alcohol. Bacterial spores are resistant, as are non-enveloped viruses. Washing hands with soap and water is effective for inactivating or removing a broader spectrum of pathogens than alcohol-based hand gel and should be performed whenever possible.

Anesthesia provider hands have also been associated with intraoperative bacterial transmission and contamination of environmental surfaces in studies by Loftus et al. [38]. The authors provide evidence for within-case contamination and also cross-case contamination associated with anesthesia provider hands indicating particularly poor compliance with hand hygiene by anesthesia providers.

The previously identified barriers to hand hygiene compliance in the operating room included difficult access to a hand sanitizer and lack of reminders to perform hand hygiene. To address these barriers, replacing wall-mounted hand sanitizer with ones on the anesthesia machine resulted in statistically significant but clinically limited improvement in hand hygiene compliance [39]. Similarly, electronic visual reminders every 15 min resulted in modest improvement in hand hygiene compliance [40]. The most effective strategy for improving anesthesia provider hand hygiene compliance was the use of personal wearable hand hygiene devices with audible reminders. When compared to traditional wall-mounted gel dispensers, the use of a personal hand hygiene device with audible reminders significantly increased the frequency of hand hygiene events [41, 42]. The use of the same wearable hand hygiene device also significantly reduced the incidence of ventilator associated pneumonia in the intensive care unit [41]. The Society for Healthcare Epidemiology of America (SHEA) expert guidance on infection prevention in the anesthesia work area recommended consideration of the use of personal hand hygiene devices [43]. The same recommendation was re-emphasized in the context of infection prevention precautions for routine anesthesia care during the SARS-CoV-2 pandemic [44]. Although the wearable hand hygiene device that was previously studied is not commercially available, there are other wearable hand hygiene devices that are commercially available (Fig. 39.3).

Some anesthesia providers are concerned that very frequent hand hygiene with alcohol-based gel can cause skin irritation [45]. A possible solution to this problem is to apply gel directly over exam gloves (see below).

Gloving

The use of non-sterile exam gloves became widespread among anesthesia providers after being adopted as a part of "universal precautions" (also known as "standard precautions") in response to the HIV epidemic. Three different surveys administered to anesthesiologists in New Zealand, United States, and the United Kingdom between 1995 and 2006 indicated that anywhere from 55 to 86% of respondents frequently or always wore gloves [46–48].

Anesthesia providers often wear non-sterile gloves to protect themselves from a patient's body fluids. Standard

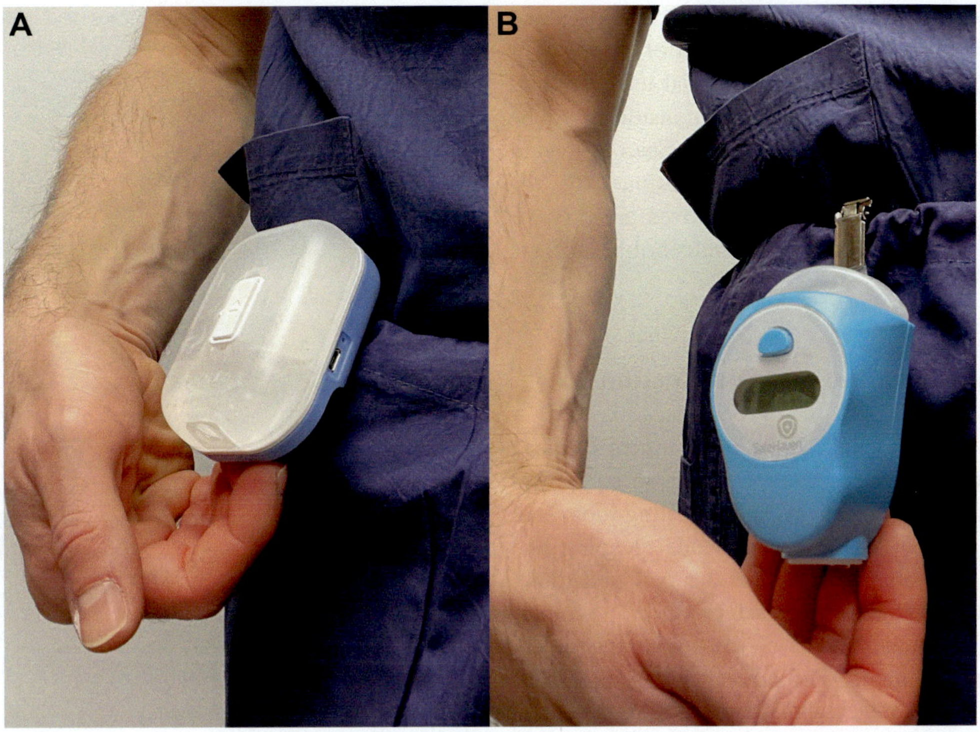

Fig. 39.3 Personal, wearable hand hygiene devices that clip to scrub pants. A. GelAuto (Blink DC, Seattle, WA), B. SafeHaven (Georgia-Pacific Professional, Atlanta, GA)

precautions recommend wearing non-sterile gloves to prevent contact with a patient's body fluids that could contain blood-borne pathogens such as HIV and hepatitis B virus (HBV). Non-sterile gloves serve as a barrier that prevents blood-borne pathogen transmission via skin breaks on the hands. There are reports of healthcare workers becoming infected with HIV after non-needle stick exposures. Although it is difficult to determine the exact mechanism of HIV transmission, these healthcare workers had their ungloved hands exposed to HIV-infected blood.

Whether gloving by healthcare workers protects patients from infection is difficult to know. A meta-analysis examining the effect of "universal gloving" on HAIs reflects this ambiguity [49]. Although the pooled results of meta-analysis showed a significant association between universal gloving and a decrease in HAIs, the association was no longer statistically significant when limiting the analysis to randomized controlled trials. A multicenter study showed that the use of gloves and gowns for all patient contact did not prevent the acquisition of MRSA and VRE when compared to usual care. The risk of infection for the patient may be similar if operating room staff touches the patient after washing their hands with soap and water or alcohol-based gel versus wearing clean non-sterile gloves.

One of the concerns with wearing non-sterile gloves is the risk of environmental contamination if the gloves are used for patient contact and then remain on the providers hands while touching surfaces or handling objects in the anesthesia work area. Soiled gloves should be removed when an episode of patient contact is completed, and hand hygiene performed with alcohol-based gel. Given the frequency of contacts with patients and their bodily fluids, anesthesia providers should be changing gloves frequently.

Double gloving has been suggested as a method for reducing contamination of the anesthesia work area during airway management. The outer gloves are removed and discarded immediately following placement of an endotracheal tube or supraglottic airway, and the presumably cleaner inner gloves are worn until the episode of care is completed. Simulation-based studies of double gloving during intubation showed a reduction in the spread of fluorescent dye from the airway of a manikin to the anesthesia work area [50, 51]. Although the evidence for double gloving is not strong, double gloving has minimal impact on anesthesia provider workflow and has the potential to impact intraoperative pathogen transmission.

Another approach to gloving is to wear gloves continuously during anesthesia care and apply alcohol-based gel to the gloves rather than to bare hands. This approach may be particularly useful for providers who develop skin irritation from frequent hand hygiene. Although concern has been expressed that alcohol-based hand gel might degrade glove material resulting in increased permeability, there is evidence that gloves continue to function as a barrier despite repeated application of gel [52]. Another concern about wearing gloves continuously is the problem of distinguishing clean from dirty gloves. In the traditional use of gloves during standard precautions, gloves are considered to be dirty, while bare hands are considered to be clean following hand hygiene. When gloves are worn continuously, the provider has to remember whether the gloves are dirty or clean following the application of alcohol-based gel (Table 39.3).

39.4.4 Surface Cleaning and Disinfection

The operating room is a challenging environment to clean and disinfect[4] since it contains multiple pieces of equipment and is occupied by multiple patients and operating room staff throughout the day. The CDC recommends cleaning and disinfecting the operating room before the first procedure, between procedures and after the last procedure (i.e., terminal clean).[5] The primary focus of these cleaning procedures are non-critical items. The critical and semi-critical items that come into contact with the patient require specialized disinfection as described in Table 39.4 [53].

The choice of disinfectant is critical when cleaning surfaces and floors and will determine if the most resistant pathogens will be eliminated or not. Some of the most resistant pathogen to disinfectants include *Clostridium difficile* spores, *Mycobacteria*, non-enveloped viruses such as norovirus, and fungi. Only sterilization reliably destroys all pathogens. High-level disinfection will destroy all pathogens except for some bacterial spores, while low-level disinfection is the least effective and will not destroy the most resistant pathogens [53]. Most hospitals prefer to clean high-touch surfaces with low-level disinfectant such as hypochlorite, quaternary ammonium compounds, and hydrogen peroxide based products. Sporicidal products which allow for high-level disinfection were rarely used unless patients were under contact precautions. Standard bleach is typically avoided as a sporicidal agent since it is corrosive, irritant, and leaves visible residue when dry. However, a commercial bleach spray formula was shown to be an effective sporicidal agent without the unwanted effects. Based on the evidence from the outside of the operating room, high-touch surfaces and floors in the operating room would benefit from addition of sporicidal agents to low-level disinfection to ensure effective cleaning and reduced transmission of most pathogens (Table 39.5).

Table 39.3 Recommended adult doses and redosing intervals for commonly used antimicrobials for surgical prophylaxis

Antimicrobial	Adult dose	Redosing interval (h)
Ampicillin-sulbactam	3 g (ampicillin 2 g/sulbactam 1 g)	2
Ampicillin	2 g	2
Aztreonam	2 g	4
Cefazolin	2, 3 g for pts weighing ≥ 120 kg	4
Cefuroxime	1.5 g	4
Cefotaxime	1 g	3
Cefoxitin	2 g	2
Cefotetan	2 g	6
Ceftriaxone	2 g	NA
Ciprofloxacin	400 mg	NA
Clindamycin	900 mg	6
Ertapenem	1 g	NA
Fluconazole	400 mg	NA
Gentamicin	5 mg/kg	NA
Levofloxacin	500 mg	NA
Metronidazole	500 mg	NA
Moxifloxacin	400 mg	NA
Piperacillin-tazobactam	3.375 g	2
Vancomycin	15 mg/kg	NA
Erythromycin base	1 g	NA
Metronidazole	1 g	NA
Neomycin	1 g	NA

Adapted from Bratzler DW, Dellinger EP, Olsen KM, Perl TM, Auwaerter PG, Bolon MK, Fish DN, Napolitano LM, Sawyer RG, Slain D, Steinberg JP, Weinstein RA; American Society of Health-System Pharmacists (ASHP); Infectious Diseases Society of America (IDSA); Surgical Infection Society (SIS); Society for Healthcare Epidemiology of America (SHEA). Clinical practice guidelines for antimicrobial prophylaxis in surgery. Surg Infect (Larchmt). 2013 Feb;14(1):73–156

The current cleaning and disinfecting practices in the hospital setting have not properly addressed the contamination of environmental surfaces [54]. The relationship between environmental contamination and HAI is not well understood. Microbiological surveys of the hospital environment with comparison of pathogens found in the environment with those isolated from patients are not routinely performed. Methods frequently used for surveillance of environmental contamination such as fluorescent markers and adenosine triphosphate bioluminescence assays are crude techniques that lack specific information about the type and quantity of pathogens.

[4] Cleaning refers to removal of dirt and organic matter from surfaces using soap or detergents. Disinfection refers to killing viruses and bacteria on surfaces using chemicals.

[5] CDC Best Practices for Environmental Cleaning in Healthcare Facilities available at https://www.cdc.gov/hai/prevent/resource-limited/cleaning-procedures.html.

Table 39.4 Decontamination methods of patient care items and environmental surfaces

Process	Level of pathogen inactivation	Method	Healthcare application
Sterilization[d]	Eliminates all pathogens including bacterial spores	High temperature Low temperature Liquid immersion	Heat-tolerant and heat-sensitive critical[a] and semicritical[b] items
High-level disinfection	Eliminates all pathogens except some bacterial spores	Heat-automated pasteurization Liquid immersion	Heat-sensitive semi-critical items
Low-level disinfection	Eliminates some pathogens but not mycobacteria or spores	Liquid contact	Non-critical[c] items or surfaces with no visible blood

[a]Critical patient care items are objects that enter sterile tissue or the vascular system and include surgical instruments, cardiac and urinary catheters, and implants

[b]Semi-critical patient care items are objects that come in contact with intact mucous membranes and non-intact skin and include respiratory therapy equipment, endoscopes, bronchoscopes, laryngoscope blades and handles, etc.

[c]Non-critical patient care items are objects that come in contact with intact skin but not mucous membranes and include monitoring equipment (blood pressure cuffs, pulse oximeters), bedpans, infusion pumps, etc.

[d]Prions are resistant to conventional chemical and physical decontamination methods and are not readily inactivated by conventional sterilization procedures

Adapted from Rutala WA, Weber DJ. Disinfection, sterilization, and antisepsis: An overview. Am J Infect Control. 2019 Jun;47S:A3–A9

Anesthesia Machines

Anesthesia machines are difficult to clean given the complexity of surfaces, the presence of drawers and numerous items inside the drawers. Enhanced cleaning of anesthesia machines between and during procedures as part of an infection prevention bundle significantly reduced postoperative HAIs [55]. Anesthesia machines and monitors were wiped with a cloth soaked in quaternary ammonium compound before each procedure, after induction of anesthesia and after each procedure. Instead of enhanced cleaning, others have proposed redesigning the anesthesia machine altogether to improve the cleaning and disinfection. Although a simulation-based study did not find a significant difference in the number of cleaned sites between conventional and redesigned anesthesia machines [56], design improvements of anesthesia machines and other pieces of operating room equipment could facilitate more effective cleaning.

Another approach to reducing equipment contamination is the use of disposable plastic covers specifically designed for anesthesia machines, monitors, keyboards, and other equipment that are difficult to clean. Intraoperative use of an anesthesia machine covers significantly decreased the bacterial contamination on the anesthesia machine [57]. The use of anesthesia machine covers and enhanced cleaning and disinfection between cases and at the end of the day with particular focus on "high-touch" surfaces has been recommended in several publications [43, 44, 58].

Anesthesia Carts

The traditional anesthesia cart may be the most challenging piece of operating room equipment from the standpoint of infection prevention, since it has multiple drawers containing supplies and equipment intended to serve multiple patients. Anesthesia providers are repeatedly accessing anesthesia cart drawers, often with contaminated hands or gloves. The contamination level of the anesthesia cart has not been studied, and its role in pathogen transmission is not well understood. Proper cleaning and disinfection of the inside of the anesthesia cart would require enormous resources and time, even if it was performed only at the end of the day, similar to terminal cleaning. A better strategy would be to prevent contamination of the anesthesia cart in the first place, with anesthesia providers performing hand hygiene prior to accessing the drawers. This approach was studied as part of an anesthesia work area CLABSI prevention bundle intended to reduce infection rates of central venous catheters placed in the intensive care unit which were then used for intravenous access during anesthesia [59]. The CLABSI prevention bundle consisted of a standardized intravenous line starting kit, a drug administration manifold attached to an intravenous pole, hand sanitizer on the anesthesia cart, anesthesia work area divided into "dirty" and "clean" areas, with the anesthesia cart included in the "clean" area, and a room turnover cleaning checklist. The rate of CLABSI was reduced, but implementation and compliance with this practice was challenging.

A more transformative approach might be to replace the traditional anesthesia cart with a single patient anesthesia case pack, similar to the surgical case packs. These packs would contain commonly used anesthesia supplies needed for a single case, unlike the anesthesia cart that contains supplies for multiple patients.

Laryngoscopes

Reusable laryngoscopes are semi-critical devices that require high-level disinfection. Laryngoscope blades can

Table 39.5 Recommended infection prevention precautions for anesthesia providers

Suggested practice	Comments
Provider	
Adhere to the WHO five moments of hand hygiene	Alcohol-based hand gel source needs to be close to provider or personal, wearable hand gel devices should be used. Frequent hand hygiene is essential for personal protection and protects patients from HAIs
Perform hand hygiene first before accessing anesthesia cart drawers	Contents of anesthesia cart are easily contaminated and difficult to clean
Wear eye protection at all times during anesthesia care	Required by United States department of labor, occupational safety and health administration standard 1910.1030
Consider wearing respirator during anesthetic care	Given the risk of airborne pathogens especially when increased infectious risk during epidemics and pandemics, consider wearing N-95 or FFP-2 filtering facepiece respirator
Wear double gloves for airway management	Discard the outer glove immediately following airway management to limit surface contamination
Surfaces	
Wipe anesthesia machine and cart "high-touch" areas with hospital-designated disinfection wipes during procedure (if not covered with plastic covers)	"High-touch" areas of anesthesia machine have been shown to be frequently contaminated
Single-use plastic covers for parts or all of anesthesia machine, computers, keyboards, and monitors	Covers can reduce bioburden on contaminated, difficult to clean surfaces
Administer drugs only through closed injection ports which have been decontaminated with alcohol-based wipe, scrub, or cap	Conventional open lumen stopcocks are difficult to disinfect and have been shown to be frequently contaminated
Wipe cell phones and other personal communications devices with disinfection wipes compatible with electronic devices	Cell phones have been shown to be contaminated with antibiotic resistant pathogens during use in the hospital
Use high-level disinfection or sterilization for reusable standard and video laryngoscopes	Recommended by CDC. Consider single-use standard and video laryngoscopes if available and cost-effective. Be aware that some video laryngoscopes cannot undergo high-level disinfection or sterilization
Air	
Place HEPA filter on exhalation side of anesthesia circuit (at least) and/or between the airway and the Y of the circuit (to filter gas in both directions)	HEPA filter effectively filters small particles including viruses
Manage endotracheal tubes to minimize aerosolization following placement	Place HEPA filter on open lumen of double lumen tube during single lung ventilation
Consider surgical smoke evacuation	Risk of infection of providers by surgical smoke is unknown, but surgical smoke evacuation was a recommended practice prior to the COVID-19 pandemic
Consider discussing respiratory infection prevention measures during the "time out" (surgical safety checklist)	The risk of airborne pathogen transmission should be discussed with operating room staff and appropriate precautions should be taken if the risk is elevated. Surgical team should consider whether to vacate the operating room during airway management

WHO—World Health Organization, HAI—Healthcare-associated infection
Adapted from Bowdle A, Jelacic S, Shishido S, Munoz-Price LS. Infection Prevention Precautions for Routine Anesthesia Care During the SARS-CoV-2 Pandemic. Anesth Analg 2020; 131: 1342–1354

easily undergo high-level disinfection, but laryngoscope handles typically require disassembly and removal of electrical components prior to high-level disinfection or sterilization. Contaminated laryngoscopes have been associated with infectious outbreaks due to inadequate cleaning and disinfection [60]. Despite the available evidence of infectious risks associated with low-level disinfection, conventional laryngoscope and videolaryngoscope handles often do not undergo proper high-level disinfection or sterilization. Furthermore, some videolaryngoscope handles cannot undergo high-level disinfection or sterilization per the manufacturer's recommendations [44]. Videolaryngoscopes have been recommended by some authors in preference to standard laryngoscopes in the airway management for patients infected with SARS-CoV-2, raising further concerns about proper disinfection. Single-use conventional laryngoscopes and videolaryngoscopes may be cost-effective alternatives to high-level disinfection of reusable equipment [43].

Injection Ports

Contaminated intravenous line injection ports are associated with intraoperative bacterial transmission and patient mortality [7, 8]. One of the strategies to reduce injection port contamination is improved hand hygiene [61]. Another strategy is the use of closed injection ports, the surface of which can be decontaminated with relative ease. By contrast, conventional open lumen stopcocks that are often used in anesthesia practice are difficult or impossible to disinfect with either alcohol wipes or alcohol-based scrub.

Stopcocks with closed injection ports covered with alcohol-containing caps as part of the catheter care bundle were associated with significant reduction in stopcock lumen contamination, 30-day postoperative infections, and phlebitis when compared to stopcocks with standard caps [62]. The use of alcohol-containing caps that remain on injection ports at all times instead of alcohol-based wipes or scrubs are the preferred option in the anesthesia setting because of the need to immediately inject drugs during anesthesia care. Anesthesia providers usually do not have time to wipe or scrub the surface of closed injection ports prior to each use. Based on the available evidence, the use of closed injection ports and disinfection of the port surface prior to drug administration was recommended by the SHEA expert guidance for both central and peripheral venous catheters [43]. Open stopcocks should not be used by anesthesia providers to inject drugs. Drugs should only be injected into closed ports with the injection surface covered by an alcohol-containing cap at all times, or scrubbed with alcohol before each use (Fig. 39.4).

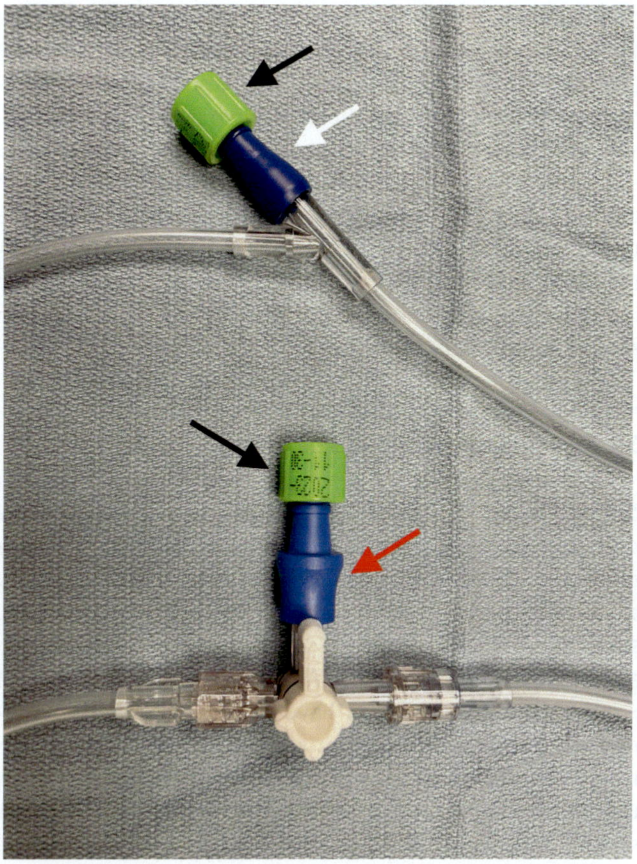

Fig. 39.4 Three-way stopcock with a closed injection port (red arrow) and alcohol-containing cap (black arrow) and an in-line closed injection port (white arrow) with alcohol-containing cap (black arrow)

39.4.5 Intravascular Catheters

Central venous catheters are a well-recognized source of bloodstream infection and, therefore, are managed with a standardized set of infection prevention measures.[6] Although arterial and peripheral venous catheters have not received as much attention, they may also be important sources of bloodstream infection.

Peripheral intravenous catheters are routinely used in perioperative care. Most anesthesia providers consider peripheral intravenous catheters as having relatively low risk of causing bloodstream infections. However, the potential of peripheral intravenous catheters for producing bloodstream infections may be underestimated. A systematic review suggested that peripheral venous catheters accounted for 23% of catheter-related bloodstream infections [63]. A single institution implemented a bundle of practice changes to reduce the incidence of peripheral intravenous catheter-related bloodstream infections in 2003 and observed a substantial decrease in peripheral venous catheter-related bloodstream infections during the next 13 years [64]. One of the practice changes implemented was the use of sterile gloves for peripheral intravenous catheter placement instead of non-sterile exam gloves.

A systematic review and meta-analysis of bloodstream infections related to arterial catheters suggested that infection rates were similar to central venous catheters [65]. Published guidelines recommend using a placement bundle for arterial catheters similar to that for central venous catheters, including sterile gloves and a sterile drape.[7]

[6] CDC Checklist for CLABSI prevention available at https://www.cdc.gov/hai/pdfs/bsi/checklist-for-CLABSI.pdf.

[7] CDC Guidelines for the Prevention of Intravascular Catheter-Related Infections (2011): Summary of Recommendations available at https://www.cdc.gov/infectioncontrol/guidelines/bsi/recommendations.html.

It is likely that all intravascular catheters have a similar potential for producing bloodstream infection and should be placed using aseptic technique after careful skin decontamination. The femoral site should be avoided whenever possible because of higher infection rates compared to other sites. Anesthesia providers should clean skin with chlorhexidine and consider using sterile gloves for the placement of peripheral intravenous catheters. All catheters should be inspected during the perioperative period and the ones that are no longer needed or show any sign of infection should be promptly removed.

39.4.6 Respiratory Precautions

Surgical masks as part of standard precautions are worn by operating room staff primarily for splash protection and to reduce contamination of the surgical field from respiratory droplets (especially from coughs and sneezes). However, surgical masks do not provide adequate protection from airborne pathogens because they do not form a tight seal around the face and do not have efficient filtering, in comparison with respirators (such as N-95 and similar filtering facepiece respirators). Given the growing concern about transmission of respiratory pathogens, operating room staff should consider adopting routine respiratory precautions in addition to standard precautions [44]. Operating room staff may be at increased risk for infection by airborne pathogens since they frequently perform or are in close proximity to aerosol-generating procedures, are exposed to aerosols produced by the surgical procedure including smoke, and are working in close contact with multiple providers for prolonged periods of time. The American Society of Anesthesiologists, the American Association of Nurse Anesthetists, the Anesthesia Patient Safety Foundation, the American College of Surgeons, and the Academy of Otolaryngology-Head and Neck Surgery have recommended that operating room staff routinely wear filtering facepiece respirators (such as N-95 respirators) at least during periods when community prevalence of transmissible respiratory pathogens is high (such as the SARS-CoV-2).

The centerpiece of respiratory precautions is the filtering facepiece respirator (e.g., N-95). However, the current design of filtering facepiece respirators has significant limitations, including frequently poor fit, resistance to breathing, discomfort, single-use, and limited filtering efficacy (typically around 95%). There is a need for innovative, improved design of both disposable and reusable respirators (such as elastomeric and powered air-purifying respirators, PAPRs) [66]. An adhesive respirator shown in Fig. 39.5 is just one example of an innovative design to improve respirator fit and comfort.

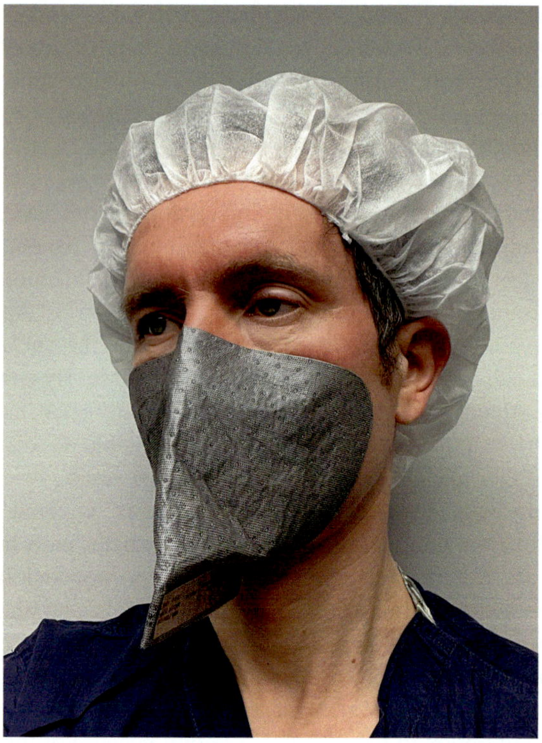

Fig. 39.5 Strapless N-95 respirator attached to the face with adhesive to improve user fit of the author (SJ) who failed fit test with conventional N-95 respirator (Avery Dennison, Glendale, CA)

Another component of respiratory precautions is the routine use of surgical smoke evacuators. The Occupational Safety and Health Administration (OSHA) does not specifically mandate the use of surgical smoke evacuators, but both the National Institute of Occupational Safety and Health (NIOSH) and the Association of periOperative Registered Nurses (AORN) have recommended their use.[8] A review concerning surgical smoke also strongly recommended the use of filtering facepiece respirators (such as N-95) in addition to smoke evacuation systems (Fig. 39.6) [22].

Operating room airflow follows complex patterns, with implications for infection prevention that are poorly understood. Hospital rooms that are occupied by patients with airborne respiratory infections may have negative pressure airflow which is intended to prevent contaminated air from entering adjacent hallways and rooms. Operating rooms have positive airflow; air which is not evacuated from the room through return ducts may be forced into adjacent hallways and rooms. This is of particular concern when

[8] Occupational Safety and Health Administration recommendations can be found at https://www.osha.gov/laser-electrosurgery-plume. National Institute of Occupational Safety and Health recommendations can be found at https://www.cdc.gov/niosh/topics/healthcarehsps/smoke.html. Association of periOperative Registered Nurses recommendations are limited to members only.

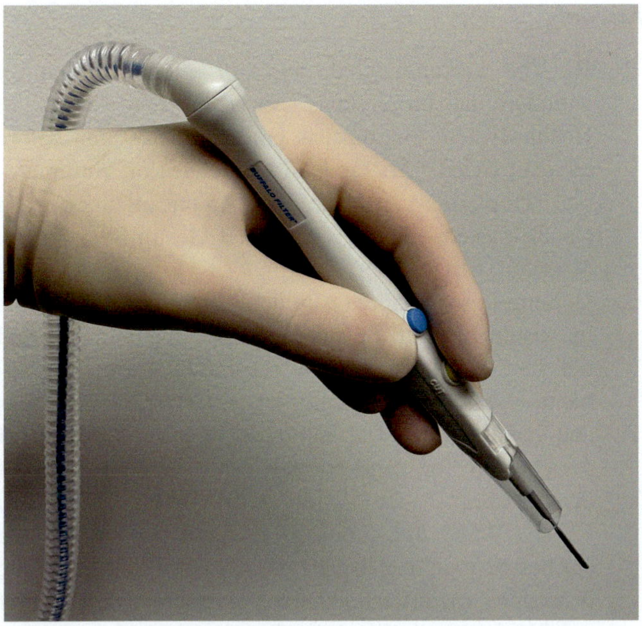

Fig. 39.6 Example of surgical smoke evacuator (PlumePen Pro, Buffalo Filter, Lancaster, NY)

patients are infected with airborne pathogens. A possible approach to this problem is the use of portable HEPA air purification units in operating rooms for use during intubation and extubation. This recommendation was initially part of the CDC guidelines but was removed from the updated guidelines in 2005 [67].

The use of negative pressure instead of positive pressure operating rooms for patients with airborne respiratory diseases has been proposed as a solution for minimizing the spread of airborne pathogens outside of operating room and into surrounding areas. Some hospitals during the SARS and MERS outbreaks converted operating rooms into negative pressure rooms to facilitate procedures in patients with SARS and MERS infections and in anticipation of future respiratory disease outbreaks. Whether the use of negative pressure operating rooms would increase the risk of surgical wound infection is unknown.

39.4.7 Vaccinations

Perioperative vaccination recommendations for pediatric patients recommend vaccination with an inactive vaccine at least 1 week before an elective procedure and with live attenuated vaccine at least 3 weeks before a procedure [68]. The German equivalent of CDC (Robert Koch Institute) recommends even shorter waiting times; 3 days for inactive vaccine and 14 days for live attenuated vaccine. The Society of Thoracic Surgeons Workforce on Critical Care has issued a guideline recommending coronavirus disease vaccine for all elective cardiothoracic surgery patients [69].

Intraoperative Bacterial Transmission and Mortality

The association between operating room environmental contamination, postoperative HAIs, and mortality is difficult to establish but has been previously reported. Although one of the few single-center studies evaluating this association found that contaminated stopcocks were not associated with HAIs, the contaminated stopcocks were associated with higher mortality [7]. The association between contaminated stopcocks and mortality was also observed in a multicenter study [8]. Furthermore, interventions such as the use of a wearable hand hygiene device significantly decreased the incidence of HAIs [61]. The same wearable hand hygiene device was shown to significantly reduce ventilator associated pneumonia in the intensive care unit [41]. Finally, an infection prevention bundle including improvements in perioperative hand hygiene, vascular care, environmental cleaning, and patient decolonization efforts significantly reduced HAIs [55].

39.5 Questions and Answers

Questions (Choose the Most Appropriate Answer)

1. What is the recommended time of administration of antimicrobial prophylaxis per American Society of Health-System Pharmacists guideline?
   A. 30 min before incision
   B. 60 min before incision
   C. 120 min before incision
   D. At the time of anesthesia induction
2. What is the minimum appropriate level of disinfection for semi-critical items?
   A. Low-level disinfection
   B. Sterilization
   C. High-level disinfection
   D. Cleaning
3. The WHO five moments of hand hygiene include performing hand hygiene
   A. Before touching another healthcare worker
   B. Before entering patient room
   C. Before and after touching the patient
   D. Before medication preparation
4. Standard antibiotic prophylaxis in surgical patients with a history of rash from penicillin is
   A. Vancomycin instead of cefazolin
   B. Levofloxacin instead of cefazolin
   C. Vancomycin and cefazolin
   D. Cefazolin

5. For coverage of methicillin-susceptible staph, the best prophylactic antibiotic coverage would be
   A. Vancomycin
   B. Cefazolin
   C. Levofloxacin
   D. Sulbactam
6. The most important function of surgical masks worn in the hospital is
   A. Protecting health care workers from splashes with potentially infectious body fluids
   B. Protecting health care workers from airborne respiratory viruses
   C. Protecting patients from airborne respiratory viruses
   D. Capturing droplets produced by sneezing or coughing
7. Filtering facepiece respirators such as N-95
   A. Are interchangeable with surgical masks for protection from airborne particles
   B. Provide better source protection (protect others from particles exhaled by the wearer) than PAPRs
   C. Do not require fit testing
   D. Do not allow any small particles to pass through the filtering material
8. SARS-CoV-2
   A. Is spread primarily by contact
   B. Is spread primarily by droplets
   C. Is spread primarily by airborne particles
   D. Transmission can be reliably prevented by wearing surgical masks
9. Laryngoscopes
   A. Are semi-critical devices that require high-level disinfection prior to reuse
   B. Are semi-critical devices that can be wiped off with hospital germicidal wipes prior to reuse
   C. Are non-critical devices that can be wiped off with hospital germicidal wipes prior to reuse
   D. Are critical devices that require sterilization prior to reuse

10. Safe handling of IV injection ports includes
    A. Gel hands prior to handling, use only closed ports and cover the closed port with an isopropyl alcohol cap between uses
    B. Gel hands prior to handling and use stopcocks with open ports
    C. Gel hands prior to handling, use only stopcocks with open ports, and scrub the stopcock with alcohol prior to each use
    D. Use only stopcocks with open ports, keep the IV tubing off the floor, and If the stopcock touches the floor, scrub it with alcohol prior to use

Answers

1. **B.** The recommended time of administration of antimicrobial prophylaxis per American Society of Health-System Pharmacists guideline is 60 min before incision (ASHP Therapeutic Guidelines on Antimicrobial Prophylaxis in Surgery. American Society of Health-System Pharmacists. Am J Health Syst Pharm. 1999;56(18):1839–1888).
2. **C.** Semi-critical patient care items are objects that come in contact with intact mucous membranes and non-intact skin and include respiratory therapy equipment, endoscopes, bronchoscopes, laryngoscope blades and handles, etc. The minimum appropriate level of disinfection for semi-critical items is high level of disinfection.
3. **C.** The WHO five moments of hand hygiene include (1) before touching a patients, (2) before clean/aseptic procedure, (3) after body fluid exposure risk, (4) after touching a patient, and (5) after touching patient surroundings.
4. **D.** Patients with a history of minor penicillin allergy such as a rash, can safely receive cephalosporins. Only when there is a history of a serious reaction to penicillin, such as anaphylaxis, should cephalosporins be withheld. Because cephalosporins are considerably more effective against methicillin susceptible S. aureus than the antibiotics which are used as substitutes, cephalosporins should not be withheld because of a minor reaction to penicillin.
5. **B.** Cephalosporins such as cefazolin are considerably more effective against methicillin susceptible S. aureus than the antibiotics which are used as substitutes.
6. **A.** The most important function of surgical masks worn in the hospital is protecting healthcare workers from splashes with potentially infectious body fluids. Surgical masks are not tight fitting and do not have filtering material to protect healthcare workers and patients from airborne respiratory viruses. For the same reasons, surgical masks do not capture droplets produced by sneezing or coughing.
7. **B.** Filtering facepiece respirators such as N-95 provide better source protection (protect others from particles exhaled by the wearer) than PAPRs since PAPRs are not tight fitting and release exhaled air out into the environment due to positive pressure. Filtering facepiece respirators are not interchangeable with surgical masks since respirators do provide protection from airborne particle while surgical masks do not. Respirators such as N-95 require fit testing and do not filter all small particles due to their 95% filtering efficiency; 5% of small particles will not be filtered.

8. **C.** Although early during the COVID-19 pandemic, SARS-CoV-2 was thought to be spread by droplets, the growing evidence for spread primarily by airborne particles supported the airborne route of transmission. Surgical masks are inadequate for respiratory protection due to lack of tight fit and proper filtering material.
9. **A.** Laryngoscopes are semi-critical devices since they come in contact with patient mucosa and therefore, require high-level disinfection prior to reuse.

10. **A.** Safe handling of IV injection ports includes gelling hands prior to handling, use of only closed ports and covering the closed port with an isopropyl alcohol cap between uses as recommended by the SHEA expert guidance.

Appendix

Wound classification criteria used by the CDC National Healthcare Safety Network (NHSN) and Healthcare Infection Control Practices Advisory Committee (HICPAC)*

Clean Procedure—An uninfected operative wound in which no inflammation is encountered and the respiratory, alimentary, genital, or uninfected urinary tracts are not entered. In addition, clean wounds are primarily closed and, if necessary, drained with closed drainage. Operative incisional wounds that follow non-penetrating (blunt) trauma should be included in this category if they meet the criteria.

Clean-Contaminated Procedure—Operative wounds in which the respiratory, alimentary, genital, or urinary tracts are entered under controlled conditions and without unusual contamination. Specifically, operations involving the biliary tract, appendix, vagina, and oropharynx are included in this category, provided no evidence of infection or major break in technique is encountered.

Contaminated Procedure—Open, fresh, accidental wounds. In addition, operations with major breaks in sterile technique (e.g., open cardiac massage) or gross spillage from the gastrointestinal tract and incisions in which acute, non-purulent inflammation is encountered are included in this category.

Dirty or Infected Procedure—Includes old traumatic wounds with retained devitalized tissue and those that involve existing clinical infection or perforated viscera. This definition suggests that the organisms causing postoperative infection were present in the operative field before the operation.

*Adapted from Bratzler DW, Dellinger EP, Olsen KM, Perl TM, Auwaerter PG, Bolon MK, Fish DN, Napolitano LM, Sawyer RG, Slain D, Steinberg JP, Weinstein RA; American Society of Health-System Pharmacists (ASHP); Infectious Diseases Society of America (IDSA); Surgical Infection Society (SIS); Society for Healthcare Epidemiology of America (SHEA). Clinical practice guidelines for antimicrobial prophylaxis in surgery. Surg Infect (Larchmt). 2013 Feb;14(1):73–156.

References

1. Watkins RR, Gowen R, Lionakis MS, et al. Update on the pathogenesis, virulence, and treatment of *C. auris*. Pathog Immun. 2022;7(2):46–65.
2. Kumar J, Eilertson B, Cadnum JL, et al. Environmental contamination with Candida species in multiple hospitals including a tertiary care hospital with a *C. auris* Outbreak. Pathog Immun. 2019;4(2):260–70.
3. Loftus RW, Koff MD, Brown JR, et al. The epidemiology of *S. aureus* transmission in the anesthesia work area. Anesth Analg. 2015;120(4):807–18.
4. Loftus RW, Koff MD, Brown JR, et al. The dynamics of Enterococcus transmission from bacterial reservoirs commonly encountered by anesthesia providers. Anesth Analg. 2015;120(4):827–36.
5. Loftus RW, Brown JR, Patel HM, et al. Transmission dynamics of gram-negative bacterial pathogens in the anesthesia work area. Anesth Analg. 2015;120(4):819–26.
6. Munoz-Price LS, Weinstein RA. Fecal patina in the anesthesia work area. Anesth Analg. 2015;120(4):703–5.
7. Loftus RW, Koff MD, Burchman CC, et al. Transmission of pathogenic bacterial organisms in the anesthesia work area. Anesthesiology. 2008;109(3):399–407.
8. Loftus RW, Brown JR, Koff MD, et al. Multiple reservoirs contribute to intraoperative bacterial transmission. Anesth Analg. 2012;114(6):1236–48.
9. Kluytmans JA, Mouton JW, Ijzerman EP, et al. Nasal carriage of *S. aureus* as a major risk factor for wound infections after cardiac surgery. J Infect Dis. 1995;171(1):216–9.
10. von Eiff C, Becker K, Machka K, et al. Nasal carriage as a source of *S. aureus* bacteremia: study group. N Engl J Med. 2001;344(1):11–6.
11. Wertheim HF, Vos MC, Ott A, et al. Risk and outcome of nosocomial *S. aureus* bacteraemia in nasal carriers versus non-carriers. Lancet. 2004;364(9435):703–5.
12. Sherertz RJ, Bassetti S, Bassetti-Wyss B. "Cloud" health-care workers. Emerg Infect Dis. 2001;7(2):241–4.
13. Deshpande A, Cadnum JL, Fertelli D, et al. Are hospital floors an underappreciated reservoir for transmission of health care-associated pathogens. Am J Infect Control. 2017;45(3):336–8.
14. Donskey CJ. Beyond high-touch surfaces: portable equipment and floors as potential sources of transmission of health care-associated pathogens. Am J Infect Control. 2019;12:47SA90–5.
15. Koganti S, Alhmidi H, Tomas ME, et al. Evaluation of hospital floors as a potential source of pathogen dissemination using a nonpathogenic virus as a surrogate marker. Infect Control Hosp Epidemiol. 2016;37(11):1374–7.
16. Han Z, Pappas E, Simmons A, et al. Environmental cleaning and disinfection of hospital rooms: a nationwide survey. Am J Infect Control. 2021;49(1):34–9.

17. Hambraeus A, Malmborg AS. The influence of different footwear on floor contamination. Scand J Infect Dis. 1979;11(3):243–6.
18. Munoz-Price LS, Birnbach DJ, Lubarsky DA, et al. Decreasing operating room environmental pathogen contamination through improved cleaning practice. Infect Control Hosp Epidemiol. 2012;33(9):897–904.
19. Lidwell OM, Lowbury EJ, Whyte W, et al. Effect of ultraclean air in operating rooms on deep sepsis in the joint after total hip or knee replacement: a randomised study. Br Med J. 1982;285(6334):10–4.
20. Chow TT, Kwan A, Lin Z, et al. Conversion of operating theatre from positive to negative pressure environment. J Hosp Infect. 2006;64(4):371–8.
21. Park J, Yoo SY, Ko JH, et al. Infection prevention measures for surgical procedures during a middle east respiratory syndrome outbreak in a tertiary care hospital in South Korea. Sci Rep. 2020;10(1):325.
22. Bree K, Barnhill S, Rundell W. The dangers of electrosurgical smoke to operating room personnel: a review. Workplace Health Saf. 2017;65(11):517–26.
23. El-Boghdadly K, Wong DJN, Owen R, et al. Risks to healthcare workers following tracheal intubation of patients with COVID-19: a prospective international multicentre cohort study. Anaesthesia. 2020;75(11):1437–47.
24. Judson SD, Munster VJ. Nosocomial transmission of emerging viruses via aerosol-generating medical procedures. Viruses. 2019;11(10):940.
25. Tran K, Cimon K, Severn M, et al. Aerosol generating procedures and risk of transmission of acute respiratory infections to healthcare workers: a systematic review. PLoS ONE. 2012;7(4): e35797.
26. Nestor CC, Wang S, Irwin MG. Are tracheal intubation and extubation aerosol-generating procedures. Anaesthesia. 2021;76 (2):151–5.
27. Berríos-Torres SI, Umscheid CA, Bratzler DW, et al. Centers for disease control and prevention guideline for the prevention of surgical site infection. JAMA Surg. 2017;152(8):784–91.
28. Long DR, Alverdy JC, Vavilala MS. Emerging paradigms in the prevention of surgical site infection: the patient microbiome and antimicrobial resistance. Anesthesiology. 2022;137(2):252–62.
29. Loftus RW, Koff MD, Birnbach DJ. The dynamics and implications of bacterial transmission events arising from the anesthesia work area. Anesth Analg. 2015;120(4):853–60.
30. Bratzler DW, Dellinger EP, Olsen KM, et al. Clinical practice guidelines for antimicrobial prophylaxis in surgery. Surg Infect. 2013;14(1):73–156.
31. Franklin S. A safer, less costly SSI prevention protocol-Universal versus targeted preoperative decolonization. Am J Infect Control. 2020;48(12):1501–3.
32. Septimus EJ, Schweizer ML. Decolonization in Prevention of health care-associated infections. Clin Microbiol Rev. 2016;29 (2):201–22.
33. Phillips M, Rosenberg A, Shopsin B, et al. Preventing surgical site infections: a randomized, open-label trial of nasal mupirocin ointment and nasal povidone-iodine solution. Infect Control Hosp Epidemiol. 2014;35(7):826–32.
34. Long DR, Bryson-Cahn C, Pergamit R, et al. 2021 Young investigator award winner: anatomic gradients in the microbiology of spinal fusion surgical site infection and resistance to surgical antimicrobial prophylaxis. Spine. 2021;46(3):143–51.
35. Biddle C, Shah J. Quantification of anesthesia providers' hand hygiene in a busy metropolitan operating room: what would Semmelweis think. Am J Infect Control. 2012;40(8):756–9.
36. Krediet AC, Kalkman CJ, Bonten MJ, et al. Hand-hygiene practices in the operating theatre: an observational study. Br J Anaesth. 2011;107(4):553–8.
37. Munoz-Price LS, Riley B, Banks S, et al. Frequency of interactions and hand disinfections among anesthesiologists while providing anesthesia care in the operating room: induction versus maintenance. Infect Control Hosp Epidemiol. 2014;35(8):1056–9.
38. Loftus RW, Muffly MK, Brown JR, et al. Hand contamination of anesthesia providers is an important risk factor for intraoperative bacterial transmission. Anesth Analg. 2011;112(1):98–105.
39. Munoz-Price LS, Patel Z, Banks S, et al. Randomized crossover study evaluating the effect of a hand sanitizer dispenser on the frequency of hand hygiene among anesthesiology staff in the operating room. Infect Control Hosp Epidemiol. 2014;35(6):717–20.
40. Rodriguez-Aldrete D, Sivanesan E, Banks S, et al. Recurrent visual electronic hand hygiene reminders in the anesthesia work area. Infect Control Hosp Epidemiol. 2016;37(7):872–4.
41. Koff MD, Corwin HL, Beach ML, et al. Reduction in ventilator associated pneumonia in a mixed intensive care unit after initiation of a novel hand hygiene program. J Crit Care. 2011;26(5):489–95.
42. Koff MD, Brown JR, Marshall EJ, et al. Frequency of hand decontamination of intraoperative providers and reduction of postoperative healthcare-associated infections: a randomized clinical trial of a novel hand hygiene system. Infect Control Hosp Epidemiol. 2016;37(8):888–95.
43. Munoz-Price LS, Bowdle A, Johnston BL, et al. Infection prevention in the operating room anesthesia work area. Infect Control Hosp Epidemiol. 2019;40(1):1–17.
44. Bowdle A, Jelacic S, Shishido S, et al. Infection Prevention Precautions for Routine Anesthesia Care During the SARS-CoV-2 Pandemic. Anesth Analg. 2020;131(5):1342–54.
45. Birnbach DJ, McKenty NT, Rosen LF, et al. Does adherence to world health organization hand hygiene protocols in the operating room have the potential to produce irritant contact dermatitis in anesthesia providers. Anesth Analg. 2019;129(6):e182–4.
46. El Mikatti N, Dillon P, Healy TEJ. Hygienic practices of consultant anaesthetists: a survey in the North-West region of the UK. Anaesthesia. 1999;54(1):13–8.
47. Ryan AJ, Webster CS, Merry AF, et al. A national survey of infection control practice by New Zealand anaesthetists. Anaesth Intensive Care. 2006;34(1):68–74.
48. Tait AR, Tuttle DB. Preventing perioperative transmission of infection: a survey of anesthesiology practice. Anesth Analg. 1995;80(4):764–9.
49. Chang NN, Kates AE, Ward MA, et al. Association between universal gloving and healthcare-associated infections: a systematic literature review and meta-analysis. Infect Control Hosp Epidemiol. 2019;40(7):755–60.
50. Birnbach DJ, Rosen LF, Fitzpatrick M, et al. A new approach to pathogen containment in the operating room: sheathing the laryngoscope after intubation. Anesth Analg. 2015;121(5):1209–14.
51. Birnbach DJ, Rosen LF, Fitzpatrick M, et al. Double gloves: a randomized trial to evaluate a simple strategy to reduce contamination in the operating room. Anesth Analg. 2015;120(4):848–52.
52. Birnbach DJ, Thiesen TC, McKenty NT, et al. Targeted use of alcohol-based hand rub on gloves during task dense periods: one step closer to pathogen containment by anesthesia providers in the operating room. Anesth Analg. 2019;129(6):1557–60.
53. Rutala WA, Weber DJ. Disinfection, sterilization, and antisepsis: an overview. Am J Infect Control. 2019;343:47SA3–9.
54. Carling PC, Parry MF, Von Beheren SM, et al. Identifying opportunities to enhance environmental cleaning in 23 acute care hospitals. Infect Control Hosp Epidemiol. 2008;29(1):1–7.
55. Loftus RW, Dexter F, Goodheart MJ, et al. The effect of improving basic preventive measures in the perioperative arena on *S. aureus* transmission and surgical site infections. JAMA Netw Open. 2020;12:3e201934.

56. Schmidt E, Dexter F, Herrmann J, et al. Assessment of anesthesia machine redesign on cleaning of the anesthesia machine using surface disinfection wipes. Am J Infect Control. 2020;48(6):675–81.
57. Biddle CJ, George-Gay B, Prasanna P, et al. Assessing a novel method to reduce anesthesia machine contamination: a prospective, observational trial. Can J Infect Dis Med Microbiol. 2018;2018:1–7.
58. Bowdle A, Munoz-Price LS. Preventing infection of patients and healthcare workers should be the new normal in the era of novel coronavirus epidemics. Anesthesiology. 2020;132(6):1292–5.
59. Martin LD, Rampersad SE, Geiduschek JM, et al. Modification of anesthesia practice reduces catheter-associated bloodstream infections: a quality improvement initiative. Paediatr Anaesth. 2013;23 (7):588–96.
60. Call TR, Auerbach FJ, Riddell SW, et al. Nosocomial contamination of laryngoscope handles: challenging current guidelines. Anesth Analg. 2009;109(2):479–83.
61. Koff MD, Loftus RW, Burchman CC, et al. Reduction in intraoperative bacterial contamination of peripheral intravenous tubing through the use of a novel device. Anesthesiology. 2009;110(5):978–85.
62. Loftus RW, Brindeiro BS, Kispert DP, et al. Reduction in intraoperative bacterial contamination of peripheral intravenous tubing through the use of a passive catheter care system. Anesth Analg. 2012;115(6):1315–23.
63. Mermel LA. Short-term peripheral venous catheter-related bloodstream infections: a systematic review. Clin Infect Dis. 2017;65 (10):1757–62.
64. Saliba P, Hornero A, Cuervo G, et al. Interventions to decrease short-term peripheral venous catheter-related bloodstream infections: impact on incidence and mortality. J Hosp Infect. 2018;100 (3):e178–86.
65. O'Horo JC, Maki DG, Krupp AE, et al. Arterial catheters as a source of bloodstream infection. Crit Care Med. 2014;42(6):1334–9.
66. Bowdle TA, Jelacic S, Munoz-Price LS, et al. Elastomeric respirators for COVID-19 and the next respiratory virus pandemic: essential design elements. Anesthesiology. 2021;135(6):951–62.
67. Jensen PA, Lambert LA, Iademarco MF, et al. Guidelines for preventing the transmission of *Mycobacterium tuberculosis* in health-care settings, 2005. MMWR Recomm Rep. 2005;54:1–141.
68. Lin C, Vazquez-Colon C, Geng-Ramos G, et al. Implications of anesthesia and vaccination. Pediat Anesth. 2021;31(5):531–8.
69. Merritt-Genore H, Moosdorf R, Gillaspie E, et al. Perioperative coronavirus vaccination—timing and implications: a guidance document. Ann Thoracic Surg. 2021;112(5):1707–15.

Principles of Patient Safety

40

Ian R. Slade and Yulia Obelcz

Abstract

Patient safety focuses on reducing risk of accidental injury from healthcare delivery. Despite decades of attention, medical errors still harm hundreds of thousands of patients annually. Most errors are attributable to a combination of human factors with failure points of complex systems, rather than individual lapses. Safe systems aim to improve by fostering a culture of psychological safety that supports worker willingness to openly report errors and near-miss events without fearing retribution. Medication errors are frequent and often preventable. Direct observation of anesthesia professionals in the operating room has shown an error reaching one in 20 medication administrations, such as wrong dose or swapping syringes. Recommended prevention methods include eliminating look-alike vials, using pre-filled syringes, standardizing labeling and color coding, bar code administration, and smart infusion pumps. When errors occur, patients expect timely and honest disclosure. In response to fear that disclosure increases risk of a liability judgment, many U.S. states have enacted apology laws to protect certain elements of disclosure from being used as evidence in litigation. Some evidence suggests that health systems that support early disclosure, sometimes with offers of compensation, may have lower incidence of malpractice claims. Anesthesiologists should be familiar with local risk management expectations and should have an active role in disclosure of perioperative adverse events. Awareness of general disclosure principles and practice in simulated patient scenarios is helpful preparation for real-life disclosure conversations.

Keywords

Patient safety • Human factors • Safety culture • Medication error • Medication error prevention • Medical error disclosure • Risk management

Key Points

1. Most errors are attributable to a combination of human factors and failure points in complex systems, rather than individual lapses.
2. A systems-focused approach, rather than one focused on individual blame, has the greatest potential to improve safety over time.
3. Systems with a strong culture of safety acknowledge that failure can still occur and support healthcare workers in reporting vulnerabilities.
4. Self-reporting of adverse events and near-misses is an important contribution to understanding how human factors interact with complex systems.
5. Self-reporting systems, while a critical component of safety, result in underreporting, as errors and near-misses may be unrecognized by the provider or considered non-substantial.
6. Patients and families expect timely and transparent disclosure of errors, but many physicians feel underprepared for the disclosure process.
7. Errors and adverse events have impacts on the psychological well-being of healthcare workers, and these impacts should be considered in comprehensive plans for risk management and disclosure.
8. Disclosure offers a chance for expressions of empathy and apology, and may bring physicians a sense of relief from having an open and honest discussion.
9. Many jurisdictions have enacted "apology laws" to promote disclosure by protecting elements of that process from being admitted as evidence in a liability claim.

I. R. Slade (✉) · Y. Obelcz
Department of Anesthesiology & Pain Medicine, Harborview Medical Center, University of Washington, 325 9th Ave, Box 359724 Seattle, WA 98104, USA
e-mail: islade@uw.edu

Y. Obelcz
e-mail: ivashy@uw.edu

M. Argalious et al. (eds.), *Basic Sciences in Anesthesia*,
https://doi.org/10.1007/978-3-031-60203-0_40

10. Many hospitals include just-in-time disclosure coaching for physicians as part of a comprehensive Risk Management program, as well as providing follow-up support.

40.1 Introduction

Patient safety is a familiar concept in modern health care. The objective to "do no harm" has been an aspiration of physicians for centuries, and this goal of non-maleficence remains a central component in medical ethics. Despite this guiding principle, medical errors continue to cause harm to hundreds of thousands of patients per year, and the deaths of at least tens of thousands of patients every year in the United States alone, as highlighted in the Institute of Medicine's (IOM) landmark 1999 publication *To Err Is Human: Building a Safer Health System* [1]. This publication framed patient safety from the perspective of patients as the desire to have "freedom from accidental injury." While recognizing the duty of everyone in healthcare to act in good faith, the IOM highlighted that complex systems' interaction with human factors are at the root of most medical errors.

The complexity of health systems makes it impossible to anticipate and train workers in avoiding every potential error. A systems-focused approach, rather than one focused on individual blame, has the greatest potential to improve safety over time. Systems can be intentionally designed (and redesigned) to promote patient safety via process simplification, standardization, and understanding human factors to build in opportunities for capturing potential errors before they reach the patient. Safe systems want to promote a culture where individual workers feel safe reporting errors and near-miss events, thereby facilitating continuous process improvement.

It is useful to review a few definitions of terms used in this chapter:

Medication error: Failure to give the right patient the intended drug in the correct dose, via the correct route at the correct time.

Near-miss: An event with potential for error that was intercepted, either by an individual or system, before it reached a patient.

Adverse event (AE): An undesired medical occurrence or finding during healthcare delivery that affects a patient. Not all AEs result from error, just as not all errors cause AEs.

Sentinel event: A subgroup of AEs that result in death, permanent harm, or severe temporary harm with intervention required to sustain life. Sentinel events require immediate attention of the healthcare organization and often have associated requirements for reporting to regulatory bodies [2].

Medication errors and near-misses are highly prevalent in general medicine as well as the practice of anesthesiology, carrying a high potential for harm, and therefore will be a focus of this chapter. We will also review the principles of bioethics that drive the process for disclosure of any type of medical error.

40.2 Medication Errors: Assessment and Prevention

The incidence of medical errors may vary, depending on the timing, location, and specific situation. Some report it to be the third leading cause of death in the United States [3]. While others have challenged this estimation, medical errors present a major problem in health care [4]. Medication errors constitute an important part of all medical errors and often are preventable.

40.2.1 Error Detection and Contributing Factors

Evaluating the incidence of incorrect drug administration in anesthesia practice is challenging, partly because the approaches to incident detection vary widely [5]. The most common error detection methods include voluntary reporting, chart review, direct observation, and automated computer technologies [6]. The self-reporting system often results in underreporting, with 50–60% of silent incidents because errors are either not recognized by the provider or considered non-substantial [7, 8]. Incidence of medication-related errors based on surveys alone was shown as low as 0.84% of all anesthetics [9]. Error detection based on direct observation in the operating room is significantly higher, with an error reaching one in 20 medication administrations (or every second surgical procedure), with or without an adverse drug effect [8]. When all the different detection methods are combined, the incidence of medication error approaches 6.7% of all hospital drug administrations [10].

Sources of medication errors can be either human (active failures) or system-related (latent conditions) (see Fig. 40.1), though a combination of both factors is common [11–13]. Active failure is further classified in Fig. 40.2 [14].

The main predisposing factors for medication errors are lack of vigilance, inattention, failure to read labels, and distraction [13, 15]. Inexperience, stress, and increased workload also elevate the potential for errors; their incidence increases when the anesthetic includes more than 13 different drug administrations [8, 16]. A survey by Orser demonstrated a cognitive bias when the majority of anesthesiologists

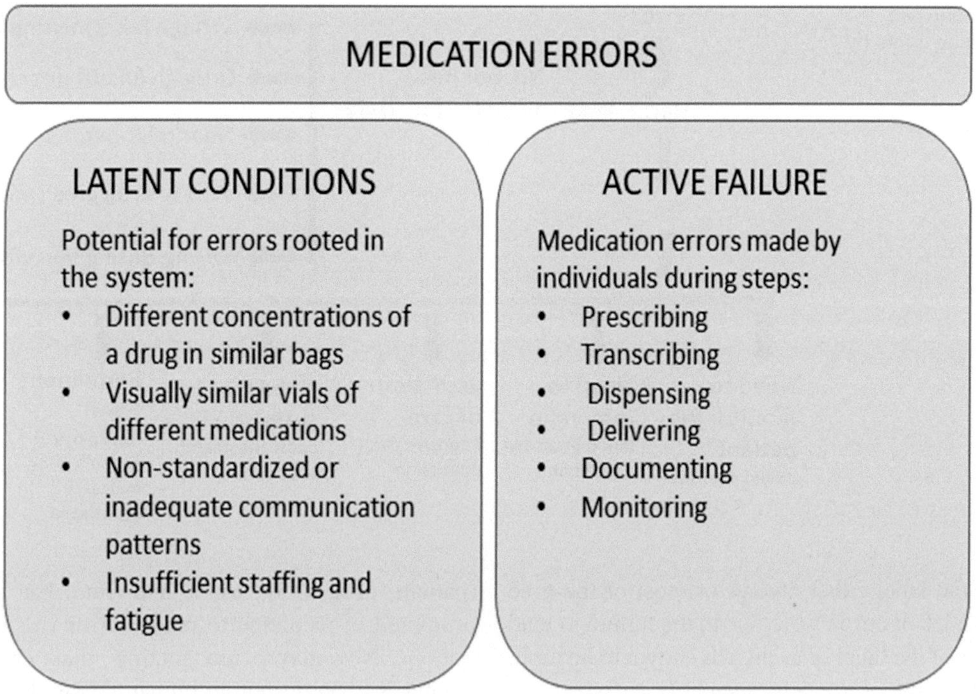

Fig. 40.1 Classification of medication errors by type: system-based versus individual-based

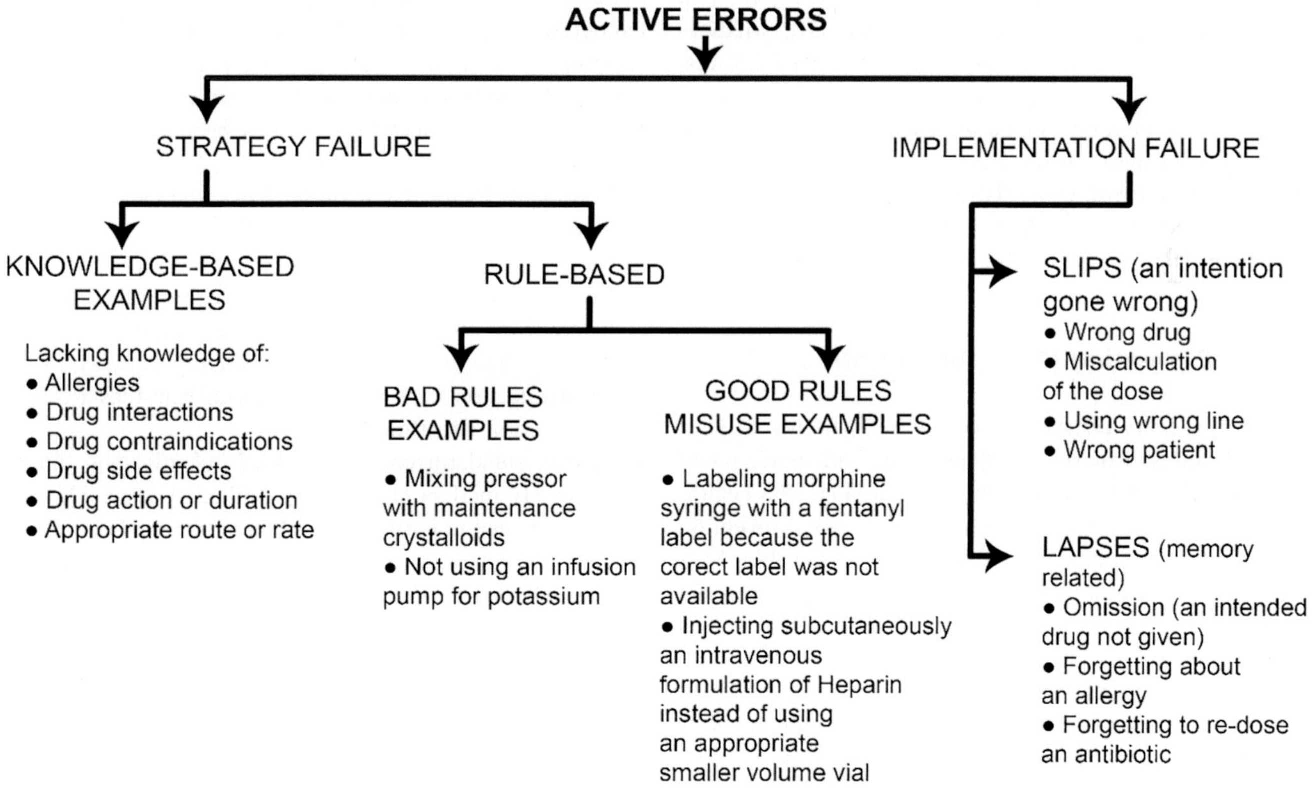

Fig. 40.2 Classification of errors by Active Failure. Adapted from JK Aronson, Medication errors: definitions and classification [14]

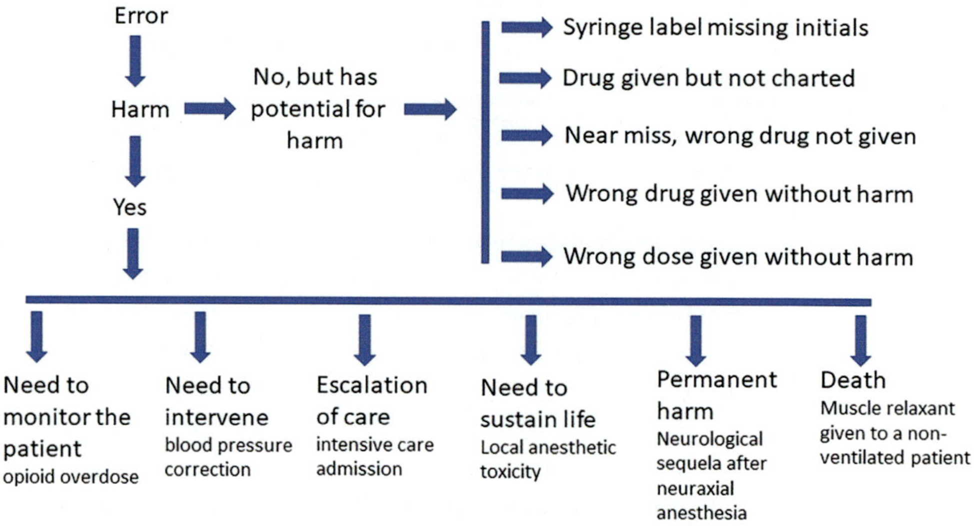

Fig. 40.3 Classification and examples of medication errors by harm potential

reported reading the label either always or most of the time but admitted that 53% of errors were due to the failure to read the label; the color of the label or a cap was shown to be more important than the name of the substance [17].

Drug errors most frequently occur during the administration phase. The most common mishaps, in decreasing order of frequency, are the wrong dose, drug substitution (syringe swap), and omission of the medication [9, 18, 19]. Similar findings apply to pediatric anesthesia [20]. Medications most often misused are antibiotics, muscle relaxants, and opioids [21].

Not all errors result in harm. However, one third of anesthetic medication errors carry potential harm, and two thirds of the harmful events are serious but non-life-threatening [8]. The potential of the medication errors to cause harm is presented in Fig. 40.3.

40.2.2 Preventing Medication Errors

Most, if not every anesthesiologist will experience at least one medication error during their career with potential to harm patients and financial consequences [17]. The healthcare system is continuously developing error prevention structures that are effective, efficient, and sustainable. System safety is strongest in an environment where practitioners are alert to the high error probability in their workflow and feel safe to report incidents and near-misses.

On an individual level, individuals administering medications can promote safety by the seemingly simple act of carefully reading the labels every time. Since lack of experience was shown as a factor contributing to errors, involving a second person in the verification process may be useful for new providers, and some recommend it as a general principle [16, 22]. The simple rule of the five "rights" (patient, drug, dose, route, and time) has been historically promoted in medicine to reduce error risk in drug administration. Nowadays, recognizing that errors still occur, emphasis is on designing human factors-based structures for medication administration practices to further reduce the incidence of human error.

It has been over two decades since *To Err Is Human: Building a Safer Health System* proposed creating a Center for Patient Safety to research why errors occur and to build the scientific foundation for safer practice [1]. Since that time, a variety of simple and more sophisticated methods to reduce the incidence of medication errors have been proven effective:

- Report all incidents of drug errors and near-misses to identify the system weaknesses that may create foundation for errors [6].
- Eliminate look-alike vials and ampules from the locations where they could be easily confused. Figures 40.4 and 40.5 illustrate examples of the similarity between different medication vials accessible during anesthesia care in the authors' department.
- Utilize standardized, color-coded, clearly and unambiguously marked labels and pre-filled syringes [22–24].
- Use medication templates to standardize medication syringe placement at the anesthesia workstation across all sites where anesthesia care is delivered [25].
- Implement bar code medication administration (BCMA) systems to use with both single administration and infusions. Scan medications directly *before* administration [26–28].
- Use smart pumps with standardized drug libraries and pre-set hard limits to prevent calculation and dosage errors. Connect infusions to the IV port most proximal to the patient. Administer boluses through a different line [29–31].

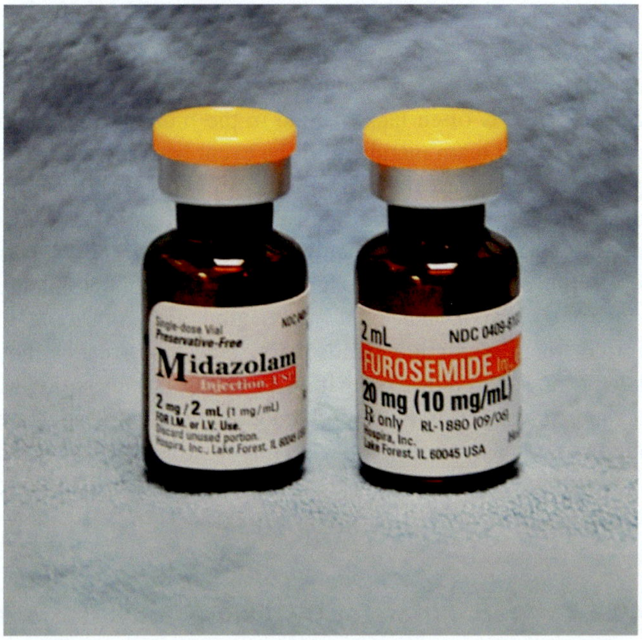

Fig. 40.4 Look-alike vials of midazolam and furosemide: same size and color

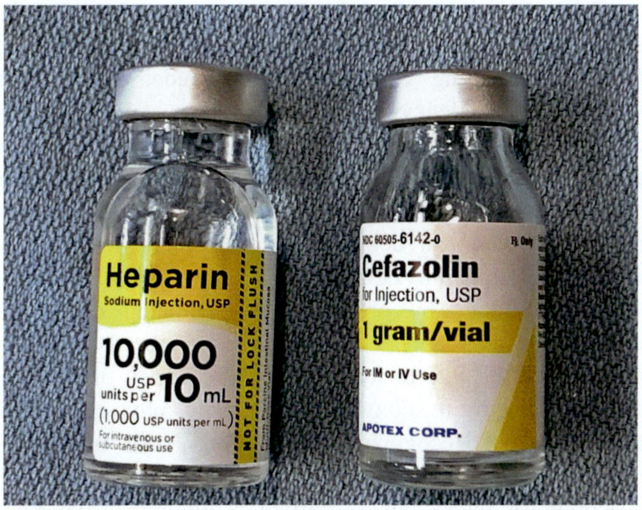

Fig. 40.5 Look-alike vials of heparin and cefazolin: same size and color

40.3 Disclosure of Errors to Patients

Despite the best intentions and vigilance of healthcare professionals, unanticipated poor outcomes still occur, and even robustly designed systems are vulnerable to periodic failure when errors will reach patients. Errors may cause temporary or permanent harm and often lead to needing further care. Beyond providing this additional treatment, physicians have a moral duty to understand the patient and family impacts and to engage in a supportive disclosure process. Errors also personally impact the involved healthcare workers, whose confidence and sense of professional competence is often shaken when they realize they are not immune to making mistakes; support for the well-being of providers must also be included in comprehensive plans for risk management and disclosure.

40.3.1 Ethical Principles Guiding Disclosure

When adverse events happen, whether caused by medical error or not, the four guiding principles of modern bioethics are a helpful foundation on which a disclosure process can be built to meet the needs of the involved patient and their support network [32]. These elements, and a description of how each pertains to disclosure, are included here:

- Autonomy—Respect for individuals and their rights to be informed and make their own decisions that impact their well-being. Most patients want to know about an unexpected event that affected or potentially affected their health. Different patients may want a greater or lesser amount of detail about the circumstances of the error, but emphasis should be on transparency and providing as much information as the patient can reasonably request [33].
- Beneficence—The desire to engage in decision-making and care that are consistent with a patient's goals. Disclosure emphasizes a shared understanding of the patient's goals and how the healthcare team acted to honor those priorities in the context of the event, such as describing the diligent efforts taken in response to minimize further risk of harm.
- Non-maleficence—The desire to "do no harm"—a reflection of the professional commitment of those providing care to use their best judgment and follow accepted standards to avoid harm. This can involve stating the concerns of the people involved in the error and its discovery, describing what went wrong, expressing regret and apologizing for the error.
- Justice—The goal that no individual or group bears a disproportionate share of the burdens or benefits of medical care. For disclosure conversations, this can manifest as an expressed desire of the individuals and system to learn from the error by adapting processes and behaviors in ways that lead to improved safety for other patients, reducing the risk of recurrence. Patients may justifiably wish to be compensated if the unexpected outcome resulted from error, and failure to divulge crucial information may deprive them of this right.

40.3.2 Addressing Barriers to Disclosure

The idea of disclosing errors to patients can bring up many barriers for physicians: discomfort with or lack of support for the process, embarrassment, fear of reputation loss, and fear of litigation. These barriers are so strong that the culture of medicine in the United States historically promoted an environment where physicians paternalistically decided what information to share with patients, with a tendency to conceal errors and avoid disclosure conversations [34].

Disclosure may also bring many physicians a sense of relief from having an open and honest discussion, offering a chance for expressions of empathy and apology for the impacts of unexpected events on patients and their families. Fortunately, the culture in medicine has begun to shift, both from external and internal pressures, and there is now broad support for disclosure of serious errors [35]. Regulations such as The Joint Commission's Sentinel Event Policy promote disclosure [2].

A major barrier has been fear that apologizing or expressing regret for an error in a disclosure conversation could be used as evidence in a liability claim. Addressing this concern and promoting patient-centered care has been central in "apology laws" that have been enacted in at least 40 U.S. states and the District of Columbia. These laws aim to promote transparency of disclosure by protecting specific types of communication shared with patients or families in a disclosure process from being admitted as evidence in a liability claim. Laws vary by jurisdiction, and the reader is encouraged to become familiar with the specific protections in their area of practice [36]. Evidence supports that hospitals implementing a disclosure program, which includes early disclosure and, in certain cases, offers of compensation, have been associated with a reduction in malpractice claims [37].

40.3.3 Disclosure Considerations in Anesthesiology

Anesthesiology has several unique circumstances compared to other specialties that can impact planning a disclosure conversation. First, relationships with patients are often formed over a very short time preoperatively, and often there has been no contact with other family members. This isolation from not having a longer-term relationship can compound the distress felt by anesthesiologists after an adverse event. Second, as the only specialty that routinely handles all immediate aspects of prescribing, procuring, preparing, administering, and monitoring the effects of different medications, when there is an error, it can feel automatically ascribed as a personal failure. In reality, there frequently have been numerous systematic failures that enabled the error.

When adverse events occur in the team-based perioperative setting, there may be an incomplete understanding of contributing factors that can lead to a misattributed root cause. There is often lack of time in the moment to debrief with the other team members. If the event has resulted in the patient needing escalated care, the surgeon may become available to meet with the family while the anesthesiologist is still tending to the patient. Despite the surgeon's best intentions and sense of urgency, disclosure at this premature stage can lead to inaccurate messaging and contribute to further distress for the family, who may lose trust if they later hear a different explanation from the anesthesiologist. As much as possible, careful coordination between team members is essential so that all involved parties have an opportunity to engage in a timely, accurate, and supportive disclosure process [38].

40.3.4 Preparation for Disclosure Conversations

Despite the widespread acknowledgment that disclosure is vital, it is natural for physicians to remain uncomfortable with the process. Adequate preparation is key to a successful conversation, and importantly, to avoid a poorly executed interaction, which can make matters worse. Disclosure training is increasingly included in medical schools and residency programs. This may take the form of simulation scenarios involving adverse events, with trained actors portraying patients or family members who react in different ways depending on the simulation scenario, and who can debrief with the trainee to improve their preparation. Physicians can benefit from role modeling opportunities by observing or practicing disclosure discussions with physicians more experienced in these processes. Still, due to the relative infrequency of needing to have disclosure conversations, many physicians feel underprepared. Recognizing the varying levels of experience, many hospitals include just-in-time disclosure coaching for physicians as part of a comprehensive Risk Management program, as well as providing follow-up support [39].

Preparation for disclosure conversations ideally starts *before* any adverse event, by establishing rapport with the patient and/or family preoperatively whenever possible. This is one of many reasons to take time and care in establishing a trustworthy relationship in advance of providing care. Consideration of the timing, setting, and participants in a disclosure scenario is important, and will vary depending on circumstances. In general, once an adverse event or error is identified, it is better to disclose this earlier versus later to have the best chance of preserving some bonds of trust.

40.3.5 Leading a Successful Disclosure Conversation

Conversations may take many forms depending on the needs of the patient and/or family, and approaches may need to be adapted based on circumstances of the particular interaction. Physicians who lead successful disclosure sessions typically seek to understand what the patient/family has already heard, use reflective listening, employ non-medical terminology as appropriate, describe next steps, and show transparency while still acknowledging uncertainty or areas where information is incomplete. It is appropriate to offer an apology when a mistake was made, and to express empathy and regret for the effects of the adverse event, while pledging to continue supportive care and making plans for follow-up as more information is available. This can help keep avenues of communication open for later questions.

Responses of patients and family members vary widely, even if faced with similar scenarios, and it is important to anticipate this. Common reactions can include shock, denial, overwhelm, sadness, and anger. In some cases, responses will be surprisingly positive, with expressions of gratitude for acknowledging an error, sharing of appreciation for transparency, and even asking about the personal well-being of the care team after the event.

Factual documentation of the disclosure conversation in the medical record is often appropriate but may vary in jurisdictions that do not have robust apology laws. In discussing causes, it is important to avoid speculation and to be careful not to cast blame on other individuals. Consultation with local risk management personnel is recommended before documenting conversations in the chart.

40.4 Conclusion

Medical errors continue to harm far too many patients, and are usually attributable to vulnerabilities in system design, rather than individual failures. Safe systems are deliberately designed to reduce risk and improve likelihood that errors will be intercepted before causing permanent harm. These systems analyze and adapt in response to errors, near-misses, AEs, and sentinel events. A culture of reporting and psychological safety are essential components in designing safer systems over time.

Medication errors are one of the most frequent high-impact adverse events in the practice of anesthesiology. While individual vigilance remains fundamental, human factors considerations inform the design of systems to promote safe care, with many examples in the realm of medication safety, such as labeling systems, BCMA, and smart infusion pumps.

When adverse events happen, safe systems favor early disclosure and apology. Timeliness and transparency are desired by patients and the general public, and now these ideas are finding broad support among medical professionals, representing a major cultural shift over the last few decades. The disclosure process is patient-centered and guided by fundamental bioethical principles. Effective disclosure processes may reduce medicolegal repercussions of error. Apology laws in most states also offer good legal protection for physicians to be able to apologize without the apology itself being admissible in a subsequent legal claim. Empathic follow-up interactions with patients and families after an adverse event supports healing for all parties involved and is an extension of anesthesiologists' professional commitment to system improvement in enhancing patient safety.

Multiple-Choice Questions

1. After induction of general anesthesia, a patient is given twice the intended dose of rocuronium. The surgical procedure takes four hours, and no harm is evident to the patient. This circumstance is best described as:
   a. Medication error
   b. Near-miss
   c. Adverse event
   d. Sentinel event
2. Which of the following scenarios represents a medication error?
   a. A patient with no history of allergy is given rocuronium and develops anaphylaxis.
   b. A patient with history of anaphylaxis to aspirin is unintentionally given ketorolac and has no evidence of allergic reaction.
   c. A patient with a history of anaphylaxis to penicillin is given morphine and develops anaphylaxis.
   d. A patient with renal failure is given fentanyl and requires naloxone to reverse respiratory depression.
3. Medication errors most frequently occur during which phase?
   a. Deciding/prescribing which drug should be given to the patient.
   b. Preparing/diluting the drug.
   c. Administering the drug to the patient.
   d. Documenting what drug was given.
4. Methods demonstrated to be effective in reducing the likelihood of medication errors include:
   a. Report all incidents of drug errors and near-misses.
   b. Eliminate look-alike vials and ampules from locations where they could be easily confused.
   c. Use smart infusion pumps with standardized drug libraries and pre-set dosing limits.

   d. All of the above.
5. Which of the following behaviors would be most likely to reduce the chance of a drug error?
   a. Use a bar code system to scan drug syringes after administration.
   b. Use standardized, color-coded, clearly and unambiguously marked labels.
   c. Develop personalized systems of medication syringe placement at the anesthesia workstation.
   d. All of the above.
6. Which of the following events should be disclosed to a patient?
   a. You give a dose of medication from a partially filled drug syringe into your patient's IV tubing; later you discover the same syringe had been used for your previous patient.
   b. While setting up an infusion pump, you discover that you prepared the infusion bag in the wrong concentration, and you prepare a new bag.
   c. You inadvertently pick up a syringe of ephedrine instead of phenylephrine and give a dose to a hypotensive patient; the hypotension is corrected.
   d. All of the above
7. You have a patient who is to receive a 1-g vancomycin infusion preoperatively over 60 min. You are working with a new trainee who prepares a vial of vancomycin powder and administers 1 g via rapid IV push preoperatively. The patient develops an infusion reaction, feels flushed, appears bright red, and reports a headache and intense itching. The system-level response that would be most likely to reduce the likelihood of event recurrence is:
   a. Educate the trainee about how to administer IV vancomycin and the risks of rapid infusion.
   b. Include the trainee in a patient conversation to disclose and apologize for the event.
   c. Invite the new trainee to present the event at an internal department meeting.
   d. Work with the pharmacy to remove powdered vancomycin from the anesthesia work area and replace it with premixed infusion bags.
8. A newly hired anesthesiologist is caring for an elderly patient having elective endovascular repair of a non-ruptured abdominal aortic aneurysm under general anesthesia. The patient has a single 20-gauge peripheral IV and an arterial line. During the anesthetic, the patient suddenly becomes very hypertensive and moves, then becomes profoundly hypotensive. The surgeon is concerned for aneurysm rupture and wants to perform a laparotomy to attempt open repair, but there is a delay in getting the right surgical instruments. Despite aggressive resuscitation efforts, the patient expires in the operating room. The most appropriate response to this event is:
   a. Place the new anesthesiologist on probation for having inadequate IV access for the planned procedure.
   b. Disciplinary action for the anesthesiologist for the patient having moved during surgery, possibly causing aneurysm perforation.
   c. Disciplinary action for the nursing staff for not having the right equipment immediately available for laparotomy.
   d. Coordinated internal event review to determine contributing factors to the intraoperative course and outcome.
9. You are providing a break to a colleague during elective laparoscopic cholecystectomy in an ASA II 65-year-old patient. The next blood pressure cycle reveals a blood pressure of 74/48 mmHg. You take a pharmacy pre-filled phenylephrine syringe from the top of the anesthesia cart and administer one milliliter of the drug, which equals 100 mcg of phenylephrine per your hospital's standards. In 30 s, the patient's heart rate is 150 per minute, and the blood pressure is 210/130 mmHg. You look at the presumed phenylephrine syringe and realize that it is epinephrine in dilution 1:10,000, in a pre-filled syringe that features a purple label, like the phenylephrine one. The most effective way to prevent such a medication error is:
   a. Handing over all medications when providing or receiving a break.
   b. Asking the pharmacy to change the label color of the epinephrine syringes.
   c. Reading the drug label every time prior to administration.
   d. All of the above.
10. Which of the following examples of phenylephrine administration could be considered a lack-of-knowledge drug error:
   a. During Cesarean section under spinal anesthesia, continue administering IV boluses of 100–200 mcg with each new mean arterial blood pressure value below 60 mmHg per non-invasive blood pressure monitor after a cumulative dose of 1000 mcg of phenylephrine has already been given.
   b. Starting a post-induction infusion at 0.5 mcg/kg/min in an octogenarian patient on chronic beta-blocker therapy with a blood pressure of 90/48 mmHg and a heart rate of 46 beats per minute.
   c. Intraosseous administration in a two-year-old polytrauma patient with hypotension.
   d. Starting an infusion at 0.5 mcg/kg/min in a healthy 27-year-old patient with mean arterial blood pressure of 52 mmHg undergoing a free-flap reconstructive surgery after a degloving injury to the upper extremity.

Answers

1. a. Medication error. Medication error is defined as the failure to give the right patient the intended drug in the correct dose, via the correct route at the correct time. The error reached the patient, so it was not a near-miss. Neither an adverse drug effect nor a need for rescue action occurred because of the dosing error, so it would not be described as an adverse event or sentinel event.
2. b. Giving a patient a drug in the same class as one to which they have a history of anaphylaxis (in this example, both are non-steroidal anti-inflammatory drugs) is a medication error, even if no apparent harm results. Not all medication errors result in adverse events. The other three answer options all describe adverse events that are not associated with medication error. Not all adverse events are the result of error.
3. c. Most drug errors occur during the administration phase. The most common mishaps, in decreasing order of frequency, are the wrong dose, drug substitution (syringe swap), and omission of the medication.
4. d. Reporting adverse events and near-misses is a vital component of identifying system vulnerabilities to improve safety. Analysis of human factors shows that look-alike drug containers are a high-risk circumstance that can lead to preparation of the wrong drug. Smart infusion pumps can reduce the likelihood of calculation and dosing errors.
5. b. Standardized labeling systems are demonstrated to reduce the likelihood of drug error by improving readability and reducing the consequences of same-class drug substitution. When bar code systems are used, scanning should occur before administration, not afterward. Medication syringe placement at the anesthesia workstation may reduce error when standardized across an organization, rather than personalized by each practitioner.
6. a. Even when used to inject only into IV tubing, a syringe may be contaminated with biologic material including bloodborne pathogens, potentially causing infectious exposure to the second patient. The second patient should be informed of the event and risk; the first patient may need to be informed as well to seek their consent to test for bloodborne pathogens. The infusion concentration example is a near-miss, as it was detected and corrected before reaching the patient. The ephedrine versus phenylephrine event was a same-class drug substitution that fortunately had an equivalent therapeutic response and would not typically be disclosed. However, you should still reflect and report the event internally to determine what individual and system factors could be addressed to reduce the chance of recurrence.
7. d. This system-level change would make it difficult to prepare a concentrated syringe of vancomycin that could be administered by IV push. By having only premixed infusion bags, although they could possibly be infused rapidly, there is a greater likelihood that the infusion would be used with a smart infusion pump that would guide the user in programming the correct duration. Educating the trainee is important, as lack of knowledge was a likely contributor. While this would reduce the likelihood of the individual making the same error, it is not a system-level change. Inclusion of the trainee in the disclosure process is an important part of professional development, but again is not a system-level change. Inviting the trainee to present at an internal department meeting may reduce the likelihood that others (especially other junior trainees) at that meeting would make the same error but would also not be a system-level change.
8. d. There are many factors that combined to lead to this undesired outcome, and an internal review is most appropriate to understand how each factor contributed and what system-level changes could improve safety. While there may have been individual gaps in judgment, the context for these decisions needs to be better understood. The options of punitive action for individuals involved in the patient's care are not the most appropriate responses.
9. c. Failure to read the label is one of the main factors contributing to medication errors. The color of the label provides a strong visual cue to the class of the medication given but does not eliminate the need to read the medication name and dose. Double-checking the label with a team member is another measure to promote safety, especially in stressful situations.
10. d. Phenylephrine has been associated with higher fetal pH than ephedrine during Cesarean delivery under spinal block and is the preferred treatment for hypotension in healthy pregnant women. The intraosseous administration of vasopressors could be lifesaving when intravenous access is impossible. Phenylephrine can decrease the heart rate and should be used cautiously in patients with baseline bradycardia; however, its use is not contraindicated. In free-flap reconstructive procedures, phenylephrine-induced vasoconstriction could compromise flap blood flow and jeopardize flap viability, and therefore could be considered an inappropriate drug administration in this context.

References

1. Institute of Medicine. To err is human: building a safer health system. Washington, DC: The National Academies Press; 2000.
2. The Joint Commission. Sentinel event policy and procedures. https://www.jointcommission.org/resources/patient-safety-topics/sentinel-event/sentinel-event-policy-and-procedures/ (2022). Accessed 9 Aug 2022.
3. Makary MA, Daniel M. Medical error-the third leading cause of death in the US. BMJ. 2016;353: i2139. https://doi.org/10.1136/bmj.i2139.
4. Jarry J. Medical error is not the third leading cause of death. https://www.mcgill.ca/oss/article/critical-thinking-health/medical-error-not-third-leading-cause-death (27 Aug 2021). Accessed 9 Aug 2022.
5. Institute of Medicine. Preventing medication errors. Washington, DC: The National Academies Press; 2007.
6. Murff HJ, Patel VL, Hripcsak G, Bates DW. Detecting adverse events for patient safety research: a review of current methodologies. J Biomed Inform. 2003;36(1–2):131–43. https://doi.org/10.1016/j.jbi.2003.08.003.
7. World Health Organization. Reporting and learning systems for medication errors: the role of pharmacovigilance centres. Geneva: World Health Organization; 2014.
8. Nanji KC, Patel A, Shaikh S, Seger DL, Bates DW. Evaluation of perioperative medication errors and adverse drug events. Anesthesiology. 2016;124(1):25–34. https://doi.org/10.1097/ALN.0000000000000904.
9. Yamamoto M, Ishikawa S, Makita K. Medication errors in anesthesia: an 8-year retrospective analysis at an urban university hospital. J Anesth. 2008;22(3):248–52. https://doi.org/10.1007/s00540-008-0624-4.
10. Elden NM, Ismail A. The importance of medication errors reporting in improving the quality of clinical care services. Glob J Health Sci. 2016;8(8):54510. https://doi.org/10.5539/gjhs.v8n8p243.
11. Reason J. Human error: models and management. BMJ. 2000;320(7237):768–70. https://doi.org/10.1136/bmj.320.7237.768.
12. Sameera V, Bindra A, Rath GP. Human errors and their prevention in healthcare. J Anaesthesiol Clin Pharmacol. 2021;37(3):328–35. https://doi.org/10.4103/joacp.JOACP_364_19.
13. Tariq RA, Vashisht R, Sinha A, Scherbak Y. Medication Dispensing Errors And Prevention. StatPearls. Treasure Island (FL)2022.
14. Aronson JK. Medication errors: definitions and classification. Br J Clin Pharmacol. 2009;67(6):599–604. https://doi.org/10.1111/j.1365-2125.2009.03415.x.
15. Chopra V, Bovill JG, Spierdijk J, Koornneef F. Reported significant observations during anaesthesia: a prospective analysis over an 18-month period. Br J Anaesth. 1992;68(1):13–7. https://doi.org/10.1093/bja/68.1.13.
16. Cooper L, DiGiovanni N, Schultz L, Taylor RN, Nossaman B. Human factors contributing to medication errors in anaesthesia practice. ASA. 2009:A614.
17. Orser BA, Chen RJ, Yee DA. Medication errors in anesthetic practice: a survey of 687 practitioners. Can J Anaesth. = J Can d'anesth. 2001;48(2):139–46. https://doi.org/10.1007/BF03019726.
18. Webster CS, Merry AF, Larsson L, McGrath KA, Weller J. The frequency and nature of drug administration error during anaesthesia. Anaesth Intensive Care. 2001;29(5):494–500. https://doi.org/10.1177/0310057X0102900508.
19. Eichhorn JH. "Syringe swaps" in OR still harming patients. APSF Newslett. 2008;23(4):49–76
20. Lobaugh LMY, Martin LD, Schleelein LE, Tyler DC, Litman RS. Medication errors in pediatric anesthesia: a report from the wake up safe quality improvement initiative. Anesth Analg. 2017;125(3):936–42. https://doi.org/10.1213/ANE.0000000000002279.
21. Cooper L, Nossaman B. Medication errors in anesthesia: a review. Int Anesthesiol Clin. 2013;51(1):1–12. https://doi.org/10.1097/AIA.0b013e31827d6486.
22. Merry AF, Anderson BJ. Medication errors–new approaches to prevention. Paediatr Anaesth. 2011;21(7):743–53. https://doi.org/10.1111/j.1460-9592.2011.03589.x.
23. Benhamou D, Piriou V, De Vaumas C, Albaladejo P, Malinovsky JM, Doz M, et al. Ready-to-use pre-filled syringes of atropine for anaesthesia care in French hospitals—a budget impact analysis. Anaesth Crit Care Pain Med. 2017;36(2):115–21. https://doi.org/10.1016/j.accpm.2016.03.009.
24. Litman RS. How to prevent medication errors in the operating room? Take away the human factor. Br J Anaesth. 2018;120(3):438–40. https://doi.org/10.1016/j.bja.2018.01.005.
25. Grigg EB, Martin LD, Ross FJ, Roesler A, Rampersad SE, Haberkern C, et al. Assessing the impact of the anesthesia medication template on medication errors during anesthesia: a prospective study. Anesth Analg. 2017;124(5):1617–25. https://doi.org/10.1213/ANE.0000000000001823.
26. Poon EG, Keohane CA, Yoon CS, Ditmore M, Bane A, Levtzion-Korach O, et al. Effect of bar-code technology on the safety of medication administration. N Engl J Med. 2010;362(18):1698–707. https://doi.org/10.1056/NEJMsa0907115.
27. Thompson KM, Swanson KM, Cox DL, Kirchner RB, Russell JJ, Wermers RA, et al. Implementation of bar-code medication administration to reduce patient harm. Mayo Clin Proc Innov Qual Outcomes. 2018;2(4):342–51. https://doi.org/10.1016/j.mayocpiqo.2018.09.001.
28. Bowdle TA, Jelacic S, Nair B, Togashi K, Caine K, Bussey L, et al. Facilitated self-reported anaesthetic medication errors before and after implementation of a safety bundle and barcode-based safety system. Br J Anaesth. 2018;121(6):1338–45. https://doi.org/10.1016/j.bja.2018.09.004.
29. Wahr JA, Abernathy JH 3rd, Lazarra EH, Keebler JR, Wall MH, Lynch I, et al. Medication safety in the operating room: literature and expert-based recommendations. Br J Anaesth. 2017;118(1):32–43. https://doi.org/10.1093/bja/aew379.
30. Ohashi K, Dalleur O, Dykes PC, Bates DW. Benefits and risks of using smart pumps to reduce medication error rates: a systematic review. Drug Saf. 2014;37(12):1011–20. https://doi.org/10.1007/s40264-014-0232-1.
31. Pinkney S, Trbovich P, Fan M, Rothwell S, Cafazzo JA, Easty A. Do smart pumps actually reduce medication errors? Biomed Instrum Technol. 2010;44(s1):64–9. https://doi.org/10.2345/0899-8205-44.s1.64.
32. Beauchamp T, Childress J. Principles of biomedical ethics, 8th ed. Oxford University Press; 2019.
33. Gallagher TH, Waterman AD, Ebers AG, Fraser VJ, Levinson W. Patients' and physicians' attitudes regarding the disclosure of medical errors. JAMA. 2003;289(8):1001–7. https://doi.org/10.1001/jama.289.8.1001.
34. Gallagher TH, Studdert D, Levinson W. Disclosing harmful medical errors to patients. N Engl J Med. 2007;356(26):2713–9. https://doi.org/10.1056/NEJMra070568.
35. Gallagher TH, Garbutt JM, Waterman AD, Flum DR, Larson EB, Waterman BM, et al. Choosing your words carefully: how physicians would disclose harmful medical errors to patients. Arch Intern Med. 2006;166(15):1585–93. https://doi.org/10.1001/archinte.166.15.1585.
36. Ross NE, Newman WJ. The role of apology laws in medical malpractice. J Am Acad Psychiatry Law. 2021;49(3):406–14. https://doi.org/10.29158/JAAPL.200107-20.

37. Kachalia A, Kaufman SR, Boothman R, Anderson S, Welch K, Saint S, et al. Liability claims and costs before and after implementation of a medical error disclosure program. Ann Intern Med. 2010;153(4):213–21. https://doi.org/10.7326/0003-4819-153-4-201008170-00002.
38. Souter KJ, Gallagher TH. The disclosure of unanticipated outcomes of care and medical errors: what does this mean for anesthesiologists? Anesth Analg. 2012;114(3):615–21. https://doi.org/10.1213/ANE.0b013e3182228604.
39. Shapiro J, Robins L, Galowitz P, Gallagher TH, Bell S. Disclosure coaching: an ask-tell-ask model to support clinicians in disclosure conversations. J Patient Saf. 2021;17(8):e1364–70. https://doi.org/10.1097/PTS.0000000000000491.

Substance Abuse in Anesthesiology: Implications for Patients and for Anesthesiologists

41

Dmitry Sharakou

Abstract

This chapter examines the prevalence and implications of substance abuse in the context of anesthesia. It highlights the significant challenges posed by intoxicated patients, emphasizing the importance of thorough preoperative assessment, including history-taking and physical examination, to identify substance use. Intraoperative management involves adjusting anesthesia dosages based on the patient's intoxication status, with considerations for both acute and chronic effects of various substances. The chapter underscores the necessity for anesthesiologists to adapt their approach based on the specific substance involved and the patient's individual circumstances, prioritizing patient safety throughout the perioperative period.

Key Points

- 30–35% of emergent and trauma cases may present with acute intoxication.
- Alcohol and cannabis are the most commonly abused substances in the United States.
- Opioids and benzodiazepines are the most commonly abused prescription substances.
- Thorough history-taking and physical examination are essential components of the preoperative assessment of acutely intoxicated patients.
- Toxicological screening is typically only necessary in case of unclear history or if polysubstance is suspected.
- In acute intoxication, elective surgery should be postponed until sobriety is achieved.
- Rapid sequence induction is a preferred method of induction in the emergency setting.
- Alcohol is one of the most commonly abused substances in the United States and is involved in the majority of trauma cases. Acute alcohol intoxication decreases MAC; chronic alcohol use has opposite effect. Alcohol withdrawal typically presents in 24–48 h, and its onset may be delayed up to 5 days.
- Benzodiazepine withdrawal is very similar to alcohol withdrawal and presents in a similar timeframe.
- Opioids are the most commonly abused prescription medications in the United States. Withdrawal is not life threatening but may be very challenging in postoperative period.
- Buprenorphine is commonly used to treat chronic pain or opioid dependence and due to its partial agonism/antagonism mechanism of action may present unique challenges in postoperative pain management.
- Methadone causes QT interval prolongation and in combination with many anesthetic and antiemetic agents may lead to torsades de pointes.
- Acute cocaine intoxication lasts for 30–120 min.
- In cocaine-induced hypertensive crisis, β-blockers are not recommended due to the potential unopposed α-effect.
- Patients acutely intoxicated with 3,4-methylenedioxymethamphetamine (MDMA) may present with hyponatremia. In severe cases, MDMA intoxication may cause serotonin syndrome.
- The incidence of substance abuse is around 3% among anesthesiology residents and around 1% in staff anesthesiologists.
- Alcohol and opioids are the two most commonly abused substances among anesthesia providers.
- Substance abuse leads to a specific behavioral pattern in anesthetists.
- In most of the United States, substance abuse in anesthesiologists is reportable to the anesthesiology boards.
- Substance abuse treatment and rehabilitation are typically not covered by insurance and present significant financial burden for the treated.

D. Sharakou (✉)
Department of General Anesthesiology and ICR, Cleveland Clinic, Cleveland, OH, USA
e-mail: shrakd@ccf.org

M. Argalious et al. (eds.), *Basic Sciences in Anesthesia*,
https://doi.org/10.1007/978-3-031-60203-0_41

- In anesthesiologists with opioid dependence, return to practicing anesthesiology is associated with a high relapse rate.

41.1 Introduction

Globally, over 300 million surgeries are performed per year, and over 50 million of those are performed in United States alone [1]. Approximately 30–35% of trauma and emergency surgery patients may be intoxicated [2], and it is also very common to have multiple substances involved [3]. Up to 60% of patients with traumatic brain injury (TBI) are intoxicated during the traumatic event [4, 5]. The most commonly implicated intoxication agents include, but are not limited to: alcohol, opioids, benzodiazepines, cocaine, amphetamines, hallucinogens, and marijuana.

Common effects of drug abuse include: physical and mental health problems, overdose or withdrawal, injuries under the influence, blood born infections (HIV, HCV, HBV, TB), psychiatric problems, intellectual impairment, personality deterioration, high-risk behavior, legal complications, and financial losses.

41.2 General Considerations

41.2.1 Preoperative Assessment

Emergency and trauma surgeries are most likely to be associated with intoxicated patients. Certain patient populations (Table 41.1) are more likely to be intoxicated prior to anesthesia, and hence, more detailed assessment might be needed.

Table 41.1 Populations at risk and predisposing factors to intoxication

• Demographic factors (poor socioeconomical conditions status, homelessness, unemployment, low level of education, parental drug abuse, etc.)
• Peer pressure
• Changing of social roles, increasing stress and alteration in the lifestyle
• Genetic predisposition (especially for alcohol)
• Certain professions (sex workers, transportation workers, and healthcare workers)
• Availability and easy access to the drugs (induction of synthetic drugs and legalization of previously illicit drugs)

Commonly used drugs:

Cannabinoids: Hashish, marijuana
Stimulants: Amphetamine, cocaine
Depressants: Barbiturates, benzodiazepines, alcohol
Opioids: Opium, morphine, heroin, codeine, buprenorphine
Hallucinogens: LSD, phencyclidine, mescaline, psilocybin
Volatile solvents: Varnish, eraser fluids, petroleum
Others: Muscle relaxants, painkillers, antihistamines, antiemetics, antidepressants.

Frequently, urine or blood drug screenings are performed in symptomatic patients; however, it is not a mandatory test for every admitted surgical patient, and hence, appropriate history collection and physical examination are essential during preoperative anesthesiologic assessment of all patients. Although some patients may attempt to hide their intoxication status, the majority will admit to substance use when asked directly. The following questions can be used to assess the history of substance use or abuse, including: "Do you sometimes drink beer wine or other alcoholic beverages?" "How many times during the past year have you had four or more alcoholic drinks on a single occasion?", "Have you used any recreational or illicit substances over the past year?" [6]. In cases where questioning alone is not reliable or cannot be performed, rapid urine drug screening is a valuable tool that can be utilized in order to rule in or out intoxication.

Physical examination should include a basic neurologic assessment (Glasgow coma scale (GCS)), airway exam, heart and lung exam, and skin assessment if regional anesthesia is considered. Signs that may suggest possible intoxication include tachy- or bradycardia, miosis or mydriasis, diaphoresis, agitation, lethargy, or hallucinations. Some signs that might suggest chronic substance abuse include track marks, extreme tooth decay (meth mouth), and chronic skin infections.

Some of general considerations in patients confirmed or suspected of being acutely intoxicated: altered mental status (AMS), seizures, respiratory abnormalities, full stomach with delayed gastric emptying and the consequent risk of aspiration, unstable and variable hemodynamics (hypo and hypertension), dehydration(hypovolemia), fluid overload, arrhythmias, and electrolyte imbalance, etc.

In patients who are long-term users of illicit and recreational substances, chronic changes may be present, including higher prevalence certain diseases (HIV, HCV, HBV, TB, and various skin infections); potential poor IV access; cardiovascular diseases; dental problems; malnutrition of various degree; psychological or psychiatric problems; and possible withdrawal.

Both chronic and acute intoxication, depending on the specific abused substance, may alter sensitivity to anesthetics, change elimination and context-sensitive half-times, increase or decrease induction and emergence times, or even lead to potentially lethal interactions between intoxicating and anesthetic agents.

41.3 Depressants

41.3.1 Alcohol

Alcohol is the most abused substance in the world. According to National Institute on Alcohol Abuse and Alcoholism, over 55% of US adults over 18 years of age drink alcohol regularly (once a month or more), over 23% admit binge drinking, and over 8% drink heavily [7].

41.3.2 Preoperative Assessment

Chronic alcohol consumption is associated with multiple comorbidities, functional and psychological changes in patients. The most prevalent is alcoholic liver disease (over 50% of liver disease-related deaths are due to alcoholic liver disease [7]). Chronic alcohol consumption causes cognitive impairment; cardiovascular disease (including cardiomyopathy, HTN, PVD); acute or chronic pancreatitis; chronic kidney disease, and malnutrition. Acute alcohol intoxication is frequently present in trauma patients and may be associated with AMS (altered mental status), full stomach, unstable hemodynamics, and altered hemostasis [8].

41.3.3 Intraoperative Management

Elective surgery should be delayed until acute intoxication is resolved, and the patient is sober. Acutely intoxicated patients should be treated as having a full stomach (EtOH is known to delay gastric emptying in non-dose dependent fashion) [9]. Alcohol also nullifies informed consent.

In emergent cases, rapid sequence induction should performed in case of general anesthesia (stomach most likely full with food and alcohol). In patients under the influence of alcohol, drug dose necessary for induction and maintenance of anesthesia is lower than in general population [10]. In patients who are hypotensive or in shock, induction drugs should be titrated under careful hemodynamic monitoring to avoid cardiovascular collapse. In many cases, invasive hemodynamic monitoring may be necessary. The required minimum alveolar concentration (MAC) of volatile anesthetics is also decreased for acutely intoxicated patients.

In patients who chronically misuse alcohol, but are not acutely intoxicated, induction and maintenance doses of anesthetics may be increased due to enzyme induction or cross-tolerance. Hepatotoxic agents such as acetaminophen should be avoided, since they may cause toxicity even at lower doses. Neuromuscular blocking agents (NMB) should be titrated to effect, since pharmacokinetics of some muscle relaxants such as rocuronium may be altered (longer onset and prolonged effect) [11].

Emergence and extubation of patients acutely intoxicated with alcohol can be delayed in cases of severe intoxication, since on emergence patients may have prolonged recovery or become combative. There is also a high probability of severe postoperative nausea and vomiting (PONV) in acutely intoxicated patients and therefore a higher risk of aspiration.

41.3.4 Postoperative Management

Depending on chronicity and timeline of alcohol ingestion, various challenges are to be expected in postoperative management of this patient population. In acutely intoxicated patient, delayed emergence is very common. Patients may experience severe PONV. Patients who chronically consume alcohol on a daily basis may go into acute withdrawal if they stayed abstinent for longer than 24 h prior to surgery. If alcohol withdrawal is suspected, patients should be monitored in the ICU settings and managed accordingly (typically acute alcohol withdrawal is managed with benzodiazepines, barbiturates, dexmedetomidine, or valproic acid).

41.3.5 Benzodiazepines

Benzodiazepines (BZD) are very similar in action and symptomology to alcohol. Most commonly abused benzodiazepines include alprazolam, diazepam, lorazepam, clonazepam, and chlordiazepoxide (over 50 different agents). If used as prescribed, BZD rarely lead to significant side effects. When misused or used in combination with other depressants such as alcohol and/or opioids, BZD may cause significant respiratory depression, stupor or coma, and hemodynamic collapse. In chronic BZD users, significant risk of withdrawal exists in case of abrupt cessation and abstinence for more than 2–3 days. Symptoms of withdrawal (agitation, restlessness, insomnia, seizures, tremors, and diaphoresis) typically present on day 4–5 of abstinence, but may occur as soon as 1 day or as late as one week after cessation [12].

41.3.5.1 Preoperative Assessment

For patients presenting for elective surgery and taking prescribed benzodiazepines, no further assessment is typically required as long as patients are asymptomatic and are taking their BZD as prescribed. For patients demonstrating symptoms of overdose or misuse of prescribed BZDs, further assessment is needed, and an elective case may be delayed until the patient is no longer symptomatic.

In emergent surgery, patients should be treated as a full stomach. If respiratory depression, coma, or hemodynamic instability present, flumazenil can be used as a reversal agent; however, it is short half-life should be considered since its effect may wear off before the effects of BZD (4–8 min until flumazenil redistribution and 40–80 min of terminal half-life, which is significantly shorter than most benzodiazepines [4]). Another concern of utilization of flumazenil is that in chronic users it may trigger withdrawal seizures in BZD users or seizures in patients who are chronically on anti-seizure medications [12]. Along with flumazenil, intranasal naloxone is frequently utilized since simultaneous use of opioids and BZD is not infrequent.

Rapid UDS is helpful in preoperative assessment for determination of any other potentially used intoxicating agents. Using UDS for sole purpose of BZD intoxication diagnosis, however, has poor sensitivity and specificity, since it may be positive in patients who had exposure a few days prior to testing or be falsely negative in patients who used clonazepam, lorazepam, midazolam, or alprazolam [12].

41.3.5.2 Intraoperative Management

As in case of other depressants such as alcohol, patients who are acutely intoxicated with benzodiazepines are more susceptible to the sedative effects of anesthetic agents and typically require lower doses on induction. Hemodynamic compromise may be observed in patients who are intoxicated with multiple sedatives in addition to benzodiazepines, and in such patients, invasive hemodynamic monitoring may be necessary prior to induction. Patients acutely intoxicated with BZD should be treated as having a full stomach, and therefore, RSI is the preferable method of induction in trauma or emergency surgery. Induction drugs dosing should be adjusted according to the patient's mentation. Maintenance anesthetics doses typically are lower in acute BZD inebriety. On the contrary, patients who are chronically using benzodiazepines will require higher induction as well as higher maintenance anesthetic doses. Chronic users are also at a higher risk of perioperative awareness, which should be taken into consideration when choosing modality of anesthesia and in monitoring anesthetic depth (e.g., processed EEG monitoring) [13].

41.3.5.3 Postoperative Management

Patients in acute benzodiazepine intoxication may experience delayed emergence and, in such case, need prolonged postoperative observation. Although some BZD have been shown to have antiemetic effect (midazolam, remimazolam, etc. [14, 15]), due to the high likelihood of preexisting full stomach, patients should be treated as such.

Chronic benzodiazepines users are at risk perioperative recall, postoperative anxiety, and agitation in which cases anxiolytics should be utilized. Patients who are chronic users but stayed abstinent for a few days prior to surgery (typically 2–5 days) may suffer symptoms of withdrawal, experiencing anxiety, tremors, disturbances of perception, psychosis, and seizures. Treatment for BZD withdrawal is BZD. Typically, the intravenous route of administration is preferred. In severe cases of withdrawal, adjunctive therapies such as dexmedetomidine, neuroleptics, or barbiturates may be necessary [12].

41.3.6 Opioids

Over the past 20 years, opioid-related death in the United States are steadily increasing, reaching a staggering 80,411 deaths in 2021 [16]. Despite ongoing efforts, the number of opioid users is rising and creates a heavy economic burden on the country—over 150 billion USD in direct losses due to opioid overdoses in addition to over 870 billion of indirect losses. During COVID-19 pandemic, number of opioid related death was going up by 18–40% per year [17].

41.3.6.1 Opiates and Opioids

Opiates extracted from the poppy plant (*Papaver Somniferum*) have been used recreationally and medicinally for millennia. Opiates belong to the larger class of drugs, the opioids, which include synthetic and semi-synthetic drugs. Naturally occurring opiates include opium, morphine, and codeine. Semisynthetic agents include heroin, hydromorphone, oxycodone, hydrocodone. Synthetic opioids include meperidine, fentanyl, alfentanil, sufentanil, pentazocine, remifentanil, butorphanol, etc.

41.3.6.2 Acute Intoxication

Typical symptoms of acute opioid intoxication include altered mental status (somnolence, stupor, and coma); respiratory depression (both respiratory rate and tidal volumes are decreased); miotic pupils that are hyporeactive to light (effect may vary when meperidine is the intoxicating agent or stimulants are used in conjunction with opioids); and decreased bowel sounds. In addition to common symptoms, side effects of cutting agents (substances used to either dilute opioids or to increase intoxicating effect) may be observed (sugar, starch, acetaminophen, procaine, benzocaine, quinine, steroids, β2-adrenergic agonist—clenbuterol, fentanyl, etc.), such as arrhythmias, QTC and QT prolongation, Torsade de Pointes, psychosis, severe vasospasm at the site of injection, and serotonin syndrome.

41.3.6.3 Preoperative Considerations

Patients who are on chronic opioid therapy are typically not required to stop taking their prescription drugs. If adherent to prescribed regimen, such patient population is generally considered safe to proceed with the surgery.

Chronic use of methadone or partial agonists–antagonists, such as buprenorphine, necessitate additional changes in anesthesia plan. Methadone prolongs QT interval, and preoperative ECG is necessary in order to determine safety of other anesthetic agents and development of antiemetic plan for postoperative management. Buprenorphine is a partial agonist of mu receptor and weak antagonist of kappa receptor that can cause unique difficulties in management of postoperative pain with opioids in patients undergoing moderate and major surgeries, since opioid efficacy is decreased [18].

In patients with acute opioid overdose ABC is priority. In comatose and apneic patients, endotracheal intubation is warranted. RSI is preferred method of induction since any patient with acute intoxication is considered having a full stomach. If opioid overdose is confirmed or suspected, naloxone is the reversal agent of choice. Typical dose of naloxone is 0.05–1 mg IV or IM, to a total of 5–10 mg, depending on severity of symptoms. If maximum dose is reached but reversal of symptoms is not achieved, consider an alternative diagnosis.

41.3.6.4 Intraoperative Management

Chronic opioid use dramatically increases tolerance within this class of drugs. Use of over 90 OME mg/day (oral morphine equivalents) is considered lowest high dose threshold [19]; however, in some cases daily dose may exceed several grams of OME. In patients on high daily opioid doses, intraoperative analgesic requirements are significantly higher than in general population, and, therefore, dosing should be adjusted and titrated to effect. If fentanyl patch is present, it should be removed prior to the induction as the absorption may vary significantly depending on peripheral perfusion and skin temperature. In acute intoxication, on the other hand, opioid analgesics should be given very cautiously, and potential prolonged effect of illicit substances should be taken in consideration. Acute opioid intoxication, whether on its own or with possible ingestion of other psychoactive substances, potentiates other anesthetic agents (both volatile and IV), and hence, dose should be carefully titrated to effect. In addition to above, variability of illicit formulations; active metabolites; may complicate an already challenging to manage case.

41.3.6.5 Postoperative Management

Postoperative management presents several challenges. Acutely intoxicated patients are at risk of delayed emergence, prolonged mechanical ventilation, significant PONV and aspiration, and AMS. Duration and settings (i.e., PACU vs ICU) should be considered in postoperative planning.

In patients who chronically use opioids, there is a high potential for withdrawal. Typically, withdrawal onset is 6–24 h after cessation. Classic opioid withdrawal presents with uncontrolled severe pain, tachycardia, chills, shivering, diarrhea, mydriasis, anxiety, sweating, and tremors. Severity can be assessed based on the clinical opioid withdrawal scale [20] and is typically treated with opioid analgesia in the postoperative period. Patient-controlled analgesia modality is frequently utilized, as well as symptomatic and supportive treatment (beta-blockers, antisialagogues, antiemetics, dexmedetomidine, and benzodiazepines). Pain control is a major challenge in postoperative management of patients who are on chronic opioid therapy. It is important to understand that in patients who are chronically opioid dependent, regional analgesia is typically insufficient when used alone, and high doses narcotics may be needed to prevent or alleviate symptoms. Patient-controlled analgesia and multimodal approach (acetaminophen, NSAIDs, gabapentin, ketamine, etc.) in general have good effect in postoperative pain management. Opioid agonists–antagonists, such as nalbuphine, should not be given as they may precipitate withdrawal. In challenging cases, pain or palliative services should be involved to facilitate transition to outpatient regimen of treatment.

41.3.7 Cannabis

According to 2021 World Health Organization, close to 150 million people (over 2.5% of total world population) use cannabis, which makes it the most used illicit substance worldwide [21]. According to CDC, close to 50 million people regularly use marijuana in the United States [22]. Although in United States cannabis is classified as schedule I (not currently accepted medical use and a high potential for abuse), 30 states decriminalized marijuana, and 18 states have allowed retail sale and possession of recreational marijuana (2022 data).

41.3.7.1 Preoperative Assessment

In acute intoxication, patients present with anxiety, confusion, depression, delusions, dulled reflexes, nystagmus, ataxia, tachycardia, increased blood pressure, orthostatic hypotension, conjunctival injection, and dry mouth. Chronic use can produce reactive airway or even pneumothorax and can lead to myocardial depression and, in rare cases, seizures. Cannabis may have a sympathomimetic effect (hence avoid ketamine, atropine, pancuronium, etc.). Severe intoxication is fairly rare and, unless another illicit or recreational substance was used, often presents with mild to moderate symptoms.

As opposed to prior practice, due to wide spread of medicinal use of marijuana, acute cannabis intoxication does not necessarily have to precipitate cancelation of the elective procedure. The decision to proceed with elective surgery in the presence of cannabis intoxication is based on a risk/benefit analysis and is typically left to the discretion of anesthesia and surgical team, with the patients' safety at the center of the decision-making. Current ASA and ASRA research indicates that patients who regularly use cannabinoids are more likely to have myocardial ischemia postoperatively and are more likely to experience worse postoperative pain and PONV compared to nonusers [23, 24].

41.3.7.2 Intraoperative Management

As with other substances of abuse, in emergency settings, patient should be treated as full stomach and need RSI. There are no specific anesthetic agents that are contraindicated or preferred in acute THC intoxication, but any drug should be titrated to effect, to avoid over or underdosing. As with other depressants, cannabis produces increased sensitivity in acute intoxication and increased tolerance in chronic intoxication to the anesthetic agents. Acute THC intoxication may potentiate stimulatory effects of amphetamines and cocaine on one hand and increase depressant effects of alcohol and benzodiazepines on the other. Cardiovascular effects of marijuana are biphasic: Low doses result in sympathetic stimulation with tachycardia and slight hypertension; high doses can inhibit sympathetic activity with unopposed parasympathetic activity leading to bradycardia and hypotension [25].

41.3.7.3 Postoperative Management

Patients acutely intoxicated with THC may experience delayed emergence, delirium, have difficulties with pain control [24]. Withdrawal is rare, and symptoms are very mild. Managements are supportive and symptomatic.

41.4 Stimulants

41.4.1 Cocaine

Cocaine is extracted from the leaves of *Erythroxylon Coca* and produces euphoria by prolongation of dopamine activity in limbic system and cerebral cortex, and it also stimulates sympathoadrenal axis. Pure cocaine was first produced in 1880s and was initially broadly used in eye and nasal surgery as a local anesthetic. According to National Survey on Drug Use and Health, over 5 million of Americans are current cocaine users, and cocaine overdose is one of the leading causes of drug-related ED visits in United States [26].

Onset of action is typically within minutes of use (nasal, IV, smoking, and oral), and duration may be from 30 to 120 min. Symptoms of acute cocaine intoxication include agitation, euphoria, restlessness, mydriasis, and diaphoresis. Toxic effects of the drug are: agitation, seizures or coma, intracranial hemorrhage, hyperthermia, headaches, nausea and vomiting, psychosis, tachycardia, hypertension, cardiac ischemia (due to coronary vasoconstriction and increased myocardial oxygen demand), heart failure, and arrhythmias. When vaporized and smoked, cocaine can cause pharyngeal burns, angioedema, alveolar hemorrhage, pulmonary edema, pneumothorax, and pulmonary infarction. Some other toxic effects include perforative ulcer, bowel ischemia, metabolic acidosis, spleen or kidney infarcts, CK elevation, hyperkalemia, and many more [27]. In long-term users, nasal septum and soft palate atrophy and necrosis may be present. Crack smokers may develop pulmonary hypertension due to crack lung.

In cases of acute intoxication, elective surgery should be postponed until the patient is sober and rescheduled when, ideally, patient stayed abstinent for at least a week. In case of emergent surgery, symptoms of acute cocaine intoxication should be treated accordingly. Agitation and hemodynamic changes are most frequent presentations of acutely intoxicated patients. For agitated patients, benzodiazepines are utilized until agitation is controlled. For uncontrolled hypertension, benzodiazepines and phentolamine are considered treatments of choice. Beta blockade is NOT recommended in hypertension associated with cocaine use, since unopposed alpha-adrenergic stimulation with use of beta-blockers with cocaine may result in coronary vasoconstriction and severe systemic hypertension [28]. For patients who present with myocardial ischemia, nitroglycerine, aspirin, and phentolamine are used. In case of metabolic acidosis with ECG changes present, sodium bicarbonate is recommended for correction of acidemia.

41.4.1.1 Intraoperative Management

RSI is induction method of choice in acutely intoxicated with cocaine patients. Succinylcholine, however, is not recommended for facilitation of endotracheal intubation, since both cocaine and succinylcholine are metabolized by plasma cholinesterase, and cocaine metabolism may be decreased, hence prolonging its toxic effects [26]. During intubation, anesthetesiologist should be aware of potentially reactive airways and possible necrosis of the palate. Preoperative premedication with benzodiazepines is considered safe and beneficial. Invasive blood pressure monitoring is necessary in most cases in order to identify and manage extreme intraoperative hemodynamic swings. Cocaine may cause both, severe hypertension or vasopressor-resistant hypotension. For hypertension management, phentolamine, nitroprusside, and nitroglycerine are most commonly used vasodilators. After the acute intoxication subsides, depletion of adrenergic receptors may precipitate significant hypotension, which, when paired with vasodilatory effects of anesthetics, is very difficult to control. For vasopressor-resistant hypotension, vasopressin is commonly utilized if other agents are ineffective. In hemodynamically stable patients, most anesthetic agents such as propofol, midazolam, etomidate, volatile anesthetics, and nondepolarizing NMB's are considered safe. For mechanical ventilation, especially in patients who smoke cocaine, lung protective modality should be used in order to prevent further lung injury and baro- and volutrauma.

41.4.1.2 Postoperative Management

Most of postoperative complications are associated with cardiovascular system effects and potential withdrawal. The management approach hemodynamic instability is the same as described in preoperative and intraoperative management. Postoperative hemodynamic and cardiac monitoring for 24–48 h is recommended. Cocaine withdrawal typically presents with anxiety, irritability, depression, loss of concentration, fatigue, hypersomnia, and paranoia. Treatment for cocaine withdrawal is mostly supportive. Pharmacologic treatment of withdrawal includes buspirone, ondansetron, and propranolol.

41.4.2 Amphetamines

Include amphetamine, methamphetamine, and dextroamphetamine, which are derivatives of phenethylamine. In clinical practice, amphetamines are used to treat AHDH, narcolepsy, and short-term treatment of obesity. According to the National Institute on Drug Abuse, over 5 million Americans misuse amphetamines and over 1.6 million can be considered chronic methamphetamine users. In 2021, over 32,000 died from overdose of stimulants other than cocaine [29].

The onset of action of amphetamines is fairly fast and, depending on the route of administration, may be from seconds (smoking) to minutes (enteral), and the duration of effect is over 24 h. Clinical presentation of acute amphetamine intoxication is very variable and may span from no symptoms to psychosis, seizures, sympathomimetic crisis, cardiovascular collapse, etc. Most commonly patients are hypertensive, tachycardic, delirious and agitated, hyperthermic, and hyperkalemic and may have kidney failure and metabolic acidosis.

41.4.2.1 Preoperative Assessment

Elective cases should be canceled if patient is found to be acutely intoxicated with amphetamines. In emergent circumstances, BMP and ABG are essential to adequately approach anesthetic management. Rapid UDS to determine other potentially used drugs. Chronic amphetamine users are typically malnourished and may have abrupt changes in behavior and significant mood swings, paranoia. HEENT exam is significant for mydriasis, mucosal injuries and extensive teeth decay, also known as "meth mouth". While acutely intoxicated, majority of patients are hypertensive and tachycardic (may present with various tachyarrhythmias), tachypneic and diaphoretic. Prolonged methamphetamine use can lead to pulmonary hypertension and edema. Amphetamines may induce nausea, vomiting, and diarrhea [30, 31].

41.4.2.2 Intraoperative Management

As in all other cases of acute intoxication, RSI is preferred modality of induction. During intubation, anesthetist should be aware of "meth mouth" and potential dental injury. In general, intraoperatively patient should be approached very similar to the patients who are acutely intoxicate with cocaine. This includes monitoring, hemodynamic instability management, and choice of and anesthetic agents. Contrary to cocaine intoxication, beta-blockade is considered safe in patients who are under influence of amphetamines and can be utilized in severely hypertensive patients. General anesthesia is preferred over regional due to concern about unopposed sympathectomy.

41.4.2.3 Postoperative Management

The main postoperative considerations are post anesthesia delirium, hemodynamic instability, and pulmonary edema/hypertension in patients with preexisting meth lung and withdrawal. As in the case with cocaine, most of the management is symptom-based; however, due to significantly longer duration of amphetamines effects, patients may need ICU admission postoperatively for appropriate monitoring and treatment.

41.4.3 Ecstasy/MDMA

3,4-methylenedioxymethamphetamine is a synthetic drug which is similar to amphetamines and mescaline. Initially was developed as appetite suppressant, now used as a "party drug". Common effects include euphoria, disinhibition, excitement, and intimacy [32].

Common acute intoxication symptoms are agitation, hypertension, tachycardia, and hyperthermia. Extasy intoxication commonly causes hyponatremia, and more rarely patients may present with seizures or even serotonin syndrome. Intoxication may last for over 6 h.

41.4.3.1 Preoperative Management

Elective surgery should be postponed until patient is sober. In emergent cases, ECG, BMP, glycemia, EtOH level, and

UDS screening need to be done. CK levels and LFTs should be assessed prior to surgery if time allows. Preoperatively agitation is usually treated with benzodiazepines. Hyponatremia is caused by excessive water consumption under the influence of MDMA, and, unless symptomatic, should be treated with fluid restriction. If patients develop seizures in the settings of hyponatremia, 3% saline in 100 ml boluses are used (up to 3) until symptom resolution. It is important to monitor for signs of serotonin syndrome (anxiety, disorientation, delirium, diaphoresis, hyperthermia, vomiting, diarrhea, hypertension, tremor, myoclonus, hyperreflexia, and muscle rigidity) [33].

41.4.3.2 Intraoperative Management

Standard RSI is an appropriate method of induction. In hyperthermic patients, antipyretics should NOT be utilized since potential liver toxicity may be precipitated; instead, active cooling and benzodiazepines or cyproheptadine are the treatment of choice [34]. Medications should be titrated to effect. Severe hypertension in MDMA intoxication has a central and peripheral component, the central component resolves with sedation, and the peripheral component can be successfully treated with sodium nitroprusside. Fluid management in most cases should be restrictive, due to hyponatremia described above.

41.4.3.3 Postoperative Management

In cases of moderate and severe toxicity, it is appropriate manage patients postoperatively in the intensive care unit settings, primarily due to concerns for serotonin syndrome, hemodynamic instability, hyponatremia, and potential liver toxicity.

41.4.4 Hallucinogens

Most commonly used hallucinogens include LSD, psylocibin, mescaline, salvia, PCP, ketamine, etc. According to US department of health, approximately 1.7 million people in United States are current hallucinogens users [35]. LSD and psylocibin are prevailing among the users; however, there is growth in popularity of designer and club drugs in recent years.

41.4.4.1 Preoperative Assessment

Symptoms broadly vary depending on the drug and include euphoria, distorted sense of time, out of the body experience, blending of senses, panic reactions, and dysphoria. In some occasions, psychosis may occur. Cardiovascular symptoms are mostly mild and include hypertension and tachycardia. Patients also may have tachypnea and hyperthermia. Less common but more worrisome is the potential for serotonin syndrome which will require management is the ICU settings [34].

In case of elective surgery, case should be canceled or postponed until the hallucinogen effect wears off. In emergent surgery, preoperative treatment is symptomatic and mostly supportive.

41.4.4.2 Intraoperative Management

Approach to mild and moderate intoxication does not vary significantly from conventional anesthetic management of the specific case. In severe intoxication treatment is symptomatic and includes benzodiazepines, antihypertensives, and IV resuscitation. In case of development of serotonin syndrome, treatment includes antihypertensives, benzodiazepines, active cooling, and the antiserotonergic cyproheptadine [36]. Intraoperative management may vary depending on whether patient co-ingested other illicit substances. Patients under influence of hallucinogens may experience delayed emergence or be agitated during emergence.

41.4.4.3 Postoperative Management

Patients under influence of hallucinogens should be recovered in a calm and quiet environment in order to avoid exacerbation of hallucinations. In cases of multiple substance use or moderate and severe symptoms, patients should be monitored for at least 24 h postoperatively. Management is supportive and symptomatic.

41.4.5 Substance Abuse in Anesthesia Providers

The problem of misuse and abuse of various substances is also present among physician anesthesiologists. According to a survey conducted across multiple centers over a 10 year period, the prevalence of substance abuse in anesthesiologists in the United States is 3.7% among residents and 1.16% among faculty. The most commonly abused substances are alcohol, opioids, and propofol. Prevalence of specific substance varies among faculty physicians and residents. In faculty physicians, 50% abuse alcohol, 23.7%—opioids, and 26.3%—all other substances. In residents, prevalence of abused substances is as follows—opioids 39%, propofol 20.3%, and alcohol 15.2% [37]. Other substances of abuse include ketamine, nitrous oxide, volatile agents, and thiopental [38]. In the early 2000s, 80% of anesthesia residencies programs reported problem of resident impairment and 19% reported pretreatment fatalities in residents [39]. Some of the precipitating factors incriminated for the higher prevalence of substance abuse among anesthesia providers access to high quantities of addictive substances, the high stress environment, workplace and interpersonal challenges, and a high burnout rate [40].

41.4.5.1 Etiology

A plethora of theories on origins of substance dependence and abuse exist, and most popular are biochemical, genetic, psychiatric, exposure related, etc. [40]. Despite multiple theories, there is no consensus on which one is the correct one. Since 1956, alcoholism has been considered an illness by American Medical Association, and since 1987 any substance dependence is considered to be an illness [41]. Genetic theory is the result of multiple studies that demonstrated that some genotypes are more predisposed to substance abuse than others [42–44]. Biochemical theory hypothesizes that the release of dopamine in the mesolimbic system of the brain provides strong reinforcements of drug-seeking behaviors, which may be associated with many drugs of abuse [45, 46]. Psychiatric theory suggests that there is a strong association between substance dependence and other psychopathology, and according to some of the studies, 57% of patients with substance abuse disorder also have various psychiatric and personality disorders (there is also a thought that in some cases substance abuse is a form of self-medicating for psychological or psychiatric disorders) [47]. Exposure-related theory is based on presumption that increased risk of addiction for certain subspecialties is related to exposures that sensitize reward pathway to promote substance use (substance abuse may change levels of neurotransmitters required to trigger work pathway) [48].

41.4.5.2 Clinical Presentation

In addition to clinical symptomology described in the first part of the chapter, there are also psychological aspects of substance abuse manifestation. One of the prevalent problems with substance abuse in physicians is a denial of the problem. The denial itself may present a significant obstacle to treatment and rehabilitation. If the physician does not recognize the presence of an issue, the treatment is less likely to be successful [49]. The denial originates from the idea of invulnerability and inability to resist addiction and ultimately lead to loss of autonomy. It is clear now that denial is not just limited to the addicts; coworkers, family, and friends may ignore or often make excuses to not see the issue as well [50].

Specific behavioral patterns are very important in recognition of substance abuse in physicians. Because of unique accessibility to the potential drugs of abuse, behavior that normally would be deemed acceptable may arouse concerns in anesthesia providers. Suspicious activities include: Spending more time in the hospital, even off duty; volunteering for extra call; refusing release for lunch or breaks; wasting higher than normal amounts of narcotics or administration of inappropriate doses of narcotics for a given case; documenting administration higher dosed of narcotics on Fridays; withdrawal from family friends and regular activity; frequent mood swings, with alternating periods of euphoria and depression; episodes of anger, hostility, irritability; weight loss and pale skin [51]. The timeframe for these symptoms to become apparent varies depending on the substance of abuse. Alcohol abuse may take years or even decades to manifest, whereas abuse of short acting opioids, volatile agents, or propofol may become apparent within months of initiation. Addiction may be so powerful that it will alter providers anesthetic management entirely; for instance, in order to save opioids for self, addicted anesthesia providers will chart appropriate or excessive administration of opioids, but in reality may run the entire cases on just volatile anesthetics and beta-blockers [52]. Reports exist of anesthesia providers substituting syringes containing opioids with syringes containing lidocaine and esmolol (and that way diverting substances for personal use); some providers have been noted to search through sharp containers looking for syringes with remaining substances of abuse. In some cases, anesthesia providers with substance dependence were noted to draw out of bags with opioid containing medications in PCAs. Physicians suffering from addictions quickly become proficient in bypassing security measures in automatic drug dispensing machines.

41.4.5.3 Legal Problems

In addition to behavioral and social changes, a variety of legal issues may arise. Potential issues include, but are not limited to fraud, controlled substance diversion, license loss, etc. It is important to understand legal actions that may vastly vary from state to state, specifically in regard to variability in physician record confidentiality, reportability to specialty boards, and maintaining of medical license. Because of the potential legal issues, consultation with legal counsel in most institutions is mandatory. In case of confirmation of substance abuse in physician, depending on the state, physician's license may be suspended or revoked, or even criminal charges may be instituted against the individual. Many states require enrollment of affected physician into rehabilitation programs in order to maintain their license.

The American Board of Anesthesiology requires an active license to practice medicine in at least one of the 50 states and currently does not restrict practice of a physician who is in rehabilitation program if the state the physician practicing in allows that physician to practice medicine while being rehabilitated [53].

41.4.5.4 Treatment

Substance abuse is diagnosed and treated by addiction psychiatrist. Once the diagnosis has been established, the physician has an option to go through treatment and rehabilitation therapy. Most commonly, physicians are referred to an inpatient facility that specializes in the treatment of physicians, and it is thought that such facility may help in developing support from similar group of people [54]. Treatment consists of detoxication, education, monitoring of abstinence, group therapy, and psychotherapy. Typically, the therapy is provided as an inpatient, in order to provide controlled environment and to remove the individual from daily stress. Typically, initial therapy may last between 8 and 12 weeks and 6–12 months. Such therapy may not always be covered by insurance and can cost as much as 3000–5000 $ per week [52]. After discharge from the inpatient setting, patients undergo long (sometimes years) rehabilitation and recovery therapy that may include halfway houses, group therapy, and sobriety monitoring. Depending on severity of addiction and the course of inpatient therapy, most states allow return to practice for recovering physicians, as long as these physicians are supervised by designated organizations. Supervision and monitoring lasts at a minimum for 5 years. During this period, abstinence monitoring is one of the most essential components of the program. Frequent UDS testing is used to monitor sobriety of the patients, although mandated, the cost of testing comes out of pocket and can be as much as 90–150$ per test. In addition to testing, patients with opioid addiction might be required to be on naltrexone, in order to prevent relapsing.

41.4.5.5 Prognosis

Controversy exists about whether anesthesia providers who abused opioids should return to practicing in the OR setting. On one hand, there is a fear that exposure to opioids may lead to relapse, and on the other, attending anesthesiologist might not have many options for employment. Current consensus is that decisions should be made on case-by-case basis. In anesthesiology residents, however, the prevailing recommendation is to retrain to an alternative specialty since the reported relapse rate may be as high as 66% [54]. Factors that increase risk of relapse include use of opioids, family history of drug abuse, and the presence of psychiatric disorder. Faculty anesthesiologists who are allowed to reenter the specialty are frequently required to sign work reentry contracts, which will outline the physician's responsibilities and limitations. In most cases, reentry contract prohibits such physician to work weekends and nights for a certain period of time [55].

Questions

1. What are 2 the most abused substances in the United States?
   - Alcohol and cannabis
   - Cocaine and opioids
   - Alcohol and opioids
   - Benzodiazepines and cannabis
2. Which substances can lead to life threatening withdrawal (select all that apply)?
   - Cocaine
   - Alcohol
   - Opioids
   - Methadone
   - Benzodiazepines
   - Cannabis
   - Methamphetamine
3. Which substances of abuse can potentially lead to life-threatening arrhythmias (select all that apply)?
   - Cannabis
   - Cocaine
   - Alcohol
   - Methadone
   - Benzodiazepines
   - Methamphetamine
4. Which prescription drug makes postoperative pain management especially challenging?
   - Methadone
   - Buprenorphine
   - Hydromorphone
   - Oxycodone
   - Naloxone
5. Which antihypertensive is recommended against use in acute cocaine intoxication?
   - Hydralazine
   - Nicardipine
   - Metoprolol
   - Amlodipine
6. Which electrolyte abnormality is most concerning in acute methylenedioxymethamphetamine intoxication?
   - Hypokalemia
   - Hyperkalemia
   - Hyponatremia
   - Hypernatremia
   - Hypercalcemia
7. What is the most common period of time until onset of EtOH and BZD withdrawal?
   - 12–24 h
   - 24–48 h
   - 3–4 days
   - 5–6 days
8. What is typical duration of acute cocaine intoxication?
   - 10–15 min
   - 30–120 min
   - 2–3 h
   - 4–8 h
9. Which substances decrease MAC in acute intoxication (select all that apply)
   - Alcohol
   - Benzodiazepines
   - Opioids
   - Cocaine

- Methamphetamine
- MDMA

10. Which substances increase MAC in acute intoxication (select all that apply)
    - Alcohol
    - Benzodiazepines
    - Opioids
    - Cocaine
    - Methamphetamine
    - MDMA
11. What is most commonly abused substance by resident anesthesiologists?
    - Propofol
    - Alcohol
    - Opioids
    - Volatile anesthetics
    - Thiopental
    - Ketamine
12. What is most commonly abused substance in attending anesthesiologists?
    - Propofol
    - Alcohol
    - Opioids
    - Volatile anesthetics
    - Thiopental
    - Ketamine
13. Is returning to practicing anesthesiology recommended for anesthesia providers with opioid substance abuse disorder?
    - Yes
    - No
    - Yes, only for anesthesia residents
    - Yes, only for attending anesthesiologists
    - Return to practicing anesthesia should be reviewed on case-by-case basis
14. How long anesthesiologists have to be monitored and screened for relapse after treatment for substance abuse disorder other than opioid abuse?
    - 1 year
    - 2 years
    - 3 years
    - 4 years
    - 5 years
    - 10 years
15. Who pays for inpatient treatment for substance abuse, rehabilitation and UDS testing in anesthetists with substance abuse disorder?
    - Health insurance
    - Hospital where physician works
    - State
    - ABA
    - Out of pocket

Answers

1. A—alcohol and cannabis are the most abused substances in the United States. According to national institute of alcohol abuse and alcoholism, over 55% of United States adults over 18 years of age drink alcohol regularly (once a month or more), over 23% admit binge drinking, and over 8% drink heavily. According to CDC close to 50 million people regularly use marijuana in the United States.
2. Alcohol and benzodiazepines abstinence in dependent individuals may lead to potentially life-threatening withdrawals.
3. Cocaine, methamphetamine, and methadone frequently cause arrhythmias. Cocaine and methamphetamine have arrhythmogenic effect through adrenergic stimulation. Methadone can cause significant QT prolongation and cause torsades de pointes especially when used in combination with other QT-prolonging substances.
4. Buprenorphine is μ-Opioid receptor partial agonist and κ and δ -Opioid receptor antagonist. Due to antagonistic effects, buprenorphine significantly decreases efficacy of other opioids, making managing postoperative pain, especially in moderate and major procedures, very challenging. In patients who undergo major surgeries while on buprenorphine multimodal analgesic approach is especially important.
5. Current recommendations are against use of metoprolol in patients with acute intoxication with cocaine. It is thought that use of β-blockers may cause unopposed α-stimulation and hence severe hypertension.
6. Intoxication with MDMA leads to excessive water consumption, hemodilution, and hyponatremia.
7. Onset of minor alcohol withdrawal symptoms (agitation, tremotrs, sweating, HTN, tachycardia, hyperthermia, and nausea) typically start in 6–12 h. Onset of hallucinosis is 12–24 h. Alcohol and BZD withdrawal seizures start in 24–48 h after cessation. Delirium tremens (hyperactive autonomic activity that may lead to cardiogenic shock) 48–72 h.
8. Duration of acute cocaine intoxication is between 30 and 120 min and depends on the rout of administration of the drug.
9. Alcohol, BZD, and opioids in the settings of acute intoxication decrease MAC.
10. Cocaine, methamphetamine, and MDMA increase MAC in the settings of acute intoxication.
11. Among resident anesthesiologists, opioids are most commonly abused (39% of anesthesia residents with substance abuse disorder were abusing opioids)
12. Among attending anesthesiologists who had substance abuse disorder, 50% were abusing alcohol.

13. Current consensus is that decisions should be made on case-by-case basis. In anesthesia residents, however, the prevailing recommendation is to retrain to alternative specialty as the reported relapse rate may be as high as 66%.
14. Current recommendation is that anesthesiologists with substance abuse disorder should be monitored at least for 5 years. That includes supervised practice and mandatory frequent UDS.
15. Most of the time, cost of the treatment, rehabilitation, and testing comes out of the patient's pocket. Inpatient rehabilitation may last from 8–12 weeks up to a year and costs on average 3000–5000$ per week. UDS can cost 90–150$.

References

1. Dobson GP. Trauma of major surgery: a global problem that is not going away. Int J Surg. 2020;81:47–54.
2. Carrigan TD, et al. Toxicological screening in trauma. Emerg Med J. 2000;17:33–7.
3. Anitescu M. The patient with substance use disorder. Curr Opin Anaesthesiol. 2019;32(3):427–37.
4. Lowenfels AB, Miller TT. Alcohol and trauma. Ann Emerg Med. 1984;13(11):1056–60. [PubMed] [Google Scholar].
5. Tien HC, Tremblay LN, Rizoli SB, et al. Association between alcohol and mortality in patients with severe traumatic head injury. Arch Surg. 2006;141(12):1185–91; discussion 92. [PubMed] [Google Scholar].
6. Chapman R, Plaat F. Alcohol and anaesthesia. Contin Educ Anaesth, Crit Care Pain. 2009;9(1):10–3.
7. National institute of alcohol abuse and alcoholism. https://www.niaaa.nih.gov/alcohols-effects-health/alcohol-topics/alcohol-facts-and-statistics/alcohol-use-united-states
8. Eismann H, et al. Influence of alcohol consumption on blood coagulation in rotational thromboelastometry (ROTEM): an in-vivo study. Korean J Anesthesiol. 2020;73(4):334–41.
9. Franke A, Nakchbandi IA, Schneider A, et al. The effect of ethanol and alcoholic beverages on gastric emptying of solid meals in humans. Alcohol Alcohol. 2005;40(3):187–93.
10. Adams C. Anaesthetic implications of acute and chronic alcohol abuse. S Afr J Anaesthesiol Analg. 2010;16:42–9.
11. Khalil M, et al. Pharmacokinetics and pharmacodynamics of rocuronium in patients with cirrhosis. Anesthesiology. 1994;80 (6):1241–7.
12. UpToDate. https://www.uptodate.com/contents/benzodiazepine-poisoning-and-withdrawal?search=benzodiazepine%20intoxication&source=search_result&selectedTitle=1 ~ 50&usage_type=default&display_rank=1
13. Practice advisory for intraoperative awareness and brain function monitoring: a report by the American society of anesthesiologists task force on intraoperative awareness. Anesthesiology. 2006;104:847–864.
14. Yi F, Xiao H, Zhu T, et al. Prevention of postoperative nausea and vomiting after gynaecological day surgery under remimazolam general anesthesia: a randomized double-blind controlled study. BMC Anesthesiol. 2022;22:292.
15. Ross JE, et al. Midazolam's effect on post operative nausea and vomiting and discharge times in outpatients undergoing cancer related surgery. AANA J. 2019;87(3):179–83.
16. National institute on Drug abuse. Drug overdose statistics. https://nida.nih.gov/research-topics/trends-statistics/overdose-death-rates
17. Florence C, Luo F, Rice K. The economic burden of opioid use disorder and fatal opioid overdose in the United States, 2017. Drug Alcohol Depend. 2021;1(218): 108350.
18. Kintz P. A new series of 13 buprenorphine-related deaths. Clin Biochem. 2002;35(7):513–6.
19. Richards GC, Mahtani KR, Muthee TB, et al. Factors associated with the prescribing of high-dose opioids in primary care: a systematic review and meta-analysis. BMC Med. 2020;18:68.
20. Clinical opioid withdrawal scale. https://nida.nih.gov/sites/default/files/ClinicalOpiateWithdrawalScale.pdf
21. UpToDate. https://www.uptodate.com/contents/cannabis-marijuana-acute-intoxication?search=canabis%20intoxication&source=search_result&selectedTitle=1 ~ 16&usage_type=default&display_rank=1
22. CDC data and statistics. https://www.cdc.gov/marijuana/data-statistics.htm#: ~ :text=Marijuana%20is%20the%20most%20commonly,at%20least%20once%20in%202019
23. Goel A, McGuinness B, Jivraj NK, et al. Cannabis use disorder and perioperative outcomes in major elective surgeries: a retrospective cohort analysis. Anesthesiology. 2020;132(4):625–35.
24. ASRA Pain Medicine. All patients should be screened for cannabis use before surgery. First U.S. Guidelines Recommend; 2023.
25. Huson HB, Granados TM, Rasko Y. Surgical considerations of marijuana use in elective procedures. Heliyon. 2018;4(9): e00779.
26. Center for Behavioral Health Statistics and Quality. Results from the 2019 national survey on drug use and health: detailed tables. Rockville, MD: Substance Abuse and Mental Health Services Administration; Department of Health and Human Services; 2020.
27. UpToDate. https://www.uptodate.com/contents/cocaine-acute-intoxication?search=cocaine%20intoxication&source=search_result&selectedTitle=1 ~ 57&usage_type=default&display_rank=1
28. Richards JR, Garber D, Laurin EG, et al. Treatment of cocaine cardiovascular toxicity: a systematic review. Clin Toxicol (Phila). 2016;54(5):345–64.
29. National Institute on Drug abuse. https://nida.nih.gov/publications/research-reports/methamphetamine/what-scope-methamphetamine-misuse-in-united-states. https://nida.nih.gov/news-events/news-releases/2018/04/five-million-american-adults-misusing-prescription-stimulants
30. Meredith CW, Jaffe C, Ang-Lee K, Saxon AJ. Implications of chronic methamphetamine use: a literature review. Harv Rev Psychiatry 2005;13(3):141–54.
31. McCarthy E, McClain E. Methamphetamine-induced lung injury. Eur J Case Rep Intern Med. 2019;6(6): 001067.
32. Wu LT, Parrott AC, Ringwalt CL, et al. The variety of ecstasy/MDMA users: results from the National epidemiologic survey on alcohol and related conditions. Am J Addict. 2009;18:452–61.
33. UpToDate. https://www.uptodate.com/contents/serotonin-syndrome-serotonin-toxicity?search=mdma%20intoxication&topicRef=302&source=see_link
34. Callaway CW, Clark RF. Hyperthermia in psychostimulant overdose. Ann Emerg Med. 1994;24:68–76.
35. Substance Abuse and Mental Health Services Administration. Key substance use and mental health indicators in the United States: results from the 2020 national survey on drug use and health. Rockville, MD: United States Department of Health and Human Services; 2021.
36. Graudins A, Stearman A, Chan B. Treatment of the serotonin syndrome with cyproheptadine. J Emerg Med 1998;16(4):615–9.
37. Survey Details Substance Abuse Among Anesthesiologists. Anesthesiology News 04/12/2019.

38. Wischmeyer PE, Johnson BR, Wilson JE, Dingmann C, Bachman HM, Roller E, Tran ZV, Henthorn TK. A survey of propofol abuse in academic anesthesia programs. Anesth Analg. 2007;105: 1066–71.
39. Collins GB, McAllister MS, Jensen M, Gooden TA. Chemical dependency treatment outcomes of residents in anesthesiology: results of a survey. Anesth Analg. 2005;101:1457–62.
40. Gold MS, Byars JA, Frost-Pineda K. Occupational exposure and addictions for physicians: case studies and theoretical implications. Psychiatr Clin North Am. 2004;27:745–53.
41. Lettieri DJ. Drug abuse: a review of explanations and models of explanation. In: Stimmel B editor. Alcohol and substance abuse in adolescence. New York: Haworth; 1985, pp. 9–40.
42. Mohn AR, Yao WD, Caron MG. Genetic and genomic approaches to reward and addiction. Neuropharmacology. 2004;47:101–10.
43. Lesch KP. Alcohol dependence and gene x environment interaction in emotion regulation: is serotonin the link? Eur J Pharmacol. 2005;526:113–24.
44. Hiroi N, Agatsuma S. Genetic susceptibility to substance dependence. Mol Psychiatry. 2005;10:336–44.
45. Picciotto MR, Zoli M, Rimondini R, Lena C, Marubio LM, Pich EM, Fuxe K, Changeux JP. Acetylcholine receptors containing the β2 subunit are involved in the reinforcing properties of nicotine. Nature. 1998;391:173–7.
46. Wang JC, Hinrichs AL, Stock H, Budde J, Allen R, Bertelsen S, Kwon JM, Wu W, Dick DM, Rice J, Jones K, Nurnberger JI Jr, Tischfield J, Porjesz B, Edenberg HS, Hesselbrock V, Crowe R, Schuckit M, Begleiter H, Reich T, Goate AM, Bierut LJ. Evidence of common and specific genetic effects: association of the muscarinic acetylcholine receptor M2 (CHRM2) gene with alcohol dependence and major depressive syndrome. Hum Mol Genet. 2004;13:1903–11.
47. Udel MM. Chemical abuse/dependence: physicians' occupational hazard. J Med Assoc Ga. 1984;73:775–8.
48. Sekine Y, Minabe Y, Ouchi Y, Takei N, Iyo M, Nakamura K, Suzuki K, Tsukada H, Okada H, Yoshikawa E, Futatsubashi M, Mori N. Association of dopamine transporter loss in the orbitofrontal and dorsolateral prefrontal cortices with methamphetamine-related psychiatric symptoms. Am J Psychiatry. 2003;160:1699–701.
49. White RK, Kitlowiski EJ. Physicians in recovery. Md Med J. 1998;37:183–9.
50. Silverstein JH, Silva DA, Iberti TJ. Opioid addiction in anesthesiology. Anesthesiology. 1993;79:354–75.
51. Berry AJ, Arnold WP. Chemical dependence in anesthesiologists: what you need to know when you need to know it. Park Ridge, Illinois: American Society of Anesthesiologists Task Force on Chemical Dependence of the Committee on Occupational Health of Operating Room Personnel; 1998 Park Ridge, Illinois, American Society of Anesthesiologists Task Force on Chemical Dependence of the Committee on Occupational Health of Operating Room Personnel.
52. Bryson EO, Silverstein JH, Warner DS, Warner MA. Addiction and substance abuse in anesthesiology. Anesthesiology 2008;109:905–17.
53. Hankes L, Bissell L. Health professionals, substance abuse: a comprehensive textbook. In: Lowinson JH, Ruiz P, Millman RB, editors. Baltimore: Williams & Wilkins; 1992, pp. 897–908.
54. Menk EJ, Baumgarten RK, Kingsley CP. Success of reentry into anesthesiology training programs by residents with a history of substance abuse. JAMA. 1990;263:3060–2.
55. Revocation of ABA certification. ABA News. 2006;19(1):4.

Advance Directives

42

Ashley Miller and Silvia Perez-Protto

Abstract

This chapter highlights the growing importance of advance care planning (ACP) in health care, particularly in pre-anesthesia settings. It discusses the legal framework, prevalence rates, and disparities in ACP completion. Key interventions, such as proactive ACP discussions and strategies to overcome barriers, are explored. Additionally, the chapter emphasizes the role of anesthesiologists in facilitating ACP discussions, ensuring patient preferences are respected, and documenting code status decisions effectively. Overall, it underscores the need for proactive engagement and effective communication to align patient care with their values and preferences.

Keywords

Advance directives • Healthcare power of attorney • Living will • Perioperative code status • Goals of care • Advance care planning

Key Points

1. Advance directives are legal documents that provide written instructions by the person in the eventuality of becoming incapacitated, preserving autonomy in medical decision-making.
2. A healthcare power of attorney also known as a, healthcare proxy, is a type of advance directive in which a person chooses a surrogate decision-maker for healthcare decisions.
3. A living will is a type of advance directive that allows patients to specify the care they would want in the event they become incapacitated and terminally ill.
4. Full code by default may not be goal concordant, nor in the best interest of high-risk surgical patients.
5. Automatic suspension of do-not-resuscitate orders before surgery violates patients' right to self-determination and medical autonomy.
6. Code status changes in the perioperative period should be clearly documented, including the time or event trigger for resuming previous code status.

42.1 Introduction

Advanced care planning has become an increasingly vital component of health care in the past thirty years since the Patient Self Determination Act was enacted in 1991 [1, 2]. This act emphasized the right of the patient to make decisions regarding their medical care and placed responsibility on healthcare institutions to provide patients with information on advance directives [3].

Advance directives are legally binding documents that allow individuals to exercise medical autonomy if deemed incapacitated. This is commonly in the form of a healthcare power of attorney (also called healthcare proxy) and living will. A systematic review published in 2017 found that 36.7% of US adults completed an advance directive document [4]. Prevalence of advance directives is higher in older age, higher education and income, and less frequent among non-white responders [5]. Advance care planning has evolved overtime, shifting from the emphasis on legal documents to the importance of goals of care conversations documentation. In 2017, a large Delphi panel defined advance care planning as "a process that supports adults at

A. Miller
Department of Intensive Care and Resuscitation,
Department of General Anesthesiology, Cleveland Clinic,
Cleveland, OH, USA
e-mail: MILLERA78@ccf.org

S. Perez-Protto (✉)
Department of Intensive Care and Resuscitation,
Department of General Anesthesiology, Cleveland Clinic,
Cleveland, OH, USA
e-mail: perezs2@ccf.org

M. Argalious et al. (eds.), *Basic Sciences in Anesthesia*,
https://doi.org/10.1007/978-3-031-60203-0_42

any age or stage of health in understanding and sharing their personal values, lifegoals, and preferences regarding future medical care. The goal of advance care planning is to help ensure that people receive medical care that is consistent with their values, goals, and preferences during serious and chronic illness." [6] The prevalence of advance care planning has been increasing over time up to 50% among older adults, with only 10–20% having discussed their wishes with clinicians. However, disparities are also seen with a prevalence of only 20% of advance care planning among racial and ethnic minorities, with limited health literacy, LGBTQIA, homeless, and incarcerated populations [7].

42.2 Advanced Care Planning in the Pre-anesthesia Clinic

Preoperative advance care planning involves alternate decision-maker identification by the patient since losing capacity is guaranteed during anesthesia. It is important to encourage patients to share their values with the appointed surrogate, as preparation for the potential need to make decisions on the patient's behalf. In a retrospective chart review, Sinha and collaborators found a prevalence of 16% of patients with advance directives scanned in the electronic medical record after preoperative clinic visits, with a higher prevalence among older patients, and those with congestive heart failure [8].

At Cleveland Clinic, we established a system to proactively approach all patients during the pre-anesthesia visit to help them to complete advance directive documents [9]. The prevalence of documents among patients initially was around 20%, higher in white compared with black patients. After the intervention that included information about advance directives and assistance in completion of the documents, the completion rate increased to 80% regardless of race Fig. 42.1.

Advance care planning preoperatively also includes goals of care conversations for patients that are seriously ill or undergoing high-risk procedures. These conversations are conducted by surgery, anesthesiology or both teams depending on the local culture. Goals of care conversations are voluntary discussions for clinicians to explore how much information the patient wants to receive to adapt how to share prognosis. They are followed by exploration of what matters most to the patient, what are the biggest fears and worries about the future of their health, developing a collaborative care plan [10]. For preoperative advance care planning, the goal of the procedure itself should be clearly stated for the patient and the team as the context to discuss code status during surgery. Unfortunately, conducting advance care planning conversations is not the norm at the pre-anesthesia clinic, and it is debatable among the medical community who is responsible to do so. Ankuda and collaborators studied patterns and predictors of deficiencies in shared decision-making including advance care planning in preoperative patients. Not surprisingly, they found that patients who are not native English speakers or have low educational level have high risk of experiencing incomplete and possible ineffective decision-making process. They were twice as likely to want to talk more about surgery and advance care planning. They are also more anxious about surgery. The study suggests the need for interventions to identify vulnerable populations to address their needs that in turn will decrease health disparities [11, 12].

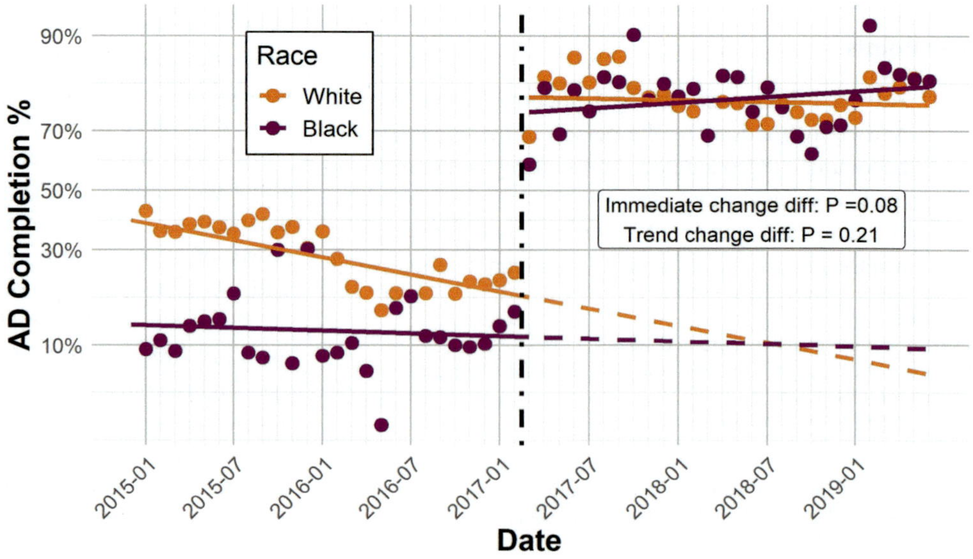

Fig. 42.1 Advance directives at Cleveland Clinic Pre-anesthesia Clinic. Trends by race

Surgeons and anesthesiologists predominantly discuss technical and logistical aspects of the surgery, sparing discussions about values, preferences, long-term postoperative risks, and quality of life [13]. In a recent study to quantify the frequency of preoperative advance care planning discussion and documentation for older patients undergoing major surgery found that only 6% included the goas of care discussion. The investigators conducted a post-surgical survey in a subset of patients who experienced significant postoperative complications reporting feeling unprepared for serious complications [14]. There are multiple barriers for perioperative communication such as lack of time during preoperative visits or on the day of surgery, inadequate training to conduct difficult conversations, fear of "taking away hope" for recovery, among others [15]. It has been also described that surgeons have an implied covenant with the patient once consented for surgery to endure every treatment to avoid death [16]. Cooper and collaborators conducted small pilot study applying structured conversations to facilitate advance care planning discussions to overcome these barriers. Most of the patients enrolled would recommend the conversation and felt less worried about surgery; however, the low recruitment for the study suggests the difficulties of implementation. Grimaldo and collaborators conducted a randomized controlled trial offering a 10-min informative session by an anesthesiologist about advance directives and the importance of communication between patients and their designated proxies regarding end-of-life care as well as information regarding life-sustaining therapies. The intervention significantly increased in advance directives completion as well as discussions between patients and their surrogates [17]. Interprofessional approach could offer an opportunity to improve perioperative goals of care conversations with involvement of geriatricians or palliative care providers for specific patient populations. Other innovative options to promote advance care planning preoperatively are video-based decision aids that may increase education about treatment options, as well as paper-based decision aids that may increase document completion [18]. It is uncommon for surgeons to discuss prolonged life support with patients undergoing high-risk surgeries. It is particularly important to establish realistic expectations for the postoperative intensive care period as well as to promote sharing goals with surrogates. Video-aids may offer standardized information delivery as a complement to the discussion with their clinicians [19].

As a summary, the pre-anesthesia visit is an opportunity to conduct advance care planning including identification of the alternate decision-maker of the patient, encouraging adults to complete advance directives documents. Coaching patients to share their values and wishes with their appointed agent helps patients to keep their autonomy while they are incapacitated. Conducting goals of care conversations with seriously ill patients or those undergoing high-risk surgery completes the advance care planning process, including setting expectations for postoperative care and quality of life. Implementation of such conversations is challenging and entails multi-professional coordination.

42.3 Preoperative Code Status Approach

The approach to code status is one of the items to consider in the plan of care before surgery, including when it is indicated to elicit treatment preferences related to cardiopulmonary resuscitation.

In general, full code by default is assumed for all patients that do not have a do-not-resuscitate (DNR) order. However, default options are only appropriate if they preserve patient's autonomy by allowing individuals to deviate from the norm without barriers, and promoting the best interest of most patients affected. Default options are discouraged when no single decision is clearly optimal for the majority of the patients. Allen and collaborators established a protocol to guide clinicians when it is appropriate to assume a full code by default versus conduct a code status discussion during preoperative evaluation. This proposed protocol takes into consideration the physical status of the individual and the effect that this may have not only on postoperative outcomes, but also on long-term outcomes after cardiopulmonary resuscitation. Based on mortality prediction authors recommend conducting code status discussion preoperatively in patients older than 75 years of age (especially those older than 85), those with functional impairment or frailty, and American Society of Anesthesiologists Physical Status 4 or greater [20]. This approach is in concordance with recently implemented standards in geriatric surgery by the American College of Surgeons [21]. At a minimum, this vulnerable patient group must be informed of the default code status being full attempt at resuscitation and be offered an explanation of the risks and benefits of cardiopulmonary resuscitation. Discussion should take place with the patient, or surrogate decision-maker in case the patient is incapacitated by the anesthesiologist, in collaboration with the surgeon if possible. Preferences for other life-sustaining therapies such as mechanical ventilation, feeding tubes, hemodialysis, and blood transfusions are guaranteed, when intensive care admission is planned for postoperative care [21]. In an emergency, goals of care and resuscitation preference discussion may not be feasible in which case full code by default remains appropriate. Documentation of an unsuccessful attempt to establish a code status is recommended.

The American Society of Anesthesiologists published guidelines in 1993 pertaining to the practice of automatic suspension of a DNR order in patients undergoing surgery. This practice was deemed to go against patients' autonomy in medical decision-making. Burkle and collaborators found that 30% of anesthesiologists, surgeons, and internists surveyed believed that DNR orders should automatically be suspended intraoperatively, while 92% of the patients believed a discussion should occur [22]. The ethical guidelines for the anesthesia care of patients with DNR orders by the American Society of Anesthesiologists provide three alternatives: (a) full attempt at resuscitation, (b) limited attempt at resuscitation with regard to specific resuscitative procedures like chest compressions or defibrillation, and (c) limited attempt at resuscitation defined with regard to the patient's goals and values allowing the anesthesiologist to use clinical judgment. It also states the need for documentation and inclusion of other physicians involved in the care [23]. The American College of Surgeons statement requires surgeons to reconsider advance directives and DNR orders before surgery, to document and convey the information to the rest of the operating room team, and to find an alternate team member to replace an individual who has an ethical or professional conflict with the decision [24]. The Association of Perioperative Registered Nurses also published guidelines revised in 2020 including the need for goals of care discussion and reconsideration of DNR orders as an integral component of the care of surgical patients [25].

It is recommended for anesthesiologist to conduct goals of care discussion with the patient or surrogate decision-maker if patient is incapacitated detailing the type of anesthesia, what is routinely involved, and the anticipated potential complications. For example, if the patient has a do-not-intubate order but would like to proceed with a type of surgery that necessitates general anesthesia, it is essential to offer information about the airway approach for the procedure and alternative options. In addition to the type of anesthesia and surgical procedure, it is vital to consider the patient's health status to share prognosis and possible clinical postoperative course. It is of benefit to have the patient's surgeon and primary care provider participate, if able. When patients or their surrogates request to fully suspend DNR orders, it is of utmost importance to clearly document the discussion and elucidate at what point in the patient's care the suspension will end. Often, this occurs when the patient recovers from anesthesia and is discharged from the post-anesthesia care unit, although it may be reasonable to consider waiting until certain postoperative events occur. Some patients may choose to place intraoperative limitations on resuscitative measures. A valid option is for the patient to allow the perioperative team to use clinical judgment in resuscitative efforts guided by understanding of the patient's wishes. An example of this would be treating an easily reversible condition caused by the effects of anesthesia, however, not to embark in prolonged resuscitation efforts. As with any perioperative change in code status, the details must be documented with the timeline of reinstating the previous code status. Maintaining a DNR order throughout surgery is also an option for patients with the understanding that the type of procedures and anesthetics may be limited within those constraints. Again, clear communication to assure understanding is important, as is documentation.

42.4 Conclusion

Emphasis on advance care planning has grown since the early 1990s. There is growing opportunity for anesthesiologists in the pre-anesthesia clinic and on pre-anesthesia evaluation to ensure that patients receive goal concordant care. Anesthesiologists have an obligation, in conjunction with the surgeon or proceduralist, to review existing advance directives, establish who the patient's surrogate is, and discuss goals of care including alternatives to intraoperative full attempt at resuscitation for seriously ill patients. In the event that a patient wishes to proceed with surgery with code status limitations, it should be clearly documented along with the anticipated timing of reinstatement, and everyone present in the operating room should be made aware.

Questions

1. Which of the following patients should you explore and document the legal decision-maker in the pre-anesthesia clinic?
   a. 87-year-old female with history of atrial fibrillation undergoing a total knee arthroplasty
   b. 19-year-old male with history of cystic fibrosis undergoing endoscopic retrograde cholangiopancreatography (ERCP)
   c. 34-year-old female with history of anemia undergoing cesarean section at term.
   d. All the above
2. An elderly appearing male presents to the emergency department after a motor vehicle collision. He is hemodynamically unstable, and the trauma surgeon prepares the operating room for an emergent exploratory laparotomy. What is the most appropriate approach to code status?
   a. Do not resuscitate
   b. Review prior code status
   c. Limited attempt at resuscitation
   d. Full code by default
3. Which of the following patient demographics is most likely to be associated to have advance directive documents completed?
   a. Black race
   b. Highly educated

c. Latino ethnicity
d. Low income

4. What is the least appropriate course of action when a patient presents for elective surgery with a pre-existing do-not-resuscitate order?
   a. Discuss code status with patient, surrogate, and surgeon
   b. Discuss code status with surgeon
   c. Proceed with surgery without code status discussion
   d. Share with the patient the probability of cardiac arrest during surgery
5. Which of the following is a type of advance directive?
   a. Do-not-resuscitate order
   b. Living will
   c. Healthcare power of attorney
   d. All the above
   e. B and C
6. A 76-year-old female with history of severe aortic stenosis, hypertension, and chronic kidney disease presents to the pre-anesthesia clinic prior to scheduled transcatheter aortic valve replacement. She has a pre-existing do-not-resuscitate order. After discussion, she wishes to suspend this code status for surgery and opts for full attempt at resuscitation. When should her code status return to DNR?
   a. When she leaves the operating room
   b. When she leaves the post-anesthesia care unit
   c. When she chooses based on discussion regarding suspension of the do-not-resuscitate
   d. When she is discharged from the hospital
7. The anesthesiologist on duty has an ethical conflict with providing anesthesia for a patient requiring emergency surgery and wishing to maintain do-not-resuscitate order during surgery. What is the most appropriate action?
   a. Proceed with surgery keeping the do-not-resuscitate order while awaiting relief from another anesthesiologist
   b. Refuse to provide anesthesia
   c. Change code status to full code
   d. Delay surgery until another anesthesiologist is available
8. A patient must be full code to proceed with general anesthesia
   a. True
   b. False

Answers

1. D—All the above is the best choice. All patients have the right to choose their decision-maker for health care, considering that not always the person chosen by the patient is the one per State Law hierarchy. It is responsibility of the anesthesiologist, who will induce the patient into a status of incapacity during general anesthesia, to explore who the patient wants to make healthcare decisions.
2. D—Full code by default is correct. In medical emergencies, consent is implied based on patient's best interest. Since this is a medical emergency, there is no sufficient time to review previous code status (which may or may not be up-to-date) and identify a surrogate decision-maker to discuss what the patient would want.
3. B—Higher education and higher income populations are more likely to have completed an advance directive. Moreover, advance directives are more prevalent in white people comparing with other races and Latino population.
4. C—Proceed without discussion of code status is the least appropriate option. It goes directly against the patient's right to autonomy in medical decision-making. The best course of action is to discuss goals of care with patient or his/her legal representative for healthcare decisions if the patient does not have capacity, including the surgeon or proceduralist. This discussion also includes sharing information about the probability of a cardiac arrest happening during surgery, risks and benefits of resuscitation, and offering different options to approach code status during and after surgery.
5. E—Living will, and healthcare power of attorney are both a type of advance directive. They are documents signed by the person or principal stating preferences of future medical care. Do-not-resuscitate is a medical order, signed by the physician or advance medical provider. Do-not-resuscitate orders are not advance directives, because they do not require the signature of the patient.
6. C—The discussion between the anesthesiologists, surgeon and/or proceduralist and the patient guides the decision about the timing of reinstating code status limitation after suspension for surgery. This may be time or event triggered.
7. A—Proceed with surgery in the case of an emergency honoring patient's wishes. Ideally, relief is arranged and occurs during the surgery. In the case of an elective procedure, replacement with another anesthesiologist without ethical conflicts may be arranged beforehand.
8. B—False. Patients with pre-existing do-not-resuscitate orders may choose to continue with that order through the perioperative period, or alter particular limitations based on goals of care discussion with healthcare providers.

References

1. Galambos CM. Preserving end-of-life autonomy: the patient self-determination act and the uniform health care decisions act. Health Soc Work. 1998;23(4):275–81.
2. Tinetti ME. The retreat from advanced care planning. JAMA. 2012;307(9):915–6. https://doi.org/10.1001/jama.2012.229.
3. La Puma J, Orentlicher D, Moss RJ. Advance directives on admission. Clinical implications and analysis of the patient self-determination act of 1990. JAMA. 1991;266(3):402–5. https://doi.org/10.1001/jama.266.3.402
4. Yadav KN, Gabler NB, Cooney E, Kent S, Kim J, Herbst N, et al. Approximately one in three US adults completes any type of advance directive for end-of-life care. Health Aff (Millwood). 2017;36(7):1244–51. https://doi.org/10.1377/hlthaff.2017.0175.
5. Rao JK, Anderson LA, Lin FC, Laux JP. Completion of advance directives among U.S. consumers. Am J Prev Med. 2014;46 (1):65–70. https://doi.org/10.1016/j.amepre.2013.09.008
6. Sudore RL, Lum HD, You JJ, Hanson LC, Meier DE, Pantilat SZ, et al. Defining advance care planning for adults: a consensus definition from a multidisciplinary Delphi panel. J Pain Symptom Manage. 2017;53(5):821–32 e1. https://doi.org/10.1016/j.jpainsymman.2016.12.331
7. McMahan RD, Tellez I, Sudore RL. Deconstructing the complexities of advance care planning outcomes: what do we know and where do we go? A scoping review. J Am Geriatr Soc. 2021;69 (1):234–44. https://doi.org/10.1111/jgs.16801.
8. Sinha S, Gruber RN, Cottingham AH, Nation B, Lane KA, Bo N, et al. Advance care planning in a preoperative clinic: a retrospective chart review. J Gen Intern Med. 2019. https://doi.org/10.1007/s11606-018-4744-8.
9. Perez-Protto SE, Rowbottom JR, Taylor MA. Wishes unknown": a case report. A A Pract. 2019;13(5):188–9. https://doi.org/10.1213/XAA.0000000000001030.
10. Bernacki RE, Block SD, American College of Physicians High Value Care Task F. Communication about serious illness care goals: a review and synthesis of best practices. JAMA Intern Med. 2014;174(12):1994–2003. https://doi.org/10.1001/jamainternmed.2014.5271
11. Ankuda CK, Block SD, Cooper Z, Correll DJ, Hepner DL, Lasic M, et al. Measuring critical deficits in shared decision making before elective surgery. Patient Educ Couns. 2014;94(3):328–33. https://doi.org/10.1016/j.pec.2013.11.013.
12. Allen MB, Siddiqui S, Nwokolo O, Kuza CM, Sadovnikoff N, Mann DG, Souter MJ. Reviewing ethical guidelines for the care of patients with do-not-resuscitate orders after 30 years: rethinking our approach at a time of transition. Anesthesiol. 2024;141(3):584–97.
13. Yefimova M, Aslakson RA. Preoperative conversations about postoperative risks, outcomes, and quality of life-time to start thinking outside the box. JAMA Netw Open. 2020;3(11):e2024048. https://doi.org/10.1001/jamanetworkopen.2020.24048.
14. Kalbfell E, Kata A, Buffington AS, Marka N, Brasel KJ, Mosenthal AC, et al. Frequency of preoperative advance care planning for older adults undergoing high-risk surgery: a secondary analysis of a randomized clinical trial. JAMA Surg. 2021;156(7): e211521. https://doi.org/10.1001/jamasurg.2021.1521.
15. Cooper Z, Corso K, Bernacki R, Bader A, Gawande A, Block S. Conversations about treatment preferences before high-risk surgery: a pilot study in the preoperative testing center. J Palliat Med. 2014;17(6):701–7. https://doi.org/10.1089/jpm.2013.0311.
16. Cassell J, Buchman TG, Streat S, Stewart RM, Buchman TG. Surgeons, intensivists, and the covenant of care: administrative models and values affecting care at the end of life. Crit Care Med. 2003;31(4):1263–70. https://doi.org/10.1097/01.CCM.0000059318.96393.14.
17. Grimaldo DA, Wiener-Kronish JP, Jurson T, Shaughnessy TE, Curtis JR, Liu LL. A randomized, controlled trial of advanced care planning discussions during preoperative evaluations. Anesthesiology. 2001;95(1):43–50; discussion 5A.
18. Aslakson RA, Schuster AL, Reardon J, Lynch T, Suarez-Cuervo C, Miller JA, et al. Promoting perioperative advance care planning: a systematic review of advance care planning decision aids. J Comp Eff Res. 2015;4(6):615–50. https://doi.org/10.2217/cer.15.43.
19. Aslakson RA, Isenberg SR, Crossnohere NL, Conca-Cheng AM, Moore M, Bhamidipati A, et al. Integrating advance care planning videos into surgical oncologic care: a randomized clinical trial. J Palliat Med. 2019;22(7):764–72. https://doi.org/10.1089/jpm.2018.0209.
20. Allen MB, Bernacki RE, Gewertz BL, Cooper Z, Abrams JL, Peetz AB, et al. Beyond the do-not-resuscitate order: an expanded approach to decision-making regarding cardiopulmonary resuscitation in older surgical patients. Anesthesiology. 2021;135(5):781–7. https://doi.org/10.1097/ALN.0000000000003937.
21. A Quality Program of the American College of Surgeons. Optimal resources for Geriatric Surgery; 2019.
22. Burkle CM, Swetz KM, Armstrong MH, Keegan MT. Patient and doctor attitudes and beliefs concerning perioperative do not resuscitate orders: anesthesiologists' growing compliance with patient autonomy and self determination guidelines. BMC Anesthesiol. 2013;13:2. https://doi.org/10.1186/1471-2253-13-2.
23. Ethical guidelines for the anesthesia care of patients with do-not-resuscitate orders or other directives that limit treatment; 2018.
24. Statement on advance directives by patients: "Do Not Resuscitate" in the operating room; 2014.
25. AORN position statement on perioperative care of patients with do-not-resuscitate or allow-natural-death orders; 2019.

Informed Consent

43

Joe Salloum and Piyush Mathur

Abstract

This chapter delves into the considerations surrounding informed consent in anesthesiology practice, emphasizing its legal, ethical, and clinical dimensions. It underscores the necessity of informed consent, especially in anesthesiology, where procedures carry unique risks separate from surgery itself. Key points include the need for thorough verbal discussions and written documentation, addressing do-not-resuscitate orders in the perioperative period, navigating pediatric anesthesia consent with surrogate decision-makers, and the complexities of obstetric anesthesia consent. The chapter also highlights the importance of informed consent in research, aligning with principles outlined in the Belmont Report. Overall, the chapter emphasizes that informed consent should extend beyond a mere signature, embodying comprehensive discussions that respect patient autonomy and safeguard against potential risks.

Keywords

Informed consent • Anesthesiology • Do-not-resuscitate orders • Perioperative period • Surrogate decision makers • Belmont Report • Ethical principles • Autonomy • Electronic consent • Clinical care • Consent process

43.1 Introduction

While the principle of informed consent has been an important consideration in the practice of anesthesiology for the past few decades, there continues to be dialogue on how to best apply informed consent for various clinical situations. Of note, anesthesiology involves a plethora of procedures and medical interventions with varying degrees of invasiveness and risk to patients. These procedures include but are not limited to tracheal intubations, invasive lines, peripheral nerve blocks, neuraxial procedures, and blood transfusions. The induction and maintenance of a general or regional anesthetic in itself carries significant risks including pulmonary aspiration, cerebral vascular accident, myocardial infarction, cardiac arrest, and death. While anesthesia is required to facilitate essential surgical procedures, a proper informed consent regarding anesthetic-specific risks is essential to maintain a patient's medical autonomy. The application of informed consent for anesthesia varies greatly between countries and medical institutions, and special considerations need to be applied for specific patient populations.

J. Salloum · P. Mathur (✉)
Divisions of General Anesthesiology and ICR,
Department of Anesthesiology, Cleveland, OH, USA
e-mail: mathurp@ccf.org

Key Points

- Anesthesiology involves a plethora of procedures and medical interventions with varying degrees of invasiveness and risk to patients.
- Informed consent must be treated as both a legal obligation by the anesthesiologist and involve both a verbal discussion and written documentation.
- Do-not-resuscitate orders do not usually specify a patient's consent for resuscitative measures that are routine for anesthesia including endotracheal intubation.
- It is important for the anesthesia team to specifically address a patient's desire to conditionally suspend certain aspects of a do-not-resuscitate order for the perioperative period.
- The anesthesia team should communicate that cardiac arrests encountered perioperatively are usually caused by reversible causes with better chances at resuscitation and give the patient the option to withhold or initiate CPR in such scenarios.
- In pediatric anesthesiology, parents or legal guardians function as surrogates to provide consent to patients who

M. Argalious et al. (eds.), *Basic Sciences in Anesthesia*,
https://doi.org/10.1007/978-3-031-60203-0_43

are not considered autonomous due to age and limited cognitive development.
- There remain few guidelines on situations where a child refuses a procedure that parents had consented to. Clinician should ascertain the relative necessity of the procedure and patient's age and understanding of the situation.
- Anesthesiologists should communicate risks to both mother and fetus when discussing anesthetic plans to obstetric patients. Most states allow pregnant minors to provide consent for procedures involving their pregnancy
- It is recommended to obtain a written consent for regional anesthesia, as with other forms of anesthesia. Providers should include major complications, albeit rare, as part of their discussion.
- Informed consent for research should include information on research procedures, potential risks, potential benefits, right to decline to participate, assurance on confidentiality, and compensation for participating.

43.2 The History of Informed Consent

Although the topic of medical ethics has been discussed thoroughly over the past several centuries, the concept of informed consent is a relatively new construct. Popular documents on medical ethics in history, including Thomas Percival's *Medical Ethics* (1803) [1] and Hippocrates' writings (fourth century B.C.) focused primarily on avoiding "upsetting" medical disclosures to patients as opposed to the current standard of informing and respecting a patient's autonomy to make their own medical decisions [2]. Over the past few decades, a few key court cases laid the legal foundation of informed consent. *Salgo v. Leland Stanford Jr. University Board of Trustees* (1957) established that providers have a duty to explain the risks and alternatives of a given treatment [3]. The court of this trial placed a particular emphasis on obtaining an "adequately informed" consent. Then in 1972, three court cases further established informed consent as law: *Wilkinson v Vesey*, *Canterbury v. Spence*, and *Cobb v. Grant* [4]. These rulings further emphasized the importance of patients having adequate information and understanding as a prerequisite to giving consent. In the years following these 1972 court cases, there grew an established belief that researchers and physicians have a moral and legal obligation to obtain consent for certain procedures [2].

43.3 The Principles of Informed Consent

Principles of informed consent in health care include the following [5]:

1. Assessment of the patient or surrogate's understanding of pertinent medical information.
2. Discuss possible management options for the disease including implications of treatment or not and possible complications.
3. Documentation of the discussion related to informed consent.

43.4 Informed Consent in Anesthesiology

As the practice of anesthesiology carries its own unique risks apart from surgery, it is imperative for anesthesia providers to ensure informed consent is obtained prior to proceeding with a procedure. Currently, hospital policies in the United States differ on whether there needs to be a separate surgical and anesthetic consent done. At many medical centers, consent for anesthesia and its associated procedures is implied under the surgical consent obtained from a proceduralist. However, as surgeons and proceduralists usually do not have specialized training in anesthesia, they may not be able to adequately inform a patient of all the risks, benefits, and alternatives that are unique to anesthesiology [5].

It is important to note that the anesthetic risks and benefits can vastly vary from patient to patient based on their medical comorbidities. As highlighted by Marcucci et al., there are even situations in which a patient may be able to provide consent for a surgical procedure but is unable to provide consent for anesthesia due to cognitive limitations [6]. In one legal case involving lack of informed consent, a patient undergoing general anesthesia for exploratory laparotomy filed a claim against an anesthesiologist after experiencing cardiac arrest with physical and cognitive sequelae from failure to establish an airway after induction [7]. In this case, the patient signed a surgery informed consent form but was not given an explanation of the risks and alternatives of general anesthesia by the anesthesiologist. Initially, the court dismissed the claim, but the decision was later reversed by a superior court because they ruled a "reasonably prudent person" in the patient's position could have made the decision for an alternative form of anesthesia (regional, local, or no anesthesia) if presented with the risks and benefits of general anesthesia [7]. In summary, informed consent should be treated as both a legal and ethical obligation by the anesthesiologist and involve both a verbal discussion and written documentation.

43.5 Do-Not-Resuscitate Orders in the Perioperative Period

General anesthesia, by its nature, creates temporary and reversible hemodynamic changes such as respiratory depression and hypotension. These changes along with the hemodynamic effects of procedures necessitate invasive procedures and resuscitative measures. Do-not-resuscitate orders do not usually specify a patient's consent for these resuscitative measures during perioperative events. For this reason, it is important for the anesthesia team to specifically address the patient's desire to temporarily suspend certain aspects of the do-not-resuscitate order during the perioperative period. Otherwise, certain procedures, many that are palliative in nature for terminally ill DNR patients, cannot be done without the ability of the anesthesia team to respond to the expected hemodynamic changes of the anesthetic and procedure.

A landmark paper by Dr. Robert Truog specifically addressed whether patients with DNR orders should be resuscitated if they suffer cardiac arrest while under anesthesia [8]. Dr. Truog notes that cardiac arrests suffered intraoperatively are usually related to reversible causes (e.g., pneumothorax from a procedure) that are more amenable to CPR and resuscitative measures than cardiac arrests suffered spontaneously on the ward or ICU. For this reason, he recommends that medical teams have a detailed discussion with their patients regarding the possibility and reversibility of cardiac arrest during a procedure. In addition, Dr. Truog calls attention to the unpredictability of pulmonary recovery after a procedure and the need to communicate the possibility of continued invasive mechanical ventilation in the days following a procedure [8]. He specifically recommends creating a preoperative plan with patients to continue mechanical ventilation for as long as the patient shows continued improvement in pulmonary function with the option to later withdraw care if clinical improvement is not seen. In a separate publication in 1999, Dr. Truog advocated for a goal-directed approach to reconciling DNR orders as opposed to a focus on individual procedures [9]. In this approach, the decision of what procedures need to be performed during intraoperative events is left to the judgment of the clinician with the guidance of the patient's established values and goals. No matter the approach, it is the anesthesiologist's duty to thoroughly discuss and document a patient's consent for procedures during the perioperative period that may otherwise conflict with a preexisting DNR order.

43.6 Informed Consent in Pediatric Anesthesiology

Informed consent for pediatric anesthesiology has its own unique considerations as it involves surrogate decision-makers. In the case of pediatric anesthesia, parents or legal guardians function as surrogates to provide consent for the patient, who are not considered autonomous agents due to their age and limited cognitive development. As with consent for an adult patient, the consent for a pediatric patient should include a description of the anesthesia plan, the benefits, risks, and alternatives. One cross-sectional observational study at a tertiary pediatric hospital involving 97 discussions with 41 different anesthesia providers found that 70% of the discussions included a description of the plan, mention of risks, and mention of benefits, but only 18% of the discussions included the solicitation of a decision by the parents [10]. A unique scenario arises when a child refuses a procedure which their parent has consented to. One survey from 453 anesthesiologists by Lewis et al. revealed 45% of clinicians had canceled a case due to child refusal in their career and that 12 years of age was the median age at which respondents would respect a child's desire to cancel a procedure [11]. The AAP suggests that children can give or refuse informed assent for a treatment "when appropriate"; however, there remain few guidelines on situations where a minor refuses assent for a surgery (especially for elective procedures) [12]. When determining whether to respect a child's refusal of anesthesia for a surgical procedure, clinicians should ascertain the relative consequences of forgoing a treatment and the patient's level of understanding of this consequence.

43.7 Informed Consent in Obstetric Anesthesiology

Obstetric anesthesiology poses its own unique consent challenges including the care of pregnant minors, the capacity for a parturient to give consent during active labor, and the maternal–fetal balance. With regards to capacity to give consent during active labor, there is a concern that the stress and pain of labor may distract a woman from being an active participant in the decision-making process. While an imperfect marker for the capacity to give consent, the ability to recall details of the consent at a later time is tied to patient comprehension. Research shows that level of education, age, previous epidural experience, pain level, and opioid premedication do not improve recall [13]. Also of note, women in labor were found to recall information as well as other patient populations: 37% recalling at least three risks for epidural analgesia, 66% recalling two risks, and 87% recalling one risk [14]. Another important consideration with obstetric patients is the balance of respecting maternal autonomy as well as fetal rights. As court decisions regarding reproductive rights are dynamic in nature and vary from state to state, clinicians should try to say informed on how legal implications may affect the care they provide. Anesthesiologists should continue to communicate the risks to both mother and fetus for various anesthetic plans, especially the risk of general versus regional anesthetics. After communicating these risks and alternatives, clinicians need to defer to the parturient's autonomy on making these decisions. With regards to pregnant minors, most states allow the patient to provide consent to procedures involving her pregnancy [13]. In states where a legal guardian is required to give consent, clinicians should still strive to attain assent from the minor.

43.8 Informed Consent for Regional Anesthesia

Despite an increase in adoption of regional anesthesia techniques, the risk of a major complication which usually guides the informed consent is low (1:10,000–1:100,000) [15]. These major risks include spinal hematoma, peripheral neuropathy, paralysis, seizures, respiratory failure, cardiac arrest, and death. These risks have been analyzed globally including in a study of American Society of Regional Anesthesia and Pain Medicine (ASRA) members in USA and through the The Third National Audit Project (NAP-3) from the UK [16, 17].

Most of the anesthesiology societies such as the American Society of Anesthesiologists, the Canadian Anesthesiologists Society, American Association of Nurse Anesthetists, and the Association of Anaesthetists of Great Britain and Ireland suggest that pertinent elements of the informed consent discussion should be documented by the physician on the patient's chart based on prior legal actions [16]. Despite the patients wanting to know the major risks, surveys such as those by ASRA have found that these are much less likely to be discussed compared to minor temporary risks such as headache, local pain, and infection [16].

A descriptive approach to informing the patients of the risk incidence is consistent with what many practitioners commonly use when obtaining informed consent for regional anesthesia [16]. It is recommended that at least some form of written documentation, whether using patient signed form or physician documentation alone should be performed in every case. Many have also recommended that detailed description of risks and benefits is provided in a written form to the patient (e.g., pamphlets) or documented with language well understood by the patients [18].

43.9 Informed Consent for Research

Similar to the rationale of informed consent for clinical care delivery, informed consent acts as a safeguard for potential research. Potential research participants need to be informed about the research procedures; the potential risks, possible benefits; autonomy or right to decline to participate or withdraw without being penalized following agreement to participate; assurance on confidentiality issues; reimbursement, compensation and incentives for participating; and the contact information of the researchers should the participant have any concerns about the study [19].

The Belmont Report attempts to summarize the basic ethical principles identified by the National Commission for the Protection of Human Subjects of Biomedical and Behavioral Research Commission for conducting research that involve human participants and expounds guidelines to assure these principles are to be abided throughout the research process [20]. The basic ethical principles summarized in this report include respect for persons, beneficence, and justice to the human research participants.

Based on the principles provided by the Belmont Report, information regarding the proposed research is generally disclosed through a participant information sheet coupled with the participant's written informed consent document or more recently through electronic consent process before participating in the study. In general, the use of electronic informed consent has been associated with increased comprehension among the research participants and hence enhanced beneficence [21].

43.10 Conclusion

Adequate consent for anesthesia remains essential given the significant risks and possible alternatives to a given anesthetic plan. Aside from the legal foundation of informed consent, clinicians should always consider the ethical basis of the consenting process, especially beneficence, non-maleficence, and autonomy. To respect the rights of a patient, an adequate consent should go well beyond a signed document to involve a thorough discussion with a qualified clinician. While the consent for anesthesia is often implied in the procedural consent, anesthesia and its associated procedures carry their own unique risks. For this reason, an anesthesiologist is best suited to obtain their own separate consent from surgeons as anesthesiologists are more capable of discussing anesthetic-specific risks as well as alternatives to an anesthetic plan. Certain patient populations and clinical situations require extra attention to patient consent. In patients considering surgery with an active do-not-resuscitate order, clinicians should initiate a thorough discussion and document the patient's wishes for specific procedures and resuscitative measures. In pediatric patients, child refusal of informed assent may be considered if the situation is appropriate to withhold treatment and the child is deemed mature enough to understand the consequences of their decision. In obstetric patients, women in labor have demonstrated the ability to recall information despite the stress and pain associated with labor and should therefore be treated as having capacity to make medical decisions. For pregnant minors, state laws vary on the capacity of giving consent, but providers should always strive to include both the parturient and guardians in the decision-making process. Informed consent principles equally apply to research participants and patients undergoing clinical care.

Questions

1. **Can consent for anesthesiology be included as part of the verbal and written consent obtained by a surgeon or proceduralist?**
   A. **Yes, it can be.**
   B. **No, a separate informed consent needs to be obtained for anesthesia care.**
   C. **No consent required.**
   (Answer: B)
   Anesthesiologists should obtain their own informed consent as anesthetic plans and procedures carry their own unique individual risks which vary from patient to patient based on medical comorbidities. As the focus of a surgical consent is usually on surgical complications, a thorough discussion of major/minor anesthetic risks and potential alternatives is often missed.
2. **Should an anesthesiologist cancel a surgery because a terminally ill patient refuses to suspend their do-not-resuscitate order?**
   A. **Yes, without suspension of do-not-resuscitate order, anesthesia care cannot be delivered.**
   B. **No, do-not-resuscitate order and various options related to it should be discussed with the patient and based on patients wishes, surgery performed.**
   C. **Proceed with surgery with local only.**
   (Answer: B)
   No. As part of the informed consent process, an anesthesiologist should ascertain a patient's goals and values and specifically discuss whether a patient is amenable to certain medical procedures or interventions that are common practice in anesthesiology. For example, a patient may be ok with an elective intubation to help facilitate general anesthesia, but refuse the placement of invasive lines/hemodynamic monitoring in the case of hemodynamic instability. A discussion specific to whether or not to initiate CPR during the perioperative setting (when CPR has better chances of good outcomes) is essential. All their wishes should be documented.
3. **A pregnant 15-year old female unaccompanied by a parent or legal guardian is requesting an epidural to help control labor pain, how would you proceed with obtaining informed consent?**
   A. **Yes, go ahead obtain informed consent and place the epidural.**
   B. **Decline to provide an epidural.**
   C. **Based on state law decide how to proceed with an informed consent, encourage shared decision-making along with the parents.**
   (Answer: C)
   Most states allow pregnant minors to give consent for procedures related to their pregnancy. Check whether your local state laws allow the clinician to directly obtain consent from the minor. As with any patient: ensure the patient has adequate cognitive ability to understand the risks/benefits/alternatives communicated in order to make an informed decision. Respect the patient's confidentiality, but at the same time, encourage minors to allow sharing of medical information and shared decision-making with supportive family members.
4. **A 14-year old boy refuses to undergo anesthesia for a pectus excavatum repair despite his parents' desire to go forward with the surgery after obtaining both surgical and anesthesia informed consent. How should the anesthesiology team proceed?**
   A. **Respect the minor's decision. Encourage shared decision-making among the family members and along with the surgical team.**
   B. **Decline to proceed with the surgery.**
   C. **Give Midazolam to the patient and proceed with the surgery considering parental consent.**
   (Answer: A)
   If the 14 year old boy demonstrates ability to comprehend risks/benefits/alternatives without any obvious factors which may limit his capacity to make an informed decision, the anesthesiologist may respect this patient's refusal to give assent, especially if this surgical procedure is considered mainly elective/cosmetic in nature.
5. **A surgeon has to convert a laparoscopic surgery to an open laparotomy due to unanticipated surgical bleeding. The anesthesiologist feels the patient may benefit from a transversus abdominus plane (TAP) block before emerging the patient from anesthesia. They did not previously discuss this plan with the patient. Should they proceed with this procedure?**
   A. **TAP block is low risk and routinely performed, so go ahead with the block.**
   B. **No, do not perform the block without informed consent from the patient or responsible party.**
   C. **Have the surgeon take the risk and do the block.**

(Answer: B)

No. Although the risk of major complications from regional anesthesia procedures are rare and the patient might benefit from having the block done under anesthesia before waking up with significant post-surgical pain, the application of informed consent applies equally to regional anesthesia. The provider should obtain the patient's/responsible party's consent before proceeding.

References

1. Thomas percival (1740–1804) codifier of medical ethics. *JAMA: The Journal of the American Medical Association*. 1965;194(12). https://doi.org/10.1001/jama.1965.03090250053021
2. Beauchamp TL. Informed consent: its history, meaning, and present challenges. Camb Q Healthc Ethics. 2011;20(4):515–23. https://doi.org/10.1017/S0963180111000259.
3. *Salgo v. Leland Stanford Jr. University Board of Trustees*; 1957.
4. *Canterbury v. Spence, 464 F.2d 772 (D.C. Cir. 1972); Cobbs v. Grant, 104 Cal. Rptr. 505, 502 P.2d 1(1972); Wilkinson v. Vesey, 295 A.2d 676 (R.I. 1972).*
5. *Informed consent*. American Medical Association. (n.d.). https://www.ama-assn.org/delivering-care/ethics/informed-consent
6. Marcucci C, Seagull FJ, Loreck D, Bourke DL, Sandson NB. Capacity to give surgical consent does not imply capacity to give anesthesia consent: implications for anesthesiologists. Anesthesia Analgesia 2010;110(2). https://journals.lww.com/anesthesia-analgesia/Fulltext/2010/02000/Capacity_to_Give_Surgical_Consent_Does_Not_Imply.54.aspx
7. Pascarella MR, Walls JD, Liu R, Chen L. Anesthesia providers are obligated to give patients the alternatives to general anesthesia when obtaining informed consent 1;2014.
8. Truog RD. "Do-not-resuscitate" orders during anesthesia and surgery. J Am Soc Anesthesiol. 1991;74(3):606–8.
9. Truog RD, Waisel DB, Burns JP. DNR in the OR: a goal-directed approach. Anesthesiology. 1999;90(1):289–95. https://doi.org/10.1097/00000542-199901000-00034.
10. Gentry KR, Lepere K, Opel DJ. Informed consent in pediatric anesthesiology. Paediatr Anaesth. 2017;27(12):1253–60. https://doi.org/10.1111/pan.13270.
11. Lewis I, Burke C, Voepel-Lewis T, Tait AR. Children who refuse anesthesia or sedation: A survey of anesthesiologists. Paediatric Anaesthesia 2007;17(12). https://doi.org/10.1111/j.1460-9592.2007.02331.x
12. Informed consent, parental permission, and assent in pediatric practice. Committee on Bioethics. J Child Fam Nurs. 1998;1(1).
13. Broaddus BM, Chandrasekhar S. Informed consent in obstetric anesthesia. Anesthesia Analgesia 2011;112(4). https://doi.org/10.1213/ANE.0b013e31820e777a
14. Affleck PJ, Waisel DB, Cusick JM, van Decar T. Recall of risks following labor epidural analgesia. J Clin Anesthesia 1998;10(2). https://doi.org/10.1016/S0952-8180(97)00258-4
15. Tierney S, Perlas A. Informed consent for regional anesthesia. Curr Opin Anaesthesiol. 2018;31(5):614–21.
16. Brull R, Wijayatilake DS, Perlas A, et al. Practice patterns related to block selection, nerve localization and risk disclosure: a survey of the American Society of Regional Anesthesia and Pain Medicine. Reg Anesth Pain Med. 2008;33(5):395–403.
17. Cook TM, Counsell D, Wildsmith JA, Royal College of anaesthetists third national audit P. Major complications of central neuraxial block: report on the third national audit project of the Royal College of Anaesthetists. Br J Anaesth. 2009;102(2):179–90.
18. White SM. Consent for anaesthesia. J Med Ethics. 2004;30(3):286–90.
19. Mduluza T, Midzi N, Duruza D, Ndebele P. Study participants incentives, compensation and reimbursement in resource-constrained settings. BMC Med Ethics 2013;14(Suppl 1):S4.
20. The Belmont Report. Ethical principles and guidelines for the protection of human subjects of research. J Am Coll Dent. 2014;81(3):4–13.
21. Bharucha AE, Rhodes CT, Boos CM, Keller DA, Dispenzieri A, Oldenburg RP. Increased utilization of virtual visits and electronic approaches in clinical research during the COVID-19 pandemic and thereafter. Mayo Clin Proc. 2021;96(9):2332–41.

Index

M. Argalious et al. (eds.), *Basic Sciences in Anesthesia*,
https://doi.org/10.1007/978-3-031-60203-0